OPERATIVE NERVE REPAIR AND RECONSTRUCTION

VOLUME **I**

OPERATIVE NERVE REPAIR AND RECONSTRUCTION

RICHARD H. GELBERMAN, MD

Professor of Orthopaedic Surgery
Harvard Medical School
Chief of Hand Surgery Service
Department of Orthopaedic Surgery
Massachusetts General Hospital
Boston, Massachusetts

126 Contributors
with illustrations by Elizabeth Roselius

J. B. LIPPINCOTT COMPANY
Philadelphia
New York
London Hagerstown

Acquisitions Editor: Darlene Barela Cooke
Developmental Editor: Delois Patterson
Project Editor: Elizabeth A. Durand
Indexer: Sandi Schroeder
Designer: Doug Smock
Production Manager: Caren Erlichman
Production Coordinator: Kevin P. Johnson
Compositor: Tapsco, Incorporated
Printer/Binder: Arcata Graphics/Halliday

Library of Congress Cataloging-in-Publication Data

Operative nerve repair and reconstruction/[edited by] Richard H. Gelberman.
p. cm.
Includes bibliographical references.
Includes index.
ISBN 0-397-51074-8 (set)
ISBN 0-397-51174-4 (Vol. 1)
1. Nerves, Peripheral—Surgery. 2. Nerves, Peripheral—Regeneration. 3. Nerves, Peripheral—Wounds and injuries.
I. Gelberman, Richard H.
[DNLM: 1. Nerve Regeneration. 2. Peripheral Nerves—injuries. 3. Peripheral Nerves—surgery. WL 500 061]
RD595.064 1991
617.4'83059—dc20
DNLM/DLC
for Library of Congress 90-13297
CIP

6 5 4 3 2 1

The authors and publisher have exerted every effort to ensure that drug selection and dosage set forth in this text are in accord with current recommendations and practice at the time of publication. However, in view of ongoing research, changes in government regulations, and the constant flow of information relating to drug therapy and drug reactions, the reader is urged to check the package insert for each drug for any change in indications and dosage and for added warnings and precautions. This is particularly important when the recommended agent is a new or infrequently employed drug.

For Sarah
And For Courtney, David, and Amanda

CONTRIBUTORS

Edward E. Almquist, MD
Clinical Professor
Department of Orthopaedics
University of Washington
Seattle, WA

Peter C. Amadio, MD
Associate Professor of Orthopedic Surgery
Mayo Medical Foundation
Rochester, MN

Harlan C. Amstutz, MD
University of California, Los Angeles
Division of Orthopaedic Surgery
Los Angeles, CA

Gregory A. Antoine, MD
Georgetown University Medical Center
Division of Plastic Surgery
Washington, DC

Marie A. Badalamente, PhD
Associate Professor
Director, Cell Biology/Structure Research Lab
Department of Orthopaedics
State University of New York at Stony Brook
Stony Brook, NY

William F. Blair, MD
Division of Hand and Microsurgery
Department of Orthopaedic Surgery
University of Iowa
Iowa City, IO

F. William Bora, Jr, MD
Professor of Orthopaedic Surgery
University of Pennsylvania School of Medicine
Chief of Hand Surgery
Hospital of the University of Pennsylvania
Consultant in Orthopedic Surgery
Children's Hospital of Philadelphia
Veteran's Administration Hospital of Philadelphia
MCMC Fitzgerald Mercy Hospital
Darby, PA

Michael J. Botte, MD
Chief, Hand and Microvascular Surgery
Division of Orthopaedic Surgery and Rehabilitation
University of California, San Diego
San Diego, CA

Richard M. Braun, MD
Associate Clinical Professor of Orthopaedic Surgery
University of California, San Diego
Instructor of Orthopaedic Surgery
Rancho Los Amigos Hospital
University of Southern California
San Diego, California

Warren C. Breidenbach, MD
Assistant Clinical Professor of Surgery (Plastic and Reconstructive)
University of Louisville
Active Staff
Jewish Hospital, Norton Hospital,
Humana Hospital—University of Louisville, and Humana Hospital—Audubon
Louisville, KY

Francesco Brunelli, MD
Associate Surgeon
Institut Français de la Main
Consultant Surgeon in Orthopaedic Unit
Cochin Hospital
Paris, France

Giorgio A. Brunelli, MD
Professor and Chairman
Department of Orthopaedics
Brescia University Medical School
Brescia, Italy

Thomas M. Brushart, MD
Assistant Professor of Orthopaedics and Neurology
Johns Hopkins University
Attending Surgeon, Raymond M. Curtis Hand Center
Lutherville, MD

William E. Burkhalter, MD
Professor and Associate Chairman for Clinical Affairs
Chief, Division of Hand Surgery
University of Miami
Jackson Memorial Medical Center
Miami, FL

Patricia M. Byron, MS OTR/L
Private Practice
Glenside, Pennsylvania
Adjunct Instructor
Department of Orthopaedic Surgery
Jefferson Medical College
Thomas Jefferson University
Formerly Clinical Director
Hand Rehabilitation Center
Philadelphia, PA

Edward R. Calkins, MD
Section of Plastic and Reconstructive Surgery
University of Michigan Medical Center
Ann Arbor, MI

Daniel B. Carr, MD
Co-Director, Anesthesia Pain Unit
Massachusetts General Hospital
Associate Professor of Anesthesiology and Medicine (Endocrinology)
Harvard Medical School
Boston, MA

Margaret Carter-Wilson, OTR, HT
Director, Hand Rehabilitation Unit
Hand Surgery Associates
Phoenix, AZ

Alan W. Christensen, MD
Assistant Professor of Surgery
Uniformed Services University of the Health Sciences (USUHS)
Bethesda, MD

William P. Cooney III, MD
Professor of Orthopedic Surgery
Mayo Medical School
Consultant, Department of Orthopedics
Chief, Section of Hand Surgery
Mayo Clinic
Rochester, MN

Daniel E. Cooper, MD
Clinical Instructor, Department of Orthopaedics
University of Texas Health Science Center
Southwestern Medical School
Attending Physician
W. B. Carroll Memorial Clinic
Orthopaedic Staff
Baylor University Medical Center
Dallas, TX

Lars B. Dahlin, MD, PhD
Assistant Professor, Resident in Hand Surgery
University of Göteborg
Sahlgren Hospital
Malmö, Sweden

Nils Danielsen, MD, PhD
Associate Professor
Department of Anatomy
University of Göteborg
Göteborg, Sweden

Gudarz Davar, MD
Massachusetts General Hospital
Laboratory of Pain Physiology
Spalding Rehabilitation Hospital
Boston, MA

Paul C. Dell, MD
Department of Orthopaedics
University of Florida Medical Center
Gainesville, FL

A. Lee Dellon, MD, FACS
Associate Professor
Johns Hopkins University School of Medicine
Division of Plastic Surgery
Department of Neurological Surgery
Division of Rehabilitation Medicine
Baltimore, MD

Jeanne L. DelSignore, MD
Clinical Instructor
Department of Orthopaedics
University of Rochester
School of Medicine
Rochester, NY

Edward Diao, MD
Assistant Professor of Orthopaedic Surgery
Hand Center of Western New York
Millard Fillmore Hospital
Buffalo, NY

Harold M. Dick, MD
Frank E. Stinchfield Professor and Chairman
Department of Orthopaedic Surgery
College of Physicians and Surgeons
Columbia-Presbyterian Medical Center
New York, NY

James H. Dobyns, MD
Professor (Emeritus) Orthopedic Surgery
Mayo Medical School
Rochester, MN

Andrew Dowd, MD
Assistant Professor
Department of Orthopaedics
State University of New York at Stony Brook
Stony Brook, NY

Joseph P. Dutkowsky, MD
Assistant Professor of Orthopaedic Surgery
University of Tennessee Center for Health Sciences
Active Staff, Campbell Clinic
Memphis, TN

Richard G. Eaton, MD
Director, Hand Center, Roosevelt Hospital
Professor of Clinical Surgery
Columbia College of Physicians and Surgeons
New York, NY

William W. Eversmann, Jr, MD
Senior Hand Surgeon
Iowa Medical Clinic
Active Staff Mercy Medical Center and Saint Luke's Hospital
Cedar Rapids, IA

Richard L. Fabian, MD, FACS
Director, Head and Neck Surgical Services
Department of Otolaryngology—Head and Neck Surgery
Massachusetts Eye and Ear Infirmary
Massachusetts General Hospital
Associate Professor
Department of Otolaryngology
Harvard Medical School
Boston, MA

Paul R. Fassler, MD
Clinical Instructor
Department of Orthopedics
University of Cincinnati
Cincinnati, OH

Donald C. Ferlic, MD
Associate Clinical Professor
University of Colorado Health Science Center
Staff Physician, St. Joseph Hospital
Denver, CO

Gary K. Frykman, MD
Clinical Professor of Orthopaedic Surgery
Loma Linda University School of Medicine
Loma Linda, CA

Gerard T. Gabel, MD
Assistant Professor
Division of Orthopedic Surgery
Baylor College of Medicine
Houston, TX

James A. Galbraith, PhD
Peripheral Nerve Research Group
University of California, San Diego
La Jolla, CA

William E. Garrett, Jr, MD, PhD
Duke University Medical Center
Durham, NC

Harris Gellman, MD
University of Southern California
Associate Clinical Professor, Orthopaedic Surgery
San Diego, California
Director, Spinal Cord Injury Upper Extremity Service
Rancho Los Amigos Medical Center
Downey, CA

Alain Gilbert, MD
Institut Francais de la Main
Paris, France

Paul W. Gorman, MD
Watauga Orthopaedic Professional Association, Inc.
Johnson City, TN

John S. Gould, MD
Professor and Chairman
Department of Orthopaedic Surgery
Medical College of Wisconsin
Director of Orthopaedics
Milwaukee Regional Medical Center
Milwaukee, WI

Brent Graham, MD, FRCS(C)
Fellow, Christine M. Kleinert Institute for Hand and Micro Surgery
Louisville, KY

Kevin Gramyk, MD
Fellow, Hand Surgery
Department of Orthopaedics
Loma Linda University Medical Center
Loma Linda, CA

Nortin M. Hadler, MD, FACP
Professor of Medicine and Microbiology/Immunology
School of Medicine
University of North Carolina at Chapel Hill
Attending Rheumatologist
University of North Carolina Hospitals
Chapel Hill, NC

Leo T. Happel, PhD
Department of Neurosurgery, Neurology and Physiology
Louisiana State University Medical Center
New Orleans, LA

Steven J. Heithoff, DO
Orthopedic Associates of Port Huron
Assistant Clinical Professor of Orthopedic Surgery
College of Osteopathic Medicine
Michigan State University
Port Huron, MI

Vincent R. Hentz, MD
Professor of Surgery
Stanford University
Chief, Division of Hand Surgery
Stanford University Medical Center
Stanford, CA

James H. Herndon, MD
David Silver Professor and Chairman
Department of Orthopaedic Surgery
University of Pittsburgh School of Medicine
Pittsburgh, PA

Alfred V. Hess, MD
Senior Resident
Department of Orthopaedics
University of Pittsburgh
School of Medicine
Pittsburgh, PA

Philip Heyman, MD
Clinical Fellow, Hand Surgery
Harvard Medical School
Assistant in Orthopedic Surgery
Massachusetts General Hospital
Boston, MA

H. Mark Hoffer, MD
Professor and Chief of Orthopedic Surgery
University of California at Irvine
Chief, Children's Orthopedics
Rancho Los Amigos Hospital
Downey, CA

Lawrence C. Hurst, MD
Associate Professor
Chief, Division of Hand and Microsurgery
Department of Orthopaedics
State University of New York at Stony Brook
Stony Brook, NY

Michael E. Jabaley, MD, FACS
Clinical Professor of Surgery (Plastic) and Orthopaedics
University of Mississippi Medical Center
Jackson, MS

Anthony W. Jevans, PhD
Clinical Chemist, Department of Pathology
Jewish Hospital
Clinical Assistant Professor
Department of Pathology
University of Louisville School of Medicine
Louisville, KY

Frank W. Jobe, MD
Clinical Professor
Department of Orthopaedics
University of Southern California
School of Medicine
Los Angeles, CA

Jesse B. Jupiter, MD
Associate Orthopaedic Surgeon
Massachusetts General Hospital
Assistant Professor of Orthopaedic Surgery
Harvard Medical School
Boston, MA

James R. Kasser, MD
Associate Chief of Orthopaedic Surgery
Children's Hospital
Assistant Professor
Harvard Medical School
Boston, MA

Mary Ann E. Keenan, MD
Chairman, Department of Orthopaedic Surgery
Albert Einstein Medical Center
Professor of Orthopaedic Surgery
Temple University School of Medicine
Philadelphia, PA

William B. Kleinman, MD
Associate Clinical Professor of Orthopaedic Surgery
Indiana University School of Medicine
Indianapolis, IN

David G. Kline, MD
Professor and Chairman
Department of Neurosurgery
Louisiana State University Medical Center
Staffs of Charity, Ochsner, Hotel Dieu, Southern Baptist and Touro Hospitals
Consultant, New Orleans VA Hospital and Kessler Air Force Base Hospital
New Orleans, LA

L. Andrew Koman, MD
Associate Professor
Section on Orthopaedic Surgery
Wake Forest University
The Bowman Gray School of Medicine
Winston-Salem, NC

Michael K. Kwan, PhD
Division of Orthopaedics and Rehabilitation
Department of Surgery
University of California, San Diego
La Jolla, CA

David Harlan Lang, MD
Private Practice
Milwaukee, Wisconsin
Formerly Hand Fellow
Christine Kleinert Institute for Hand Surgery
Louisville, KY

Ulrich Lanz, MD
Professor for Surgery
Chief, Hand Surgery Service
Department of Surgery
Wurzburg University
Federal Republic of Germany

Robert Leffert, MD
Chief of the Surgical Upper Extremity Rehabilitation Unit
Massachusetts General Hospital
Associate Professor of Orthopaedic Surgery
Harvard Medical School
Boston, MA

Graham D. Lister, MB, ChB, FRCS, FACS, MD
University of Utah Medical Center
Primary Children's Medical Center
Veteran's Administration Medical Center
Holy Cross Hospital
Shriner's Hospital
Salt Lake City, UT

Dean Sherwood Louis, MD
Professor of Surgery
Chief, Orthopaedic Hand Service
University of Michigan Hospitals
Ann Arbor, MI

Wallace E. Lowry, Jr, MD
Director, Division of Orthopaedic Surgery
Scott & White Clinic and Hospital
Texas A & M College of Medicine
Temple, TX

Göran N. Lundborg, MD, PhD
Professor and Head, Department of Hand Surgery
Malmö General Hospital
Lund University
Malmö, Sweden

Raymond Maciewicz, MD, PhD
Director, Cancer Pain Center
Neurology Service
Massachusetts General Hospital
Associate Professor of Neurology and Neuroscience
Harvard Medical School
Boston, MA

Evelyn J. Mackin, PT
Director, Hand Rehabilitation Foundation
Philadelphia, PA

Henry J. Mankin, MD
Edith M. Ashley Professor of Orthopaedic Surgery
Harvard Medical School
Chief of Orthopaedic Surgery
Massachusetts General Hospital
Boston, MA

Ralph T. Manktelow, MD, FRCSC
Chairman, Division of Plastic Surgery
University of Toronto
Head, Division of Plastic Surgery
Toronto General Hospital
Toronto, Ontario, Canada

Roy A. Meals, MD
Associate Professor of Orthopaedic Surgery
Chief of the Hand Surgery Service
University of California at Los Angeles Medical Center
Los Angeles, CA

Bryan J. Michelow, MD, FRCS (Ed & Glasg)
Senior Microsurgery Fellow
Microsurgical Research Center
Eastern Virginia Graduate School of Medicine
Norfolk, VA

Lewis H. Millender, MD
Clinical Professor of Orthopaedic Surgery
Tufts University Medical School
Assistant Chief, Hand Service
New England Baptist Hospital
Boston, MA

Hanno Millesi, MD
Professor of Plastic Surgery
University of Vienna Medical Faculty
Director of Ludwig Boltzmann Institute of Experimental Plastic Surgery
Vienna, Austria

Takaya Mizuseki, MD, PhD
Chief of Hand Division
Hiroshima Prefectural Rehabilitation Center
Taguchi, Saijyo
Higashi-Hiroshima City
Japan

Robert R. Myers, PhD
Professor of Anesthesiology
Professor of Pathology (Neuropathology)
Associate Research Career Scientist
Department of Veterans Affairs
University of California, San Diego
La Jolla, CA

Algimantas D. Narakas, MD
Associate Professor at the Medical School of the University of Lausanne
Consultant at the University Hospital for Reconstructive Surgery of the Hand, Upper Limb and Peripheral Nerves
Consultant at the Children's University Hospital
Berne, Switzerland
Chief Surgeon
Clinique Longeraie
Lausanne, Switzerland

Edward R. North, MD
Clinical Associate Professor
Department of Orthopaedic Surgery
University of Washington School of Medicine
Seattle, Washington
Evergreen Hospital
Kirkland, Washington
Overlake Hospital
Bellevue, WA

James A. Nunley, MD
Associate Professor of Surgery
Division of Orthopaedic Surgery
Duke Medical Center
Durham, NC

George E. Omer, Jr, MD, MS, FACS
Professor of Orthopaedics and Chairman
Department of Orthopaedics and Rehabilitation
Professor of Surgery and Anatomy
Co-Chief, Division of Hand Surgery
Medical Director, Physical Therapy Degree Program
School of Medicine
The University of New Mexico
Albuquerque, NM

A. Lee Osterman, MD
Associate Professor, Hand and Orthopaedic Surgery
Penn Hand Center
University of Pennsylvania
Philadelphia, PA

Clayton A. Peimer, MD
Associate Professor of Orthopaedic Surgery
Clinical Assistant
Professor of Anatomical Sciences
Professor of Rehabilitation Medicine
School of Medicine and Biomedical Sciences
University of Buffalo
State University of New York
Buffalo, NY

Gary G. Poehling, MD
Professor and Chairman
Department of Orthopaedic Surgery
Bowman Gray School of Medicine
Winston-Salem, NC

Robin R. Richards, MD, FRCS(C)
Associate Professor of Orthopaedic Surgery
University of Toronto
Head, Division of Orthopaedic Surgery
St. Michael's Hospital
Toronto, Ontario, Canada

Andrew E. Rosenberg, MD
Department of Pathology
Harvard Medical School
Massachusetts General Hospital
Boston, MA

Bjorn L. Rydevik, MD, PhD
Associate Professor of Orthopaedic Surgery
University of Gothenburg
Sahlgren Hospital
Gothenburg, Sweden

Roger E. Salisbury, MD
Professor of Surgery
Chief, Plastic and Reconstructive Surgery
New York Medical College
Director, Burn Center
Westchester County Medical Center
Valhalla, NY

C. Andrew Salzberg, MD
Assistant Professor of Surgery
New York Medical College
Valhalla, New York
Chief, Plastic Surgery
Veterans Administration Medical Center
Castle Point, NY

Thomas D. Schmalzried, MD
Orthopaedic Biomechanics Laboratory
Massachusetts General Hospital and Harvard Medical School
Boston, MA

Professor Dr. med. Hans-Martin Schmidt
Anatomisches Institut der Universitat Bonn
Bonn, Federal Republic of Germany

Lawrence H. Schneider, MD
Clinical Professor of Orthopaedic Surgery
Jefferson Medical College of Thomas Jefferson University
Director, Division of Hand Surgery
Department of Orthopaedic Surgery
Thomas Jefferson University Hospital
Philadelphia, PA

David B. Siegel, MD
Assistant Professor
Department of Orthopaedic Surgery
Bowman Gray School of Medicine
Winston-Salem, NC

John M. Siliski, MD
Department of Orthopaedic Surgery
Massachusetts General Hospital
Harvard Medical School
Boston, MA

James B. Steichen, MD
Clinical Professor of Orthopaedic Surgery
Indiana University School of Medicine
Indianapolis, Indiana
Assistant Clinical Professor of Plastic Surgery
University of Kentucky Medical Center
Lexington, KY

David R. Steinberg, MD
Clinical Fellow in Hand Surgery
Harvard Medical School
Assistant in Orthopaedic Surgery
Massachusetts General Hospital
Boston, MA

Peter J. Stern, MD
Clinical Professor of Orthopaedic Surgery
University of Cincinnati College of Medicine
Cincinnati, OH

Curtis M. Steyers, Jr, MD
Associate Professor
Division of Hand and Microsurgery
Department of Orthopaedic Surgery
University of Iowa
Iowa City, IA

James W. Strickland, MD
Clinical Professor, Orthopaedic Surgery
Indiana University School of Medicine
Chief, Section of Hand Surgery
St. Vincent's Hospital
Indianapolis, IN

Robert M. Szabo, MD
Associate Professor
Chief, Hand and Microvascular Surgery
Department of Orthopaedics
University of California, Davis
School of Medicine
Sacramento, CA

Julia K. Terzis, MD, FRCS (C), PhD
Director, Microsurgery Program
Microsurgical Research Center
Associate Professor
Department of Plastic and Reconstructive Surgery
Eastern Virginia Medical School
Norfolk, VA

Donald P. Todd, MD
Anesthetist (Senior Staff)
Massachusetts General Hospital
Associate Professor of Anaesthesia
Harvard Medical School
Boston, MA

Thomas E. Trumble, MD
Associate Professor
Department of Orthopaedics
Chief, Hand and Microvascular Surgery Service
University of Washington
Seattle, WA

Kenya Tsuge, MD
Emeritus Professor, Department of Orthopaedics
Hiroshima University School of Medicine
Director of the Hiroshima Prefectural Rehabilitation Center
Higashi-Hiroshima, Japan

Jack W. Tupper, MD
Clinical Professor of Orthopaedic Surgery
Chief, Hand Service
Children's Hospital Medical Center
Chief, Hand Surgery
Sam Medritt Hospital
Oakland, CA

Mark A. Urban, MD
Chief Resident in Orthopaedic Surgery
Hospital of the University of Pennsylvania
Philadelphia, PA

James R. Urbaniak, MD
Professor and Chief
Division of Orthopaedic Surgery
Duke University Medical Center
Durham, NC

Allen L. Van Beek, MD
Clinical Associate Professor
University of Minnesota
Department of Surgery
Edina, MN

Frank R. Voss, MD
Senior Resident, Orthopaedic Surgery
Massachusetts General Hospital
Harvard Medical School
Boston, MA

Robert L. Waters, MD
Professor of Orthopaedic Surgery
University of Southern California
Medical Director
Rancho Los Amigos Medical Center
Downey, CA

Andrew J. Weiland, MD
Surgeon-in-Chief
The Hospital for Special Surgery
Professor of Orthopaedic Surgery and Plastic Surgery
Cornell University Medical College
New York, NY

E. F. Shaw Wilgis, MD
Chief, Division of Hand Surgery
Union Memorial Hospital
Associate Professor of Plastic Surgery
Associate Professor of Orthopaedic Surgery
The Johns Hopkins School of Medicine
Lutherville, MD

Bruce S. Wolock, MD
Instructor, Orthopaedic Surgery
The Johns Hopkins University School of Medicine
The Johns Hopkins Hospital
Baltimore, MD

S.L-Y. Woo, PhD
Professor of Surgery and Bioengineering
Orthopaedic Bioengineering Laboratory
University of California, San Diego
Veterans Administration Medical Center
San Diego, CA

Michael B. Wood, MD
Professor, Department of Orthopedic Surgery
Mayo Medical School
Consultant, Section of Hand Surgery
Mayo Clinic/Mayo Foundation
Rochester, MN

Lewis A. Yocum, MD
Assistant Clinical Professor
University of Southern California
School of Medicine
Orthopaedic Surgery
Kerlan/Jobe Orthopaedic Clinic
Los Angeles, CA

Norman P. Zemel, MD
Associate Clinical Professor
Department of Orthopaedic Surgery
University of Southern California
School of Medicine
Associate, Kerlan-Jobe Orthopaedic Clinic
Los Angeles, CA

Neal B. Zimmerman, MD
Instructor in Orthopaedic Surgery
Johns Hopkins University School of Medicine
Attending Hand Surgeon
Raymond M. Curtis Hand Center
Union Memorial Hospital
Baltimore, MD

PREFACE

Peripheral nerve surgery has undergone important changes over the past 15 years. As innovations in a variety of areas have significantly broadened the scope of practice in nerve repair and reconstruction, it has become increasingly necessary for the peripheral nerve surgeon to have a reference to consult that contains an organized, systematic discussion of the problems with which patients present for treatment.

Such an expansion in scope dictates the need for a complete and comprehensive reference that is also practical and readable. *Operative Nerve Repair and Reconstruction* is intended to fill this need. While the book discusses traditional methods of management, it emphasizes innovative methods and techniques, making the assumption that the reader is an experienced surgeon with basic skills and knowledge who is looking for "state of the art" information.

This text is designed primarily to provide the technical details required to perform intricate peripheral nerve repair and reconstructive procedures in an accomplished manner. However, emphasis is also placed on the underlying principles upon which the diagnosis, treatment plan, and surgery are based, as well as the complications encountered during operative and postoperative care. Contributors have written tightly focused chapters, describing the applied anatomy, operative exposure, and preferred methods for performing specific operations. In addition, they provide an important introductory segment entitled "Author's Key Points" that is designed to help the reader focus on those specific issues the author considers most relevant. As *Operative Nerve Repair and Reconstruction* is designed primarily for clinicians, authors of introductory basic science chapters have included "Clinical Significance" statements in order to relate current scientific thinking to the practical aspects of peripheral nerve surgery.

This work is divided into two volumes, the first of which is devoted primarily to problems associated with nerve regeneration. The second volume addresses nerve compression and, in addition, includes a group of related topics: brachial plexus injury in adults and children, spinal cord injury, brain injury and stroke, and cerebral palsy. The concluding segments are devoted to the management of pain and to peripheral nerve tumors.

Where there are a variety of commonly used operative techniques for managing specific clinical problems, the most common are presented in detail. In that regard, six chapters are devoted to techniques for decompressing the ulnar nerve at the elbow. To put these chapters in perspective, other chapters are devoted to the operative decision-making process, to common pitfalls in management, and to complications associated with ulnar nerve decompression. In individual chapters, authors indicate the reasons their techniques are preferred along with the specific operative methods considered optimal.

The authors of *Operative Nerve Repair and Reconstruction*, an elite group drawn from academic and private practice, have contributed to a definitive reference and resource for day-to-day patient care. While considerable effort has been made to be as comprehensive as possible, the quickly changing basic concepts and practical applications in this rapidly growing field require practitioners to utilize other educational techniques for maintaining the knowledge and skill necessary to provide their patients with optimal methods of care.

Richard H. Gelberman, MD

ACKNOWLEDGMENTS

A number of individuals have made substantial contributions of time and effort to the completion of this book. As this two-volume text represents a compilation of individual efforts, I wish to extend my deep appreciation to them.

To the more than 100 contributing authors, whose intense efforts are apparent in these pages, I am deeply grateful. These doctors, the most accomplished clinicians and researchers in peripheral nerve surgery, have given of their time and have made great efforts to create a comprehensive current text.

I am also very grateful to the many other people who made completion of this book possible:

My wife, Sarah, for her unfailing support and her valuable insight.

Darlene Cooke, Editor-in-Chief/Medical Books, whose enthusiasm, energy and organizational skills have made her a delightful publisher.

Elizabeth Roselius, who, in creating 200 original schematic drawings, showed great intelligence, artistic skill, and thorough anatomical knowledge.

Delois Patterson, Associate Editor/Medical Books; Paul Monteforte, Administrative Assistant; and Elizabeth Durand, Project Editor, whose editorial assistance was invaluable.

Finally, my mentors Drs. Goldner and Urbaniak at Duke University, Henry Mankin and my colleagues at the Massachusetts General Hospital, and Wayne Akeson and my colleagues at the University of California, San Diego, who have allowed me to gain the knowledge and experience to undertake a project of this scope.

CONTENTS

VOLUME ONE

Part I.

MORPHOLOGY AND PHYSIOLOGY OF PERIPHERAL NERVE 1

1. Structure and Function of Peripheral Nerve **3**
   Goran Lundborg
   Lars B. Dahlin
2. Impulse Conduction **19**
   James A. Galbraith
   Robert R. Myers
3. Biomechanical Properties of Peripheral Nerve **47**
   Michael K. Kwan
   Savio L-Y. Woo
4. Biochemical Properties of Peripheral Nerve **55**
   Lawrence C. Hurst
   Marie A. Badalamente
5. The Neuromuscular Junction **73**
   William E. Garrett, Jr.
6. Sensory Receptors **85**
   Julia K. Terzis
   Bryan J. Michelow

Part II.

INJURY, DEGENERATION, AND REGENERATION 107

7. Injury, Degeneration, and Regeneration **109**
   Göran Lundborg
   Nils Danielsen

Part III.

CLINICAL EVALUATION 133

8. Sensibility Testing **135**
   A. Lee Dellon

9. Motor Testing **159**
William F. Blair

10. Electrophysiological Testing **171**
Allen L. Van Beek
Philip Heyman

11. Pitfalls in Interpretation of Electrophysiological Testing **185**
A. Lee Dellon

12. Anomalous Innervation of the Upper Extremity **197**
Roy A. Meals
Edward R. Calkins

Part IV.
ALIGNMENT 213

13. The Mechanical and Humoral Control of Specificity in Nerve Repair **215**
Thomas M. E. Brushart

14. Internal Topography of Peripheral Nerves as Related to Repair **231**
Michael E. Jabaley

15. Electrical Nerve Stimulation in the Awake Patient **241**
Michael E. Jabaley

16. Histochemical and Biochemical Aids to Nerve Repair **259**
David H. Lang
Graham D. Lister
Anthony W. Jevans

Part V.
OPERATIVE TECHNIQUE 273

17. Instrumentation for Nerve Repair **275**
Paul W. Gorman
Paul C. Dell

18. Techniques of Epineural and Group Fascicular Repair **287**
E. F. Shaw Wilgis

19. Fascicular Repair **295**
Jack W. Tupper

20. Sutureless Methods of Nerve Repair **305**
Edward Diao
Clayton A. Peimer

21. Modified Techniques of Nerve Repair: Epineurial Splint **315**
Michael E. Jabaley

22. New Approaches in Nerve Suture **327**
Kenya Tsuge
Takaya Mizuseki

23. Partial Nerve Injuries **335**
Lawrence C. Hurst
Andrew Dowd

Part VI.
APPLIED ANATOMY, OPERATIVE EXPOSURE, RESULTS OF REPAIR 347

24. Factors Affecting the Results of Peripheral Nerve Repair **349**
David R. Steinberg
L. Andrew Koman

25. Median Nerve: Applied Anatomy and Operative Exposure **365**
David B. Siegel
Richard H. Gelberman

26. Median Nerve Repairs: The Results of Treatment **379**
William P. Cooney

27. Radial Nerve: Applied Anatomy and Operative Exposure **393**
David B. Siegel
Richard H. Gelberman

28. Radial Nerve—Results **409**
Curtis M. Steyers

29. Ulnar Nerve: Applied Anatomy and Operative Exposure **413**
David B. Siegel
Richard H. Gelberman

30. Ulnar Nerve Repair **425**
James W. Strickland
Richard S. Idler
Jeanne L. DelSignore

31. Axillary Nerve **437**
James A. Nunley
Gerard Gabel

32. Spinal Accessory Nerve **445**
Gerard Gabel
James A. Nunley

33. Digital Nerves **453**
John S. Gould

34. Facial Nerve Paralysis **461**
Richard L. Fabian

35. Peripheral Nerve Injuries to the Lower Extremity **489**
Michael B. Wood

Part VII.
NERVE GRAFTING 505

36. Overcoming Defects in Peripheral Nerves **507**
Thomas Trumble

37. Indications and Techniques of Nerve Grafting **525**
Hanno Millesi

38. Donor Nerves for Grafting **545**
James A. Nunley

39. Results of Nerve Grafting **553**
Gary K. Frykman
Kevin Gramyk

40. Vascularized Nerve Grafts **569**
Warren C. Breidenbach
Brent Graham

41. Nerve Grafting Through Resorbable Tubes **587**
Mark A. Urban
F. William Bora, Jr.

Part VIII.
NERVE LESIONS IN CONTINUITY 599

42. Nerve Lesions in Continuity **601**
Leo T. Happel
David G. Kline

Part IX.
NERVE INJURY ASSOCIATED WITH FRACTURES AND OTHER TRAUMA 617

43. Peripheral Nerve Injuries Associated with Fractures and Dislocations **619**
David B. Siegel
Richard H. Gelberman

44. Nerve Injury Associated With Fractures in Children **635**
Joseph P. Dutkowsky
James R. Kasser

45. Nerve Injuries Associated With Gunshot Wounds of the Extremities **655**
George E. Omer, Jr.

46. Thermal Injury of Peripheral Nerve **671**
C. Andrew Salzberg
Roger E. Salisbury

47. Nerve Injury Associated with Devascularizing Trauma **679**
Jesse B. Jupiter

Part X.
OPERATIVE RECONSTRUCTION FOR IRREPARABLE PERIPHERAL NERVE INJURIES (Excluding Brachial Plexus) 687

48. Principles of Tendon Transfers **689**
Edward E. Almquist

49. Tendon Transfer for Radial Nerve Palsy **697**
Lawrence H. Schneider

50. Median Nerve Palsy **711**
William W. Eversmann

51. Ulnar Nerve Palsy **729**
William E. Burkhalter

52. Tendon Transfers for Combined Nerve Injuries **747**
George E. Omer, Jr.

53. Lower Extremity Nerve Palsies **763**
John M. Siliski
Frank Voss

54. Free Muscle Transfer for Functional Reconstruction **775**
Ralph T. Manktelow

55. Direct Muscular Neurotization **783**
Giorgio A. Brunelli

56. Free Flaps for Providing Sensibility to the Hand **793**
Alain Gilbert
Francesco Brunelli

Part XI. REHABILITATION 811

57. Rehabilitation Following Nerve Repair **813**
Evelyn J. Mackin
Patricia M. Byron

58. Sensory Re-Education **827**
Margaret Carter-Wilson

VOLUME II

Part XII. PERIPHERAL NERVE COMPRESSION 845

59. Pathophysiology of Nerve Compression **847**
Lars B. Dahlin
Björn Rydevik

Part XIII. MEDIAN NERVE COMPRESSION—DISTAL 867

60. Carpal Tunnel Syndrome—General **869**
Robert M. Szabo

61. Anatomy of the Median Nerve in the Carpal Tunnel **889**
Hans-Martin Schmidt
Ulrich Lanz

62. Carpal Tunnel Release **899**
   A. Open Release of Transverse Carpal Ligament **899**
   Richard H. Gelberman

   B. Endoscopic Carpal Tunnel Release **913**
   Edward R. North

63. Treatment of Severe Compression of the Median Nerve **921**
Wallace E. Lowry, Jr.

64. Tendon Transfers for Severe Carpal Tunnel Syndrome **927**
Richard M. Braun

65. Acute Carpal Tunnel Syndrome **939**
Richard H. Gelberman

66. Cumulative Trauma, Carpal Tunnel Syndrome in the Workplace—Epidemiological and Legal Aspects **949**
Nortin M. Hadler

67. Evaluation and Treatment of Median Neuropathy Associated With Cumulative Trauma **957**
Dean S. Louis

68. Carpal Tunnel Release in Patients With Peripheral Neuropathy **963**
James H. Dobyns

69. Complications of Treatment of Carpal Tunnel Syndrome **967**
James R. Urbaniak

Part XIV.
MEDIAN NERVE COMPRESSION—PROXIMAL 981

70. Anterior Interosseous Nerve Compression Syndrome **983**
Peter J. Stern
Paul R. Fassler

71. Pronator Syndrome **995**
Peter J. Stern
Paul R. Fassler

Part XV.
RADIAL NERVE COMPRESSION 1003

72. Posterior Interosseous Nerve Compression Syndrome **1005**
James B. Steichen
Alan W. Christensen

73. Radial Tunnel Syndrome **1023**
Graham D. Lister

74. Radial Sensory Nerve Entrapment **1039**
A. Lee Dellon

Part XVI.
ULNAR NERVE COMPRESSION 1053

75. Clinical Assessment and Conservative Treatment of Cubital Tunnel Syndrome **1055**
Donald C. Ferlic

76. In Situ Decompression of the Ulnar Nerve at the Elbow **1063**
Donald C. Ferlic

77. Anterior Intramuscular Transposition **1069**
William B. Kleinman

78. Anterior Subcutaneous Transposition **1077**
Richard G. Eaton

79. Medial Epicondylectomy **1087**
Steven J. Heithoff
Lewis H. Millender

80. Submuscular Transposition/Ulnar Nerve Decompression in Athletes **1097**
Norman P. Zemel
Frank W. Jobe
Lewis A. Yocum

81. Treatment and Complications of Failed Decompression of the Ulnar Nerve at the Elbow **1107**
Peter C. Amadio
Gerard T. Gabel

82. Perspectives on the Operative Treatment of Cubital Tunnel Syndrome **1121**
James R. Urbaniak
Gerard T. Gabel

83. Ulnar Tunnel Syndrome **1131**
Richard H. Gelberman

Part XVII.
OTHER COMPRESSION AND TRACTION NEUROPATHIES 1145

84. Compression and Traction Neuropathies About the Shoulder and Arm **1147**
Algimantas O. Narakas

85. Thoracic Outlet Syndrome **1177**
Robert D. Leffert

86. Compressive Neuropathies of the Lower Extremity **1197**
Michael B. Wood

87. Double Crush and Multiple Compression Neuropathy **1211**
A. Lee Osterman

88. Nerve Injury Associated With Patient Positioning in the Operating Room **1231**
Daniel E. Cooper

Part XVIII.
BRACHIAL PLEXUS INJURY IN ADULTS 1243

89. Nerve Injury and Total Hip Arthroplasty **1245**
Thomas P. Schmalzried
Harlan C. Amstutz

90. Brachial Plexus—Applied Anatomy and Operative Exposure **1255**
Bruce Wolock
Hanno Millesi

91. Assessment and Monitoring of Brachial Plexus Injury in the Adult **1273**
Neal B. Zimmerman
Andrew J. Weiland

92. Brachial Plexus Injury in Adults: Operative Repair **1285**
Hanno Millesi

93. Operative Treatment for Irreparable Lesions of the Brachial Plexus **1303**
Robin R. Richards

94. Neurotization in the Treatment of Brachial Plexus Injuries **1329**
Algimantas O. Narakas

Part XIX.
BRACHIAL PLEXUS INJURY IN CHILDREN 1359

95. Assessment and Natural History of Brachial Plexus Injury in Children **1361**
H. Mark Hoffer

96. Operative Repair of the Brachial Plexus in Infants and Children **1369**
Vincent R. Hentz

Part XX.
SPINAL CORD INJURY 1385

97. Spinal Cord Injury/Tetraplegia **1387**
Harris Gellman
Robert L. Waters

Part XXI.
BRAIN INJURY AND STROKE 1413

98. Brain Injury and Stroke **1415**
Michael J. Botte
Mary Ann E. Keenan

Part XXII.
CEREBRAL PALSY 1453

99. Cerebral Palsy **1455**
Richard H. Gelberman

Part XXIII.
PAIN 1477

100. Pain Pathways and Responses to Pain **1479**
Gudarz Davar
Raymond Maciewicz

101. Pain Dysfunction Syndrome **1489**
James H. Dobyns

102. Reflex Sympathetic Dystrophy **1497**
L. Andrew Koman
Gary G. Poehling

103. Neuromas **1525**
James H. Herndon
Alfred V. Hess

104. Treatment of the Painful Injured Nerve In-Continuity **1541**
John S. Gould

105. Chronic Pain Treatment With Direct Electrical Nerve Stimulation **1551**
William P. Cooney III

106. Therapeutic Blocks and Continuous Infusion in the Treatment of Chronic Pain **1563**
Daniel B. Carr
Donald P. Todd

Part XXIV. PERIPHERAL NERVE TUMORS 1571

107. Principles of Soft-Tissue Tumor Management **1573**
Henry J. Mankin

108. Benign and Malignant Tumors of Peripheral Nerve **1587**
Andrew E. Rosenberg
Harold M. Dick
Michael J. Botte

I

MORPHOLOGY AND PHYSIOLOGY OF PERIPHERAL NERVE

1 Structure and Function of Peripheral Nerve

2 Impulse Conduction

3 Biomechanical Properties of Peripheral Nerve

4 Biochemical Properties of Peripheral Nerve

5 The Neuromuscular Junction

6 Sensory Receptors

1

Structure and Function of Peripheral Nerve

Goran Lundborg
Lars B. Dahlin

AUTHORS' KEY POINTS

- Nerve fibers are extended processes of proximally located nerve cell bodies. The viability of axons depends on the intracellular anterograde and retrograde axonal transport of essential products, as well as nutrition provided by an intraneural microvascular system.
- The basic connective tissue elements of the nerve trunk are the endoneurium, perineurium, and epineurium. The *epineurium* protects nerve from compression and, ultimately, from stretch. The diffusion barrier of the *perineurium* maintains a positive endoneural fluid pressure and an optimal intrafascicular environment. The *endoneurium* provides a framework of support for individual nerve fibers.
- The blood vessels of peripheral nerve extend longitudinally within the epineurium. In the perineurium, vascular plexi are formed with longitudinal vessels extending for considerable distances between cellular layers. The endoneural microvascular network consists of arterioles and venules, and a longitudinally oriented segmental capillary network. Endoneural blood vessels possess a blood–nerve barrier.
- While well-developed anastomoses ensure adequate blood flow to peripheral nerve following considerable direct extrinsic trauma, blood flow is inhibited significantly by relatively low levels of longitudinal stretch.

STRUCTURE OF PERIPHERAL NERVE

Peripheral nerve is a composite structure consisting of a number of cellular and tissue elements. Its connective tissue coats provide protection of and nutrition to the functional units, the nerve fibers. The nerve fibers are extended processes of cell bodies located in the spinal cord (motor neurons), dorsal root ganglia (sensory neurons), or sympathetic ganglia (sympathetic neurons). Each fiber is embedded in loose *endoneural* connective tissue.

Bundles of fibers are collected in *fascicles*; each fascicle is protected by an external membranous structure, the *perineurium*. The perineurium, because it possesses a diffusion barrier to a number of extrinsic macromolecules, maintains an optimal intrafascicular environment. Fascicles are embedded in a well-vascularized areolar connective tissue membrane, the *epineurium*. The epineurium protects nerve fibers from compression and ultimately from stretch deformation. Nerve fiber function depends on a local energy supply provided by a longitudinally oriented intraneural microvascular system, the main channels of which are located in the epineurium. Through a well-developed system of anastomoses located throughout all connective tissue layers, the vascular supply to nerve is well maintained.

The assessment and treatment of nerve injuries is based on an understanding of the composition and function of the various tissue components of nerve, the fundamental characteristics of which are presented in this chapter.

Nerve Fibers

Nerve fibers, or *axons*, are extended processes of nerve cell bodies situated in the spinal cord, dorsal root ganglion, and sympathetic ganglia. The ratio between the size of a cell body and its axon is considerable, as axons may extend over distances corresponding to many thousands of times the cell body diameter (Fig. 1-1). A consequence of this

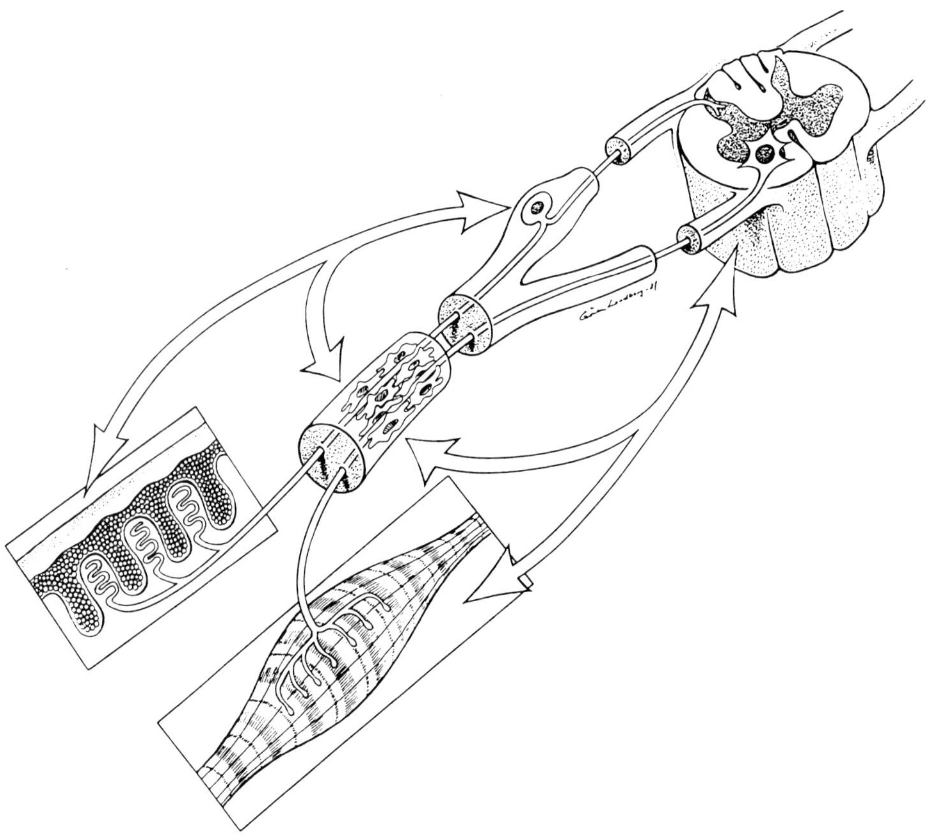

Figure 1–1. *The neuron with its nerve cell body located in the ventral horn in the spinal cord or in dorsal root ganglion and the extended process (axon) extending out to the periphery (muscle and skin). The target organs are influenced trophically from the nerve cell bodies and are also dependent on a constant supply of neuronotrophic factors from the target organ or the Schwann cells. These factors are transported up to the cell bodies. (From Lundborg G. Nerve injury and repair. Edinburgh: Churchill-Livingstone, 1988:2, with permission.)*

extremely specialized cellular composition is that the axon contains more than 90% of the total cytoplasmic volume of the nerve cell (neuron). Since the axon represents one nerve cell in continuity over a very long distance, a localized lesion to an axon has serious structural and functional consequences for survival of the whole neuron, including the nerve cell body.[3,4,18,24,41–43,106]

Nerve fibers are either *myelinated* or *nonmyelinated* (Fig. 1-2).[104] While both myelinated and nonmyelinated axons are surrounded by a chain of Schwann cells arranged end to end, the specific relationship between the Schwann cell and axon differs. The myelinated nerve fiber consists of one axon, which is associated with only one Schwann cell at any one level. The membrane of the Schwann cell, the *myelin sheath*, is wrapped spirally around the axon, creating a multilaminate sleeve of lipids and proteins (Fig. 1-3). In nonmyelinated fibers, Schwann cells accumulate large numbers of axons, which are located in internal troughs (Fig. 1-4). The Schwann cells, arranged in a longitudinal sequence, approach each other at the *nodes of Ranvier*, where fingerlike cellular processes interdigitate. At these locations there is an exchange of ions between the axon and the surrounding extracellular fluid, allowing saltatory propagation of impulses from node to node to occur (see Chap. 2). This allows for the rapid propagation of impulses in myelinated fibers. Between the nodes of Ranvier, the compact myelin and cytoplasm within a Schwann cell are arranged in a series of concentric subcellular compartments surrounding the axon. This insulates the Schwann cell both morphologically and physiologically from the endoneurium. The axon has a core of axoplasm surrounded by a

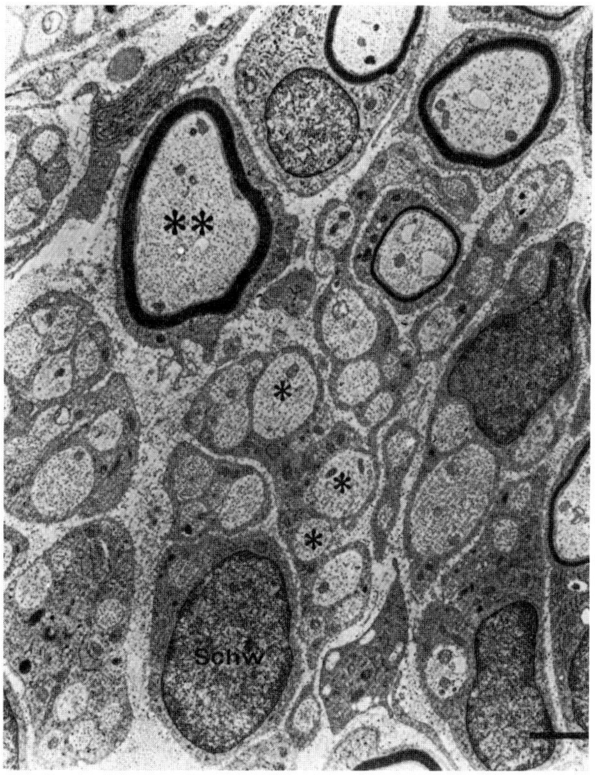

Figure 1–2. *Ultrastructural appearance of cross section of nerve fibers of rat sciatic nerve. Myelinated fibers (**) with myelin sheath are seen among numerous nonmyelinated fibers (*). (Schw = Schwann cell. The length of the bar is 1 μm.) (From Lundborg G. Nerve injury and repair. Edinburgh: Churchill-Livingstone, 1988:36, with permission.)*

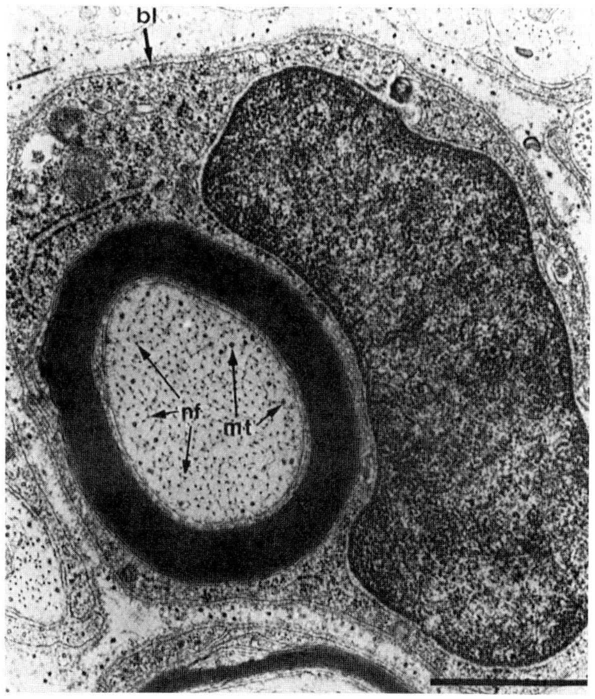

Figure 1–3. *One myelinated nerve fiber with its myelin sheath created by the Schwann cell. The Schwann cell is surrounded by a basal lamina (bl). A part of the cytoskeleton of the nerve fiber is visible. (mt, microtubulus; nf, neurofilaments. The length of the bar is 1 μm.) (From Lundborg G. Nerve injury and repair. Edinburgh: Churchill-Livingstone, 1988:37, with permission.)*

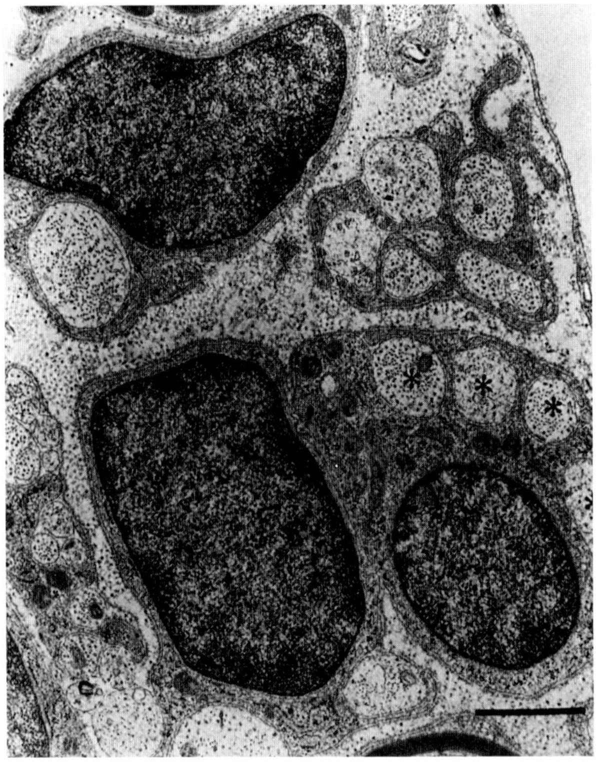

Figure 1–4. *Nonmyelinated nerve fibers with several fibers enclosed in troughs in the cytoplasm of one Schwann cell. (The length of the bar is 1 μm.) (From Lundborg G. Nerve injury and repair. Edinburgh: Churchill-Livingstone, 1988: 38, with permission.)*

continuous plasma membrane—the axolemma. In nonmyelinated fibers the ion exchange is continuous, giving a lower impulse velocity. The Schwann cells of the myelin sheath are bounded peripherally by a continuous Schwann cell plasma membrane. The basal lamina, the Schwann cell membrane, and the reticular and collagen fibrils of the endoneurium provide a framework of support for the nerve fiber. The resulting channel is labeled the *endoneural tube.*[64]

Ultrastructurally, axoplasm contains a variety of proteins and cytoskeletal elements, among which *microtubules* and *neurofilaments* (see Fig. 1-3) are the most prominent. Microtubules, consisting of polymerized α- and β-tubulin, are located centrally in the axon together with neurofilaments.[29,62,89,110] Proteins associated with microtubules appear as fine filamentous structures on the surfaces of the microtubule. The latter consist of three proteins with different molecular weights. Microfilaments, composed of actin and other proteins, are approximately 6 nm wide and are located mainly just beneath the axolemma.

Clinical Significance

Conduction properties of peripheral nerve are related to the structure of the axon and myelin sheath. Schwann cells interdigitate at the nodes of Ranvier, allowing for saltatory propagation of impulses in myelinated fibers. Protection of nerve fibers is provided by the epineurium and the perineurium.

Nerve Fiber Types

Erlanger and Gasser classified nerve fibers into three groups, based on the relationship between the shape of the compound axon potential and the fiber size.[21] Group A fibers are the largest and have the fastest conduction velocities. These fibers are myelinated somatic afferents and efferents. Myelinated autonomic and preganglionic fibers belonging to Group B and Group C fibers are thin, slowly conducting nonmyelinated visceral and somatic afferent fibers. Postganglionic, autonomic efferents are also in Group C. It is through the thin nonmyelinated C fibers (0.1–1 μm) that the sensation of deep burning pain is transferred. Group A fibers are further subdivided according to fiber size into A-α (15–20 μm), A-β (8–15 μm), and A-δ (2–5 μm). Efferent motor fibers, which have a large diameter, belong to the A-α fiber group. A-δ fibers transfer the sensation of sharp, pricking pain and temperature, while the A-β fibers are associated with touch.

Clinical Significance

Nerve fiber types are related to specific functions (eg, burning pain, sharp pain, temperature, touch, etc).

Axonal Transport

The neuron consists of a nerve cell body and one or more extended processes. The axon depends on the nerve cell body for both survival and function. Within the axon there is a continuous bidirectional transport system. Axonal transport of a wide range of substances and organelles, including proteins, membranous vesicles, neurotransmitters, lipids, mitochondria, and RNA, occurs. Transport from the nerve cell body down the axon is known as *anterograde transport*; transport in the opposite direction is termed *retrograde transport*.

While the transport of various substances is a phenomenon seen in many cells, the transport system of neurons is unique. Materials are transported within the axons to their sites of function over distances that are many times the diameter of their cell bodies.

Anterograde Transport

Essential materials are provided to axons from synthesis sites in the nerve cell body. There is a steady loss of constituents as they are carried peripherally, with the result that only 70% of such materials reach the axon terminal. Five groups of anterograde transport based on transport rates have been established (Table 1-1).[25,31,36,37,115] *Fast axonal transport* (20–410 mm/day; Groups I and II) consists of the passage of material that is membrane-bound and material associated with membranes of subcellular organelles, such as small vesicles and secretory granules, as well as soluble materials and transmitter-associated enzymes.[25,31] Fast transport is critically dependent on an adequate supply of energy. It is blocked by anoxia, metabolic inhibitors,[12,13,38,74] and a number of toxic substances.[61] The inhibitors of axonal transport and neurotransmitters and neurotransmitter-associated enzyme delivery have a profound effect on synaptic transmission.[17]

While *slow axonal transport* has a considerably lower velocity (0.1–30 mm/day) than fast axonal transport, the amount of proteins transported is greater and the protein composition is different. Unlike fast transport, which is relatively constant from one type of neuron to another, slow transport rates vary with different nerves and with the substances being transported.[11,73] There are three components of slow transport. Component a (SCa), or group V (0.1–1 or 12–15 mm/day), consists of cytoskeletal elements (eg, subunit proteins of microtubules [α- or β-tubulin]) and three neurofilament subunit proteins (Fig. 1-5).[10,11,28,29,37,40,44,62] Slow component b (SCb, group IV) is more complex in composition, containing elements of axoplasmic or microtrabecular matrix (eg, actin, clathrin, and

Table 1–1 *Components of Axonal Transport*

Component	*Velocity*	*Composition*
ANTEROGRADE		
Fast		***Membrane-Associated Materials***
Groups I and II	20–410 mm/day	Membrane constituents, transmitter-associated enzymes, various small-molecular-weight materials (eg, amino acids)
Group III	4–8 mm/day	Polypeptides (eg, myosin-like actin-binding polypeptide)
Slow		***Cytoskeletal and Associated Proteins***
Group IV (SCb)	2–30 mm/day	Elements of axoplasmic or microtrabecular matrix (eg, actin, clathrin)
Group V (SCa)	0.1–15 mm/day	eg, tubulin, neurofilament triplet
RETROGRADE		
Fast	≤300 mm/day	"Recycled materials," neuronotrophic factors (eg, NGF)
Slow	3–8 mm/day	Single protein

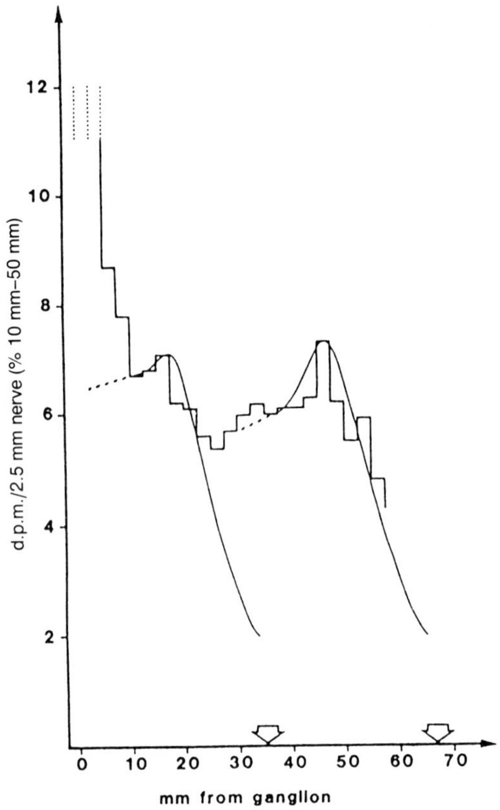

Figure 1–5. *Diagram showing two waves of slow axonal transport in rabbit vagus nerve. The nerve cell bodies in the nodose ganglion are labeled by injection with a radioactive amino acid; the amino acid is incorporated in proteins and thereafter transported in the axon. After an appropriate time the nerve is taken out and transected in 2.5-mm pieces. Each nerve piece is processed and the amount of radioactivity is measured. The y axis shows the amount of radioactivity, and the x axis shows the length of each nerve piece from the nodose ganglion. Two clear waves of slow axonal transport (corresponding to SCb and SCa) are seen with a velocity of 12–15 mm/day and 25–30 mm/day, respectively. (Reproduced by kind permission of Journal of Neurological Sciences 1986.)*

calmodulin) (see Fig. 1-5).[10,11,37,44,60,62] The velocity of SCb is higher (2–4 or 25–30 mm/day) than that of SCa. The third component (4–8 mm/day, group III) contains a myosin-like polypeptide.[11,118] Slow transport depends on a constant supply of materials from the nerve cell body.

Most of the theories on the mechanism of anterograde transport provide an important role for *microtubules*.[25] Recent data demonstrating the close relationship between microtubules and the fast axonal transport system emphasize the fundamental concept that anterograde axonal transport is an energy-requiring process.[14]

Retrograde Transport

Transport from the periphery to the nerve cell body is called *retrograde transport*. The velocity of this transport system (as great as 300 mm/day) is considerably lower than that of fast transport.[7] There seems to be a slow component in retrograde transport (1–2 mm/day).[22,23] The protein composition of retrograde transport is similar to that of fast transport. The materials transported include multivesicular and multilamellar organelles (prelysosomal and lysosomal structures).[107] Viruses such as herpes simplex may be incorporated at axon terminals and transferred through the axon to the nerve cell body by retrograde transport. In this way, retrograde transport of certain agents may have profound negative effects on the cell body. Material originally transported by anterograde transport to the axon terminal is transported back to the nerve cell body. The "recycling process" of materials, one function of retrograde transport, is based on a reversal process that takes place at the terminal.[15] It appears that at least 50% of fast-transported proteins in motor neurons are transported back to the nerve cell body.[8] Materials returned to the cell body are either degraded or re-used.

An important function of retrograde transport is the transfer of information regarding the status of the axon, its terminals, its target cells, and its environment.[8,112] That information is transferred by special factors (neuronotrophic factors), which are proteins supplied by the target territory, incorporated by the axon terminals, and transported by retrograde transport to the nerve cell body. It is there that modulatory effects are exerted.[112] The first specialized factor described is *nerve growth factor* (NGF).[39,102] Neuronotrophic factors (NTF) are important for nerve survival and the lack of these factors is probably responsible for the functional and structural nerve cell body changes that take place after injury.[9,16,24,26]

Retrograde transport's transmission mechanism is similar to that of anterograde transport and requires energy.[14] Substances that interfere with the metabolism of axons[20] and injuries that cause isch-

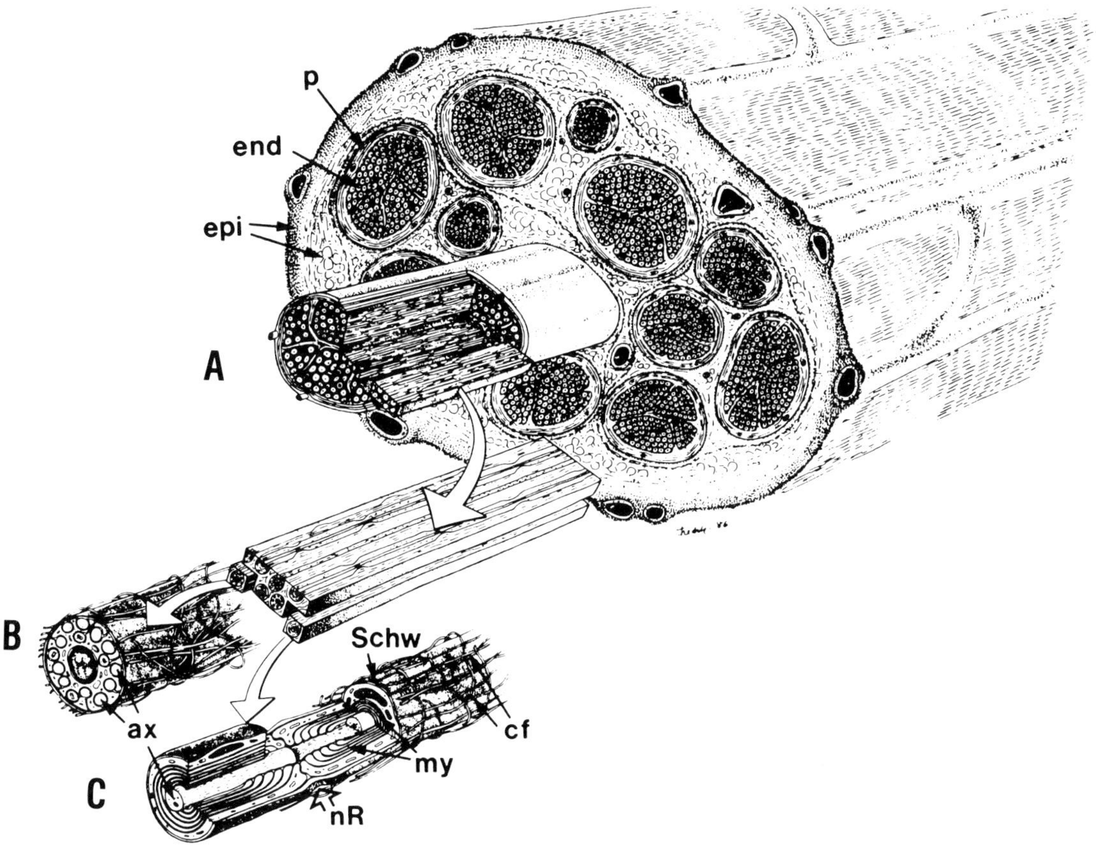

Figure 1–6. *Schematic drawing of the microanatomy of the peripheral nerve trunk with all its components. (**A**) The fascicles of the peripheral nerve surrounded by the perineurium (p) and embedded in a loose connective tissue—the epineurium (epi). The intrafascicular tissue elements surrounding the nerve fibers are called the endoneurium (end). (**B**) Nonmyelinated nerve fibers (ax) enclosed in troughs in one Schwann cell. (**C**) One axon around which one Schwann cell (Schw) is wrapped spirally. The place where two adjacent Schwann cells meet is called the node of Ranvier (nR). (From Lundborg G. Nerve injury and repair. Edinburgh: Churchill-Livingstone, 1988:33, with permission.)*

emia can block retrograde transport.[34,108] It appears that retrograde transport does not depend on continuity with the cell body, since transport continues within isolated nerve segments until Wallerian degeneration occurs.

Clinical Significance

Anterograde and retrograde axonal transport are energy-dependent functions of nerve that provide nutrients and cytoskeletal elements to the periphery by anterograde, and recycling and information transfer by retrograde axonal transport. Injury to the nutritional or structural components of nerve can interfere with axonal transport.

Perineurium

Inside fascicles, nerve fibers are collected in a loose collagenous matrix containing fibroblasts, mast cells, a capillary network, and the endoneurium (Fig. 1-6). As nutrients passing from capillaries to axons, as well as waste products passing in the opposite direction, extend over fairly large extracellular spaces, the vital nutritive process becomes susceptible to certain pathological states, such as endoneural edema.

Each fascicle is surrounded by a dense, mechanically strong multilamellar sheath, the *peri-*

neurium.[32] The perineurium is composed of flattened cells with a basement membrane on both outer and inner aspects. The number of lamellae varies with the diameter of the fascicle, with up to 15 layers surrounding fascicles of mammalian nerve trunks. Adjacent cells are closely related to each other by interdigitations of cell processes, the gaps between which are extremely narrow.[94–97,105] The spaces separating the perineural lamellae contain longitudinally and obliquely oriented collagen fibers and elastic fibers.[103] These spaces also contain vessels that run longitudinally over long distances before they enter the endoneural space (Fig. 1-7).

Although the endoneural space is isolated by perineural cells, this isolation is not total. Individual blood vessels pass through the perineurium accompanied by a perineural sleeve. The perineurium is not closed all the way to the periphery—it terminates as an open-ended sleeve just proximal to the motor endplates. This may be a critical point for the entry into the endoneural space of substances that otherwise could not penetrate the perineurium along the course of the nerve.

While Thomas and Jones[103] claim that the perineurium includes only concentric cellular lamellae, other investigators feel that the term "perineurium" includes these cell layers as well as the connective tissue layer located immediately outside the cellular lamellae.[64,100] The distinction is of clinical importance when considering the technical aspects of group fascicular repair (see Chap. 18).

The perineurium is a mechanically strong membrane; in experimental studies it has sustained elevations of intrafascicular pressure of up to levels of 300 to 750 mm Hg before rupturing.[93] It also protects the contents of the endoneural space, acting as a mechanical barrier to external trauma, and serves as a diffusion barrier, which makes it important for preserving the specific internal environment of the endoneurium.

Perineural Diffusion Barrier

The perineurium constitutes a diffusion barrier to numerous substances (eg, large proteins),[49,52,57,59,64,85,99,105] small molecular proteins,[33,77,78,86,99] and ferritin.[76,113] The barrier function works in both directions—from outside the fascicle to the inside, as well as from inside outward. While endoneural edema occurs due to the tight mechanical junction that exists between individual perineural cells, the perineural membrane acts as a metabolically active diffusion barrier.[105] Perineural cells show high activity for different diphosphore-relating and oxidative enzymes. ATP has been demonstrated intracellularly in micropinocytotic vesicles, as well as in basement membranes.[72,91,94]

The perineural diffusion barrier is important in maintaining osmosis as well as an electrolytic equilibrium around axons. It is believed that the perineural diffusion barrier is an important component

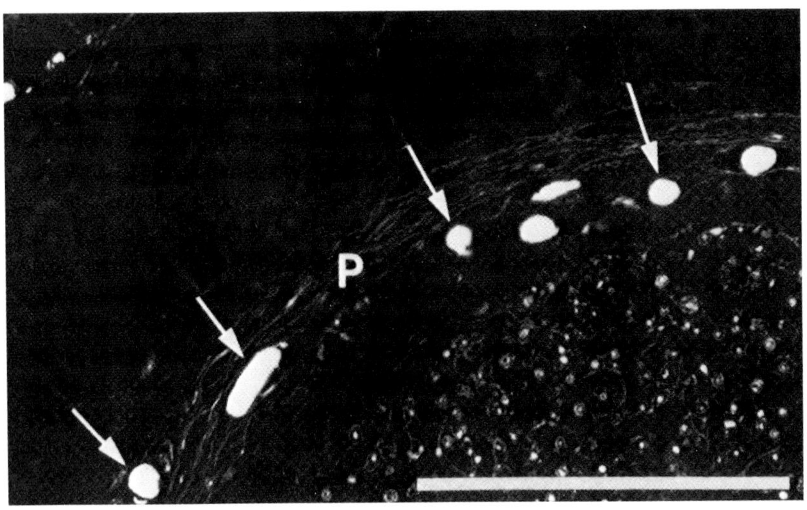

Figure 1–7. *Cross section of perfused human median nerve showing vessels running longitudinally (arrows) between lamellae at various steps of the perineurium (p). (The length of the bar is 0.1 mm.) (From Lundborg G. Nerve injury and repair. Edinburgh: Churchill-Livingstone, 1988:45, with permission.)*

in the regulation and maintenance of the "internal milieu" of the endoneural space. Together with the diffusion barrier made by the walls of endoneural capillaries (the blood–nerve barrier), the perineurium protects the endoneurium from external influences by providing an effective filter against the influx of ions, proteins, and other potentially hazardous agents. This special endoneural environment is believed to be of the utmost importance for optimal nerve fiber function—a suggestion supported by the fact that impaired nerve function is seen in association with experimental barrier damage.[84]

The perineural barrier is important in protecting nerve fibers from associated damage. As the perineurium is remarkably resistant to mechanical trauma, the diffusion barrier works properly even after profound nerve injury.[54] It has been shown experimentally that external compression of magnitudes as great as 400 to 600 mm Hg for several hours fails to interfere with the barrier function (see Chap. 59).[88] On the other hand, local crush injuries cause a deterioration of the barrier function that may persist for prolonged periods.[84]

Clinical Significance

The perineurium, a distinct multilamellated sheath, has a protective function as well as a barrier function in order to maintain a constant and adequate internal milieu for nerve fibers.

Intrafascicular Tissue Pressure

The stiffness of nerve fascicles is attributed to a slightly positive intrafascicular tissue pressure. Tissue pressure within the fascicle, termed *endoneural fluid pressure* (EFP), is normally +1.2–1.5 mm Hg,[46,47,71] slightly greater than levels seen in other tissues (eg, muscle tissue has an EFP of −2 mm Hg).[27] Once the perineural tube is transected, endoneural contents bulge at the free nerve ends, a phenomenon called *mushrooming*. After nonpenetrating injuries (eg, ischemia, compression, cryogenic insult), EFP increases dramatically.[52,56,70] Since protein cannot escape peripherally through the perineurium, a compartment syndrome in miniature occurs, which interferes with the integrity of the intrafascicular microvascular system.[54]

Epineurium

The epineurium is a loose, soft connective tissue layer that embeds and protects the fascicles, cushioning them during movements of the extremity and protecting them against external trauma. It acts as a protective cushion for the functional units of nerve. It contains a well-developed vascular plexus with numerous longitudinal main vascular channels that feed the endoneural capillary plexus. The deep layers of epineurium simultaneously separate fascicles and keep them loosely together. Superficially, the connective tissue is condensed to a sheath, delimiting nerve from surrounding structures to which it is very loosely attached by a layer resembling the conjunctiva. This allows a great deal of motion.

The amount of epineurium relative to nerve cross-sectional area varies with specific nerves and nerve levels.[100,101] Near joints, epineurium is more abundant than elsewhere, constituting up to 75% of the cross section of nerves, probably due to the fact that nerves are subjected to friction and compression at these sites. Histologically, the epineurium resembles other types of loose connective tissue that contain fibroblasts, macrophages, and mast cells.

An important function of the epineurium, and of extraneural connective tissue, is the provision of a certain amount of gliding of nerve with movement of the extremity. The excursion of nerve trunks may be as great as 50 mm (level of the brachial plexus). The values given for the median and ulnar nerves just proximal to the elbow are 7.3 mm and 9.8 mm, respectively, during full elbow flexion and extension (see Chap. 18).[117] Proximal to the carpal tunnel, excursion of the same nerves is 14.5 mm and 14.8 mm, respectively. Distal to the carpal tunnel the values are 6.8 mm and 6.5 mm, respectively.

The longitudinal movement of nerve trunks is made possible by the special arrangement of the interface layers between nerve and surrounding tissues.[35,63,111] Superficial to the epineurium, an adventitia of loose connective tissue allows a great deal of neural gliding. There is also a gliding layer located more deeply inside the nerve trunk that allows fascicles to slide within the deeper layers of the epineurium. A specialized vascular anatomical

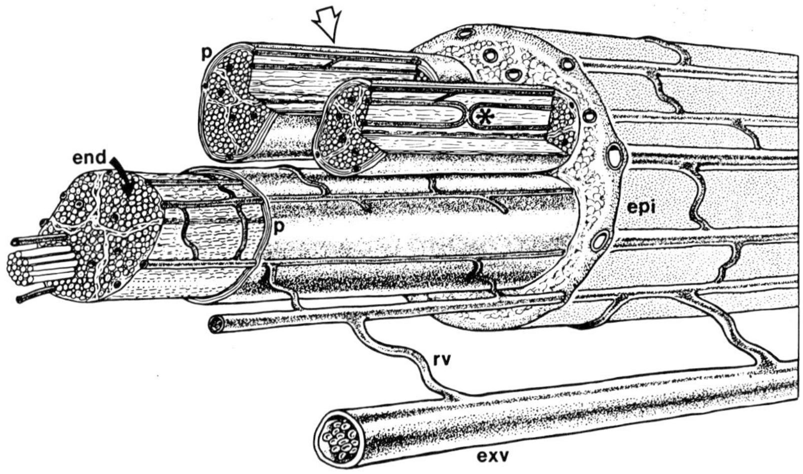

Figure 1–8. *Schematic drawing of the microvascular architecture in a peripheral nerve. Vascular plexi in the epineurium (epi) are led via regional vessels (rv) from extrinsic vessels (exv). There are vascular plexi in the superficial and deep layers of the epineurium, perineurium (p), and endoneurium (end). Note the oblique course of the vessels penetrating the perineurium (open arrow). An intrafascicular double-loop formation is indicated by *. (From Lundborg G. Nerve injury and repair. Edinburgh: Churchill-Livingstone, 1988:43, with permission.)*

arrangement, both inside and outside nerve, allows considerable neural excursion without loss of nutrition.

Clinical Significance

Functions of the epineurium include protection of nerve against compression and provision of extraneural gliding, a function that may be inhibited by scarring associated with nerve injury.

INTRANEURAL MICROVASCULAR SYSTEM

Architecture

Peripheral nerves are well-vascularized structures with separate but extensively interconnected microvascular systems in the epineurium, perineurium, and endoneurium. For surgeons treating nerve injuries, the role of the intraneural microvascular system is important with regard to the effects of chronic irritation, compression, mobilization, stretching, and transection. Since the development of microsurgical techniques, intraneural dissections have become common, and the effects of intraneural vascular damage secondary to such procedures must be considered. An adequate energy supply, which is provided by intraneural microvessels, is essential for nerve function and axonal transport.[1,5,6,19,49–52] The microvascular system within nerve is characterized by vessels that extend longitudinally within the epineurium (Fig. 1-8). Along the course of nerve, this vascular system is reinforced by *segmental regional vessels of extrinsic origin.* These regional vessels travel in a loose adventitia of connective tissue that surrounds nerve, allowing it to slide longitudinally in its bed with movements of the extremity.

The main longitudinal vessels of the "intrinsic" vascular system of nerve are located in the epineurium. In the deeper layers, prominent vessels provide anastomoses segmentally to fascicles. Vascular plexi are then formed within the perineurium (see Figs. 1-7, 1-8). Longitudinal microvessels extend for long distances between the individual cellular layers of the perineurium. Such vessels course over long distances before piercing the inner perineural layer. They enter the endoneural space in a characteristic oblique way. The oblique passage of microvessels through the inner membrane of the perineurium may create a valve mechanism whereby increases in intrafascicular tissue pressure reduce lumen size, impeding fascicular blood flow (Fig. 1-9).[49,50,69] The intrinsic and extrinsic systems are in equilibrium with each other, each being able to compensate for functional disturbances in the other.

Within fascicles there is an endoneural microvascular network consisting mainly of capillaries but also including arterioles and venules. The longitudinally oriented capillary system is formed throughout the fascicles of the nerve. Segmental endoneural capillary systems are linked together like components of a chain by "double U-loop" anastomoses (see Fig. 1-8). They also are linked to extrafascicular epineural vessels by transperineural

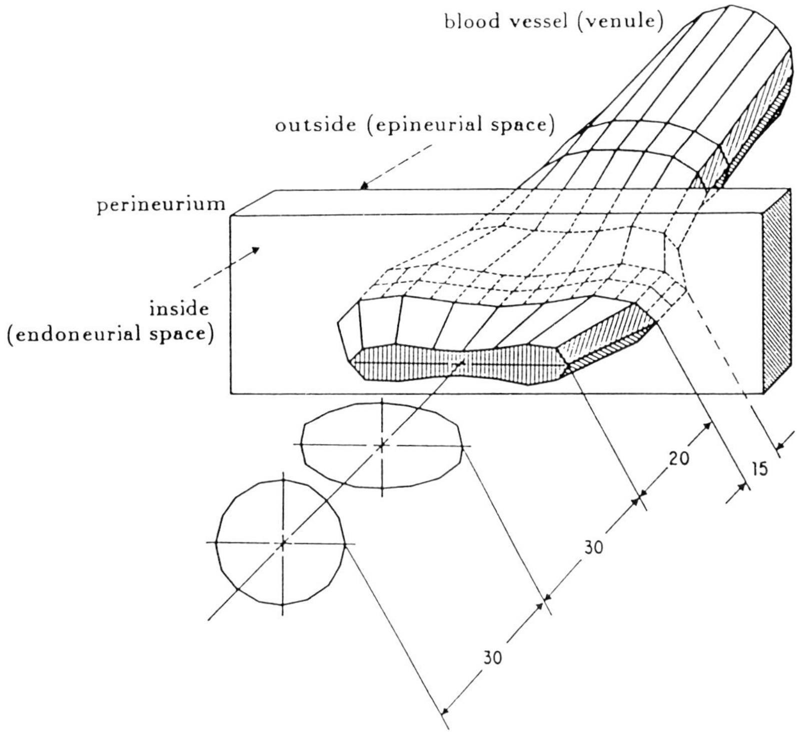

Figure 1–9. *Three-dimensional computer analysis of deformation of the cylindrical blood vessels that pass obliquely through the perineurium into a fascicle where edema is present. Tissue properties are well defined and are believed to represent pathophysiological values present in edematous neuropathies and with an endoneurial fluid pressure of 6 mm Hg. The perspective of the drawing is from inside the endoneurium. (From Myers RR, Murakami H, Powell HC. Reduced nerve blood flow in edematous neuropathies: A biochemical mechanism. Microvascular Res 1986;32:147, with permission.)*

anastomoses. There is a considerable reserve capacity for blood flow in nerve due to the presence of longitudinal vessels that can compensate for loss of regional extrinsic vessels as nerve is mobilized over considerable distances.[49,50]

Intraneural Microcirculation

Recent studies[49,50,55] have shown that the anastomoses between vessels in different layers of nerve are extremely well developed and that no single direction of blood flow in endoneural vessels is predominant in any segment of the nerve trunk. The direction of blood flow in individual endoneural vessels can change immediately if slight compression is applied to the surface of the nerve or if a regional feeding artery is damaged.

Intravital microscopic techniques have been used to observe the capillary function of fascicles directly under various experimental conditions.[49,50,55] While the well-developed anastomoses between layers of nerve help ensure adequate blood flow when extrinsic regional vessels are damaged or nerve is transected, longitudinal tension interferes with intraneural microvascular flow at fairly low levels of strain.[57] If tension is applied to a nerve trunk, regional segmental vessels are stretched and extrinsic vascular inflow is inhibited. When tibial nerves were stretched experimentally, 8% impairment of venular blood flow was noted.[57] When stretch was 15%, a complete loss of intraneural circulation was noted.[57,65,66,75] In addition, tension narrows fascicles, contributing to the obliteration of intrafascicular capillaries (see Chap. 3). This phenomenon may occur as extremities are manipulated into extreme positions (eg, ulnar nerve below the medial epicondyle when the elbow is maximally flexed, nerves sutured under excessive tension, [90] etc.) (see Chap. 36). Intraneural blood flow is reduced initially when ulnar nerves are mobilized and transferred anteriorly to the medial epicondyle.[75]

The ratio of blood flow to metabolic activity in peripheral nerve is high compared to that seen in the brain. In the sciatic nerve of rats the value for nerve blood flow (NBF) is 14 to 16 ml/min/100 g. [48,68] The NBF in diabetic rats is lower, about 8.7 ml/min/100 g.[45,109] This is important when considering the relationship between diabetic neuropathy and nerve trauma (see Chap. 68).

Clinical Significance

The nerve's microvascular system is both segmental and longitudinal in orientation. This anatomical arrangement allows for extensive longitudinal dissection of nerve without significant injury to intraneural perfusion. Intrafascicular vessels possess a barrier function (blood–nerve barrier).

"Nervi Nervorum"

In the wall of epineural vessels are fine nerve endings from the sympathetic nervous system.[2,49] These adrenergic nerve fibers, originating from fibers running inside nerve trunks, represent a system through which nerve regulates its own microcirculation. In animal experiments, stimulation of the lumbar sympathetic chain is followed by an immediate decrease in intraneural microcirculation due to vasoconstriction.[92] It also has been reported that there are other nerve fibers, mainly nonmyelinated ones, running longitudinally or spirally in the epineurium. Free nerve endings in all connective tissue layers, including the perineurium, have been observed.[30]

Blood–Nerve Barrier

The diffusion barrier of the perineurium maintains an optimal osmotic and electrolytic environment around axons within fascicles. The blood–nerve barrier (BNB) corresponds to the blood–brain barrier of the central nervous system. Its structural and functional features allow for the creation of a barrier to several substances, including macromolecules, circulating in the blood. While substances easily pass through the endothelium of vessels in the epineurium, little or no leakage is seen through endoneural microvessels.[50,52,78–82,86,114]

Due to tight junctions between extremely closely apposed endothelial cells,[5,86] the BNB is structurally analogous to junctions noted between individual cells in the perineural membrane. Together with the diffusion barrier provided by the perineurium, the BNB is essential for maintaining a unique endoneural environment. Changes in the barrier function of the endoneural vessels and perineurium also occur in association with traumatic nerve injuries and some surgical procedures. Like other well-vascularized tissues in the body, peripheral nerve responds to trauma with an inflammatory reaction, including an increase in vascular permeability and a leakage of proteins from the blood into the interstitium. The epineural vessels do not contain a BNB, and they respond very early to even a slight trauma by increasing their permeability. Following physical or chemical trauma, or trauma due to ischemia, the BNB permeability increases and endoneural edema occurs.[53,58,67,70,83,87] Intrafascicular vascular perfusion may then be jeopardized. Increases in the permeability of endoneural capillaries following trauma may be due to direct mechanical injury or the result of released endogenous chemical mediators (eg, histamine and serotonin, located in mast cells in the nerve).[79–82] The endoneural space lacks lymphatic vessels.[98,100]

Moderate trauma to a nerve trunk may damage epineural blood vessels long before endoneural capillaries are affected. Epineural vessels, lacking a BNB, leak macromolecules in response to trauma. Increased vascular permeability in nerves occurs not only as an immediate response to trauma, but also as a second wave, peaking about 2 weeks after the injury. While the resulting epineural edema does not penetrate the perineurium, microvascular thrombus formation may occur and fibroblast invasion may take place if the traumatic episode is either severe or extends over a wide interval. Prolonged irritation may result in fibrosis of the epineurium, a condition seen in chronic nerve entrapment syndromes.

More severe crush or compression injuries may interfere directly with the BNB or the endoneural vessels, resulting in intrafascicular edema. Due to the barrier function of the perineurium, edema does not escape through the perineural membrane. Considerable increases in endoneural fluid pressure (EFP) may occur, creating a closed compartment syndrome in miniature.[56,70] As the endoneural space lacks lymphatic vessels, the drainage of endoneural edema depends on the slow interstitial bulk flow of fluid in a proximal–distal direction within the endoneurium.[116] Fluid drains from the endoneural space at the most distal part of nerve trunks where the perineurium terminates adjacent to nerve endings.

If endoneural edema is longstanding, as in severe chronic nerve compression, invasion by connective tissue elements occurs and fibrosis results. Endoneural fibrosis represents an extremely difficult clinical situation that cannot be ameliorated by surgery (see Chap. 63).

REFERENCES

1. Adams WE. The blood supply of nerves. I. Historical review. J Anat (London) 1942; 76:323–341.
2. Appenzeller O, Dithal KK, Cowen T, Burnstock G. The nerves to blood vessels supplying blood nerves: The innervation of vasa nervorum. Brain Res 1984; 304:383–386.
3. Archer DR. Axonal transport and related responses to nerve injury. Doctoral Thesis, University of Liverpool, 1987.
4. Barron KD. Comparative observations on the cytologic reactions of central and peripheral nerve cells to axotomy. In: Kao CC, Bunge RP, Reier PJ, eds. Spinal cord reconstruction. New York: Raven, 1983:7–40.
5. Bell MA, Weddell AGM. A morphometric study of intrafascicular vessels of mammalian sciatic nerve. Muscle Nerve 1984; 7:524–534.
6. Bell MA, Weddell AGM. A descriptive study of the blood vessels of the sciatic nerve in the rat, man and other mammals. Brain 1984; 107:871–898.
7. Bisby MA. Retrograde axonal transport. In Fedoroff S, Hertz L, eds. Advanced Cellular Neurobiology, vol 1. New York: Academic Press, 1980: 69–118.
8. Bisby MA. Functions of retrograde axonal transport. Federation Proceedings 1982; 41:2307–2311.
9. Bisby MA. Retrograde axonal transport and nerve regeneration. In: Elam JS, Cancalon P, eds. Axonal transport in neuronal growth and regeneration. Advances in neurochemistry, vol 6. New York/London: Plenum, 1984:45–67.
10. Black MM, Lasek RJ. Slow components of axonal transport: Two cytoskeletal Networks. J Cell Biol 1980; 86:616–623.
11. Brady ST, Lasek RJ. The slow components of axonal transport: Movements, compositions and organization. In: Weiss DG, Ed. Axoplasmic transport. Berlin: Springer-Verlag, 1982:206–217.
12. Brady ST, Lasek RJ, Allen RD. Fast axonal transport in extruded axoplasm from squid giant axon. Science 1982; 218.
13. Brady ST, Lasek RJ, Allen R. Videomicroscopy of fast axonal transport in extruded axoplasm: A new model for study of molecular mechanisms. Cell Motility 1985; 5:81–101.
14. Bray D. Fast axonal transport. Nature 1985; 315: 178–179.
15. Bray JJ, Kon CM, Breckenridge BM. Reversed polarity of rapid axonal transport in chicken motoneurons. Brain Res 1971; 33:560–564.
16. Cragg BH. What is the signal for chromatolysis. Brain Res 1970; 23:1–21.
17. Dahlström A. Axoplasmic transport and synaptic transmission. In: Weiss DG, Gorio A, eds. Axoplasmic transport in physiology and pathology. Berlin: Springer-Verlag, 1982:16–20.
18. Ducker TB. The central cell body and axonal regeneration. In: In: Gorio A, Millesi H, Mingrino S, eds. Post-traumatic peripheral nerve regeneration: Experimental basis and clinical implications. New York: Raven, 1981:7–11.
19. Edshage S. Peripheral nerve suture. Acta Chir Scand 1964; suppl 331:1–104.
20. Edström A, Hanson M. Retrograde axonal transport of proteins in vitro in frog sciatic nerves. Brain Res 1973; 61:311–320.
21. Erlanger J, Gasser H. Electrical signs of nervous activity. Philadelphia: University of Pennsylvania Press, 1937.
22. Fink DJ, Gainer H. Axonal transport of proteins: A new view using in vivo covalent labeling. J Cell Biol 1980; 85:175–186.
23. Gainer H, Fink DJ. Evidence for slow retrograde transport of serum albumin in rat sciatic nerve. Brain Res 1982; 233:404–408.
24. Grafstein B. The nerve cell body response to axotomy. Exp Neurol 1975; 48:32–51.
25. Grafstein B, Forman DS. Intracellular transport in neurons. Phys Rev 1980; 60:1167–1283.
26. Grafstein B, McQuarrie IG. Role of the nerve cell body in axonal regeneration. In: Cotman CW, ed. Neuronal plasticity. New York: Raven, 1978:155–195.
27. Hargens AR, Akeson WH, Mubarak SJ, et al. Fluid balance within the canine anterolateral compartment and its relationship to compartment syndromes. J Bone Joint Surg [Am] 1978; 60:499–505.
28. Hoffman PN, Lasek RJ. Identification of major structural polypeptides of the axon and their generality among mammalian neurons. J Cell Biol 1975; 66:351–366.
29. Hollenbeck PJ. The transport and assembly of the axonal cytoskeleton. J Cell Biol 1989; 108:223–227.
30. Hromada J. On the nerve supply of the connective tissue of some peripheral nervous system components. Acta Anat 1963; 55:343–351.
31. Karlsson JO. Axonal transport in retinal ganglion cells. In: Osborne NN, Chader GJ, eds. Progress

in retinal research, vol 3.Pergamon, 1984:105–123.
32. Key A, Retzius G. Studien in der Anatomie des Nervensystems und des Bindegewebes. Stockholm: Samson & Wallin, 1876.
33. Klemm H. Das Perineurium als Diffusionsbarriere gegenüber Peroxydase bei epi- und endoneuraler Applikation. Zeitschrift der Zellforschung 1970; 108:431–445.
34. Kristensson K, Olsson Y, Sjöstrand J. Axonal uptake and retrograde transport of exogenous proteins in the hypoglossal nerve. Brain Res 1971; 32:399–406.
35. Lang J. Ueber das Bindegewebe und die Gefässe der Nerven. Zeitschrift der Anatomische Entwicklung 1962; 123:61–79.
36. Lasek RJ. The dynamic ordering of neuronal cytoskeletons. Neurosci Res Program Bull 1981; 19: 7–32.
37. Lasek RJ, Garner JA, Brady ST. Axonal transport of the cytoplasmic matrix. J Cell Biol 1984; 99: 212–221.
38. Leone J, Ochs S. Anoxic block and recovery of axoplasmic transport and electrical excitability of nerve. J Neurobiol 1978; 9:229–245.
39. Levi-Montalcini R. The nerve growth factor—target cells interactions, a model system for the study of directed axonal growth and regeneration. Birth Defects Original Article Series 1983; 19:3–22.
40. Levine J, Willard M. The composition and organization of axonally transported proteins in the retinal ganglion cells of the guinea pig. Brain Res 1980; 194:137–154.
41. Lieberman AR. The axon reaction: A review of the principal features of perikaryal responses to axon injury. Int Rev Neurobiol 1971; 14:49–124.
42. Lieberman AR. Some factors affecting retrograde neuronal responses to axonal lesions. In: Bellaris R, Gray EG, eds. Essays on the nervous system. Oxford: Clarendon, 1974:71–105.
43. Lieberman AR. Sensory ganglia. In: Landon DN, ed. The peripheral nerve. London: Chapman & Hall, 1976:188–278.
44. Lorenz T, Willard M. Subcellular fractionation of intra-axonally transported polypeptides in rabbit visual system. Proc Nat Acad Sci 1978; 75:505–509.
45. Low PA, Ward K, Schmelzer J, Brimijoin S. Ischemic conduction failure and energy metabolism in experimental diabetic neuropathy. Am J Physiol 1985; 248:E457–E462.
46. Low PA, Dyck PJ. Increased endoneurial fluid pressure in experimental lead neuropathy. Nature 1977; 269:427–428.
47. Low P, Marchand G, Know F, Dyck PJ. Measurement of endoneurial fluid pressure with polyethylene matrix capsules. Brain Res 1977; 122:373–377.
48. Low PA, Nukada H, Schmelzer JD, Tuck RR, Dyck PJ. Endoneurial oxygen tension and radial topography in nerve edema. Brain Res 1985; 341:147—154.
49. Lundborg G. Ischemic nerve injury. Experimental studies on intraneural microvascular pathophysiology and nerve function in a limb subjected to temporary circulatory arrest. Scand J Plast Reconstr Surg 1970; suppl 6:1–113.
50. Lundborg G. Structure and function of the intraneural microvessels as related to trauma, edema, formation and nerve function. J Bone Joint Surg [Am] 1975; 57:938–948.
51. Lundborg G. The intrinsic vascularization of human peripheral nerves: Structural and functional aspects. J Hand Surg 1979; 4:34–41.
52. Lundborg G. Nerve injury and repair. Edinburgh: Churchill-Livingstone, 1988:.
53. Lundborg G, Dahlin LB, Danielsen N, Hansson HA, Necking LE, Pyykkö I. Intraneural edema following exposure to vibration. Scan J Work Environ Health 1987; 13:326–329.
54. Lundborg G, Nordborg C, Rydevik B, Olsson Y. The effect of ischemia on the permeability of the perineurium to protein tracers in rabbit tibial nerve. Acta Neurol Scand 1973; 49:287–294.
55. Lundborg G, Brånemark PI. Microvascular structure and function of peripheral nerves: Vital microscopic studies of the tibial nerve in the rabbit. Adv Microcirc 1968; 1:66–88.
56. Lundborg G, Myers R, Powell H. Nerve compression injury and increase in endoneurial fluid pressure: A miniature compartment syndrome. J Neurol Neurosurg Psychiatry 1983; 46:1119–1124.
57. Lundborg G, Rydevik B. Effects of stretching the tibial nerve of the rabbit: A preliminary study of the intraneural circulation and the barrier function of the perineurium. J Bone Joint Surg [Br] 1973; 55:390–401.
58. Lundborg G, Schildt B. Microvascular permeability in irradiated rabbits. Acta Radiol 1971; 10:311–320.
59. Martin KH. Untersuchungen über die perineurale Diffusionsbarriere and gefriergetrockneten Nerven. Zeitschrift der Zellforsch 1964; 64:404–428.
60. McLean WG. Slow axonal transport of actin and regeneration rate in non-myelinated sensory nerve. Brain Res 1985; 333:255–260.
61. McLean WG, Frizell M, Sjöstrand J. Pathology of axonal transport. In: Lajtha A, ed. Handbook of neurochemistry, vol 9. New York: Plenum, 1985: 67–86.

62. McLean WG, McKay AL, Sjöstrand J. Electrophoretic analysis of axonally transported proteins in the rabbit vagus nerve. J Neurobiol 1983; 14:227–236.
63. Millesi H. Nerve grafting. Clin Plast Surg 1984; 11:105–113.
64. Millesi H, Terzis J. Nomenclature in peripheral nerve surgery: Committee report of the International Society of Reconstructive Microsurgery. Clin Plast Surg 1984; 11:3–8.
65. Miyamoto Y, Tsuge K. Effects of tension on intraneural microcirculation in end-to-end neurorrhaphy. In: Gorio A, Millesi H, Mingrino S, eds. Post-traumatic peripheral nerve regeneration: Experimental basis and clinical implications. New York: Raven, 1981:281–291.
66. Miyamoto Y, Watari S, Tsuge K. Experimental studies on the effects of tension in intraneural microcirculation sutured peripheral nerves. Plast Reconstr Surg 1979; 63:398–403.
67. Myers RR, Powell HC, Heckman HM, Costello ML, Katz J. Biophysical and pathological effects of cryogenic nerve lesion. Ann Neurol 1981; 10: 478–485.
68. Myers RR, Mizisin AP, Powell HC, Lampert PW. Reduced nerve blood flow in hexachlorophene neuropathy: Relationship to elevated endoneurial fluid pressure. J Neuropathol Exp Neurol 1982; 41:391–399.
69. Myers RR, Murakami H, Powell HC. Reduced nerve blood flow in edematous neuropathies: A biochemical mechanism. Microvascular Res 1986; 32:145–151.
70. Myers RR, Powell HC. Endoneurial fluid pressure in peripheral neuropathies. In: Hargens A, ed. Tissue fluid pressure and composition. Baltimore: Williams & Wilkins, 1981:193–207.
71. Myers RR, Powell HC, Costello ML, Lambert LW, Zweifach BW. Endoneurial fluid pressure: Direct measurement with micropipettes. Brain Res 1978; 148:510–515.
72. Novikoff AB, Quintana N, Villaverde H, Forshirm R. Nucleoside phosphatase and choline esterase activities in dorsal root ganglia and peripheral nerve. J Cell Biol 1966; 29:525–545.
73. Ochs S. Rate of fast axoplasmic transport in mammalian nerve fibres. J Physiol (Lond) 1972; 227: 627–645.
74. Ochs S. Energy metabolism and supply of ~P to the fast axoplasmic transport mechanism in nerve. Federation Proceedings 1974; 33:1049–1058.
75. Ogata K, Naito M. Blood flow of peripheral nerve: Effects of dissection, stretching and compression. J Hand Surg [Br] 1986;11:10–14.
76. Oldfors A. Permeability of the perineurium of small nerve fascicles: An ultrastructural study using ferritin in rats. Neuropathol Appl Neurobiol 1981; 7:183–194.
77. Oldfors A, Johansson BR. Barrier and transport properties of the perineurium. An ultrastructural study with ^{125}I-labelled albumin and horseradish peroxidase in normal and protein-deprived rats. Acta Neuropathol (Berl) 1979; 47:139–143.
78. Oldfors A, Sourander P. Barriers of peripheral nerve towards exogenous peroxidase in normal and protein-deprived rats. Acta Neuropathol (Berl) 1978; 43:129–134.
79. Olsson Y. Studies on vascular permeability in peripheral nerves. I. Distribution of circulating fluorescent serum albumin in normal, crushed and sectioned rat sciatic nerve. Acta Neuropathol (Berl) 1966; 7:1–15.
80. Olsson Y. Studies on vascular permeability in peripheral nerves. 2. Distribution of circulating fluorescent serum albumin in rat sciatic nerve after local injection of 5-hydroxy-tryptamine, histamine and compound 48/80. Acta Physiol Scand 1966; 69(suppl):284.
81. Olsson Y. Mast cells in the nervous system. Int Rev Cytol 1968; 24:27–70.
82. Olsson Y. Topographical differences in the vascular permeability of the peripheral nervous system. Acta Neuropathol (Berl) 1968; 10:26–33.
83. Olsson Y. The involvement of vasa nervorum in diseases of peripheral nerves. In: Bruyn V, ed. Handbook of clinical neurology, part II, vol 12, Vascular diseases of the nervous system. 1972: 641–664.
84. Olsson Y, Kristensson K. The perineurium as a diffusion barrier to protein tracers following trauma to nerves. Acta Neuropathol (Berl) 1973; 23:105–111.
85. Olsson Y, Kristensson K, Klatzo I. Permeability of blood vessels and connective tissue sheaths in the peripheral nervous system to exogenous proteins. Acta Neuropathol (Berl) ; suppl V:61–69.
86. Olsson Y, Reese TS. Inaccessibility of the endoneurium of mouse sciatic nerve to exogenous proteins. Anat Rec 1969; 63:722–728.
87. Powell HC, Myers RR, Zweifach BW, Lampert PW. Endoneurial fluid pressure in hexachlorophene neuropathy. Acta Neuropathol (Berl) 1978; 41:139–148.
88. Rydevik B, Lundborg G. Permeability of intraneural microvessels and perineurium following acute, graded experimental nerve compression. Scand J Plast Reconstr Surg 1977; 11:179–187.
89. Soifer D. Assembly and disposition of microtubule proteins: Some boundary conditions for possible role of microtubules in axonal transport. In: Weiss

DG, ed. Axoplasmic transport. Berlin: Springer Verlag, 1982:81–90.

90. Samii H, Wallenborn R. Tierexperimentelle Untersuchungen über den Einfluss der Spannung auf den Regenerationserfolg nach Nervennath. Acta Neurochir 1972; 27:87–110.
91. Schlaepfer WW, La Valle MC, Torack RM. Cytochemical demonstration of nucleoside phosphorase activity in myelinated nerve fibers in the rat. Histochemistry 1969; 18:281–291.
92. Selander D, Månsson LG, Karlsson L, Svanvik J. Adrenergic vasconstriction in peripheral nerves of the rabbit. Anesthesiol 1985; 62:6–10.
93. Selander D, Sjöstrand J. Longitudinal spread of intraneurally injected local anesthetics. Acta Anaest Scand 1978; 22:622–634.
94. Shantaveerappa TR, Bourne GH. The "perineurial epithelium," a metabolically active continuous protoplasmic cell barrier surrounding peripheral nerve fasciculi. J Anat 1962; 96:527–536.
95. Shantaveerappa TR, Bourne GH. The perineurial epithelium of sympathetic nerves and ganglia and its relation to the pia arachnoid of the central nervous system and perineural epithelium of the peripheral nervous system. Zeitschrift der Zellforschung 1964; 61:742–753.
96. Shantaveerappa TR, Bourne GH. Enzyme histochemical properties of the perineurial epithelium following nerve transection. Anat Rec 1964; 150: 35–47.
97. Shantaveerappa TR, Bourne GH. Perineural epithelium: A new concept of its role in the integrity of the peripheral nervous system. Science 1966; 154:1464–1467.
98. Shdanow DA. Die Lymphwege des peripherischen und Zentralnervensystems. Anatomischer Anzeiger 1931; 71:231–245.
99. Söderfeldt B, Olsson Y, Kristensson K. The perineurium as a diffusion barrier to protein tracers in human peripheral nerve. Acta Neuropathol (Berl) 1973; 25:120–126.
100. Sunderland S. Nerves and nerve injuries. Edinburgh/London/New York: Churchill-Livingstone, 1978.
101. Sunderland S, Bradley K. The cross-sectional area of peripheral nerve trunks devoted to nerve fibres. Brain 1949; 72:428–439.
102. Thoenen H, Barde YA. Physiology of nerve growth factor. Physiol Rev 1980; 60:1284–1335.
103. Thomas PK, Jones B. The cellular response to nerve injury. J Anat 1967; 100:45–55.
104. Thomas PK, Ochoa J. Microscopic anatomy of peripheral nerve fibres. In: Dyck PJ, Thomas PK, Lambert EH, Bunge MB, eds. Peripheral neuropathy. Philadelphia: WB Saunders, 1984:39–96.
105. Thomas PK, Olsson Y. Microscopic anatomy and junction of the connective tissue components of peripheral nerve. In: Dyck PJ, Thomas PK, Lambert EH, Bunge MB, eds. Peripheral neuropathy. Philadelphia: WB Saunders, 1984:97–120.
106. Torvik A. Central chromatolysis and the axon reaction: A reappraisal. Neuropathol Appl Neurobiol 1976; 2:423–432.
107. Tsukita S, Ishikawa H. The movement of membranous organelles in axons: Electron microscopic identification of anterogradely and retrogradely transported organelles. J Cell Biol 1980; 84:513–530.
108. Tuček S, Hanlíková V, Stráníková D. Effect of ischemia on axonal transport of choline acetyltransferase and acetylcholinesterase and on ultrastructural changes of isolated segments of rabbit nerves in situ. J Neurol Sci 1978; 36:237–245.
109. Tuck RR, Schmelzer JD, Low PA. Endoneurial blood flow and oxygen tension in the sciatic nerves of rats with experimental diabetic neuropathy. Brain 1984; 107:935–950.
110. Vallee RB, Bloom GS, Theurkouf WE. Microtubule associated proteins: Subunits of the cytomatrix. J Cell Biol 1984; 99:38s–44s.
111. Van Beek A, Kleinert HE. Practical microneurorrhaphy. Orth Clin North Am 1977; 8:377–386.
112. Varon S, Adler R. Nerve growth factors and control of nerve growth. Curr Top Dev Biol 1980; 16: 207–252.
113. Waggener JD, Bunn SM, Beggs J. The diffusion of ferritin within the peripheral nerve sheath: An electron microscopy study. J Neuropathol Exp Neurol 1965; 24:430–443.
114. Waksman BH. Experimental study of diphtheric polyneuritis in the rabbit and guinea pig. III. The blood–nerve barrier in the rabbit. J Neuropathol Exp Neurol 1961; 21:35–77.
115. Weiss DG, Gross GW. The microstream hypothesis of axoplasmic transport; characteristics, predictions and compatibility with data. In: Weiss DG, ed. Axoplasmic transport. Berlin: Springer-Verlag, 1982:362–383.
116. Weiss P, Wang H, Taylor AC, Edds MV Jr. Proximo-distal fluid convection in the endoneurial spaces of peripheral nerves, demonstrated by colored and radioactive (isotope) tracers. Am J Physiol 1945; 143:521–540.
117. Wilgis S, Murphy R. The significance of longitudinal excursions in peripheral nerves. Hand Clin 1986; 2:761–768.
118. Willard M. The identification of two intra-axonally transported polypeptides resembling myosin in some respects in the rabbit visual system. J Cell Biol 1977; 75:1–11.

2

Impulse Conduction

James A. Galbraith
Robert R. Myers

AUTHORS' KEY POINTS

- Nerve is composed of a membrane that is selectively permeable to potassium at rest. Therefore, its resting potential is near the potassium equilibrium potential.
- Voltage-sensitive channels, or pores, within the membrane selectively control the flow of ions.
- During excitation, nerve becomes permeable to sodium and depolarizes to near the sodium equilibrium potential. It recovers when the sodium channels close and potassium channels open.
- Passive nerve acts as an electrical cable.
- Structural changes induced by injury or disease alter the action potential spatially and temporally.

One of the major functions of the nervous system is to relay information throughout the body in response to external stimuli. This is done through a specialized network of cells that generate and transmit electrical impulses over long distances in fractions of a second with no loss of information. Small ionic exchanges across the neuronal membrane lead to these impulses. Once a critical level of excitation is reached, the membrane's ionic permeabilities change to produce a transient reversal of membrane potential and an impulse that is a self-propagating, constant-amplitude signal called the *action potential*. This chapter presents the underlying mechanisms of impulse generation and propagation in order to better interpret the responses obtained in the course of nerve injury and repair. This is done in a rigorous format based on the detailed mathematical constructs developed to describe the observed ionic and electrical properties of the tissue. However, since the function of the nervous system is so tightly linked to its structure, the structural basis for impulse conduction is also presented before concluding with descriptions of electrophysiological dysfunctions of the system secondary to clinically observed abnormalities.

The vertebrate nervous system is divided into the central, peripheral, and autonomic nervous systems. Although the roles of these systems differ, they have in common the propagation of single action potentials as their principal means of communication. The peripheral nervous system, in particular, is a series of signal conductors that form the transmission lines responsible for conducting signals. In fact, understanding nervous system impulse conduction is built on electrical engineering knowledge of transmission lines and cable theory. Biological systems have evolved specialized circuitry that lends itself to this type of engineering analysis, which contributes to an understanding of the molecular process linking the structure and function of the nervous system.

SYSTEM OVERVIEW

The unit building block of the nervous system, the neuron, has a structure and function similar to that of the entire nervous system. It is made up of a cell body (soma) and a large number of emanating branches (dendrites). The soma contains the nucleus, which is responsible for integrating inputs from other cells and subsequently generating a response in much the same way as the central nervous system does at a higher level. Other nerve cells supply inputs to the neuron through junctions, or synaptic connections, on the dendrites and the soma. While many dendrites are short, tapered offshoots, in most neurons there is one process that is longer and more uniform than the others, the axon (Fig. 2-1). The axon is responsible for transmitting outgoing signals from the cell and is considered analogous to the peripheral nervous system.

Nerves, like all cells, consist of a plasma membrane and cytoplasm. The cytoplasm, or axoplasm, is a long cylindrical core enveloped by the excitable membrane of nerve. While ions flow through axoplasm with relative ease, the opposite is true of the surrounding membrane. It acts as the ionic barrier between the interior and exterior of the cell that is responsible for the asymmetric distribution of ions between the inside and outside of the axon. It manifests a concentration ratio from outside to inside the axon of 9:1 for sodium and 1:20 for potassium.

The slowest type of conducting fibers are small and unmyelinated. Only the smallest fibers in ver-

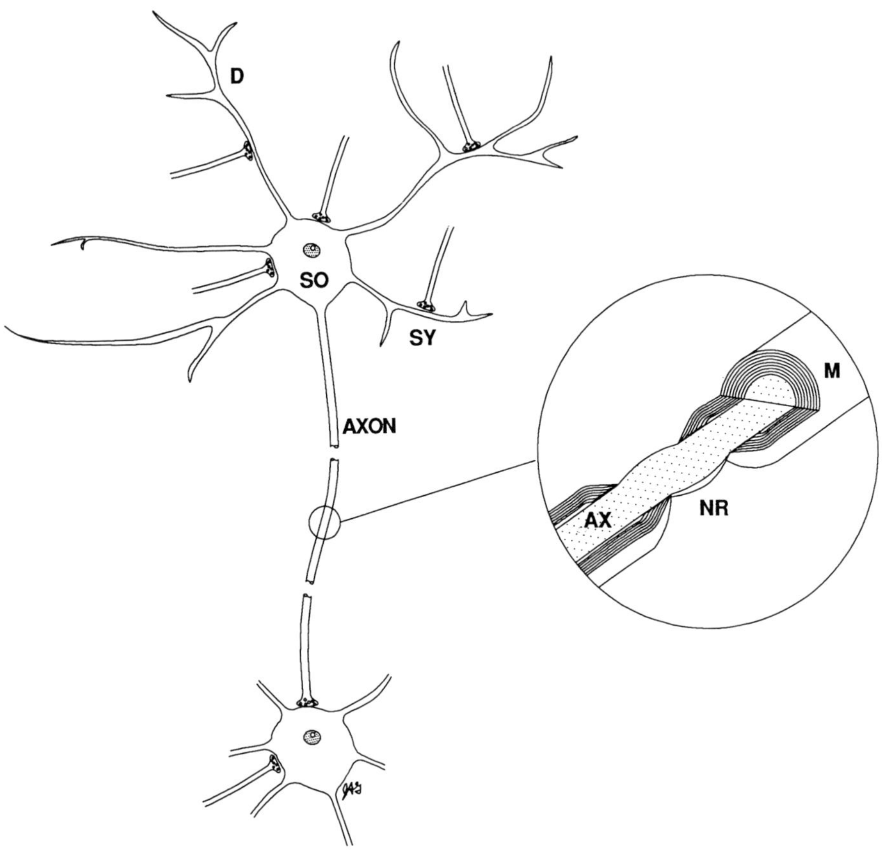

Figure 2–1. *Structural components of a neuron. D, dendrite; SO, soma; SY, synapse; AX, axon; NR, node of Ranvier; M, myelin.*

tebrates lack myelin, while most invertebrate nerve fibers are unmyelinated. In the peripheral nervous system, unmyelinated nerves are surrounded by an outer wrapping of Schwann cells. One Schwann cell may encase several small axons or only part of a very large fiber. Myelinated nerves are normally faster-conducting than their unmyelinated counterparts. Myelin, elaborated on these axons by Schwann cells, encircles the axon repeatedly to form a concentric wrapping in proportion to axonal diameter.[28,89] Void of Schwann cell cytoplasm, myelin changes the electrical properties of the nerve considerably in this region. Approximately every millimeter along the fiber, the myelin sheath is interrupted between longitudinally adjacent Schwann cells, and a 1-μm region of excitable membrane is exposed to extracellular fluid (see Fig. 2-1). This region, known as the node of Ranvier, gives rise to the rapid conduction properties of myelinated nerves.

Clinical Significance

The anatomical construction that allows saltatory conduction to occur is the interruption, at approximately 1-mm intervals, of the multilaminated myelin sheath that insulates the axon. This exposes the excitable nerve membrane at regions known as the node of Ranvier.

PHYSICAL PRINCIPLES

Demonstrated abnormalities of nervous system electrical activity are diagnostic of various pathologic conditions. Because the activity occurs in an electrical network, an understanding of some basic electrical terms and concepts is important for interpreting electrophysiological data.

Matter is composed of two differently charged particles: protons, which are positively charged particles in the nucleus of atoms, and electrons, which are negatively charged and orbit the nucleus. Most materials have an equal number of electrons and protons and are thus electrically neutral; however, electrons can be added or removed from an atomic orbit to cause a charge imbalance. When such an imbalance exists, the object is electrically charged and will attract material that is oppositely charged, while repelling materials of similar charge. The unit used to quantify charge, the *coulomb* (C), is defined as 6.24×10^{18} protons of positive charge. One proton has a charge of 1.6×10^{-19} C. A quantity used when dealing with charge is *Faraday's constant* (F), named after the British physicist Michael Faraday. Faraday's constant is defined as the charge on one mole of any single-valence–charged ions. Since each mole contains Avogadro's number of atoms (6.02×10^{23}), one mole of protons has 9.6×10^{4} C/mol of charge.

When a net amount of charge moves from one location to another, *current* (I) flows between these locations. Current is the net number of charges that move past a point during a given period of time. It is expressed more precisely as dq/dt, the time rate of change of charge. The unit of measure for current is *amperes* (abbreviated A or amps), after the French physicist André Ampère. If one coulomb of charge moves past a point in 1 second, the current is one amp (1 coulomb/1 second). In electrical networks, positive current flow is the direction of movement of positive charges.

There are two fundamental points to remember about current. The first is that it is directional; that is, if the same net number of charges flow from A to B as from B to A, then the magnitude of these currents will be the same, but their polarity will be opposite. The second is that the net charge, not the total number of charges, is important. If 1000 charges move between A and B, while at the same time 1000 charges move from B to A, both the net amount of charge and the current are zero.

For current to flow, work must be done to cause the charges to move. The amount of work required to move a unit amount of positive charge from one location to another is the *voltage* (V) or potential difference between the two points. If the potential difference between A and B is one volt, it will take one joule of energy to move one coulomb of charge between these points. To move a charge from a region of lower potential to one of higher potential requires that energy be put into the system, whereas energy is liberated when the charge travels in the opposite direction, down the potential field. Voltage is always expressed in terms of two points. Any point can be assigned as a reference point; the earth is commonly used, and thus voltage is often expressed with respect to ground.

Conductance (g) is the second parameter that determines the amount of current flowing between two points. It gives an indication of the effort required for current to flow in a material. Consider two electrodes placed in an electrolyte solution with a voltage applied across them. Current flows from the electrode with the higher potential to the one with lower potential. If an insulating barrier is placed between the electrodes, it is more difficult for the charges to move from one electrode to the other. In other words, less charge is conducted, and the conductance of the solution is lowered. Conductance is expressed by the simple relationship $g = I/V$ and has the derived units of amps per volt or *siemens* (S). This equation is known as *Ohm's law*, after the German physicist Georg Ohm. It states that the current in a conducting material is equal to a proportionality constant, the conductance, times the voltage. It is also commonly written as $V = IR$, where R is the reciprocal of the conductance and is known as *resistance*, which is measured in ohms (Ω).

When resistive elements are connected in series, the total resistance is obtained by adding the individual resistances. When resistors are connected in parallel, the total resistance is given by the sum of the individual conductances.

If a pair of conductors or plates is separated by an insulating material, charge on one side is trapped and cannot traverse the gap. To get to the other side it must move through some external pathway. Such a configuration, called a *capacitor*, has electrical properties that are important in neurophysiology. When a small amount of charge, $-\Delta q$, is removed from the top plate of a capacitor via some parallel pathway to the lower plate, there is $+\Delta q$ charge on the top plate and $-\Delta q$ on the bottom plate. Because work is required to separate these unlike charges, a small voltage change takes place, and the top plate is raised $+\Delta V$ volts. More concisely, the migrating charge, q, is proportional to the potential difference between the plates: $q = CV$, where the constant of proportionality, C, is capacitance measured in coulombs/volt or Farads (F). As current runs through a capacitor, it transfers charge from one plate to the other while keeping the total net charge the same. Since the definition of current is the time rate of change of charge, the current–voltage relationship for a capacitor can be obtained from the equation $q = CV$. Current through a capacitor is proportional to the rate of change of the voltage across it: $I = CdV/dt$. The proportionality constant is determined by several physical characteristics of a capacitor, including the area of the plates, the distance between the plates, and the effectiveness of the insulating material in the gap between the plates. Finally, capacitors combine according to rules that are opposite those used for resistances. Parallel capacitors add, while the total capacitance of capacitors in series is equal to the reciprocal of the individual capacitors.

Clinical Significance

The activity of neurons is governed by fundamental electrical concepts, and understanding the relationships between current, voltage, conductance, and capacitance aids in interpreting electrophysiological data. These principles explain how axons conduct signals and how these signals can be recorded.

RECORDING TECHNIQUES

The simplest and most common technique used to observe signals generated by nerves is electronic amplification and display. Because the signal generated by nerve may be only a few millivolts, it is necessary to amplify it to a voltage level that instruments can display. Commercial amplifiers accomplish this by transistor networks, the details of which are unimportant to this discussion. However, several key points should be kept in mind regarding amplifiers.

In order to ensure that the voltage displayed is the voltage measured, it is necessary to know the input resistance or input impedance of the amplifier. *Impedance* is a combination of resistance and capacitance into an equivalent element whose value is frequency dependent. Since the electrode used to measure the cell's activity has resistance to current flow, and it is connected in series with a measuring device that has it own internal resistance, some voltage drop will occur across each because they are connected in series. To illustrate this, suppose that the electrode's resistance is 1000 ohms and the input resistance of the amplifier is also 1000 ohms. If there is a one-volt signal at the tip of the electrode, then 0.5 milliamps (mA) will flow through the electrode and amplifier. According to Ohm's law, the 0.5 mA of current through 1000 ohms induces a 0.5-volt drop at the input to the amplifier, only half of the initial voltage of the cell. If the input resistance of the amplifier is instead 1,000,000 ohms, and the calculation is repeated, the voltage is 0.9990 volts at the input to the amplifier, a much more acceptable value.

A final consideration in amplifier selection is noise level. *Noise* is random electrical oscillation and is inherent in any circuit. It is desirable to use an amplifier with a noise level that is much less than that of the signal to maximize the signal-to-noise ratio, so that the signal will not be lost in the noise.

Once the signal is amplified, the time-varying voltage is displayed on an *oscilloscope*, which consists of a sealed glass vacuum tube with an electron beam that can be controlled in both the x and y axes. The x axis is used as a time base to sweep the beam across the face of the oscilloscope, while the y-axis deviation of the beam is proportional to the signal amplitude. Alternately, a more recent method of data manipulation uses a digital representation of the signal and allows storage in a computer for off-line analysis. The *analog-to-digital convertor* used in this method generates discrete values at distinct times that represent the analog, or continuously varying signal. These convertors freeze the signal for a brief instant, compare it to the discrete levels that are internally available, and generate a digital code representative of the closest level.

There are two basic types of electrical recording techniques used with nerves, *extracellular* and *intracellular*. As the names imply, extracellular electrodes use a recording electrode located on the outer surface of the nerve, while intracellular electrodes use a recording electrode inside the cell (Fig. 2-2). However, both use an extracellular reference electrode. The first intracellular recording that measured the transmembrane potential across the cell membrane was performed by Hodgkin and Huxley in 1939.[43] They inserted a 100-μm glass cannula down the center of the unmyelinated squid giant axon and found a resting potential of approximately −60 mV. Upon stimulation they were able to record the dynamic behavior of the membrane, the action potential. This signal reversed polarity and caused the inside of the nerve to become positive with respect to the outside before it reversed itself again and recovered to its resting level.

Most cells, however, are not large enough for a 100-μm electrode, and it was not until 1949 that Ling and Gerald developed an acceptable method for use in smaller cells.[74] They heated small glass capillary tubes in the middle and pulled the ends apart to cause the center to taper into a fine tip. This *microelectrode*, filled with isotonic KCl and an Ag/AgCl wire, was inserted into the large end and attached to an amplifier (see Fig. 2-2*A*). The tip of the microelectrode, less than 0.5 μm, did not disturb the normal function of the cell it impaled.

While intracellular readings are easier to interpret, they are still technically difficult to accomplish and often are not even feasible. Therefore, extracellular electrodes are used commonly for stimulating and recording. If a section of nerve is mobilized and several pairs of silver wires are placed beneath it, it is possible to elicit and record an electrical response. One pair of wires is connected to a stimulator that produces a brief electrical pulse, and another pair of wires at the opposite end is connected to a high input resistance amplifier that records the response. As the fiber is stimulated, a wave of excitation travels down the nerve, generating a signal with an initial upward deflection followed by a downward deflection on the display. This signal is known as a *biphasic action potential* because of its polarity changes (see Fig. 2-2*B*). The polarity of the nerve's membrane is reversed at the peak of an action potential and, as the signal passes under one electrode, it is opposite in polarity to the second electrode.

A variation of this technique involves crushing the recording end of the nerve and placing the most distal electrode under that point; the resulting signal is a *monophasic action potential*. It shows a single polarity peak since it cannot propagate past the injury site.

The recording just discussed could have come from a single nerve fiber or from a bundle of hundreds of fibers. When it is obtained from a bundle, the signal is known as a *compound action potential* because hundreds of axons are stimulated

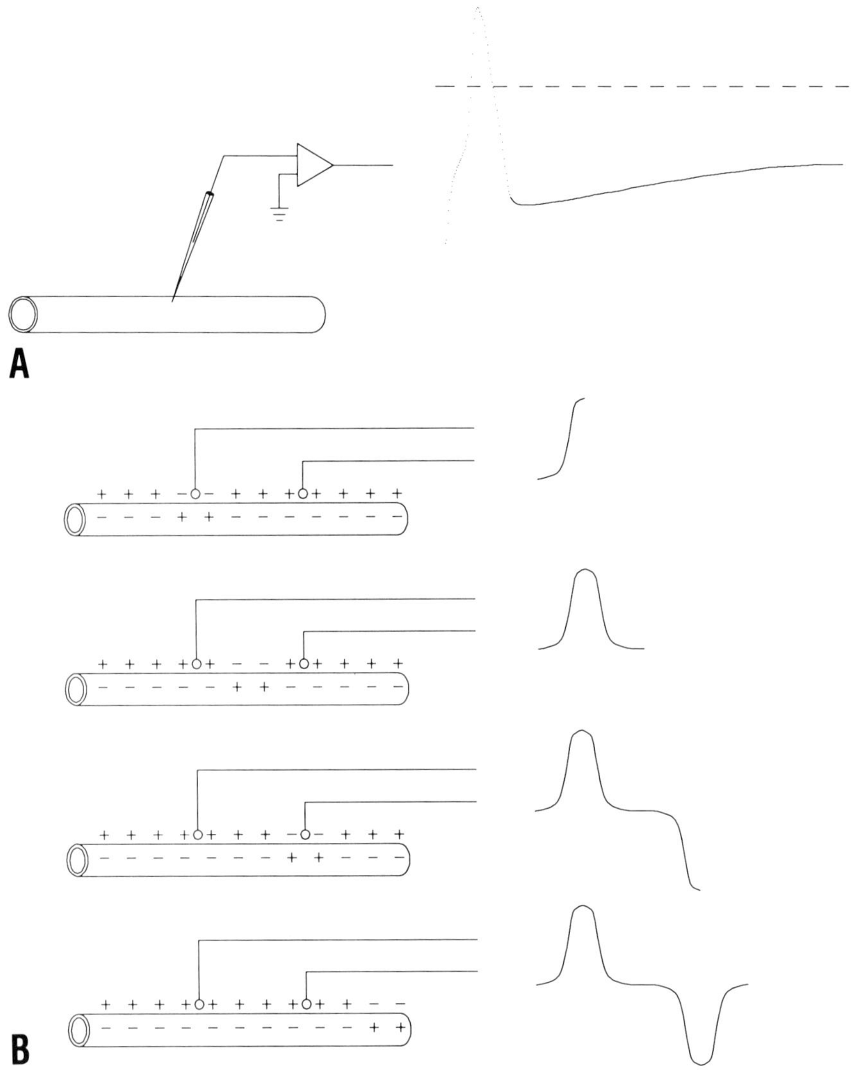

Figure 2–2. *Electrical signals recorded during impulse conduction. (**A**) Intracellular recording of membrane potential and action potential from a single nerve fiber. (**B**) Extracellular recording of biphasic action potential. At rest the inside of the nerve is negative relative to the outside. As the signal passes underneath the first electrode, the polarity of this region of membrane is reversed, and a negative deflection is observed. While the signal is between the electrodes there is no deflection, and when the signal reaches the second electrode, the polarity is reversed and a positive deflection results.*

in synchrony and a composite result is recorded (Fig. 2-3). While an individual axon produces an all-or-none action potential, a compound action potential grows in a graded fashion. It increases in amplitude, and the strength of the stimulus pulse is enlarged as more single axon responses contribute to the signal. However, while this is true for a bundle of identical fibers, most bundles contain a variety of fiber sizes. This gives rise to multiple monophasic peaks as a result of the lower threshold and higher conduction velocity of larger fibers.[25] Because these signals travel at different speeds, the

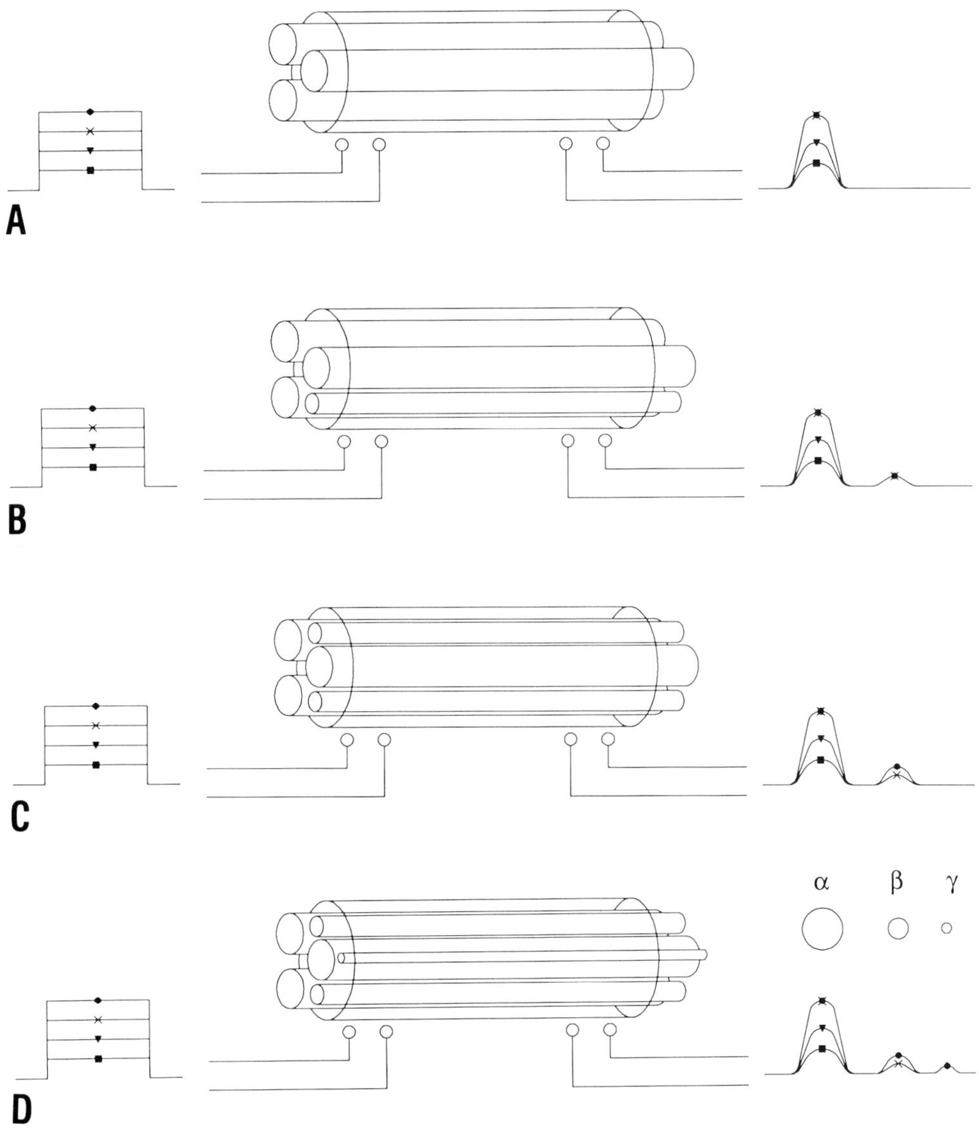

Figure 2–3. *Contribution of different fiber sizes to compound action potential. Four stimulus levels are shown on the left side, and the nerve's corresponding electrical activity is shown on the right side. (**A**) In a bundle with identical axons, α, more axons will be stimulated as the amplitude of the pulse is increased, and the recorded waveform will grow in a graded fashion. When all the axons are stimulated, the recorded signal will not get any larger. (**B**) A smaller diameter fiber, β, is added to the original bundle. It has a larger threshold for excitation and a slower conduction velocity because of its smaller size. This results in a second peak that appears at a larger stimulus level and is delayed in time. (**C**) Increasing the number of β fibers results in a graded response in the second peak as well. (**D**) The addition of a third fiber, γ, produces a third peak further delayed in time. Due to their very small size, the γ fibers have the highest threshold of the three groups and appear only with the largest stimulus pulse. The overall response of the fiber can then be summarized as follows. The largest fibers will be most easily excited, and their response will be observed first. As the amplitude of the stimulus pulse is increased, more α fibers will be recruited and the signal will grow in size. In addition, the response of smaller fibers will begin to appear with peaks that are delayed in time. Continuing to increase the stimulus after all the fibers are stimulated will not increase the amplitude of the recorded signal.*

width of the compound action potential lengthens with increased separation of the stimulating and recording electrodes.

Clinical Significance

Stimulation of a segment of peripheral nerve by extracellular electrodes will result in a compound electrical response that can be recorded with a second set of electrodes. The signal from each axon is called the action potential. It will be *biphasic* if the signal propagates past both electrodes and *monophasic* if it passes only one. As the stimulus intensity is increased, more fibers will generate action potentials, and the compound signal will increase in amplitude. The precise shape of the compound action potential depends on the different fiber sizes and their varying conduction velocities.

MEMBRANE STRUCTURE

When a microelectrode penetrates a cell, the potential difference between it and a reference electrode in the bath suddenly jumps to a new level between −60 and −90 millivolts. While this implies that a barrier has been crossed, what evidence is there to suggest that a separate membrane exists at the surface of the nerve? Several experiments on the squid giant axon provide support for a specialized surface structure. Hodgkin and Keynes introduced radioactive potassium onto the surface of an axon and found that it entered very slowly; after 2 hours about 10% of the internal potassium was labeled.[52] They then measured the movement of labeled potassium through the axoplasm and found that it was only a few percentage points slower than in water. This implied that a surface barrier was restricting passage of ions between the external medium and axoplasm, since the potassium ion's movement was similar inside and outside the axon.

Another indication that a specialized membrane structure surrounds nerve came from the fact that the central core of the axon can be bored out and replaced with an artificial solution without loss of electrical function.[5,6] On the other hand, slight damage to the surface results in a loss of excitability. In addition, studies of the passive electrical properties of nerve indicate that it behaves as if it were an electrical cable (a center conductor surrounded by an insulating film). From these and other experiments, the *membrane theory* was developed. Cells are surrounded by a selectively permeable plasma membrane that regulates the internal environment of the cell.

This membrane, which contains some carbohydrates, is composed predominantly of lipids and proteins (Fig. 2-4). The idea that lipids play a role in the cell's membrane was first suggested by Overton in 1899 when he observed that materials soluble in lipids pass through the cell membrane more easily than those that are insoluble.[81] The lipids that have a phosphate group are more properly called phospholipids. They also have a polar head, which is hydrophilic, and a hydrocarbon tail, which is hydrophobic. When they are added to the surface of water, a monolayer forms, with the polar heads associating with the water and the tails orienting away from the water.

The idea that the cell membrane is a double thickness monolayer, or *bilayer*, was suggested by Gorter and Grendel in 1925.[32] They extracted lipids from erythrocytes, using them to form monolayers, which had an area roughly twice the cell's surface area. By forming a bilayer, the lipids created a more stable, low-energy configuration. Their hydrophobic tails became sequestered from the watery environment on either side. Subsequently, electron microscopy of cell membranes stained with osmium tetroxide by Robertson showed a pair of dark lines, 20 Å thick, separated by 35 Å. Since the stain was preferential to polar material, this was consistent with a lipid bilayer structure, which he called the *unit membrane*.[88]

Calorimetry measurements of phospholipid membranes indicate that they are in a more fluid than solid state.[99] The experiments of Frye and Edidin (1970) showing that fluorescent antibodies could move laterally within the membrane provided more evidence of the membrane's "fluidity."[27] From this information, Singer and Nicolson proposed the current conceptual model of the membrane, the *fluid mosaic model*.[96] In this model the term "fluid" refers to the ability of the phospholipids and proteins to move laterally, as if the membrane were a viscous fluid, and the term "mosaic" refers to the random dispersal of proteins throughout the membrane.

While the idea of proteins adsorbed on the surface of the membrane was not new,[21] the fluid mo-

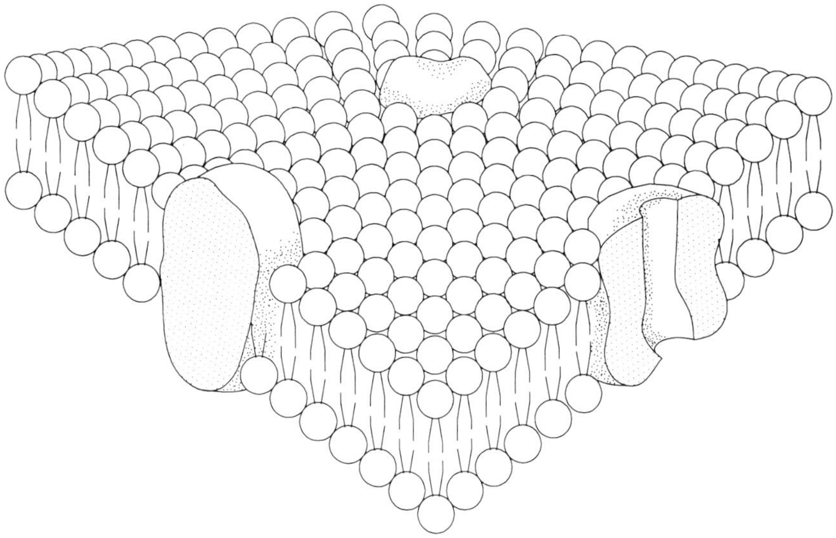

Figure 2–4. *Schematic representation of fluid mosaic model after Singer and Nicolson (see reference 96). The polar heads of the bilayer face the watery environment, while the hydrophobic hydrocarbon tails are contained in the center of the membrane. Proteins located in the membrane either span it (intrinsic) or simply penetrate part of the way through it (extrinsic). These proteins can move laterally throughout the fluid membrane. Specialized proteins, such as the one on the right side, are responsible for the passage of ions across the membrane and hence the electrical excitability of nerve.*

saic model expanded it to include two classes of proteins: intrinsic and extrinsic. Intrinsic proteins were considered integral to the membrane, spanning from one side to the other, with their polar groups outside the membrane and their hydrophobic region anchored in the center. Extrinsic proteins were anchored in the membrane but did not bridge the bilayer.

The fluid state of the membrane allows the phospholipids to move.[24,62,82,91] Sophisticated techniques such as electron spin resonance, nuclear magnetic resonance, and fluorescence photobleaching indicate that the movement can be lateral either within the plane of the membrane or across it, a trans-bilayer flip-flop. Lateral motion occurs much more often than flip-flops, since it takes a great deal of energy for the polar head of the molecule to traverse the hydrophobic portion of the membrane. As a result of this low rate of traversing the membrane, most bilayers tend to be asymmetric in structure.

Pure lipid bilayers are impermeable to almost all ions, regardless of size.[62,77] Biological membranes, however, have a much higher ionic conductance. In fact, it is their conductance to specific ions that provides the basis for neural activity. Within biological membranes it is generally assumed that function-specific proteins are responsible for many complex cell actions, such as enzymatic, immunologic, and electrophysiological responses. Proteins can move in the membrane, just as phospholipid molecules exhibit a lateral motion.[24,62,76,91] Due to their size, the diffusional rates are obviously much lower, and some may be unable to move at all if they are anchored to the underlying cytoskeleton. Flip-flop of proteins does not appear to occur.

Clinical Significance

Nerves are surrounded by an insulating phospholipid membrane. Inserted into this membrane are function-specific proteins that make it selectively permeable to various ions and give rise to the nerve's excitable behavior.

CONCENTRATION GRADIENTS, PERMEABILITIES, AND POTENTIALS

Neural membranes derive their unique properties from the inclusion of specialized proteins in an otherwise impermeable membrane. These proteins control the passage of ions and, in conjunction with the nerve's local environment, are responsible for the transmembrane potential. This selective permeability does not allow the intracellular and extracellular ion concentration differences to be eliminated by simple diffusion. Normally, when two different concentrations of an ion are present in a bath, they mix until the concentration is uni-

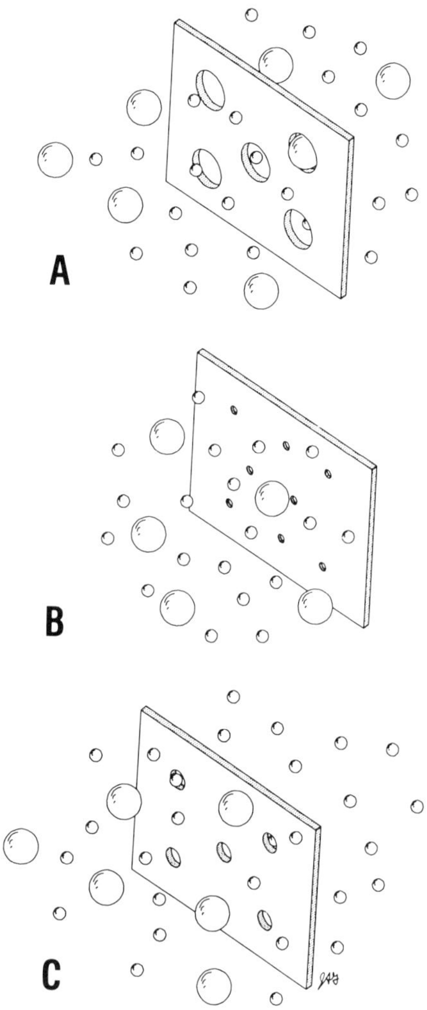

Figure 2–5. *Permeability of different membranes. When two solutions containing different concentrations of a salt solution are present in a bath, they will mix or diffuse until the concentration is uniform everywhere. If a membrane is interspersed between the two solutions, this process is modified. (**A**) In membranes whose pores are large enough for both ions to traverse the membrane down their concentration gradients, the ion with the larger mobility will move slightly faster. This will create a transient diffusion potential due to the slight separation of charge. (**B**) When the holes in the membrane are too small for any ions to pass through, no diffusion will occur, and no potential difference arises across the membrane. (**C**) A selectively permeable membrane allows only one species of ion to pass; this will create a charge imbalance between the two sides of the membrane. Eventually, an equilibrium condition will be reached, and the forces due to the concentration and electrical gradient will balance each other. The potential that is developed at equilibrium is known as the Nernst potential.*

form everywhere. This process is known as diffusion. Higher concentrations of ions diffuse down their concentration gradients toward lower levels to bring about equilibrium.

If electrodes are placed on either side of a porous membrane that separates two differing concentrations of a salt solution such as KCl, the movement of ions across the membrane is impeded, and an electrical potential arises. However, even if the membrane has pores through which both species of ions freely pass, a *diffusion or junction potential* is created because the chloride ion has greater mobility and is therefore moving slightly faster than the potassium ion. This occurs despite the fact that there is an equal driving force for both ions (Fig. 2-5*A*). This results in a small charge imbalance, which causes the dilute solution to become electrically negative with respect to the concentrated solution. The charge imbalance impedes the motion of additional negatively charged chloride ions while it accelerates positive charges. A 10:1 concentration difference yields a 1-mV diffusion potential, which is transient and eventually disappears as the potassium concentrations equilibrate.

At the other extreme is the situation where the pores are too small to allow either ion to pass. No potential difference is generated because there is no concentration gradient (Fig. 2-5*B*). However, if water can traverse the membrane, it will attempt to do so in response to the osmotic forces present.

The case with intermediate-sized pores is more applicable to neural membranes (Fig. 2-5*C*). If a membrane has pores large enough to allow one ion to pass, but not others, it is said to be *selectively permeable*. Since the potassium ion in this example has a smaller radius than the chloride ion, it will move through the pores in the membrane and diffuse down its concentration gradient, while the chloride ion will not (provided there are not other overriding forces). However, two driving forces control the movement of ions: the concentration gradient and the electrical field. The differential movement of charge causes the more dilute solution to become electropositive with respect to the concentrated solution. As the process continues, the electrical gradient eventually opposes the concentration gradient, and the two forces balance. The potential across the membrane is then given by the *Nernst equation*:

$$V_m = \frac{RT}{F} \ln\left(\frac{C_o}{C_i}\right) \quad (1)$$

Since RT/F is about 25 mV, a 10:1 concentration difference will generate a 58.2-mV equilibrium potential. This is almost 60 times greater than the 1-mV diffusion potential that is generated for the same concentration differences.

Clinical Significance

With the same concentration gradient, a membrane that is selectively permeable has a membrane potential many times greater than the simple diffusion potential of a nonselective membrane.

ORIGIN OF THE RESTING POTENTIAL

While a concentration gradient can generate a small electrical potential, a membrane that can discriminate between two ionic species will generally induce a much greater potential. This situation exists in nerve, except that the membrane is selectively permeable to more than one ionic species. Obtaining an expression for the resting potential in this type of membrane requires the Nernst-Planck equation and several assumptions. The first assumption is the *independence relation*, which states that one ion does not interfere with the movement of another ion either in terms of direct physical action or through its electrical field. The second assumption, the *constant field* assumption, states that the potential field in the membrane is a linear function of distance. When these assumptions are applied to the Nernst-Planck equation, the *Goldman–Hodgkin–Katz (GHK) equation*[29,51] for membrane potential is obtained:

$$E = \frac{RT}{F} \ln\left(\frac{P_{Na}[Na_o] + P_K[K_o] + P_{Cl}[Cl_i]}{P_{Na}[Na_i] + P_K[K_i] + P_{Cl}[Cl_o]}\right) \quad (2)$$

This is essentially a weighted Nernst equation, with the importance of each ion's contribution to the resting potential determined by its permeability. Additional ions could have been included simply by adding their corresponding permeabilities and concentrations to the numerator and denominator of equation 2.

The original hypothesis regarding the ionic basis of a cell's resting potential was suggested by Bernstein, who thought that the cell's membrane was permeable exclusively to potassium but upon excitation became uniformly permeable to all ions.[8] However, if this were the case, a linear change in external potassium would yield a corresponding linear response in membrane potential according to the Nernst equation. At high concentrations of potassium, the membrane potential behaves as a linear function of potassium concentration, but at lower levels it deviates significantly. When the GHK equation is used to fit this data, the curve agrees very well.

Another interesting point about selectively permeable membranes is that membrane potential can be varied as much as 129 mV, from the potassium equilibrium potential to the sodium equilibrium potential, simply by varying its permeability. The significance of this observation was pointed out by Hodgkin and Katz when they found that the resting potential of the squid axon could be accounted for by a P_K:P_{Na}:P_{Cl} equal to 1:0.04:0.45, while at the peak of the action potential this ratio would have to change to 1:20:0.45.[51]

Studies using radioactive sodium and potassium movement into and out of the axon have been used to determine the membrane's resting permeability to these ions. In these experiments an imbalance was observed between the inward and outward permeability values. This implied that an active process was aiding the movement of ions.[53–55]

Subsequently the *sodium pump*, which moves sodium out of the axon and potassium into the axon against their concentration gradients through an ATP-dependent mechanism, was discovered.[97] This pump is electrogenic, meaning that it does not perform a 1:1 exchange of ions. Instead, it generates a net movement of charge in which roughly three sodium ions pumped out of the axon bring two potassium ions back (Fig. 2-6).[10,22,106] As might be expected, this pump's operation depends on both the internal sodium concentration and the external potassium concentration.[54,56] If the pump is shut down, sodium and potassium will ultimately move down their concentration gradients, and the resting potential will become zero, as the GHK equation predicts. This process may take several hours, however, during which time excitability is unaffected and the axon will still be able to fire tens of thousands of action potentials.

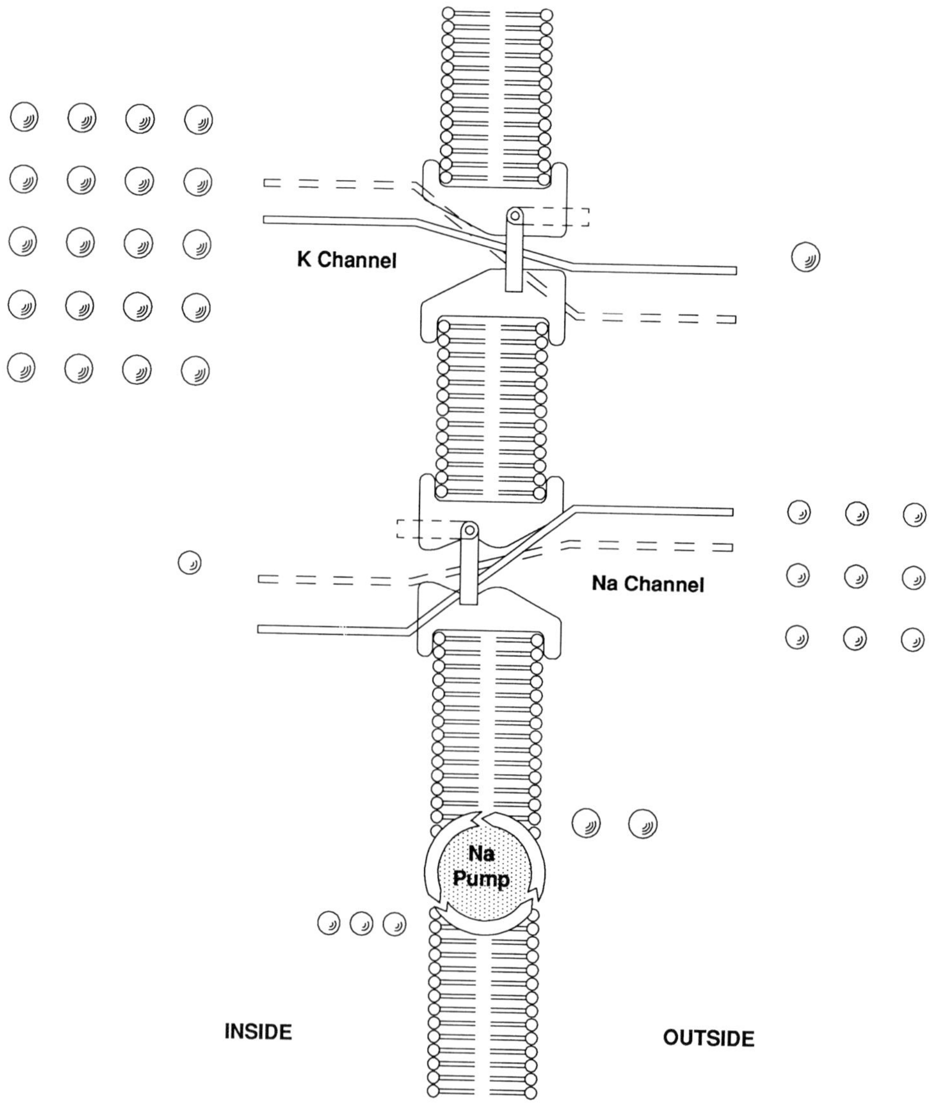

Figure 2–6. *Ion pathways, concentrations, and electrochemical gradients for the major ions involved in impulse conduction. The sodium concentration is nine times higher outside than inside the membrane, and potassium is 20 times more concentrated inside than outside. The resting membrane potential is close to the potassium equilibrium potential; therefore, the electrochemical potential (solid lines) is small for potassium but large for sodium. At the peak of the action potential (dashed lines) the membrane potential approaches the sodium equilibrium potential. The sodium pump exchanges sodium and potassium against their concentration gradients through an ATP-dependent mechanism. The inward movement of potassium is coupled to the outward movement of sodium in a 3:2 ratio.*

Clinical Significance

The resting potential of the nerve is due to the membrane's selective permeability to several ions. At rest the membrane is more permeable to potassium than sodium, while at the peak of the action potential the opposite is true. The sodium pump is ATP-driven and maintains the resting potential of the nerve by the movement of sodium and potassium against their concentration gradients. The pump has a margin of safety against conditions affecting energy substrate delivery such as ischemic conduction failure. Diabetics, for instance, have an increased resistance to ischemic conduction failure that is thought to be related to abnormal increases in neural stores of glucose.

THE PASSIVE AXON: THE NERVE AS AN ELECTRIC CONDUCTOR

Small electrical impulses or subthreshold stimuli do not excite the membrane but cause a small depolarization or hyperpolarization that dies out after the stimulus is removed. Single subthreshold stimuli do not involve the generation of an action potential and are termed *passive* or *electrotonic* responses that simply dissipate energy. When they were first discovered, it was thought that these small changes in polarization were incompatible with an all-or-none response from the nerve, but since then it has been shown that they are critical in determining how active signals spread.[31–34,57,65,92,93]

To generate an electrical model for the axon's behavior, the axon is divided into small patches, and the movement of ions is followed from patch to patch. From an ion's point of view, the membrane represents a barrier to its movement and therefore is a high-resistance pathway, while both the external media and the axoplasm are low-resistance pathways that allow it to move parallel to the inside and outside of the membrane with relative ease. To complete the model, since the membrane separates two conductors, it also acts as a capacitor that is in parallel with the resistance (Fig. 2-7*A*).

In many ways this system is similar to a submerged electrical cable that has a central core conductor surrounded by an insulator. The use of cable theory to explain nervous signal propagation was first proposed by Hermann after it was originally derived by Lord Kelvin for the transatlantic telegraph cable.[33,66] Note that although the nerve acts like a cable, it is a very leaky one. A typical value for the resting membrane resistance is 1500 Ω/cm, while that for the axoplasm is 50 Ω/cm, a ratio of 30:1. For a copper wire, this same ratio may be as high as 10^{20}:1.

The *cable equation* describes the voltage as a function of both time and position:

$$V = \left(\frac{r_m}{r_i + r_o}\right)\frac{\delta^2 V}{\delta x^2} - (r_m c_m)\frac{\delta V}{\delta t} \qquad (3)$$

The two bracketed terms have special significance in signal propagation and are redefined as follows:

$$\lambda^2 = \frac{r_m}{r_i + r_o} \qquad \tau = r_m c_m \qquad (4)$$

Lambda (λ) is known as the *space constant*, and it determines how far a signal spreads. Note that if the membrane resistance is assumed to be constant, then a low internal resistance yields a large space constant and vice versa. Often, for purposes of discussion, the external resistance is considered negligibly small. Tau (τ) is known as the *time constant*, and it indicates how quickly the membrane responds to signals. The time constant includes the membrane's capacitance because capacitors respond only to dynamic signals, not to static levels. The importance of these constants can be demonstrated by considering the response of the axon to a current step from a microelectrode (see references 57 and 61 for derivation). At very long times a steady state is reached, and the solution shows that voltage decays exponentially traveling farther from the injection site. However, while most of the resulting current flows down the axis of the fiber, at each patch of membrane a small percentage of ions will exit the axon. At the next patch of membrane, once again the same percentage of the remaining ions will depart. This continues down the length of the axon until the signal eventually dies out (Fig. 2-7*B*). A smaller space constant causes the signal to decay more rapidly; a larger one allows the signal to spread quite far down the axon.

Another limiting case is the response at the injection site ($x = 0$). Here the function is qualitatively similar to a rising exponential; however, it rises at a faster rate. For example, at $t/\tau = 1$ it is roughly 20% closer to its final value. As the time constant increases, the response of the signal is delayed. Generally, the larger the time constant, the more slowly the signal will rise. Thinking of the ions flowing down the axon, the fewer ions that reach successive patches of membrane must also first charge up the capacitors of the preceding patches.

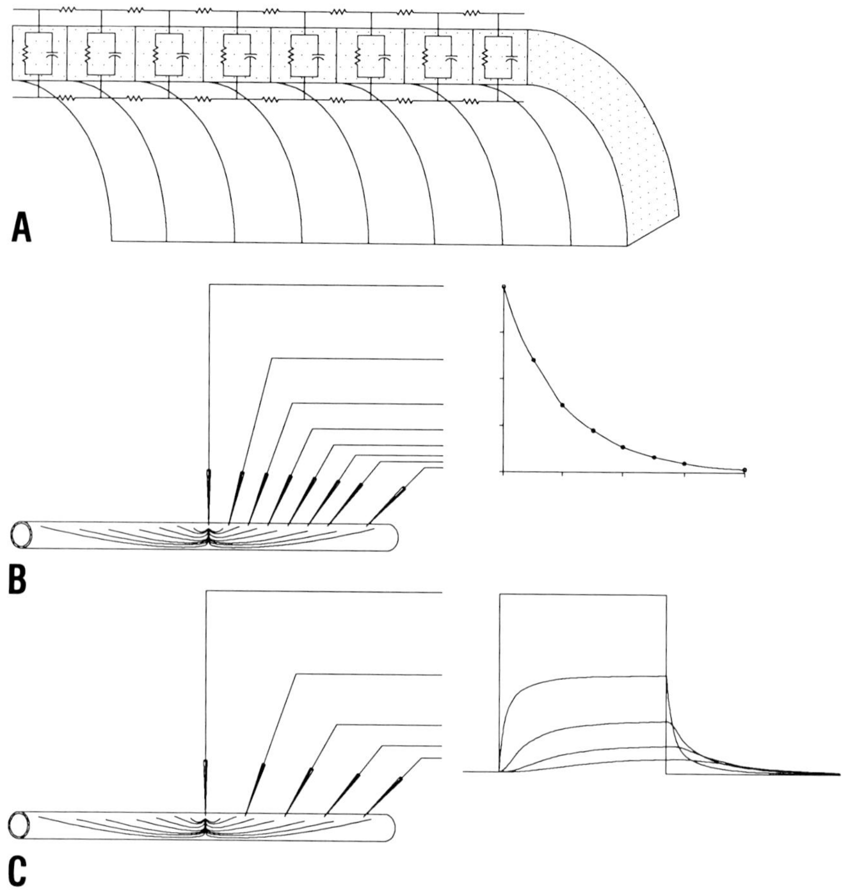

Figure 2–7. *The passive or electrotonic properties of the nerve. (**A**) For subthreshold passive spread of signals, the nerve behaves much like an electrical cable, and each small patch of the nerve's membrane can be modeled as a series of interconnected parallel RC circuits. (**B**) When a steady, small current is injected into the nerve for a long period of time, an equilibrium is reached. Readings of the voltage away from the electrode show that it decays exponentially. (**C**) The passive response of the axon to a subthreshold step. The voltage is measured away from the injection site and slowly rises to reach a finite value.*

The axon's response far from the electrode is mathematically complicated, but it can be qualitatively described rather simply: the farther from the microelectrode, the greater the delay in the appearance of the signal, the more slowly the response rises to its final value, and the greater the exponential decay of the steady-state value (Fig. 2-7*C*).

The resistances and capacitance in the previous discussion have been expressed in terms of a unit length of nerve. This does not give any indication of how these parameters vary with the diameter of the axon or, more appropriately, per square centimeter. When this conversion is done, we see that while the time constant is unrelated to fiber size, the space constant scales as the square root of diameter. This indicates why larger fibers conduct faster than smaller ones: for the same stimulus, a longer portion of the membrane is brought to a level above threshold. A more rigorous argument based on cable theory was presented by Hodgkin when he speculated that if the membrane's properties remain constant, then such a square root relationship would be expected.[40] However, while the behavior of some axons fits with this analysis, that of others does not.[30,35,41,58,83,94,103,107] While the exact dependence of signal propagation on fiber size is unknown, conduction velocity does increase with diameter.

Clinical Significance

The nerve behaves like an electrical cable whose conduction properties vary with its resistance and capacitance. Conduction velocity varies directly with axon diameter.

THE ACTIVE AXON: THE NERVE AS A SIGNAL CONDUCTOR

Cable theory provides a good model for subthreshold responses and supports the membrane theory. However, the purpose of the nerve is to conduct electrical impulses over distances far greater than those that can be achieved with a simple passive mechanism alone. Preceding the action potential, it is the electrotonic response that brings the membrane up to threshold. Since the distance ahead of the action potential depends on the space constant, a local region of membrane will actively generate an action potential that will, in turn, passively raise the next section of membrane to threshold, and so on down the axon. Current advances in *local circuits* (Fig. 2-8A). Its connection to signal propagation was demonstrated in several experiments by Hodgkin.[36,37] By applying either pressure or cold to a small portion of nerve, Hodgkin was able to block the propagation of the action potential beyond that point. When a signal was initiated at the proximal end of the nerve, small depolarizations, or "extrinsic potentials," arose beyond the barrier. These potentials decayed exponentially with distance from the block, as did almost identical signals

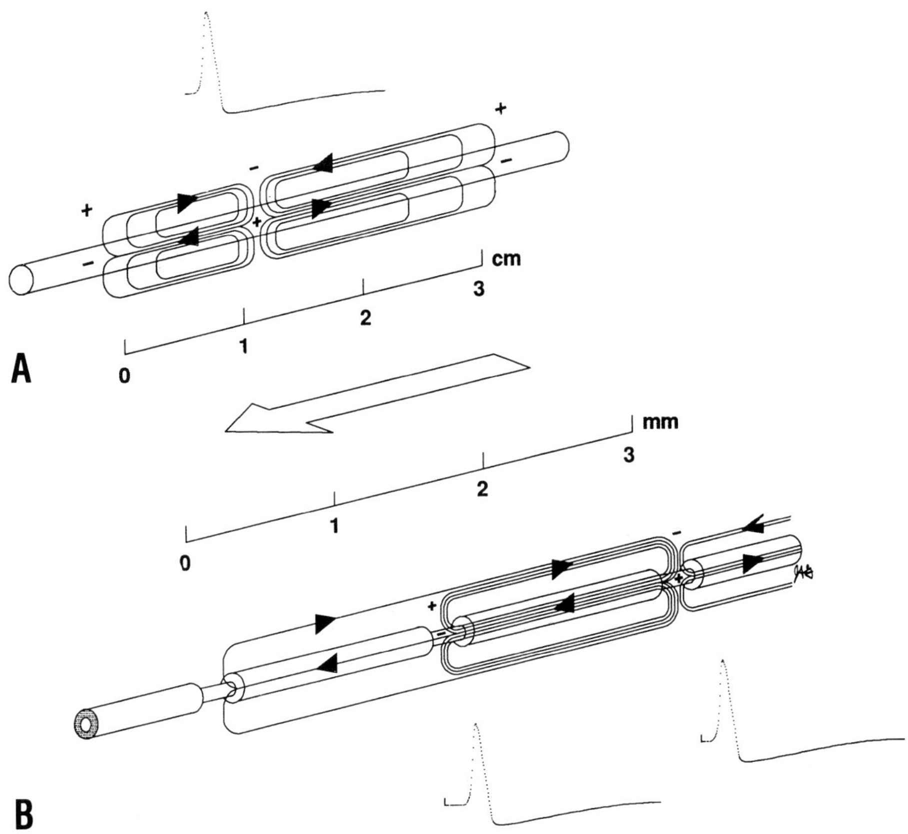

Figure 2–8. *Signal conduction in unmyelinated and myelinated nerves. The large arrow indicates the direction of propagation of the action potentials from right to left. (**A**) In unmyelinated nerves conduction takes place uniformly and successively along the axon. Small patches of membrane are brought to threshold immediately ahead of the action potential by the local circuit currents. The solid arrows indicate the direction of current flow. (**B**) In myelinated fibers the myelin sheath is an effective insulator that causes the local currents to flow down the center of the nerve and exit only at the node of Ranvier. This results in saltatory or jumping conduction from one node to the next; as a consequence, the action potential is delayed farther along the axon. The scales next to each axon indicate the approximate distance the local circuit currents are active at any instance in time during propagation. Note that the radial scale is slightly exaggerated: the unmyelinated axon may be 0.5 mm in diameter while the myelinated nerve may have a diameter of 0.015 mm.*

that were generated by a stimulator placed immediately before the block. In addition, the excitability on the distal side of the block was higher, indicating that the membrane had already been somewhat depolarized. In another series of experiments Hodgkin showed that by increasing or decreasing the external resistance, propagation velocity could be correspondingly altered.[39] This was consistent with the electrotonic properties of nerve and its function in impulse conduction.

Up to this point the model has been based on an unmyelinated fiber that has uniform properties along its length with action potentials appearing in uniform temporal and spatial progression at all points on the fiber. In myelinated fibers, a tight wrapping of Schwann cells envelops the axon. Considering the axon as an electrical cable, the addition of myelin adds to the radial resistance while at the same time reducing the capacitance of the cable. The overall effect of myelin is to make a more effective channel for flow of ions down the center core (the radial-to-axial resistance ratio increases from 30:1 to 5×10^6:1). The breaks in this cable insulation provide exit points for the current so that the signal appears to jump from one node to the next. This process is known as *saltatory conduction*.

Lillie first suggested that this type of periodic insulation restricts the movement of ions to a specific pathway, increasing the transmission speed of nervous signals.[73] He based his theory on an iron wire model immersed in nitric acid. With this model, electrical activity spread up and down the wire. When glass tubing was used to insulate the wire in a fashion analogous to a myelinated fiber, the signal jumped from one uninsulated region to the next.

When single myelinated fibers were first isolated by Kato, it was demonstrated that their thresholds were lowest near nodes and greatest in internodal regions.[63,64] In addition, application of local anesthetics was effective only when placed on nodes.[101–103] This pointed toward the node as the excitable region responsible for signal transmission.

However, demonstration of the insulating effect of myelin and proof of saltatory conduction was provided by measurement of the radial currents at different points along the length of the fiber. By judicious placement of insulating barriers to isolate the nodal and internodal regions, current from these two sections was measured. In the internodal segment only an outward current was recorded, while at the node, the outward current was followed by an inward current indicative of an action potential.[59,60,104,105] This is precisely the response that is expected from a cable structure: the capacitors in the internodal region discharge with the passing signal, but in the node there is an additional inwardly directed current from the active signal.

To demonstrate that the return path in the local circuit included the extracellular fluid, the undissected proximal and distal portions of the nerve were placed in two distinct pools with an isolated internode positioned in air between them. When there was no electrical connection between the pools, conduction failed in the fiber. However, if a moistened thread was used to bridge the gap, conduction was restored.

These experiments provided another argument for cable theory involvement in signal propagation and demonstrated that the local circuit is extended to the nodes in myelinated fibers (Fig. 2-8*B*). Current flows from one node down the axoplasm to the next node, where it exits and returns to the starting node through the external solution. Due to the insulating properties of the myelin, electrotonic spread in such a system brings several nodes beyond the first up to threshold. Tasaki showed that when two nodes are rendered inexcitable, signal propagation can continue past the local block. When three nodes are blocked, however, conduction ceases. Another way of thinking of this scheme is to consider that voltage generated by the action potential is larger than the minimum required for the next node to reach threshold. Tasaki found that this safety factor was roughly five; that is, the voltage at the starting node is five times larger than is necessary to excite the next node.[102,103]

Clinical Significance

Myelin significantly increases conduction velocity by forcing current to flow down the center of the axon and exit only at the nodes of Ranvier. This permits the action potential to jump between nodes and allows a small diameter axon to conduct as rapidly as a large unmyelinated fiber. The Schwann cells that elaborate peripheral myelin are extremely sensitive to ischemic or mechanical injury. Conduction failure can result in myelinated nerves if the myelin is interrupted or a local anesthetic disrupts excitation over several nodes.

THE IONIC BASIS OF EXCITATION

To this point, the action potential has been discussed only in general terms. It has been shown that the basis of the resting potential lies in the semipermeable membrane. If permeabilities change, a complete reversal of the membrane's polarity can occur. It has also been shown that passive electrical properties and the geometry of myelinated and unmyelinated fibers aid in signal transmission. This section will examine the underlying ionic basis of the action potential, which is the active nonlinear process that is the underpinning of all nervous system signaling.

One of the first mechanisms proposed for the action potential was Bernstein's hypothesis that there was a generalized breakdown of membrane permeability to all ions. This idea gained support from the work of Cole and Curtis, who investigated the electrical characteristics of the squid axon both at rest and during an action potential.[16] Using a Wheatstone bridge they were able to show that the cell had a low resistance interior surrounded by a membrane consisting of a parallel capacitance and resistance. During the course of an action potential, they found that the impedance of the membrane changed dramatically (Fig. 2-9*A*). At rest the membrane resistance was 1000 Ω cm^2. When the membrane was active, it dropped to about 25 Ω cm^2, but its capacitance shifted by less than 2%.

The first successful recording of intracellular action potentials raised doubts about Bernstein's theory when it was found that the peak of the action potential was nearly 40 mV positive (Fig. 2-9*B*).[19,20,43,44] A generalized breakdown would yield an action potential that rose to only 0 mV, rather than one that reversed polarity by over 40 mV. Hodgkin and Katz provided the sodium hypothesis as a solution to this puzzle.[51] They suggested that during excitation, the membrane rapidly becomes permeable selectively to sodium, rather than all ions. Due to the large concentration gradient, sodium streams into the axon, causing the membrane potential to reverse and approach the sodium equilibrium potential. In order for the membrane to repolarize, potassium moves outward, down its concentration gradient, leaving the axon and returning the membrane to its original resting potential (Fig. 2-9*C*).

This hypothesis was verified by altering the external concentration of sodium in the bathing solution and finding that both the amplitude and rate of rise of the action potential varied with concentration as predicted by such a mechanism, much like the membrane resting potential's dependence on the external potassium concentration. Later studies of perfused axons in which the internal sodium concentration was changed also supported this conclusion.[6]

Because the membrane becomes transiently permeable to sodium ions, it should be possible to measure the flux of ions across the membrane with each action potential. A simple calculation provides an estimate of approximately one picomole. Measurements of ionic flux using radioactive tracers after stimulation have shown a sodium influx of 3.7 picomoles/cm^2 and a 4.3 picomoles/cm^2 efflux of potassium.[67,68,90] Since these quantities are larger than the predicted values, they are certainly adequate to produce the action potential, especially since the calculation assumed that only one ionic species would move to create the potential difference. At the peak of the action potential, the membrane's permeability is high to both sodium and potassium, and a 1:1 exchange between the two that would not alter the membrane potential could occur.

In addition to suggesting that the membrane becomes selectively permeable to sodium during an action potential, the sodium hypothesis makes the implicit assumption that specialized mechanisms exist in the membrane for the passage of sodium and potassium. A more powerful technique for quantifying the ionic fluxes across the membrane and establishing separate pathways for sodium and potassium was introduced by Marmot and Cole: the *voltage clamp* (Fig. 2-10).[15,49,50,75] Since an action potential induces capacitive and ionic currents that cause temporal and spatial changes along the fiber, the voltage clamp simplifies the problem of analysis by measuring the flow of current over a region of membrane where the voltage is uniform and controlled and hence fixes the space and volt-

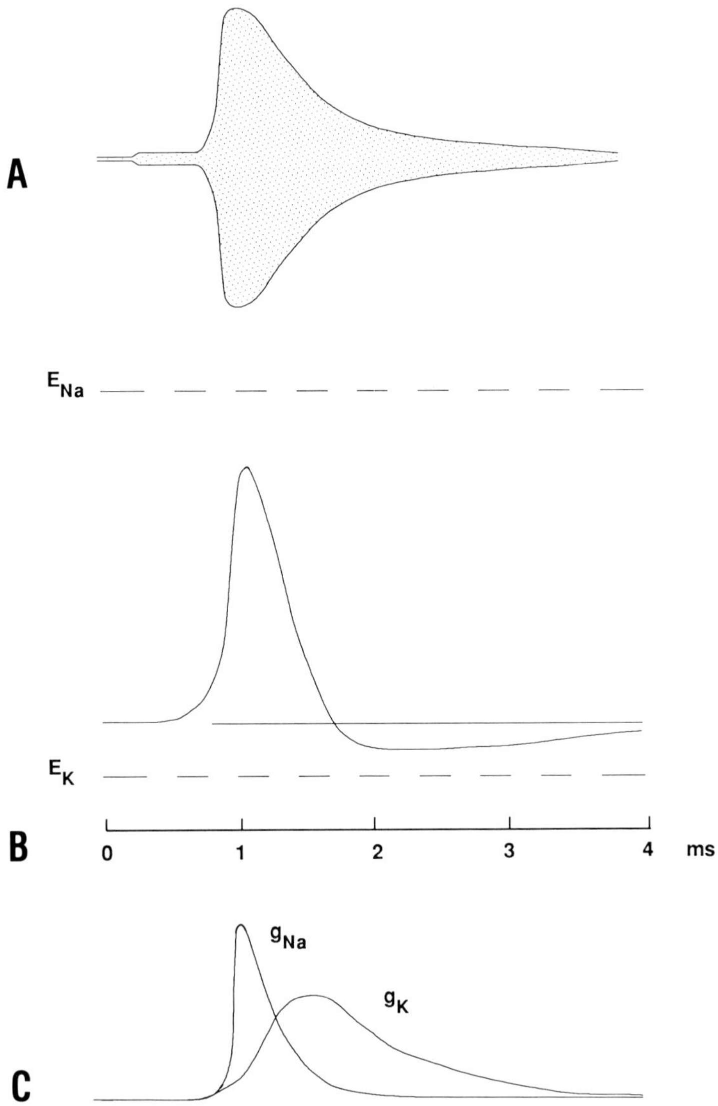

Figure 2–9. *Time course of the events underlying the action potential. (**A**) Membrane impedance after results of Cole and Curtis (see reference 16). They found that these impedance changes were a result of the membrane changing conductance during an action potential. (**B**) Intracellular action potential. Once the membrane reaches threshold, a rapid depolarization occurs; it reverses the polarity of the membrane potential and brings it near the sodium equilibrium potential. This condition is then reversed and the membrane repolarizes after a brief overshoot. (**C**) Sodium and potassium conductances of the membrane. Initially there is a sharp change in the membrane's permeability to sodium, which accounts for the depolarization. This permeability change is transient and rapidly dissipates. The membrane also independently increases its permeability to potassium with a slower time course. This causes the axon to repolarize to its resting level.*

age variables. In the case of the squid axon, a long wire is placed down its axis, causing the interior to become equipotential. This same wire is also used to inject current into the axon to force the membrane potential to match a desired control voltage. This operation of clamping the membrane requires the use of electronic feedback circuitry, which is rapid enough to sense any error induced by permeability changes between the membrane potential and the control voltage. The circuit then generates an output current signal that is equal in magnitude, but opposite in polarity, to the currents in the membrane.

The technique was applied by Hodgkin and Huxley in 1952 to record the currents generated when various-sized voltage steps were applied to the nerve.[45–47] Application of a voltage step has the advantage that the membrane's capacitive current flows only during the time that the voltage is changing and the ionic current component flows when the voltage is constant. During hyperpolarizing steps, a nearly imperceptible inward current is present, but for depolarizing steps these ionic currents are dramatically different: a substantial inward current is followed by a slower, longer-lasting outward current, and if the clamp voltage

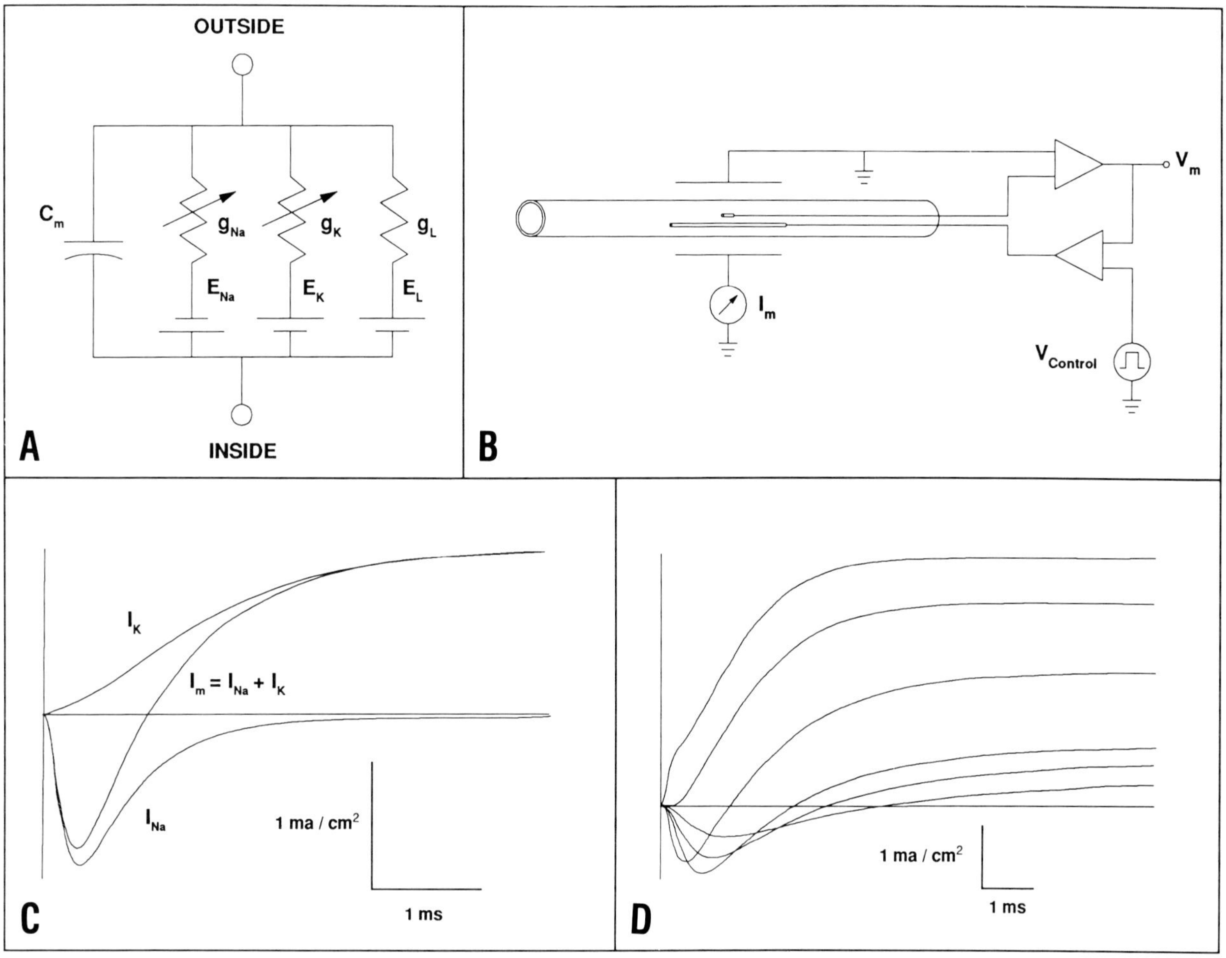

Figure 2–10. *Membrane currents responsible for impulse conduction. (**A**) Equivalent circuit proposed by Hodgkin and Huxley for the nerve membrane. In addition to the membrane's capacitance, three parallel pathways are available for ionic flow: the sodium channel, the potassium channel, and the leakage pathway. The sodium and potassium channels have voltage- and time-dependent conductances, indicated by the arrows. The leakage pathway is a small voltage-independent conductance. (**B**) Schematic of circuit used to voltage-clamp an axon. Membrane potential is measured and compared against a preset control level. Any difference between the two signals is corrected by the circuit, and the current that flows as a result of this is recorded. (**C**) The two major components of membrane current are the sodium and the potassium currents. The sodium current, a rapid inward current (downward deflection), gives way to the slower, longer-lasting outward potassium current (upward deflection). The sodium current is responsible for the depolarization of the nerve during an action potential while the potassium current repolarizes it. (**D**) A family of voltage clamp current records. Control voltage steps from the holding potential (−70 mV) to −30, −10, 10, 30, 50, and 70 mV were imposed. Note that as the voltage step approaches the sodium equilibrium potential, the current is outward because there is no driving force on the sodium ions.*

is large enough, there is a complete abolition of this inward current.

Hodgkin and Huxley were able to separate the ionic current into several parts. They found that in normal seawater, this early current reversed its polarity when the voltage step was approximately at the sodium equilibrium potential. In addition, by varying the external sodium concentration, the early inward current could be almost completely eliminated, and the remaining late current was outward regardless of clamp potential. Both these facts suggested that this early current was carried by sodium ions that were running down a concentration gradient and that the late current probably was a result of potassium doing the same. Since removal of sodium from the bathing media left the potassium current, to isolate the sodium current the current traces obtained in low sodium were subtracted from the currents recorded in normal seawater. In addition to the two major currents, I_{Na} and I_K, they also found a small voltage-independent component of indeterminate ionic origin and termed it the leakage current, I_L.

Hodgkin and Huxley not only recorded the ionic currents responsible for excitation but also provided an analytic framework to represent them.[48] Their derivation for the mechanism is a nonunique empirical fit of their data that uses mathematical functions that describe the behavior of the ionic currents as a function of both voltage and time. They introduced individual parallel pathways (later known as channels) for each ionic species to cross the membrane. They concluded that the changes in ionic current taking place in the membrane could be considered proportional to the conductance of the membrane. Since the Nernst potentials are known for each ion, and the separate currents were measured, the individual conductances could be easily obtained.

The sodium conductance is a two-step process that starts from a low value and, after a brief delay, quickly rises to a peak before it then decreases back to its initial value. The turn-on of this conductance is known as *activation* and is sharply voltage-dependent. To counteract this, a second, slower process, *inactivation*, occurs to turn off the sodium conductance. Inactivation has precedence over activation and must be completely removed before the channels can be re-activated. The potassium conductance, which also starts from a small value, rises much more slowly but then maintains its level with no subsequent reduction. Both of these conductances have maximal values, which are reached if a large enough voltage step is imposed.

Hodgkin and Huxley fit these conductances to the following mathematical expressions:

$$g_{Na} = \bar{g}_{Na} m^3 h \qquad g_K = \bar{g}_K n^4 \tag{5}$$

where the barred quantities are the maximum values of the conductance and the other three parameters, m, n, and h, are dimensionless voltage- and time-dependent variables that vary between 0 and 1. These equations yield smooth continuous functions for the conductances. Note that while the potassium conductance requires only one term to describe its response, the sodium conductance requires a second term to account for its inactivation.

Hodgkin and Huxley also proposed that these conductance or permeability changes of the channels were controlled by *independent gating particles or charges* in the membrane. When these particles were all in the proper position, the channel would be open, and ions would pass. For this to occur implies that some work must be done to move the charges in the membrane, which will generate a small current. Although the existence of these gating currents was postulated solely from an empirical fit of the data, they have since been measured.[2,3,69]

In the case of the potassium channel, four such particles were required to fit the data, each with a probability n of being in the correct place, and hence a probability of n^4 that all of them were located correctly. To describe the transition of the n gating particles between correct and incorrect positions, a first-order equation was used with two voltage-dependent rate constants: α_n and β_n. A similar scheme was also used to describe the two components of the sodium conductance. Three gating particles were needed to describe the activation of the sodium current, while a separate particle was required to account for its inactivation. It should be noted that the inactivation particle h describes the probability of the channel being closed rather than open, since its function is to turn off the flow of ions. In addition, m and h are independent of each other and are functions dependent only on time and voltage. First-order equations and voltage-dependent rate constants similar to those used for potassium describe the transitions of the sodium gating particles. This series of equations describes the behavior of the conductances as a function of both time and voltage. To obtain the total current across the membrane, the individual currents through each pathway are summed:

$$I = I_c + I_{Na} + I_K + I_L \quad (6)$$

or equivalently, with the Hodgkin–Huxley parameters included:

$$I = C_m \frac{dV}{dt} + \bar{g}_{Na}m^3h(V - V_{Na}) + \bar{g}_K n^4(V - V_k) + g_L(V - V_L) \quad (7)$$

As would be expected for an empirical fit, if these equations are solved for a given voltage, the temporal current functions are nearly identical to those recorded experimentally. The ultimate test of the model, once the conductance's dependence on voltage and time were known, was the reconstruction of an action potential by removing the constraints on voltage and space. This attempt was successful and also accurately reproduced membrane impedance changes, supra- and subthreshold responses, the net flux of individual ionic species, and other conduction phenomena.[18,30,48,70]

Over the ensuing years, researchers using a variety of improved techniques have been able to more clearly isolate these currents and the pathways responsible for them. The idea has been firmly established of separate transmembrane proteins with gates that open to form a long aqueous pore for the passage of ions and a narrower region within the pore that discriminates among various ions.[34]

However, the most significant advances have come in using microscopic approaches to the problem of dissecting out the various current-carrying pathways. Pharmacologic agents have provided clear confirmation of individual ion-selective pores or channels. The external application of nanomolar quantities of tetrodotoxin, TTX, a paralytic poison found in the puffer fish, blocks impulse conduction. When applied to an axon under voltage-clamp conditions, the early current is completely eliminated while the late current is unchanged. Hence, TTX selectively blocks sodium channels while having no effect on the potassium or leakage pathways.[79] Other agents, such as local anesthetics, also block the sodium channel but are not as uniquely specific. While the effect of TTX is to plug the channel from the outside so that no ions can enter, if pronase, a combination of proteolytic enzymes, is perfused internally, sodium channel inactivation is removed without affecting other membrane responses.[4]

A complementary channel blocker is tetraethylammonium, TEA, which extends the time required for repolarization of the action potential. When TEA is applied intracellularly, it selectively blocks the potassium channel, leaving the sodium channel unaffected.[1] Other potassium channel blockers include Ba^{+2}, Cs^+, and 4-aminopyridine. This independent blocking of specific ionic conductances, along with the most recent advance, the patch clamp that examines the electrical activity of single channels, leaves no doubt as to the existence of ion-selective channels as the means by which ions traverse the membrane.[34,80]

Voltage-clamp analysis has also been applied to the currents from myelinated nerve fibers, and it has been found that only slight modifications are necessary to model their ionic currents. Both of the activation parameters, m and n, require smaller coefficients, and the relationship between membrane permeability and current is changed to a derivation based on the Goldman equation rather than the simple Ohm's law relationship.[23,26,98] In addition to its slower activation, the potassium channel has an inactivation component that requires a second gating parameter, k, for its description. Although potassium channels are present, their role in the action potential is minimal, with much smaller peak conductances than in the squid axon. In fact, if TEA is used to block the channels, the action potential only doubles its duration, and in the mammalian peripheral nervous system the voltage-dependent potassium response that is seen in the squid is nearly absent.[14,95] This lack of activity occurs because the leakage pathway is much larger than Hodgkin and Huxley found and can repolarize the membrane without the aid of the potassium channels.

Although an in-depth discussion of the techniques and results currently used in attempts to determine the structure of the excitable membrane's channels is beyond the scope of this section, one final point that bears mentioning is the distribution of ionic channels in myelinated and unmyelinated nerve fibers.[7,11] Channels in the squid giant axon are uniformly distributed, with estimates of the sodium channel density ranging from 200 to 600/μm^2 and potassium channels estimated at a density of less than 100/μm^2.[17,72,100] In much the same way that the conduction properties of myelinated fibers differ from unmyelinated nerves, so too do the distribution and density of channels. In the nodal region, sodium channels number approximately 12,000/μm^2 depending on the technique used.[86,87] This high density produces the large inward current needed to depolarize the internodal region. Potassium channels, as might be expected from the minimal currents present, are relatively sparse in the nodal region, numbering in the hundreds at most. The situation in the internode is diametrically opposite to that in the node. When the myelin sheath is removed, it is found that there are no sodium currents present, only potassium currents.[13,86] There are also indications of the existence of sodium and potassium channels in the surrounding Schwann cells of unmyelinated fibers, although their interaction with the axons is not yet clear.[12]

To summarize the findings of this section, when a depolarizing pulse occurs, sodium ions flow into the axon. If enough sodium ions flow into the axon to overcome the equal flow of potassium ions out of the axon, the sodium channels are activated and the membrane depolarizes. A reinforcing or positive feedback system then causes the depolarizing membrane to open more sodium channels and further increase the membrane potential. This process does not go on indefinitely since at the same time, and independently, sodium channel inactivation begins and the slower potassium channels, which allow potassium ions to flow out of the axon and repolarize the membrane, begin to open.

Clinical Significance

In the membrane there are specific ion pathways or channels for the individual ionic species of importance to nerve conduction. Sodium channels are responsible for the initial depolarization of the membrane, and potassium channels cause the repolarization of the membrane. These channels are evenly distributed in unmyelinated fibers, but in myelinated fibers sodium channels are concentrated at the node of Ranvier and potassium channels are concentrated in the adjacent internodal region. Specific toxins that can bind to these ion channels have been a useful tool in basic biophysical studies. Local anesthetics block sodium channels as a mechanism producing conduction failure. Demyelination can expose potassium channels and in conjunction with the loss of internodal insulation can cause nerve dysfunction.

FACTORS AFFECTING IMPULSE CONDUCTION

This chapter has provided a basis for understanding the normal functioning of nervous tissue. More often than not, however, abnormal functioning of the nervous system is of more interest. From the principles and explanation presented earlier, pathological function can be predicted. Likewise, abnormal electrophysiological function can be correlated with structural injury.

Variations in the cross-sectional area of a fiber as a function of axial position can change the shape and velocity of the propagated signal.[31,70] In regions where there are dramatic radius changes, such as in a compressed region, the internal resistance is raised and a larger current density will exist across the membrane. Conversely, when the radius suddenly increases, fewer ions will cross the membrane and propagation may fail if threshold is not reached.

Myelinated fibers gain their conduction velocity advantage from the addition of a myelin sheath, but for a given outside diameter, what is the best ratio of axoplasmic to myelin cross-section? As the myelin thickness increases, internal resistance of the fiber increases due to the smaller axoplasmic radius. This means the space constant (equation 4) is reduced, as is the axial current flow, since it is easier for ions to flow across the membrane than down its center core. The theoretical optimum value of this ratio is approximately 0.6 to 0.7; interestingly, this number is found throughout fibers in nature, although it decreases slightly in very small fibers.[30,41,59–61,78,94,107]

In addition to the electrical properties of the myelin sheath, the spacing of the periodic interruptions in it is another variable parameter. For a fiber with a large space constant, the nodes can be farther apart since there will still be sufficient current to bring them to threshold. Hence, larger fibers generally have proportionally larger internodal distances since their internal resistance is lower and their corresponding space constant larger. The optimum proportionality constant for this function has been found to range between 100 and 200 depending on the species.[30,61,78,85] Note that a closer than optimal spacing can have the effect of slowing, or delaying, transmission of the signal. At some point the advantages of myelination are no longer overwhelming, and unmyelinated axons can conduct as quickly. Comparing the theoretical square root velocity–diameter relationship of unmyelinated fibers to the linear velocity–diameter relationship of myelinated fibers indicates that the crossover point occurs at a diameter between 0.2 and 1.0 μm.[94,107]

One final design consideration is the optimal number of channels to attain maximum conduction velocity. If there are too many channels, an increased capacitance results from the movement of the gating charges. For the squid axon, Hodgkin calculated this number to be approximately 500/μm^2, which is very close to that actually measured.[42]

As biological variability demonstrates, slight changes in morphology will still permit conduction, but at less than maximal rates. However, if these parameters are altered too much, impulse conduction will be significantly impaired. An example of this is fibers that have undergone injury and subsequent demyelination. This process tends to remove the myelin sheath and therefore increases the capacitance and reduces the radial resistance of the axon. This means that the time constant increases while the space constant decreases. In terms of signal transmission, these effects are complementary in slowing and reducing the propagated signal. The node beyond the demyelinated section will be charged more slowly and to a lesser level than normal and thus may not reach threshold. This occurs because there are more capacitors to charge in the internode. The lower radial resistance means that more current will flow out of the demyelinated portion. If the internodal distance is reduced because only parts of the internode are removed or because of remyelination, propagation is correspondingly slowed.[9,70,71,85] Since propagation depends on both passive cable properties and ion channels, it is important to remember that these properties may change with disease or injury. Some continuous conduction has been observed where action potentials propagate along the bare internodal region as if it were a normal unmyelinated fiber.[9,108] There are also indications that sodium channels in the internodal region may allow for signal propagation, but at a slower rate. The origin of these channels, and whether they are synthesized or redistributed, is unclear.[9,12,86] The important point to remember is that if the next functional node can be brought up to threshold, then propagation will continue beyond the affected region with only a temporal delay in signal conduction.

Modification of the nerve's microenvironment can also alter impulse conduction in otherwise normal fibers. Elevated temperatures will increase conduction velocities, since not only are the kinetics of the ion channel temperature-sensitive (with a Q_{10} of approximately 3), but the axoplasmic resistance also is influenced by temperature.[48,78,84] Altering the nerve's ionic milieu leads to changes in the resting potential of the fiber, as predicted by the GHK equation, which in turn affects the activity of the voltage-dependent channels. It is well known that the converse is also true: cold will block signal conduction. In addition, channel activity can be blocked or otherwise altered by pharmacologic agents.

Note that when a local block at a node occurs, the entire fiber has been functionally removed from the bundle because there is no propagation beyond that point.[84] The implications of fiber loss on a larger scale would be observed as a reduction in the amplitude of the compound action potential, since fewer fibers would be available to contribute to the response, but those which did contribute would have normal velocities. However, since there is a far greater number of fibers than the minimum necessary to accomplish most tasks, it is only when a relatively large quantity of fibers is removed that a deficit will appear.

Clinical Significance

Clinical measures of conduction velocity reveal only major abnormalities in nerve function because of the duplicity of signals recorded. Since temperature directly affects conduction velocity and electrode separation is divided by latency to obtain velocity, both must be carefully controlled to avoid errors in interpretation.

REFERENCES

1. Armstrong CM. Time course of TEA$^+$-induced anomalous rectification in squid giant axons. J Gen Physiol 1966;50:491–503.
2. Armstrong CM, Bezanilla F. Currents related to movement of the gating particles of the sodium channels. Nature 1973;242:459–461.
3. Armstrong CM, Bezanilla F. Charge movement associated with the opening and closing of the activation gates of the Na channels. J Gen Physiol 1974;63:533–552.
4. Armstrong CM, Bezanilla F, Rojas E. Destruction of sodium conductance inactivation in squid axons perfused with pronase. J Gen Physiol 1973;62: 375–391.
5. Baker PF, Hodgkin AL, Shaw TI. Replacement of the axoplasm of giant nerve fibres with artificial solutions. J Physiol (Lond) 1962;164:330–354.
6. Baker PF, Hodgkin AL, Shaw TI. The effects of changes in internal ionic concentrations on the electrical properties of perfused giant axons. J Physiol (Lond) 1962;164:355–374.
7. Barchi RL. Probing the molecular structure of the voltage-dependent sodium channel. Ann Rev Neurosci 1988;11:455–495.
8. Bernstein J. Untersuchungen zur Thermodynamik der bioelektrischen Ströme. Pflüg Arch 1902;92: 521–562.
9. Bostok H, Sears TA. The internodal axon membrane: Electrical excitability and continuous conduction in segmental demyelination. J Physiol (Lond) 1978;280:273–301.
10. Caldwell PC, Hodgkin AL, Keynes RD, Shaw TI. The effects of injecting "energy-rich" phosphate compounds on the active transport of ions in the giant axons of *Loligo*. J Physiol (Lond) 1960;152: 561–590.
11. Catterall WA. Genetic analysis of ion channels in vertebrates. Ann Rev Physiol 1988;50:395–406.
12. Chiu SY. Sodium currents in axon-associated Schwann cells from adult rabbits. J Physiol (Lond) 1987;386:181–203.
13. Chiu SY, Ritchie JM. Evidence for the presence of potassium channels in the internode of frog myelinated nerve fibres. J Physiol (Lond) 1982;322: 485–501.
14. Chiu SY, Ritchie JM, Rogart RB, Stagg D. A quantitative description of membrane currents in rabbit myelinated nerve. J Physiol (Lond) 1979;292:149–166.
15. Cole KS. Dynamic electrical characteristics of the squid axon membrane. Arch Sci Physiol 1949;3: 253–258.
16. Cole KS, Curtis HJ. Electrical impedance of the squid giant axon during activity. J Gen Physiol 1939;22:649–670.
17. Conti F, DeFelice LJ, Wanke E. Potassium and sodium ion current noise in the membrane of the squid giant axon. J Physiol (Lond) 1975;248:45–82.
18. Cooley I, Dodge FA. Digital computer solutions for excitation and propagation of the nerve impulse. Biophys J 1966;6:583–599.
19. Curtis HJ, Cole KS. Membrane action potentials from the squid giant axon. J Cell Comp Physiol 1940;15:147–157.
20. Curtis HJ, Cole KS. Membrane resting and action potentials from the squid giant axon. J Cell Comp Physiol 1942;19:135–144.
21. Danielli JF, Davson H. A contribution to the theory of permeability of thin films. J Cell Comp Physiol 1935;5:495.
22. De Weer P, Geduldig D. Electrogenic sodium pump in squid giant axon. Science 1973;179: 1326–1328.
23. Dodge FA, Frankenhaeuser B. Membrane currents in isolated frog nerve fibre under voltage clamp conditions. J Physiol (Lond) 1958;143:76–90.
24. Edidin M. Translational and rotational diffusion in membranes. Ann Rev Biophys Bioeng 1974;3: 179–201.
25. Erlanger J, Gasser HS. Electrical signs of nervous activity. Philadelphia: University of Pennsylvania Press, 1937.
26. Frankenhaeuser B. Quantitative description of sodium currents in myelinated nerve fibers of *Xenopus laevis*. J Physiol (Lond) 1960;151:491–501.
27. Frye CD, Edidin M. The rapid mixing of cell surface antigens after formation of mouse–human heterokayrons. J Cell Sci 1970;7:319–332.
28. Geren BB. The formation from the Schwann cell surface of myelin in the peripheral nerves of chick embryos. Exp Cell Res 1954;7:558–562.
29. Goldman DE. Potential, impedance and rectification in membranes. J Gen Physiol 1943;27:37–60.
30. Goldman L, Albus JS. Computation of impulse conduction in myelinated fibers; theoretical basis of the velocity-diameter relation. Biophys J 1968;8:596–607.
31. Goldstein SS. Models of conduction in nonuniform axons. In: Waxman SG, ed. Physiology and pathobiology of axons. New York: Raven Press, 1978: 227–236.

32. Gorter E, Grendel F. On bimolecular layers of lipoids on the chromocytes of the blood. J Exp Med 1925;41:439–443.
33. Hermann L. Beitrage zur Physiologie und Physik des Nerven. Pflüg Arch 1905;109:95–144.
34. Hille B. Ionic channels of excitable membranes. Massachusetts: Sinauer Associates Inc., 1984.
35. Hodes R. Linear relationship between fiber diameter and velocity of conduction in giant axon of squid. J Neurophysiol 1953;16:145–154.
36. Hodgkin AL. Evidence for electrical transmission in nerve. Part I. J Physiol (Lond) 1937;90:183–210.
37. Hodgkin AL. Evidence for electrical transmission in nerve. Part II. J Physiol (Lond) 1937;90:211–232.
38. Hodgkin AL. The subthreshold potentials in a crustacean nerve fibre. Proc R Soc Lond [B] 1938;126:87.
39. Hodgkin AL. The relation between conduction velocity and the electrical resistance outside a nerve. J Physiol (Lond) 1939;94:560–570.
40. Hodgkin AL. A note on conduction velocity. J Physiol (Lond) 1954;125:221–224.
41. Hodgkin AL. The conduction of the nervous impulse. Liverpool: University Press, 1964.
42. Hodgkin AL. The optimum density of sodium channels in an unmyelinated nerve. Phil Trans R Soc Lond [B] 1975;270:297–300.
43. Hodgkin AL, Huxley AF. Action potentials recorded from inside a nerve fibre. Nature 1939;144: 710–711.
44. Hodgkin AL, Huxley AF. Resting and action potentials in single nerve fibres. J Physiol (Lond) 1945;104:176–195.
45. Hodgkin AL, Huxley AF. Currents carried by sodium and potassium ions through the membrane of the giant axon of *Loligo*. J Physiol (Lond) 1952;116:449–472.
46. Hodgkin AL, Huxley AF. The components of membrane conductance in the giant axon of *Loligo*. J Physiol (Lond) 1952;116:473–496.
47. Hodgkin AL, Huxley AF. The dual effect of membrane potential on sodium conductance in the giant axon of *Loligo*. J Physiol (Lond) 1952;116:497–506.
48. Hodgkin AL, Huxley AF. A quantitative description of membrane current and its application to conduction and excitation in nerve. J Physiol (Lond) 1952;117:500–544.
49. Hodgkin AL, Huxley AF, Katz B. Ionic currents underlying activity in the giant axon of the squid. Arch Sci Physiol 1949;3:129–150.
50. Hodgkin AL, Huxley AF, Katz B. Measurement of the current voltage relations in the membrane of the giant axon of *Loligo*. J Physiol (Lond) 1952;116:424–448.
51. Hodgkin AL, Katz B. The effects of sodium ions on the electrical activity of the giant axon of the squid. J Physiol (Lond) 1949;108:37–77.
52. Hodgkin AL, Keynes RD. The mobility and diffusion coefficient of potassium in giant axons from *Sepia*. J Physiol (Lond) 1953;119:513–528.
53. Hodgkin AL, Keynes RD. Movements of cations during recovery in nerve. Symp Soc Exp Biol 1954;8:423–437.
54. Hodgkin AL, Keynes RD. Active transport of cations in giant axons from *Sepia* and *Loligo*. J Physiol (Lond) 1955;128:28–60.
55. Hodgkin AL, Keynes RD. The potassium permeability of a giant nerve fibre. J Physiol (Lond) 1955;128:61–88.
56. Hodgkin AL, Keynes RD. Experiments on the injection of substances into squid giant axons by means of a microsyringe. J Physiol (Lond) 1956; 131:592–616.
57. Hodgkin AL, Rushton WAH. The electrical constants of a crustacean nerve fibre. Proc R Soc Lond [B] 1946;133:444–479.
58. Hursh JB. Conduction velocity and diameter of nerve fibers. Am J Physiol 1939;127:131–151.
59. Huxley AF, Stämpfli R. Evidence for saltatory conduction in peripheral myelinated nerve fibres. J Physiol (Lond) 1949;108:315–339.
60. Huxley AF, Stämpfli R. Saltatory transmission of the nervous impulse. Arch Sci Physiol 1949;3:435.
61. Jack JJB, Noble D, Tsien RW. Electric current flow in excitable cells. London: Oxford University Press, 1983.
62. Jain MK. Introduction to biological membranes. John Wiley & Sons, 1988.
63. Kato G. The microphysiology of nerve. Tokyo: Maruzen, 1934.
64. Kato G. On the excitation, conduction and narcotization of single nerve fibres. Cold Spring Harbor Symp Quant Biol 1936;4:202.
65. Katz B. Experimental evidence for a non-conducted response of nerve to subthreshold stimulation. Proc R Soc Lond [B] 1937;124:244–276.
66. Kelvin WT. On the theory of the electric telegraph. Proc R Soc 1855;7:382–399.
67. Keynes RD. The ionic movements during nervous activity. J Physiol (Lond) 1951;114:119–150.
68. Keynes RD, Lewis PR. The sodium and potassium content of cephalopod nerve fibers. J Physiol (Lond) 1951;114:151–182.

69. Keynes RD, Rojas E. Kinetics and steady-state properties of the charged system controlling sodium conductance in the squid giant axon. J Physiol (Lond) 1974;239:393–434.
70. Khodorov BI. The problem of excitability. Electrical excitability and ionic permeability of the nerve membrane. New York: Plenum Press, 1974.
71. Koles ZJ, Rasminsky M. A computer simulation of conduction in demyelinated nerve fibres. J Physiol (Lond) 1972;227:351–364.
72. Levinson SR, Meves H. The binding of tritiated tetrodotoxin to squid giant axons. Philos Trans R Soc Lond [Biol] 1975;270:349–352.
73. Lillie RS. Factors affecting transmission and recovery in the passive iron nerve model. J Gen Physiol 1925;7:473–507.
74. Ling G, Gerard RW. The normal membrane potential of frog sartorius fibers. J Cell Comp Physiol 1949;34:393–396.
75. Marmot G. Studies on the axon membrane. I. A new method. J Cell Comp Physiol 1949;34:351–382.
76. McCloskey M, Poo M. Protein diffusion in cell membranes: Some biological implications. Int Rev Cytol 1984;87:19–81.
77. Montal M, Mueller P. Formation of biomolecular membranes from lipid monolayers and a study of their electrical properties. Proc Natl Sci USA 1972;69:3561–3566.
78. Moore LW, Joyner RW, Brill MH, Waxman SD, Najar-Joa M. Simulations of conduction in uniform myelinated fibers. Biophys J 1978;21:147–160.
79. Narahashi T, Moore JW, Scott WR. Tetrodotoxin blockage of sodium conductance increase in lobster axons. J Gen Physiol 1964;47:965–974.
80. Neher E, Sakmann B. Single-channel currents recorded from membrane of denervated frog muscle fibres. Nature 1976;260:799–802.
81. Overton E. Uber die allgemeinen osmotischen Eigenschaften der Zelle, ihre vermutlichen Ursachen und ihre Bedeutung für die Physiologie. Vjschr Naturforsch Ges Zurich 1899;44:88–135. Repr. in Branton D, Park RR, eds. Papers on biological membrane structure. Boston: Little Brown, 1968: 45–52.
82. Peters R, Brunger A, Schulten K. Continuous fluorescence microphotolysis: A sensitive method for study of diffusion processes in single cells. Proc Natl Acad Sci USA 1981;78:962–966.
83. Pumphrey RJ, Young JZ. The rates of conduction of nerve fibres of various diameters of cephalopods. J Exp Biol 1938;15:453–466.
84. Rasminsky M. The effects of temperature on conduction in demyelinated single nerve fibers. Arch Neurol 1973;28:287–292.
85. Rasminsky M, Sears TA. Internodal conduction in undissected demyelinated nerve fibers. J Physiol (Lond) 1972;227:323–350.
86. Ritchie JM. The distribution of sodium and potassium channels in mammalian myelinated nerve channels. In: Ritchie JM, Keynes RD, Bolis L, eds. Ion channels in neural membranes. New York: Alan R Liss, 1986:105–122.
87. Ritchie JM, Rogart RB. Density of sodium channels in mammalian myelinated nerve fibers and nature of the axonal membrane under the myelin sheath. Proc Natl Acad Sci USA 1977;74:211–215.
88. Robertson JD. The molecular structure and contact relationship of cell membranes. Progr Biophys 1960;10:343–418.
89. Robertson JD. Myelinating and non-myelinating nerve fibers during development: A new component of the endoplasmic reticulum of Schwann cells. J Physiol 1960;153:40P.
90. Rothenberg MA. Studies on permeability in relation to nerve function. II. Ionic movement across axonal membranes. Acta Biochem Biophys 1950;4: 96.
91. Rothman JE, Lenard J. Membrane asymmetry. Science 1977;195:743–753.
92. Rushton WAH. A new observation in the excitation of nerve and muscle. J Physiol (Lond) 1932;75: 16–17P.
93. Rushton WAH. The initiation of the propagated disturbance. Proc R Soc Lond [B] 1937;124:201–243.
94. Rushton WAH. A theory of the effects of fibre size in medullated nerve. J Physiol (Lond) 1951;115: 101–122.
95. Schmidt H, Stämpfli R. Die Wirkung von Tetraäthylammoniumchlorid auf den einzelnen Ranvierschen Schnurring. Pflüg Arch 1966;287:311–325.
96. Singer SJ, Nicolson GL. The fluid mosaic model of the structure of cell membranes. Science 1972;175:720–722.
97. Skou SJ. Enzymatic basis for active transport of Na^+ and K^+ across cell membranes. Physiol Rev 1965;45:596–617.
98. Stämpfli R, Hille B. Electrophysiology of the peripheral myelinated nerve. In: Llinas R, Precht W, eds. Frog neurobiology: A handbook. New York: Springer-Verlag, 1976:3–32.
99. Steim JM, Tourtellotte ME, Reinert JC, McElhaney RN, Rader RL. Calorimetric evidence for the liquid

crystalline state of lipids in a biomembrane. Proc Natl Acad Sci USA 1969;63:104–109.
100. Strichartz GR, Rogart RB, Ritchie JM. Binding of radioactively labeled saxitoxin to the squid giant axon. J Memb Biol 1979;48:357–364.
101. Tasaki I. Electric stimulation and the excitatory process in the nerve fibre. Am J Physiol 1939;125: 380.
102. Tasaki I. The electro-saltatory transmission of the nerve impulse and the effect of narcosis upon the nerve fibre. Amer J Physiol 1939;127:211.
103. Tasaki I. Physiology and electrochemistry of nerve fibers. New York: Academic Press, 1982.
104. Tasaki I, Takeuchi T. Der am Ranvierschen Knoten entstehende Aktionsstrom und seine Bedeutung für die Erregungsleitung. Pflüg Arch 1941;244: 696–711.
105. Tasaki I, Takeuchi T. Weitere Studien über den Aktionsstrom der markhaltigen Nervenfaser und ueber die elektrosaltatorische Ubertragung des Nervenimpulses. Pflüg Arch 1942;245:764–782.
106. Thomas RC. Electrogenic sodium pump in nerve and muscle cells. Physiol Rev 1972;52:563–594.
107. Waxman SG, Bennett MVL. Relative conduction velocities of small myelinated and non-myelinated fibers in the central nervous system. Nature [New Biol] 1972;238:217–219.
108. Waxman SG, Brill MH. Conduction through demyelinated plaques in multiple sclerosis: Computer simulations of facilitation by short internodes. J Neurol Neurosurg Psychiatry 1978;41: 408–417.

3

Biomechanical Properties of Peripheral Nerve

Michael K. Kwan
Savio L-Y. Woo

AUTHORS' KEY POINTS

- Peripheral nerve, which is flexible, exhibits nonlinear stress–strain behavior when placed under tension. Initially the nerve has a low modulus, and after a large toe region the modulus increases with increasing strain.
- In situ peripheral nerve is under significant strain, but the corresponding in situ stress is minimal (less than 0.05 MPa).
- In situ strain of peripheral nerve varies with limb position, but is not likely to exceed the limit beyond which significant tension (or stress) is developed in the nerve.
- Perineurium is the major tensile load-carrying connective tissue component of peripheral nerve.
- As axons themselves contribute little to the tensile strength of peripheral nerve, the proximal and distal segments of transected nerve have the same mechanical properties as normal nerve.
- The maintenance of small amounts of in situ stress suggests that sustained increases in tension could be an important factor adversely affecting electrophysiological properties of nerve.
- Peripheral nerve, like most soft tissues, exhibits time-dependent viscoelastic behavior, including creep (ie, gradual elongation of the nerve with time when the tissue is placed under a fixed tension) and stress relaxation (ie, relaxation of tension in the nerve after it is stretched to a fixed elongation).
- Significant alterations of conduction properties may result from a small amount of mechanical stretch, 6% above the in situ length.

Understanding the biomechanical properties of peripheral nerve is essential for characterization of the effects of stretch on the conduction properties of neural tissue. Trauma to the extremities, such as high-energy traction to the brachial plexus, and clinical situations such as nerve repair under tension often cause stretch injuries to nerve and result in disability in forms of motor and sensory impairment as well as pain.[16,23,24] It is generally assumed that, within certain limits, nerve can adapt to stretch with only transient functional changes. However, data on the biomechanical properties of peripheral nerve (such as the amount of tensile strain that causes structural damages) are limited and inconsistent. Early published data indicate that failure strain ranges from 11% to 100%.[5,9,10] These wide variations are believed to have been caused by difficulties in mechanical testing of very flexible nerve tissues. In the literature there is also disagreement regarding which structural component of peripheral nerve is responsible for its tensile strength.[7,26] Recently, with modern and improved techniques, the mechanical properties as represented by tensile stress–strain curves have been assessed.[13,22] Further, these properties are correlated with the structural damage to the peripheral nerve under tension. This chapter discusses the in situ stress and strain in peripheral nerve, the stress–strain properties of peripheral nerve, the viscoelastic properties of peripheral nerve, and the correlation of these biomechanical findings to nerve stretch injuries and repair.

IN SITU STRESS AND STRAIN IN PERIPHERAL NERVE

Nerve, like many soft connective tissues, is under certain amounts of stress and strain when in the body, so-called in situ stress and strain. The existence of in situ stress and strain is believed not only to be relevant to the strength and integrity of tissue, but also to be important for its homeostasis, ie, maintenance of size, mass, shape and function.[6] Findings on in situ stress and strain in peripheral nerve have not been well documented, however. Only recently has a method been developed to measure the in situ stress and strain of rabbit tibial nerve.[13]

Authors' Preferred Method of Studying Nerve Stress and Strain

With the knee and ankle joints fixed at 90° of flexion, rabbit tibial nerve is exposed. Generally, the length of the nerve varies with the angle of flexion at these joints. Care is taken to avoid trauma to the nerve. The nerve is irrigated with 0.9% normal saline solution to prevent dehydration during the preparation. It is then marked by placing two parallel black lines (using Verhoff stain) 1 cm apart on its exposed surface. A reference measuring scale is placed alongside the nerve specimen on the same plane as the nerve surface. The distance between the black lines, representing the in situ length of nerve, is measured by using a video dimensional analyzer (VDA) and the reference scale. The VDA system is an accurate and noncontacting method for length (or strain) measurement. It has been used effectively in testing soft connective tissues such as articular cartilage, tendons, and ligaments.[32,33]

A nerve specimen approximately 5 cm long between the ankle and the knee is then excised. The width and thickness of the isolated nerve specimen are measured for computation of cross-sectional area. One end of the specimen is wrapped in saline-soaked gauze and mounted in a self-tightening clamp. The clamped nerve is then suspended and allowed to hang freely for 5 minutes. The length of the nerve at this point, with no external load (defined as zero-load length), is measured by the VDA and used as gauge length. The amount of retraction in length is used to calculate the in situ strain ([in situ length − gauge length]/gauge length). The in situ strain of rabbit tibial nerve is 11.0 ± 1.5% (n = 9), which is relatively large compared to many other soft connective tissues. The in situ stress, on the other hand, is determined as the stress corresponding to the in situ strain on the tensile stress–strain curve determined for nerve. The in situ stress is discussed with the tensile properties of peripheral nerve in the next section.

TENSILE PROPERTIES OF PERIPHERAL NERVE

Studies on the tensile properties of peripheral nerve date back to the early works of Wertheim (1847), which were concerned primarily with the "breaking point" of stretched nerve.[31] Values ranging from 18 to 165 kg for sciatic nerve and 20 to 50 kg for median nerve were reported by Takimoto in 1917.[27] Later, experimental studies on popliteal nerve showed that elongation of 11% or more caused severe, extensive damage.[9] Significantly different results were reported by Denny-Brown and coworkers,[5] who claimed that peripheral nerve segments could be extended 100% without structural damage, while Hoen and associates[10] indicated that 25% to 50% elongation without damage was possible. Liu and colleagues,[14] on the other hand, concluded that peripheral nerve could be damaged if stretched more than 4%. Sunderland and coworkers[26] later measured the "strength and elasticity" of peripheral nerve and reported that the tensile strength varied from 0.5 to 3.1 kg/mm^2 (or 4.9–30.4 MPa). The strain at the "elastic limit" ranged from 8% to 20%, and the maximal strain (at failure) was approximately 30%. These ranges of variation were thought to be due to the nonhomogeneous structure of nerve trunks, which consist of a complex variety of elements with different strengths and elasticity.

In our laboratory, the stress–strain characteristics and structural damage of rabbit tibial nerve under tension have been assessed.[13,22] These characteristics are determined in a tensile test, where the excised nerve is clamped and set at its gauge length (ie, zero-load length), and then loaded to failure at an extension rate of 1 cm/min (or strain rate of 0.5%/sec). By measuring the load with a sensitive load cell (accuracy: 0.005 N) and tensile strain with the VDA, the load-elongation (structural properties) and stress–strain (mechanical properties) curves are determined.

Peripheral nerve is easily extensible initially, as a minimal amount of tension is required to stretch it (Fig. 3-1). Rabbit tibial nerve can be elongated approximately 6 mm with very little tension. With further elongation, nerve stiffens as the slope of the curve rises steadily. The increase in stiffness is due to the stretching of connective tissues within nerve. The rabbit tibial nerve has an ultimate elongation of 16.3 ± 0.7 mm and an ultimate load of 9.52 ± 0.47 N.[13] For human ulnar nerves the ultimate load is reported to be 65 to 155 N, and for human median nerve, 73 to 220 N.[24] It should be noted that these data refer to normal nerves;

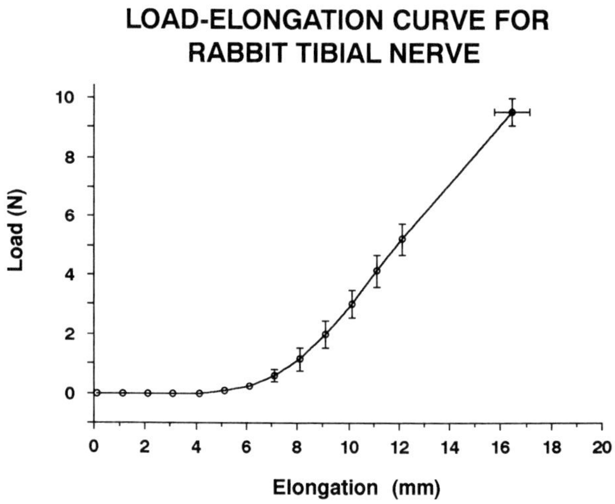

Figure 3-1. *The load-deformation curve for rabbit peripheral tibial nerve. A 1-cm long nerve can be stretched from its zero-load length by about 3.5 mm before appreciable tension develops in it.*

chronically injured nerves may have altered biomechanical properties such as increased stiffness.[2]

In the limited literature regarding the biomechanical behavior of peripheral nerve, nerve is often described as a linearly elastic material, and terms such as elastic (or Young's) modulus and limit of elasticity, among others, are used. Peripheral nerve, in fact, exhibits *highly nonlinear stress–strain behavior* (Fig. 3-2).[13] The stress–strain behavior follows the general characteristics of the load-elongation curve. It has a large initial toe region (i.e. low-stiffness region), demonstrating that the nerves may stretch up to 15% strain under minimal stress. Much of the strain within the toe region is due to the removal of the slack in nerve fascicles, as well as in the nerve trunk as a whole. With further application of tensile strain, nerve fibers and endoneural tubes, as well as the perineurium, are recruited and begin to lengthen. This results in gradual increases in the modulus of nerve. The modulus reaches a maximal value at about 20% strain and then remains fairly constant until failure. With further stretching, the endoneural tubes may rupture, and a disorganization of the endoneurial contents may occur inside still-intact perineural sheaths. At the point of failure, rupture of the perineurium of nerve fascicles occurs. For rabbit tibial nerve, the tensile strength and ultimate strain are

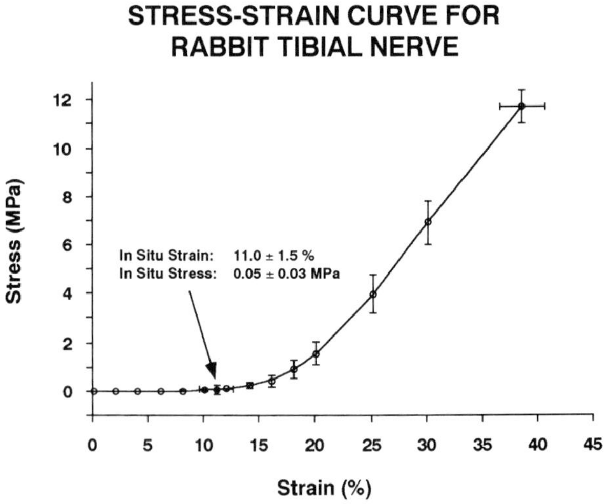

Figure 3–2. *The stress–strain curve for rabbit tibial nerve. The nerve exhibits a low stiffness toe region of about 15% and begins to retain significant tension as the strain increases beyond 20%.*

found to be 11.7 ± 0.7 MPa and 38.5 ± 2.0%, respectively.

The toe region, as seen in Figure 3-2, extends well past the in situ strain of nerve (ie, 11.0 ± 1.5%), which corresponds to a very small in situ stress of 0.05 ± 0.03 MPa. While in situ nerve is under relatively large strain, it is under minimal stress. The in situ strain generally varies with angles of flexion of joints. It is unlikely that it would exceed the toe region; thus the stress in nerve remains small. In other words, within physiological range of motions, peripheral nerve is flexible without developing significant amounts of tension. The maintenance of a small amount of in situ stress also suggests that sustained increases in stress could be an important factor adversely affecting the functional properties of nerves.

It has been observed that when peripheral nerve fails mechanically, it often appears grossly intact.[12] This striking observation may have clinical relevance (ie, it may not be reliable to assess the structural integrity of a nerve trunk through visual examination only). Histological study of failed specimens reveals that while there are multiple ruptures of perineural sheaths along the course of failed nerve specimens, there is no noticeable structural damage of any other connective tissue components (Fig. 3-3). This suggests that the perineurium of the nerve fascicles is a major load-carrying connective tissue component. The perineural sheath does not rupture at one given point in the nerve, but rather along the nerve over some distance. Therefore, stretch injuries to peripheral nerve may not be a localized phenomenon.

In failed nerve, nerve fibers within fascicles also appear intact. The fibers do not seem to contribute significantly to the tensile strength of peripheral nerve. This observation is supported by the fact that the distal segment of a severed nerve, with its nerve fibers that have undergone Wallerian degeneration, has the same mechanical properties as normal nerve.[26]

Clinical Significance

Under normal conditions, while peripheral nerve is under considerable strain, in situ stress is low. The major intraneural structure resisting stress is the perineurium. This connective tissue coat may rupture at a point at which both axons and the epineurium remain intact. Thus, gross inspection of nerve after stretch injury may not reveal significant intraneural disorganization.

VISCOELASTIC PROPERTIES OF PERIPHERAL NERVE

Like most connective tissues, peripheral nerve exhibits time-dependent viscoelastic behavior.[8,11,30] This behavior includes creep (ie, gradual elongation of nerve with time when the tissue is placed under a fixed tension) and stress relaxation (ie, relaxation of tension in nerve when it is stretched to a fixed point of elongation). Viscoelastic behavior is an important property for nerve in that its initial elongation on loading can be limited. In other words, the high degree of tension in nerve, when mechanically stretched, can be relieved. These properties for peripheral nerve are not well described, as available reports in the literature are rather limited. Hartung and coworkers observed stress relaxation in nerve when testing the tissue under cyclic loading.[8] Kendall reported creep phenomenon for rabbit sciatic nerve, but did not mention the strain level and rate of strain used in the study.[11]

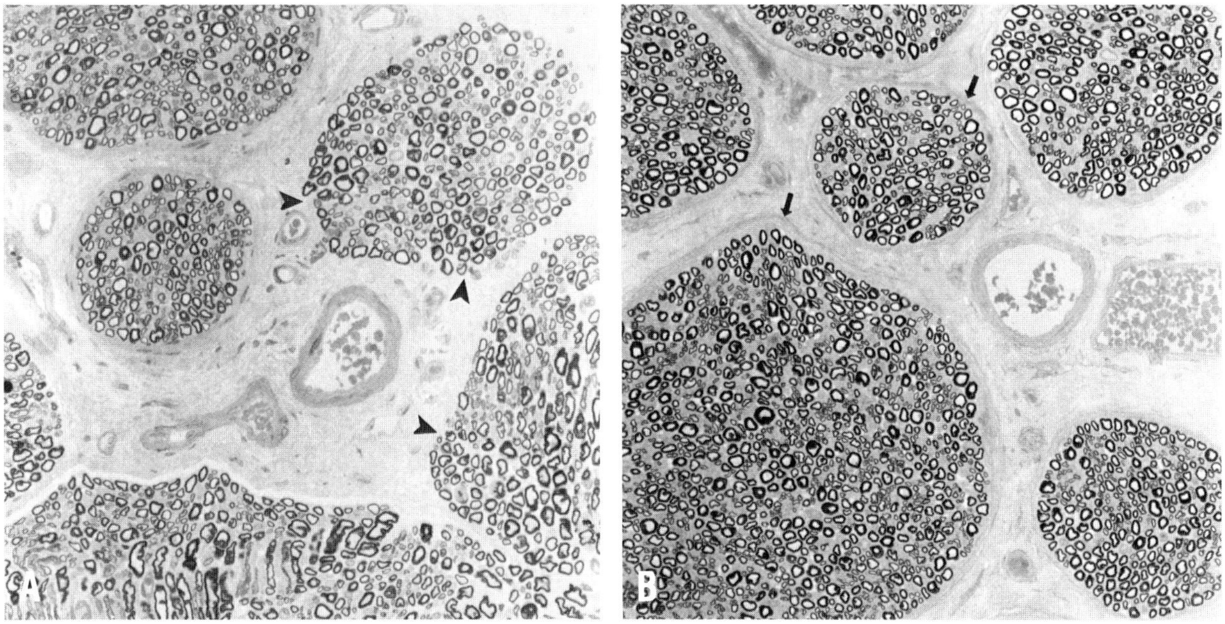

Figure 3–3. *(**A**) Transverse section of normal rabbit tibial nerve. Note discrete fascicles bounded by intact perineurium (arrows). The loose connective tissue of the epineurium contains several vessels. Paraphenylenediamine (original magnification 200×). (**B**) Transverse section of stretched rabbit tibial nerve. The perineurium is disrupted and absent in some fascicles (arrow heads), permitting direct communication between the endoneurium and the epineurium. Note also that the epineurium contains erythrocytes outside the blood vessels. Paraphenylenediamine (original magnification 200×).*

Most recently in our laboratory, the stress relaxation behavior of rabbit tibial nerve at various stress levels was investigated.[30] Nerves were stretched at 3%/sec, held at either 6%, 9%, or 12% above the in situ strain level, and then allowed to stress relax for 1 hour. The results showed that the peak tensions for the 6%, 9%, and 12% groups were 0.86 ± 0.49 N, 2.17 ± 0.64 N, and 3.14 ± 0.79 N, respectively. The tension in the nerves decreased rapidly during the first 10 minutes, to 64% to 74% of peak values (Fig. 3-4), and more slowly thereafter for the remainder of the experiment, to 52% to 67% at the end of 1 hour. Generally, less stress relaxation occurs at higher strain levels. However, the difference between 9% and 12% was insignificant.

The knowledge of nerve viscoelasticity is of fundamental importance to microsurgeons involved in nerve repair. When approximating the ends of transected nerve, for example, nerve stretch should be slow enough to avoid high initial peak tension. It should be gradual to allow sufficient attenuation of the developed stress.

Clinical Significance

Nerve, exhibiting viscoelastic behavior, can be elongated significantly by slow stretch.

FUNCTIONAL CHANGES IN PERIPHERAL NERVE DUE TO STRETCHING

The mechanical properties of peripheral nerve are important for protection of nerve fascicles and the integrity of their physiological functions. The perineurium, for instance, is the principal load-carrying connective tissue component of nerve. It also has the important function of maintaining the specific environment of the endoneural space by acting as

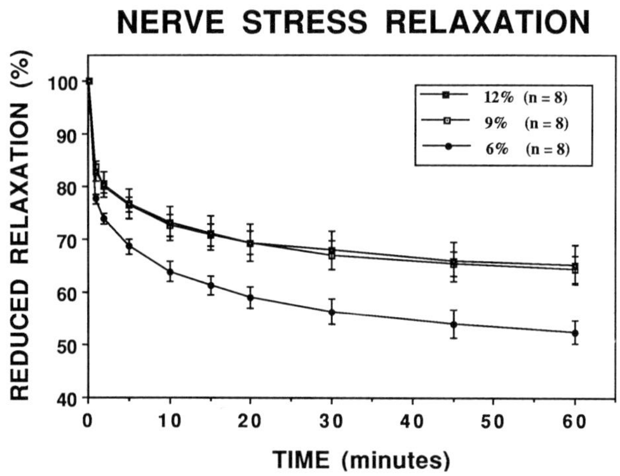

Figure 3-4. *The stress relaxation (normalized by the peak value) for rabbit tibial nerve at strain levels of 6%, 9%, and 12%.*

a diffusion barrier against several macromolecular substances.[19,20,29] Changes in its diffusion properties, or structural damage caused by stretching, may lead to pronounced acute or long-term impairment of nerve function.[15,16,21] The precise effects of elongation on the diffusion properties of the perineurium, and on the function of nerve, are not well understood. In fact, although mechanical deformation has been long known to cause functional changes in peripheral nerve, the data regarding the point at which these changes occur are scanty and conflicting.[1,3–5,9,10,18,25,27,28] Mitchell,[18] for example, reported that peripheral nerve may be stretched up to 25% strain without interruption of conduction, while Denny-Brown and associates[5] reported 100% and Highet and colleagues[9] reported 11%. These conflicting data may have been caused, in part, by insufficient and inconsistent data regarding the biomechanical properties of peripheral nerve available at that time (see Chap. 36).

In a later study of in vivo intraneural blood flow in the rabbit tibial nerve during gradual stretching, it was shown that impairment of venular blood flow was induced when nerve was stretched 8% beyond in vivo length.[17] Complete intraneural ischemia was induced at 15% beyond in vivo length. As described earlier, structural injury to the perineural sheath occurs at 27% beyond the in situ strain.[13] Thus a sequence of changes takes place when peripheral nerve is stretched beyond its in situ dimensions.

In a more recent study, we have investigated the effects of different strain levels on conduction properties of rabbit tibial nerve.[30] In this study, the tibial nerves of anesthetized rabbits were stretched to either 0% (sham), 6%, or 12% beyond the in situ strain for 1 hour, and then relaxed for a 1-hour recovery period. During the stretch and recovery periods, the compound nerve action potential (CNAP) was continuously measured and compared with initial baseline data to determine the effects of applied strain. The results show that at 6% strain, the CNAP amplitude remains stable for 20 minutes and then gradually decreases to about 40% of baseline values at the end of the 1-hour stretch (Fig. 3-5). Upon release of strain, the CNAP amplitude recovered to near baseline values within 30 minutes. At 12% strain, the CNAP amplitude decreased rapidly to 50% of baseline values in 10 minutes and was completely blocked by the end of the 1-hour stretch. When strain was re-

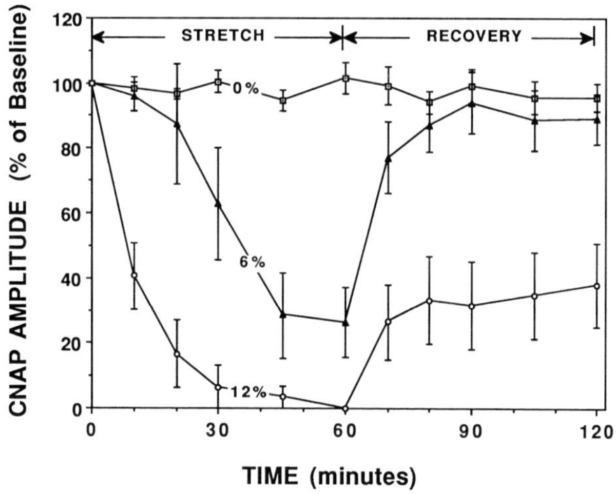

Figure 3-5. *The amplitude of the compound nerve action potential (CNAP), expressed as a percentage of the baseline values prior to nerve stretch. Significant decreases with 6% and 12% strains are seen. Upon release of the strains, the 6% group shows good recovery, while the 12% group shows incomplete recovery.*

leased, the amplitude recovered to 40% of baseline values in 30 minutes and plateaued thereafter.

These data are important, as they clearly demonstrate the sensitivity of peripheral nerve to mechanical stretching beyond its in situ dimension. Significant alterations of conduction properties may result from small amounts of strain, in the range of 6%. Since impairment of venular blood flow is not induced until nerve is stretched to 8%, the conduction loss seen at lower strain levels may be due primarily to mechanical deformation.[17]

Clinical Significance

The conduction properties of peripheral nerve are affected significantly by applications of longitudinal stress (irreversible changes occur in the range of 12% strain). Study of the effects of stretch on the morphologic characteristics of peripheral nerve, compared to perfusion, provides insight as to the fundamental cause of nerve conduction failure.

REFERENCES

1. Adey WR. The nervous system of the earthworm megascolex. J Comp Neurol 1951;94:57–93.
2. Beel JA, Groswald DE, Luttges MW. Alterations in the mechanical properties of peripheral nerve following crush injury. J Biomech 1984;17:185–193.
3. Bullock TH. Functional organization of the giant fiber system of lumbricus. J Neurophysiol 1945;8: 55–71.
4. Carlson A. The effects of stretching the nerve on the rate of conduction of the nervous impulse. Am J Physiol 1910;27:323–330.
5. Denny-Brown D, Doherty MM. Effects of transient stretching of peripheral nerve. Arch Neurol Psychiat 1945;54:116–122.
6. Fung YC. Cellular growth in soft tissues affected by the stress level in service. In: Skalak R, Fox CF, eds. Tissue engineering. New York: Alan R Liss, 1988: 45–50.
7. Haftek J. Stretch injury of peripheral nerve: Acute effects of stretching on rabbit nerve. J Bone Joint Surg [Br] 1970;52:354–365.
8. Hartung C, Arnold G. Histomechanicsche eighenschaften peripherer nerven. Nervenarzt 1973;44: 80–84.
9. Highet WB, Sanders FK. The effects of stretching nerves after suture. Br J Surg 1943;30:355–371.
10. Hoen TI, Brackett CE. Peripheral nerve lengthening. I. Experimental. J Neurosurg 1956;13:43–48.
11. Kendall JP, Stokes IAF, O'Hara JP, Dickson RA. Tension and creep phenomena in a peripheral nerve. Acta Scand Orthop 1979;50:721–725.
12. Kwan MK, Rydevik BL, Myers RR, et al. Stretch injury of rabbit peripheral nerve: A biomechanical and histological study. Proc 35th Ann Mtg, Orth Res Soc 1988;13:430.
13. Kwan MK, Wall EJ, Weiss JA, Rydevik BL, et al. Analysis of rabbit peripheral nerve: *In situ* stresses and strains. Biomechanics Symposium, American Society of Mechanical Engineers/AMD 1989;98: 109–112.
14. Liu CT, Benda CE, Lewey FH. Tensile strength of human nerves. Arch Neurol 1948;59:322.
15. Lundborg G. Structure and function of the intraneural microvessels as related to trauma, edema formation and nerve function. J Bone Joint Surg [Br] 1975;57:938–948.
16. Lundborg G. Nerve injury and repair. Edinburgh: Churchill-Livingstone, 1988.
17. Lundborg G, Rydevik B. Effects of stretching the tibial nerve of the rabbit: A preliminary study of the intraneural circulation and the barrier function of the perineurium. J Bone Joint Surg [Br] 1973;55: 390–401.
18. Mitchell SW. Injuries of nerves and their consequences. Philadelphia: JB Lippincott, 1872.
19. Oldfors A. Permeability on the perineurium of small nerve fascicles: an ultrastructural study using ferritin in rats. Neuropathol Appl Neurobiol 1981;7:183–194.
20. Olsson Y, Reese TS. Inaccessibility of the endoneurium of mouse sciatic nerve to exogenous proteins. Anat Rec 1969;63:722–728.
21. Rydevik B, Lundborg G. Permeability of intraneural microvessels and perineurium following acute, graded experimental nerve compression. Scand J Plast Reconstr Surg 1977;11:179–187.
22. Rydevik BL, Kwan MK, Myers RR, et al. An in vitro mechanical and histological study of acute stretching on rabbit tibial nerve. J Orthop Res 1990;8:694–701.
23. Seddon H. Surgical disorders of the peripheral nerves. Edinburgh: Churchill-Livingstone, 1972.
24. Sunderland S. Nerves and nerve injuries, ed. 2. Edinburgh: Churchill-Livingstone, 1978.
25. Sunderland S. Stretch-compression neuropathy. Clin Exp Neurol 1981;18:1–13.

26. Sunderland S, Bradley KC. Stress–strain phenomena in denervated peripheral nerve trunks. Brain 1961;84:125–127.

27. Takimoto G. Ueber die nervendehnung. Experimentelle und klinische unterung. Mitt Med Fak K Jap Univ 1917;16:73–136.

28. Turner RS. The rate of conduction in stretched and unstretched nerves. Physiol Zool 1951;24:323–329.

29. Waggener JD, Bunn SM, Beggs J. The diffusion of ferritin within the peripheral nerve sheath: an electron microscopy study. J Neuropathol Exp Neurol 1965:24:430–443.

30. Wall EJ, Kwan MK, Garfin SR, Woo SL-Y. Stress relaxation of a peripheral nerve. Proc 36th Ann Mtg, Orth Res Soc 1990;15:579.

31. Wertheim MG. Memoire sur l'elasticité et la adhesion des principaux tissues du corps humanin. Ann Chim Phys 1847;21:385–414.

32. Woo SL-Y, Akeson WH, Jemmott GF. Measurement of nonhomogeneous directional mechanical properties of articular cartilage in tension using a video dimensional analyzer. J Biomechanics 1976;9:785–791.

33. Woo SL-Y, Gomez MA, Seguchi Y, et al. Measurement of mechanical properties of ligament substance from a bone–ligament–bone preparation. J Orthop Res 1983;1:22–29.

4

Biochemical Properties of Peripheral Nerve

Lawrence C. Hurst
Marie A. Badalamente

AUTHORS' KEY POINTS

- A nerve cell (neuron) is composed of a cell body (perikaryon), dendrite branches, and one axon branch from the cell body. The neuron is a specialized impulse-conducting cell with a special problem: it cannot divide after injury.
- Axoplasmic transport is the mechanism that moves cytoplasmic organelles and macromolecules in the axon via the cell's cytoskeleton. There are fast and slow neurochemical components. This transport is critical to routine protein turnover both during the normal state and after injury.
- The neuronal membrane (neurolemma) is important in the maintenance of ionic gradients. After nerve injury or repair, the most damaging ion shift is the influx of calcium ions into neuroplasm and axoplasm. This triggers activation of the enzyme calpain. This phenomenon also occurs in skeletal muscle after axotomy and repair. Calpain degrades proteins in nerve and muscle after injury.
- After axotomy and repair, the tips of axon sprouts, called the *growth cone,* appear to require growth-associated proteins transported from the cell body, growth factors supplied by Schwann cells or target tissues, and an oriented "pathway" made of extracellular matrix molecules.
- To enhance functional recovery after nerve repair in humans, sophisticated biochemical manipulations that affect how regenerating axons choose their pathway and attach to their target tissues is necessary. The completeness and efficiency of axon regeneration also needs to be influenced at the molecular level.

This chapter emphasizes the biochemical properties of peripheral nerve physiology. Aspects of peripheral nerve neurochemistry that are altered by nerve injury and recovery are also summarized. (For a more extensive review of neurochemistry, see references 4, 15, 80, and 88.) The concepts presented here have been developed by neuroscientists who have studied multiple in vitro and in vivo animal models; little work has been done in human tissue.

THE NEURON

The neuron is a cell that metabolizes the same carbohydrates, lipids, proteins, and nucleic acids as do all other cells. Also like other cells, the neuron carries out biological oxidation reactions to make energy for such energy-dependent activities as active transport and impulse conduction. Unlike many other cells, however, a neuron cannot divide after injury.

The neuron has a cell membrane (neurolemma), cytoplasm (neuroplasm), neuroplasmic organelles, a specialized cytoskeleton, and a nucleus with nucleoli. The chromatin of the nucleus is composed of deoxyribonucleic acid (DNA), which contains the code for numerous specialized neuroproteins. The nucleoli are composed of ribonucleic acid (RNA). A neuron may have many dendrite branches but usually has only one axon branch, which extends over a great length. In the axon (axon cylinder) the neuroplasm is called axoplasm.[4,15,45,59] The organelles contained in the perikaryon (cell body) of the neuron are mitochondria, ribosomes, Golgi apparatus, lysosomes, and endoplasmic reticulum.[1] There are two types of endoplasmic reticulum—rough and smooth. The rough endoplasmic reticulum is involved with protein synthesis; the smooth endoplasmic reticulum stores and secretes calcium in order to maintain intercellular calcium at a low level.[4,49,59]

A special organelle found in all neurons is the *Nissl substance* in the cell body. This structure, originally studied by light microscopy, has been shown by electron microscopy to be a combination of rough endoplasmic reticulum, free ribosomes, and clustered ribosomes.[66] The RNA-rich ribosomes of the Nissl substance are one of the principal organelles of protein synthesis in the cell body.[4,59] After proteins are synthesized in the Nissl substance, some travel via the endoplasmic reticulum to the Golgi apparatus. The Golgi apparatus, composed of aggregates of smooth-walled cisternae and vesicles, is responsible for concentrating proteins and packing them in vesicles for axoplasmic transport and also for making primary lysosomes.[4,59,66]

The primary lysosome is an ovoid or spherical organelle whose principal function is the degradation of unneeded cellular proteins, RNA, and DNA. To function, the primary lysosome fuses with a waste-containing phagosome and injects hydrolytic enzymes.[4,66] Lysosomes contain several calcium-activated proteases that are sensitive to the intracellular calcium levels. Lysosomes also contain acid and alkaline hydrolase enzymes.[4,66]

The mitochondria of the neurons are located in the cell body, in the axon near the node of Ranvier, and at nerve endings.[66] The mitochondria perform the two important functions of oxidative phosphorylation (aerobic metabolism) and storage of calcium. Mitochondria process glucose and oxygen through the Krebs cycle to synthesize ATP from ADP.[4,59,66]

Axonal proteins are produced in the cell body by two metabolic pathways. The first is the *membranous* route, and the second is the *cytoskeleton* route. Membranous protein structures are vesicles and secretory granules. They are produced by the rough endoplasmic reticulum and enveloped by a membrane at the Golgi apparatus. These microstructures may be transported antegrade (away from the cell body) or retrograde (toward the cell body) in an axon by *fast axoplasmic transport.* After retrograde transport, proteins are often degraded in the cell body by lysosomes. The proteins of the second cytoskeletal route are synthesized by free ribosomes. Cytoskeletal components are transported by slow axoplasmic transport and undergo enzyme degradation in the cytoplasm of the axon terminal.[49]

Clinical Significance

Proteins are synthesized in Nissl substance, concentrated and packed in vesicles in the Golgi apparatus, and carried to the periphery by the axonal transport system. On return to the cell body, proteins are degraded by lysosomes containing calcium-activated proteases, and acid and alkaline hydrolases.

CELL MEMBRANE

The cell body and its axon are covered by a cell (plasma) membrane. The surface of the axon relative to the cell body is enormous: 90% to 95% of the neuron cell surface is on the axon.[15,59] The cell membrane of the neuron is a bilayer of phospholipids (Fig. 4-1).[1,2,4,15,59] Each phospholipid is composed of a glycerophosphorylester and two fatty acids.[1] The hydrophobic ends of these lipids face each other, and the hydrophilic ends face the exterior and interior of the neuron, respectively.[59] The lipids are combined with protein and carbohydrates. The resultant structure is a living flexible barrier that controls but does not stop the movement of water, ions, and proteins.[1,4,15]

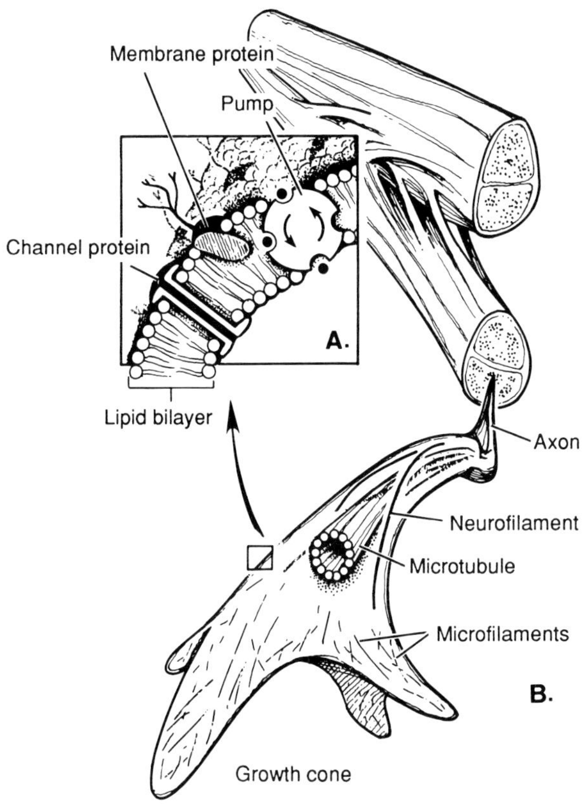

Figure 4-1. *(**A**) A portion of the axon membrane is enlarged to show the structure of the cell membrane. Ninety-five percent of the cell membrane covers the axon, not the cell body. Note the lipid bilayer, channel proteins, membrane proteins, transport pump, and unlabeled surface glycoproteins. (**B**) Enlarged axon shows the microtubule with its 13 protofilaments, the neurofilaments, and the microfilaments in the growth cone area.*

There are two types of membrane proteins, the intrinsic or integral and the peripheral or associated proteins. The integral proteins extend through the lipid layer. These proteins are the structural basis of the ionic channels, the transport pumps, the receptor sites, and the symport and antiport systems. These structures mediate the interaction between the extracellular matrix and the cytoskeleton. They also control mechanical functions such as cell shape and exocytosis.[2] The lipid bilayer is covered externally by a thin glycocalyx, which is composed of glycoprotein (carbohydrates). These glycoproteins are important adhesion and recognition molecules. The adhesion molecules are called neural cell adhesion molecules.[1,2,4,15,59]

One of the important functions of the neural membrane is to control ion concentrations and transmembrane gradients. The ionic gradients, particularly the sodium and potassium gradients, across the neural membrane are a source of potential energy.[2] This potential energy is the source of the nerve action potential (see Chap. 2). This potential energy is also used for controlling intracellular pH, ATP synthesis, and nutrients and other metabolic concentrations.[2,4] The disruption and subsequent reestablishment of ionic balance is also critical to understanding axonal degeneration and regeneration after nerve repair.

Ionic balance is controlled in the neural membrane by ion channels, gated ion channels, antiporters and symporters (obligatory coupled transporters), and ATP-coupled active transporters (sodium–potassium pump).[2,4] Channels allow very rapid ion movements along diffusion gradients. The antiporter and symporter move coupled ions or molecules in opposite or identical directions respectively.[2] The primary regulator of the sodium–potassium gradients is the sodium–potassium pump, which is a transmembrane protein called Na^+,K^+ATPase. This protein is composed of two alpha subunits that have sodium and ATP binding sites inside the neural membrane and potassium binding sites outside the membrane. The two beta subunits are glycoproteins.[2,15] The pump represents a coupled sodium–potassium active transport mechanism.[28] It is now generally accepted that a sodium–potassium activated adenosine triphosphatase (ATPase) is involved in effecting this transport.[87] For every molecule of ATP split, three sodium ions are pumped out and two potassium ions are taken in. The activity of the pump is increased by increases in internal sodium concentration.[82] Two other factors known to influence the rate of pumping are external sodium (a decrease increases the rate of pumping) and temperature (at low temperatures the pump is inhibited).[82]

In the peripheral nervous system, the sodium–potassium pumps are concentrated at the nodes of Ranvier and axon tips.[2] The sodium channels are also concentrated at the nodes of Ranvier, while the potassium channels are concentrated primarily at the internode area of the axon membrane.[44,45]

Clinical Significance

Ionic balance across the semipermeable phospholipid neural membrane is controlled by an ATP-dependent sodium pump. The pump is activated by high concentrations of intraneural sodium and low concentrations of extraneural sodium.

REGULATION OF CALCIUM CONCENTRATION

The concentration of intracellular calcium is important because it regulates intraneuronal signals, regulates other ion channels (sodium), acts in the second messenger system, and participates in neurotransmitter release.[1] The two major systems for regulating calcium ion concentration are the calcium ATPase pump and the sodium–calcium antiporter.[56] Both are located in the plasma membrane. The process of calcium efflux is regulated by the calcium ATPase pumps and the sodium–calcium antiporter. Exchange studies show that the latter exchange transports three ions of sodium into the cell for every calcium ion pumped out.[1,2] Additionally, there are specific calcium channels located in the plasma membrane that are regulated by binding proteins such as calmodulin.[1,2] Calmodulin, with a molecular weight of 17,000, contains 148 amino acids. It has four calcium binding sites. After calcium binding occurs, calmodulin is very resistant to denaturation and is in the active state. This intracellular calcium receptor protein has many functions: it is involved in enzyme modulation, calcium transport, exocytosis of neurotransmitters, cell division, microtubule assembly and disassembly, DNA synthesis, and axoplasmic transport.[39,59]

THE SCHWANN CELL, MYELIN, AND THE EXTRACELLULAR MATRIX

Schwann cells are the oligodendrocytes of the peripheral nervous system. They produce the sheath of myelinated neurons and provide the neurolemma of unmyelinated nerves.[4,15,59,88] In addition to myelin, Schwann cells produce axon-promoting components of the extracellular matrix, such as collagen, laminin, and fibronectin.[77] The specialized Schwann cells at the motor terminals of the axons are called *teloglia*.[91]

Each Schwann cell provides myelin insulation for a given segment of axon. The unmyelinated area between Schwann cells is the *node of Ranvier*. Concentrations of mitochondria increase at the nodes. The distance from one node to the next is proportional to the axon diameter, varying from 50 μm to 1500 μm.[59] The node has close proximity to extracellular fluids and provides the axon with fast saltatory conduction in myelinated nerves. Velocities in these fibers are proportional to the fiber diameter.[15] In the unmyelinated neuron, velocity is proportional to the square root of the diameter.[58,59]

Myelination of axons by Schwann cells is a complicated process. First, a trough of neurolemma partially surrounds the axon and forms the mesaxon.[3] Like a jelly roll, spiral wrappings develop and compact to form a multilamellar myelin sheath of variable thickness. Pockets of cytoplasm called *Schmidt-Lantermann clefts* are left in the compact myelin.[58,59] The sheath has an intermediate degree of liquidity that reduces membrane permeability.[15] Myelin normally has a water content of 40%, a 70% to 85% lipid content, and a 15% to 30% protein content[58,83,84] and has a layered (protein-lipid-protein-lipid) structure.[59] Myelin lipids in peripheral nerves include cholesterol, cerebrosides, sphingomyelin, glycerolipids, lecithin, sulfatides, ethanolamine phosphatides, and the phosphatidyls—serines and inositols. There is proportionally more sphingomyelin and less cerebroside and sulfatide in the peripheral nervous system than in the central nervous system.[59] Myelin protein content studies in peripheral nerve show that a single glycoprotein, P_0 (molecular weight, 30,000), accounts for more than half of the myelin protein.

Another myelin protein is *myelin-associated glycoprotein* (100 kDa).[94] Myelin-associated glycoprotein is located in the periaxonal membrane of the Schwann cells, Schmidt-Lantermann clefts, the paranodal loops, and outer mesaxon. These locations suggest that myelin-associated glycoprotein is involved in maintaining normal myelin membrane spacing. Myelin also contains *myelin basic proteins* and enzymes that synthesize and transport enzymes such as neural protease.[59] Myelin basic proteins are located on the cytoplasmic face of the myelin membranes. The major myelin basic protein in human peripheral nerve is the 17.2-kDa form.[58]

Once an axon segment is myelinated, the Schwann cell axon is covered by an external basal lamina, which is also synthesized by the Schwann cell.[69] Additional extracellular matrix macromolecules are also synthesized by the Schwann cells.[69] Some of these are the molecules of the endoneural and perineural basement membrane such as laminin, an 800-kDa glycoprotein; fibronectin, a 440-kDa protein; neural cell adhesion molecule, a 170-kDa glycoprotein; and entactin, a 150-kDa protein.[13,69,86] Schwann cells in vitro have been shown to synthesize these substrates as well as Type IV and V collagen. Heparin sulfate proteoglycan is also synthesized by Schwann cells.[13,46]

The Schwann cells also contain, and probably produce, apolipoprotein E, a 37-kDa protein involved in packing and transporting cholesterol esters and fatty acids.[38,91] In addition, the Schwann cells can make nerve growth factor (NGF) and express NGF receptors.[40]

Clinical Significance

Schwann cells are responsible for producing the multilaminated lipoprotein myelin sheath, which is invaginated at the nodes of Ranvier to allow saltatory conduction. Schwann cells also produce the external basal lamina, laminin, fibronectin, NGF, and other protein substances.

THE CYTOSKELETON

An exciting area of cell biology is the study of cytoskeletal structure and function. Present in all eukaryotic cells, the cytoskeleton is a major structural component of the mitotic spindle and of organelles, like cilia.[83] In the neuron there are three cytoskeletal elements: the microfilament, the neurofilament, and the microtubule (Figs. 4-1, 4-2).[4,15,26,83,88]

Microfilaments (5–7 nm in diameter) are composed of double-stranded helical actin and are located in the cell body, axon, and axon growth cone. Microfilaments are more randomly oriented than the neurofilaments or microtubules and can interact with myosin. In the cell body, microfilaments control movements of materials in the cell membrane, anchor membrane structures, and form a cell body cytoskeleton that dictates organelle movements.[4,15,26,83,88]

The neurofilaments (10 nm in diameter) are the intermediate-size cytoskeletal elements located in the cell body and axon. They are composed of three proteins (polypeptides): a core protein of 70 kDa and two side-arm proteins, one 140 kDa and one 220 kDa. These proteins can be disrupted by calcium-activated neutral protease (calpain). The side-arms of all neurofilaments can form cross-bridges to adjacent neurofilaments.[15,26,88] The neurofilaments provide structural rigidity, especially in the axon cylinder area.

Microtubules (neurotubules, 24 nm in diameter) are composed of 13 protofilaments (diameter 5 nm). The protofilaments are made of alpha and beta dimers of the globular protein tubulin (molecular weight, 120,000). They provide mechanical control of cell shape and are the proposed "railroad

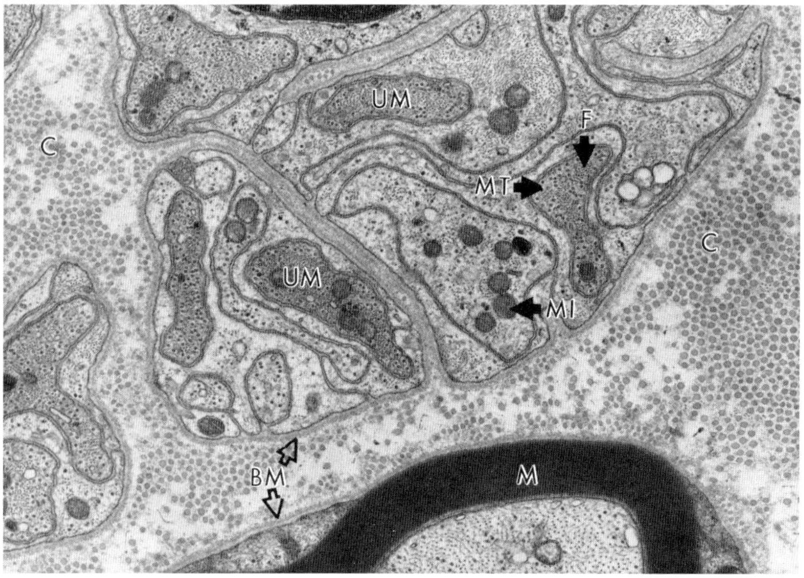

Figure 4–2. *Electron micrograph of an opponens pollicis nerve in a capuchin (Cebus) monkey. This cross section shows several unmyelinated axons (UM) and one myelinated axon (M) within endoneurial collagen (C). A thin basement membrane (BM) surrounds small fascicles of the unmyelinated axon as well as the myelinated axon. The axons have cytoskeletal (micro- and neuro-) filaments (F) and microtubules (MT). Some axons show mitochondria (MI). (×20,000)*

tracks" of the axoplasmic transport system.[15,26,88] The tubulin of the microtubule is associated with a unique group of proteins called microtubule-associated protein, a guanosine-5′-diphosphate that may be an ATPase protein that can cause sliding of these unique molecules.[15]

Clinical Significance

Microfilaments are cytoskeletal structures that control intracellular organelle movement. Neurofilaments provide structural rigidity to the axon, while microtubules provide a guide for axonal transport and a mechanism for controlling cell shape.

AXOPLASMIC TRANSPORT

Impulse conduction is the primary function of the neuron, but without axoplasmic transport this primary function could not be sustained. Routine protein turnover requires the cell body to produce numerous proteins and organelles that are needed in the axon. Axoplasmic transport, the mechanism that moves these cellular components to their functional sites, is critical to neuron survival.[78] Axoplasmic transport is also critical to the embryologic development of the neuron and to regeneration after axotomy and repair.

The early classic works on axoplasmic transport defined two broad categories based on speed: fast and slow axoplasmic transport (Fig. 4-3).[4,15,27,48,59,61] Recent data have suggested that there are at least five rate categories of axoplasmic transport.[15] These velocity-based categories may be parts of a continuum of axoplasmic transport velocities. However, the traditional concept of fast and slow axoplasmic transport is important to the current understanding of the various mechanisms of axoplasmic transport.[59,61]

Fast Axoplasmic Transport

Fast axoplasmic transport, also called membranous or microtubule-dependent transport (see Fig. 4-3), moves proteins along the microtubules at 400 mm/day. In preparation for fast axoplasmic transport, protein, phospholipids, glycoprotein, and glycolipids all pass through an initiation sequence in the cell body. Molecules move from the rough endoplasmic reticulum to the smooth endoplasmic reticulum to the Golgi apparatus, where they are

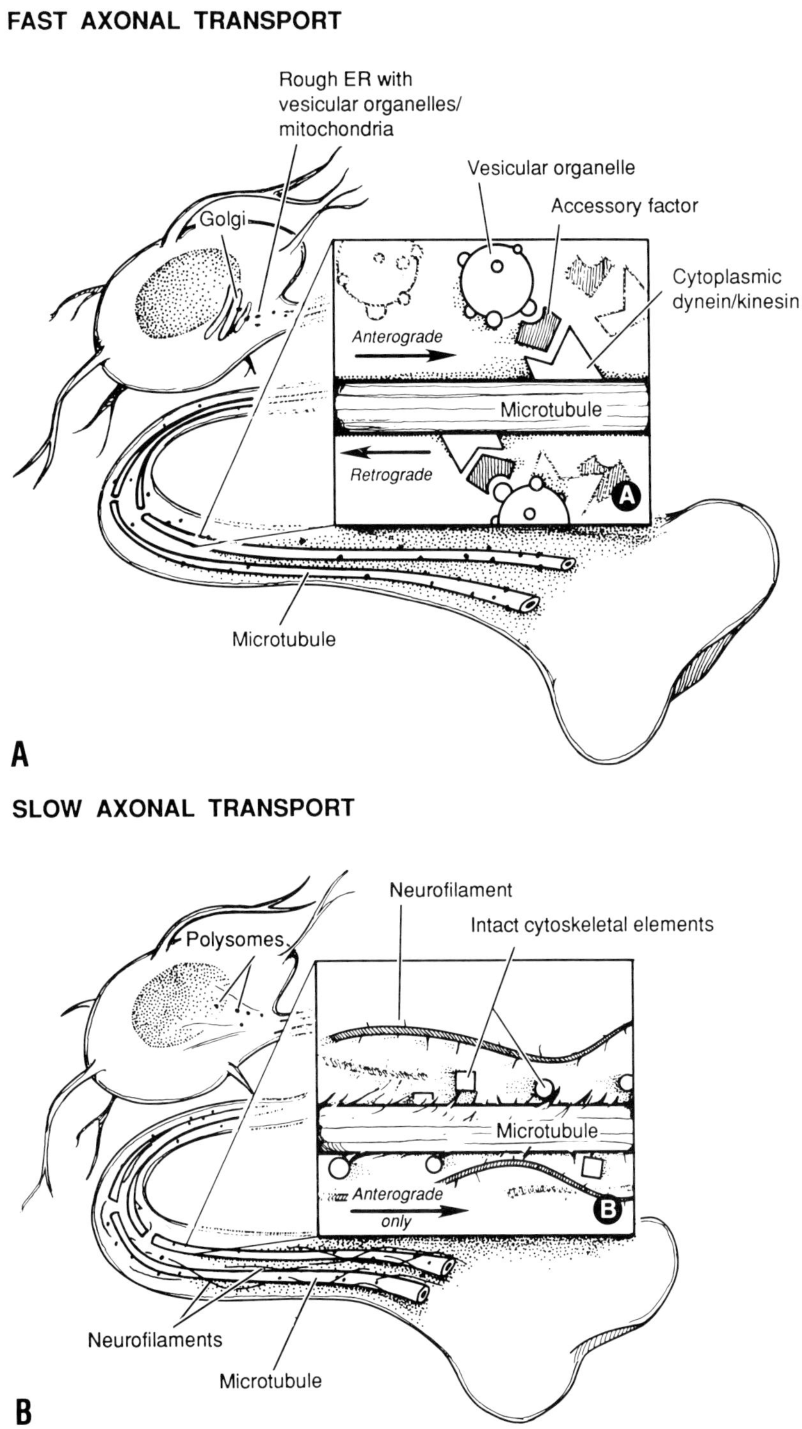

Figure 4–3. *(**A**) Fast axon transport materials are prepackaged by the Golgi apparatus (GA) and the rough endoplasmic reticulum (ER). The vesicular organelles are moved distally (antegrade) by cytoplasmic kinesin's interaction with the microtubule. Kinesin's motor activity is modulated by the accessory factors. The retrograde motor is dynein. (**B**) Slow axon transport materials are prepared for antegrade transport by the polysomes. Neurofilament subunits and other cytoskeletal elements move slowly along the microtubule. There is no retrograde slow axon transport.*

made into membrane-bound vesicles and where proteins acquire carbohydrate or sulfate side chains.[27] These vesicles become the vesiculotubular elements that are pooled prior to leaving the cell body to enter the axon.[27,59] This initiation process is very sensitive to calcium and sodium levels.[27,43]

Plasma membrane precursors, the synaptic vesicles, and smooth endoplasmic reticulum vesicles are the quickest movers, at 410 mm/day. The mitochondria move more slowly.[22] Despite the overall speed, the vesicular or mitochondrial organelles progress by *saltatory movement*, characterized by stops and changes in velocity along a single microtubule.[22] This has been demonstrated by Allen's video-enhanced contrast optical microscopy.[26] It is also apparent from Allen's and other studies that fast axoplasmic transport can move vesicles in both anterograde and retrograde directions.[15,59,61]

The biochemical mechanistic models of fast axoplasmic transport are complex and constantly changing as new experimental data improve the understanding of transport regulation.[59] In 1971, Ochs proposed the transport filament model in which proteins, polypeptides, vesicles, and mitochondria are carried along the microtubule attached by side-arm connections.[61] This mechanism required that glucose be used to produce ATP via axon glycolysis, calmodulin activation, and Mg-Ca ATPase. Sheetz, Steuer, and Schroer have recently summarized an advanced view of the fast axoplasmic transport mechanism and regulation, showing that fast microtubule-dependent organelle transport is based on an organelle translocation complex.[78] This complex has three components: motors that are enzymes that power the transport, accessory proteins that modulate motor activity, and membrane-binding sites on the microtubules that determine organelle direction along the microtubule.[22,61,78] The motor or translocation protein for antegrade fast axoplasmic transport is *kinesin*. The retrograde fast axoplasmic transport motor is cytoplasmic *dynein*.[22,61,78] Kinesin is a microtubule-activated ATPase composed of four 101-kDa and one 80-kDa subproteins. It can be inhibited by 5′-adenylyl imidodiphosphate (AMP-PNP). Dynein is also a protein component of the microtubule with ATPase activity.[22]

Slow Axoplasmic Transport

Slow axoplasmic transport differs from fast transport in its speed, its initiation process, the materials it carries, and its unidirectional (antegrade) character.[4,26,27,48,49] In general, slow axoplasmic transport carries a more limited and specific group of proteins than fast axoplasmic transport. Slow axoplasmic transport is further divided into three types: slow component a (SCa), with a transport velocity of 1 mm/day; slow component b (SCb), with a transport velocity of 2 to 4 mm/day; and intermediate slow component, with a transport velocity of 4 to 8 mm/day.[26,48] These velocities vary with the type of neuron tested, the temperature, and the stage of neuron development.[26]

Slow transport proteins are synthesized by the "free" ribosomes of the cell body. The SCa carries principally five polypeptides: alpha and beta tubulin and three other subunits that are probably parts of the neurofilament.[21,48,59] SCa activity is evenly distributed through the cross-sectional area of the axon.[11] SCb carries about 200 different proteins and functions mostly near the axolemma.[11] Some of the proteins carried by SCb are actin, clathrin, calmodulin, and metabolic enzymes such as creatinine phosphokinase.[48]

The most accepted mechanism of slow axoplasmic transport is the structural hypothesis proposed in the early 1980s by Lasek and Brady, who hypothesized that "proteins are actively transported in the axon either as an integral part of a moving cytological structure or in a long-term association with these structures."[48] The basic tenet of this hypothesis is that assembled cytoskeletal parts are transported. Bamburg pointed out some theoretical problems with this hypothesis.[11] Weisenberg demonstrated slow component particles containing unassembled cytoskeletal components translocated on the tubule at a rate similar to SCa.[11] The mechanisms of slow axoplasmic transport and fast axoplasmic transport may be more similar than previously recognized.

Clinical Significance

Current concepts of fast axonal transport include enzymes for energy, accessory proteins for motor activity, and microtubular-binding sites for determining organelle direction. Fast axon transport (up to 410 mm/day) is bidirectional, while slow transport (1–8 mm/day) is unidirectional (antegrade).

NEUROTROPHIC FACTORS

Just as the neurochemistry of myelin implies that impulse conduction is really a two-cell system (the neuron and the Schwann cell), the neurochemistry of trophic factors implies that healthy impulse conduction is really a three-cell system, consisting of the neuron, the Schwann cell, and the target cell.

One of the most thoroughly studied trophic growth factors is the protein NGF, originally described in the early 1950s.[50] NGF, with a molecular weight of 26,000, is a 131.5-kDa protein made up of alpha, beta, and gamma subunits. The 44-kDa beta subunit appears to be the only neuroactive component.[3,83,95] In target tissues, NGF is present only in minute amounts. The major source of NGF in the laboratory is the mouse submaxillary gland, but the mouse and the human genes for beta NGF have been cloned and there is a 90% homology.[10,90]

Two major roles have been defined for NGF and NGF cell surface receptors. The first occurs during axonal development. NGF determines the number of sympathetic and sensory neurons that innervate appropriate targets during embryogenesis. However, it is not clear that routine neural survival is totally dependent on NGF, despite the fact that some have shown that it regulates growth and neurotransmitter production throughout life.[52,91]

The second role of NGF is its sensory and sympathetic axon-promoting function after neural damage such as axotomy. NGF does not affect motor axon regeneration. The mechanism of the limited axon promotion is unknown, but retrograde transport of exogenous NGF has been demonstrated.[16,18,90] What NGF does at the cell body is unclear. Current evidence suggests that it effects phospholipid metabolism by rapid stimulation of methylation, increases the synthesis of nerve growth protein B50, affects the synthesis of glycoprotein, and initiates ruffling of the cell membrane.[18]

Clinical Significance

NGF determines the number of sensory and sympathetic neurons innervating target organs embryologically and promotes the growth of axons following transection. NGF is being studied as an adjunctive therapy following nerve repair.

Other Neurotrophic Factors

Several other neurotrophic factors have been identified. These can be divided into four categories. *Survival factors* increase the number of neurons surviving in vitro, *neurite-promoting factors* increase the percentage of neurons growing neurites, and *substrate binding factors* and *developmental factors* influence the type and growth of neurons but not the extent of growth.[18] Some examples of these other neurotrophic factors are brain-derived neurotrophic factor, ciliary neurotrophic factor, neuroleukin, apolipoprotein E, laminin, fibronectin (ICAM or intercellular adhesion molecules), insulin-like growth factors (IGF I and II), glia-derived nexin factor, fibroblast growth factor, and epidermal growth factor.[3,18,88,90,91] Neuroleukin has been considered a novel trophic factor, but two recent studies have reported that it is equivalent to the cytoplasmic enzyme glucose-6-phosphate isomerase.[12]

PROTEASES

Enzymes (proteases) and protease inhibitors appear to play a role in axonal regeneration.[57,70] Also, the normal function of axons and target tissues, such as skeletal muscle, appears to be partially modulated by proteases.[6–10,17,31–33,41,42] Recent data suggest a balance between cell-derived proteases and inhibitors that modulate neurite elongation and regeneration.[57] During axonal regeneration, the tips of the axon sprouts, called the growth cone, rapidly extend and retract microspikes in adhesion to and de-adhesion from the extracellular matrix. Proteases are thought to dictate the interactions of the microspikes with their environment, thus controlling motility, or forward movement, of the growth cone. Plasminogen activators[57] and a calcium-dependent protease[64] are two of the enzymes that have been identified in growth cone motility. The actions of the proteases in the growth cone are also modulated by protease inhibitors. The two protease inhibitors glia-derived nexin and urokinase have also been detected in association with the growth cone.[57]

Proteases regulate normal protein turnover in the axon and peripheral tissues, such as skeletal muscle. Cytoskeletal components of the axon, such as microfilaments, neurofilaments, and microtubules, appear to be degraded by calcium-activated neutral protease (calpain), as do axonal membrane proteins such as spectrin.[88] The susceptibilities of myofibrillar proteins to various proteases are complicated. Myosin, actin, alpha actinin, C, M, and Z proteins, troponin T, troponin I, and tropomyosin are all degraded by calpain. Myosin and actin are also degraded by alkaline proteases and cathepsins B, D, and L.[7,60] An understanding of proteases and protease inhibitors is important to the concepts of how axons and their target tissues respond after denervation and nerve repair.

GANGLIOSIDES

Gangliosides are glycosphingolipids. There are 60 known types of gangliosides. They are synthesized in the cell body and transported by fast axoplasmic transport. Functionally, one ganglioside (GM1) has been shown to promote synaptogenesis, neurite formation, and sprouting. Gangliosides may also enhance NGF activity. At the cell membrane they have also been shown to increase sodium pump activity.[23,24,80] However, the effects of gangliosides in promoting axon regeneration are unconfirmed.[7]

Clinical Significance

A predictable sequence of biochemical events occurs following nerve transection. There is an ingress of sodium ions and a loss of potassium ions. There is also an influx of calcium ions, which results in the activation of proteases, upsetting intra-axonal equilibrium. As a result, microfilaments, neurofilaments, and microtubules are degraded rapidly.

LOCAL RESPONSE OF AXONS TO INJURY

When an axon is cut, cellular damage becomes apparent after a few hours when healthy tissue begins to show signs of degradation. This rapid degeneration occurs at both the proximal and distal stumps. Degradation is initially mediated by ionic shifts across the axon membrane.[19] After nerve injury some ion shifts, such as the ingress of chloride ions into axoplasm, may do no harm, but most shifts, such as influx of sodium ions and massive loss of potassium ions, are quite damaging (Fig. 4-4).[19,74–76]

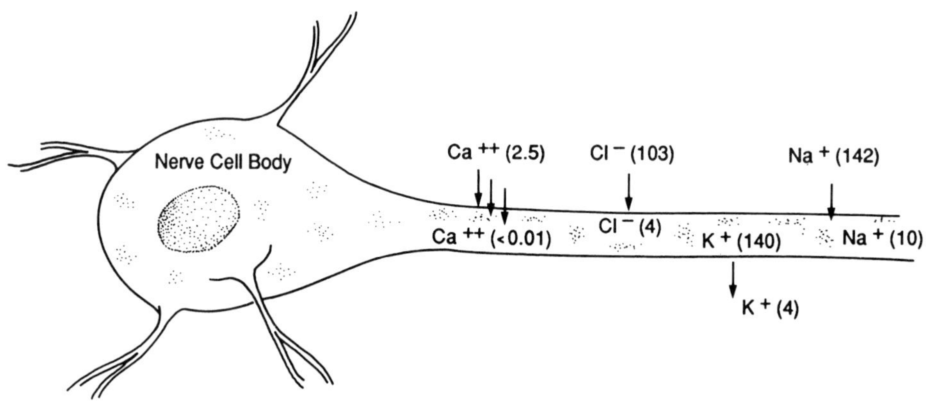

Figure 4–4. *Ion shifts, after damage to the axon membrane, are shown by the arrows. Ion concentrations in millimoles are shown in parentheses in the intra- and extra-axonal environment. (From deMedinaceli L, Seaber AV. Experimental nerve reconnection: Importance of initial repair. Microsurgery 1989, 10:59, with permission.)*

Perhaps the most damaging of the ionic shifts that occur after an axon is severed is the influx of calcium ions.[63,74–76] The influx of the calcium ion into a damaged peripheral nerve triggers the activation of a specific intra-axonal enzyme known as calcium-activated neutral protease (calpain or CANP).[6,8–10] There are two forms of calpain: one requires millimolar calcium for activation, the other is activated by micromolar calcium.[17] It is postulated that calpain plays a role in normal neurofibrillar proteolysis. The rate of synthesis of axonal microfilaments, neurofilaments, and microtubules is in a state of equilibrium with the rate of calpain-mediated proteolysis. However, once the enzyme is activated by an influx of excess calcium ions due to an injury, the normal state of equilibrium shifts, and the rate of intra-axonal proteolysis of filaments and tubules exceeds the rate of protein synthesis.

Other local axonal changes after axotomy include ischemia and proliferation of Schwann cells and macrophages.[71,72] Schwann cells and macrophages are known to phagocytose cellular debris, including myelin, at the site of injury.[77] Further, collagen scar (neuroma) develops at the site of nerve transection.[14,47,92] The formation of a neuroma has been described as a result of metabolically active fibroblasts.[14] However, a more recent report suggests that myofibroblasts also contribute to collagen proliferation and neuroma formation at the site of injury.[5]

RETROGRADE AND REGENERATIVE CHANGES

Just proximal to the site of injury, the axon displays similar degenerative changes. These may extend from one node of Ranvier (in the case of a mild crush) to a few millimeters or several centimeters above the lesion (as in the case of axotomy). Anterior horn (motor) and posterior (sensory) cell bodies in the spinal cord, as well as dorsal root ganglia (sensory) cell bodies, also reflect the injury with a complex series of anatomical, biochemical, and physiological changes known collectively as the retrograde axon reaction.[51] Histologic changes, termed *chromatolysis*, include swelling of the cell body (perikaryon), dispersal of Nissl substance into dendrites, enlargement and movement of the nucleus to the periphery of the cytoplasm, and swelling of mitochondria.[13,67] The more proximal the site of axotomy, the more intense are these changes. By 2 to 3 weeks the reaction generally peaks, and the cell body either dies or shows a gradual recovery that often lasts many months.

The retrograde axon reaction is, in many ways, a preparation of the cell body for regeneration.[25] For example, the synthesis of RNA and protein increases. Several proteins that are ordinarily not found in the cell body or are found in small amounts are produced in large quantities following axotomy for transport in regenerating axons; these include the growth-associated proteins. The literature suggests that eventual guidance of regenerating axons for elongation is partially governed by the growth cone that forms at the distal tip of growing axon sprouts. It is becoming apparent that growth cones in injured peripheral nerves in mammals contain specific growth-associated proteins, the synthesis of which is increased 20- to 100-fold during successful regeneration.[79,81]

Several growth-associated proteins have been identified. One, GAP-43, is a soluble 37-kDa membrane-associated phosphoprotein that is produced in the cell body and delivered by the fast component of axonal transport.[29] Another protein, apolipoprotein E, has been implicated in the mobilization of lipid-rich myelin debris and in the reuse of lipid by both Schwann cells for new myelin sheath membranes and by growth cones in the local assembly of axonal membranes.[37,38] Axonal elongation at growth cones also correlates to the expression of the protein tubulin, which is delivered after injury by the slow component of axoplasmic transport.[30] Other types of secreted or cell-associated proteins have been identified in innervated peripheral nerve. Four of these proteins (37 kDa, 44 kDa, 70 kDa, and 90 kDa) show enhanced rates of synthesis 2 weeks after injury, while six (27 kDa, 38 kDa, 39 kDa, 45 kDa, 51 kDa, and 54 kDa) show decreased rates of synthesis.[79] The exact roles that these and various other proteins play in the molecular response to nerve injury has not been clearly defined.

Growth cones are guided during their elongation by undefined growth factors in the distal segments of injured peripheral nerve and by growth influences from target tissues. One of the best-studied growth factors is NGF, which also plays a role as an axon-promoting factor after damage such as axotomy.[50] NGF flows *from* the targets, into nerve terminals and by retrograde flow along the axons to the cell body. If the flow of NGF is disrupted, as by injury, regeneration of axons will be affected. However, peripheral nerve damage leads to a prompt induction of NGF and NGF receptor protein synthesis by Schwann cells at the site of injury, presumably providing an immediate source of NGF to reestablish retrograde flow and support the proximal stump. Retrograde flow is initiated by binding and internalization of NGF to its low-affinity receptor, a single 83-kDa glycosylated acetylated peptide chain. In the distal stump, Schwann cells also synthesize and secrete NGF and NGF receptor in a process regulated by the secretion of interleukin-1 by invading macrophages. Growth cone chemotaxis has also been demonstrated both in vitro and in vivo for NGF.[52]

Another growth factor, brain-derived growth factor, also appears to enhance the initial onset of axonal regeneration of sensory (dorsal root ganglion) neurons in vitro.[52] Ciliary neurotrophic factor is a growth factor that has been shown in vitro to promote the survival of parasympathetic ciliary ganglion neurons. Ciliary neurotrophic factor, a 22- to 23-kDa protein, is found in a variety of tissues.[93] High ciliary neurotrophic factor protein content and activities have been shown in animal skeletal muscle and peripheral nerve.[20]

The possible clinical use of NGF, brain-derived growth factor, or ciliary neurotrophic factor for enhancement of recovery following peripheral nerve repair will require additional experimentation both in vitro and in vivo to determine the long-term effects of these growth factors. Recent reports also suggest that the gangliosides, particularly GM1, may have effects similar to those predicted for NGF.[23,24] Gangliosides may promote axonal regeneration by acting on neuronal membrane receptors for growth factors, enhancing their uptake.

Clinical Significance

Peripheral nerve transection induces the production of NGF by Schwann cells at the injury site. NGF guides the growth cone into the distal stump.

THE DISTAL STUMP

When an axon is cut or crushed, the distal portion degenerates in all known vertebrate nerve in a process called *wallerian degeneration.*[92] The axon breaks into ellipsoidal fragments of progressively smaller size. During wallerian degeneration there is a rapid loss of myelin lipids within 1 to 2 weeks. Loss of myelin proteins proceeds even more rapidly, and the disappearance of the major P_0 glycoprotein may precede slightly the loss of the myelin basic proteins.[84] The biochemical mechanisms underlying axonal degeneration are not fully understood; however, influx of calcium ions produces axon disaggregation and proteolysis of actin, tubulin, and neurofilaments. This process is mediated by the enzyme calpain[6,8–10,31,33] and the lysosomal cathepsins. Proliferating Schwann cells and macrophages phagocytose cellular debris and myelin fragments by about 1 month after injury.

Schwann cells also play an important role in the distal stump of an injured peripheral nerve because they synthesize components of an oriented extracellular matrix that provides conditions conducive for axonal regeneration.[34–36,69] This phenomenon has been called contact guidance, referring to the fact that the regenerating growth cone adheres preferentially to certain substrates. A properly synthesized, oriented, and intact extracellular matrix is essential in guiding axonal outgrowth. The organization of the extracellular matrix with Schwann cells in the distal nerve stump is also termed the *bands of Bungner.* Schwann cells in the distal stump undergo complex changes associated with the myelin ensheathement of regenerating axons.

On contact with axonal growth cone sprouts, Schwann cells proliferate, express surface cerebrosides, and down-regulate surface NGF receptors and cell adhesion molecules. If the regenerating axon reaches a sufficient diameter, the Schwann cell synthesizes myelin-associated glycoprotein, myelin P_0 protein, and myelin basic proteins to remyelinate the sprouts.[71,72]

TROPIC AND TROPHIC FACTORS

Axonal regeneration is influenced by neurotropism and neurotrophism. *Neurotropism* is the finding in

Y-tube models that a nerve will regenerate preferentially toward a distal nerve rather than other tissue.[65] *Neurotrophism* is the concept that an axon will regenerate preferentially to an appropriate distal receptor such as the neuromuscular junction of skeletal muscle.[53–55] Trophic influence on regenerating motor axons by skeletal muscle has been well demonstrated.[89] In vitro, skeletal muscle extracts are known to promote neurite outgrowth. This phenomenon has been attributed to two undefined proteins, one with a molecular weight less than 30 kDa and the other 35 kDa.[62,85]

However, no specific trophic substance for motor axons has been completely characterized, as in the case of NGF. It has been suggested that the processes leading to motor axon regrowth after peripheral nerve injury depend on two mechanisms that regulate induction and inhibition.[68] The first mechanism is peripheral and involves growth-promoting factors such as the oriented extracellular matrix, target-derived factors such as the 30-kDa and 35-kDa skeletal muscle factors, products of degeneration such as myelin, and Schwann cell activity. These act directly on axon sprouts and nerve endings to induce their growth. The second mechanism is central and suggests that, similar to NGF, axon growth can be induced in the motor nerve cell body by target-derived molecules that are continuously transported to the cell body by retrograde axonal flow, where they exert inhibitory influences on growth.[68] One remarkable finding is that axons reinnervating skeletal muscle show a remarkable preference for their original synaptic sites.[73] This topographic neurotrophic contact guidance has in part been attributed to the extracellular matrix. The postsynaptic cell itself apparently need not be present for the axons to recognize their appropriate target site; however, the extracellular matrix basement membrane must be present.[16,73]

When a motor axon is cut, its target skeletal muscle atrophies. This complex enzymatic biochemical event involves a variety of muscle proteins, including the contractile proteins myosin and actin; the major regulatory proteins tropomyosin and troponins C, I, and T; the minor regulatory proteins M, C, F, and I, and actinins; and the scaffold proteins, connectin, Z protein, and desmin.[60] As in peripheral nerve, it appears that calpain activation by excess calcium ion influx is a major event in initiating skeletal muscle degradation (Figs. 4-5, 4-6).[6–10,31,33,96] The following enzymes degrade muscle proteins: alkaline protease, serine protease, calcium-activated neutral protease (calpain), and the lysosomal, acidic cathepsins A, B, C, D, and L.[60] Most interestingly, calpain has been immu-

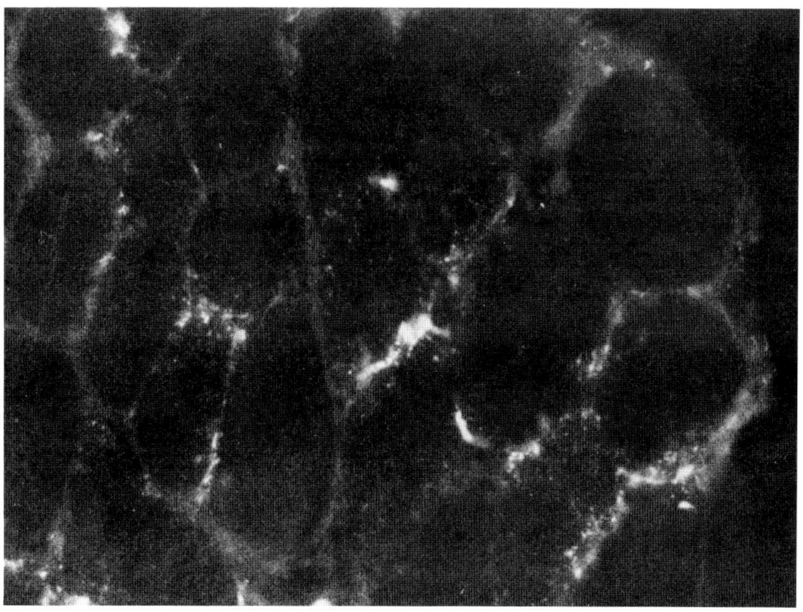

Figure 4–5. *Cross section of an opponens pollicis muscle from a capuchin monkey. Fluorescent immunochemical reaction for calcium-activated neutral protease (calpain) shows association with endomysial collagen, the myofiber membrane, and a slight reaction within the cells (×440).*

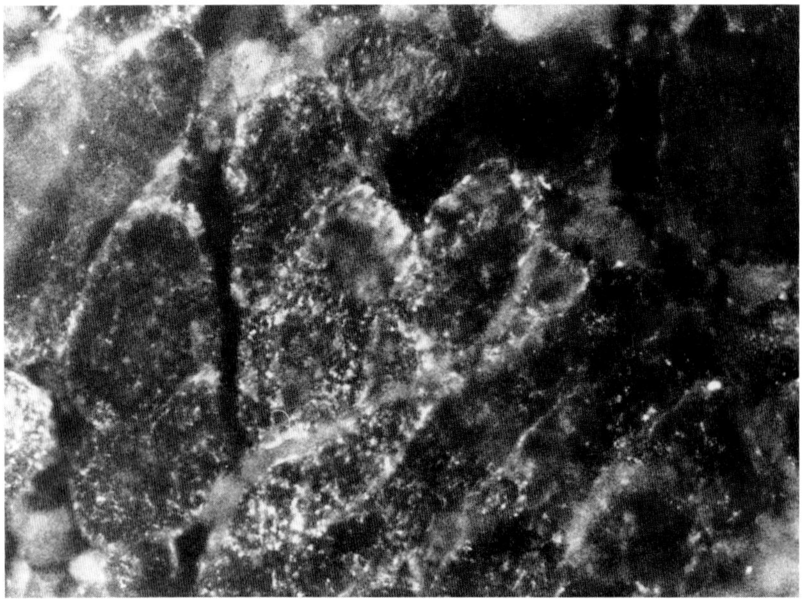

Figure 4–6. *Cross section of an opponens pollicis muscle from a capuchin monkey 3 months after median nerve repair at the wrist. Fluorescent immunochemical reaction for calpain shows that the enzyme is widely dispersed in the endomysin and within denervated myofibers (×440).*

nochemically localized in association with Z lines of the myofiber, basement membrane and sarcolemma of myofibers, and basement membrane of the neuromuscular junction in normal and denervated muscle.[9] Thus, calpain appears to be situated intracellularly to degrade the Z band, an event that may help to trigger disassembly of myofibrils. The localization of calpain in or near the sarcolemma suggests that the enzyme may also play a role in altering membrane structure.

The hypothesis now being tested in our laboratory involves the inhibition of calpain by specific inhibitors such as leupeptin for enhancement of neuromuscular recovery following nerve repair. Our hypothesis proposes that if the proteolytic breakdown of end-target skeletal muscle (with its basement membrane) as well as the basement membrane of the neuromuscular junction can be delayed or prevented, then reinnervation will occur more efficiently, since the neurotrophic target is retained.

Clinical Significance

Following transection, peripheral nerve demonstrates *neurotrophic capability* (preferential regeneration to appropriate distal receptors) and *neurotropic activity* (preferential regeneration toward a distal nerve segment over that of other tissues, such as tendon or muscle).

SUMMARY

Although many unanswered questions remain, it appears likely that the limiting factor in functional restoration following nerve injury and microsurgical repair is not only the inability of axons to regenerate completely. Improvements in operative microsurgical techniques have aided regeneration by providing an improved pathway, but it is still partially inaccurate. Therefore, current techniques do not translate into full functional recovery. There appear to be two types of *specificity* expressed during axonal embryogenesis that would need to be invoked in the regenerating nerve after nerve repair in order to ensure proper target tissue reinnervation. The first is *correctness of pathfinding* from the site of injury to the region of the target tissue. The second is the *selection of the appropriate postsynaptic target* from several that might be available in the same vicinity.

The influence of trophic substances and growth-promoting factors could be used to enhance the degree of regeneration in nerve-injury patients. However, the most well-defined growth factor, NGF, is known to promote sprouting of axons only in sensory and sympathetic neurons. Additional trophic factors that may support the survival of both motor and sensory neurons or enhance axonal outgrowth are the subjects of intensive research. However, if it is true that the real difficulty lies not only in the ability of axons to fully regenerate, but also in the specificity with which the regenerating axons choose where they will grow and where they will attach to a target, then much more sophisticated biochemical manipulations will be necessary to enhance functional recovery after microsurgical nerve repair.

REFERENCES

1. Albers R. Cell membrane structure and functions. In: Siegel G, Agranoff B, Albers R, Molinoff P, eds. Basic neurochemistry. New York: Raven Press, 1989:35–48.
2. Albers R, Siegel G, Stahl W. Membrane transport. In: Siegel G, Agranoff B, Albers R, Molinoff P, eds. Basic neurochemistry. New York: Raven Press, 1989:49–70.
3. Arenander A, de Vellis J. Development of the nervous system. In: Siegel G, Agranoff B, Albers R, Molinoff P, eds. Basic neurochemistry. New York: Raven Press, 1989:479–508.
4. Atwood H, MacKay W. Essentials of neurophysiology. Toronto and Philadelphia: BC Decker 1989: 1–64.
5. Badalamente M, Hurst L, Ellstein J, McDevitt C. The pathobiology of human neuroma: An electron microscopic and biochemical study. J Hand Surg [Br] 1985; 10:49–53.
6. Badalamente M, Hurst L, Paul S, Stracher A. Enhancement of neuromuscular recovery after nerve repair in primates. J Hand Surg [Br] 1987; 12:211–217.
7. Badalamente M, Hurst L, Stracher A. Effects of pharmacological agents on neuromuscular recovery after nerve repair. In: Carraro U, Angelini C, eds. Cell biology and clinical management in functional electrostimulation of neurones and muscles. Padova: Cleup Editore, 1985:19–22.
8. Badalamente M, Hurst L, Stracher A. Calcium-induced degeneration of the cytoskeleton in monkey and human peripheral nerves. J Hand Surg [Br] 1986; 11:337–340.
9. Badalamente M, Hurst L, Stracher A. Localization and inhibition of calcium-activated neutral protease (CANP) in primate skeletal muscle and peripheral nerve. Exp Neurol 1987; 98:357–369.
10. Badalamente M, Hurst L, Stracher A. Neuromuscular recovery using calcium protease inhibition after median nerve repair in primates. Proc Natl Acad Sci 1989; 86:5983–5987.
11. Bamburg J. The axonal cytoskeleton: Stationary or moving matrix? Trends in Neurosciences 1988; 11: 248–249.
12. Barde Y. What, if anything, is a neurotrophic factor? Trends in Neurosciences 1988; 11:343–346.
13. Barron K. Comparative observations on the cytologic reactions of central and peripheral nerve cells to axotomy. In: Bunge R, Reier P, eds. Spinal cord regeneration. New York: Raven Press, 1983:7–40.
14. Bora F, Pleasure D, Didizian N. A study of nerve regeneration and neuroma formation after nerve suture by various techniques. J Hand Surg 1976;1: 138–143.
15. Bradford H. Chemical neurobiology: An introduction to neurochemistry. New York: WH Freeman, 1986:1–495.
16. Bunge M, Johnson M, Ard M, Kleitman N. Factors influencing the growth of regenerating nerve fibers in culture. In: Seil F, Herbert E, Carlson B, eds. Neural regeneration. Amsterdam, New York, and Oxford: Elsevier, 1987:61–74.
17. Dayton W, Schollmeyer J. Localization of calcium-activated neutral protease in skeletal muscle. J Cell Biol 1981; 87:267–272.
18. Dekker A, Gispen W, de Wied L. Minireview: Axonal regeneration, growth factors and neuropeptides. Life Sciences 1987; 41:1667–1678.
19. DeMedinacelli L, Seaber A. Experimental nerve reconnection: Importance of initial repair. Microsurg 1989; 10:56–70.
20. Ebendal T. Comparative screening for ciliary neurotrophic activity in organs of the rat and chicken. J Neurosci Res 1987; 17:19–24.
21. Filliatreau G, Denoulet P, deNechaud B, Di-Giamberardino L. Stable and metastable cytoskeletal polymers carried by slow axonal transport. J Neurosci 1988; 8:2227–2233.
22. Forman D. Fast axonal transport: Recent developments. In: Seil F, Herbert E, Carlson B, eds. Neural regeneration. Amsterdam, New York, and Oxford: Elsevier, 1987:103–112.
23. Gorio A. Gangliosides as a possible treatment affecting neuronal repair processes. Adv Neurol 1988; 47:523–530.
24. Gorio A, Marini P, Zanoni R. Motor neuron sprouting capacity enhancement by exogenous gangliosides. Neurosci 1983; 8:417–429.
25. Grafstein B, McQuarrie I. Role of the nerve cell body in axonal regeneration. In: Cotam C, ed. Neural plasticity. New York: Raven Press, 1978; 155–195.

26. Hammerschlag R, Brady S. Axonal transport and the neuronal cytoskeleton. In: Siegel G, Agranoff B, Albers R, Molinoff P, eds. Basic neurochemistry. New York: Raven Press, 1989; 457–478.
27. Hammerschlag R, Stone G. Prelude to fast axonal transport: Sequence of events in the cell body. In: Iqbal Z, ed. Axoplasmic transport. Boca Raton: CRC Press, 1986:21–34.
28. Hodgkin A, Keynes R. Active transport of cations in giant squid axons from Sepia and Loligo. J Physiol 1955; 128:28–60.
29. Hoffman P. Expression of GAP-43, a rapidly transported growth-associated protein, and class II beta tubulin, a slowly transported cytoskeletal protein, are coordinated in regenerating neurons. J Neurosci 1989; 9:893–897.
30. Hoffman P, Cleveland D. Neurofilament and tubulin expression recapitulates the developmental program during axonal regeneration: Induction of a special beta tubulin isotope. Proc Natl Acad Sci USA 1988; 85:4530–4533.
31. Hurst L, Badalamente M, Ellstein J, Stracher A. Inhibition of neural and muscle degeneration after epineural neurorrhaphy. J Hand Surg [Am] 1984; 9:564–571.
32. Hurst L, Badalamente M, Paul S. Nerve injuries in the upper extremity. In: Dee R, Mango E, Hurst L, eds. Principles of orthopaedic practice. New York: McGraw-Hill, 1988:666–689.
33. Hurst L, Badalamente M, Stracher A. Localization of calcium-activated neutral protease (CANP) in denervated human skeletal muscle and peripheral nerve. Neuro-Orthopedics 1987; 4:55–61.
34. Ide C. Nerve regeneration and Schwann cell basal lamina: Observations of long-term regeneration. Archives of Histology (Japan) 1983; 46:243–257.
35. Ide C. Nerve regeneration through the basal lamina scaffold of the skeletal muscle. Neurosci Res 1984; 1:379–391.
36. Ide D, Tohyaja K, Yokota R, Nitatori T, Onodera S. Schwann cell basal lamina and nerve regeneration. Brain Res 1983; 288:61–75.
37. Ignatius M, Gebicke-Haerter P, Pitas R, Shooter M. Apolipoprotein E in nerve injury and repair. In: Seil F, Herbert E, Carlson B, eds. Neural regeneration. Amsterdam, New York, and Oxford: Elsevier, 1987: 177–184.
38. Ignatius M, Gebicke-Haerter P, Schilling J, et al. Characterization of a 37-kDa protein resembling apolipoprotein E that may facilitate lipid degradation, storage and reutilization in an injured nerve. Intl Symposium on Neural Regeneration 1985; 46.
39. Iqbal Z. Calmodulin and its role in axoplasmic transport. In: Iqbal Z, ed. Axoplasmic transport. Boca Raton: CRC Press, 1986:45–56.
40. Johnson EJ, Taniuchi M, DiStefano P. Expression and possible function of nerve growth factor receptors on Schwann cells. Trends in Neurosciences 1988; 11:299–304.
41. Kamakura K, Ishiura S, Fujita T, Nonaka I, Sugita S. Localization of calcium-activated neutral protease in the peripheral nerve. Muscle Nerve 1985; 8:380–382.
42. Kamakura K, Ishiura S, Sugita H, Toyokura Y. Identification of calcium-activated neutral protease and its effect on neurofilament degeneration. J Neurochem 1983; 40:908–913.
43. Kanje M. Ionic requirements for fast axonal transport. In: Iqbal Z, ed. Axoplasmic transport. Boca Raton: CRC Press, 1986:35–44.
44. Kocsis J, Waxman S. Ionic channel organization of normal and regenerating mammalian axons. In: Seil F, Herbert E, Carlson B, eds. Neural regeneration. Amsterdam, New York, and Oxford: Elsevier, 1987: 89–102.
45. Kocsis J, Waxman S. Membrane organization and myelin remodeling in regenerating axons. Advances in Neurology 1988; 47:31–50.
46. Lander A, Fujii D, Gospodarowicz D. Characterization of a factor that promotes neurite outgrowth: Evidence linking activity to a heparin sulfate proteoglycan. J Cell Biol 1982; 94:574–585.
47. Lane J, Bora F, Pleasure D. Neuroma scar formation following peripheral nerve transection. J Bone Joint Surg [Am] 1978; 60:197–203.
48. Lasek R, Garner J, Brady S. Axonal transport of the cytoplasmic matrix. J Cell Biol 1984; 99:212–221.
49. Lasek R, Katz M. Mechanisms of the axon tip regulate metabolic processes critical to axonal elongation. In: Seil F, Herbert E, Carlson B, eds. Neural regeneration. Amsterdam, New York, and Oxford: Elsevier, 1987:49–60.
50. Levi-Montalcini R, Angeletti P. Nerve growth factor. Physiol Review 1968; 48:534–569.
51. Lieberman A. The axon reaction: A review of the principle features of perikarial responses to axon injury. Intl Rev Neurobiol 1971; 14:49–124.
52. Lindsay R. Nerve growth factors (NGF) (BGNF) enhance axonal regeneration but are not required for survival of adult sensory neurons. J Neurosci 1988; 8:2394–2405.
53. Lundborg G. Nerve injury and repair. Edinburgh: Churchill-Livingstone, 1988:149–195.
54. Lundborg G, Dahlin L, Danielsen N, Nanchemson A. Tissue specificity in nerve regeneration. Scand J Plast Reconstr Surg Hand Surg 1986; 20:279–283.
55. MacKinnon S, Dellon A, Lundborg G, Hudson A,

Hunter D. A study of neurotrophism in a primate model. J Hand Surg [Am] 1986; 11:888–894.
56. McBurney R, Neering I. Neuronal calcium homeostasis. Trends Neurosci 1987; 10:164–169.
57. Monard D. Cell-derived proteases and protease inhibitors as regulators of neurite outgrowth. Trends in Neurosciences 1988; 11:541–544.
58. Morell P, Quarles R, Norton W. Formation, structure, and biochemistry of myelin. In: Siegel G, Agranoff B, Albers R, Molinoff P, eds. Basic neurochemistry. New York: Raven Press, 1989:109–136.
59. Noback C, Demarest R. The human nervous system: Basic principles of neurobiology, ed 3. New York: McGraw-Hill, 1981:49–123.
60. Obinata T, Maruyama K, Sugita H, Kohama K, Egbasi S. Dynamic aspects of structural proteins in vertebrate skeletal muscle. Muscle Nerve 1981; 4: 456–488.
61. Ochs S. A brief history on present status of transport mechanism models. In: Smith R, Bisby M, eds. Axonal transport. New York: Alan R Liss, 1987:1–14.
62. Oppenheim R, Haverkamp L, Prevette D, McManaman J, Appel S. Reduction of naturally occurring motoneuron death in vivo by a target-derived neurotrophic factor. Science 1988; 240:919–922.
63. Pant H, Gainer H. Properties of a calcium-activated protease in squid axoplasm which selectively degrades neurofilament protein. J Neurobiol 1980; 11: 1–12.
64. Pittman R. Release of plasminogen activator and a calcium-dependent metalloprotease from cultured sympathetic and sensory neurons. Dev Biol 1985; 110:91–101.
65. Politis M. Specificity in mammalian peripheral nerve regeneration at the level of the nerve trunk. Brain Res 1985; 328:271–276.
66. Raine C. Neurocellular anatomy. In: Siegel G, Agranoff B, Albers R, Molinoff P, eds. Basic neurochemistry. New York: Raven Press, 1989:3–34.
67. Ramon y Cajal S. Degeneration and regeneration of the nervous system, edited and translated by May R. New York: Hafner, 1968.
68. Rotshenker S. Multiple modes and sites for the induction of axonal growth. Trends Neurosci 1988; 8:363–366.
69. Rutka J, Apodaca G, Stern R, Rosenblum M. The extracellular matrix of the central and peripheral nervous systems: Structure and function. J Neurosci 1988; 69:155–170.
70. Saito Y, Kawashima S. Enhancement of neurite outgrowth in PC12h cells by a protease inhibitor. Neurosci Letters 1988; 89:102–107.
71. Salzer J, Bunge R. Studies of Schwann cell proliferation: An analysis in tissue culture of proliferation during development, Wallerian degeneration and direct injury. J Cell Biol 1980; 84:739–752.
72. Salzer J, William A, Glaser L, Bunge R. Studies of Schwann cell proliferation: Characterization of the stimulation and specificity of the response to a neurite membrane fraction. J Cell Biol 1980; 84:753–766.
73. Sanes J, Marshall L, McMahan U. Reinnervation of muscle fiber basal lamina after removal of myofibers: Differentiation of regenerating axons at original synaptic sites. J Cell Biol 1978; 13:519–565.
74. Schlaepfer W, Hasler M. Characterization of the calcium-induced disruption of neurofilaments in rat peripheral nerve. Brain Res 1979; 168:299–309.
75. Schlaepfer W, Micko S. Chemical and structural changes of neurofilaments in transected rat sciatic nerve. J Cell Biol 1978; 78:369–378.
76. Schlaepfer W, Micko S. Calcium-dependent alterations of neurofilament proteins of rat peripheral nerve. J Neurochem 1979; 32:211–219.
77. Selzer M. Nerve regeneration. Semin Neurol 1987; 7:88–96.
78. Sheetz M, Steuer E, Schroer T. The mechanism and regulation of fast axonal transport. Trends Neurosci 1989; 12:474–478.
79. Shooter E. Molecular responses to nerve injury. Intl Symposium Neural Regeneration 1985; 25.
80. Siegel G, Agranoff B, Albers R, Molinoff P. Basic neurochemistry, ed 4. New York: Raven Press, 1989:1–984.
81. Skene J. Axonal growth-associated proteins. Ann Rev Neurosci 1989; 12:127–156.
82. Skou J. The (Na + K) activated enzyme system and its relationship to transport of sodium and potassium. Q Rev Biophys 1975; 7:401–434.
83. Smith E, Hill R, Lehman I, Lefkowitz R, Handler P, White A. Principles of biochemistry: Mammalian biochemistry, ed 7. New York: McGraw-Hill, 1983: 243–272.
84. Smith M, Benjamins J. Model systems for study of myelin metabolism. In: Morell P, ed. Myelin. New York: Plenum Press, 1984:441–487.
85. Smith R, Appel S. Extracts of skeletal muscle increase neurite outgrowth and cholinergic activity of fetal rat spinal motor neurons. Science 1983; 219: 1079–1081.
86. Sorkin B, Hoffman S, Edelman G, Cunningham B. Sulfation and phosphorylation of the neural cell adhesion molecule, N-CAM. Science 1984; 225: 1477–1478.
87. Stahl W. The Na,K,ATPase of nervous tissue. Neurochem Intl 1986; 8:449–476.
88. Steward O. Principles of cellular, molecular, and

developmental neuroscience. New York: Springer-Verlag, 1989:1–257.
89. Sunderland S. Nerve and nerve injury. Baltimore: Williams & Wilkins, 1968:69–133.
90. Varon S, Manthorpe M, Davis G, Williams L, Skaper S. Growth factors. Adv Neurol 1988; 47:493–521.
91. Walicke P. Novel neurotrophic factors, receptors, and oncogenes. Ann Rev Neurosci 1989; 12:103–126.
92. Waller A. Experiments on the section of the glossopharyngeal and hypoglossal nerves of the frog: An observation on the alterations produced thereby in the structure of their primitive fibers. Edinburgh Med Surg J 1851; 76:369–376.
93. Watters D, Hendry I. Purification of a ciliary neurotrophic factor from bovine heart. J Neurochem 1987; 49:705–713.
94. Willison H, Trapp B, Bacher J, Quarles R. The expression of myelin-associated glycoprotein in regenerating cat sciatic nerve. Brain Res 1988; 444: 10–16.
95. Yankner B, Shooter E. The biology and mechanism of nerve growth factor. Ann Rev Biochem 1982; 51:845–868.
96. Zeman R, Kameyama T, Matsumoto K, Bernstein P, Etlinger J. Regulation of protein degradation in muscle by calcium. J Biol Chem 1986; 260:13619–13624.

5

The Neuromuscular Junction

William E. Garrett, Jr.

AUTHOR'S KEY POINTS

- Excitation of electrically active membranes in nerve and muscle is not continuous across the neuromuscular junction. Rather, there is a chemical process by which acetylcholine is released by the nerve, diffuses, and initiates the process of electrical conduction in the muscle membrane.
- The chemical transmission process is susceptible to a variety of pharmacologic and physiological influences. Pharmacologic agents can affect function at the level of the nerve membrane, the muscle membrane, or the synaptic cleft. Neuromuscular transmission is also sensitive to ischemia.
- Intact nerve fibers can sprout to innervate denervated fibers. The sprouts enter the degenerated axon and follow the course of the axon to the pre-existing synapse.
- Even in previously denervated muscle, regenerating nerve fibers preferentially form synapses at the site of the previous neuromuscular junction.

The essential purpose of the neuromuscular junction is to transfer action potentials traveling along axons to similar action potentials in muscle fibers. This occurs in the absence of electrical or structural continuity between nerve and muscle, and is accomplished in an elegant and ordered manner. The present understanding of this process has evolved over several hundred years, with the greatest advances occurring in the mid-20th century. For their contributions to our understanding of neuromuscular transmission, four scientists have received Nobel prizes: Sir Henry Dale and Otto Loewi (1936), Sir John Eccles (1963), and Bernard Katz (1971).

STRUCTURE

The motor nerves to skeletal muscle traverse the entire distance from the spinal cord to muscle. The cell bodies of efferent motor nerves, residing in the spinal cord, give rise to axons, the basic neural element of peripheral nerve. A single cell body and its axon provide innervation to a variable number of muscle fibers. The cell body, its axon, and all of the muscle fibers innervated by that axon are called collectively a *motor unit*. The size of a motor unit varies from fewer than 10 to more than 1000 muscle fibers innervated by a single axon. Axons of motor nerves are myelinated. Within the substance of the muscle the axons ramify to supply single branches to each muscle fiber that is a part of the motor unit. The motor nerves ramify and make their way to indentations on the surface of the muscle fiber. The terminal branches end in distinctive structural specializations of nerve and underlying muscle that are collectively called the *motor end plate.*[1]

The motor end plate has been well characterized structurally. In vertebrates, a normal muscle fiber usually contains only one motor end plate. These motor end plates occur in a distinctive location along the muscle fibers, at the approximate center of the muscle fiber length.[5] Since muscle fibers are arranged regularly within a muscle, the whole muscle displays a distinct band of motor end plates when stained by techniques that localize neuromuscular junctions (eg, histochemical cholinesterase stains). Localization of the stain is related to the architecture of muscle fibers and the tendons of origin and insertion. Exceptions to the general staining pattern include the sartorius and gracilis muscles: both contain muscle fibers that may not extend the entire length between tendons of origin and insertion.

The histologic appearance of the motor end plate is characterized by an oval-shaped specialization of nerve, Schwann cells, and underlying muscle. The surface of the muscle cell is specialized to form a mound of cytoplasm with many nuclei and mitochondria. This specialization is called the *sole plate.*[2] The terminal nerve ending indents the muscle cytoplasm, and the glial cells or Schwann cells cover the motor end plate (Fig. 5-1).

Electron microscope studies have provided considerable detail of the neuromuscular junction.[16,30] The axon branch loses its myelin cover near its termination. The axon terminals lie adjacent to the sarcolemma of muscle in an indentation in the surface of the muscle fiber. This surface indentation is called the *primary synaptic cleft.* A space of about 50 nm always separates the cell surface of the nerve from that of the muscle. The muscle surface is further folded into a series of secondary synaptic clefts. These primary and secondary membrane foldings greatly amplify the surface membrane area of the specialized postsynaptic region of muscle. While the Schwann cell processes do not penetrate the primary and secondary synaptic clefts, the basement membrane of muscle is continuous throughout this region (Fig. 5-2).

The ultrastructure of the motor end plate reveals a number of interesting features that relate to the function of neuromuscular transmission. Axon terminals are rich in mitochondria, neurofilaments, and endoplasmic reticulum. Microtubules are absent. A constant feature is the presence of many

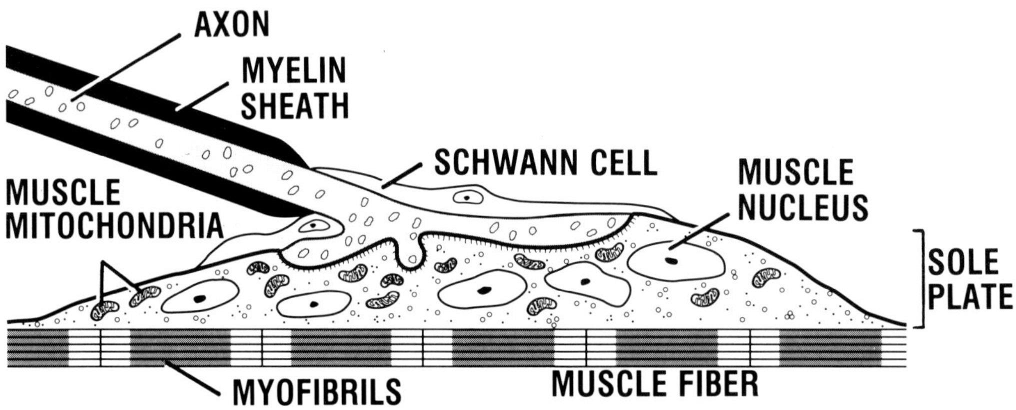

Figure 5–1. *Features of neuromuscular junction by light microscopy. The nerve terminal axon loses its myelin sheath but is still covered by a Schwann cell. The distal axon lies in an indentation in the muscle membrane. The membrane of the muscle fiber is raised in a mound, the sole plate. This area is rich in cellular organelles, although it is devoid of myofibers.*

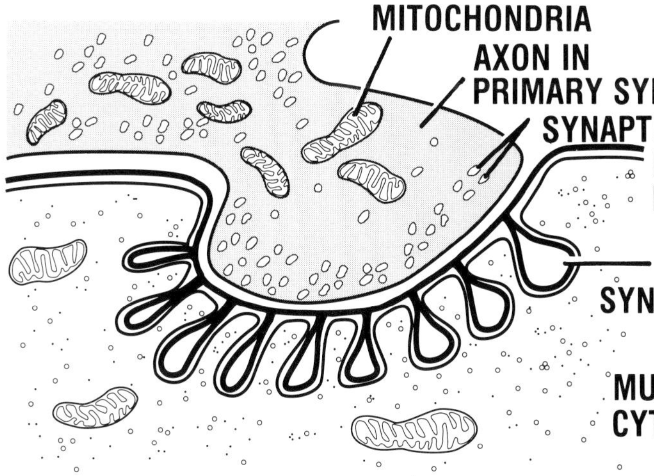

Figure 5-2. *Features of neuromuscular junction by electron microscopy. The primary synaptic cleft is further divided by a series of indentations of the muscle fiber membrane, called secondary synaptic clefts. The basement membrane of the muscle is continuous throughout the primary and secondary synaptic clefts. There are numerous synaptic vesicles in the terminal axon.*

spherical vesicles surrounded by a plasma membrane. These vesicles are 40 to 50 nm thick and contain *acetylcholine*, which acts as a chemical transmitter across the space separating the terminal axon from the muscle surface.

The synaptic vesicles, which abound in the terminal axonal processes, are concentrated near the secondary synaptic clefts. Freeze-fracture electron microscopy shows that the axonal membrane is specialized in this zone, which is thought to be the area for release of the neurotransmitter. The axonal membrane contains an ordered array of *intramembranous particles*, about 10 nm in size, which are presumed to be involved with transmitter release.[9] The postsynaptic membrane of the muscle is also highly specialized.[9] Similar intramembranous densities in the highly folded sarcolemma are involved with the process of transmission. These membranous particles, 10 nm in size, are arranged in rows. Within the cytoplasm of the muscle is a network of filaments that connects the membrane particles and other structural filaments in the muscle.

Functionally, these particles are associated with the receptors for acetylcholine. The understanding of receptor structure and localization has been enhanced greatly by the discovery of a very potent neurotoxin, alpha-bungarotoxin, which has been isolated from poisonous snake venom. This molecule binds to the acetylcholine receptor and can be labeled for electron microscope localization. The area of the postsynaptic intramembranous particles corresponds to the region of alpha-bungarotoxin localization.

When acetylcholine binds to the receptor, there is a momentary depolarization of the postsynaptic membrane. Acetylcholine function must be relatively brief to allow for repolarization of the membrane. Acetylcholine is hydrolyzed by the enzyme acetylcholinesterase. Structural studies have localized cholinesterase activity to the synaptic cleft, specifically to the basal lamina that always exists in the cleft between the pre- and postsynaptic membranes.[24]

Although many of the structural features of mammalian synapses are constant, there is some variability. The forms of primary and secondary synaptic clefts depend on the type of muscle fiber.[4]

Muscle fibers are not uniform; rather, there are distinct fiber types distinguished by histochemical, physiological, and biochemical factors. Type I fibers are physiologically characterized as slow twitch, while Type II fibers have a fast contraction speed. Type II fibers, although faster, are more susceptible to fatigue than Type I fibers. Biochemical and metabolic differences form the basis of the histochemical classification system. Mammalian studies have shown that Type II fibers have regular and deeper secondary clefts than Type I fibers. The synaptic clefts of Type IIB fibers are numerous and regular, while Type IIA fibers have deeper clefts extending close to the myofibrils in the muscle fiber, and the clefts are further apart. The extraocular muscles of some mammalian species may have a distinct structure characterized by multiple contact areas between nerve and muscle; however, neuromuscular junctions in axial skeletal muscle are of the variety discussed above.

PHYSIOLOGY

The physiology of neuromuscular transmission is more easily appreciated once the structural studies are understood. A sequence of events begins with the action potential in nerve and extends to the action potential generated in muscle. In nerve, the action potential propagates along the axon of the motor component to the region of the motor end plate. The current flow of the action potential does not propagate directly across the synaptic cleft; rather, it activates the process of chemical transmission across the junction.

Classic studies have demonstrated that the nerve action potential and the resulting depolarization cause the synaptic vesicles containing acetylcholine to fuse with the axonal membrane, thereby emptying their acetylcholine into the synaptic cleft. The acetylcholine then diffuses across the synaptic space to interact with a specific acetylcholine receptor in muscle. Depolarization of the membrane is responsible for the movement of vesicles and transmitter release. With normal depolarization, there is transmembrane movement of sodium ions into the cell. In addition, neuromuscular transmission seems to depend on calcium currents. An inward flow of calcium ions is necessary for movement of the vesicles toward the synaptic membrane, fusion of the vesicles and the membrane, and exocytosis of the vesicles. Removal of calcium or the addition of other divalent cations capable of competing with calcium blocks transmission.[23]

Once acetylcholine is released into the synaptic cleft, it reacts with the postsynaptic membrane on the muscle, initiating an action potential within the muscle. Acetylcholine itself depolarizes the muscle membrane. The resulting potential, the *end-plate potential*, is a local depolarization of the muscle fiber confined to the region of the motor end plate. The local depolarization caused by the action of acetylcholine is adequate to trigger an all-or-nothing response in the muscle membrane. (The initial changes at the end plate are due to current flow of sodium and potassium.)[13] The action potential is then propagated along the muscle membrane in a manner similar to the mechanism of the axonal membrane.

The nature of acetylcholine release at the nerve terminal has been studied in great detail during the past 30 years. The amount of depolarization induced in the end-plate potential is about 100 mV. However, electrodes placed within muscle near the end plate also demonstrate small changes in the membrane potential that are similar to the end-plate potential in shape but are very much smaller (about 0.6 mV). These miniature end-plate potentials occur spontaneously, except in muscle that has been previously denervated. It has been shown that the miniature end-plate potentials are due to the release of a single vesicle or a quantum from the nerve terminal.[6,7] The individual vesicles do not contain enough acetylcholine to cause sufficient depolarization to trigger an action potential.

These findings led to the quantal theory of transmitter release. Elegant studies showed that the end-plate potentials responsible for synaptic transmission are equivalent to the sum potential of an integral number of miniature end-plate potentials. Each miniature end-plate potential represents the quantal content of one vesicle containing acetylcholine. A normal end-plate potential has been calculated to represent about 250 quanta or vesicles.[19] It appears that each of the quanta contains about 1000 to 10,000 molecules of acetylcholine.[20,28]

Acetylcholine is synthesized in the axon terminal. The enzyme *choline acetyltransferase* transfers an acetyl group from acetyl-coenzyme A to choline to form acetylcholine, which is synthesized in the axoplasm and then concentrated in the vesicles. Its synthesis is related to the amount of neural activity present in the axon. Acetylcholine reacts with its receptor on the postsynaptic muscle membrane, initiating a change in membrane permeability, particularly to sodium ions. This process leads to postsynaptic depolarization. The receptor is associated with the particles seen in freeze-fracture electron micrographs.

Clinical Significance

The action potential is initiated by release of acetylcholine into the synaptic cleft. Acetylcholine from numerous vesicles initiates an end plate potential, triggering an all-or-none response in muscle.

Degradation of acetylcholine is also extremely important in the function of synaptic transmission. The action of the molecule is relatively short, and its hydrolysis is carried out by the enzyme *acetylcholinesterase.* In addition to this specific esterase, other less-specific enzymes can hydrolyze acetylcholine. Cholinesterase is located in the region of the synaptic clefts in the postsynaptic membrane. Acetylcholinesterase is localized to the basal lamina and is therefore extracellular. This enzyme can be affected pharmacologically (see section on Pharmacology).

Impulse Transmission (Fig. 5-3)

An action potential travels down the nerve to the terminal axon. At the presynaptic axon, membrane depolarization allows an influx of calcium current. Calcium ions are necessary for the presynaptic vesicles containing acetylcholine to fuse with the nerve membrane, releasing acetylcholine into the synaptic cleft. Acetylcholine diffuses to the postsynaptic muscle membrane and interacts with a specific acetylcholine receptor. This interaction causes depolarization, or end-plate potential, of the muscle membrane. The amount of depolarization is adequate to trigger an action potential in the muscle that then extends to the rest of the muscle. Acetylcholine is hydrolyzed by acetylcholinesterase and is thereby inactivated, which ends the perturbation and restores the synapse to its resting condition.

As might be expected, this process is slower than the simple propagation of an action potential. The synaptic delay (the time required from the arrival of the impulse in the nerve to the propagation of a potential in muscle) is about 0.2 to 0.5 msec. This time is divided into the time required for vesicle release, the time necessary for diffusion of acetylcholine, and the time needed for depolarization of muscle by the acetylcholine-receptor complex. Most of the delay appears to be in the interval needed for release of acetylcholine.[1]

Clinical Significance

Axon terminals contain vesicles of acetylcholine. Diffusion occurs across an indentation in the surface of muscle, called the primary synaptic cleft, to a specialized muscle surface called the sole plate. Acetylcholine binds to muscle receptors, depolarizing the postsynaptic membrane. This diffusion is slower than nerve conduction and leads to a slight delay in conduction. This is part of the synaptic delay sometimes reported in nerve-conduction tests.

Effect of Ischemia

Neuromuscular transmission is very susceptible to ischemia. A period of ischemia leads to a loss of muscle contraction response to nerve stimulation. The nerve and muscle fibers remain capable of propagating action potentials for some time after failure, demonstrating that the most susceptible function is that of synaptic transmission.[21]

PHARMACOLOGY

Because there are multiple physiological processes involved in neuromuscular transmission, there are many mechanisms by which pharmacologic agents may affect the process. The discoveries regarding junctional physiology have most often arisen from studies of substances effective at the neuromuscular junction. Pharmacologic substances are effective at a variety of locations, including the postjunctional muscle, the prejunctional nerve terminal, and the synaptic cleft region.

Postjunctional Drug Action

The most thoroughly investigated mechanism of pharmacologic action concerns the postjunctional membrane. This is where the interaction between acetylcholine and its receptor is altered. d-Tubocurarine, an arrow poison used by natives of the

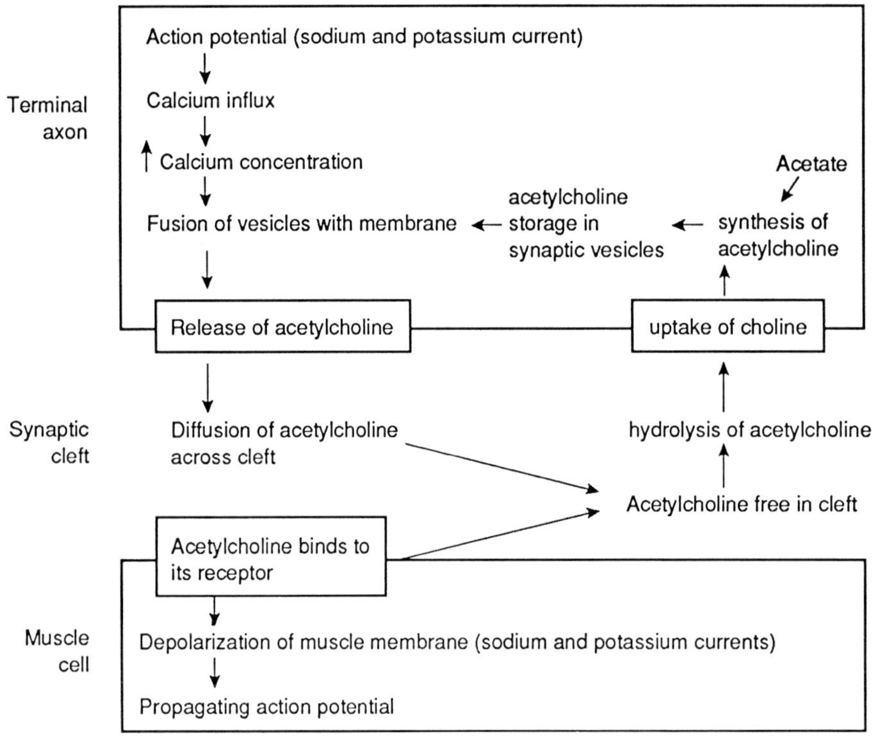

Figure 5-3. *Scheme of neuromuscular transmission*

Amazon region, provides the classic example of this mechanism. This substance, first characterized by Claude Bernard in 1850, is a purified form of curare that acts by competitive inhibition with acetylcholine.[27] For normal function, the receptor is believed to bind acetylcholine and to undergo a conformational change. The acetylcholine receptor sits within, and probably spans, the plasma membrane. Its structure makes the receptor capable of acting as an ion channel across the plasma membrane. In its resting state, the receptor blocks ion passage, but following binding of acetylcholine, the receptor undergoes a conformational change. The change allows for the passage of certain ions through the channel.[18] Cations passing through the channel create an end-plate potential in the postjunctional membrane. d-Tubocurarine binds to the receptor but does not induce the conformational change necessary to allow current flow. When d-tubocurarine rather than acetylcholine is bound to the receptor, the receptor is blocked and the membrane is not depolarized. Thus d-tubocurarine behaves as a non-depolarizing blocking agent (Fig. 5-4).

Because of its rapid onset of action and relative safety, d-tubocurarine is a favorite anesthetic agent. Other non-depolarizing blocking agents are pancuronium and gallamine.

There is also a group of compounds that act on the acetylcholine receptor, causing the conformational change in the receptor that allows depolarization. These depolarizing blockers are usually structural analogs of acetylcholine. Succinylcholine, the most studied of these, is widely used in anesthesia. When administered intravenously, succinylcholine induces depolarization, and muscle contractions normally follow. However, the activation of muscle is transient and paralysis soon follows. While succinylcholine continues to cause depolarization at the end plate, the adjacent muscle membrane accommodates in such a way that it no longer propagates the end-plate potential as a muscle action potential.[32] Succinylcholine is active for about 1 minute after intravenous infusion, and

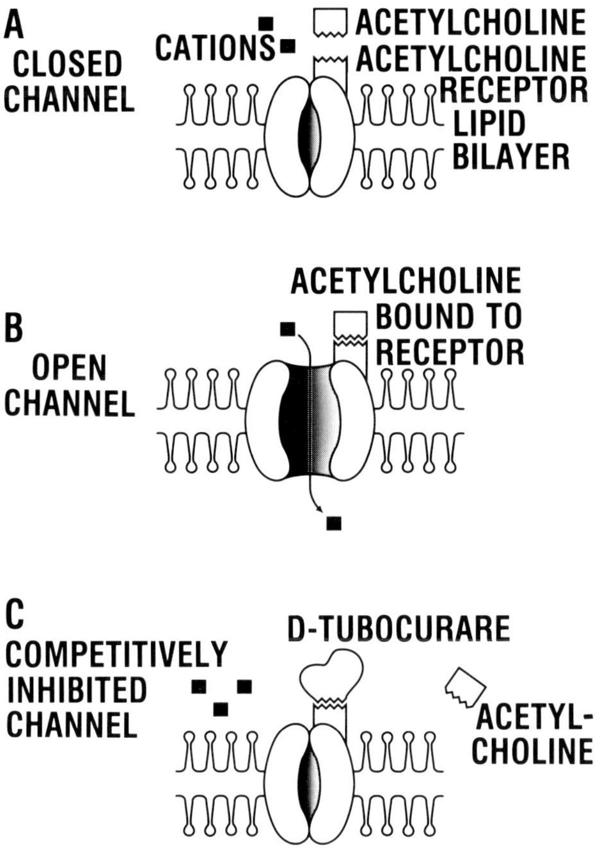

Figure 5–4. *Pharmacology of acetylcholine receptor. (**A**) In the resting state, the receptor traverses the lipid bilayer of the cell membrane. Its channel is closed and cations cannot pass. (**B**) When acetylcholine binds to the receptor, the receptor undergoes a conformational change and can transmit cations from the cell exterior into the interior. (**C**) Competitive inhibitors such as d-tubocurare reversibly bind to the receptor. The receptor does not change conformation and does not allow passage of cations. The bound competitor prevents acetylcholine from binding to the active site of the receptor.*

its effect lasts about 15 minutes. The rapid decay of its activity is due to hydrolysis by plasma cholinesterase. The rapid onset and recovery of action makes succinylcholine extremely useful in anesthesia. A number of undesirable effects are connected with transient muscle activation, including increased intra-abdominal pressure, which may induce vomiting, and postanesthetic muscle soreness due to mild muscle injury incurred during the initial contractions. Another depolarizing blocking agent, decamethonium, is not in common clinical use.

Junctional Drug Action

Another site of pharmacologic action after the postsynaptic membrane is the synaptic cleft. Anticholinesterase drugs inhibit the function of acetylcholinesterase, enhancing the effect of acetylcholine released at the synapse. They act more as potentiators than blockers. Most anticholinesterase drugs bind to acetylcholinesterase, preventing binding and subsequent hydrolysis of acetylcholine. Most of these drugs compete with acetylcholine for the active site on the esterase. To be useful clinically, the inhibitor should provide reversible inhibition of cholinesterase. Physostigmine (eserine) is a naturally occurring inhibitor. The agents that are most useful clinically include pyridostigmine (Nestinon), neostigmine (Prostigmine), and endrophonium (Tensilon). These drugs are useful in the diagnosis and treatment of myasthenia gravis and glaucoma.

Other extremely potent cholinesterase inhibitors—the organophosphorus anticholinesterase inhibitors—differ from the above compounds in that their effects are irreversible. These highly toxic inhibitors have been used as chemical warfare agents, the so-called nerve gases. When these compounds react with acetylcholinesterase they phosphorylate the enzyme, thereby inactivating it permanently. Among them, diisopropyl fluorophosphate and parathion are useful as insecticides. However, the irreversible nature of the reactions they cause makes them very toxic. Acute and chronic poisoning due to the effects of these insecticides are not uncommon.[15]

Clinical Significance

The many biological events involved with synaptic transmission offer numerous possibilities for pharmacologic intervention. Several agents act on the acetylcholine receptors. Some agents, such as d-tubocurarine, bind to the receptor without causing depolarization. Others, such as succinylcholine, bind and cause depolarization. Both classes lead to inhibition of the action of acetylcholine. Agents may also inhibit cholinesterase and potentiate the effects of acetylcholine. These include neostigmine, which binds reversibly, or toxic nerve gases, which are irreversible.

Prejunctional Drug Action

There are also compounds that affect neuromuscular transmission in the prejunctional region of the distal axon. As might be expected, these compounds can also affect acetylcholine synthesis or release mechanisms. Hemicholinium limits the amount of acetylcholine within the axon by blocking the uptake of choline from the extracellular region. Botulinus toxin, the potentially deadly substance from some cases of food poisoning, stops the release of acetylcholine, thereby blocking neuromuscular transmission.

Other compounds act more proximally in the terminal nerve axon. Tetrodotoxin prevents propagation of the action potential by blocking the sodium ion channel, stopping neuromuscular transmission by preventing the propagation of the action potential to the terminal axon.

EFFECTS OF NERVE INJURY ON THE MOTOR END PLATE

Acute Changes

Profound changes occur at the neuromuscular junction in response to a more proximal nerve injury. The axon distal to an axonotmetic or neurotmetic injury undergoes wallerian degeneration. The processes of degeneration and loss of function at the neuromuscular junction are not instantaneous, but are dependent on time and on the distance between the axonal lesion and the synapse. Failure of synaptic transmission is delayed by a few hours to several days. The length of time until failure depends on the length of the nerve distal to the lesion; a longer distal segment allows more time before synaptic failure occurs.[25] For each centimeter of distal axon, there is an estimated 45-minute delay in axonal failure. The first site of failure is at the junction rather than in the axon. The axon can transmit an action potential for some time after failure of synaptic transmission.[14,26]

Structural studies show that changes in the axon correspond to the failure of transmission, proceeding from disorganization to structural breakdown to dissolution. Initially, changes are not prominent in muscle juxtaposed to the axon, but with time, as the motor end plate degenerates, changes occur in the entire muscle. While a detailed analysis of these changes in the muscle is beyond the scope of this chapter, certain relevant features deserve mention.

Physiological changes in muscle are prominent; resting membrane potential falls, and the localization of the acetylcholine receptor changes dramatically.[12] Innervated muscle contains the receptor in the postjunctional synaptic region. Following denervation the receptor can be found over a wide area of the muscle membrane. As a result, the muscle membrane becomes susceptible to the action of acetylcholine in extrajunctional regions. The muscle membrane exhibits action potentials that occur spontaneously in single fibers. These potentials, called *fibrillations*, arise near the site of the motor end plate and do not appear until about 2 to 3 weeks after denervation. Their presence is often the basis of the diagnosis of acute denervation by electromyography.[26]

Clinical Significance

After significant nerve injury, acetylcholine receptors lose their specific localization at the end plate and diffuse over the cell membrane. The muscle membrane becomes less stable at about this time, and spontaneous action potentials or fibrillations occur. These changes occur after 2 to 3 weeks.

Recovery Following Injury

Following denervation, some recovery is possible. If continuity is not lost, or if continuity is restored to nerve, axonal regeneration occurs. If denervation is only partial, recovery can occur without regeneration of the primary axons. The process of nerve regeneration, covered in detail in Chapter

7, will be addressed here as it relates to synapse formation.

The phenomenon of nerve regeneration is well studied. Ramon y Cajal first showed that axons sprout from the proximal nerve stump and grow into the distal portion of the nerve that is undergoing wallerian degeneration.[29] The rate of regeneration varies but approaches 2 to 3 mm/day. The axonal growth cones grow along the distal nerve and form synapses with the denervated muscle fibers. As with normal synaptic relations, there is usually only one synapse per fiber. Some of the muscle fibers may have more than a single motor end plate, but about 90% of the fibers have only a single motor end plate.[3]

In some species, such as the salamander, a regenerating nerve can reestablish synapses with its original muscle fibers. That is not the case with mammalian regeneration, where the reestablished synapses are not selective. This leads to abnormalities in the recovery of neuromuscular function. Interestingly, although nerves do not establish precise connections with their original muscles, the site of new synapses is usually the same as that of the previous synapse. Part of this ability is due to the basal lamina, which remains intact after denervation and can function as a recognition site for sprouts or regenerating fibers.[22]

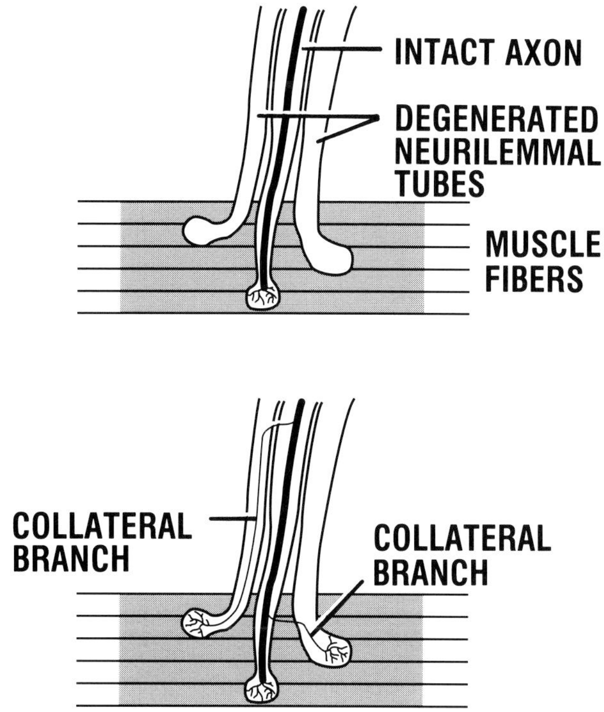

Figure 5–5. *Collateral sprouting in reinnervation of muscle fibers. (**A**) A partially denervated muscle. Two fibers have undergone degeneration, leaving an empty neurilemmal tube. A third fiber is normal. (**B**) Reinnervation by sprouts. Sprouts have arisen from the intact axon and have entered the neurilemmal tubes previously degenerated. The sprouts travel down the tubes and establish new synapses at the site of previous neuromuscular junctions.*

Sprouting

There is another mechanism for restoring innervation to denervated fibers in partially denervated muscles. Rather than awaiting outgrowth from the proximal stump, intact axons can sprout and form synapses with denervated fibers.[10] Sprouts occur from axons that are relatively close to the muscle fibers from the intramuscular portion of the nerve. Sprouts may come from the terminal nonmyelinated portion of the axon (terminal sprouts) or from axonal segments at the nodes of Ranvier (nodal sprouts).[8] These sprouts usually enter the perineural sheath of a degenerated axon and travel to the site of the previous motor end plate (Fig. 5-5).[17,26] Their course may be more circuitous than normal, and their relatively small diameter may cause a slower nerve conduction velocity (that is, the action potential is slower to reach the muscle fibers innervated by sprouts than the muscle fibers of the original motor unit). The course of the action potential is spread out over time, and there may be several reversals of potential in the electrical recordings of the new motor units. These polyphasic action potentials provide electromyographic evidence of reinnervation.

Factors that influence sprouting have been investigated in detail. Electrical stimulation of nerves enhances their sprouting,[18] younger animals produce more sprouts than older ones,[11] and fast-twitch muscles develop sprouts more quickly.[16] While factors that initiate sprouting have been investigated extensively, a single well-defined mechanism that explains the initiation of the sprouting process has not been identified. Factors released from the degenerating distal nerve stump are possible sources of sprouting stimulus. Lack of muscle activity, induced by a variety of means, can induce sprouting even in the absence of a degenerating axon. Other factors are also possible.[26]

Sprouts are affected by a variety of chemical, structural, and physiological factors. Even when muscle fibers are allowed to degenerate and then are irradiated to prevent regeneration, sprouts still make contact with the original synapses. This indicates that the intact basement membrane may be important in the restoration of synapses.[31]

Clinical Significance

Nerves reestablish their original connections with muscle fibers, forming synapses in the same location as previous ones. This is due to the preservation of basal lamina, which guides axon sprouts to regenerating fibers.

SUMMARY

Concepts regarding the neuromuscular junction have been developed steadily over the past century. Elucidation of the process of transmission of an electrical potential from nerve to muscle membrane has provided insight into some of the most interesting physiological and pharmacologic discoveries of the century. There is now great interest in determining the reparative and regenerative processes of neuromuscular junctions. While there are many technical and surgical limitations to recovery following nerve injury and repair, the physiological inability of neuromuscular connections to reform precisely is a significant impediment to the recovery of function after nerve injury.

REFERENCES

1. Aidley DL. The physiology of excitable cells. New York: Cambridge University Press, 1971:93–127.
2. Bloom W, Fawcett DW. A textbook of histology. Philadelphia: WB Saunders, 1975:311–313.
3. Brown MC, Ironton R. Sprouting and regression of neuromuscular synapses in partially denervated mammalian muscles. J Physiol (London) 1978; 278: 325–348.
4. Carry MR, Morita M. Structure and morphogenesis of the neuromuscular junction. In: Brumback RA, Gerst J, eds. New York: Futura, 1984:25–63.
5. Coers C, Woolf AL. The innervation of muscle: A biopsy study. Oxford: Blackwell, 1959:12–41.
6. Del Castillo J, Katz B. Quantal components of the end-plate potential. J Physiol (London) 1954; 124: 560–573.
7. Del Castillo J, Moore JW. On increasing the velocity of a nerve impulse. J Physiol (London) 1959; 148: 665.
8. Edds MV. Experiments on partially deneurotized nerves. J Exp Zool 1949; 111:211–226.
9. Ellisman MH, Rash JH, Staehlin AL, Porter KR. Studies of excitable membranes. II. A comparison of specializations at neuromuscular junctions and nonjunctional sarcolemmas of mammalian fast and slow twitch muscle fibers. J Cell Biol 1976; 68:744–752.
10. Exner S. Die Innervation des Kehlkopfes. S B Akad Wiss Wien 1984; 89:63–118.
11. Fagg GE, Scheff SW, Cotman CW. Axonal sprouting at the neuromuscular junction of adult and aged rats. Exp Neurol 1981; 74:847–854.
12. Fambrough DM. Control of acetylcholine receptors in skeletal muscle. Physiol Rev 1979; 59:165–225.
13. Fatt P, Katz B. An analysis of the end-plate potential recorded with an intracellular electrode. J Physiol (London) 1951; 115:320–369.
14. Gilliat RW, Fowler TJ, Rudge P. Peripheral neuropathy in baboons. Adv Neurol 1975; 10:253–272.
15. Goth A. Medical pharmacology: Principles and concepts, ed 5. St. Louis: CV Mosby, 1970:49–74.
16. Heuser JE, Reese TS. Structure of the synapse. In: Brookhart JM, Mountcastle VB, Kandel ER, eds. The nervous system. Bethesda, Maryland: American Physiology Society, 1979:261–294.
17. Hoffman H. Local reinnervation in partially denervated muscle: A histophysiological study. Aust J Exp Biol Med Sci 1950; 28:383–397.
18. Hoffman H. Acceleration and retardation of the process of axon-sprouting in partially denervated muscles. Aust J Exp Biol Med Sci 1952; 30:541–566.
19. Hubbard JI, Wilson DF. Neuromuscular transmission in a mammalian preparation in the absence of blocking drugs and the effect of d-tubocurarine. J Physiol 1973; 228:307–325.
20. Katz B, Miledi R. The statistical nature of the acetylcholine potential and its molecular components. J Physiol 1972; 224:665–699.
21. Krnjevic K, Miledi R. Failure of neuromuscular propagation in rats. J Physiol 1958; 140:440–461.

22. Letinsky MS, Fischbeck KH, McMahon VJ. Precision of reinnervation of original postsynaptic sites in frog muscle after a nerve crush. J Neurocytol 1976; 5:691.

23. McArdle JJ. Overview of the physiology of the neuromuscular junction. In: Brumback RA, Gerst J, eds. The neuromuscular junction. New York: Futura, 1984:203–355.

24. McMahan J, Sanes J, Marshall L. Cholinesterase is associated with the basal lamina at the neuromuscular junction. Nature 1978; 271:172–174.

25. Miledi R, Slater CR. On the degeneration of rat neuromuscular junctions after nerve section. J Physiol 1970; 207:507–528.

26. Miller RG. The effects of nerve injury on the neuromuscular junction. In: Brumback RA, Gerst J, eds. The neuromuscular junction. New York: Futura, 1984:203–255.

27. Pelouze M, Bernard C. Recherches sur le curare. C R Acad Sci 1850; 533–537.

28. Potter LT. Synthesis, storage, and release of [^{14}C] acetylcholine in isolated rat diaphragm muscles. J Physiol 1970; 206:145–166.

29. Ramon y Cajal S. Studies on degeneration and regeneration of the nervous system. Translated and edited by May RM. London: Oxford University Press, 1928:265–280.

30. Robertson JD. The ultrastructure of a reptilian myoneural junction. J Biophys Biochem Cytol 1956; 2:381–394.

31. Sanes JR, Marshall LM, McMahan UJ. Reinnervation of muscle fiber basal lamina after removal of myofibers. J Cell Biol 1978; 78:176–198.

32. Standaert FG. Pharmacology of the neuromuscular junction. In: Brumback RA, Gerst J, eds. The neuromuscular junction. New York: Futura, 1984:203–255.

6

Sensory Receptors

Julia K. Terzis
Bryan J. Michelow

AUTHORS' KEY POINTS

- *Sensation* is the perception of an external stimulus. Sensibility of a target tissue is related to the density of innervation and the type and number of mechanoreceptors present. *Sensory receptors* are the transducers that convert mechanical stimuli into electrical impulses.
- Sensory receptors can be broadly categorized into two groups, encapsulated or unencapsulated receptors. *Unencapsulated* receptors are free nerve endings concerned with the modalities of temperature and pain. *Encapsulated* mechanoreceptors are innervated by the larger nerve fibers and can be further classified on the basis of their response characteristics and their rate of adaptation to a steady stimulus.
- *Quickly adapting* (phasic) receptors are detectors of movement and produce a burst of impulses at the onset and upon removal of a continuous monotonic stimulus.
- *Slowly adapting* (tonic) receptors best respond to constant touch and sustained pressure and discharge throughout the duration of the stimulus. Two classes can be distinguished, according to their pattern of discharge.
- Slowly adapting type one receptors (SA I) have little or no spontaneous discharge in the resting state. SA I receptors are most sensitive to vertical displacement and have less response to skin stretch.[8]
- Slowly adapting type 2 receptors (SA II) maintain a slow, regular discharge in the absence of stimulation. SA II receptors are more sensitive to stretch than to vertical displacement.[4]
- The afferent fibers that subserve peripheral sensibility have been identified to be primarily from groups A and C.[25]

HISTORY

The body's ability to exist in an ever-changing environment depends on its ability to maintain internal homeostasis. Mechanisms to sense environmental changes are therefore vital so that appropriate homeostatic adjustments can be made. Interpretation of these changes is made possible by sensory receptors, the function of which is to code sensory information into a form that is intelligible to the brain.[32] Specially developed sensory endings have developed for four of the senses (vision, hearing, taste, and smell). The fifth sense, which is located in the skin, was named "touch" by Aristotle, but the multitude of different sensations from this organ has led to the use of the term "general sensation," which includes sensation from the skin, joints, and viscera.[71] Cutaneous sensation has been studied for many years, but it was only at the beginning of the 19th century that philosophical argument gave way to scientific investigation.

In 1838, in an attempt to explain these phenomena, Muller proposed his theory of "specific energies" and "specific irritability" of nerves.[59] According to the theory of specific energies, a nerve possesses specific properties such that when stimulated by different stimuli, it always results in the same kind of sensation. This was thought to be due not to an anatomical or physiological difference between nerves, but rather to something intrinsic to the nerve axon or its central connection. By "specific irritability," Muller meant that the terminal ends of the nerve were in some way specialized to react preferentially to specific stimuli. Muller concluded that each sensation has a specific receptor, a specific nerve pathway, and a specific central locus of perception.

At the same time, von Helmholtz introduced the term "sensory modality" to designate "a class of sensations connected by qualitative continua."[7] For example, tone is a single modality because in hearing, there is a continuous series of tones with no qualitative gaps. This concept gained popularity, and the four major sensory categories of touch, warm, cold, and pain were promoted to the status of "modality." The cutaneous sense, however, was not considered a single modality, since several types of sensations were present.[71]

In the few years that followed, it became generally accepted that there existed a series of specific nerve fibers providing either well-defined sensations or groups of sensations. Warm and cold sensations were thought to be served by the same end organ. Hering, in 1879, suggested that the same nerve responded to warm or cold in different ways.[39] Riley argued that hot and cold were relative terms, with their receptors influenced in a way analogous to the effect light or darkness had on the rod receptors of the eye (ie, heat and cold were to temperature what light and darkness were to sight).[65]

In 1884, Blix discovered a multitude of tiny "spots" in normal skin that reacted preferentially to touch, cold, warm, or pain.[5] The spots for warm and those for cold were clear-cut and easily separable. The different anatomical distribution of warm spots and cold spots in the skin confirmed the individuality of these modalities. The spots for touch were more numerous, and those for pain were so closely set that Blix became doubtful of their individuality.[5]

After Perkin's discovery of aniline in 1856, staining methods became available, and with improvements in microscopic technique, histological study of the skin became feasible.[71] In addition to free nerve endings found in all areas of skin, six types of anatomically differentiated nerve endings were soon described: Pacinian corpuscles (1834),[62] Meissner corpuscles (1853),[51] Krause end bulbs (1859),[46] Merkel cell–neurite complex (1875),[53] and Ruffini endings (1891).[66]

Von Frey suggested that under each sensory spot, there was an end organ or group of end organs specialized to respond to a particular type of stimulus.[80] This specialized end organ was connected to a fiber that conveyed the impulses to the brain, where they were appropriately interpreted. Von Frey postulated that the specialization of the end organ would be anatomically distinct, and he allocated each of the four established modalities to one of the known end organs as follows: pain to free nerve endings, cold to the Krause end bulbs, warm to the Ruffini endings, and touch to the Meissner corpuscles.[71,81]

Von Frey did not go unchallenged: Goldscheider criticized the inclusion of pain as a modality.[27] Pain was unique in that any type of stimulus, in excess, could produce it, he argued. Aristotle, according to Sinclair, considered pain to be a "passion of the soul, the opposite of pleasure; a state of mind rather than a sensation."[71] Pain is not quite the same sensation as touch, warm, or cold, since it can be separated into two components, the sensation itself and the emotional reaction to the sensation.[14] Sinclair quotes Leriche: "Physical pain is not a simple affair of an impulse travelling along a nerve at a fixed rate. It is the resultant of a conflict between a stimulus and the whole individual."

Von Frey was also criticized because the four sensory experiences he described did not explain experiences such as roughness, hardness, clamminess, or stickiness.[70] Alrutz was unsuccessful in trying to explain these as blends of the four modalities.[2] The inadequacy of von Frey's theory was realized when both Goldscheider,[29] in 1884, and Donaldson[21] in 1885, demonstrated cold and warm spots in areas where only free nerve endings were found.

Sherrington, in the early 1900s, took a less rigid view of end-organ specificity and proposed that a nerve fiber might be stimulated by a number of stimuli but that each fiber was more sensitive to a particular stimulus.[69]

In 1905, Head introduced the theory of sensory duality.[38] After sectioning a cutaneous sensory nerve on the dorsum of his own arm and studying the return of sensation, he concluded that there were two anatomically distinct systems of nerve fibers, each associated with its own end organs. The first group, which mediated extremes of temperature and pain, he called the "protopathic system." It was concerned with unpleasant sensations and was the first to return after injury. The second, the "epicritic system," subserved light touch and temperature discrimination. The inconsistency of this system was demonstrated by Carr in 1916; much debate followed.[11]

Research by Erlanger and Gasser, in 1924, indicated that sensory specificity was in some way related to fiber size.[25] Large fibers were associated with touch and small fibers with pain, but these were not mutually exclusive.

In 1928, Adrian proposed the "all-or-none" law: in response to a stimulus, an axon either transmitted or nothing happened.[1] Technical advances and the development of microrecording electrodes enabled examination of electrical charges within individual cells, confirming that this law applied to the axon but that graduated responses were the rule in the cell bodies of the central nervous system.[71]

In 1965, Melzack and Wall introduced the gate control theory.[52] Painful stimuli excite small myelinated A delta and unmyelinated C fibers. These excite second-order neurons, which reach the cortex and thus the level of consciousness. Skin receptors, when stimulated by rubbing the skin for example, excite large fibers that are inhibitory to the second-order neurons. Whether or not the second-order neurons transmit onwards depends on the balance of large and small fiber input to the second-order neurons. Small-fiber activity "opens" the gate; large-fiber activity "closes" it.

This led to research into the use of counterstimulation as a means to block pain.[26,84] Nathan pointed out inconsistencies in the theory[61] and further research lead to the discovery of enkephalins and enkephalinergic receptors in the midbrain, pons, and medulla.[22,30,40]

GENERAL CHARACTERISTICS OF SENSORY RECEPTORS

Sensation is the perception of afferent volleys from the periphery. *Sensibility* of a target tissue is related to the density of innervation and the type and number of mechanoreceptors present. *Stereognosis* is the ability to perceive and understand the form and nature of objects by the sense of touch. *Sensory receptors* are the transducers that convert mechanical stimuli into electrical impulses that are transmitted to the brain. The frequency and pattern of these impulses constitute the *neural code*.[58]

A receptor responds to a stimulus by initiating a characteristic output. The output depends on the speed (rapid or slow) with which the receptor adapts to the stimulus. Adaptation, therefore, refers to the characteristic response of the receptor to a steady stimulus (Fig. 6-1).

Quickly adapting (phasic) receptors produce impulses that progressively decrease to zero or to a baseline value in response to a continuous steady stimulus (Table 6-1).

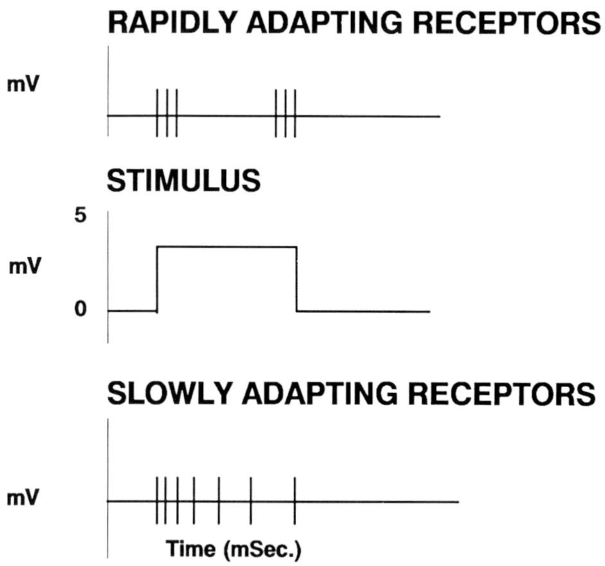

Figure 6-1. *Characteristic response of a rapidly adapting and a slowly adapting receptor to a steady stimulus.*

Slowly adapting (SA) receptors continue their pulse response throughout the duration of the stimulus. These receptors respond to a steady stimulus with a dynamic and static phase. The onset of a stimulus initiates the dynamic phase, during which these receptors respond with a high rate of discharge. The static phase begins at the end of active receptor displacement and is marked by an exponential fall in the output frequency, followed by a slow decrease in rate, until an irregular, low rate of discharge is maintained for the duration of the stimulus.[10,37]

Two classes of SA receptors can be distinguished on the basis of their patterns of discharge:

SA type 1 (SA I) receptors have little or no spontaneous discharge in the resting state. During the dynamic phase, high rates of discharge (up to 1500/sec) occur. SA I receptors are most sensitive to vertical displacement and have less response to skin stretch.[8]

SA type 2 receptors (SA II) maintain a slow, regular discharge in the absence of stimulation. The maximal frequency of output of the SA II receptor (up to 300/sec) occurs during the dynamic phase of the monotonic stimulation, and the static phase has a regular rate of discharge that remains above baseline. SA II receptors are more sensitive to stretch than to vertical displacement.[4] Thus, SA II receptors provide more sensory information about pressure and position than SA I receptors.

Stimulus intensity is encoded by the impulse frequency of a given receptor and the number of receptors activated. A stronger stimulus generates a correspondingly greater frequency of receptor impulses from a greater number of receptors. These two parameters are then centrally processed to quantitate the stimulus.

If a mechanical stimulus changes in magnitude (increases or decreases), the quickly adapting (QA) receptor responds by a burst of impulses at the time of the stimulus change; however, SA receptors respond by a change in the frequency of the output (Fig. 6-2).[34]

Table 6–1. *Encapsulated Mechanoreceptors in Glabrous and Hairy Skin*

Skin Type	*Adaptation*	*Sensory Receptor*
GLABROUS SKIN	Fast →	Meissner corpuscle
	→	Pacinian corpuscle
	Slow → SA I →	Merkel cell–neurite complex
	→ SA II →	Ruffini end organ
HAIRY SKIN	Fast →	Hair receptor
	→	Pacinian corpuscle
	Slow → SA I →	Merkel cell–neurite complex
	→ SA II →	Ruffini end organ

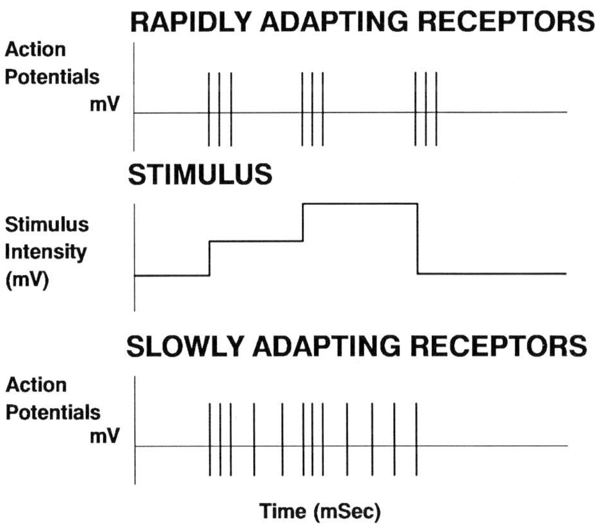

Figure 6-2. *Characteristic response of a rapidly adapting and a slowly adapting receptor to a change in stimulus magnitude.*

AFFERENT NERVE FIBERS

The afferent fibers innervating the sensory receptors have been identified as primarily from groups A and C, as defined by Erlanger and Gasser.[25]

Group A beta fibers carry very sensitive information with a high degree of spatial resolution. These are relatively large, myelinated fibers with fast conduction velocities (30–70 m/sec) and they provide innervation to the encapsulated nerve endings.

Group A delta fibers transmit sensory information with low spatial resolution. These are the smallest of the myelinated fibers and conduct at 5 to 30 m/sec. They are associated with unencapsulated free nerve endings sensitive to cooling, pricking pain, and tickling.

Group C fibers are unmyelinated and conduct at 2 m/sec. They are associated with unencapsulated free nerve endings serving the sensations of warmth, cold, pain, and itch.[21]

The ratio of A to C fibers in peripheral nerves varies from 1:1 in areas of the face and hand to 1:5 in nerves innervating the trunk. This provides an understanding of the differential sensitivity to stimuli of different parts of the body. The innervation of sensory receptors is also organized so that the more important, high-quality sensibility is conveyed by larger, rapidly conducting myelinated fibers, informing the brain of a stimulus change without undue delay. The less important, poor-resolution sensibility is transmitted along smaller, unmyelinated fibers.[33]

CLASSIFICATION OF SENSORY RECEPTORS

Sensory receptors can be categorized as those subserving *special senses* (vision, hearing, taste, and smell) and those addressing *somatic sensation.* The latter include receptors specialized to cutaneous sensation (eg, touch), visceral sensation, and proprioception (eg, joint position). Sherrington coined the terms exteroceptors, interoceptors, and proprioceptors, respectively, to define these receptors.[69]

This chapter focuses on cutaneous receptors that have selective sensitivity to natural stimuli. For a detailed discussion of the receptors for special senses, visceral sensation, and proprioception, the reader is referred to specific texts on the subject.[35,57]

The cutaneous receptors are specialized to sense external stimuli and can be classified functionally according to the nature of the stimulus to which they are most sensitive. *Mechanoreceptors* detect physical distortions of the skin, *thermoreceptors* register changes in skin temperature, and *nociceptors* are activated by potentially harmful physical or chemical stimuli.[42,47,56] Cutaneous mechanoreceptors can be further differentiated on the basis of functional and morphological differences.

Functionally, mechanoreceptors differ in the manner in which they respond to a continuing, steady mechanical stimulus (ie, in the rate of adaptation). Some are detectors of transients only (QA mechanoreceptors) while others respond to the onset of the mechanical stimulus with a high-frequency discharge but continue to fire during the stimulus application with a frequency determined by the magnitude of the external stimulus. The latter are the SA mechanoreceptors.

Morphologically, the differences are limited to the type of association of the neurite with the non-nervous tissue elements. When the association is extensive, as in the case of the lamellated receptors, a large surface area of contact is provided between the neurites and the layered cellular investment. Such associations impart the functional characteristics of a QA mechanoreceptor.[77]

When the specialized contact between neurites and non-nervous tissue elements is on a more limited basis, a more graded response is produced. Such morphological associations correspond to the response characteristics of a SA mechanoreceptor.

Finally, there is a category of fibers where there is no obvious morphological association between neurites and non-nervous tissue elements.

On the basis of these morphological attributes, cutaneous mechanoreceptors can be classified as follows:[77]

1. *Lamellated* mechanoreceptors have extensive specialized contact between neurites and non-nervous tissue elements and a QA response. Examples are Pacinian corpuscles, Meissner corpuscles, and hair cells.
2. *Nonlamellated* mechanoreceptors have limited specialized contact between neurites and non-nervous tissue elements and a slowly adapting response. Examples are Merkel cell–neurite complexes and Ruffini organs.
3. *Free neurite terminals* have no obvious specialized contact with non-nervous tissue elements. Examples are free nerve endings.

The anatomical location of the receptors enables the receptors to be categorized into those existing in glabrous skin (non–hair-bearing), hairy skin, mucocutaneous skin, and muscles and joints.[77]

Both myelinated and unmyelinated sensory nerves are present in glabrous and hair-bearing skin. These nerve fibers end either as free nerve endings or innervate specific encapsulated end organs. The encapsulated mechanoreceptors in glabrous and hairy skin are listed in Table 6-1.

There is essentially no difference between glabrous skin and hair-bearing skin in terms of location and function of the free nerve endings. The encapsulated Pacinian corpuscles, Merkel cell–neurite complexes, and Ruffini end organs are also present in both locations.[13,77] Particular to hair-bearing skin are the hair receptors; Meissner corpuscles are particular to glabrous skin.[77]

Free Nerve Endings

Free nerve endings constitute the majority of sensory receptors in the skin. Found in abundance in both glabrous and hairy skin, they are assumed to be responsible for sensations of cold and warm, the nociceptive response of pain, and vague sensations of itch and tickle. Derived from unmyelinated axons, the basal lamina of the Schwann cell fuses with the basal layer of the epidermis, and the bare axon enters the epidermis.[57] These free nerve ending are extensions of slowly adapting A delta or C fibers.[57] Cold gnosis has been associated with A delta myelinated fibers. Warmth receptors have been associated with unmyelinated C fibers.[34] Both types of receptors are slowly adapting and have a temperature-dependent continuous discharge.

Tickle and itch sensations are not caused by mild stimulation of pain fibers as was previously thought, but rather by specific receptors.[85] These are found exclusively in the superficial layers of the skin and are innervated by very small C fibers.

Glabrous Skin Receptors

Glabrous (nonhairy) skin of humans has the highest peripheral innervation density and is represented by one of the largest areas of the sensory homunculus in the cortex. The relative thickness of the epidermis and its unique ridged character influence the mechanical deformation of the skin surface and thereby modulate tactile sensitivity.

Knibestol and Vallbo first demonstrated that glabrous skin in humans has four types of morphologically distinct mechanoreceptors for which functional correlates have been identified with some certainty.[45] These include two QA receptors (Meissner and Pacinian corpuscles) and two SA units (the Merkel cell–neurite complex [SA I] and the Ruffini ending [SA II]). These identical receptors were previously demonstrated in subhuman primates.[23,24,77]

Quickly Adapting Receptors

The Pacinian corpuscle, which is large enough to be visible to the naked eye, was understandably the first anatomical structure to be associated with cutaneous sensation (Fig. 6-3).[72] It lies in the deep dermis and subcutaneous tissue, is innervated by a single group A beta fiber, and exists singly or multiply. Three distinct microanatomical areas can be defined: the inner core, the middle zone, and the capsule.

The axon enters the corpuscle and loses its myelin sheath. The terminal two nodes of Ranvier are intracorpuscular. Distal to the last node, the unmyelinated axon thickens and is filled with multiple mitochondria, neurofilaments, and neurotubules. Layers of concentric flattened Schwann cells, each with its own basal lamina, surround the nerve ending, forming an inner core. The middle zone separates the inner core from the outer capsule and consists of a subcapsular space filled with amorphous ground substance. The outer capsule is an extension of the perineural sheath of the afferent nerve supplying the corpuscle.[39,48] It consists of 20 to 30 lamellae of simple squamous epithelium. More than a third of the estimated 2000 Pacinian corpuscles in the human skin are in the digits; more than 100 are in a single finger (Fig. 6-3).[38,70]

The corpuscle is sensitive to mechanical displacement, particularly vibration. Acting as a filtered transducer, the outer capsule acts to dampen low-frequency vibrations from the central end organ, virtually eliminating any vibration less than 100 Hz. The Pacinian corpuscle is maximally re-

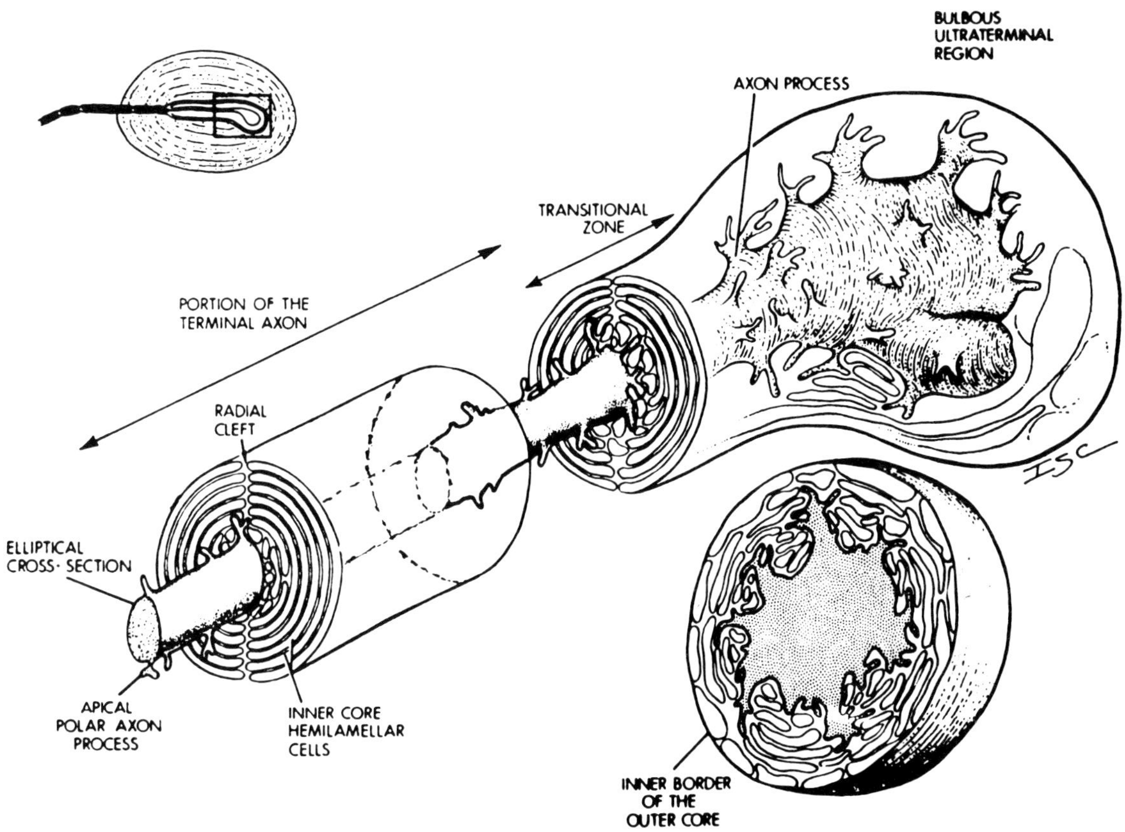

Figure 6-3. *Diagram of a portion of a Pacinian corpuscle (indicated by the boxed area in the upper-left diagram) illustrating the terminal neurite and inner core ultrastructure. (From Spencer PS, Schaumburg HH. An ultrastructural study of the inner core of the Pacinian corpuscle. J Neurocytol 1973;2:217, with permission.)*

sponsive at 250 to 300 Hz.[57] The fast-adapting core and lamellae structure provide the basis for the sensation of high-frequency vibrations and moving touch.

The Meissner corpuscle, found within the dermal papillae, is the terminal end of several group A beta fibers encapsulated by what appears to be modified Schwann cells folded into multiple lamellae (Fig. 6-4). The lamellar cell of the Meissner corpuscle is similar to the lamellar cell of the Pacinian corpuscle.[12] The lamella cells are stacked as sheets, one upon another, with scanty intercellular tissue. The unmyelinated terminal part of the nerve fibers weaves among the lamellae.[71] Fine collagen fibrils extend from the lamellar cells and are attached to the surrounding basal layer of the epidermis by semidesmosomes.[4] This mechanical link between skin and corpuscle enables small stimuli to be transferred to the more central portions of the multilamellated structure (see Fig. 6-4). Five to nine axons innervate a single corpuscle, but it is uncertain if these fibers are from the same nerve.[44,77]

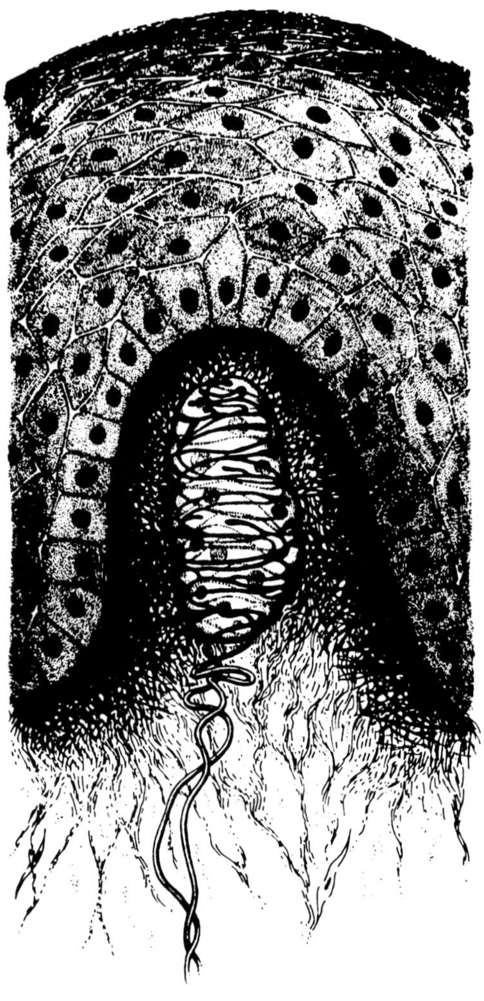

Figure 6-4. *The Meissner corpuscle, located in the dermal papillae of glabrous skin, is a rapidly adapting encapsulated mechanoreceptor serving the modality of low-frequency vibration. (From Dykes RW. Sensory receptors. In: Daniel RK, Terzis JK, eds. Reconstructive microsurgery. Boston: Little, Brown & Co, 1977:329, with permission.)*

When viewed in longitudinal section, a similarity to lanceolate endings in hair follicles is noted. Both Meissner corpuscles and hair follicles are quickly adapting; one may speculate that this corpuscle is the glabrous skin analog of the hair receptor.

Under sustained pressure, an impulse is produced only at the onset, removal, or change of the magnitude of the stimulus; hence, this is a velocity or acceleration sensor and is "tuned" to receive optimal vibrations of 30 to 40 Hz.[57] The sensory submodality subserved by this QA receptor is low-frequency flutter-vibration and moving touch.[75]

Slowly Adapting Receptors

The Merkel cell–neurite complex is found in the basal region of the epidermis, at the dermal–epidermal junction (Fig. 6-5).[23] Groups of five or ten such complexes are interspersed among the basal layer cells, forming an Iggo dome.[42] The afferent nerve, a group A beta fiber, loses its Schwann cell covering and ends in a spray of unmyelinated terminals (neurites), each enclosed by a specialized epithelial cell with clear cytoplasm that is possibly of neural crest derivation—the Merkel cell.[60] One Merkel cell–neurite complex may receive more than one nerve terminal, and a given nerve fiber may supply more than one complex.[71] The presence of multiple cytoplasmic processes, containing microvilli, lying between the cells of the adjacent epidermis are characteristic of this complex (Fig. 6-5).

The Merkel cell–neurite complex is an SA mechanoreceptor of the type 1 variety. This enables the receptor to sense constant touch or pressure and is largely responsible for tactile gnosis of

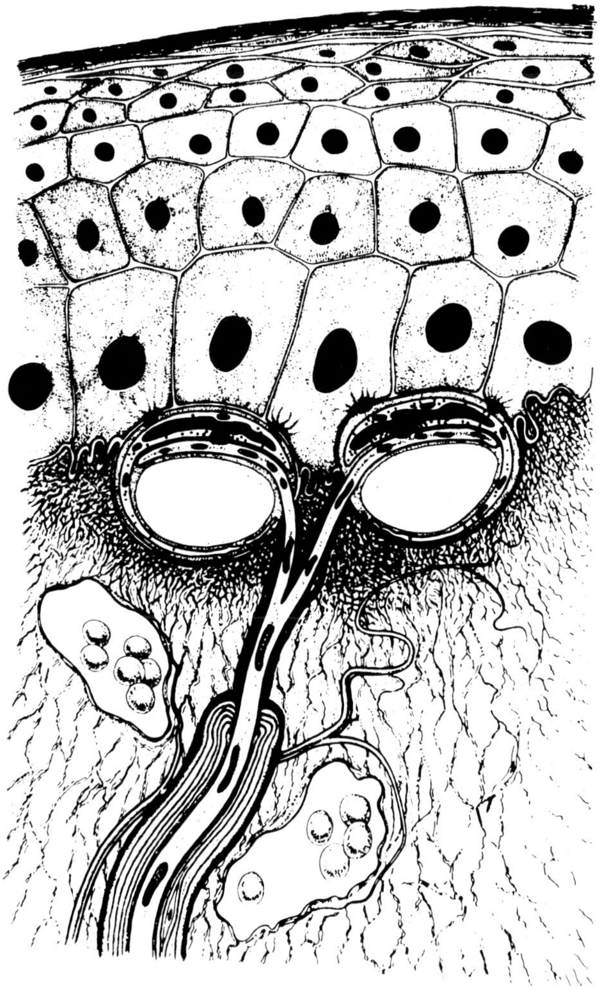

Figure 6-5. *The Merkel cell–neurite complex is composed of epithelial cells that surround the nerve terminals of a myelinated fiber. The cells are located at the base of the intermediate ridges in glabrous skin or, in hairy skin, in raised domes called touch domes. This is a slowly adapting (SA I) mechanoreceptor serving the modality of constant touch. (From Dykes RW. Sensory receptors. In: Daniel RK, Terzis JK, eds. Reconstructive microsurgery. Boston: Little, Brown & Co, 1977:323, with permission.)*

static objects.[19] It produces an output that exhibits dynamic and static phases. During the dynamic phase, the receptor responds to both the velocity and the magnitude of the stimulus with a high impulse rate (up to 1500/sec).

The discharge frequency of the Merkel cell–neurite complex is temperature-dependent. Cooling the skin causes receptor excitation; warming inhibits discharge.[44]

The Ruffini end organ (SA II receptor) is spindle-shaped, 1 to 2 mm long, and located within the dermis. It is also present near joints. The receptor consists of the terminal unmyelinated branch of a group A beta fiber ensheathed by a specialized endoneurial cell capsule, within which is a fluid-filled space.[77] Collagen fibrils pass through this space and connect subcutaneous and dermal layers with the receptor core, thus providing a mechanical link between receptor and surrounding tissue.[4]

Each Ruffini ending is innervated by a single myelinated axon, which may innervate several adjacent endings. There is a continuous background discharge in the absence of mechanical stimulation, the frequency of which increases with stimulation (SA type II receptor). During unvarying stimulation, the discharge frequency declines to a plateau above baseline and a regular low-frequency output is maintained for the duration of the stimulus. As with SA I receptors, the baseline background discharge of the SA II receptors is altered by skin cooling (excitation) or warming (inhibition).

Ruffini endings respond maximally to skin stretch and less to direct vertical displacement. Stretch of the collagen fibers stretches the core of the receptor because of the mechanical link, thus providing an assessment of tissue tension.[77]

Clinical Significance

In glabrous skin, two QA and two SA receptors are found. The QA Meissner corpuscle senses low-frequency vibration, and the Pacinian corpuscle senses high-frequency vibratory input. The SA Merkel cell–neurite complex (SA I) senses constant touch; the Ruffini end organ (SA II) senses skin stretch. Free nerve endings sense warm, cold, and pain.

Hairy Skin Receptors

The hair itself is a specialized component of the cutaneous receptor mechanism. Mountcastle estimated that 80% of small myelinated fibers in a cutaneous nerve terminate in relation to hairs.[57] A group A beta fiber extensively branches and innervates several follicles (Fig. 6-6). Several myelinated fibers (five to nine in humans) encircle the

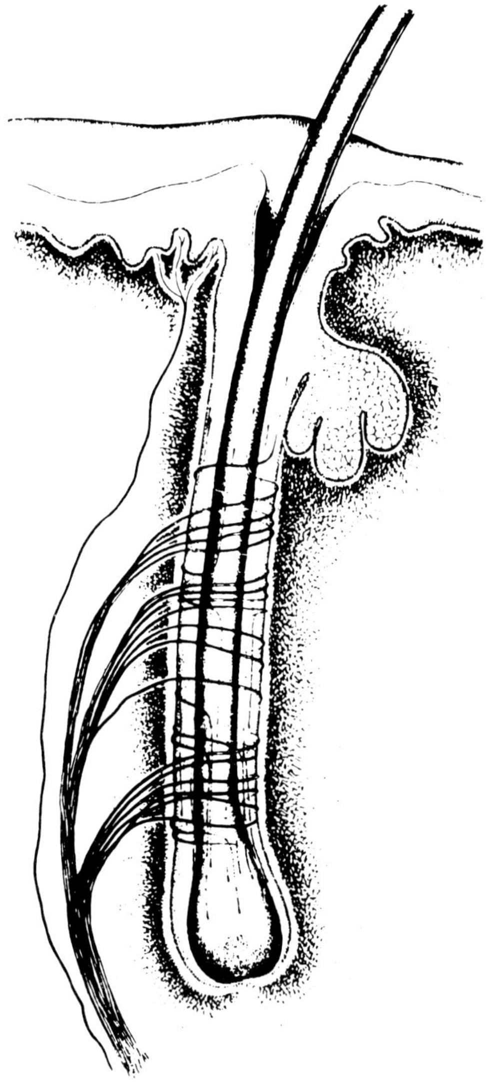

Figure 6-6. *The hair follicle is innervated by several myelinated fibers entwined around the hair shaft. Distortions of the hair shaft due to hair movement are transmitted to this rapidly adapting mechanoreceptor. (From Dykes RW. Sensory receptors. In: Daniel RK, Terzis JK, eds. Reconstructive microsurgery. Boston: Little, Brown & Co, 1977: 325, with permission.)*

follicle just below the sebaceous gland.[82] Within the dermal sheath of the follicles, the nerve fiber loses its myelin sheath, becomes spindle-shaped, and proceeds along the basal lamina. The term "lanceolate" has been used to describe these flattened nerve terminals containing numerous mitochondria.[3,4] A second cluster of spindle-shaped nerve endings found just deep to the sebaceous glands are supplied by myelinated fibers that ascend along the hair shaft. Thirdly, papillary endings are found within the basal lamina of the epidermis and are innervated by an unmyelinated fiber.[23]

Hair movement is transmitted to these receptors. The impulse is transient, as the receptor complex is quickly adapting and responds to vibratory or moving stimuli. The receptor is a functional analog of the Meissner corpuscle in glabrous skin.[19,77] The maximal stimulation occurs at vibrations of 30 to 40 Hz, which is similar to the Meissner corpuscle.[57]

Clinical Significance

In hairy skin, two QA and two SA sensory receptors are present. The QA hair receptor senses hair movement and corresponds to the Meissner corpuscle found in glabrous skin. The QA Pacinian corpuscle senses high-frequency vibration. The SA Merkel cell–neurite complex (SA I) senses constant touch; the SA Ruffini end-organ (SA II) senses skin stretch. As in glabrous skin, free nerve endings provide warm, cold, and pain sensibility.

Mucocutaneous Receptors

The transitional zone between hairy skin and mucous membrane possesses a sensory ending not seen in the other areas. The *Krause end bulb* has a terminal neurite complex resembling tangled yarn. The ending is not encapsulated. Also known as the genital end bulb, it is found in structures such as the glans penis, clitoris, lip, eyelid, and perianal region. Originally described as a cold receptor, the Krause end bulb is probably a Meissner corpuscle variant with no apparent functional difference and similar functional properties.[71] In addition to the encapsulated nerve receptors, free nerve endings are the most common receptors found in genital skin.[44]

Muscle and Joint Receptors

Several types of receptors provide position sense, stretch, tension, and "deep sensibility." These include muscle spindles, Golgi tendon organs, the encapsulated joint receptors, and nociceptive free nerve endings.[9,67]

The *muscle spindle* is a fusiform encapsulated receptor found within skeletal muscle. Specialized muscle fibers (intrafusal) are enclosed by a multilayered capsule innervated by gamma efferent (fusimotor) fibers. The configurations of the intrafusal nuclei differentiate these fibers into two types: nuclear bag (clustered around the cell center) or nuclear chain (axially distributed fibers).[50]

Primary afferent (type 1 alpha, heavily myelinated, large, quickly conducting) fibers and *secondary afferent* (myelinated type 1 beta) fibers enter the spindle through the capsule. The primary endings (type 1 alpha) surround the intrafusal fibers at the nuclear bag or chain with a series of anulospiral terminals. The secondary afferents (type 1 beta) are smaller and are located on either side of the primary endings. This anatomical arrangement of fibers has functional significance: both primary and secondary endings are activated when the whole muscle is stretched. Primary endings behave much like QA receptors, being most responsive during the moving phase of the stretch. Secondary endings respond best to prolonged stretch.[54]

Unlike other receptors, gamma efferent fusimotor fibers provide an external influence on these receptors. By maintaining a constant intrafusal fiber length over a wide range of muscle lengths, the intrafusal fiber can modulate the sensitivity of the sensory receptors.[31]

Free nerve endings have also been found in muscle spindles and are of fiber type C. The Golgi tendon organ is found within tendinous structures and ligaments. It is an SA receptor structurally similar to Ruffini endings. It responds in a linear fashion with maximal output frequencies at times of maximum tension.[34] Free nerve endings of fiber type C, which are also present in capsules and ligaments, are presumed to be nociceptive.

Clinical Significance

Muscle and joint receptors include muscle spindles, Golgi tendon organs, the encapsulated joint receptors, and nociceptive free nerve endings. These provide position sense, stretch, tension, and deep sensibility.[57]

SENSORY RECEPTOR INNERVATION

With the aid of precise neurohistology, coupled with single-unit electrophysiology, defining the relationship between the sensory receptors and their innervation has been possible (Table 6-2). A typical peripheral nerve consists of closely packed nerve fibers, ectodermally derived specialized supportive cells, connective tissue elements, lymphatics, and blood vessels.[15] The peripheral branches of sensory nerves supplying the skin enter the subcutaneous tissue and form a subcutaneous plexus.[79] From this plexus, the deeply located receptors (Pacinian corpuscles and Ruffini endings) are innervated (Fig. 6-7).

Nerves then penetrate the dermis and form a dermal plexus beneath the epidermal ridges, from

Table 6–2. *Innervation of Glabrous and Hairy Skin*

Receptor	*Modality*	*Nerve Fiber*	*Conduction Velocity*	*Response*
Meissner corpuscle	Flutter, low-frequency vibration	A beta	30–70 m/sec	Phasic
Pacinian corpuscle	High-frequency vibration	A beta	30–70 m/sec	Phasic
Merkel cell–neurite complex	Constant touch	A beta	30–70 m/sec	Phasic and tonic
Ruffini end organ	Stretch	A beta	30–70 m/sec	Tonic
Hair	Hair movement	A beta	30–70 m/sec	Phasic
Free nerve ending	Cold	A delta	5–30 m/sec	
	Warm, pain	C fibers	<2 m/sec	

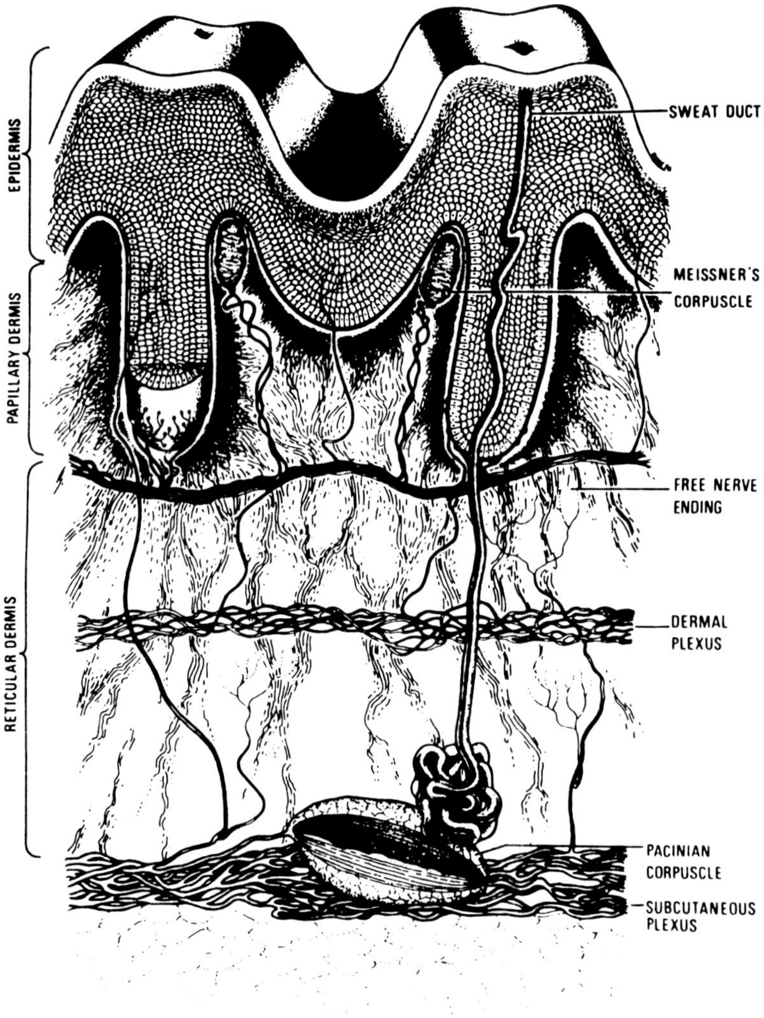

Figure 6-7. *Terminal branches of cutaneous nerves form the subcutaneous nerve plexus. From this plexus, the deeply located Pacinian and Ruffini endings are innervated. The nerves then form the dermal plexus from which the superficial Meissner corpuscles and Merkel cell–neurite complexes receive their neural elements. Note the abundance of free nerve endings. (From Dykes RW. Sensory receptors. In: Daniel RK, Terzis JK, eds. Reconstructive microsurgery. Boston: Little, Brown & Co, 1977:322, with permission.)*

which the superficial receptors are innervated (Meissner corpuscles and Merkel cell–neurite complexes). From this second plexus, free nerve endings enter the dermal papillae and epidermis (Fig. 6-7). Each plexus also contains sympathetic postganglionic fibers that supply the blood vessels, sweat glands, and erector pili muscles of the skin.

Consideration of the location of the receptors in the skin provides further evidence regarding receptor function. Located superficially within the skin, at the dermal–epidermal junction, are the QA Meissner corpuscles and the SA Merkel cell–neurite complexes (SA I). At a deeper level are the QA Pacinian corpuscles and the SA Ruffini endings (SA II).

Janig postulated that the smaller the distance between the skin surface and the nerve ending, the greater the stimulus required to generate an action potential at the periphery of the receptive field.[43] The implication is that the receptive field of the Meissner corpuscles and the Merkel cell–neurite complexes has sharp boundaries that thus provide for *accurate localization* and *accurate spatial discrimination.*[77]

The more deeply located Pacinian corpuscles are each innervated by a single afferent fiber, and each receptive field thus has a single peak of maximal sensitivity. Being QA receptors, they are most sensitive to high-frequency vibration and are less suitable for spatial discrimination. Pacinian corpuscles are also found in the proximity of joints and fibrous capsules and may have a proprioceptive function.

The Ruffini endings (SA II), also located in the deep dermis, are oriented along the axis of dermal fibrous strands. Skin stretch directed along the longitudinal axis of the capsule will increase the axonal discharge. The spontaneous activity of this receptor may be an indicator of the tension of fibrous tissue in relation to various joint movements, thus serving a proprioceptive function as well.

The density of innervation of various skin regions requires consideration. Why are the fingertips so exquisitely sensitive to fine touch, but the skin of the palm is not? Bolton[6] and Sinclair[71] have demonstrated an increased density of Meissner corpuscles in the fingertips compared to the palms. Cauna and Mannan have shown an even distribution of Pacinian corpuscles and Ruffini endings (SA II) in the hand.[12] The fingertips, therefore, have a high density of sensory units with small, distinct receptive fields particularly suitable for tactile acuity.[77]

These concepts indicate that the response of a receptor to stimulation is not merely a result of its anatomical structure alone, but rather that the response is determined by numerous functional factors, including stimulus intensity, stimulus type (lateral vs vertical skin displacement), and spatial and temporal patterns of afferent impulses elicited from different mechanoreceptors. It thus becomes important to study innervation patterns and responses of a whole population of mechanoreceptor units so as to better understand the perception of touch.[75]

SENSORY TRANSDUCTION

Transformation of Stimuli in Receptors

A stimulus is an objectively measurable quantity, such as mechanical deformation of skin. Each receptor responds optimally to one stimulus type. This property is called *specificity of receptors.* The stimulus that is effective in each case is called the *adequate stimulus* for the receptor.[57] For example, light is the adequate stimulus for the retinal rod receptors.

Generator Potentials

All mechanoreceptors respond to distortion of their structures. When an adequate stimulus stimulates a receptor by distorting its structure, the receptor membrane permeability changes.[34] An increase in membrane conductance for all small ions (Na^+, K^+, Ca^{2+}, Cl^-) results. When the receptor is the termination of the nerve fiber, as in free nerve endings, depolarization sets off a nerve action potential. If a specialized non-neural receptor cell is deformed, a potential, known as a generator potential, develops at the terminal neurite. As the generator potential rises above the threshold level, action potentials are initiated and propagated along the afferent nerve fiber. The larger the generator potential, the greater the frequency of action potentials (Fig. 6-8).

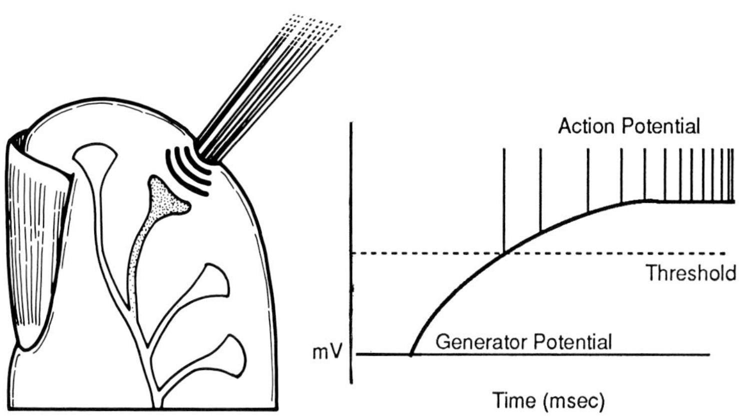

Figure 6-8. *Sensory transduction. Distortion of the non-neural elements of the mechanoreceptor by an adequate stimulus alters membrane permeability in the terminal neurite, creating a generator potential. Above threshold an action potential is initiated, the frequency of which depends on the magnitude of the generator potential.*

Receptive Field

The receptive field is the skin area over which a single nerve fiber responds to an adequate stimulus. The size of the field depends on the branching and distribution of the neurites of the afferent fiber. A Meissner corpuscle may be innervated by numerous nerve fibers, and a single nerve fiber may innervate numerous Meissner corpuscles. The receptive field of an individual fiber, therefore, may be quite large and overlap that of other fibers. A stronger stimulus is needed at the periphery than in the center of the field to elicit the same response. When stimulating a point on the skin, the afferent response will be greater from the receptive field that has the stimulus at its center when compared to the adjacent receptive field, which is stimulated near its periphery (Fig. 6-9). Thus, when stimulating a point in a receptive field, different neurites will be stimulated to a different degree depending on the stimulus location. By analyzing the pattern of discharges from the afferent fibers, the exact position of the stimulus within a receptive field can be accurately determined. With overlapping fields, the system is less vulnerable should an afferent fiber be injured.

Clinical Significance

The phenomenon of overlapping receptive fields provides a mechanism to accurately determine the position of the stimulus within a receptive field. A second advantage is that the system is less vulnerable should an afferent fiber be injured, since sensibility will be provided by an adjacent fiber from an overlapping field.

Phenomenon of Inhibition

A disadvantage of overlapping receptive fields is loss of sharp stimulus boundaries, since peripherally positioned neurites will be activated and blur the edge of the stimulus. To prevent this phenomenon, afferent fibers relay centrally onto local inhibitory interneurons as well as onto second-order neurons. These interneurons synapse with the adjacent second-order cells. The second-order cell in the center will thus have a larger effect on neighboring cells than the neighboring cells will have on it. The image therefore becomes sharpened (Fig. 6-10).

The mechanism of lateral inhibition is of fundamental importance and enables convergence and divergence in projection from one neuronal level to another. In this way, lateral inhibition is analogous to adaptation by reducing the redundancy of neural signals. A second advantage is the conversion from a system of impulses that are based on frequency at the receptor level to a system that is

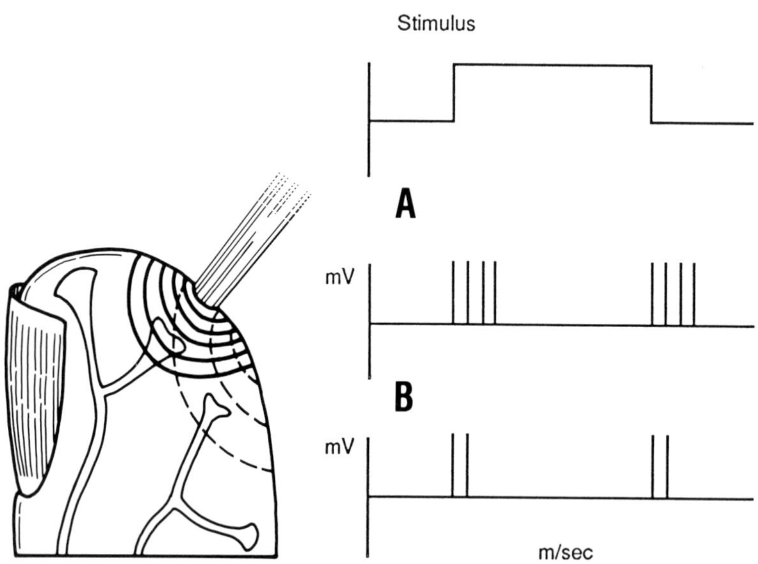

Figure 6-9. *The receptive field is the area of skin over which a single nerve fiber will respond to an adequate stimulus. The afferent response will be greater from the center of a receptive field (A) than from the periphery (B).*

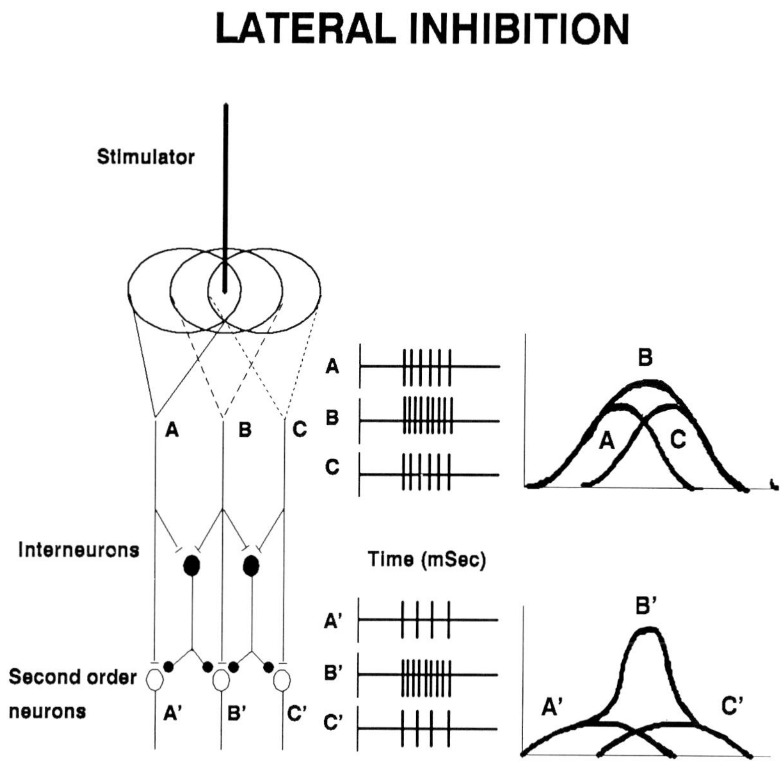

Figure 6-10. *Lateral inhibition provides a mechanism for accurate spatial discrimination and localization by making the boundaries of a stimulated receptive field sharper. It also enables conversion of sensory information based on frequency to a "pattern"-based system, thereby providing the basis for sensory coding.*

Receptive field B is stimulated near its center, resulting in a greater afferent response than in adjacent fields A and C, and in a stronger stimulus for the second-order neuron B′ compared to A′ and C′. The inhibitory interneurons, although dampening all afferent inputs to the second-order neurons, have a greater effect on the weakly stimulated second-order neurons A′ and B′. The border of the receptive field is thus made sharper.

pattern-based at the neuron level, thereby providing the basis for sensory coding.

Receptors and Their Central Connections

The afferent fibers from cutaneous receptors are bipolar cells. Their cell bodies lie in the dorsal root ganglia near the spinal cord. Axons run from the sensory endings in the skin to their terminal projections in the central nervous system (Fig. 6-11).[15] Embryologically, the dorsal root ganglia are connected in an orderly fashion to different areas of skin. The areas of skin subserved by each dorsal root ganglion defines a dermatome. The dermatomes overlap; any point on the skin surface has representation from at least three dorsal root ganglia.

The broad division of afferent fibers into two groups on the basis of size and type of ending is also reflected in their mode of termination within the central nervous system. The larger fibers from encapsulated mechanoreceptors turn rostrally soon after entering the dorsal horn of the spinal cord, forming a pair of large ascending tracts, the dorsal columns. These continue ipsilaterally up to the level of the medulla and terminate in the dorsal column nuclei (gracile and cuneate). From these nuclei, second-order fibers cross to the other side and continue up as the medial lemniscus to the ventrobasal complex of thalamic nuclei.[36] The fibers then relay through the internal capsule to the region of the cerebral cortex called the somatosensory cortex. There is preservation of the topological relationship between the various areas of the body so the somatosensory cortex consists of a map of the opposite side of the body (sensory homunculus). Distortion with exaggeration of special areas is present. Fingers and lips have large representative areas compared to the back and legs.

The smaller afferents, derived mainly from free endings and concerned with temperature, pain, and light touch, do not ascend immediately on entering the spinal cord. These synapse in the central gray matter with interneurons. The interneurons excite

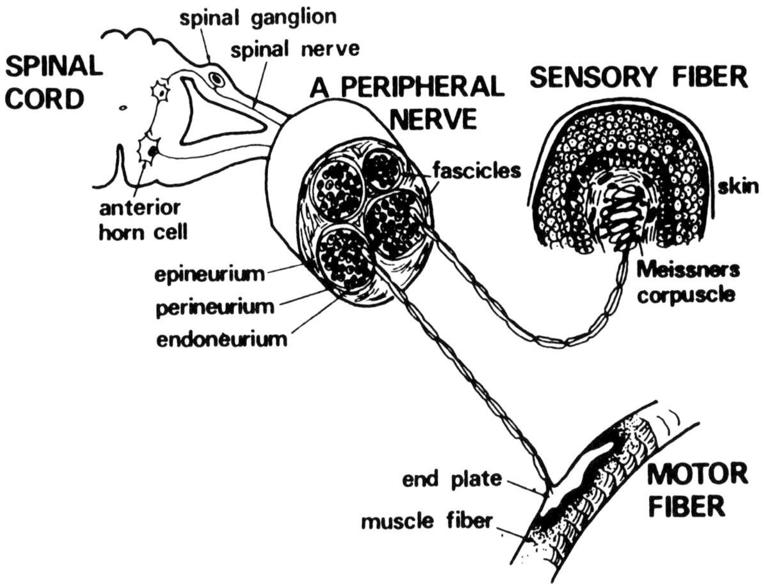

Figure 6-11. *The afferent fibers from cutaneous receptors are bipolar cells with their cell bodies in the dorsal root ganglia, near the spinal cord. Embryologically, the dorsal root ganglia innervate areas of skin (known as dermatomes) in an orderly fashion. (From Terzis JK. Structure and function of the peripheral nerve. In: Daniel RK, Terzis JK, eds. Reconstructive microsurgery. Boston: Little, Brown & Co, 1977: 297, with permission).*

third-order neurons, which cross to the other side and then pass rostrally in the spinothalamic projection. This projection is composed of an anterior and a lateral spinothalamic tract, both terminating in thalamic nuclei. This anatomical arrangement is of diagnostic value. A hemisection of the cord that interrupts all ascending fibers on one side results in a loss of deep pressure and vibration sense below the level of the lesion on one side, and loss of pain, warm and cold sensibility on the contralateral side of the body.

The dorsal column system, therefore, conveys sensations requiring rapid transmission (30–100 m/sec), a high degree of localization, and fine gradation of intensity of the stimulus. It is reserved for sensations from encapsulated mechanoreceptors. The anterolateral spinothalamic tracts transmit sensations that do not require rapid transfer (10–60 m/sec) and that lack discrete localization. It does, however, transmit a broad spectrum of sensory modalities such as pain, warm, and cold.

DENERVATION AND REINNERVATION OF SENSORY RECEPTORS

Injury may result in damage to sensory receptors and peripheral nerves. Depending on the severity of the injury, damage to the receptor may or may not be reversible. Injury to the supplying peripheral nerve depends on the severity of the trauma and the efficiency of the repair. Seddon's classification of nerve injury is as follows (see Chap. 7):

1. *Neurapraxia* is a local conduction block with preservation of axonal continuity. Morphologically, the axon exhibits local demyelination.
2. *Axonotmesis* implies axonal interruption but integrity of the connective tissue sheaths.
3. *Neurotmesis* reflects disruption of the axon, endoneurium, perineurium, and epineurium.

Intact adjacent nerves sprout into denervated regions of neighboring dermatomes in an attempt to restore innervation. Following successful nerve repair, a process of remodeling occurs in which the regenerating axons replace the adjacent sprouts, which then withdraw. The eventual sensory recovery, however, is never normal.

There is evidence that upon denervation, all encapsulated receptors undergo progressive atrophy. Dellon studied the sequence of sensory recovery in an injured nerve.[19,20] The sequence of recovery is pain and temperature first, followed by 30-cps perception, moving touch, constant touch, and lastly 256-cps vibration (see Chap. 8).

Dykes and Terzis, studying the neural events following nerve crush, demonstrated that a regenerating axon may sprout and enter two separate peripheral receptive fields with different response characteristics.[24] Dellon suggested that regenerating axons can reinnervate a different type of end organ and that the reinnervated end organs that were cross-innervated may function.[19] Protective sensation is thus re-established, although with false localization.

Encapsulated Receptors

Pacinian Corpuscle

The tightly wound lamellae of the Pacinian corpuscle degenerate over a period of time (the time course is unknown).[19] Glees and coworkers demonstrated that Pacinian corpuscles with adequate blood supply can survive for a long time.[28] It seems that in the case of the Pacinian corpuscle, the presence of a nerve fiber is not essential to the survival of the end organ, and there is no special attraction exerted by denervated corpuscles on regenerating nerve fibers.[28]

Pacinian corpuscles reinnervate with difficulty, and high-frequency vibration seems to be the last submodality to return, if it does at all. Dellon mentioned the possibility that a "mechanical block" of the injured axon prevents the reinnervation of the receptor.[19] This notion is unlikely; it is more likely that the problem is the low probability of the regenerating fiber to make the correct peripheral connection due to the 1:1 ratio between receptor and nerve fiber.[77]

Meissner Corpuscle

Meissner corpuscles undergo progressive denervation, beginning with the axon terminal and followed by atrophy of the lamellar cell complex itself.[18] In rhesus monkeys, axons of regenerating sensory nerves reinnervate the denervated Meissner corpuscles. There is no evidence that Meissner corpuscles regenerate de novo. Terzis and Dykes, in their extensive studies on reinnervation of glabrous skin in baboons following crush and transection injuries, showed the following[24,78]:

Reinnervated Meissner corpuscles exhibit response characteristics similar to controls, but the tuning curves have uniformly higher thresholds.

After reinnervation, SA fibers display stimulus response curves with elevated thresholds, and they tend to saturate at lower stimulus intensities than normal fibers.

Submodality specificity is a property of the regenerating axon.

Merkel Cell–Neurite Complex

The Merkel cell–neurite complex undergoes similar progressive atrophy postdenervation and within a short time the receptor disappears. After successful reinnervation, trophic factors from the atrophic Merkel cell–neurite complex or from the axon result in the regeneration of the fiber/receptor system, but only in the special areas in which it previously existed.

Clinical Significance

Following denervation, the neurites innervating the sensory receptors degenerate, while the capsule of the mechanoreceptors atrophies. Subsequent to nerve repair, mechanoreceptors can become reinnervated in part and have response characteristics restored but with higher thresholds.

SENSORY RECOVERY

Sunderland described good sensory recovery even after delays of 2 years.[73,74] Woodhall and Beebe reported similarly good results following long delays prior to sensory nerve repair.[83] Despite reports to the contrary,[19,68] we have seen rewarding degrees of sensory recovery even after intervals of 14 years. The tactile acuity in these cases always improved with the use of desensitization and sensory re-education protocols (see Chap. 58).

In re-innervated glabrous skin of the baboon, receptive field sizes, shapes, and thresholds returned to near-normal values following crush.[24,77] Submodality specificity was maintained and appeared to be a property of the regenerating axon.

Work on skin grafts has shed some light on this subject. The classic studies by Hutchinson, Tough, and Wyburn in 1949,[41] Ponten[63] in 1960, and Mannerfelt[49] in 1962 established conclusively that transplanted soft tissue recovers a sensory pattern more like its recipient bed than its donor site if sufficient re-innervation occurs. Early clinical psychophysical evaluations of the return of sensation to skin grafts and flaps showed that:[16,17,47]

1. The recoveries of different sensory submodalities (ie, pain, touch, and temperature) are dissociated.
2. The progress of free skin graft reinnervation is inordinately slow, requiring postoperative periods of a year or more before complete sensory recovery across even relatively small grafts is obtained.
3. The end results obtained by the use of free skin graft transfers tend to be inferior to those provided by alternative procedures (eg, the pedicle flap).

Ridley in 1970 noted that hairy skin grafts transferred to the fingertip assumed some of the anatomical configurations of normal glabrous skin, including the presence of fiber terminations reminiscent of Merkel cell–neurite complexes, which are common to both hairy and glabrous skin.[64] However, the grafts were devoid of Meissner corpuscles, indicating that the de novo regeneration of this receptor type did not occur. He also noted that a number of fibers terminating in locations normally occupied by Meissner corpuscles assumed a complex coiled configuration. The functional properties of such endings are unknown.

The physiological properties of sensory fibers reinnervating skin grafts appear to have been examined in only two studies. Terzis recorded the activity of afferent fibers that had reinnervated autografts that had been transferred from the abdomen to the rabbit ear.[76] However, observations were limited to the fiber conduction velocities. In a more recent study, Terzis, Dykes, and Turnbull reported their results following single-fiber dissection studies. Meissner-like tuning curves were observed in skin grafts in the baboon's hand in the absence of identifiable endings in glabrous skin biopsies.[79] The strong suggestion from this latter study is that the terminal fiber determines the response characteristics of the receptor, while the non-neuronal corpuscle is perhaps of little functional significance.[79]

Clinical Significance

When resurfacing a fingertip, the best sensibility is obtained if similar tissue (namely, glabrous skin containing similar receptors) is used. Hairy skin is of inferior sensory capability and is preferred coverage for areas of lesser sensory demand. Receptors do not develop de novo.

CONCLUSION

Sensory receptors are the transducers that enable interaction between the organism and its external environment. Their function is to convert external stimuli into electrical impulses. Two broad groups, encapsulated and unencapsulated sensory receptors, can be differentiated. The unencapsulated free nerve endings are ubiquitous and are primarily concerned with crude touch, temperature, and pain. Innervated by A delta and C fibers, transmission is slow (2–30 m/sec) and spatial integrity poor. These fibers synapse in the gray matter of the spinal cord and cross to the opposite anterolateral spinothalamic tract prior to ascending rostrally. Hemisection of the spinal cord therefore results in loss of the above-mentioned sensory modalities on the opposite side of the body, below the lesion.

Encapsulated sensory receptors are innervated by fast-conducting A beta fibers (30–70 m/sec). So as to promote rapid transfer of information from sensory receptor to cerebral cortex, large myelinated fibers enter the spinal cord and ascend the ipsilateral dorsal columns to the sensory nuclei in the medulla, prior to synapsing with second-order neurons.

Encapsulated sensory receptors can be further categorized by their ability to adapt quickly or slowly to a steady stimulus. QA receptors (Meissner corpuscle for flutter and low-frequency vibration; Pacinian corpuscle for high-frequency vibration) are sensitive to a changing stimulus. This function correlates well with their lamellated structure, which makes these receptors more sensitive to vertical displacement than stretch.

SA sensory receptors (Merkel cell–neurite complex for constant touch; Ruffini end organ for stretch) provide information that enables the individual to maintain posture. This is enhanced by the input from muscle and joint receptors (muscle spindles, Golgi tendon organs, and the encapsulated joint receptors). A mechanical link between these receptors and surrounding connective tissue provides a structure that lends itself to being more sensitive to stretch than vertical displacement.

The phenomenon of overlapping receptive fields provides a mechanism for accurately determining the position of the stimulus within a receptive field. A second advantage is that the system is less vulnerable should an afferent fiber be injured, since sensibility can be restored by an adjacent fiber from an overlapping field.

Lateral inhibition allows for a sharper sensory image and converts a system of impulses that are based on frequency at the receptor level to a system that is pattern-based at the neuron level.

Sensory coding, a process that maximizes communication in the sensory system, is based on receiving, transforming, transmitting, storing, and retrieving information. This is achieved by successive processes of encoding, transmission, readout, and re-encoding. The cutaneous mechanoreceptors are responsible for coding sensory events into impulse patterns in afferent nerve fibers. The transmission and modification of impulses takes place in different populations of neurons in the central nervous system.

REFERENCES

1. Adrian ED. The basis of sensation. The action of the sense organs. London: 1928.
2. Alrutz S. Stedien auf dem gebiete der temperatursinne. II. Die hitzeempfindung. Scand Arch Physiol 1900; 10:340–352.
3. Andres KH. Uber die Feinstruktur der Rezeptoren an Sinushaaren. Z Zellforsch 1966; 75:339–365.
4. Andres KH, von During M. Morphology of cutaneous receptors. In: Iggo A, ed. Handbook of sensory physiology. II: Somatosensory system. New York: Springer, 1973:3–28.
5. Blix M. Experimentella beitrage zur losung der frage uber die specifische energie der hautnerven. Z Biol 1884; 20:141–156.
6. Bolton CF, Winkelman RK, Dyck PJ. A quantitative study of Meissner's corpuscles in man. Neurology (Minn) 1966; 16:1–9.
7. Boring EG. Sensation and perception in the history of experimental psychology. New York, Appleton-Century-Crofts, 1942.
8. Burgess PR, Perl ER. Cutaneous mechanoreceptors and nocireceptors. In: Iggo A, ed. Handbook of sensory physiology. II: Somatosensory system. New York: Springer, 1973:29–78.
9. Carpenter RHS. Proprioception. In: Carpenter RHS, ed. Neurophysiology. Baltimore: University Park Press, 1984:100–114.
10. Carpenter RHS. Receptors and synapses. In: Carpenter RHS, ed. Neurophysiology. Baltimore: University Park Press, 1984:47–81.
11. Carr H. Head's theory of cutaneous sensibility. Psychol Rev 1916; 23:262–279.
12. Cauna N, Mannan G. The structure of the human digital Pacinian corpuscles (corpuscula lamellosa) and its functional significance. J Anat 1958; 92:1–20.
13. Chambers MR, Andres KH, Duering M, Iggo A. The structure and function of the slowly adapting Type II mechanoreceptor in hairy skin. Q J Exp Physiol 1972; 57:417.
14. Chapman LF, Dingman HF, Ginsberg SP. Failure of systemic analgesic agents to alter the absolute sensory threshold for the simple detection of pain. Brain 1965; 88:1011–1022.
15. Daniel RK, Terzis JK. Structure and function of the peripheral nerve. In: Daniel RK, Terzis JK, eds. Reconstructive microsurgery. Boston: Little, Brown, 1977:295–319.
16. Davis JS, Kitlowski EA. Regeneration of nerves in skin grafts and skin flaps. Am J Surg 1934; 24:501–544.
17. Davis L. The return of sensation to transplanted skin. Surg Gynecol Obstet 1934; 59:533–543.
18. Dellon AL. Reinnervation of denervated Meissner corpuscles. A sequential histological study in the monkey following fascicular nerve repair. J Hand Surg 1976; 1:98–109.
19. Dellon AL. Evaluation of sensibility and re-education of sensation in the hand. Baltimore: Williams & Wilkins, 1981:193–246.
20. Dellon AL, Curtis RM, Edgerton MT. Evaluating recovery of sensation in the hand following nerve injury. Johns Hopkins Med J 1972; 130:235.
21. Donaldson HH. On the temperature sense. Mind 1885; 10:399–416.
22. Duggan AW, Hall JG, Headly PM. Morphine, enkephalin and the substancia gelatinosa. Nature 1976; 264:456.
23. Dykes RW. Sensory receptors. In: Daniel RK, Terzis JK, eds. Reconstructive microsurgery. Boston: Little, Brown, 1977:320–333.
24. Dykes RW, Terzis JK. Reinnervation of glabrous skin in baboons: Properties of cutaneous mechanoreceptors subsequent to nerve crush. J Neurophysiol 1979; 42:1461–1478.

25. Erlanger J, Gasser HS, eds. Electrical signs of nervous activity. Philadelphia: University of Pennsylvania Press, 1937:34–78.
26. Gammon GD, Starr I. Studies on the relief of pain by counter-irritation. J Clin Invest 1941; 20:13–20.
27. Geldard FA. The human senses, ed 2. New York, 1972.
28. Glees P, Mohuiddin A, Smith AG. Transplant of Pacinian bodies in the brain and thigh of the cat. Acta Anat (Basel) 1949; 7:213–224.
29. Goldscheider A. Die specifische energie der temperaturenerven. Mh Prakt Derm 1884; 3:198–208.
30. Goldstein A. Opioid peptides (endorphins) in pituitary and brain. Science 1976; 193:1081.
31. Granit R. Muscle receptors and their reflexes. In: Granit R, ed. Receptors and sensory perception. New Haven: Yale University Press, 1967:191–233.
32. Guyton AC. Functional organization of the human body and control of the "internal environment." In: Guyton AC, ed. Textbook of medical physiology, ed 6. Philadelphia: WB Saunders, 1981:2–11.
33. Guyton AC. Organization of the nervous system. Basic function of synapses. In: Guyton AC, ed. Textbook of medical physiology, ed 6. Philadelphia: WB Saunders, 1981:560–576.
34. Guyton AC. Sensory receptors and their basic mechanisms of action. In: Guyton AC, ed. Textbook of medical physiology, ed 6. Philadelphia: WB Saunders, 1981:588–596.
35. Guyton AC, ed. Textbook of medical physiology, ed 6. Philadelphia: WB Saunders, 1981:588–592.
36. Guyton AC. Somatic sensations: I. The mechanoreceptive sensations. In: Guyton AC, ed. Textbook of medical physiology, ed 6. Philadelphia: WB Saunders, 1981:597–610.
37. Harrington T, Merzenich MM. Neural coding in the sense of touch: Human sensations of skin indentation compared with the response of slowly adapting mechanoreceptive afferents innervating the hairy skin of monkeys. Exp Brain Res 1970; 10:251.
38. Head H. The afferent nervous system from a new aspect. Brain 1905; 28:99–116.
39. Hering E. Der temperatursinin. In: Hermann's Handbook der Physiologie. III. Sinnesphysiologie. Leipzig. 1879:415–439.
40. Hughes J. Isolation of endogenous compound from the brain with pharmacological properties similar to morphine. Brain Res 1975; 88:295.
41. Hutchinson J, Tough JS, Wyburn GM. Regeneration of sensation in graft skin. Br J Surg 1949; 2:82–94.
42. Iggo A, Muir AR. The structure and function of a slowly adapting touch corpuscle in hairy skin. J Physiol (Lond) 1969; 200:763–796.
43. Janig W. Morphology of rapidly and slowly adapting mechanoreceptors in the hairless skin of the cat's hind foot. Brain Res 1968; 28:100–115.
44. Jones EG. The nervous tissue. In: Weiss L, ed. Cell and tissue biology: A textbook of histology, ed 6. Baltimore: Urban & Schwarzenberg, 1988:324–334.
45. Knibestol M, Vallbo AB. Single unit analysis of mechanoreceptor activity from human glabrous skin. Acta Physiol Scand 1970; 80:178–195.
46. Krause W. Ueber nervenendigungen. Z Rat Med 1939; 5:28–43.
47. Kredel FE, Evans JP. Recovery of sensation in denervated pedicle and free skin grafts. Arch Neurol Psychiatr 1933; 29:1203–1221.
48. Lowenstein WR. Biological transducers. Sci Am 1960; 203:98.
49. Mannerfelt L. Evaluation of functional sensation of skin grafts in the hand area. Br J Surg 1962; 15: 136–154.
50. McIntyre AK. Afferent limb of the myotatic reflex arc. Nature 1951; 168:168–169.
51. Meissner G. Beitrage zur Anatomie und Physiologie der Haut. Leipzig: Voss, 1853.
52. Melzack R, Wall PD. Pain mechanisms: A new theory. Science 1965; 150:971–979.
53. Merkel F. Tastzellen und Tastkorperchen bie den haustheiren und beim menschen. Arch Mikr Anat 1875; 11:636–652.
54. Merton PA. Slowly conducting muscles spindle afferents. Acta Physiol Scand 1953; 29:87–88.
55. Mountcastle VB. The problem of sensing and the neural coding of sensory events. In: Quarton GC, Melnechuk T, Schmitt FO, eds. The neurosciences. New York: Rockefeller University Press, 1967:6: 393–408.
56. Mountcastle VB, ed. Medical physiology, ed 13. St Louis: CV Mosby, 1974:285–306.
57. Mountcastle VB, ed. Medical physiology, ed 14. St Louis: CV Mosby, 1980:327–347.
58. Mountcastle VB, ed. Medical physiology, ed 14. St Louis: CV Mosby, 1980:336–338.
59. Muller J. Handbuch der physiologie des menschen, ed 2. Coblenz, 1838.
60. Munger BL. Patterns of organization of peripheral sensory receptors. In: Lowenstein WR, ed. Handbook of sensory physiology. I. Principles of receptor physiology. New York: Springer, 1971:524–558.
61. Nathan PW. The gate-control theory of pain: A critical review. Brain 1976; 99:123–158.

62. Pacini F. Nuovi organi scorperti nel corpo umano. Ciro, Pistoia, 1840.
63. Ponten B. Grafted skin: Observations on innervation and other qualities. Acta Chir Scand 1960 [suppl]; 257:1–75.
64. Ridley A. A biopsy study of the innervation of forearm skin grafted to the finger tip. Brain 1970; 93: 547–554.
65. Riley WH. A study of the temperature sense. J Nerv Ment Dis 1894; 21:549–566.
66. Ruffini A. Di un nuovo organo nervose terminale e sull presenza dei corpuscoli Golgi-Mazzoni nel connettivo sottocutaneo dei polpastrelli delle dita delf'uomo. Atti del Academia nazionale dei lincei (Memorie) 1891; 7:395–410.
67. Schmidt RF. Somatovisceral sensibility. In: Schmidt RF, ed. Fundamentals of sensory physiology, second corrected edition. New York: Springer, 1981:81–125.
68. Shaffer JM, Cleveland F. Delayed suture of sensory nerves of the hand. Ann Surg 1950; 131:556–563.
69. Sherrington CS. Integrative action of the nervous system. Silliman Memorial Lectures. New Haven: Yale University Press, 1906:412.
70. Sinclair DC. Cutaneous sensation and the doctrine of specific energy. Brain 1955; 78:584–614.
71. Sinclair DC, ed. Mechanisms of cutaneous sensation. New York: Oxford University Press, 1981:152–236.
72. Spencer PS, Schaumburg HH. An ultrastructural study of the inner core of the Pacinian corpuscle. J Neurocytol 1975; 2:217.
73. Sunderland S. Capacity of reinnervated muscles to function efficiently after prolonged denervation. Arch Neurol Neurosurg Psychiatry 1950; 64:755–771.
74. Sunderland S. Nerves and nerve injuries. Edinburgh: Churchill-Livingstone, 1968:366–401.
75. Talbot WH, Darian-Smith I, Kornhuber HH, Mountcastle VB. The sense of flutter vibration: Comparison of the human capacity with response patterns of mechanoreceptive afferents from the monkey hand. J Neurophysiol 1968; 31:301.
76. Terzis JK. Functional aspects of reinnervation of free skin grafts. Plast Reconstr Surg 1976; 58:142–156.
77. Terzis JK. Functional aspects of cutaneous reinnervation. PhD thesis, McGill University, 1980.
78. Terzis JK, Dykes RW. Reinnervation of glabrous skin in baboons: Properties of cutaneous mechanoreceptors subsequent to nerve transection. J Neurophysiol 1980; 44:1214–1225.
79. Terzis JK, Dykes RW, Turnbull BG. Properties of mechanoreceptive fibers serving skin grafts transferred to the hands of adult baboons (Papio anubis). J Physiol 1984; 357:1–22.
80. von Frey M. Beitrage zur physiologie des schmerzsinns. Ber Sachs Ges Wiss Math-Phys 1894; 46:185–196, 283–296.
81. von Frey M. The distribution of afferent nerve fibers in the skin. JAMA 1906; 47:645.
82. Weddell G. The anatomy of cutaneous sensibility. Br Med Bull 1945; 3:167–172.
83. Woodhall B, Beebe GW. Peripheral nerve regeneration: A follow-up study of 3635 World War II injuries. Veterans Administration Medical Monograph. Washington DC: US Govt. Printing Office 1956:309.
84. Wynn WH. Counter-irritation. Practitioner 1947; 158:185–190.
85. Zotterman Y. Touch, pain and tickling: an electrophysiological investigation on cutaneous sensory nerves. J Physiol 1939; 95:1–28.

II

INJURY, DEGENERATION, AND REGENERATION

7 Injury, Degeneration, and Regeneration

7

Injury, Degeneration, and Regeneration

Göran Lundborg
Nils Danielsen

AUTHORS' KEY POINTS

- Peripheral nerve regeneration is a complex biological process that involves not only the nerve cell but also other non-neuronal cell components such as Schwann cells, fibroblasts, endothelial cells, and macrophages.
- The survival of the neuron and the regeneration of its process, the axon, depend on certain active biomolecules. Some of these molecules have trophic influences on nerve cells; one example of such a neurotrophic factor is nerve growth factor (NGF). Other substances stimulate the neuron to produce neurites (ie, to regenerate); an example of a neurite-promoting factor is the glycoprotein laminin. Several other active biomolecules have neurotrophic or neurite-promoting effects on neurons.
- Experimental nerve repair techniques such as tubulization have proved to be very useful tools as attempts have been made to understand the complex process of nerve regeneration. Future research regarding nerve regeneration will require both in vitro and in vivo techniques.

From a biological standpoint, the issue of neuronal damage and regeneration is complex. The neuron represents one enormously elongated nerve cell, the cell body of which is situated within the central nervous system (for motor neurons in the anterior horn of the spinal cord) or in the peripheral nervous system (for sensory neurons in the dorsal root ganglion). The cell body's extended process, containing as much as 90% of its total axoplasmic volume, is situated within the peripheral nervous system. A lesion of the axon, which divides the neuron into two parts, has immediate as well as long-term consequences for the distal and proximal components, including the nerve cell body. The only method of restoring lost cellular components is by producing a new axon—a process that puts enormous requirements on the metabolic potential of the nerve cell body. Of considerable importance, this process involves the production and advancement of axonal sprouts growing towards distal targets.

When a nerve trunk is severed, all axons are divided, separating proximal and distal stumps. Since distal parts cannot survive without connection to the cell body, they disintegrate and disappear. The regeneration process does not include mitosis and proliferation of nerve cells. While the total nerve-cell number is unaltered, the existing cells do their best to regain original axoplasmic volume. However, the remaining cell components in the nerve trunk present quite another picture: Schwann cells and fibroblasts proliferate, macrophages assemble, and endothelial cells proliferate and form new intraneural vessels. Thus, two completely different cellular procedures take place simultaneously. Restoration of original neuronal microstructure occurs, and proliferation of all other cellular components takes place. This process makes healing of neural injuries unique compared to other tissues (eg, tendons, bones, and connective tissue).

While the biology of nerve regeneration is very special in terms of its complexity, the resulting functional outcome of nerve repair is often unsatisfactory. Since regenerating axons must advance over long distances to peripheral targets, delays in reinnervation result in irreversible damage to peripheral target structures. Misdirection of regenerating axons may be followed by incorrect reinnervation of targets, a phenomenon that has serious functional consequences.

Clinical Significance

The two factors of time from injury to nerve repair and axon alignment are significant with regard to the functional results of nerve repair.

COMPONENTS OF NERVE INJURIES

Considering the complex anatomy of the peripheral nerve trunk, it is natural to consider that a lesion may affect, in addition to the axon, a number of other cell and tissue components (Fig. 7-1). Inflammation of, or a slight compression injury of, a nerve trunk interferes with intraneural microcirculation, causing an anoxic or hypoxic state within the endoneural space. Thus, functional disturbances are induced in axons that are not structurally damaged. While ischemia may be reversible immediately once compression is released, if edema is induced in nerve, microvascular disturbances may persist for longer times. A more prominent compression lesion may induce local damage to myelin sheaths, resulting in conduction disturbances or conduction blocks at specific levels. The axon itself may remain intact. More severe injuries interrupt axon continuity, resulting in degeneration of the distal segment; if endoneural tubes, perineurium, or epineurium is damaged, the regeneration process may be considerably complicated.

Clinical Significance

Both functional (primarily ischemia) and structural components of neural injury can be identified. The extent of nerve recovery depends, to a large extent, on the severity of axonal and neural connective tissue disruption.

CLASSIFICATION OF NERVE INJURIES

Nerve injuries are associated with many different factors (eg, ischemia, burns, mechanical forces). A variety of classification systems of injury severity have been devised.

Seddon introduced a *functional* classification, describing three stages of nerve injury.[162–164] *Neurapraxia* refers to a local conduction block. The continuity of axons is preserved, as is the excitability of nerve structures distal to the lesion. According to Seddon's original classification, neurapraxia includes complete motor paralysis, while there is usually substantial sparing of sensory and sympathetic functions.[164] This phenomenon is explained by differences in vulnerability to compression by large and thin nerve fibers.[29,113] It corresponds to an acute local demyelinating block as seen after compression injury.[40,41,133] Examples of such nerve injuries are "Saturday-night palsy," representing high radial nerve palsy, and nerve injuries occurring after tourniquets have been inflated to excessive pressures. Such conduction

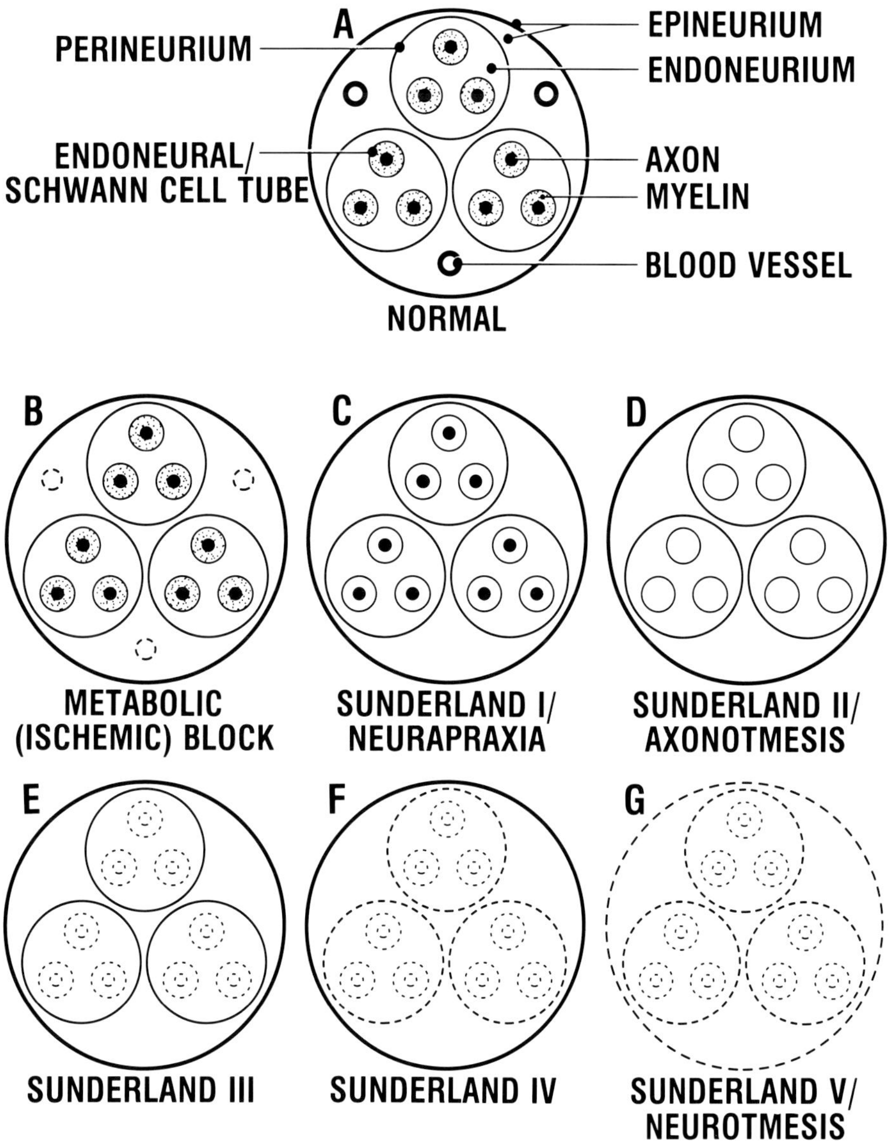

Figure 7–1. *(**A**) Normal nerve with three fascicles and three vessels. (**B**) Metabolic (ischemic) block where vessels have been obliterated but remaining structures are intact. (**C**) Sunderland class I injury; Seddon, neurapraxia. Myelin is gone but fascicles are still present. (**D**) Sunderland class II injury; Seddon, axonotmesis. Axons and myelin are gone but endoneural tubes are preserved. (**E**) Sunderland class III injury. Endoneural tubes are gone but the perineurium is preserved. (**F**) Sunderland class IV injury. Perineurium is gone but the epineurium remains. (**G**) Sunderland class V injury; Seddon, neurotmesis. All connective tissue coats of nerve, including epineurium, have been damaged.*

blocks persist until local myelin repair occurs, restoring excitability and conduction of nerve fibers over the injured segment. This process usually requires weeks to months.

The next level of nerve injury described by Seddon is termed *axonotmesis*, implying a loss of axonal continuity at the site of the lesion. The endoneural tubes, however, remain intact. Such a lesion corresponds to an advanced nerve compression injury or crush or traction injury severe enough to interrupt axonal continuity, resulting in Wallerian degeneration. In such situations the time required for functional recovery corresponds to the time required for axons to regenerate and reinnervate distal targets. In axonotmesis the endoneural tubes, guiding axonal regrowth, remain intact[62] and the prognosis for reinnervation of correct targets is good. However, irreversible damage to muscle tissue may occur prior to the time required for reinnervation.

Neurotmesis connotes total severance of nerve or destruction of its interior structures (perineurium, endoneural tubes) to the extent that the interior anatomy of the nerve trunk is totally disorganized over the area of injury.[164] Spontaneous regeneration does not occur in such situations; operative repair is required.

Injuries of peripheral nerve trunks seen in clinical practice are often of a mixed character and do not always fall within one of Seddon's definitions. Sunderland introduced a more detailed classification based on tissue pathoanatomy of the various components of the nerve trunk.[175,176] Injuries of the first and second degree correspond to Seddon's groups neurapraxia and axonotmesis, respectively. Since severe nerve trauma may result in a mixed pathoanatomical picture, depending on fascicular topography and the vulnerability of fiber groups of various size to trauma, these types may occur simultaneously.

The more severe nerve injuries (neurotmesis, according to Seddon) are divided into subgroups by Sunderland depending on the continuity or discontinuity of individual connective tissue components. Sunderland's third-degree injury connotes loss of axonal continuity as well as of continuity of endoneural tubes; the perineurium remains intact, however. Such third-degree injury may be seen following severe compression or traction trauma where the continuity and orientation of endoneural tubes are lost. Such injuries are usually accompanied by intrafascicular bleeding, edema, and ischemia resulting in the development of intrafascicular fibrosis. Sunderland's fourth-degree injury defines loss of continuity of the perineurium while the epineurium is preserved. The fifth-degree injury indicates severance of the entire nerve trunk.

PROXIMAL CHANGES

Severance of axons is followed by characteristic structural changes in corresponding cell bodies.[56,57,89,90] Since the lesion causes loss of large amounts of axoplasmic volume, the cell body has to prepare for replacement of the lost axoplasm. Changes include swelling of the cell body, displacement of the nucleus to the periphery, and disappearance of basophilic material from the cytoplasm (chromatolysis). Ultrastructurally, chromatolysis is due to the disorganization of the structure of rough endoplasmic reticulum.[57] The chemical changes include changes in RNA and protein metabolism, as demonstrated by increased RNA and protein content in regenerating neurons.[16] Since changes in protein synthesis occur, changes in axonal transport could also be expected. There is a shift of materials towards components necessary for the construction of the axon.[56] Decreased amounts of axonally transported components associated with synaptic transmission have been demonstrated.[15,53,77] Components associated with the regeneration process (ie, proteins and glycoproteins) increase.[53,54]

Several explanations have been proposed for the cell body's reaction following severance of an axon. It has been suggested that the exclusion of neurotrophic substances, normally produced by target cells and transported by retrograde axonal transport to nerve cell bodies, may produce such a reaction.[64,69,144] Theoretically, retrograde transport of substances produced by proliferating non-neuronal cells at the site of injury may also help to induce the signal.

Clinical Significance

Specific, predictable changes occur in the nerve cell body following nerve injury. The type, extent, and level of injury will directly affect the magnitude of these changes.

INITIATION AND ORGANIZATION OF AXONAL OUTGROWTH

Proximal to the lesion, axons degenerate for a distance of one or several internodal segments, leaving the corresponding "endoneural tube" (the endoneural connective tissue sheath plus the basal lamina of the Schwann cell) an empty cylinder.[147,176] Following an initial delay, varying in time with species and severity of lesion, each proximal stump sends out a number of terminal or collateral sprouts, which advance distally (Fig. 7-2).[176] *Collateral sprouts* arise from a proximal node of Ranvier where axons are still intact, advancing distally on the inside of the basal lamina along the tube. *Terminal sprouts* arise from the tip of remaining axons. The sprouts, arising from one myelinated axon and advancing inside one endoneural tube, constitute a *regeneration unit* (Figs. 7-3, 7-4).[96,122–

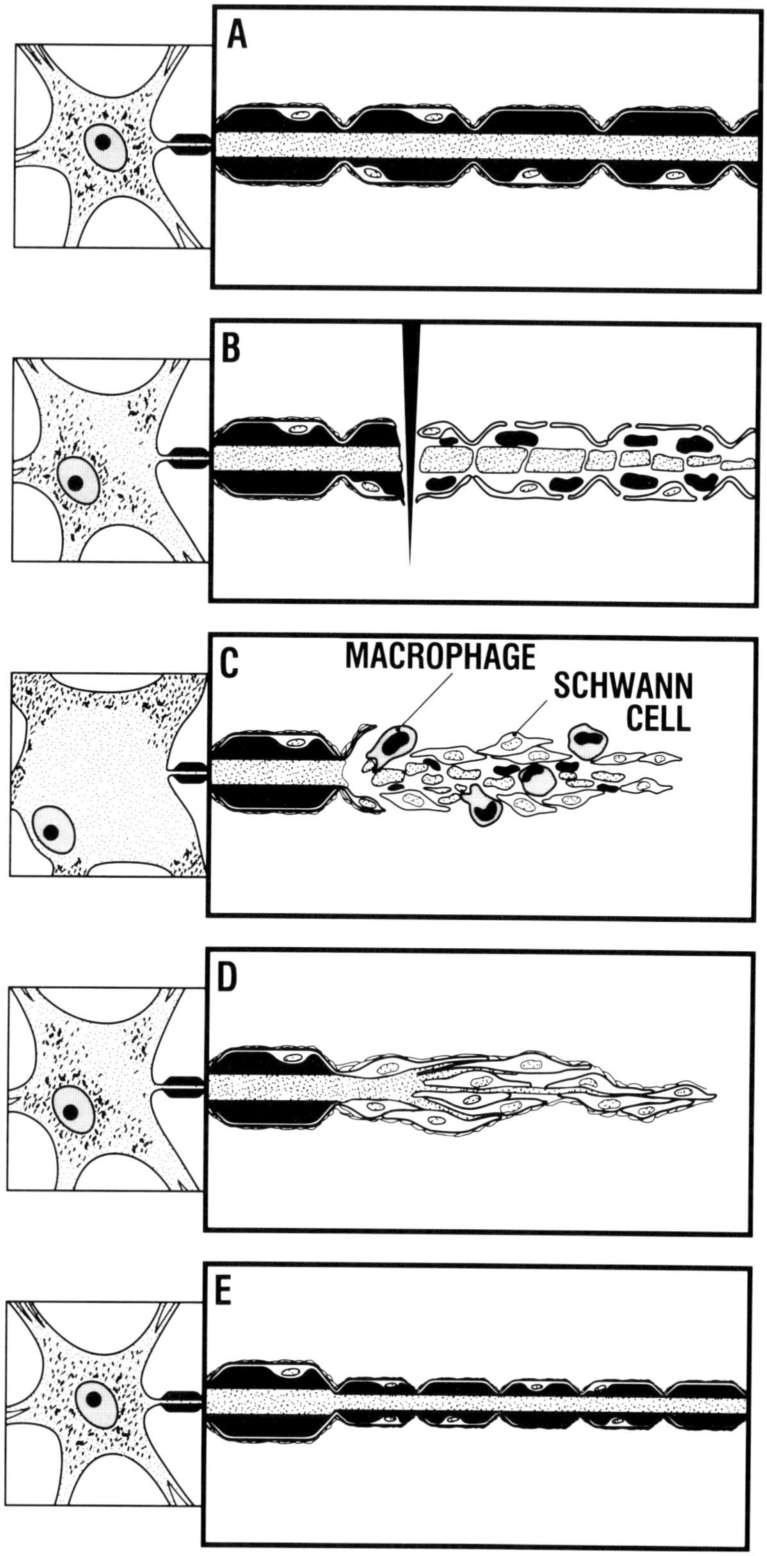

Figure 7–2. *Degeneration and regeneration of myelinated fibers. (**A**) Normal nerve. (**B**) Following transection, initial changes consist of distal fragmentation of axon and myelin sheath. Proximally, degeneration takes place to the nearest node of Ranvier. (**C**) Distally, Schwann cells proliferate. Macrophages and Schwann cells phagocytose debris. (**D**) Distally, Schwann cells occupy the endoneural tubes forming the bands of Bungner. Sprouting occurs from the proximal axonal stump. Advancing sprouts then become embedded in Schwann cell cytoplasm. (**E**) Axons make connections with their peripheral targets, and nerve fibers mature. Sprouts that do not make appropriate connections atrophy and disappear. In the cell body, changes include swelling, migration of the nucleus to the periphery, and condensation of basophilic material (chromatolysis).*

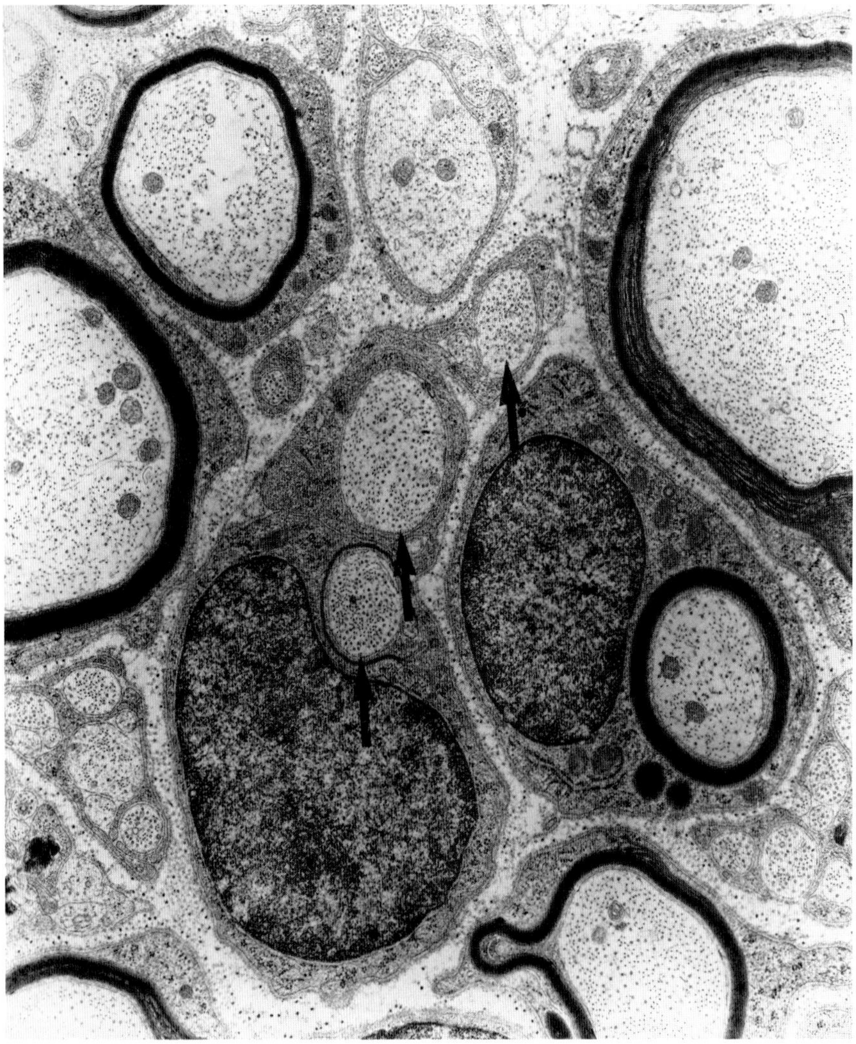

Figure 7–3. *Advancing sprouts (arrows) enclosed within one Schwann cell. One sprout is undergoing myelination.*

[124,195] Over the weeks following repair, the average number of axons within regeneration units diminishes. As regeneration proceeds, one of them usually matures and becomes myelinated, while the others disappear. The reduction in total number of sprouts occurs as some axons make connections with peripheral targets, thereby receiving trophic substances that lead to maturation.

Growth Cone

In in vitro systems, the most distal parts of neurites develop an area of swelling from which several microspikes or filopodia arise: a *growth cone.* These filopodia are constantly moving, apparently exploring the local microenvironment. The microspikes contain a considerable amount of actin, which probably plays an important role in mobility. Filopodias may extend and retract in a matter of minutes. If they adhere to a structure, the tension generated causes the growth cone to turn toward the point of attachment.[20,44,58,81,82,199] Growth cones have also been observed in vivo in certain experimental systems (for instance, in frogs).[67,112,150] The growth cones and the microspike movements play an essential role in determining the orientation and growth direction of sprouts. The adhesiveness and molecular composition of the substrate, including the presence of neurite-promoting factors, may be the determining factors.

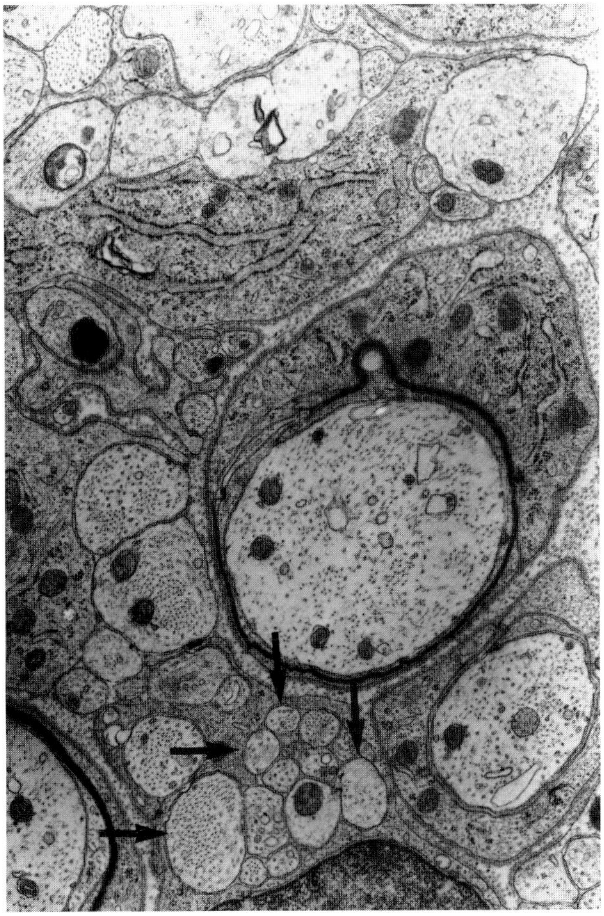

Figure 7–4. *Regenerating sprouts in the silicone chamber model. Numerous sprouts (arrows) originating from one parent axon constitute a regeneration unit.*

Clinical Significance

Terminal sprouts, regeneration units, the growth cone, and filopodia are key to orientation and growth of regenerating axons following complete nerve injury. Axons that explore the environment and make appropriate peripheral connections are stimulated to mature; others are resorbed.

Compartmentation

Close to the site of injury, the proximal stump of a severed nerve becomes separated into numerous "minifascicles" to replace original large fascicles. This phenomenon, extensively described in ultrastructural studies,[124,125] includes the encirculation of groups of fibers by endoneural fibroblasts. Perineural-like structures called minifascicles are formed. The stimulus to such compartmentation may be a disturbance of the endoneural environment due to perineural damage. It is believed that the formation of these fascicles expresses the need for rapid restitution of a normal endoneural environment. In the silicone chamber model used for nerve regeneration (a silicone tube bridging a 10-mm gap in the rat sciatic nerve), nerves regenerate but do not form minifascicles.[195] This is in contrast to similar experiments using tubes made of Gore-Tex with 5- to 30-μm pores in the tube wall; in these experiments, the regenerating nerve formed numerous minifascicles.[36] It has been concluded that the impermeable silicone chamber can act as an artificial perineural layer.

Distal Nerve Stump

When axons are transected, distal parts rapidly disintegrate, undergoing *wallerian degeneration*. The microtubuli and neurofilaments of the axoplasm disintegrate due to a proteolytic process,[95,156–159,185] a calcium-dependent process mediated by calcium-activated enzymes in the axoplasm. Probably, the increased permeability of axonal membranes to calcium, as well as the influx of calcium from the transected axonal ends, causes disintegration of neurofilaments. Although this process starts within hours after transection, morphological changes in the distal stump are visible only after 2 to 3 days. Following initial axon swelling, myelin breaks up into fragments. Over time, the myelin is phagocytized by Schwann cells and invading macrophages. Although disposal of all myelin fragments may require several months, the most obvious morphological changes take place within the first week after axotomy.

Clinical Significance

Predictable components of wallerian degeneration include initial disintegration of axons in the distal stump, followed by dissolution of myelin. Myelin is then phagocytized by Schwann cells and macrophages.

Non-Neuronal Cell Reactions

After nerve severance, increased Schwann cell mitotic activity is seen. Schwann cells proliferate rapidly, forming columns (*bands of Büngner*). The multiplication of Schwann cells peaks on the third day after injury and thereafter slowly declines during the following weeks, as long as reinnervation does not occur. A second wave of Schwann cell mitosis occurs during the regenerative phase. The Schwann cell columns are important pathways for the regenerating sprouts. Besides constituting guidelines for regenerating axons, Schwann cells also synthesize trophic factors to support neuronal survival and axonal growth.

Connective tissue cells of the distal stump change appearance and function following injury. In the endoneurium and perineurium there are extensive changes in the distribution of collagen types and fibronectin.[152] Collagen production in the endoneurium probably is due to both fibroblast activity and Schwann cell activity.[13,179] New endoneural collagen is formed external to the basal lamina of the Schwann cells, causing a thickening of the endoneural tube. With extended intervals to reinnervation, the collagen becomes denser and the endoneural tubes narrower.

Clinical Significance

Schwann cells multiply and form columns that appear to influence and stimulate the direction and magnitude of axonal growth. Endoneural collagen production increases following injury, causing progressive, time-related shrinkage of distal tubules.

Axonal Growth in the Distal Stump

The advancement of axons over the zone of injury is a critical process that may determine the success or failure of functional regeneration. Once regenerating axons reach the distal nerve stump, they may approach a Schwann cell column, grow at random into the connective tissue, or extend outside the distal nerve stump. If they do not reach a column of Schwann cells, the axons extend only a short distance. Initially, sprouts are located on the inner surface of the basal lamina. Later they are embedded in the cytoplasm of Schwann cells. The basal lamina that originally surrounds the Schwann cell column may rupture and disappear as the diameter of regenerating fibers increases.[173] Initially, the total number of axons in the distal stump may exceed the number in the proximal stump as a result of excess formation of sprouts. With time the number decreases, however, as sprouts make peripheral connections. Axons reaching their targets mature and increase in diameter, probably as a result of trophic substances supplied from target organs.[7,61,153]

Once regenerating axons reach a Schwann cell, a signal is established that initiates the myelinating procedure.[140,172] The instruction to the Schwann cell to form myelin is based on a genetic code located in the cell body of the corresponding neuron. Regenerating previously myelinated axons are ensheathed with myelin when growing into unmyelinated nerves. Previously myelinated fibers remain unmyelinated when regenerating into distal nerve stumps that originally contained myelinated fibers.[5,6,172,188–190] *Thus, each neuron is coded to be myelinated or nonmyelinated.* The instruction to the Schwann cell to form myelin requires a direct axon–Schwann cell contact.[140]

A second phase of Schwann cell proliferation occurs when regenerating axons reach Schwann cells,[136] a procedure that precedes the formation of myelin lamellae. It seems that neuronal regulation of myelinogenesis involves surface membrane interaction between the plasma membrane of the axon and the Schwann cell.[172]

The outgrowth rate of axons is different depending on level and species. After transection and suture, the outgrowth rate is always worse than after crush injury. The regeneration rate in experimental animals may be as high as 3 to 4 mm/day. The regeneration rate in humans is nonlinear, with gradually decreased regeneration rates in distal parts. The outgrowth rate in humans falls within the range of 1 to 2 mm/day.[19,164]

Clinical Significance

Once an axon reaches its target, it increases in diameter and matures. Whether it remains nonmyelinated or becomes myelinated depends on the original structure of the fiber. Axon regrowth rates depend on the magnitude and level of injury; average regrowth in adults is 1 to 2 mm/day.

FACTORS INFLUENCING AXONAL GROWTH

Axon regeneration can take place only if the nerve cell body has survived the trauma and if the substrate, or growth terrain, is suitable for axonal advancement. Also, the substrate must contain factors offering directional guidance for growth. Such conditions involve the combined action of several conditions and factors.

Neurotrophic Factors

The survival of nerve cells depends on a trophic influence from peripheral target cells. These target cells normally supply chemical signals to their innervating cells. The signals are transmitted by retrograde axonal transport along the axon and used to sustain essential activities of the nerve cell body.[143,181,182,184] Such signals are provided by neurotrophic factors, synthesized by the target tissue, or by cell components of the nerve trunk itself, such as Schwann cells.

Most studies regarding the effects of neurotrophic factors have been done in vitro. The well-known protein nerve growth factor (NGF) has formed an outstanding model for neurotrophic factors.[66,84,85,87,88,165] This factor selectively enhances the survival and outgrowth of neurites from embryonic neurons of sympathetic and sensory ganglia. Originally, NGF was isolated from sarcoma tumors in mice and the submandibular gland of adult male mice.[86–88] In vivo there is evidence that sources of NGF may be peripheral tissues innervated by sensory and sympathetic neurons,[9] as well as glial cells and Schwann cells of the nervous system.[45,183] NGF occurs normally in animal nerves.[149]

The first evidence that neurotrophic factors were present in vivo during nerve regeneration was obtained using the silicone chamber model for nerve regeneration. The chamber rapidly becomes filled with fluid. Nerve stump–derived fluid has been tested for neurotrophic activity using a combined in vivo/in vitro technique (Fig. 7-5). These experiments demonstrated that the chamber fluid contained neurotrophic activity for all three nerve components of peripheral nerve (ie, sympathetic, sensory, and spinal cord neurons).[93,94,102] The highest neurotrophic activity is noted 1 to 3 days after chamber implantation; activity declines subsequently (Fig. 7-6).

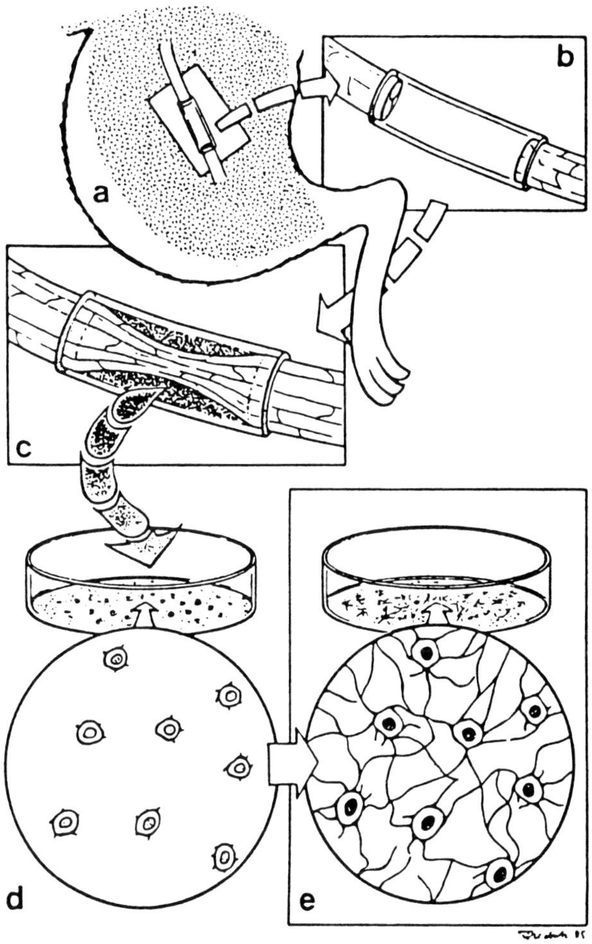

Figure 7–5. *The combined in vivo/in vitro approach. (**A, B**) Sciatic nerves of rats were transected and the nerve stumps implanted into a silicone chamber. (**C**) After varying time intervals, fluid was removed from the chamber, and dilutions of the fluid were tested on neuronal in vitro systems for (**D**) neurotrophic or (**E**) neurite-promoting activity. Similar experiments have been done to demonstrate that chamber fluid contains factors that affect Schwann cell behavior. (From Lundborg G. Nerve injury and repair. Edinburgh: Churchill-Livingstone, 1988, with permission.)*

With the introduction of immunohistochemical and molecular biological techniques, new information has been obtained regarding the occurrence and action of NGF during nerve injury and regeneration. Normally, the neuron demand for NGF is

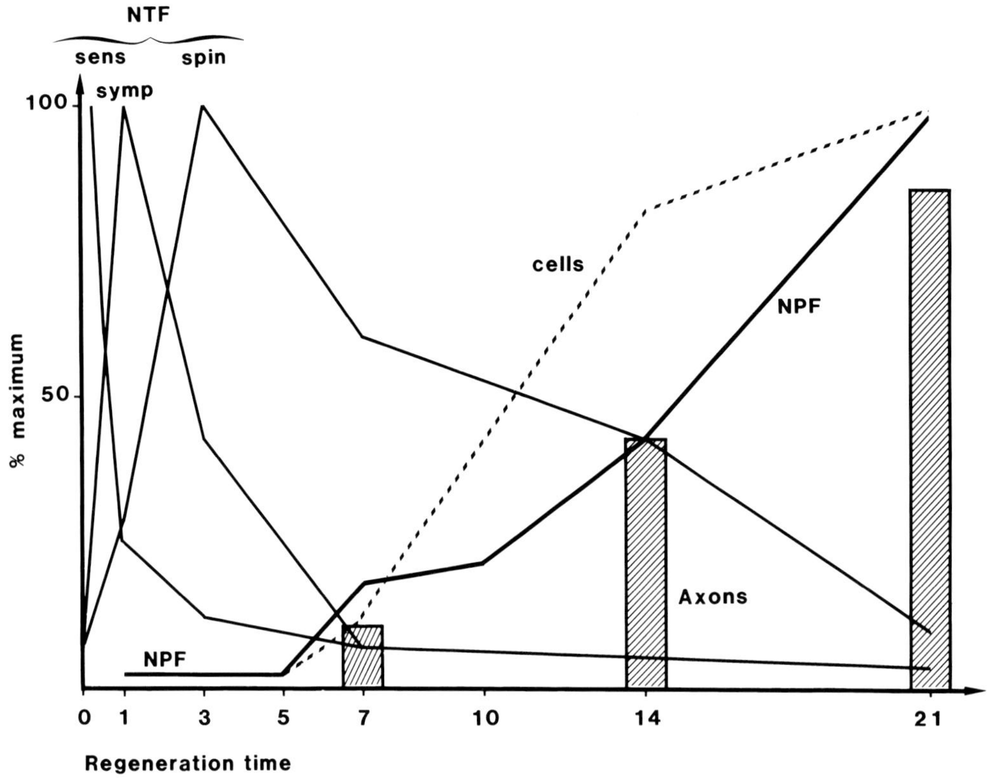

Figure 7–6. *Composite representation of temporal events in the silicone chamber model for nerve regeneration. The chamber fluid contains neurotrophic factors (NTF) for all three nerve components of the peripheral nerve: sensory (sens), sympathetic (symp), and spinal cord neurons (spin). The content of neurotrophic activity peaks within 1 to 3 days after chamber implantation. The content of neurite-promoting factors (NPF) such as laminin starts to increase after 5 to 7 days and coincides with the migration of cells into the fibrin matrix that forms between the two nerve stumps. (From Varon S, Manthorpe M, Williams LR. Neuronotrophic and neurite-promoting factors and their clinical potentials. Dev Neurosci 1984;6:73–100, with permission.)*

satisfied by synthesis within the cells of the innervation territory.[70,178] When peripheral nerve is transected, the normal supply of NGF from the innervation territory is lost. In order to replace NGF, non-neuronal cells in the distal nerve stump (and in a short segment of the proximal nerve stump) produce NGF.[71] The areas producing NGF correspond with the areas undergoing Wallerian degeneration. Increased synthesis of NGF in non-neuronal cells is triggered by interleukin-1, released from invading macrophages.[91] These findings demonstrate the important role of multipotent macrophages, cells participating in myelin degradation as well as synthesis of neurotrophic factors. Nerve transection also induces the formation of NGF receptors located on the cell surfaces of Schwann cells that form the bands of Büngner.[177]

Thus, Schwann cells can produce both the NGF molecule and its receptor, suggesting an autocrine/paracrine function of NGF. This may also be a mechanism for the presentation of the NGF molecule to regenerating axons. The receptors initiated by transection of axons bind NGF to the surface of Schwann cells. When the axons advance along the Schwann cell surface, the factors can be transferred into the interior of the growth cones. In this way the receptor-bound NGF molecules act as substrates with both neurotrophic and haptotactic (chemotaxis on a surface) effects on regenerating axons.[177] A "track" of NGF molecules, which regenerating axons can follow, is formed on the surfaces of Schwann cells.

There are several other neurotrophic factors, most of which support both the survival of nerve cells and the outgrowth of neurites. For instance, ciliary neuronotrophic factor (CNTF) has been demonstrated in the eye of chick embryos, directed toward neurons of the ciliary ganglion.[1,11,107,109,110] Other neurotrophic factors have been demonstrated in extracts from heart[116] or "conditioned media" (media collected after exposure to cultures of Schwann cells).[182]

Another growth factor, fibroblast growth factor (FGF), has neurotrophic effects on certain neurons both in vitro and in vivo.[8,126,166,186,187] It is also a potent angiogenic factor and a mitogen for fibroblasts and endothelial cells,[55] as well as for peripheral and central glial cells.[79,137,171] Another known growth factor, somatomedin-C or insulinlike growth factor-1 (IGF-1), has been demonstrated in both the proximal and distal stumps of transected rat sciatic nerves.[65]

Clinical Significance

Neurotrophic factors, synthesized by target tissues, enhance the survival and outgrowth of nerve fibers. The protein nerve growth factor (NGF) is the best-known neurotrophic factor.

Neurite-Promoting Factors

The growth of neurites requires factors that promote their extension. Neurite-promoting factors may be bound to the surface of cells or tissue structures, they may be humoral, or they may be confined to the medium within the microenvironment. Media conditioned by glial cells, skeletal and heart muscle cells, and Schwannoma cultures contain neurite-promoting factors.[2,25,68,111] In addition to supporting survival of selected neurons, NGF has a neurite-promoting effect in vitro.[21] Substances of special interest that possess neurite-promoting effects are the glycoproteins fibronectin and laminin.[12,33,38,39,108,151,198] *Laminin,* a normal component of the basal lamina surrounding Schwann cells,[180] has a particularly strong neurite-promoting effect when its substratum is bound. Since laminin, which normally occurs in peripheral nerves, has a strong neurite-promoting effect in vitro, it is tempting to assume a similar mode of action in vivo, especially since the regenerating sprouts are located on the inner surface of the basal lamina. Definitive proof of this assumption is lacking, however.

In vivo and in vitro experiments have been used to demonstrate that the fluid accumulating in the silicone chamber model contains a high activity of the neurite-promoting factor laminin 2 to 3 weeks after chamber implantation.[92] The increase in laminin content coincides with the time of cellular and axonal migration into the chamber (see Fig. 7-6). Other studies have demonstrated that chamber fluid contains factors that promote Schwann cell adhesion, migration, and proliferation.[80]

Contact Guidance

Growing axons tend to follow surfaces or interfaces between various media. *Contact guidance,* as this process is called, can be stimulated by the boundary between solid structures and liquids, or between solid structures and gases.[191] In a medium lacking definite orientation, nerve processes follow random courses. In the presence of oriented interfaces, they are guided by the direction of the interfaces.

In experimental and clinical studies, contact guidance is probably a very important factor for axonal orientation and is perhaps the only one that can be addressed by the surgeon. Of special interest is the fact that a fibrin clot always forms between the two stumps of a cut nerve. A longitudinal orientation of stretch lines occurs in such clots as they shrink. This phenomenon explains why nerve fibers sometimes can cover extended gaps, growing along tissue structures in the local environment.

Chemotaxis and Neurotropism

Forssman and Ramon y Cajal noted that the axons of the proximal nerve stump of a severed nerve exhibit preferential growth toward a nerve graft or distal nerve stump, regardless of the alignment of the nerve fibers.[49,50,146,147] It was felt that the distal degenerating nerve stump produced a substance that, by the process of diffusion and establishing a concentration gradient, attracted and guided axons toward the distal nerve stump. The term *chemotaxis*, or *neurotropism*, was introduced, indicating a directional movement of an axon toward a distant source of a chemical emanation. Over the years this concept has been the subject of considerable controversy: some authors have doubted the existence of chemotaxis,[192] while others have claimed that the phenomenon occurs under well-defined experimental conditions, provided regeneration is not disturbed by other extrinsic influences.[59,60,98,101,129,131,132,141,161]

Chemotaxis is a well-known biological phenomenon occurring in different biological systems. White blood cells are attracted by bacterial products to areas of inflammation.[155] Also, the direction of movements of bacteria is influenced by molecules that set up a concentration gradient at a distance.[78] NGF exerts a chemotactic effect on growing embryonic sympathetic and sensory axons.[22,46,83] A dramatic example of the chemotactic response to NGF in tissue culture was presented by Gundersen and Barrett[59,60] and Gundersen.[58] When a micropipette containing NGF was placed near growing axons of neurons from chick dorsal root ganglion neurons and gently moved above the median surface, the axons rapidly (within 9–21 min) altered the direction of growth in response to the gradient of NGF. The proposed mechanism by which NGF molecules bind to NGF receptors on Schwann cell surfaces is a combination of contact guidance and neurotropism.[177]

Clinical Significance

There is increasing evidence that nerve regeneration is influenced both by contact guidance and by neurotropism (chemotaxis). The latter is the process by which axons are directed to a peripheral source of chemical emanation.

EXPERIMENTAL REGENERATION IN CHAMBER MODELS

Various biological chamber systems have proved useful for the purposes of analyzing the occurrence of neurotrophic and neurite-promoting factors following nerve damage in vivo (see above). The use of chamber systems has made it possible to manipulate the local microenvironment in order to study influences on regeneration. Chamber systems have made it possible to study the intrinsic mechanisms that regulate axonal growth in vivo. In all chamber experiments, tubes of various materials (eg, silicone, polyethylene, biodegradable polymers) are used to bridge gaps between proximal and distal nerve stumps of transected nerves (most often, the rat sciatic nerve).

Spatial–Temporal Progress of Regeneration

The spatial–temporal progress of regeneration has been examined in detail using the silicone chamber model.[195] Within the first day of implantation, the chamber becomes filled with a fluid that contains both neurotrophic and neurite-promoting factors. Next, a longitudinally oriented fibrin matrix connects the two nerve stumps. This acellular fibrin matrix forms between 3 and 7 days after chamber implantation. The matrix is then invaded by cells from both nerve stumps. The first cells to migrate into the fibrin matrix are circumferential perineural-like cells, probably of fibroblast origin. They are followed by vessels and Schwann cells. The two cell fronts meet at approximately 16 to 17 days (Fig. 7-7).[30,33,128] Axons migrate into the matrix behind the Schwann cell front. Myelination is the last process to occur in this model.

In an effort to enhance the generation of early fibrin matrix formation, silicone chambers have been prefilled with a dialyzed plasma solution.[193] This has induced the formation of a longitudinally oriented matrix that bridges the gap within 24 hours. Early fibrin matrix formation has been shown to stimulate significantly the ingrowth of all cellular elements.[193]

Clinical Significance

The sequence of nerve regeneration involves the formation of fluid containing neurotropic and neurotrophic factors, the formation of a fibrin matrix, and the invasion of fibroblasts, vessels, and Schwann cells, followed by axons, which are ultimately myelinated.

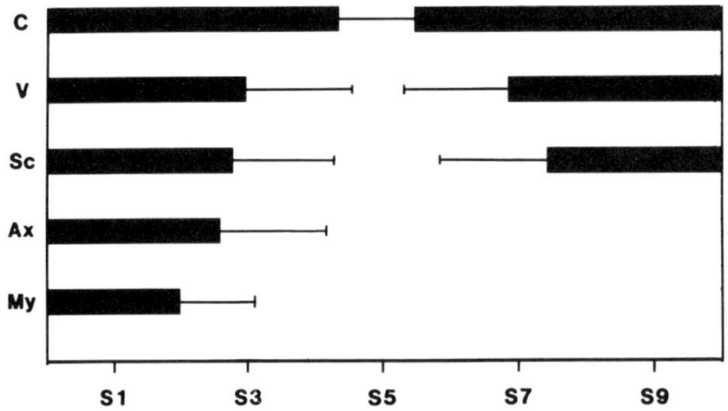

Figure 7–7. *Spatial advances of various cellular elements in phosphate-buffered saline prefilled silicone chambers. Regeneration time was 16 days. At this point the two cell fronts make contact. The silicone chamber model for nerve regeneration with a 16-day regeneration time makes it possible to test the effects of various drugs, prefillings, or other alterations of the chamber microenvironment on the migration into the chamber of each individual cell component.*[33,34,127,128,193] *Mean (n = 10) ± SD is shown. C; circumferential perineural-like cells; V, vessels; Sc, Schwann cells; Ax, axons; My, myelin. Abscissa S1 to S9 = cross-section at 1 to 9 mm from the proximal nerve stump. (From Danielsen N. Regeneration of the rat sciatic nerve in the silicone chamber model. Restor Neurol Neurosci 1990 [in press], with permission.)*

Importance of the Distal Nerve Stump

In the first experiments with the silicone chamber model, the importance of the distal nerve stump was tested.[97,100] It was found that regenerating axons bridged the chamber if the gap was 10 mm or less. Regeneration failed if the gap was increased to 15 mm or more, however. If the distal nerve stump was excluded from the chamber, regeneration was limited to only 4 to 5 mm. These findings have been confirmed in other chamber models.[32,160] It has been demonstrated that regeneration across gaps occurs only if the tissue in the distal opening is a segment of nerve.[154,196] Regeneration does not occur if the distal opening contains muscle, skin, or tendon. The influence of the distal nerve stump on regeneration is mediated by cellular or humoral factors. Schwann cell migration into the fibrin matrix is crucial for successful regeneration across gaps. Invasion of other cell types, such as fibroblasts, is insufficient to ensure regeneration.[196]

Other chamber experiments using semipermeable chambers have demonstrated that regeneration can occur in the absence of distal nerve stumps.[3] These chambers provide axons access to growth-promoting substances from the environment.

ORIENTATION OF AXONS

Tissue Specificity

Biological chamber systems have been used to investigate the question of whether regenerating axons are oriented preferentially toward nerve tissue. By the use of a modified mesothelial chamber system (a rectangular chamber, 2 × 6 × 12 mm) we demonstrated that regenerating axons cross chambers diagonally if distal nerve stumps are present.[98,101] If the distal stump is missing, axons grew only a few millimeters into the square-shaped chamber. In other studies, performed in the same time period, humoral factors were identified, emanating from the distal nerve stump. These factors had a neurotropic effect on regenerating axons.[139,141] Politis and coworkers used a Y-shaped silicone chamber system that provided regenerating axons a choice between two outlets.[139,141] In one experiment they replaced the distal nerve stump with slow-releasing pellets containing extracts from degenerating distal nerve stumps. They found that regenerating axons grew preferentially toward the pellets.

Other research groups directly challenged Weiss's old experiments with homologous aorta bifurcations by substituting Y-shaped chambers of various other materials, such as silicone. These experiments demonstrated that regenerating rat and primate axons preferred to grow toward nerve tissue.[99,103,132] A more detailed analysis using the rectangular mesothelial chamber has demonstrated that regenerating axons orient toward the distal nerve stump.[129–131]

Neurotropism exists in vivo. Nerve fibers orient and grow toward nerve tissue. Previous concepts of randomized growth and contact guidance are also supported, however, as both mechanisms (neurotropism and contact guidance) appear to be important for the orientation of regenerating axons.

Topographic Specificity

Y-chamber systems have also been used to demonstrate the phenomenon of the selective specificity of regenerating axons. Politis showed that regenerating axons of the rat peroneal nerve proximal stump preferred to grow toward the distal peroneal nerve stump rather than toward the distal tibial nerve stump.[138] Similar results have been presented by others.[161] However, experimental confirmation or demonstration of the underlying mechanisms for this phenomenon has not been provided.

End-Organ Specificity

It has been suggested that regenerating axons can discriminate between sensory and motor targets.[18] Later experiments have confirmed a preferential reinnervation of motor nerves by regenerating motor axons.[17] This phenomenon is probably due to a "pruning" mechanism in which regenerating motor axons grow toward several targets, and only those axons that reinnervate correct targets survive and mature; others are aborted.

ENHANCEMENT OF AXONAL GROWTH

Several experimental procedures other than operative manipulations have been tried to improve nerve regeneration. Both the systemic administration of substances and the local manipulation of the microenvironment have been attempted in an effort to improve nerve regrowth. In particular, biological chamber systems have proved useful in experiments where the local environment is altered.

Conditioning Lesion

If a nerve lesion is preceded by a "conditioning lesion" (crush or transection) applied 1 to 3 weeks earlier, regenerating fibers grow faster than if a conditioning lesion has not been performed.[63,117,119,120] An increase of more than 20% in axon outgrowth has followed a preliminary lesion 2 weeks earlier.[117–119,121] Forman demonstrated a stimulatory effect on sensory axons following conditioning lesions applied as recently as 2 days earlier.[48] A conditioning effect may also be induced by a chronic compression.[10]

Increases in the rate of axonal outgrowth may be explained by changes induced in cell bodies by priming lesions. A cell body response occurs that is an adaptation of intracellular metabolism to the metabolic requirements necessary for regeneration (eg, increased protein metabolism). There is also an increase in the production of rough endoplasmic reticulum, substrates containing or influencing the amount of enzymes that affect protein metabolism.[42,43] It is also possible that local events induced by the conditioning lesion account for increased axonal outgrowth,[28,47] perhaps by stimulation of non-neuronal cells and production by these cells of trophic or tropic factors.

Hormones

Experimental hyperthyroidism (administration of triiodothyronine, T_3 or L-thyroxine, T_4) has been shown to have positive effects on nerve regeneration (eg, accelerated regeneration and recovery).[24,114,115,174] However, conflicting results have been obtained indicating that experimental hyperthyroidism did not accelerate nerve regeneration.[27,52] Several of these studies can be questioned, since the doses used probably were too small to induce hyperthyroidism.[14,31] Administration of T_4 in doses adequate to induce hyperthyroidism, as indicated by reduced body growth, induced regeneration across a 15-mm gap in the rat sciatic nerve (this normally does not occur); stimulated outgrowth of axons from the proximal nerve stump was also seen.[31] Increased regeneration rates of motor fibers after T_4 administration have also been reported.[203] The mechanism by which hyperthyroidism stimulates regeneration may involve the regulation of the synthesis of specific proteins.

Other hormones have also been tested. The subcutaneous administration of growth hormone via implanted miniosmotic pumps has been shown to stimulate the regeneration rate of sensory neurons.[75] It has also been demonstrated that administration of testosterone accelerates axonal outgrowth and facilitates the regenerating fibers in reaching the distal nerve stump.[201,202,204] Testosterone probably increases the metabolic activity of hormone target neurons.

Electromagnetic Fields

It has been clearly demonstrated in various experimental systems that electrical stimulation (pulsed electromagnetic fields [PEMFs] or direct current [DC]) stimulates outgrowth of axons in vivo and in vitro.[72,134,135,142,145,167–169] The mechanism for these effects is unclear. Changes in ionic currents around growing fiber tips induced by electrical fields have been suggested as one mechanism.[51] Both direct effects on the growing neurites, and indirect effects by a stimulation of growth processes secondary to whole body exposure, have been suggested by Sisken and coworkers.[168]

The effects of electrical stimulation vary with experimental models and types and qualities of electric field. In one recent study, Sisken and associates tested the effects of PEMFs on rat sciatic nerve regeneration following the administration of a crush lesion.[168] Rats were placed between a pair of Helmholtz coils and exposed to PEMF of frequency 2 Hz and magnetic flux density of 0.3 mT. A daily treatment of 4 hours for 3 to 6 days increased the rate of initial axonal outgrowth by 22%. The stimulatory effects were independent of the direction of the field. Rats exposed to PEMF for 4 hours/day for 7 days before crush, followed by 3 days after crush without PEMF, also showed significantly increased regeneration, indicating conditioning effects induced by the field.

Alteration of Microenvironment

The first experiments with the silicone chamber model demonstrated that regeneration failed if the gap distance was 15 mm or more in rat sciatic nerves.[97] The question of inducing regeneration across gaps larger than 10 mm has been the focus of considerable study.

By prefilling silicone chambers with phosphate-buffered saline (PBS) or dialyzed plasma, regeneration across a 15-mm gap has been induced in the rat.[194] Prefilling 10-mm-gap silicone chambers with PBS stimulates fibrin matrix formation within chambers, causing generation of nerve structures three times greater, with three times more axons, than in empty chambers.[197] The number of regenerating nerve fibers also increases if the silicone chamber is made permeable by cutting holes in the chamber wall.[73]

Substance other than PBS or dialyzed plasma have been used to promote nerve regeneration. Prefilling nerve chambers with the neurite-promoting factor laminin has increased the regeneration rate.[105,106] Prefilling nerve chambers with collagen-glycosaminoglycan gels,[200] laminin-containing or collagen-containing gels,[104] or by cutting holes in the chamber walls[74] have all induced regeneration across gaps of 15 to 25 mm. Regeneration across 15-mm gaps can also be obtained by predegenerating distal nerve stumps or by preconditioning proximal nerve stumps.[28]

In other experiments, the effects of a multiple injection into chambers have been studied.[128] It was found that a mixture of laminin, testosterone, ganglioside GM_1, and catalase increased the diameter and vascularization of regenerating nerves. This mixture also stimulated the ingrowth of Schwann cells and axons from proximal nerve stumps as well as the formation of myelin. In later studies, this mixture has been redefined, with catalase omitted.[127] Individual agents have not been as effective as the catalase-lacking mixture.

Neurotrophic Factors

The effect of neurotrophic factors (growth factors) on nerve regeneration in vivo has been examined. By prefilling silicone chambers with an NGF solution, both the number of myelinated axons and the thickness of myelin sheaths were increased.[148] A mixture of NGF and collagen added to polyethylene chambers improved regeneration rates.[37] The effect of prefilling silicone chambers with NGF has also been examined in a rabbit facial nerve model.[23] Surprisingly (since motor neurons do not apparently respond to NGF) the regenerating nerves were larger and gave a higher-density distribution of axon growth.

Specially designed silicone chambers containing nitrocellulose paper strips have been used to test the effects of substrate-bound fibroblast growth factor (FGF) on nerve regeneration.[35] FGF-containing chambers demonstrated a significantly more advanced migration of perineural-like cells and Schwann cells. Nerves in these chambers also had increased vascularization compared to controls.[34] Biodegradable nerve regeneration chambers, with slow-release functions, have been used to test the effects of controlled FGF release on nerve regeneration across 15-mm gaps in rat sciatic nerves. These experiments clearly demonstrated the existence of FGF-stimulated nerve regeneration.[4] The use of polyethylene tubes containing FGF has also demonstrated increased numbers of myelinated fibers.[26]

Administration of insulinlike growth factor-1 (IGF-1) via osmotic minipumps, applied either locally at the nerve lesion or at the dorsal root ganglion level, has been shown to stimulate regeneration of nerve fibers.[76,170] Thymidine-incorporation experiments suggest that IGF-1 stimulates nonneuronal proliferation indirectly.[170] Administration of antibodies to IGF-1 inhibits regeneration.[76]

Clinical Significance

It appears that regenerated nerve has a process of selective reinnervation based on the specific distal nerve stump or peripheral target. The administration of various substances in the region between the nerve stumps influences the rate and extent of selective nerve regrowth. The clinical potential of creating a microenvironment into which neurotrophic and neurotropic substances can be added has considerable promise for the next level of advancement in clinical nerve regeneration.

REFERENCES

1. Adler R, Landa KB, Manthorpe M, Varon S. Cholinergic neuronotrophic factors: Intraocular distribution of trophic activity for ciliary neurons. Science 1979; 204:1434–1436.
2. Adler R, Manthorpe M, Skaper SD, Varon S. Polyornithine-attached neurite promoting factors (PNPFs). Culture sources and responsive neurons. Brain Res 1981; 206:129–144.
3. Aebischer P, Guénard V, Winn SR, Valentini RF, Galletti PM. Blind-ended semipermeable guidance channels support peripheral nerve regeneration in the absence of a distal nerve stump. Brain Res 1988; 454:179–187.
4. Aebischer P, Salessiotis AN, Winn SR. Basic fibroblast growth factor released from synthetic guidance channels facilitates peripheral nerve regeneration across long nerve gaps. J Neurosci Res 1989; 23:282–289.
5. Aguayo AJ, Charron L, Bray GN. Potential of Schwann cells from unmyelinated nerves to produce myelin: A quantitative ultrastructural and autoradiographic study. J Neurocytol 1976; 5: 565–573.
6. Aguayo AJ, Epps J, Charron L, Bray GN. Multipotentially of Schwann cells in cross-anastomosed and grafted myelinated and unmyelinated nerves. Brain Res 1976; 104:1–20.
7. Aitken JT. The effect of peripheral connections on the maturation of regenerating nerve fibres. J Anat 1949; 83:38–42.
8. Anderson KJ, Dam D, Lee S, Cotman CW. Basic fibroblast growth factor prevents death of lesioned cholinergic neurons in vivo. Nature 1988; 332: 360–361.
9. Angeletti PU, Vigneti E. Assay of nerve growth factor (NGF) in subcellular fractions of peripheral tissues by microcomplement fixation. Brain Res 1971; 33:601–604.
10. Arntz C, Kanje M, Lundborg G. Regeneration of the rat sciatic nerve after different conditioning lesions: Effects of the conditioning interval. Microsurgery 1989; 10:118–121.
11. Barbin G, Manthorpe M, Varon S. Purification of the chick eye ciliary neuronotrophic factor (CNTF). J Neurochem 1984; 43:1468–1478.
12. Baron van Evercooren A, Kleinman HK, Ohno S, Marangos P, Schwartz JP, Dubois-Dalcq ME. Nerve growth factor, laminin and fibronectin promote neurite growth in human fetal sensory ganglia cultures. J Neurosci Res 1982; 8:179–194.
13. Barton AA. An electron microscope study of degeneration and regeneration of nerve. Brain 1962; 85:799–808.
14. Berenberg RA, Forman DS, Wood DK, DeSilva A, Demaree J. Recovery of peripheral nerve function after axotomy: Effect of triiodothyronine. Exp Neurol 1977; 57:349–363.
15. Boyle FC, Gillespie JS. Accumulation and loss of noradrenaline central to a constriction on adrenergic nerves. Eur J Pharmacol 1970; 12:77–84.
16. Brattgård S-O, Edström J-E, Hydén H. The chem-

ical changes in regenerating neurons. J Neurochem 1957; 1:316–325.
17. Brushart TME. Preferential reinnervation of motor nerves by regenerating motor axons. J Neurosci 1988; 8:1026–1031.
18. Brushart TME, Seiler WA. Selective reinnervation of distal motor stumps by peripheral motor axons. Exp Neurol 1987; 97:289–300.
19. Buchtal F, Kühl V. Nerve conduction, tactile sensibility, and the electromyogram after suture or compression of peripheral nerve: A longitudinal study in man. J Neurol Neurosurg Psychiatry 1979; 42:436–451.
20. Bunge MB. Fine structure of nerve fibres and growth cones of isolated sympathetic neurons in culture. J Cell Biol 1973; 56:713–735.
21. Campenot RB. Local control of neurite development by nerve growth factor. Proc Natl Acad Sci USA 1977; 74:4516–4519.
22. Charlwood KA, Lamont DM, Banks BEC. Apparent orienting effects produced by nerve growth factor. In: Zaimis E, Knight J, eds. Nerve growth factor and its antiserum. London: Athlone Press, 1972: 102–107.
23. Chen Y-S, Wang-Bennett LT, Coken NJ. Facial nerve regeneration in the silicone chamber: The influence of nerve growth factor. Exp Neurol 1989; 103:52–60.
24. Cockett SA, Kiernan JA. Acceleration of peripheral nervous regeneration in the rat by exogenous triiodothyronine. Exp Neurol 1973; 39:389–394.
25. Collins F. Induction of neurite outgrowth by a conditioned-medium factor bound to the culture substratum. Proc Natl Acad Sci USA 1978; 75: 5210–5213.
26. Cordeiro PG, Seckel BR, Lipton SA, D'Amore PA, Wagner J, Madison R. Acidic fibroblast growth factor enhances peripheral nerve regeneration in vivo. Plast Reconstr Surg 1989; 83:1013–1019.
27. Cotrufo R, Dattola R, Deodato M, Pisani F, Messina C. Experimental hyperthyroidism fails to expedite reinnervation of muscles denervated by crushing sciatic nerves in rabbits. Exp Neurol 1979; 65: 271–277.
28. Dahlin LB, Danielsen N, Ochi M, Lundborg G. Axonal growth in mesothelial chambers: Effects of a proximal preconditioning lesion and/or predegeneration of the distal nerve stump. Exp Neurol 1988; 99:655–663.
29. Dahlin LB, Shyu B-C, Danielsen N, Andersson SA. Effects of nerve compression or ischaemia on conduction properties of myelinated and non-myelinated nerve fibres. An experimental study in the rabbit common peroneal nerve. Acta Physiol Scand 1989; 136:97–105.
30. Danielsen N. Regeneration of the rat sciatic nerve in the silicone chamber model. Restor Neurol Neurosci 1990; 1:253–259.
31. Danielsen N, Dahlin LB, Ericson LE, Crenshaw A, Lundborg G. Experimental hyperthyroidism stimulates axonal growth in mesothelial chambers. Exp Neurol 1986; 94:56–65.
32. Danielsen N, Dahlin LB, Lee YF, Lundborg G. Axonal growth in mesothelial chambers: The role of the distal nerve segment. Scand J Plast Reconstr Surg 1983; 17:119–125.
33. Danielsen N, Müller H, Pettmann B, et al. Rat amnion membrane matrix as a substratum for regenerating axons from peripheral and central neurons: Effects in a silicone chamber model. Dev Brain Res 1988; 39:39–50.
34. Danielsen N, Pettmann B, Vahlsing HL, Manthorpe M, Varon S. Fibroblast growth factor effects on peripheral nerve regeneration in a silicone chamber model. J Neurosci Res 1988; 20:320–330.
35. Danielsen N, Vahlsing HL, Manthorpe M, Varon S. A two-compartment modification of the silicone chamber model for nerve regeneration. Exp Neurol 1988; 99:622–635.
36. Danielsen N, Williams LR, Dahlin LB, Varon S, Lundborg G. Peripheral nerve regeneration in Gore-Tex chambers. Scand J Plast Reconstr Surg 1988; 22:207–210.
37. Da Silva CF, Langone F. Addition of nerve growth factor to the interior of a tubular prosthesis increases sensory neuron regeneration in vivo. Brazilian J Med Biol Res 1989; 22:691–694.
38. Davis GE, Engvall E, Varon S, Manthorpe M. Human amnion membrane as a substratum for cultured peripheral and central nervous system neurons. Dev Brain Res 1987; 33:1–10.
39. Davis GE, Varon S, Engvall E, Manthorpe M. Substratum-binding neurite-promoting factor: Relationship to laminin. Trends Neurosci 1985; 8:528–532.
40. Denny-Brown D, Brenner C. Paralysis of nerve induced by direct pressure and by tourniquet. Arch Neurol Psychiatry 1944; 51:1–26.
41. Denny-Brown D, Brenner C. Lesion in peripheral nerve resulting from compression by spring clip. Arch Neurol Psychiatry 1944; 52:1–19.
42. Ducker TB. Pathophysiology of peripheral nerve trauma. In: Omer G, Spinner M, eds. Management of peripheral nerve problems. Philadelphia: WB Saunders, 1980:475–486.
43. Ducker TB. The central cell body and axonal de-

generation. In: Gorio A, Millesi H, Mingrino S, eds. Post-traumatic peripheral nerve regeneration: Experimental basis and clinical implications. New York: Raven, 1981:7–11.

44. Ebendahl T. The relative roles of contrast inhibitions and contact guidance in orientation of axons extending on aligned collagen fibrils in vitro. Exp Cell Res 1976; 98:159–169.
45. Ebendahl T, Jacobson CO. Human glial cells stimulating outgrowth of axons in cultured chick embryo ganglia. Zoon 1975; 3:169–172.
46. Ebendahl T, Jacobson CO. Tissue explants affecting extension and orientation of axons in cultured chick embryo ganglia. Exp Cell Res 1977; 105: 379–387.
47. Edbladh M, Edström A. Environmental factors contribute to the enhanced regeneration of frog sciatic sensory axons by a conditioning lesion. Acta Physiol Scand 1989; 135:169–172.
48. Forman DS. The use of axonally transported radioactive proteins as markers of axonal regeneration following crush or suture. In: Jewett DL, McCarroll HR Jr, eds. Nerve repair and regeneration: Its clinical and experimental basis. St. Louis: CV Mosby, 1980:95–97.
49. Forssman J. Über die Ursachen, welche die Wachsthumsrichtung der peripheren Nervenfasern bei der Regeneration bestimmen. Beitr Z Pathol Anat 1898; 24:56–100.
50. Forssman J. Zur Kenntnis des Neurotropismus. Weiter Beiträge. Beitr Z Pathol anat 1900; 27: 407–430.
51. Freeman JA, Manis PB, Snipes GJ, et al. Steady growth cone currents revealed by a novel circularly vibrating probe: A possible mechanism underlying neurite growth. J Neurosci 1985; 13:257–283.
52. Frizell M, McLean WG. The effect of triiodothyronine on axonal transport in regenerating peripheral nerves. Exp Neurol 1979; 64:225–230.
53. Frizell M, Sjöstrand J. Transport of proteins, glycoproteins, and cholinergic enzymes in regenerating hypoglossal neurons. J Neurochem 1974; 22: 845–850.
54. Frizell M, Sjöstrand J. The axonal transport of [^{3}H]-labelled glycoproteins in normal and regenerating peripheral nerves. Brain Res 1974; 78:109–123.
55. Gospodarowicz D, Neufeld G, Schweigerer L. Fibroblast growth factor. Mol Cell Endocrinol 1986; 46:187–204.
56. Grafstein B. The nerve cell body response to axotomy. Exp Neurol 1975; 48:32–51.
57. Grafstein B, McQuarrie IG. Role of the nerve cell body in axonal regeneration. In: Cotman CW, ed. Neuronal plasticity. New York: Raven, 1978:155–195.
58. Gundersen RW. Sensory neurite growth cone guidance by substrate-absorbed nerve growth factor. J Neurosci Res 1985; 13:199–212.
59. Gundersen RW, Barrett JN. Neuronal chemotaxis: Chick dorsal root axons turn toward high concentrations of nerve growth factor. Science 1979; 206: 1079–1080.
60. Gundersen RW, Barrett JN. Characterization of the turning response of dorsal root neurites towards nerve growth factor. J Cell Biol 1980; 87: 546–554.
61. Gutmann E, Sanders FK. Recovery of fibre numbers and diameter in the regeneration of peripheral nerves. J Physiol 1943; 101:489–518.
62. Haftek J, Thomas PK. Electron-microscope observations on the effects of localized crush injuries on the connective tissues of peripheral nerve. J Anat 1968; 103:233–243.
63. Hall-Craggs EBC, Brand P. Effect of previous nerve injury on the regeneration of free autogenous muscle grafts. Exp Neurol 1977; 57:275–281.
64. Hammond GR, Smith RS. Inhibition of the rapid movement of optically detectable axonal particles by colchicine and vinblastine. Brain Res 1977; 128: 227–242.
65. Hansson HA, Dahlin LB, Danielsen N, et al. Evidence indicating trophic importance of IGF-1 in regenerating peripheral nerves. Acta Physiol Scand 1986; 126:609–614.
66. Harper GP, Thoenen H. Nerve growth factor: Biological significance, measurement and distribution. J Neurochem 1980; 34:5–16.
67. Harris WA, Holt CE, Smith TA, Gallenson N. Growth cones of developing retinal cells in vivo on cultured surfaces and in collagen matrices. J Neurosci Res 1985; 13:101–122.
68. Helfand SL, Smith GA, Wessells NK. Survival and development in culture of dissociated parasympathetic neurons from ciliary ganglia. Dev Biol 1976; 50:541–547.
69. Hendry IA. The response of adrenergic neurons to axotomy and nerve growth factor. Brain Res 1975; 94:87–98.
70. Heumann R. Regulation of the synthesis of nerve growth factor. J Exp Biol 1987; 132:133–150.
71. Heumann R, Korsching S, Bandtlow C, Thoenen H. Changes of nerve growth factor synthesis in non-neuronal cells in response to sciatic nerve transection. J Cell Biol 1987; 104:1623–1631.
72. Jaffe LF, Poo M. Neurites grow faster towards the

cathode than the anode in a steady field. J Exp Zool 1979; 209:115–128.

73. Jenq C-B, Coggeshall RE. Nerve regeneration through holey silicone tubes. Brain Res 1985; 361: 233–241.
74. Jenq C-B, Coggeshall RE. Permeable tubes increase the length of the gap that regenerating axons can span. Brain Res 1987; 408:239–242.
75. Kanje M, Skottner A, Lundborg G. Effects of growth hormone treatment on the regeneration of rat sciatic nerve. Brain Res 1988; 475:254–258.
76. Kanje M, Skottner A, Sjöberg J, Lundborg G. Insulin-like growth factor 1 (IGF-1) stimulates regeneration of the rat sciatic nerve. Brain Res 1989; 486:396–398.
77. Karlström L, Dahlström A. The effects of different types of axonal trauma on the synthesis and transport of amino storage granulas in rat sciatic nerve. J Neurobiol 1973; 4:191–200.
78. Koskland DE. Bacterial chemotaxis in relation to neurobiology. Ann Rev Neurosci 1980; 3:43–75.
79. Krikorian D, Manthorpe M, Varon S. Purified mouse Schwann cells: Mitogenic effects of fetal calf serum and fibroblast growth factor. Dev Neurosci 1982; 5:77–91.
80. Le Beau JM, LaCorbiere M, Powell HC, Ellisman MH, Schubert D. Extracellular fluid conditioned during peripheral nerve regeneration stimulates Schwann cell adhesion, migration and proliferation. Brain Res 1988; 459:93–104.
81. Letourneau PC. Possible roles for cell-to-substratum adhesion in neuronal morphogenesis. Dev Biol 1975; 44:77–91.
82. Letourneau PC. Cell-to-substratum adhesion and guidance of axonal elongation. Dev Biol 1975; 44: 92–101.
83. Letourneau, PC. Chemotactic response of nerve fibre elongation to nerve growth factor. Dev Biol 1978; 66:183–196.
84. Levi-Montalcini R. Effects of mouse tumor transplantation on the nervous system. Ann NY Acad Sci 1952; 55:330–343.
85. Levi-Montalcini R. The nerve growth factor 35 years later. In Vitro Cell Dev Biol 1987; 23:227–238.
86. Levi-Montalcini R, Booker B. Excessive growth of the sympathetic ganglia evoked by a protein isolated from mouse salivary glands. Proc Natl Acad Sci USA 1960; 46:373–384.
87. Levi-Montalcini R, Hamburger V. Selective growth-stimulating effects of mouse sarcoma on the sensory and sympathetic nervous system of the chick embryo. J Exp Zool 1951; 116:321–362.
88. Levi-Montalcini R, Hamburger V. A diffusable agent of mouse sarcoma producing hyperplasia of sympathetic ganglia and hyperneurotization of the chick embryo. J Exp Zool 1953; 123:233–288.
89. Lieberman AR. The axon reaction: A review of the principal features of perikaryal responses to axonal injury. Int Rev Neurobiol 1971; 14:49–124.
90. Lieberman AR. Some factors affecting retrograde neuronal responses to axonal lesions. In: Bellairs R, Gray EG, eds. Essays on the nervous system. Oxford: Clarendon, 1974:71–105.
91. Lindholm D, Heumann R, Meyer M, Thoenen H. Interleukin-1 regulates synthesis of nerve growth factor in non-neuronal cells of rat sciatic nerve. Nature 1987; 330:658–659.
92. Longo FM, Hayman EG, Davis GE, et al. Neurite-promoting factors and extracellular matrix components accumulating in vivo within nerve regeneration chambers. Brain Res 1984; 309:105–117.
93. Longo FM, Manthorpe M, Skaper SD, Lundborg G, Varon S. Neuronotrophic activities accumulate in vivo within silicone nerve regeneration chambers. Brain Res 1983; 261:107–117.
94. Longo FM, Skaper SD, Manthrope M, Williams LR, Lundborg G, Varon S. Temporal changes of neuronotrophic activities accumulating in vivo within nerve regeneration chambers. Exp Neurol 1983; 81:756–769.
95. Lubinska L. Pattern of Wallerian degeneration of myelinated fibres in short and long peripheral stumps and in isolated segments of rat phrenic nerve. Interpretation of the role of axoplasmic flow of the trophic factor. Brain Res 1982; 233:227–240.
96. Lugnegåard H, Berthold C-H, Rydmark M. Ultrastructural morphometric studies on regeneration of the lateral sural cutaneous nerve in the white rat after transection of the sciatic nerve. II. Regeneration after nerve suture and nerve grafting. Scand J Plast Reconstr 1984 (suppl); 20:45–104.
97. Lundborg G, Dahlin LB, Danielsen N, et al. Nerve regeneration in silicone chambers: Influence of gap length and of distal stump components. Exp Neurol 1982; 76:361–375.
98. Lundborg G, Dahlin LB, Danielsen N, Johannesson A, Hansson H-A. Regenerating nerve fibres in performed mesothelial chambers: Influence of the distal segment of a transected nerve on growth and direction. In: Lee AJC, Albrektsson T, Bråanemark P-I, eds. Clinical application of biomaterials. Advances in biomaterials, vol 4. Chichester: John Wiley & Sons, 1982:323–329.
99. Lundborg G, Dahlin LB, Danielsen N, Nachemson

AK. Tissue specificity in nerve regeneration. Scand J Plast Reconstr Surg 1986; 20:279–283.

100. Lundborg G, Gelberman RH, Longo FM, Powell HC, Varon S. In vivo regeneration of cut nerves encased in silicone tubes. Growth across a 6-mm gap. J Neuropathol Exp Neurol 1982; 42:412–422.

101. Lundborg G, Hansson H-A. Nerve lesion with interruption of continuity: Studies on the growth pattern of regenerating axons in the gap between proximal and distal nerve ends. In: Gorio A, Millesi H, Mingrino S, eds. Post-traumatic peripheral nerve regeneration. Experimental basis and clinical implications. New York: Raven, 1981:229–239.

102. Lundborg G, Longo FM, Varon S. Nerve regeneration model and trophic factors in vivo. Brain Res 1982; 232:157–161.

103. Mackinnon SE, Dellon AL, Lundborg G, Hudson AR, Hunter D. A study of neurotrophism in a primate model. J Hand Surg [Am] 1986; 11:888–894.

104. Madison RD, Da Silva CF, Dikkes P. Entubulation repair with protein additives increases the maximum nerve gap distance successfully bridged with tubular prostheses. Brain Res 1988; 447:325–334.

105. Madison R, Da Silva CF, Dikkes P, Chiu T-H, Sidman RL. Increased rate of peripheral nerve regeneration using bioresorbable nerve guides and a laminin-containing gel. Exp Neurol 1985; 88:767–772.

106. Madison RD, Da Silva C, Dikkes P, Sidman RL, Chiu TH. Peripheral nerve regeneration with entubulation repair: Comparison of biodegradable nerve guides vs polyethylene tubes and the effects of a laminin-containing gel. Exp Neurol 1987; 95:378–390.

107. Manthorpe M, Barbin G, Varon S. Isoelectric focusing of the chick eye ciliary neuronotrophic factor. J Neurosci Res 1982; 8:233–239.

108. Manthorpe M, Engvall E, Rouslathi E, Longo FM, Davis GE, Varon S. Laminin promotes neuritic regeneration from cultured peripheral and central neurons. J Cell Biol 1983; 97:1882–1890.

109. Manthorpe M, Skaper S, Adler R, Landa K, Varon S. Cholinergic neuronotrophic factors: Fractionation properties of an extract from selected chick embryonic eye tissues. J Neurochem 1980; 34:69–75.

110. Manthorpe M, Skaper SD, Williams LR, Varon S. Purification of adult rat sciatic nerve ciliary neuronotrophic factor. Brain Res 1985; 367:282–286.

111. Manthorpe M, Varon S, Adler R. Neurite-promoting factor (NPF) in conditioned medium from RN22 Schwannoma cultures. Bioassay, fractionation and other properties. J Neurochem 1981; 37:759–767.

112. Mason CA. Growing tips of embryonic cerebellar axons in vivo. J Neurosci Res 1985; 13:55–74.

113. McGregor RJ, Sharpless SK, Luttges MW. A pressure model for nerve compression. J Neurol Sci 1975; 24:299–304.

114. McIsaac G, Kiernan JA. Acceleration of neuromuscular re-innervation by triiodothyronine. J Anat 1975; 120:551–560.

115. McIsaac G, Kiernan JA. Accelerated recovery from peripheral nerve injury in experimental hyperthyroidism. Exp Neurol 1975; 48:88–94.

116. McLennan IS, Hendry IA. Parasympathetic neuronal survival induced by factors from muscle. Neurosci Lett 1978; 10:269–273.

117. McQuarrie IG. The effect of conditioning lesion on the regeneration of motor axons. Brain Res 1978; 152:597–602.

118. McQuarrie IG. Accelerated axonal sprouting after nerve transection. Brain Res 1979; 167:185–188.

119. McQuarrie IG. Acceleration of axonal regeneration in rat somatic motoneurons by using a conditioning lesion. In: Gorio A, Millesi H, Mingrino S, eds. Post-traumatic nerve regeneration. Experimental basis and clinical implications. New York: Raven, 1981:49–58.

120. McQuarrie IG, Grafstein B. Axon outgrowth enhanced by a previous nerve injury. Arch Neurol 1973; 29:53–55.

121. McQuarrie IG, Grafstein B, Gershon MD. Axonal regeneration in rat sciatic nerve: Effect of a conditioning lesion and of dbcAMP. Brain Res 1977; 132:443–453.

122. Mira JC. Effects of repeated experimental localized freezings in the distal stump of peripheral nerve. In: Terzis J, ed. Clinics in plastic surgery: Symposium on peripheral nerve microsurgery. Philadelphia: WB Saunders, 1984:17–26.

123. Morris JH, Hudson AR, Weddell G. A study of degeneration and regeneration in the rat sciatic nerve using electron microscopy. I. Traumatic degeneration of myelin in the proximal stump of the divided nerve. Z Zellforsch 1972; 124:76–102.

124. Morris JH, Hudson AF, Weddell G. A study of degeneration and regeneration in the rat sciatic nerve based on electron microscopy. II. The development of the "regenerating unit." Z Zellforsch 1972; 124:103–130.

125. Morris JH, Hudson AF, Weddell G. A study of degeneration and regeneration in the rat sciatic nerve using electron microscopy. IV. Changes in fascicular microtopography, the perineurium and en-

doneurial fibroblasts. Z Zellforsch 1972; 124:165–203.

126. Morrison RS, Sharma A, deVellis J, Bradshaw RA. Basic fibroblast growth factor supports the survival of cerebral cortical neurons in primary culture. Proc Natl Acad Sci USA 1987; 83:7537–7541.

127. Müller H. Further evaluation of the effects of laminin, testosterone, ganglioside GM1, and catalase on early growth in rat nerve regeneration chambers. Exp Neurol 1988; 101:228–233.

128. Müller H, Williams LR, Varon S. Nerve regeneration chamber: Evaluation of exogenous agents applied by multiple injections. Brain Res 1987; 413:320–326.

129. Nachemson AK. Axonal regeneration and growth direction in square-shaped mesothelial chambers. Scand J Plast Reconstr Surg 1988; 22:199–206.

130. Nachemson AK, Hansson H-A, Dahl D, Lundborg G. Visualization of regenerating nerve fibres by neurofilament immunohistochemistry. Acta Physiol Scand 1986; 126:485–489.

131. Nachemson AK, Hansson H-A, Lundborg G. Neurotropism in nerve regeneration: An immunohistochemical study. Acta Physiol Scand 1988; 133: 139–148.

132. Ochi M. Experimental study on orientation of regenerating fibres in the severed peripheral nerve. Hiroshima J Med Sci 1983; 31:389–406.

133. Ochoa J, Fowler TJ, Gilliatt RW. Anatomical changes in peripheral nerves compressed by a pneumatic tourniquet. J Anat 1972; 113:433–455.

134. Orgel MG, O'Brien WJ, Murray HM. Pulsing electromagnetic field therapy in nerve regeneration: An experimental study in the cat. Plast Reconstr Surg 1984; 73:173–182.

135. Patel N, Poo MM. Orientation of neurite growth by extracellular electric fields. J Neurosci 1982; 2:483–496.

136. Pellegrino RG, Spencer PS. Schwann cell mitosis in response to regenerating peripheral axons in vivo. Brain Res 1985; 341:16–25.

137. Pettmann B, Weibel M, Sensenbrenner M, Labourdette G. Purification of two astroglial growth factors from bovine brain. FEBS Lett 1985; 185: 102–108.

138. Politis MJ. Specificity in mammalian peripheral nerve regeneration at the level of the nerve trunk. Brain Res 1985; 328:271–276.

139. Politis MJ, Ederle K, Spencer PS. Tropism in nerve regeneration in vivo. Attraction of regenerating axons by diffusible factors derived from cells of transected peripheral nerves. Brain Res 1982; 253: 1–12.

140. Politis MJ, Spencer PS. A method to separate spatially the temporal sequence of axon-Schwann cell interaction during nerve regeneration. J Neurocytol 1981; 10:221–232.

141. Politis MJ, Spencer PS. An in vivo assay of neurotropic activity. Brain Res 1983; 278:229–231.

142. Pomeranz B, Mullen M, Markus H. Effect of applied electrical fields on sprouting of intact saphenous nerve in adult rat. Brain Res 1984; 303:331–336.

143. Prestige MC. Differentation, degeneration and the role of the periphery: Quantitative considerations. In: Schmitt FO, ed. The neurosciences second study program. New York: Rockefeller University Press, 1970:73–82.

144. Purves D, Njå A. Effect of nerve growth factor on synaptic depression following axotomy. Nature 1976; 260:535–536.

145. Raji ARM, Bowden REM. Effects of high-peak pulsed electromagnetic fields on the degeneration and regeneration of the common peroneal nerve in rat. J Bone Joint Surg [Br] 1983; 65:478–492.

146. Ramon y Cajal S. Studien über Nervenregeneration. Leipzig 1908. (Quoted by Weiss, 1941.)

147. Ramon y Cajal S. Degeneration and regeneration of the nervous system, vol. 1. London: Oxford University Press, 1928.

148. Rich KM, Alexander TD, Pryor JC, Hollowell JP. Nerve growth factor enhances regeneration through silicone chambers. Exp Neurol 1989; 105: 162–170.

149. Richardson P, Ebendahl T. Nerve growth activities in rat peripheral nerve. Brain Res 1982; 246:57–64.

150. Roberts A, Patton DT. Growth cones and formation of central and peripheral neurites by sensory neurones in amphibian embryos. J Neurosci Res 1985; 13:23–38.

151. Rogers SL, Letourneau PC, Palm SL, McCarthy J, Furcht LT. Neurite extension by peripheral and central nervous system neurons in response to substratum-bound fibronectin and laminin. Dev Biol 1983; 98:212–220.

152. Salonen V, Lehto M, Vaheri A, Aro H, Peltonen J. Endoneurial fibrosis following nerve transection. An immunohistological study of collagen types and fibronectin in the rat. Acta Neuropathol (Berl) 1985; 67:315–321.

153. Sanders FK, Young JZ. The influence of peripheral connections on the diameter of regenerating nerve fibre. J Exp Biol 1946; 22:203–212.

154. Scaravilli F. The influence of distal environment

on peripheral nerve regeneration across a gap. J Neurocytol 1984; 13:1027–1041.
155. Schiffman E, Corcoran BA, Wahl SM. N-formylmethionyl peptides as chemotactic attractants for leucocytes. Proc Natl Acad Sci USA 1975; 72: 1059–1062.
156. Schlaepfer W. Calcium-induced degeneration of axoplasm in isolated segments of rat peripheral nerve. Brain Res 1974; 69:203–215.
157. Schlaepfer W. Structural alterations of peripheral nerve induced by a calcium ionophore A23187. Brain Res 1977; 136:1–9.
158. Schlaepfer WW, Hasler MB. Characterization of the calcium-induced disruption of neurofilaments in rat peripheral nerve. Brain Res 1979; 168:299–309.
159. Schlaepfer W, Micko S. Calcium-dependent alterations of neurofilament proteins of rat peripheral nerve. J Neurochem 1979; 32:211–219.
160. Seckel BR, Chiu TH, Nyilas E, Sidman RL. Nerve regeneration through synthetic biodegradable nerve guides: Regulation by the target organ. Plast Reconstr Surg 1984; 74:173–181.
161. Seckel BR, Ryan SE, Gagne RG, Chiu TH, Watkins E Jr. Target-specific nerve regeneration through a nerve guide in the rat. Plast Reconstr Surg 1986; 78:793–798.
162. Seddon H. Three types of nerve injury. Brain 1943; 66:237–288.
163. Seddon HJ. Peripheral nerve injuries. Medical Research Council Special Report Series 282. London: Her Majesty's Stationery Office, 1954.
164. Seddon H. Surgical disorders of the peripheral nerves. Edinburgh: Churchill-Livingstone, 1972.
165. Shooter EM, Yankner BA, Landreth GE, Sutter A. Biosynthesis and mechanism of action of nerve growth factor. Rec Progr Horm Res 1981; 37:417–446.
166. Sievers J, Hausmann B, Unsicker K, Berry M. Fibroblast growth factors promote the survival of adult rat retinal ganglion cells after transection of the optic nerve. Neurosci Lett 1987; 76:157–162.
167. Sisken BF, Barr E, Estes RS. Electrical effects on nerve ganglia in vitro. In: Hunt TK, Heppenstall RB, Pines E, Rovey D, eds. Soft and hard tissue repair: Biological and clinical aspects. New York: Praeger, 1984.
168. Sisken BF, Kanje M, Lundborg G, Herbst E, Kurtz W. Stimulation of rat sciatic nerve regeneration with pulsed electromagnetic fields. Brain Res 1989; 485:309–316.
169. Sisken BF, Smith SD. The effects of minute direct electrical currents on cultured chick embryo trigeminal ganglia. J Embryol Exp Morph 1975; 33: 29–35.
170. Sjöberg J, Kanje M. Insulinlike growth factor 1 (IGF-1) as a stimulator of regeneration in freeze-injured rat sciatic nerve. Brain Res 1989; 485:102–108.
171. Skaper SD, Varon S. Ionic response and growth stimulation in rat astroglial cells: Differential mechanisms of ganglioside and serum. J Cell Physiol 1987; 130:453–459.
172. Spencer PS. Neuronal regulation of myelinating cell function. Society for Neuroscience Symposium 1979; 4:275–321.
173. Spencer PS, Politis MJ, Pellegrino RG, Weinberg HJ. Control of Schwann cell behavior during nerve degeneration regeneration. In: Gorio A, Millesi H, Mingrino S, eds. Post-traumatic nerve regeneration. Experimental basis and clinical implications. New York: Raven, 1981:411–426.
174. Stelmack BM, Kiernan JA. Effects of triiodothyronine on the normal and regenerating facial nerve of the rat. Acta Neuropathol (Berl) 1977; 40:151–155.
175. Sunderland S. A classification of peripheral nerve injuries producing loss of function. Brain 1951; 74:491–516.
176. Sunderland S. Nerves and nerve injuries, ed 2. Edinburgh: Churchill-Livingstone, 1978: 133–141.
177. Taniuchi M, Clark HB, Schweitzer JB, Johnson EM Jr. Expression of nerve growth factor receptors by Schwann cells of axotomized peripheral nerves: Ultrastructural location, suppression by axonal contact, and binding properties. J Neurosci 1988; 8:664–681.
178. Thoenen H, Bandtlow C, Heumann R, Lindholm D, Meyer M, Rohrer H. Nerve growth factor: Cellular localization and regulation of synthesis. Cell Mol Neurobiol 1988; 8:35–40.
179. Thomas PK. Changes in the endoneurial sheaths of peripheral myelinated nerve fibres during Wallerian degeneration. J Anat 1964; 98:175–182.
180. Timpl R, Rohde H, Robey PG, Rennard SI, Foidart JM, Martin GR. Laminin: A glycoprotein from basement membranes. J Biol Chem 1979; 254: 9933–9937.
181. Varon S, Adler R. Nerve growth factors and control of nerve growth. Curr Top Dev Biol 1980; 16: 207–252.
182. Varon S, Adler R. Trophic and specifying factors directed to neuronal cells. Adv Cell Neurobiol 1981; 2:115–163.

183. Varon S, Bunge RP. Trophic mechanisms in the peripheral nervous system. Ann Rev Neurosci 1978; 1:327–361.
184. Varon S, Manthorpe M, Williams LR. Neuronotrophic and neurite-promoting factors and their clinical potentials. Dev Neurosci 1984; 6:73–100.
185. Vial JD. The early changes in the axoplasm during Wallerian degeneration. J Biophys Biochem Cytol 1958; 4:551–556.
186. Walicke PA, Baird A. Neurotrophic effects of basic and acidic fibroblast growth factors are not mediated through glial cells. Dev Brain Res 1988; 40:71–79.
187. Walicke PA, Cowan WM, Keno N, Baird A, Guillemin R. Fibroblast growth factor promotes survival of dissociated hippocampal neurons and enhances neurite extension. Proc Natl Acad Sci USA 1986; 83:3012–3016.
188. Weinberg HJ, Spencer PS. Studies on the control of myelinogenesis. I. Myelination of regenerating axons after entry into a foreign unmyelinated nerve. J Neurocytol 1975; 4:395–418.
189. Weinberg HJ, Spencer PS. Studies on the control of myelinogenesis. II. Evidence for neuronal regulation of myelin production. Brain Res 1976; 113: 363–378.
190. Weinberg HJ, Spencer PS. The fate of Schwann cells isolated from axonal contact. J Neurocytol 1978; 17:555–569.
191. Weiss P. Nerve patterns: The mechanics of nerve growth. Growth (Third Growth Symposium) 1941; 5:163–203.
192. Weiss P, Taylor AC. Further experimental evidence against "neurotropism" in nerve regeneration. J Exp Zool 1944; 95:233–257.
193. Williams LR. Exogenous fibrin matrix precursors stimulate the temporal progress of nerve regeneration within a silicone chamber. Neurochem Res 1987; 12:851–860.
194. Williams LR, Danielsen N, Müller H, Varon S. Exogenous matrix precursors promote functional nerve regeneration across a 15-mm gap within a silicone chamber in the rat. J Comp Neurol 1987; 264:284–290.
195. Williams LR, Longo FM, Powell HC, Lundborg G, Varon S. Spatial–temporal progress of peripheral nerve regeneration within a silicone chamber: Parameters for a bioassay. J Comp Neurol 1983; 218: 460–470.
196. Williams LR, Powell HC, Lundborg G, Varon S. Competence of nerve tissue as distal insert promoting nerve regeneration in a silicone chamber. Brain Res 1984; 293:201–211.
197. Williams LR, Varon S. Modification of fibrin matrix formation in situ enhances nerve regeneration in silicone chambers. J Comp Neurol 1985; 231:209–220.
198. Yamada KM. Cell surface interactions with extracellular materials. Ann Rev Biochem 1983; 52: 761–799.
199. Yamada KM, Spooner BS, Wessells NK. Axon growth: Roles of microfilaments and microtubules. Proc Natl Acad Sci USA 1970; 66:1206–1212.
200. Yannas IV, Orgill DP, Silver J, Norregaard TV, Zervas NT, Schoene WC. Polymeric template facilitates regeneration of rat sciatic nerve across a 15-mm gap. Transactions of the Fifth European Conference on Biomaterials, Paris, Sept. 4–6, 1985:163.
201. Yu W-H. Effect of testosterone on the regeneration of the hypoglossal nerve in rats. Exp Neurol 1982; 77:129–141.
202. Yu W-H, Srinavasan R. Effect of testosterone and 5α-dihydroxitestosterone on regeneration of the hypoglossal nerve in rats. Exp Neurol 198; 71: 431–435.
203. Yu W-H, Srinavasan R. Effect of thyroid hormone treatment on the regeneration of the hypoglossal nerve in rats. Exp Neurol 1981; 73:325–329.
204. Yu W-H, Yu MC. Acceleration of the regeneration of the crushed hypoglossal nerve by testosterone. Exp Neurol 1983; 80:349–360.

III

CLINICAL EVALUATION

8 Sensibility Testing

9 Motor Testing

10 Electrophysiological Testing

11 Pitfalls in Interpretation of Electrophysiological Testing

12 Anomalous Innervation of the Upper Extremity

8

Sensibility Testing

A. Lee Dellon

AUTHOR'S KEY POINTS

- Understanding the relationship between nerve fibers and sensory receptors is fundamental to understanding which sensory test is appropriate in a specific clinical situation.
- The determination of when regeneration is proceeding and when operative intervention is required can be made by using the relationship *threshold is to innervation density* (in the sensory system) *as weakness is to atrophy* (in the motor system).
- The Meissner corpuscle is sensitive to a stimulus of 30 cycles per second; the Pacinian corpuscle is most sensitive to stimulation of 256 cycles per second.
- Peripheral nerve demonstrates altered function in a predictable way. For the motor system, weakness is seen first, followed by wasting. Sensory abnormalities are heralded by abnormal cutaneous vibratory thresholds (vibrometer testing) and altered cutaneous pressure thresholds (von Frey testing), followed by abnormal two-point discrimination.
- There are only three truly objective tests of sensory function: the ninhydrin test, the O'Rain skin wrinkling test, and electrophysiological testing.
- A specific pattern of sensory recovery follows nerve injury. The first recovering perception is low-frequency 30 Hz vibratory sensibility. Shortly thereafter, moving-touch stimuli are perceived. Lagging behind is the perception of constant touch. High-frequency vibration, such as 256 Hz, is the last to recover.
- In determining the timing of sensory re-education, the order of events is useful. Since the 256 Hz vibratory perception recovers last, late-phase sensory re-education is initiated when that vibratory stimulus is perceived.

My current approach to evaluating sensibility, based on neurophysiology and refined to fit the needs of both the busy hand surgeon and the precise researcher, is quick, reliable, and valid. It has evolved over more than 20 years and it continues to evolve.[8]

Historical aspects of the confusion and controversy in sensory testing have been described in detail.[11] The sensory receptors depicted in earlier texts were often inaccurate, based upon the histochemical artifacts of 19th-century histologists, while the physiological correlations enshrined in our teaching tomes (Table 8-1) represented armchair tabulations of relationships, more theoretical than real. Today, using light and electron microscopic observations of carefully fixed tissues, three-dimensional reconstructions of the glabrous skin are possible (Fig. 8-1). The basic neurophysiologic research and the correlations between the neurophysiologic research and clinical sensory testing have been reviewed previously.[9–12,21,25] These relationships, and their application to clinical evaluation of sensibility, are listed in Tables 8-2 through 8-5.

TERMINOLOGY FOR SENSIBILITY TESTING

1. **Sensibility**: the neurophysiologic substrata: nerve fibers, nerve receptors
2. **Sensation**: the conscious perception of the response of the neurophysiologic substrata to stimulation
3. **Quickly adapting**: the property of the nerve fiber-receptor response to a constant-touch stimulus in which the nerve fiber fires once or twice and then does not fire again until the stimulus is removed. Thus, the fiber-receptor system quickly adapts to a constant-touch stimulus. The quickly adapting fiber-receptor does not vary its rate of firing with difference in intensity of the stimulus.
4. **Slowly adapting**: the property of the nerve fiber-receptor response to a constant-touch stimulus in which nerve impulses continue to fire throughout the duration of the constant-touch stimulus. The slowly adapting fiber-receptor will vary its rate of firing depending on stimulus intensity.
5. **Threshold**: the level of stimulation required to initiate an impulse along the nerve fiber. Various nerve fibers have different thresholds, depending upon the nerve fiber diameter, the degree of myelination, and the nature of the stimulus.
6. **Cutaneous vibratory threshold**: the stimulus intensity, for a given stimulus frequency, necessary to initiate an impulse in the quickly adapting fiber-receptor system
7. **Cutaneous pressure threshold**: the stimulus intensity required to initiate an impulse in the slowly adapting fiber-receptor system
8. **Innervation density**: the number of nerve fiber-receptors for a given surface area. The higher the innervation density, the greater the number of nerve fiber-receptors in a given area and the greater that area's sensory "acuity" (similar to visual acuity, ie, being able to make finer sensory discriminations between object choices).
9. **Static two-point discrimination**: the classic form of two-point discrimination described by Weber[11] whereby two "points" in constant contact with the skin are discriminated based on the ability to discriminate one from two at variable distances between the two points. This is a measurement of the innervation density of the slowly adapting fiber-receptor system.
10. **Moving two-point discrimination**: measurement of the innervation density of the quickly adapting fiber-receptor system whereby a person discriminates whether one or two "points" are moving along the surface of the finger from proximal to distal.[9]

Table 8–1. *"Traditional" Sensation–Receptor Relationships*

Sensation	Receptor
Cold	Krause's end bulb
Heat	Rufini's end organ
Touch	Meissner corpuscle
Pressure	Pacinian corpuscle
Vibration	Bone

(From Dellon AL. Evaluation of sensibility and re-education of sensation in the hand. Baltimore: Williams & Wilkins, 1981, with permission.)

PERTINENT ANATOMY AND ITS IMPLICATIONS

Figure 8-1 and Tables 8-1 through 8-5 represent the relationships between the known anatomy, as determined by light and electron microscopy, and current neurophysiology. The anatomy of the gla-

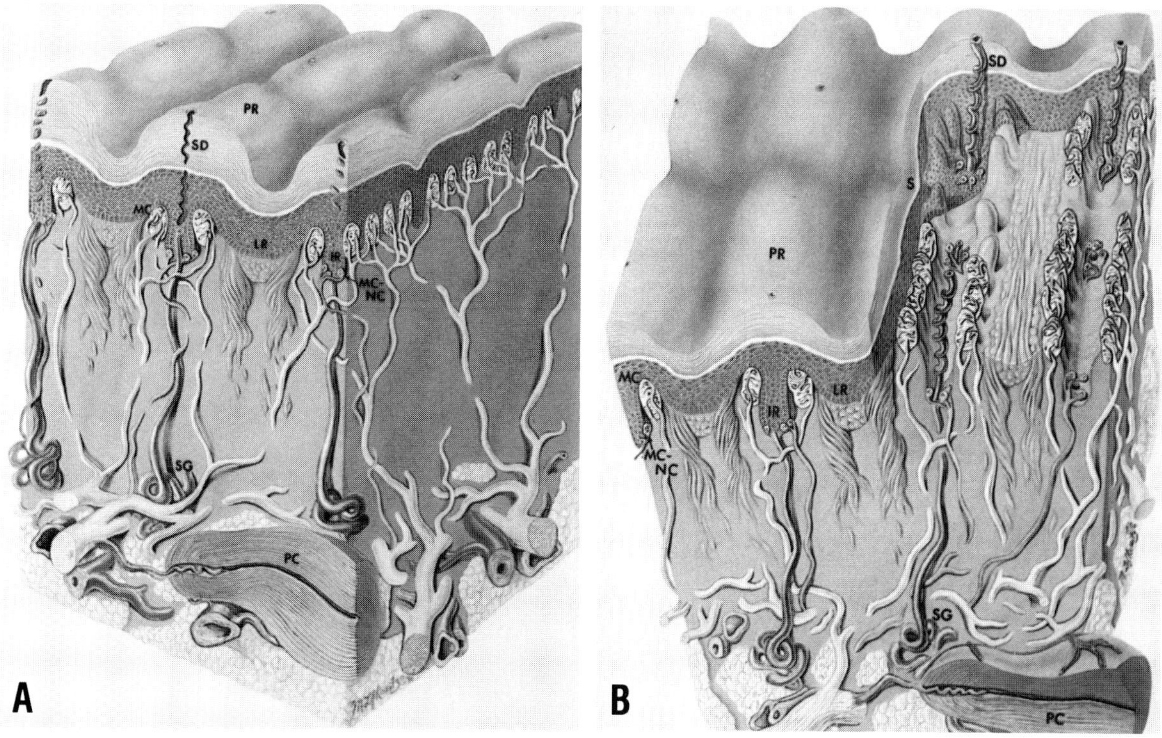

Figure 8–1. *Three-dimensional reconstruction of glabrous skin. There are three "corpuscular" endings. The Pacinian corpuscle (PC), a quickly adapting fiber, most sensitive to high-frequency stimuli, is located in deep dermis. The Meissner corpuscle (MC), a quickly adapting fiber most sensitive to low-frequency stimuli, is located in dermal papillae. The Merkel cell-neurite complex (MC-NC), a slowly adapting fiber, most sensitive to constant touch and pressure, is located at the base of an intermediate ridge (IR) at sites of sweat gland ducts. (**A**) Note relationship of papillary ridges (PR) to intermediate ridge, which transduces horizontal motion into vertical motion to maximize mechanical stimulation of sensory receptors in dermal papillae for movement detection, and direct pressure transduction to the underlying Merkel cells. Limiting ridges (LR) are bound down by collagen bundles to deep dermis. (**B**) Cutaway view to demonstrate longitudinal relationships of receptors to sweat ducts (SD) along intermediate ridges. Note multiple Merkel cells per one nerve fiber, one Pacinian corpuscle to one nerve fiber, and one Meissner cell innervated by multiple nerve fibers. (Reprinted with permission from Dellon AL. Evaluation of sensibility and re-education of sensation in the hand. Baltimore: Williams & Wilkins, 1981.)*

brous skin may be thought of as units in which the papillary ridges are linked, with each ridge having directly beneath it an intermediate ridge.[7] On either side of the intermediate ridge is a dermal papilla. On the outside of these is a limiting ridge. This smaller ridge is bound by collagen fibers to the deeper subcutaneous tissues. If pressure is placed directly downward upon a fingerprint (a papillary ridge), directly beneath this will be the intermediate ridge, and directly beneath this are the clear cells described by Merkel.[11]

Immediately adjacent to these clear cells are expanded bulb neurite endings. A group of four to six clear cells with expanded bulb endings relates to a single myelinated group A beta fiber. The clear cells are based around the circumference of a sweat duct, which enters into the base of the intermediate ridge. This entire structure maximizes the mechanical transduction of a force to this nerve fiber-receptor population. The osmium that Merkel initially used in his stain primarily stained the dopamine of the melanocytes. The so-called clear cells do, however, stain by osmium. Only by ultrastructural analysis can it be determined that these

Table 8–2. *Testing Nontouch Perceptions*

Patient Perception	***Neurophysiology***	***Clinical Test***
Pain	C fibers (unmyelinated) A delta fibers (thinly myelinated)	Pin prick
Heat	A delta fibers (thinly myelinated)	Hot water–heated end of tuning fork
Cold	A delta fibers (thinly myelinated)	Ice water–filled test tubes
Sweating	C fibers (unmyelinated)	Ninhydrin
Joint position	A beta fibers (thickly myelinated)	Joint positioning skin stretching
"Muscle tension"	A delta fibers (thinly myelinated to Golgi tendon-organ and muscle spindles)	None

clear cells contain dense bodies and are in a direct relationship to the expanded bulb neurite endings (ie, distinguishing a Merkel cell from a melanocyte). Similar relationships have been well documented in the raccoon.[51] These have been correlated by direct nerve fiber recordings and shown to be slowly adapting fiber-receptor systems. Because this system continues to fire throughout the duration of the stimulus and because this rate of firing may increase or decrease as stimulus intensity changes, it may be this system that conveys the perception of pressure.[49]

The concept of the fingerprint as a digital skin organization to maximally transduce mechanical stimuli continues with relationship to the Meissner corpuscle.[7] Meissner corpuscles are located in most dermal papillae. Between three and nine separate nerve fibers from group A beta myelinated fibers innervate an individual Meissner corpuscle. As a force moves along the surface of a fingertip, as with a movement of an object across the fingertip, the horizontal movement is translated by the papillary ridges and broken into multiple repetitive (vibratory) movements. These cause the intermediate

Table 8–3. *Testing Perception of Moving Touch: Quickly Adapting Fiber/Receptor (Meissner)*

Human Perception	***Neurophysiologic Descriptor***	***Clinical Test***
Movement	Stimulus	Finger stroking
Flutter	Stimulus	30-Hz tuning fork
Intensity	Threshold	Vibrometer
Object recognition	Innervation density	Moving two-point discrimination*

* *Recommended testing instrument: Disk-Criminator, P.O. Box 16392, Baltimore, MD 21210.*

Table 8–4. *Testing Perception of Moving Touch: Quickly Adapting Fiber/Receptor (Pacinian)*

Human Perception	***Neurophysiologic Descriptor***	***Clinical Test***
Movement	Stimulus	Finger stroking
Vibration	Stimulus	256-Hz tuning fork
Intensity	Threshold	Vibrometer
Object recognition	Innervation density	Moving two-point discrimination*

* *Recommended testing instrument: Disk-Criminator, P.O. Box 16392, Baltimore, MD 21210*

Table 8–5. *Testing Perception of Constant Touch: Slowly Adapting Fiber/Receptor (Merkel Cell)*

Patient Perception	**Physiological Descriptor**	**Clinical Test**
Nonmoving touch	Stimulus	Finger stroking
Pressure	Threshold	Semmes-Weinstein nylon monofilaments*
"Object recognition"	Innervation density	Static two-point discrimination†

* *May also be measured with the Pressure-Specifying Discriminator (NK Biotechnical Engineering, P.O. Box 26335, Minneapolis, MN 55426; telephone: 612-541-0411)*
† *Recommended testing instrument: Disk-Criminator, P.O. Box 16392, Baltimore, MD 21210*

ridge to oscillate like a pendulum between the limiting ridges, causing a force to come maximally against the Meissner corpuscles. The Meissner corpuscles are most sensitive to low-frequency stimuli, similar to what car passengers feel riding across railroad tracks: they bounce up and down each time the car crosses a track, generating a low-frequency stimulus.[50]

In contrast, the Pacinian corpuscle, deep in the dermis with onionlike layers about it, is an extremely sensitive receptor. Because the Pacinian corpuscle is so large, it was the first corpuscle to be described, and because of its size it was the first corpuscle to have its single nerve fiber recorded electrically. The Pacinian corpuscle is the paradigm of the quickly adapting fiber-receptor system. It is most sensitive to high-frequency stimulation. A high-frequency, low-intensity stimulus such as wind blowing across a finger is sufficient to set off the Pacinian corpuscle.

The Meissner corpuscle is most sensitive to a stimulus intensity of 30 cycles per second, whereas the Pacinian corpuscle is most sensitive to a stimulus of 256 cycles per second, *if both of these vibratory stimuli are of the same intensity.* Any vibratory frequency, if delivered at a high enough intensity, will set off any quickly adapting fiber. Quickly adapting fibers stop firing shortly after a touch stimulus. However, throughout the time during which a vibration is occurring, this repetitive movement can entrain impulses, and thus quickly adapting fibers can continue to fire in response to vibratory stimuli. The quickly adapting fiber-receptor system is the one best suited to transmit stimuli that are perceived as movement.

When a single nerve fiber is in contact with a single receptor (and they have a perfect relationship), the threshold for stimulation will be normal. If there is only one fiber-receptor system in a given area, however, the innervation density will be low. This arrangement allows a stimulus to be perceived at a very low intensity but does not allow the stimulus to be easily localized. Conversely, if there are many nerve fibers in an area, even if their relationship to the receptors is not normal (ie, a high threshold), there will be a high innervation density. This allows a stimulus, if it is delivered with enough intensity, not only to be perceived but also to be localized accurately because the high number of nerve fibers have overlapping peripheral receptive fields, permitting central localization.[11,14,15,38]

PATHOPHYSIOLOGY: APPLICATIONS TO TESTING SENSIBILITY

A peripheral nerve responds predictably to an alteration in its function. Because altered function is predictable and because changes in nerve function can be measured, our current understanding of pathophysiology can be used as a guide to clinical sensibility testing. Table 8-1 outlines the relationships between sensation and receptor. For muscle function, the differences are easily perceived, but it is more confusing for the sensory system. When a "motor nerve" becomes compressed and the nerve slowly begins to lose function, the first abnormality detected is weakness. Once the motor nerve has stopped functioning for a significant period of time and the muscle loses neural stimulation, then wasting or atrophy develops. Thus, with nerve compression in the motor system, weakness is seen first, followed by wasting.

With a sensory nerve, the analogous situation is heralded by diminished function. There is decreased ability to perceive that a stimulus is occurring. This is a threshold change. Thus, whereas vibration would have been perceived by a normal nerve to have a certain intensity, the same degree of stimulus intensity, applied to a nerve that has been compressed, is no longer perceived as clearly. The patient manifests this by saying that the tuning fork does not feel as "loud." By a mechanism that is not yet well understood, it appears that in the earliest stage of a nerve compression, there may be heightened perception, ie, a lowering of threshold. Thus, in very early nerve compression, the tuning fork might at first be perceived as "louder."[10,12]

Once the sensory nerve stops functioning, there is a decrease in the number of nerve fibers that carry impulses centrally, and therefore the innervation density is reduced. Innervation density is measured by two-point discrimination. Thus, in nerve compression, first there are threshold changes, and later there are two-point discrimination changes. *Therefore, abnormal two-point discrimination in the sensory system has the same implication as wasting in the motor system.* Since there is no neurophysiologic basis for group A beta fibers, which are quickly adapting, to be affected differently during nerve compression from those that are slowly adapting, there is no difference in the clinical implication of an abnormal cutaneous vibratory threshold (vibrometer testing) and a cutaneous pressure threshold (von Frey testing).

The same sequence of events occurs in acute nerve compression as in chronic nerve compression, with only one difference: the time frame (ie, the rate at which the pressure is applied). However, since acute compression causes sensory fibers to carry altered function more quickly to the conscious level, sensory testing is more effective in acute nerve compression, in terms of diagnosis, than motor testing.

In choosing whether to measure cutaneous pressure thresholds or cutaneous vibratory thresholds, the examiner determines which is the easier test to apply in the given clinical situation. If numerical quantitation of an abnormality is unnecessary, either for comparative measurements or on a research basis, but rather a clinical determination is required (ie, whether an operative decompression should be carried out in an acute compartment syndrome), then qualitative testing of the threshold with a tuning fork stimulus is indicated. These pathophysiological–clinical implications have been well documented in experimental and clinical research models for acute[26,55,60] and chronic[23,37,41,42,52] nerve compression situations, as well as in evaluation of human histopathological tissue.[22,40,43,44]

ACTUALLY TESTING SENSIBILITY

Erik Moberg, acclaimed as the "father of sensory testing," has spent more than two decades emphasizing the need for clinicians to quantitate sensation in a way that correlates with hand function.[18] He emphasized that medical school teaching was designed by neurologists to help localize a lesion in the central nervous system (Fig. 8-2). Moberg termed the traditionally taught medical school tests "academic," in contrast to "functional" tests of sensibility that help the surgeon determine what the hand can do. For example, he found that a patient's ability to determine whether he was being stimulated by something that was cold or hot or whether he could identify pain or feel cotton wool stroking across his finger has no correlation with whether the patient can carry out a specific task, such as picking up objects while blindfolded and placing them into a container.[47,48]

For Moberg, hand function was defined in terms of precision or gross sensory grips. He found that the classic Weber two-point discrimination was the best test available for correlation with precision grips. This remains a critical question, especially with regard to evaluation of impairment. Consider this recent letter:

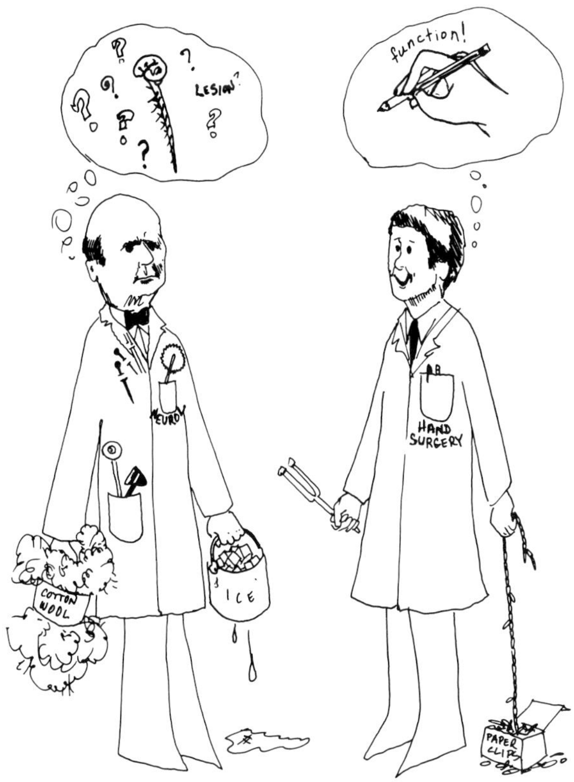

Figure 8–2. *Academic versus functional approach to sensibility testing. The traditional, or academic, approach, as typified on the left, developed as a neurologic tool to localize lesions in the central nervous system. The alternative approach attempts to answer the question, "What can the hand do?" Hand function, defined as precision or sensory grip, is best determined by measurement of two-point discrimination using the ubiquitous paper clip. Diagnosis of nerve division or entrapment is aided by the tuning fork evaluation. (Reprinted with permission from Dellon AL. Evaluation of sensibility and re-education of sensation in the hand. Baltimore: Williams & Wilkins, 1981.)*

To Mr. ———, Esquire:

I write to you because my insurance company sent me to Doctor ——— for an evaluation of my hand impairment. This doctor spent approximately four minutes examining my hand. During this time, he took an instrument that looked like a pizza-pie cutter and rolled it across my fingers. He stuck me with a pin. He asked me to squeeze his hand and then told me that he had learned all he had to know.*

* *Reinfelder, James. Letter to his lawyer, Dec. 15, 1989.*

The Clinical Assessment Committee of the American Society for Surgery of the Hand has recommended to the American Academy of Orthopaedic Surgeons that the evaluation of impairment, with regard to sensibility testing, include at least a measurement of two-point discrimination, and that this may be supplemented by documentation of threshold in the appropriate areas.[1] The testing of pain perception is not recommended. The rating of the presence of pain during an impairment evaluation is totally different, related to patient discomfort from nerve injury rather than a determination of the extent of small unmyelinated fibers transmitting the perception of pain.

How Can I Tell if a Patient Is Malingering?

There are only three truly objective tests of sensory function. By "objective," I mean that the answer to the test does not depend upon the patient's interpretation of a test. None of these three tests has any precise correlation with the degree of recovery of sensory function.

The ninhydrin test described by Moberg is one (Fig. 8-3).[47] The patient applies his fingertips to, for example, an appropriate paper, and the paper is then sprayed with a technique that will demonstrate the presence of amino acids. If a nerve is intact or has regenerated to any degree, ninhydrin will document this by the presence of sweat, which contains amino acids. If the patient says he has no perception of sensation in this finger, this is unlikely to be true if a ninhydrin test documents amino acids coming from the end of the finger.

O'Rain described a test in which a denervated finger, when placed in water, will not wrinkle.[53,54]

The third type of objective test is an electrodiagnostic test. If the patient indicates he has no perception of sensation in the finger and the distal sensory latency is normal, this indicates that the patient is malingering. (The converse is not true: patients can still have perception even when there is no response electrically.)

My preference for detecting malingering in the sensory system is to hold the patient's hand and to tell the patient I am going to determine whether

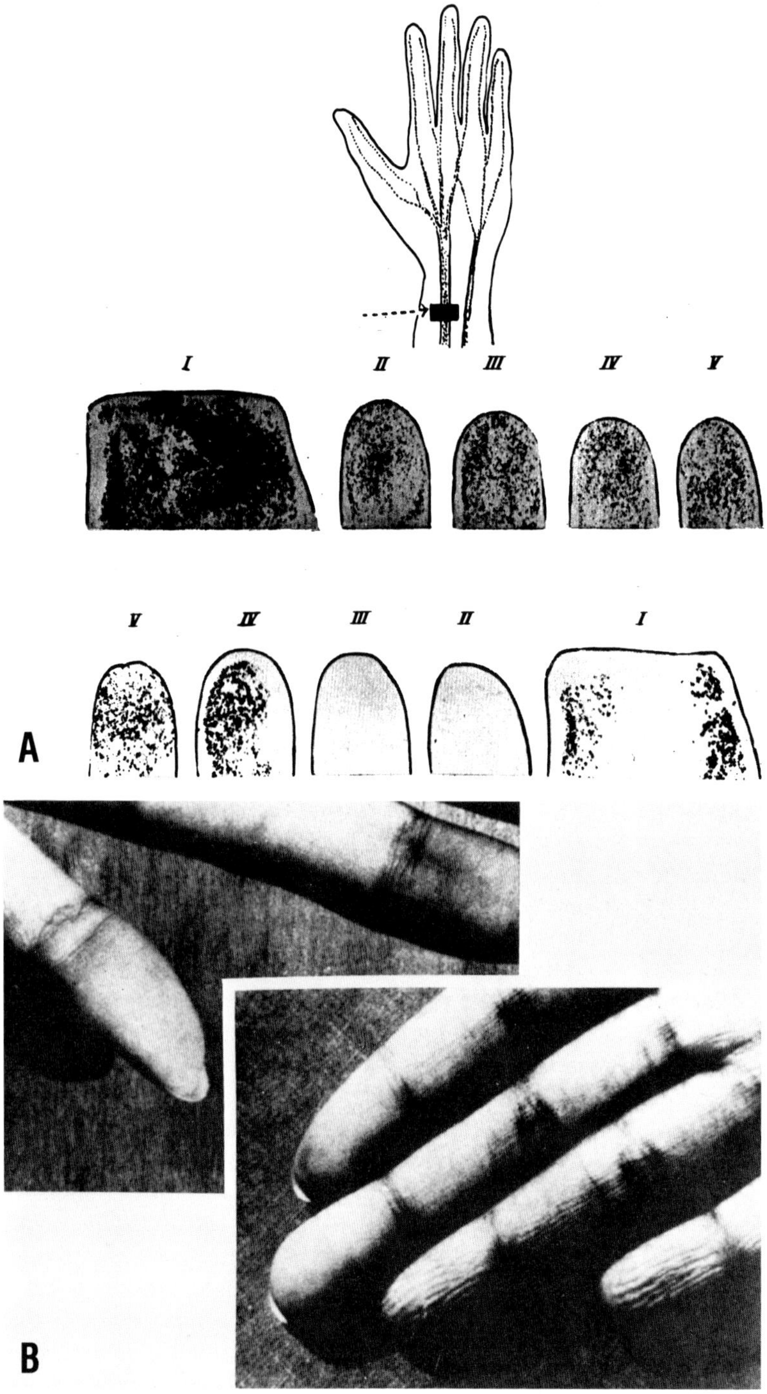

Figure 8–3. *Identifying malingerers. (**A**) Example of Moberg's ninhydrin test of both hands of patient with a median nerve division. The row of prints at the top are from the patient's uninjured hand. The prints on the bottom show no sweating in index and middle fingers, while the thumb print shows sweating on lateral borders of the thumb print from overlapping radial nerve. (**B**) Skin wrinkling phenomenon of water-immersed finger is lost after denervation. Note absence of wrinkles in thumb (upper left) and index and middle fingers (lower right). (Reprinted with permission from Moberg E. Objective methods of determining functional value of sensibility in the hand. J Bone Joint Surg [Br] 1958;40: 454–466.)*

he can feel pain. This is the only time I use pain stimulus in sensibility testing. I hold the finger with one hand while I stick it with a sterile 25-gauge needle, after having previously swabbed the fingertip with an alcohol sponge. The patient with true loss of sensation will not pull the finger away. The malingerer will pull the finger away, either just before it is touched or just after it is touched, even though he attempts to keep his facial expression neutral.

Is the Nerve Divided?

If a nerve is divided, it loses its function. When the nerve has a motor component, one checks for absence of function in muscles the nerve innervates (ie, abductor pollicis brevis with median nerve injury). For the sensory nerve, one considers the distribution of sensation. The question then becomes, "What is the best sensibility test to determine if sensation is present?"

Traditionally, a pin has been used, but my preferred technique uses a tuning fork. Since the 256-Hz tuning fork is the smallest and most easily carried (a similar small tuning fork is available in most emergency-room settings), this is the instrument of choice. A pin raises some fear in the patient being examined. Certainly a small child does not permit examination with a needle. If sensation is present, the patient's trust and confidence is quickly lost. If the patient is inebriated or hostile, a pain stimulus may elicit an unpleasant reaction toward the examiner. Use of a tuning fork obviates these problems. For the small child, I tap the tuning fork and let the child hear the sound. Then I ask the child to tell me when he can "hear" the tuning fork with his finger. The child's face is turned to the side and a hand placed between his face and his hand to be tested. When the examiner touches the child's finger with the tuning fork, if sensation is present the child often smiles or laughs. A patient who has some degree of pain in the hand from an injury perceives the vibratory stimulus if the nerve is intact. This occurs despite the presence of pain because the stimulus is relatively new and becomes apparent despite the background of pain. An additional pain stimulus, as from a needle stick, may not be perceived as readily.

In testing with a tuning fork, it is important to ask a series of questions. The first question is, "Do you feel something?" If the patient answers affirmatively, it is important to localize the perception, as the patient may be perceiving the vibratory stimulus from an area adjacent to that innervated by the nerve in question. For example, if one is concerned about the median nerve at the wrist and the thumb or index finger is being stimulated with a tuning fork, the vibratory force, being a wave, will travel along the finger. It is thus possible for the patient to perceive the stimulus through the intact radial sensory nerve despite loss of function of the median nerve. Thus, the second question is, "Where do you feel this?" If the patient answers, "Over the back of my index finger," then the examiner can be sure the median nerve is not functioning.

If vibratory stimulus is perceived, the patient is asked to compare the intensity of the stimulus over the area affected with the same area in the opposite hand. Thus, the third question is, "How does this stimulus (eg, over the index finger of the left hand) compare with this one (eg, over the index finger of the right hand)?" If the nerve is intact but injured due to bleeding or blunt trauma, it may have an altered threshold when compared with the rest of the contralateral hand. In this case, the nerve is not divided but has diminished function due to either partial nerve injury or compression.

For the digital nerves in particular, precise localization of vibratory stimulus is essential. Because there is overlap between the two digital nerves at the digital pulp, vibratory stimulation is administered over the autonomous zone for the digital nerve (ie, from the distal half of the middle phalanx to the proximal half of the distal phalanx). Since vibratory stimulation is a wave, if a single digital nerve is divided, the wave from the autonomous zone of the injured digital nerve will cross to the opposite digital nerve's territory where it is perceived. The patient's perception of diminished sensation on one side compared with the other is a "soft" neurologic sign indicative of a nonfunctional nerve.

Why Use the Wrong End of the Tuning Fork?

A final point in vibratory testing is that the double-pronged end of the tuning fork is used. When a tuning fork is struck, the entire tuning fork vibrates at the same frequency. The difference between the single-prong and double-prong end is one of intensity. Since it is essentially a screening examination, we use the stimulus at its maximum intensity as a test of the injured nerve. The double-prong end has the greatest vibration and, therefore, the greatest intensity. The tuning fork was originally used to test hearing or "bone conduction." The stimulus area was the thinly protected mastoid process or the malleolus. At these sites, the single-prong end was appropriate. When the testing area is the soft pulp of the fingertip, the greater intensity of the double-prong end is necessary (Fig. 8-4).

Is the Nerve Compressed?

During the clinical evaluation of the patient suspected of having a compressed nerve, the quickest, most reliable way of assessing nerve function is with the tuning fork (Table 8-6).[10] With nerve compression the first change in a sensory nerve is a threshold change. The first sensation that can be examined is touch perception related to the quickly or slowly adapting fibers. Threshold changes in quickly adapting fibers cause the tuning fork stimulus to be perceived less strongly.

An exception is noted in early nerve compression, where there appears to be heightened perception of the sensory stimulus so the tuning fork may seem "louder" (Tables 8-6, 8-7), but it is unusual for patients to present for evaluation this early in their degree of nerve compression.[12] One is not likely to see this phenomenon very often. There may be a brief period during which there is no change in threshold at a time when the patient's symptoms "come and go." A patient seen at this particular time with this particular history would be appropriate for "stress testing" followed by repeat tuning fork evaluation.

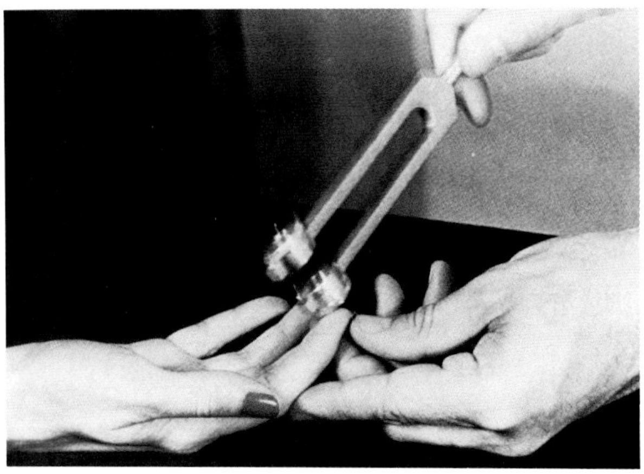

Figure 8–4. *Tuning fork use. Apply the double-prong end to the surface area to be tested. The entire tuning fork vibrates at the same frequency. The double-prong end has greater amplitude and greater stimulus intensity. For the fingertip with a padded pulp, using this end minimizes the risk of false-negative results, since it is a supramaximal stimulus. (Reprinted with permission from Mackinnon SE, Dellon AL. Surgery of the Peripheral Nerve. New York: Thieme, 1988.)*

For median nerve compression at the wrist, the appropriate stress test is the Phalen's sign, with the wrist held in flexion (see Chap. 60). For ulnar nerve compression at the elbow, the appropriate stress test is elbow flexion (see Chap. 76). For radial sensory compression in the forearm, the appropriate stress test position is performed with pronation of the forearm (see Chap. 74).[22]

The most critical step of testing sensibility with a tuning fork for detecting nerve compression is comparing it to an area innervated by a nerve not suspected of being compressed. Thus, in evaluating a patient for carpal tunnel syndrome, the perception of the 256-Hz vibratory stimulus would require comparing the patient's perception of the index finger to the little finger of the same hand or index finger of the opposite hand. If median nerve compression at the wrist and ulnar nerve compression at the elbow are suspected in one extremity, the index and little fingers are evaluated and compared with the contralateral index and little fingers.

If a patient is suspected of having bilateral median and ulnar nerve compression lesions, which may be seen following motor vehicle accidents or with diffuse peripheral neuropathy, qualitative sensory testing is unreliable. In these cases, quantitative sensory testing is most appropriate, with either cutaneous pressure threshold measurement (nylon monofilaments, the cutaneous vibratory threshold [vibrometer]) (Fig. 8-5) or the Pressure-Specifying Discriminator (Fig. 8-6).* The values obtained are compared with normative data.

Use of the tuning fork to diagnose nerve compression has a good diagnostic correlation with electrodiagnostic studies.[25,55,58] Further, the usu-

* *NK Biotechnical Engineering, P. O. Box 26335, Minneapolis, MN 55426. Telephone: 612-541-0411.*

Table 8–6. *Sensibility Testing: Pathophysiology*

	Clinical Signs/Symptoms	
	Motor System	*Sensory System*
NERVE COMPRESSION		
Early (↑ threshold)	Weakness	Abnormal perception of vibratory and pressure threshold
Late (↓ innervation density)	Wasting	Abnormal two-point discrimination
NERVE DIVISION	No function	No function
NERVE REGENERATION		
Early	Weakness	30 Hz, then 256 Hz with abnormal thresholds
Late	↑ strength; ↑ bulk (may never be normal)	Improving pressure thresholds; may never reach normal
		Two-point discrimination (moving before static, moving better than static, may never be normal)

Table 8–7. *Staging Nerve Compression Using Sensibility Testing*

	Abnormal CVT*	***256 Hz***		***Abnormal 2PD†***	
		Increased	*Decreased*	*Static*	*Moving*
CARPAL TUNNEL SYNDROME (percentage of patients)					
Early degree	0%	42%	0%	0%	0%
Moderate degree	35%	21%	70%	0%	0%
Severe degree	85%	0%	100%	48%	84%
CUBITAL TUNNEL SYNDROME (percentage of patients)					
Early degree	N/A	100%	0%	0%	0%
Moderate degree	N/A	0%	33%	0%	0%
Severe degree	N/A	0%	100%	80%	100%

* *Cutaneous vibratory threshold*
† *Static 2PD ≥ 6 mm, moving 2PD ≥ 4 mm*
(From Dellon AL. The vibrometer. Plast Reconstr Surg 1983;71:427, with permission)

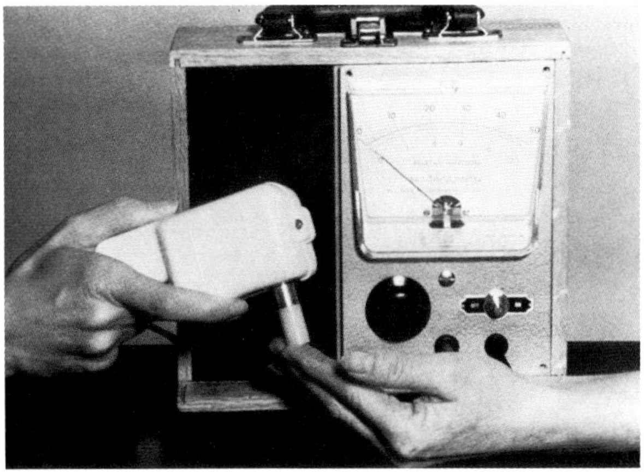

Figure 8–5. *Vibrometer. An example of a single-frequency, variable-intensity vibrometer (available through Biothesiometer, Chagrin Falls, OH 44022). Note that the top scale measures in volts, the bottom in microns of amplitude. (Reprinted with permission from Dellon AL. The vibrometer. Plast Reconstr Surg 1983;71:427.)*

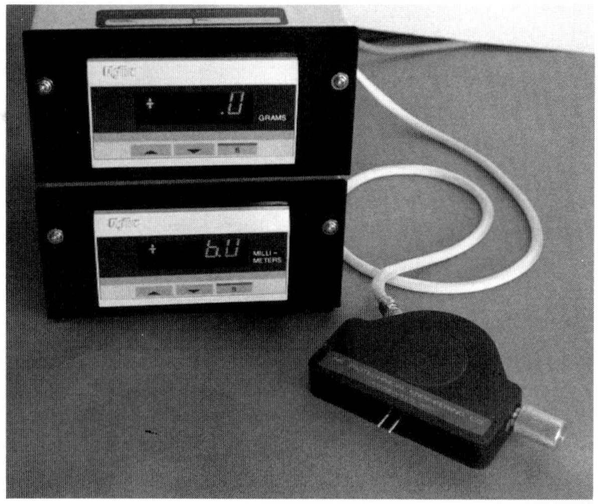

Figure 8–6. *Pressure-Specifying Discriminator. This is the prototype of an examining room model that permits digital readout of cutaneous pressure threshold in grams. It is used to determine the force applied either by a single or beneath two rounded tips. Thus, the force may be defined at which the patient perceives one versus two points, as well as determining threshold functions. (Available through NK Biotechnical Engineering, P.O. Box 26335, Minneapolis, MN 55426.) (See also Fig. 8–16.)*

ally elicited clinical sign, the positive Tinel's sign, also has an excellent correlation with vibratory perception testing using the tuning fork. The Tinel's sign, originally described as evidence of neural regeneration following nerve division, is present in nerve compression. A positive sign is seen because chronic nerve compression causes nerve degeneration.[13] With nerve compression, dorsal root ganglion cells remain viable and attempt regeneration. The presence of a positive Tinel's sign documents the presence of regenerating nerve fibers at the site of nerve compression. This has also been of value in diagnosing nerve compression in children.[27]

In summary, my preference for a sensibility testing device for the diagnosis of peripheral nerve compression, either acute or chronic, is the tuning fork. There are no advantages to using one frequency over another as long as supramaximal stimuli are achieved. If the patient indicates heightened perception in the tested area, an early nerve compression lesion is present. This correlates with intermittent symptoms and supports a nonoperative approach. If there is decreased perception of vibratory stimuli, a diagnosis of nerve compression is made with confidence if the patient's history and clinical evaluation are consistent with that. Nonoperative management is indicated if there is no muscle wasting and if two-point discrimination is normal (Table 8-8). Electrophysiological testing is not advised for routine use (see Chap. 11).

Degree of Nerve Compression

In order to determine which treatment is most appropriate, the stage of the disease is determined.

Table 8–8. *Two-Point Discrimination: Normative Values*

Location	*Static (mm)*	*Moving (mm)*
Fingertip pulp	2–6	2–3
Thumb/index web	15.9 ± 4.7	15.1 ± 4.5
Big toe pulp	8.5 ± 2.2	8.1 ± 2.4
Big/2nd toe web	16.95 ± 4.5	15.1 ± 4.5

(Data from references 5, 19, 30, 33)

There has been a generalized failure to approach nerve compression as if it were a medical problem with stages where treatment is based on the magnitude of nerve injury present. The pathophysiology of nerve compression suggests that a clinical staging system can be determined. The basis for this has been described earlier[11,12] and the concept expanded upon and applied to a given nerve compression lesion (eg, ulnar nerve entrapment at the elbow).[17] The concept has been extended to other peripheral nerve compression.[38] Table 8-6 illustrates that early nerve compression lesions cause threshold changes, while later compression, following nerve degeneration, causes a reduction in innervation density.

For the early or minimal stages of nerve compression, patients' symptoms vary. In the early stage, paresthesias are intermittent. At this stage, the only positive findings on physical examination may be increased perception of vibratory stimulation. Provocative tests, such as the Tinel's sign and the "stress tests" (ie, Phalen's sign) may be positive.

With more advanced compression, the patient's signs are more heightened, causing a greater disruption of daily activities. Perception of vibratory stimuli is usually decreased and provocative signs are generally positive. Cutaneous pressure thresholds (determined by nylon monofilaments or Force-Defined Sensory Discriminator) and cutaneous vibratory thresholds (measured by vibrometer) are reduced. In advanced compression, sensory symptoms are persistent, and innervation density changes (moving and static two-point discrimination) are elevated (Fig. 8-7). Normal values for two-point discrimination are given in Table 8-8.

For severe nerve compression as determined by sensibility testing (ie, abnormal two-point discrimination), additional operative treatment, such as an internal neurolysis, may be considered as adjunctive therapy. Microsurgical internal neurolysis has been found to be safe in the primate model[31,39] and may have additional benefit, as demonstrated in the rat model, in conditions of severe nerve compression.[45] This is controversial, however (see Chap. 63).[28,56]

Is the Nerve Regenerating?

Following nerve repair, whether primary, delayed primary, or secondary, whether perineural or epineural, or whether a reconstruction has been carried out using a nerve graft or some type of nerve conduit, in the end alive dorsal root ganglion cells attempt neural regeneration. The events of neural regeneration have been extensively reviewed recently.[19,38] The clinical pattern of recovery of sensation was described in 1972: the first sensations to recover are those perceived through the un-

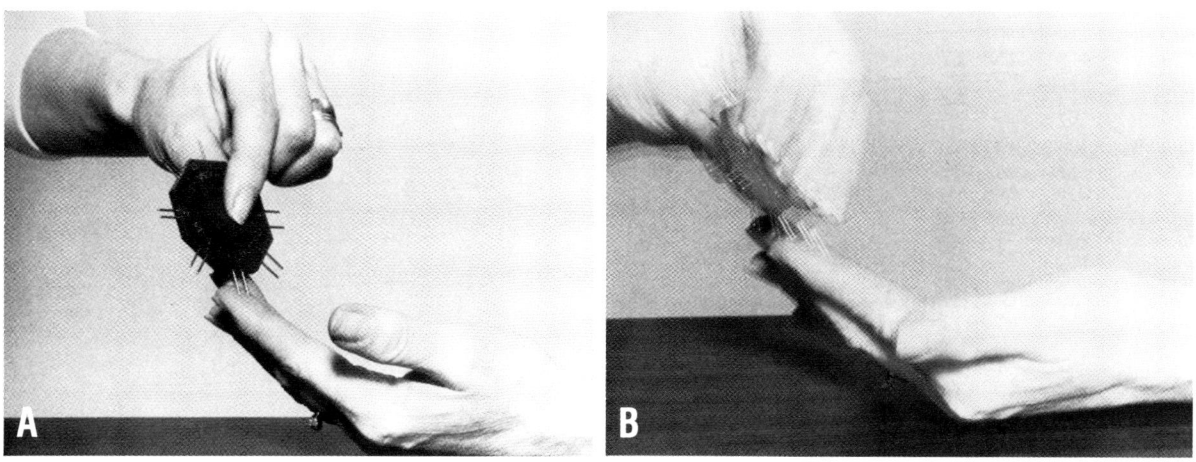

Figure 8-7. *Measurement of two-point discrimination with the Disk-Criminator. (**A**) Static two-point discrimination. (**B**) Moving two-point discrimination. (Available through Disk-Criminator™, P.O. Box 16392, Baltimore, MD 21210.)*

myelinated and small myelinated fibers, such as pain and temperature.[20] Recovering along with these is sudomotor function (ie, sweating). After even the poorest of repairs, this type of sensory recovery usually occurs. The advancing edge of regenerating fibers causes "tingling."[13] Jules Tinel made this observation originally: he noticed that those who had a tingling sign that progressed from the site of nerve injury distally eventually made some degree of recovery following nerve injury. Those who did not have a progressing sign (ie, did not have a "progressing Tinel") did not experience recovery.

The first test for determining whether a nerve is regenerating is carried out by distal-to-proximal tapping along the course of nerve regeneration until a tingling sign, with distal sensations, is elicited. Proximal-to-distal tapping, a proximal Tinel's sign, locates the site of nerve injury or repair. The distance between these two points should increase over time as the nerve regenerates. If this does not occur, regeneration is not occurring (see Fig. 8-8). The degree to which the Tinel's advances is not a prognostic sign in terms of ultimate degree of functional recovery. If the Tinel's sign does not progress, operative intervention to reevaluate the site of nerve repair or reconstruction may be indicated.

The rate of neural regeneration has been considered to be approximately 1 mm per day (or 1 inch per month). This subject has been extensively reviewed,[38] including the original works of Seddon and Sunderland.[57,59] The rate can be faster for unmyelinated nerves and younger patients (see Fig. 8-8).

Order of Sensory Recovery

The pattern of sensory recovery with respect to sensory submodalities was developed using the sensibility testing described above[20] and has been confirmed by other authors.[29] *The first perception to recover is of low-frequency 30-Hz vibratory stimuli.* Shortly thereafter, moving-touch stimuli are perceived. Lagging behind is the perception of constant touch. *High-frequency vibration, such as 256 Hz, is the last to recover.* The basis for this sequence has been related to the relationship of sensory receptors to nerve fibers.[11] Low-frequency quickly adapting fiber-receptors recover first because Meissner corpuscles are easier to reinnervate. The nerve fiber-to-receptor ratio is greater than one. It is hardest, perhaps, to reinnervate the Pacinian corpuscle, where a single nerve fiber must not only make contact with a single receptor but must also enter the receptor from a particular spot in order to arrive in the central core of the onion-like ellipsoid.

When attempting to determine the timing of sensory re-education, the order of events is useful.[11] Since the 256-Hz vibratory perception recovers last, once this stimulus can be perceived at

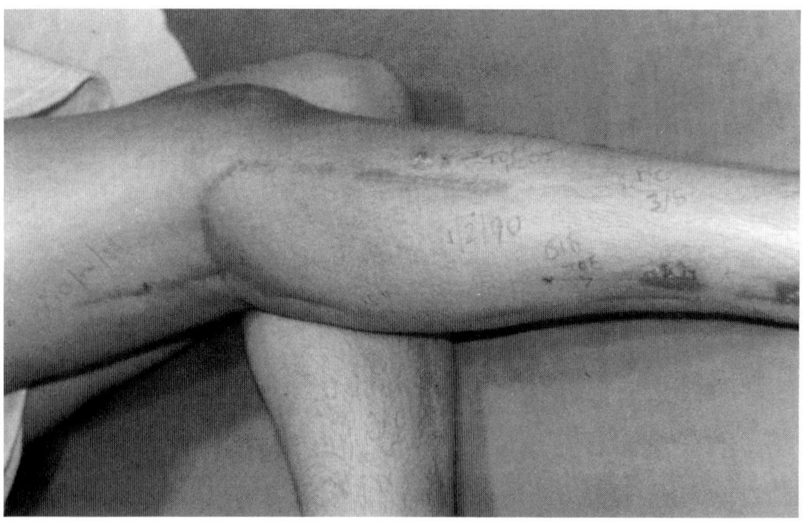

Figure 8–8. *Advancing Tinel. Postoperative view of the lower leg 3 months after a 15-cm interpositional interfascicular graft to the right posterior tibial nerve and neurolysis of the (intact) common peroneal nerve. Note "proximal Tinel" proximal to the popliteal fossa and "distal Tinel" at midcalf, where palpation elicits the perception of "toe." More anterior palpation elicits perception of "foot-dorsum," over common peroneal branches. Muscle strength of 3/5 has returned to extensor digitorum communis (DC), as the neurolysed nerve recovers more quickly than the grafted nerve. Note that 10 inches separates the proximal and distal Tinel, a rate of advancement of 3 mm/day in this 17-year-old patient.*

the fingertip it is clear that all touch submodalities have recovered and late-phase sensory re-education may begin (see Chap. 58).

In eliciting the earliest signs of regeneration, the 30-Hz tuning fork is the most useful tool. It is useful not only in evaluating patients after nerve repair but also in following the recovery of patients with severe peripheral neuropathy in whom peripheral nerve decompressions have been done (eg, diabetics). These nerves recover as if they have undergone nerve repair. Thirty-Hz perception occurs before perception of 256 Hz (Fig. 8-9).[16]

The observation that this orderly sequence of events is occurring (ie, that the pattern of sensory recovery is proceeding as above) is reassuring. Further documentation can be made once these sensory submodalities have reached a given level by switching from qualitative to quantitative measurements. At this point, threshold measurements are initiated using either the cutaneous vibratory or the cutaneous pressure threshold. Such measurements initially demonstrate a high threshold (eg, a high reading on the nylon monofilaments, representing a large force) or a high threshold for vibratory perception (eg, a high number of microns of indentation of the vibratory probe). With the passage of time and progressive neural regeneration, with maturation of the nerve fiber and receptor endings, and with sensory re-education, there is a decrease in threshold or an improvement in perception (eg, the number on the handle of the nylon monofilaments decreases and the microns of indentation required to carry out stimulation is reduced). Thus, with additional "neural regeneration," nerve fibers do not grow a greater distance, but achieve maturity between nerve fiber and receptor. This is combined with the patient's improved sensation as he experiences the neural

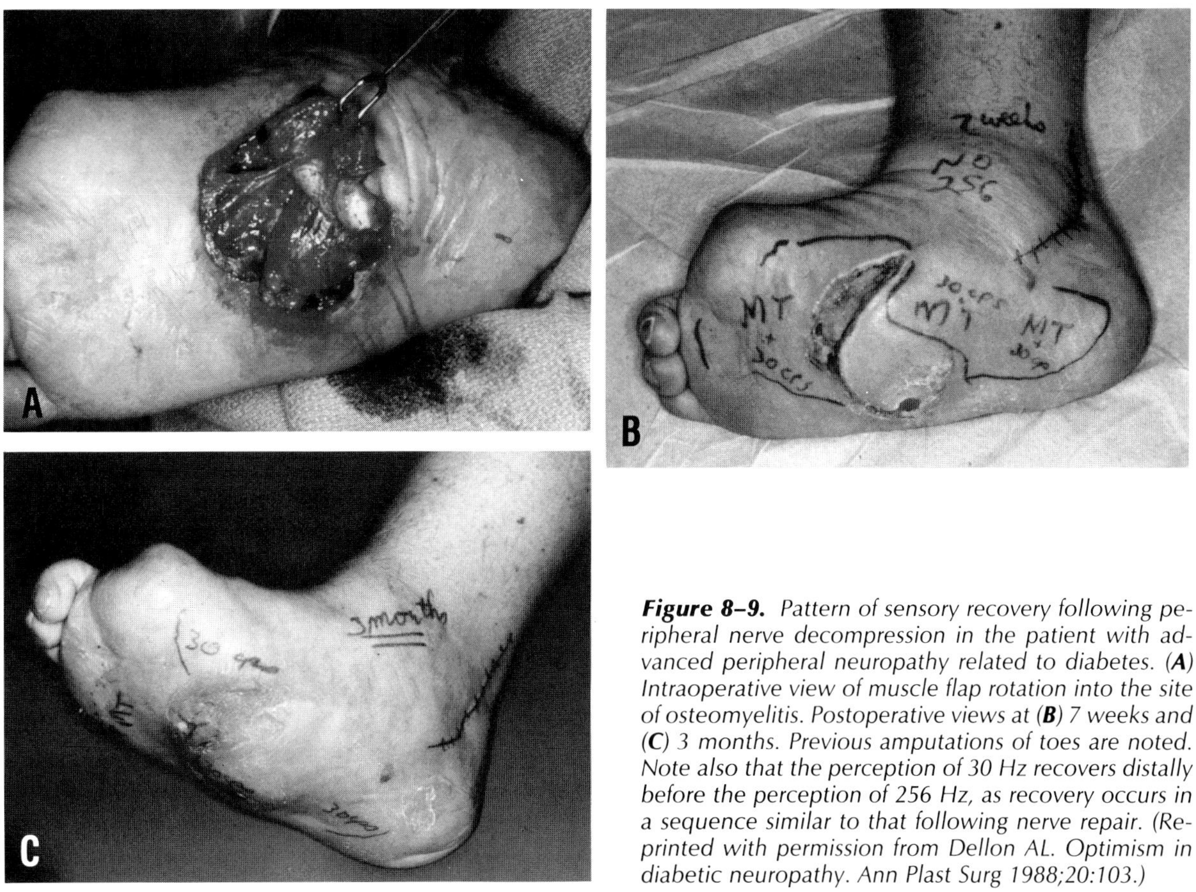

Figure 8–9. *Pattern of sensory recovery following peripheral nerve decompression in the patient with advanced peripheral neuropathy related to diabetes. (**A**) Intraoperative view of muscle flap rotation into the site of osteomyelitis. Postoperative views at (**B**) 7 weeks and (**C**) 3 months. Previous amputations of toes are noted. Note also that the perception of 30 Hz recovers distally before the perception of 256 Hz, as recovery occurs in a sequence similar to that following nerve repair. (Reprinted with permission from Dellon AL. Optimism in diabetic neuropathy. Ann Plast Surg 1988;20:103.)*

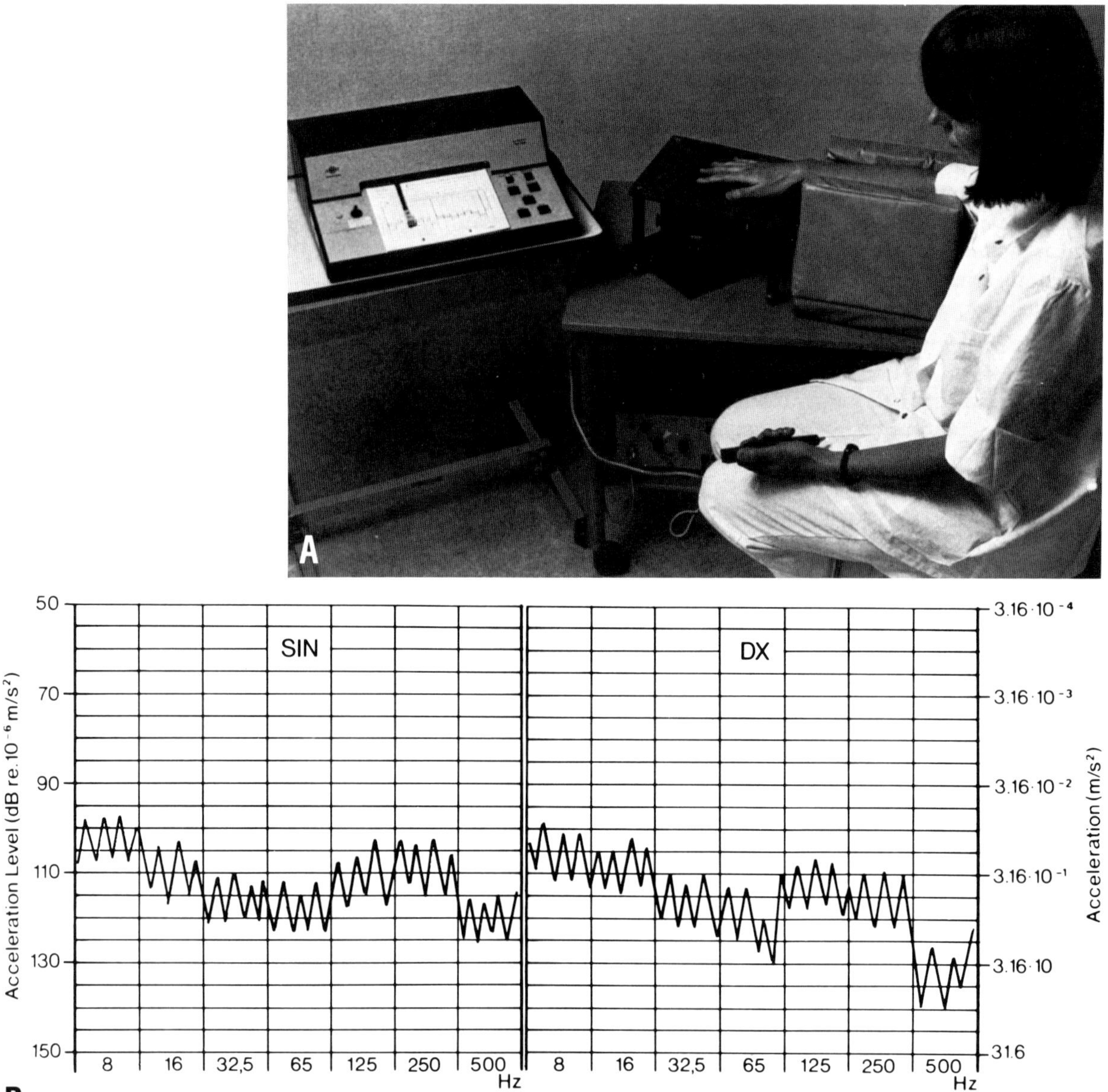

Figure 8–10. *Equipment for assessment of vibrotactile sense between frequencies 8 and 500 Hz. (**A**) The fingertip to be tested is placed on the probe of a vibration exciter (placed under a test table). The increase and decrease in vibration intensity are controlled by a switch in the patient's contralateral hand. (**B**) Vibration thresholds are shown on a vibrogram. The normal vibrogram demonstrates high vibration intensity at the bottom and low vibration intensity at the top. A low curve level indicates a high perception threshold per vibration. The curve peaks between 125 and 250 Hz, indicating a decreased perception threshold within these frequencies. (Reprinted with permission from Lundborg G. Nerve injury and repair. Edinburgh: Churchill-Livingstone, 1988 and Lundborg G, Lie-Stenstonn AK, Sollerman C, Stranberg T, Pyykko J. Digital vibrogram: A new diagnostic tool for sensory testing in compression neuropathy. J Hand Surg [Am] 1986;11:693.)*

stimuli. At this point, innervation density will still be low and two-point discrimination will not have improved.

Further neural regeneration occurs as the population of nerve fibers and receptors increases with increasing innervation density. Further, the patient with increased sensory experience (ie, through late-phase sensory re-education) (see Chap. 58) recovers both moving and static two-point discrimination.

How Is the Degree of Sensory Recovery Measured?

Once sensation has recovered and documentation of the final level is sought, measurement of innervation density and of threshold is carried out. At present, this is done with two separate measurements. The most reliable instrument for determining two-point discrimination is the Disk-Criminator[8,24,36] (see Fig. 8-7). Threshold measurements are made with either the nylon monofilament technique or the Pressure-Specifying Discriminator (see Figs. 8-6, 8-16) for the slowly adapting fiber-receptor system or with the vibrometer[12] for the quickly adapting fiber-receptor system (see Fig. 8-5). Multiple-frequency, variable-intensity vibrometers have also been described for measuring thresholds in the hand (Fig. 8-10).[34,35] A useful schema for correlating testing results has been offered by Waylett (Fig. 8-11).

What if the Electrodiagnostic Test Results Do Not Agree with Results from Clinical Sensibility Testing?

Clinical evaluation is the cornerstone of therapeutic decision making. The correlation of a patient's symptoms with findings on physical examination takes precedence over results of electrodiagnostic testing, except in situations where malingering is suspected, there are multiple peripheral nerves involved (eg, more than one extremity or if a systemic disease such as peripheral neuropathy is suspected), or if the electrodiagnostic testing

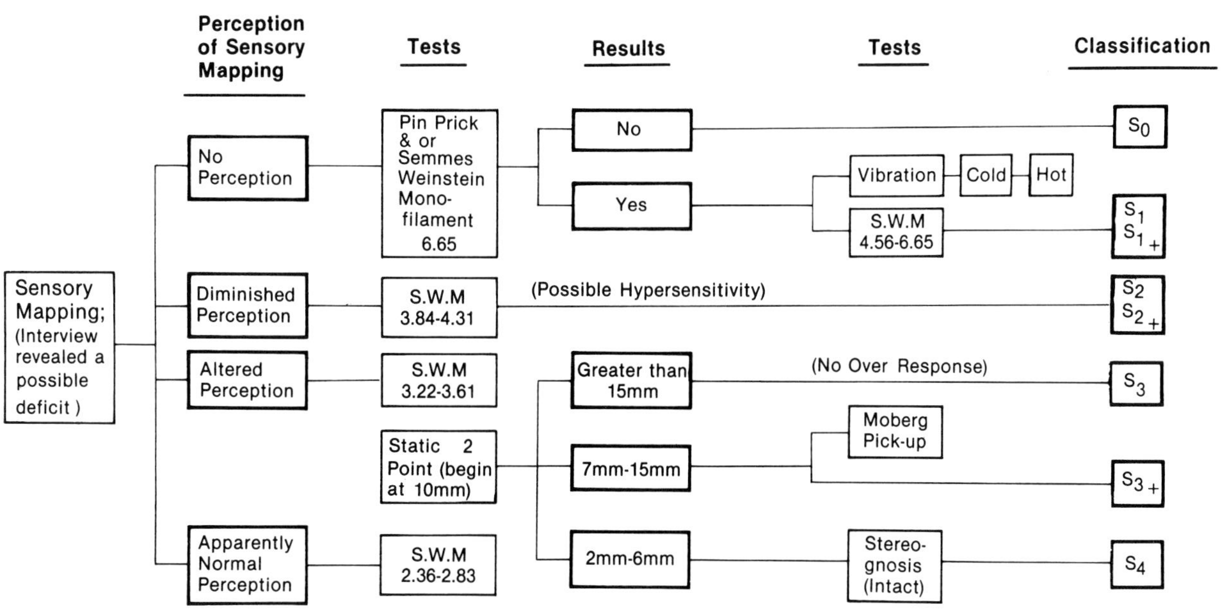

Logic Tree Format for Selection of Tests for Repaired or Grafted Nerves

Figure 8–11. *Scheme for correlating results of sensibility testing. "Logic Tree" developed by Janet Waylett, O.T.R., Loma Linda University. (Published with permission of the author.)*

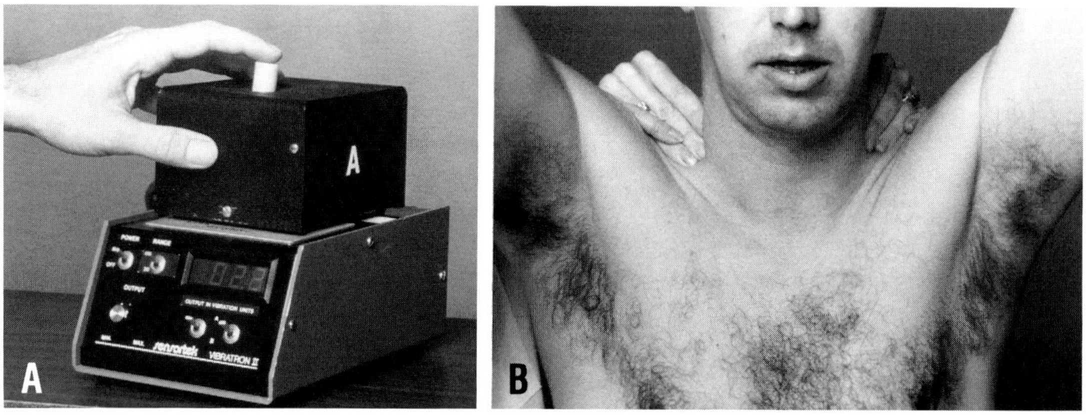

Figure 8–12. *Stress testing to elicit signs of subclinical nerve compression. (**A**) To demonstrate brachial plexus compression ("thoracic outlet syndrome"), a baseline cutaneous vibratory threshold is measured. (**B**) After the patient's symptoms are provoked by holding the hand above the head for 2 minutes, the threshold measurement is repeated. Direct pressure over the plexus may also be used as a provocative test. If significant brachial plexus compression is present, the baseline threshold value will increase (become worse). (Photographs courtesy of Susan E. Mackinnon, M.D., Toronto.)*

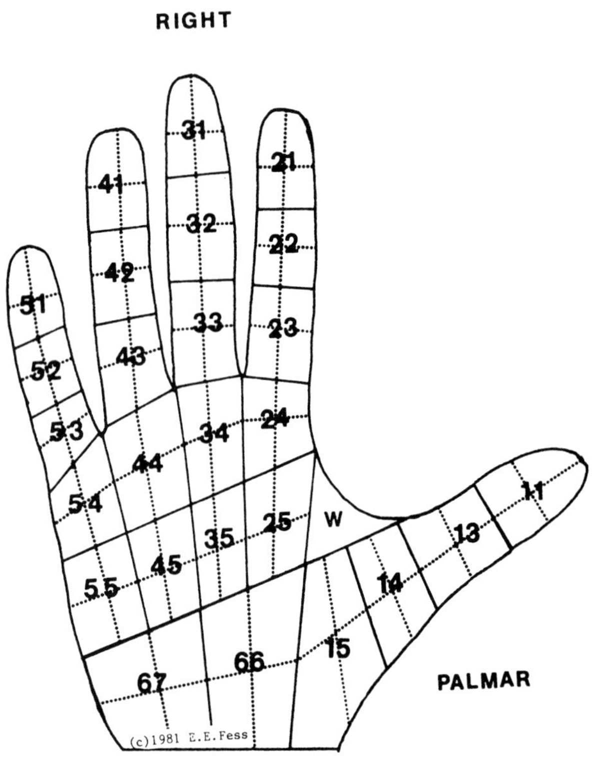

Figure 8–13. *Detailed sensory map. Completing an evaluation of sensibility in so many areas during one examination session has the potential for inherent errors related to patient and physician concentration, totally apart from instrumentation or technique errors.*

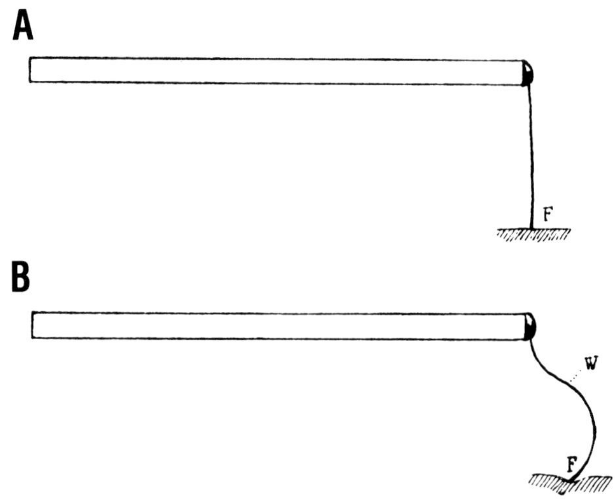

Figure 8–14. *Original von Frey "hairs," forerunner of the Semmes-Weinstein nylon monofilament, were hairs. Here they are shown glued to a candlestick. The force of application was defined by the force delivered when the hair shaft bent, this force being determined by the biochemical properties of the hair (now nylon) shaft. Dividing the force by surface area of the shaft tip gives "stress," or pressure, the appropriate value to report (see Table 8–9). Errors are possible in force application, shaft production, tip surface area, etc. These errors theoretically can be corrected by placing a "force sensor" at the base of a relatively "nondeformable" shaft (see Figs. 8–6, 8–16). (Reproduced with permission from Dellon AL. Evaluation of sensibility and re-education of sensation in the hand. Baltimore: Williams & Wilkins, 1981.)*

demonstrates either no electrical response or denervation (see Chap. 11). However, a common clinical problem is reliance on laboratory studies.

A detailed correlation was possible in a series of patients on whom electrodiagnostic testing was done by physicians referring patients for hand surgery.[38] Each patient had detailed sensibility testing. The study demonstrated that 20% of patients with clinical diagnosis of carpal tunnel syndrome of mild degree had normal electrodiagnostic testing values. Although this finding may not have been unexpected, the finding that 20% of patients with severe carpal tunnel syndrome, based on clinical grounds, also had normal electrodiagnostic testing, was surprising. Further, many clinicians have evaluated patients with unilateral complaints who have values on electrodiagnostic testing indicating bilateral involvement. In my experience, about 20% of the patients on whom I operate for carpal tunnel syndrome have values on electrodiagnostic studies that do not correlate with the clinical examination. Also, 50% of the patients on whom I operate for cubital tunnel syndrome have normal electrodiagnostic testing. This false-negative rate increases to 75% for those patients with radial sensory nerve compression in the forearm (see Chap. 74). Electrodiagnostic studies are more commonly positive with lower extremity nerve entrapment, probably because symptoms are present for a longer time prior to patients' presentation for treatment.

In summary, if the results of electrodiagnostic studies do not correlate with clinical impression, which is based on the history, understanding the mechanism of injury, and detailed sensibility testing as described in this chapter, then I rely on clinical modalities rather than electrodiagnostic testing

Table 8–9. *Force and Stress Calculations and Measurements for Semmes-Weinstein Monofilaments*

Manufacturer's Mark ($\log_{10}$ force)	Calculated Force (g)	Calculated Stress (g/mm²)	Measured Stress (g/mm²)
6.10	126	243	171
5.88	76	181	175
5.46	28	107	82
5.18	15.2	69	85
5.07	11.8	66	95
4.93	8.5	61	76
4.74	5.5	68	39
4.56	3.6	47	37
4.31	2.1	33	30
4.17	1.5	32	34
4.08	1.2	29	24
3.84	0.7	19.3	15.7
3.61	0.4	17.7	9.3
3.22	0.2	11.1	7.5
2.83	0.1	4.9	6.5
2.44	0.0	3.3	4.0
2.36	0.2	5.2	2.1
1.65	0.0	1.5	1.3

(Data from Levin LS, Pearsall G, Ruderman RJ. von Frey's method of measuring pressure sensibility in the hand—an engineering analysis of the Weinstein-Semmes pressure aesthesiometer. J Hand Surg 1978;3:311.)

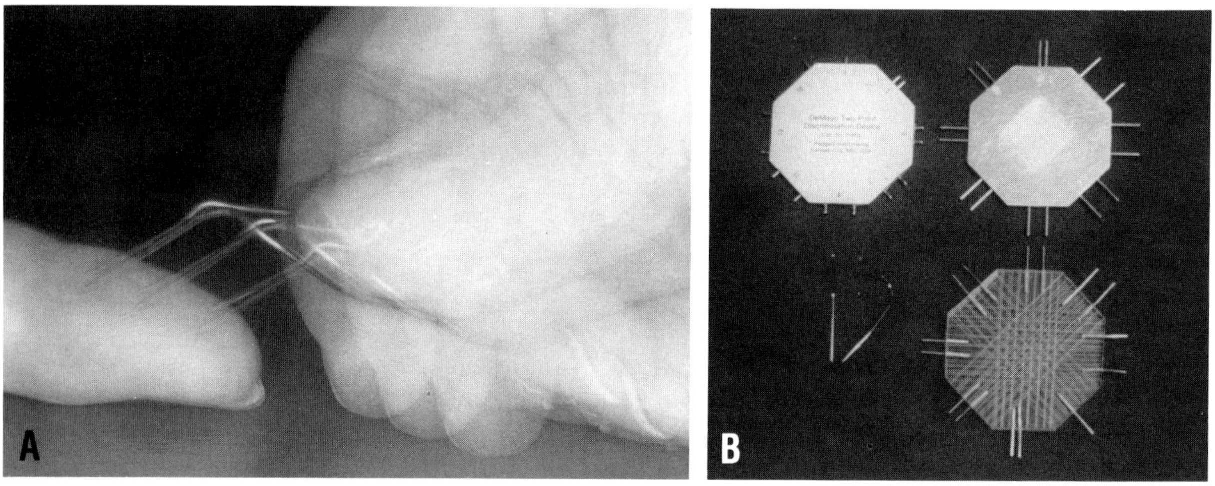

Figure 8–15. *Evolution of testing instruments from (**A**) paperclip to (**B**) Disk-Criminator. The DeMayo device (available through Padgett Instrument, 2838 Warwick Trafficway, Kansas City, MO 64108) is noted.*

(with the exception of malingering, peripheral neuropathy, or the presence of bilateral disease, which makes comparison of one hand to the other difficult).

I do not believe that sensibility testing is reliable in the presence of pain in the area to be tested, or diffuse hand pain. The patient is referred for "desensitization," a form of sensory re-education (see Chap. 58), or underlying abnormalities, such as neuromas or nerve entrapment lesions, are treated.

RECENT DEVELOPMENTS IN TESTING SENSIBILITY

Provocative tests to bring out an underlying subclinical nerve entrapment have been devised. Flexing the wrist to bring out median nerve compression, placing pressure over the median nerve or the site of suspected compression, flexing the elbow for ulnar nerve entrapment at the elbow, and pronating the forearm for radial sensory entrapment have been carried out with accurate results. A most difficult area in which to make a clinical diagnosis, thoracic outlet syndrome, has also been studied. Electrophysiological testing is not diagnostic. Symptoms are most commonly elicited by having the patient raise the arm above the head. A technique has been devised whereby the cutaneous vibratory threshold is determined with the patient's arm at the side.[46] The patient then holds the arm above the head until symptoms appear (this usually takes less than 2 minutes). The vibratory pressure threshold is measured again. If it is abnormal, brachial plexus compression is considered a likely cause of the patient's symptoms (Fig. 8-12). Similar documentation is possible by measuring the change in the cutaneous perception threshold with the Neurometer.†

One area requiring improvement in sensibility testing is the determination of the *testing end point.* One of the major concerns in the past has been the time required to carry out the sensory examination. Implicit in this is the fact that not only the patient, but the examiner as well, loses interest and perhaps precision when the sensory examination requires an extended period to conduct. One of the prime targets of criticism in this regard is detailed mapping with cutaneous pressure threshold instruments (see Fig. 8-13). The test requires the application of several testing instruments, each requiring separate judgments, which means that the entire testing process has an increased risk of error. Apart from instrumentation or technique errors, errors in patient and physician concentration may also occur.

---

† Dellon, A. L. unpublished data, 1990.

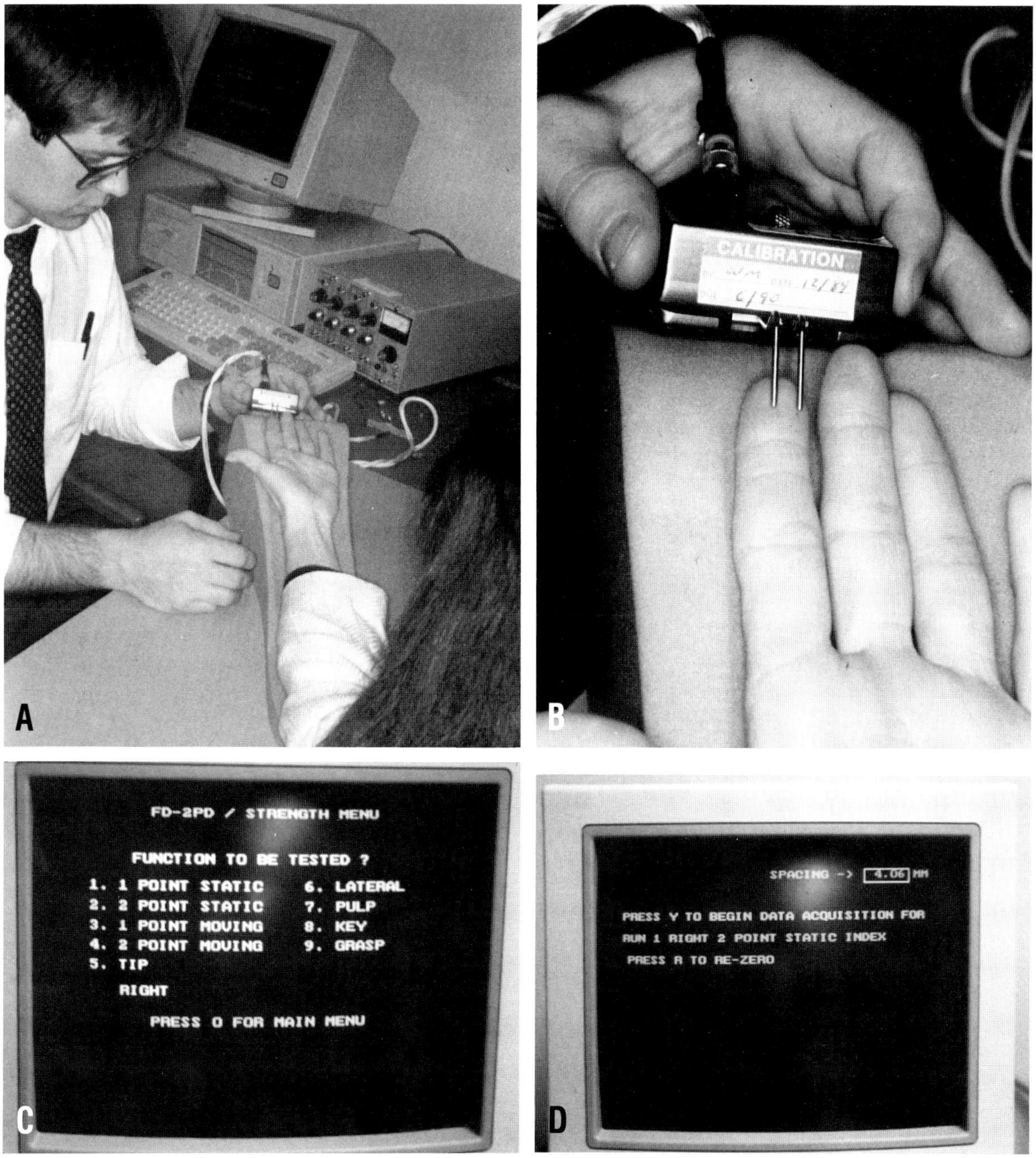

Figure 8–16. *Pressure-Specifying Discriminator. (**A**) The examiner sits in front of the personal computer and signal conditioner, holding the Pressure-Specifying Discriminator (close-up in **B**), while the patient sits with the area to be tested comfortably supported to minimize patient hand vibration. (**C**) The software program permits the choice of sensibility testing or measurement of pinch and grasp with the hand assessment system. Note that the "one-point static" measurement is a cutaneous pressure threshold measurement; thus, a von Frey measurement can be made with the instrument, and a set of nylon monofilaments is not needed. Choosing "two-point static" permits the force to be measured at which the patient can discriminate one from two "points." The same measurements are possible for moving-touch parameters. (**D**) The "re-zero" feature permits the sensitive transducers to be balanced for gravity, permitting the measurements to be done horizontally on fingers, vertically on the side of the leg, and upside down on the plantar aspect of the foot. (Available through NK Biotechnical Engineering, P. O. Box 26335, Minneapolis, MN 55426.)*

Errors have been noted with the application of specific devices. The original von Frey hairs, true hairs attached to the end of a candlestick, were applied as shown in Figure 8-14. Errors involved with this type of measuring instrument have been summarized following a detailed biomechanical evaluation:

> Variations in the buckling stress as high as the factor of eight are difficult to avoid. Gross errors arise from careless application, variations in the elastic modulus due to changes in temperature and humidity, and variations in the attachment of the fibers to handles and differences in the ends of the filaments. Interpreting results for this instrument (Semmes-Weinstein) requires an understanding of factors which can influence those results. Probes are simple to use but easy to misinterpret.[32]

A further common problem with the Semmes-Weinstein monofilaments is that the number on the handle is actually the log to the base 10 of the calculated force. Unfortunately, this number (the log to base 10, ie, 2.36 or 3.84 or 6.65) is mistakenly recorded as the actual measured force. This number cannot be added and divided and used for statistical purposes. The force actually measured with this instrument then must be divided by the cross-sectional area of the end of the filament to arrive at the measured stress (or pressure), which is grams per square millimeter (Table 8-9). Just as a series of instrument changes has brought two-point discriminator testing from the paper clip through gauge devices that had accurate interspace distances but pointed tips, to disc-shaped devices that had fixed distances with rounded tips (Fig. 8-15), so too has product development evolved into a better instrument, the Pressure-Specifying Discriminator (Figs. 8-6, 8-16), to determine cutaneous pressure threshold, eliminating the errors described above.

Extensive evaluations with the Semmes-Weinstein nylon monofilaments have been carried out, with great attention given to recording the results.[2,4,6] Bell-Krotoski identified inherent errors in using testing instruments due to the natural movements of the hands of patients and examiners during testing.[3]

Ideally, an instrument should be available that can determine the force at which a two-point discrimination test is measured. Theoretically this instrument could have one of the two points not used during the test and the same instrument, therefore, could be used to obtain a cutaneous pressure threshold. If this instrument were connected online to a computer, the average force generated after 2 seconds of continuous measurements could be obtained, allowing correction of the variability of the force/time relationships. Such an instrument, the Pressure-Specifying Discriminator, has been developed (see Figs. 8-6, 8-16). This instrument places a force-transducer beneath each rounded metal prong. Prong distance is variable to permit discrimination of two points. The force beneath either one or both prongs can be measured, with time-averaging of the force, and direct digital online computer recording.

REFERENCES

1. American Society for Surgery of the Hand, Clinical Assessment Committee Recommendations, September 1989.
2. Bell JA. Light touch—deep pressure testing using Semmes-Weinstein monofilaments. In: Hunter JM, Schneider LH, Mackin EJ, Callahan AD, eds. Rehabilitation of the hand, ed. 2. St. Louis: CV Mosby, 1984:399–406.
3. Bell-Krotoski JA, Buford WL. The force/time relationship of clinical sensory testing instruments. J Hand Ther 1988;1:76–85.
4. Bell-Krotoski JA, Tomancik E. The repeatability of testing with Semmes-Weinstein monofilaments. J Hand Surg [Am] 1987;12:155–161.
5. Brown CJ, Mackinnon SE, Dellon AL, Bain JR. The sensory potential of free flap donor sites. Ann Plast Surg 1989;23:135–140.
6. Callahan AD. Sensibility testing: Clinical methods. In: Hunter JM, Schneider LH, Mackin EJ, Callahan AD, eds. Rehabilitation of the hand, ed 2. St. Louis: CV Mosby, 1984:407–431.
7. Cauna N. Nature and functions of the papillary ridges of the digital skin. Anat Record 1954;119: 449–468.
8. Crosby PM, Dellon AL. A comparison of two-point discrimination test devices. Microsurg 1989;10: 134–137.
9. Dellon AL. The moving two-point discrimination test; clinical evaluation of the quickly-adapting fiber receptor system. J Hand Surg 1978;3:474–481.

10. Dellon AL. Clinical use of vibratory stimuli to evaluate peripheral nerve injury and compression neuropathy. Plast Reconstr Surg 1980;65:466–476.
11. Dellon AL. Evaluation of sensibility and re-education of sensation in the hand. Baltimore: Williams & Wilkins, 1981.
12. Dellon AL. The vibrometer. Plast Reconstr Surg 1983;71:427–431.
13. Dellon AL. Tinel or not Tinel. J Hand Surg [Br] 1984;9:216.
14. Dellon AL. Touch sensibility in the hand. J Hand Surg [Br] 1984;9:11–13.
15. Dellon AL. Functional sensation and its re-education. In: Terzis J, ed. Microreconstruction of nerve injuries. Philadelphia: WB Saunders, 1987:33–52.
16. Dellon AL. Optimism in diabetic neuropathy. Ann Plast Surg 1988;20:103–105.
17. Dellon AL. Review of treatment results for ulnar nerve compression at the elbow. J Hand Surg [Am] 1989;14:688–699.
18. Dellon AL. The sensational contributions of Erik Moberg. J Hand Surg [Br] 1990;15:24–29.
19. Dellon AL. Wound in healing in nerve. Clin Plast Surg 1990;17:545–570.
20. Dellon AL, Curtis RM, Edgerton MT. Evaluating recovery of sensation in the hand following nerve injury. Johns Hopkins Med J 1972;130:235–243.
21. Dellon AL, Kallman CH. Evaluation of functional sensation in the hand. J Hand Surg 1983;8:865–870.
22. Dellon AL, Mackinnon SE. Radial sensory nerve entrapment in the forearm. J Hand Surg [Am] 1986;11:199–205.
23. Dellon AL, Mackinnon SE. Human ulnar neuropathy at the elbow: Clinical, electrical and morphometric correlations. J Reconstr Microsurg 1988;4:179–184.
24. Dellon AL, Mackinnon SE, Crosby PM. Reliability of two-point discrimination measurements. J Hand Surg [Am] 1987;12:693–696.
25. Dellon AL, Munger BL. Correlation of histology and sensibility after nerve repair. J Hand Surg 1983;8:871–878.
26. Dellon AL, Schneider R, Burke R. Effect of acute compartmental pressure changes upon response to vibratory stimuli. Plast Reconstr Surg 1983;72:208–216.
27. Dellon AL, Trujak JE, Rochman GM. Medial nerve compression in Weill-Marchesani syndrome. Plast Reconstr Surg 1984;74:127–130.
28. Gelberman RH, Pfeffer GB, Galleraith RT, Szabo RM, Rydevik B, Dimick M. Results of treatment of severe carpal tunnel syndrome without internal neurolysis of the median nerve. J Bone Joint Surg [Am] 1987;69:896–903.
29. Gelberman RH, Urbaniak JR, Bright DS, Levin LS. Digital sensibility following replantation. J Hand Surg 1978;3:313–319.
30. Gellis M, Pool R. Two-point discrimination distances in the normal hand and forearm. Plast Reconstr Surg 1977;59:57–62.
31. Jiranec W, Seiler WA, Dellon AL. Teaching the technique for microsurgical intraneural neurolysis. J Reconstr Microsurg 1987;3:137–141.
32. Levin LS, Pearsall G, Ruderman RJ. von Frey's method of measuring pressure sensibility in the hand: An engineering analysis of the Weinstein-Semmes pressure aesthesiometer. J Hand Surg 1978;3:311–316.
33. Louis DS, Greene TC, Jakobsen KE, Rasmussen C, Kolowich P, Goldstein SA. Evaluation of normal values for stationary and moving two-point discrimination in the hand. J Hand Surg [Am] 1984;9:552–555.
34. Lundborg G. Nerve injury and repair. Edinburgh: Churchill-Livingstone, 1988:120–122.
35. Lundborg G, Lie-Stenstrom AK, Sollerman C, Stromberg T, Pyykko J. Digital vibrogram: A new diagnostic tool for sensory testing in compression neuropathy. J Hand Surg [Am] 1986;11:693–699.
36. Mackinnon SE, Dellon AL. Two-point discrimination tester. J Hand Surg [Am] 1985;10:906–907.
37. Mackinnon SE, Dellon AL. Experimental study of chronic nerve compression: Clinical implications. Clin Hand Surg 1986;2:639–650.
38. Mackinnon SE, Dellon AL. Surgery of the peripheral nerve. New York: Thieme, 1988:1–88.
39. Mackinnon SE, Dellon AL. Evaluation of microsurgical internal neurolysis in a primate median nerve model of chronic nerve compression. J Hand Surg [Am] 1988;13:345–351.
40. Mackinnon SE, Dellon AL, Daneshvar A. Histopathology of the tarsal tunnel syndrome: Examination of a human tibial nerve. Contemp Orthop 1984;9:43–48.
41. Mackinnon SE, Dellon AL, Hudson AR, Hunter DA. Chronic nerve compression an experimental model in the rat. Ann Plast Surg 1984;13:112–120.
42. Mackinnon SE, Dellon AL, Hudson AR, Hunter DA. A primate model for chronic nerve compression. J Reconstr Microsurg 1985;1:185–194.
43. Mackinnon SE, Dellon AL, Hudson AR, Hunter DA. Chronic human nerve compression: A histologic assessment. Neuropath Appl Neurobiol 1986;12:547–565.
44. Mackinnon SE, Dellon AL, Hudson AR, Hunter DA.

Histopathology of compression of the superficial radial nerve in forearm. J Hand Surg [Am] 1986;11: 206–209.

45. Mackinnon SE, O'Brien JP, Dellon AL, MacLean AR, Hudson AR, Hunter DA. An assessment of the effects of different treatment strategies, including internal neurolysis, on a chronically compressed rat sciatic nerve. Plast Reconstr Surg 1988;81:251–256.
46. Mackinnon SE, Patterson GA. Stress testing to diagnose thoracic outlet syndrome. Presented at the Society of Thoracic Surgeons meeting, Palm Springs, Calif., January 20, 1990.
47. Moberg E. Objective methods of determining functional value of sensibility in the hand. J Bone Joint Surg [Br] 1958;40:454–466.
48. Moberg E. Methods for examining sensibility. In: Flynn JE, ed. Hand surgery. Baltimore: Williams & Wilkins, 1966:435–449.
49. Mountcastle VB. Modality and topographic properties of single neurons of cat's sensory cortex. J Neurophys 1957;20:408–434.
50. Mountcastle VB, Darian-Smith I. A neural base for the sense of flutter-vibration. Science 1967;155: 597–600.
51. Munger BL, Pubols LM. The sensorineural organization of digital skin of the raccoon. Brain Behav Evol 1972;5:367–393.
52. O'Brien JP, Mackinnon SE, MacLean AR, Dellon AL, Hudson AR, Hunter DA. A model of chronic nerve compression in the rat. Ann Plast Surg 1987;19:430–435.
53. O'Rain S. New and simple test of nerve function in the hand. Brit Med J 1973;3:615–616.
54. Phelps PE, Walker E. Comparison of the finger wrinkling test results to established sensory tests in peripheral nerve injury. Am J Occup Ther 1977;31: 565–572.
55. Phillips JE, Mackinnon SE, Beatty E, Dellon AL, O'Brien J. Vibratory sensory testing in acute compartment syndrome: A clinical and experimental study. Plast Reconstr Surg 1987;79:796–801.
56. Rhoades CE, Mowery CA, Gelberman RH. Results of internal neurolysis of the median nerve for severe carpal tunnel syndrome. J Hand Surg [Am] 1985;10: 253–256.
57. Seddon HJ, Medawar PB, Smith H. Rate of regeneration of peripheral nerves in man. J Physiol 1943;102:191–215.
58. Spindler HA, Dellon AL. Nerve conduction studies and sensibility testing in carpal tunnel syndrome. J Hand Surg 1982;7:260–263.
59. Sunderland S. Rate of regeneration in human peripheral nerve. Arch Neurol Psych 1947;58:251–295.
60. Szabo RM, Gelberman RH, Williamson RV, Dellon AL, Yaru NC, Dimick MP. Vibratory sensory testing in acute peripheral nerve compression. J Hand Surg [Am] 1984;9:104–108.

9

Motor Testing

William F. Blair

AUTHOR'S KEY POINTS

- Each nerve and corresponding muscle has a specific test for optimal demonstration of function.
- Proximal brachial plexus injuries, in the upper roots or trunks, can be delineated accurately by testing muscles innervated by the suprascapular, dorsal scapular, and long thoracic nerves.
- Injuries at the infraclavicular brachial plexus level involve branches primarily from the cord level: the medial and lateral pectoral nerves affecting the anterior periscapular muscles, and branches from the posterior cord affecting the posterior and lateral periscapular muscles.
- Similarly, injuries to branches of the lumbosacral plexus (T12–S5) are localized by sequential muscle examination.
- Accurate motor testing depends on the absence of muscle and tendon injury, the presence of joint mobility, and patient cooperation. Despite these limitations, it is an invaluable tool for assessing the integrity of the peripheral nervous system.

GENERAL CONSIDERATIONS

Motor testing is used to determine whether specific muscles or muscle groups are capable of contraction and, to the extent possible, to assess the quality of that contraction. Muscle contraction depends on the integrity of the muscle, normal passive motion in the joints across which the muscle acts, and the quality of innervation of the muscle. For the peripheral nerve surgeon, the question of the quality of innervation is paramount.

Motor testing is used clinically to assess the extent of injury or disease.[1–4] After trauma, the results of motor testing in large part define the magnitude of the primary injury. In neuromuscular disease, motor testing defines the extent and severity of involvement. These observations form the basis of the patient's prognosis. The results of initial motor testing are the baseline against which the results of treatment are assessed. The initial, baseline motor testing evaluation must be thorough and accurate. Motor testing is especially important after peripheral nerve reconstruction, when the results are used to assess the quality and extent of reinnervation.

Muscle contraction can be assessed qualitatively, semi-quantitatively, and quantitatively. Qualitative assessment is completed by having the patient describe the muscle strength, by inspecting muscle mass and contour, and by observing voluntary motion. Semi-quantitative assessment, which is used most widely, is essentially manual motor strength testing. It is based on a grading system that requires thorough knowledge of muscle and peripheral nerve anatomy and muscle function (Table 9-1). Motor testing has the distinct advantage of providing information about either the whole nerve or specific motor branches. It is fundamental to the assessment of peripheral nerve injury and treatment. This form of testing is convenient, inexpensive, and readily repeatable in the clinic setting, so it is appropriately the primary content of this chapter.

The quantitative assessment of muscle function requires the use of one of a variety of dynamometers for testing grip and pinch strengths. Many new computer-interfaced machines measure strength, power, and endurance. However, these instruments do not isolate muscles well; therefore they are not as specific as manual motor testing in the assessment of specific nerve deficits.

The clinical task of testing a specific muscle can be done in two basic ways. In the first technique, the joints across which the muscle in question acts are positioned in neutral, and the patient is asked to produce the desired motion or to contract the tested muscle. For example, the metacarpophalangeal (MP) joint of the thumb is held in neutral and the patient is instructed to flex the tip to test the flexor pollicis longus. In this method of testing, instruction by the examiner is often most efficiently done by demonstration. The patient's ability to produce the desired motion is assessed. In the second technique, the body part is placed in the position into which the tested muscle would normally move that part. The patient's ability to maintain that position, against resistance, is assessed. For example, the patient's forearm is placed in full supination and the patient is asked to pronate against the resistance of the examiner's grasp to test the pronator teres. Practically, either or both of these test methods are used.

Table 9–1. *Muscle Power Grading*

Grade	Description
0–None	No palpable muscle contraction
1–Trace	Palpable muscle contraction, detectable by examiner
2–Poor	Active joint motion present with gravity eliminated
3–Fair	Muscle can move joint through full range of motion against gravity
4–Good	Full range of motion against gravity and some resistance
5–Normal	Full range of motion with a maximum force that is normal for that muscle

Motor testing may also be supplemented by functional testing. For example, the patient may be asked to reach above the head, or open and close a fist, or walk on the toes to elicit variations in complex motions that are characteristic of specific deficits.

UPPER EXTREMITY

Motor testing in the upper extremity is conveniently considered in terms of the brachial plexus proximally and in terms of each of the specific, major peripheral nerves distally.

Brachial Plexus

Brachial plexus injuries are among the most difficult to assess because of the complexity of the anatomy and variations in injury patterns (Fig. 9-1). It is convenient to consider brachial plexus injuries as preganglionic (Zone 1), postganglionic and supraclavicular (Zone 2), and infraclavicular (Zone 3). However, most brachial plexus injuries are complex, involving injuries that extend through the zones. Zone 1 and 2 injuries cannot be differentiated from each other on the basis of motor testing. However, injuries within Zone 1 and 2 can be con-

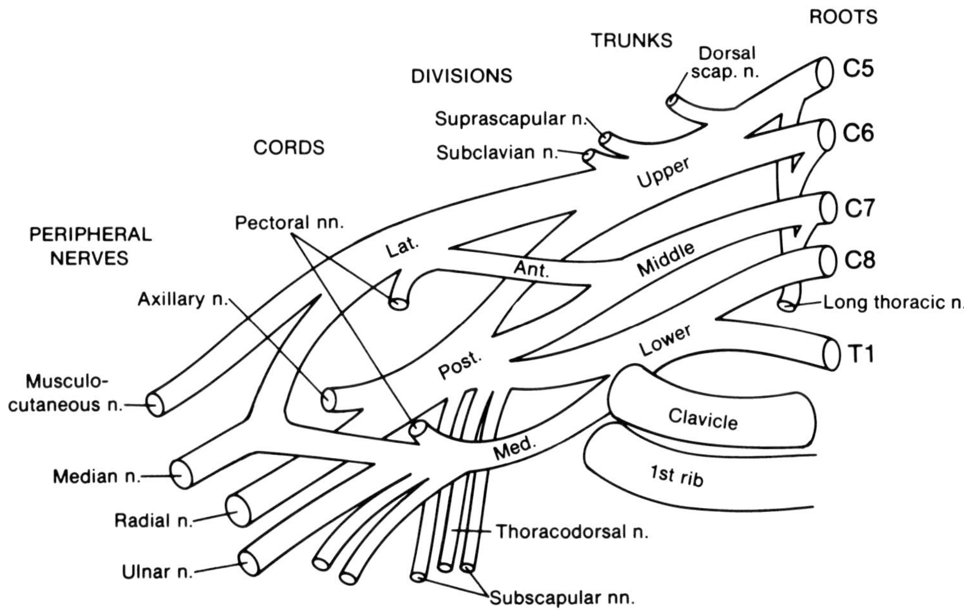

Figure 9–1. *The brachial plexus. Knowledge of plexus anatomy and motor testing helps to localize lesions in the plexus. Periscapular paralysis indicates a high level of plexus injury.*

firmed by specific supraclavicular and infraclavicular deficits.

Supraclavicular Deficits

Proximal injuries in the upper roots or trunks affect the following nerves and their corresponding motor tests.

1. Suprascapular. Supraspinatus (C5, C6) and infraspinatus muscles are tested with the patient in an upright position. The arm is at the side, and the elbow is flexed 90°. The patient externally rotates the arm against resistance. Weakness of external rotation indicates deficiency in the spinati.
2. Dorsal scapular. Rhomboid (C5) and levator (C3, C4) muscles are tested with the patient upright and observed from behind. For the rhomboid, the patient adducts or retracts the scapulae, attempting to approximate them posteriorly. For the levators, the patient shrugs the shoulders upward against downward pressure on both shoulders. Weakness of shoulder shrugging suggests levator weakness.
3. Long thoracic. The serratus anterior (C5–7) muscle is evaluated by having the patient simulate a push-up against the wall while in the standing position. If the scapula protrudes from the posterior chest wall, or wings, scapular protraction is absent, and serratus anterior function is deficient.

Infraclavicular Deficits

Injuries at this level involve branches primarily from the cords. Branches from the medial and lateral cords affect anterior periscapular musculature; branches from the posterior cord affect the posterior and lateral periscapular musculature.

1. Pectoral nerves, medial and lateral. The pectoralis major (C5–T1) and minor (C8–T1) muscles are tested with the patient upright. The arm is at the side, the elbow flexed 90°, and the hand straight ahead. The patient moves the hand toward the anterior trunk, against the examiner's resistance, which is applied at the wrist. Decreased strength of arm adduction suggests weakness of the pectoral muscles.
2. Thoracodorsal nerve. The latissimus dorsi (C6–8) muscle is best tested with the patient standing and observed from posterolaterally. The muscle is an adductor and internal rotator of the arm; it is difficult to isolate. The patient places both hands on the hips and pushes inward. Contraction of the

muscle can be inspected and palpated. Alternately, to assess the strength of contraction, the arm is held fully abducted. The patient then adducts against resistance. The latissimus dorsi is observed on the lower lateral aspect of the thorax (Fig. 9-2).

3. Subscapular nerve, upper and lower. The subscapularis (C5, C6) muscle, innervated by both subscapular nerves, is tested with the patient upright, the arm at the side, and the elbow flexed 90°. The hand is straight ahead. The patient attempts to rotate the hand to the anterior trunk, against the examiner's resistance. Decreased strength of internal rotation suggests subscapularis weakness. The lower subscapular nerve innervates the teres major muscle, which is tested in the same manner as the latissimus dorsi.

Three patterns of injury involve the supraclavicular zones. Total plexus injuries result in a flail shoulder and arm and paralysis of all muscles in the hand. An upper plexus palsy (Erb-Duchenne) results in paralysis of the rhomboids, supraspinatus, infraspinatus, deltoid, and brachialis muscles. The arm hangs at the side with the shoulder internally rotated, the elbow extended, and the forearm pronated. A lower plexus palsy (Dejerine-Klumpke) results in paralysis of the muscles of the hand and weakness of the flexor carpi ulnaris and flexor digitorum to the small finger. All four fingers are clawed, the thumb is adducted, and the palm is flattened.

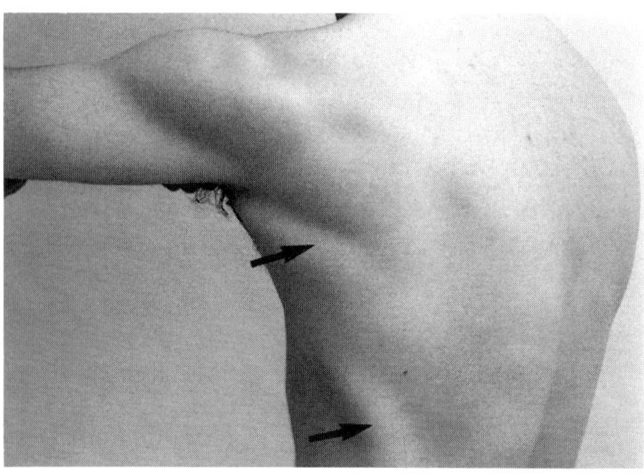

Figure 9–2. *When adducting the arm against resistance, the latissimus dorsi muscle appears as a curved contour on the lower lateral aspect of the thorax (arrow).*

Peripheral Nerves

The major peripheral nerves are considered as they exit the posterior cord (axillary, radial), lateral cord (musculocutaneous), both lateral and medial cords (median), and finally the medial cord (ulnar). The branches are best considered in terms of the muscles they innervate sequentially, from proximally to distally.

Axillary Nerves

1. Deltoid (C5, C6). The deltoid muscle is most easily tested by considering the middle portion representative. The patient is upright, the arm is at the side, and the examiner stands posteriorly and uses a hand to stabilize the acromion. The patient abducts the arm against resistance. The anterior and posterior portions of the muscle, although functionally important, are difficult to isolate from other periscapular muscles. Weakness of shoulder abduction suggests axillary nerve palsy.
2. Teres minor (C5, C6). This muscle is tested in the same manner as the supraspinatus and infraspinatus muscles, from which it cannot be readily distinguished.

Radial Nerve (Fig. 9-3)

1. Triceps (C6–8). With the patient upright, the shoulder is fully abducted and forward flexed 20°. The elbow is allowed to flex 90°. The patient attempts to extend the elbow against resistance to a horizontal position. The inability to extend the elbow indicates possible triceps denervation.
2. Brachioradialis (C5, C6). With the patient upright, the elbow is positioned in 90° of flexion. The contour of the anterolateral aspect of the elbow is inspected. The elbow is flexed against resistance while the examiner palpates and carefully observes contraction.
3. Extensor carpi radialis longus and brevis (ECRL, ECRB) (C6, C7). With the volar aspect of the forearm on the examination table and the elbow flexed 90°, the patient is instructed first to extend and then to extend and radially deviate the wrist. The ability to perform both functions indicate innervation of both muscles above the elbow level.
4. Supinator (C5, C6). With the olecranon resting on the examination table and elbow fully flexed, the

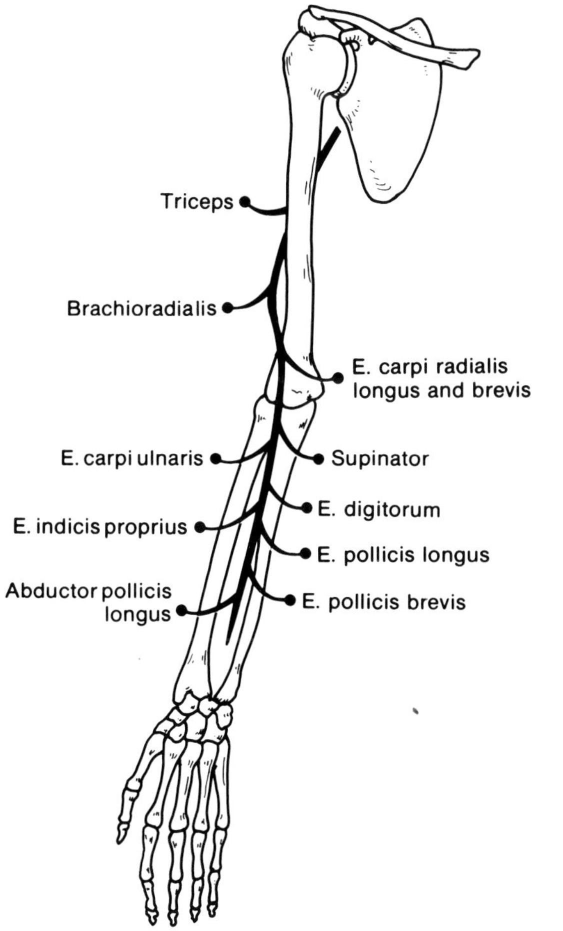

Figure 9-3. *Muscles innervated by the radial nerve, as viewed from the posterior aspect of the upper extremity. E, extensor.*

forearm is positioned in neutral. The patient supinates against the resistance of the examiner's grasp at the wrist. Weakness of supination indicates probable supinator denervation, but the biceps must also be considered and tested.

5. Extensor carpi ulnaris (ECU) (C6–8). The volar aspect of the forearm is placed on the examination table, and the elbow is flexed. The patient both extends and ulnarly deviates the wrist. If testing for both ECRL and ECU results in dorsoradial deviation of the wrist, a low radial or posterior interosseous nerve palsy is suggested.
6. Extensor digitorum communis (EDC) (C6–8). The volar aspect of the forearm rests on the examination table. The wrist is positioned in neutral. The patient is instructed to raise the fingers from the table, into hyperextension at the MP joints. The examiner provides fingertip resistance to the dorsum of the patient's finger. The strength of extension and observation of tendon tension on the dorsum of the hand indicate EDC innervation.
7. Extensor digiti minimi (C6–8). The same test is performed as for EDC, except the patient is instructed to elevate only the small finger.
8. Extensor indicis proprius (C7, C8). The same test is performed as for EDC, except the patient elevates only the index finger.
9. Extensor pollicis longus (EPL) (C7, C8). The ulnar border of the forearm is placed on the examination table. The patient is instructed to extend the thumb, to specifically demonstrate extension of the distal phalanx. The examiner may use one hand to hold the MP joint in neutral while the patient extends the thumb. With a fingertip, the examiner resists extension of the distal phalanx, confirming EPC innervation.
10. Extensor pollicis brevis (EPB) (C6, C7) (Fig. 9-4). The test is completed as if for EPL, except that the examiner secures the carpometacarpal (CMC) joint. Thumb MP extension is observed and tested by fingertip resistance.
11. Abductor pollicis longus (APL) (C6, C7). The dorsal surface of the forearm rests on the examination table, with the wrist in neutral. The patient elevates the thumb away from the table while resistance is applied to the distal and volar aspect of the metacarpal. Strength of abduction and palpation of tendon tension on the radial aspect of the wrist confirm APL contraction.

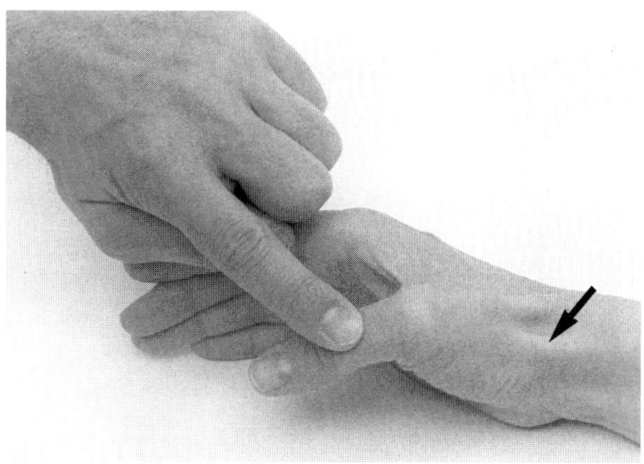

Figure 9-4. *The extensor pollicis brevis muscle (arrow) extends the thumb metacarpophalangeal joint against resistance applied dorsally.*

Musculocutaneous Nerve

1. Biceps (C5, C6). The elbow is fully extended and the forearm supinated. The patient is instructed to flex the elbow fully against the resistance of the examiner's grasp on the distal forearm. Tension in the distal tendon can be palpated between the fingertips. This finding and the visible, anterior arm muscle firmness confirm contraction.
2. Brachialis (C5, C6). The test is the same as for the biceps. The brachialis muscle emerges lateral to the biceps, where it may be palpated during active flexion.

Ulnar Nerve (Fig. 9-5)

1. Flexor carpi ulnaris (C8, T1). The dorsal surface of the forearm rests on the examination table with the wrist in neutral. The patient is instructed to flex and then to flex and ulnarly deviate the wrist. The tendon must be palpated during testing to verify its contraction, as the flexor carpi radialis and palmaris longus muscles have similar actions.
2. Flexor digitorum profundus (FDP) to the small and ring fingers (C7–T1). The dorsal surface of the forearm rests on the table. The proximal interphalangeal (PIP) joint is held in neutral. The patient is instructed to flex the distal phalanx against resistance. Flexion of the distal interphalangeal (DIP) joint can only be accomplished by the FDP.
3. Abductor digiti minimi (C8, T1). With the wrist in neutral, the dorsal surface of the hand rests on the table. The patient is instructed to abduct the little finger against the examiner's fingertip resistance. The muscle must be carefully observed and palpated during this examination.
4. Flexor digiti minimi (FDM) (C8, T1). With the wrist in neutral and the dorsal surface of the hand

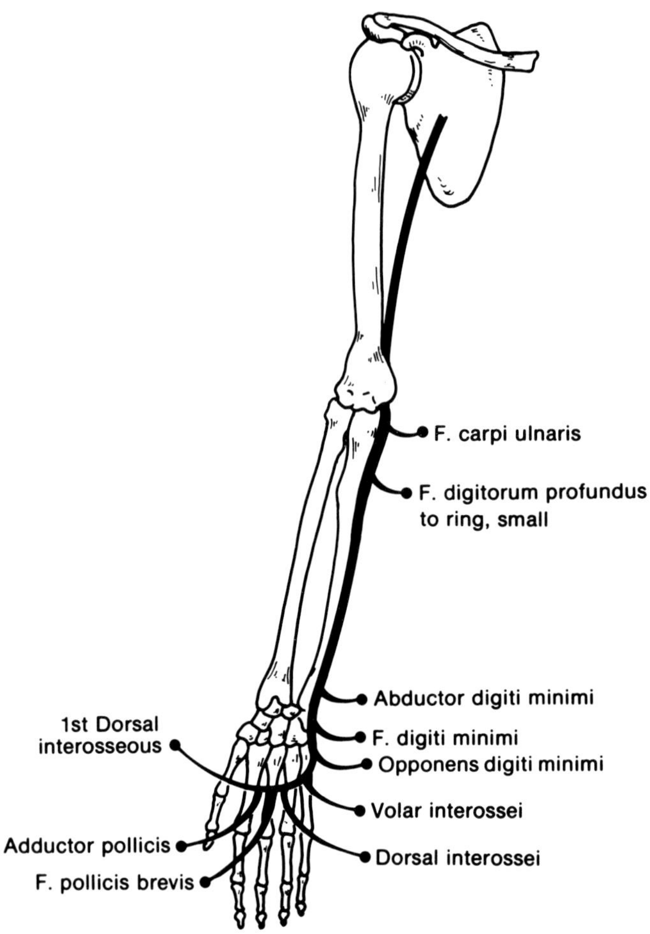

Figure 9–5. *Muscles innervated by the ulnar nerve, as viewed from the anterior aspect of the upper extremity. F, flexor.*

on the table, the small finger is positioned so that it points directly upward. The patient is asked to maintain this position against an extension force applied to the proximal phalanx.

5. Opponens digiti minimi (C8, T1). The test for opponens is essentially the same as that for FDM.
6. Volar interosseous muscles (C8, T1). The hand is positioned on the table with the palm down and the fingers resting on the surface. The patient is instructed to move the index finger medially and then to move the ring and small fingers laterally, all on the plane of the table. These active motions are toward the midline of the long finger.
7. Dorsal interosseous muscles (C8, T1). The hand is positioned on the table with the palm down and the fingers resting on the surface. The patient is instructed to move the long finger radially on the plane of the table and then to move the long and ring fingers ulnarly in the same manner. These active motions are all away from the midline of the long finger.
8. Flexor pollicis brevis (C8, T1) (Fig. 9-6). Although the superficial portion of this muscle is innervated by the median nerve and the deep portion by the ulnar nerve, all testing will be considered here under the ulnar nerve section. The ulnar border of the hand rests on the examination table. The examiner stabilizes the first metacarpal in neutral, midway between full abduction and adduction. The patient is instructed to flex the MP joint, bending the thumb toward the small finger. Active MP joint flexion, both observed and demonstrated against resistance, confirms innervation.
9. Adductor pollicis (C8, T1). The dorsal surface of the hand is placed on the table. The examiner positions the thumb in adduction. The patient is instructed to move the thumb to the palmar surface of the index MP joint, while the examiner provides resistance to the ulnar border of the distal thumb.
10. First dorsal interosseous (C8, T1) (Fig. 9-7). The hand is positioned with the palmar border resting on the table. The index finger is then positioned in abduction by the examiner, so that its side points toward the ceiling. Fingertip pressure is applied to the radial side of the index finger while the muscle mass is observed and palpated. The terminal branch of the ulnar nerve in the hand is responsible for radial deviation of the index finger.

Median Nerve (Fig. 9-8)

1. Pronator teres (C6, C7). The patient is in the upright position with the elbow flexed at 90° and resting against the side of the chest wall. The forearm is fully supinated. The examiner firmly grasps the patient's hand or wrist and asks the patient to pronate against the resistance. This test does not isolate the pronator teres from the pronator quadratus.
2. Flexor carpi radialis (FCR) (C6, C7). The forearm

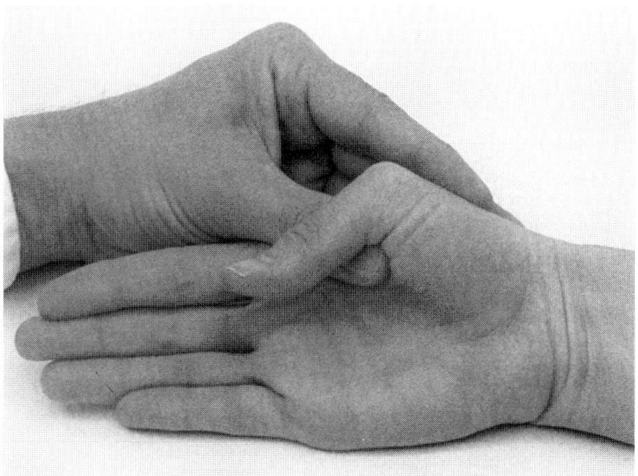

Figure 9–6. *The flexor pollicis brevis muscle flexes the thumb metacarpophalangeal joint when the first metacarpal is stabilized in a neutral position.*

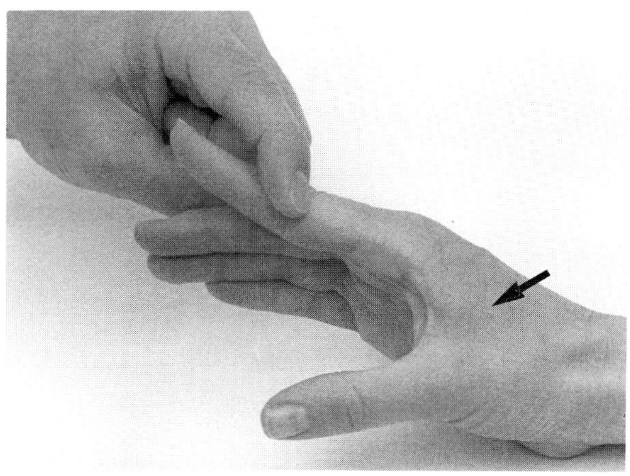

Figure 9–7. *The first dorsal interosseous muscle (arrow) radially deviates the index finger against resistance; it visibly and palpably contracts along the radial aspect of the second metacarpal.*

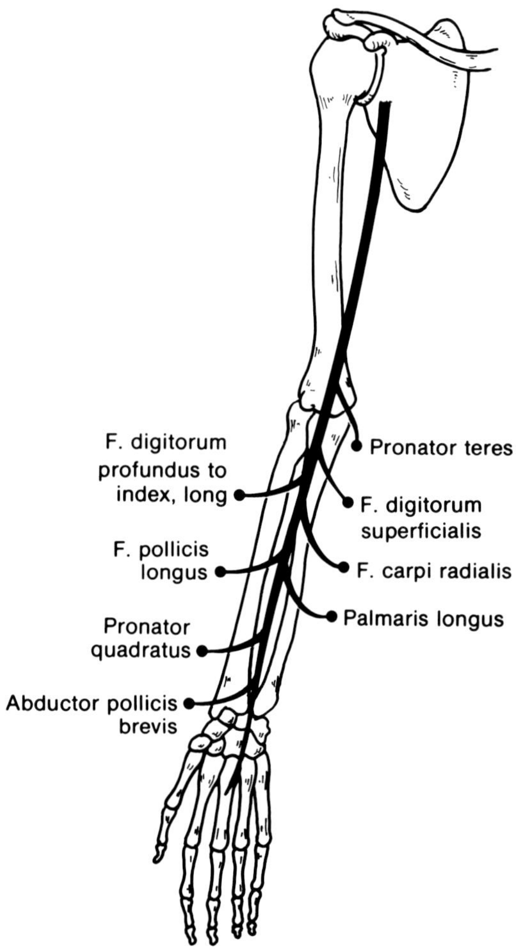

Figure 9–8. *Muscles innervated by the median nerve, as viewed from the anterior aspect of the upper extremity. F, flexor.*

is positioned with the dorsal surface on the table. The patient is instructed to flex the wrist, moving the hand toward the ceiling. Tension in the FCR tendon is observed and palpated. This test does not differentiate between the FCR and the palmaris longus, which can also be seen to contract just ulnar to the FCR.

3. Flexor superficialis (FDS) (C7–T1). This muscle sends independent tendons to each of the four fingers. Therefore, the FDS tendon to each finger can be assessed separately. The hand is positioned with the dorsal surface on the table. All fingers except the finger being tested are held in full extension on the table surface. Because the flexor digitorum profundus tendons function as a group, the maneuver pulls all FDP tendons to full length. This leaves only the FDS tendon to function. It actively flexes the proximal interphalangeal joint in the tested finger.
4. Flexor pollicis longus (FPL) (C7–T1). The ulnar border of the hand rests on the table, with the wrist in neutral. The examiner stabilizes the MP joint of the thumb. The patient is instructed to flex the terminal phalanx against fingertip resistance. Active IP flexion confirms FPL innervation in the forearm.
5. Flexor digitorum profundus to index and long fingers (C7–T1). This muscle is tested in the same manner as the small and ring fingers. The dorsal surface of the forearm rests on the table, and the PIP joints are held in a neutral position. The patient is instructed to flex the distal phalanx against resistance.
6. Pronator quadratus (C7–T1). The olecranon is placed on the table, the elbow is fully flexed, and the forearm is positioned in full supination. The examiner firmly grasps the hand and wrist and asks the patient to pronate against the resistance. Although the pronator quadratus cannot be fully isolated from the pronator teres, full flexion of the elbow will minimize the contribution from the teres.
7. Abductor pollicis brevis (C6, C7) (Fig. 9-9). The dorsum of the hand is placed on the examining table. The examiner positions the thumb in full abduction, placing it away from the plane of the palm toward the ceiling. The patient is then instructed to maintain the thumb in that position while contraction of the abductor is observed and

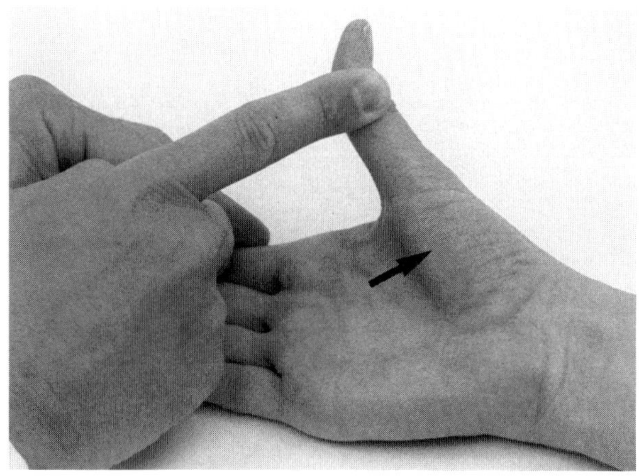

Figure 9–9. *The abductor pollicis brevis muscle (arrow) maintains an abducted position of the first metacarpal against fingertip pressure.*

palpated. Fingertip pressure is then applied to the radial aspect of the thumb, gently pushing it toward the base of the index finger. Alternately, the thumb can be placed at the base of the index finger and the patient can be asked to abduct the thumb toward the ceiling while the examiner performs the same observations.

8. Opponens pollicis (C6, C7) (Fig. 9-10). The patient is instructed to make an "O" between the thumb and the little finger. The examiner then hooks a finger in the "O" to test for its breaking strength and thus the strength of the opponens. Opponens can not be isolated from the abductor pollicis brevis or flexor pollicis brevis; testing for this muscle requires an intact opponens digiti minimi.

LOWER EXTREMITY

Lumbosacral Plexus

The lumbosacral plexus is formed by contributions from roots T12 to S5. Anatomically the lumbar plexus emerges from behind the psoas muscle. The major nerves that exit the lumbar plexus innervate the thigh. The lumbar plexus can be considered as having anterior and posterior components. The anterior component, the obturator nerve, innervates the medial aspect of the thigh, and the posterior component, the femoral nerve, innervates the anterior thigh. The sacral plexus lies on the anterior surface of the piriformis muscle and exits through the greater sciatic foramen to enter the buttock. The sacral plexus, too, can be considered as having anterior and posterior components. The anterior parts of the plexus form the tibial nerve and additional small branches to the hip rotators. The posterior parts form the common peroneal nerve and branches to the buttock.

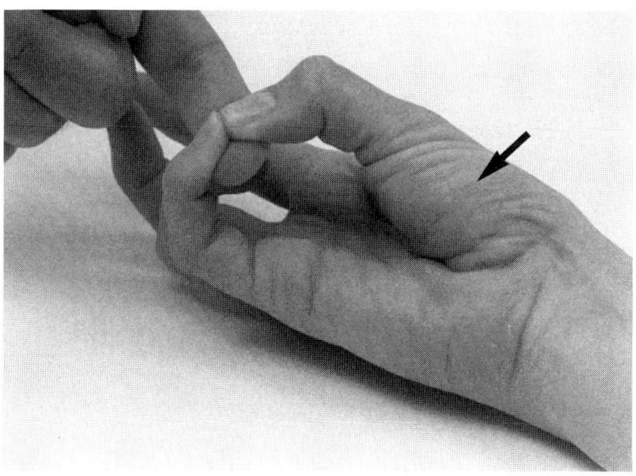

Figure 9–10. *Although difficult to isolate, the opponens muscle (arrow) is necessary to form a tight "O" with the thumb and small finger.*

Peripheral Nerves

Obturator Nerve (Fig. 9-11)

1. Adductor longus (L2, L3). The patient may be either sitting or supine, with the legs abducted. The patient is instructed to adduct the legs while resistance is applied on the medial aspect of the knees. Strong adduction indicates obturator integrity.
2. Adductor brevis (L3, L4) and magnus (L3–5). The test for these muscles is the same as for the adductor longus. These three muscles cannot be readily differentiated on clinical examination.
3. Gracilis (L3, L4). This muscle adducts the thigh and internally rotates the knee. It is tested in the same manner as the adductor group, muscles from which it cannot be isolated.

Femoral Nerve (Fig. 9-11)

1. Quadriceps (L2–4). This muscle group is best tested with the patient in the sitting position. The knee is allowed to flex fully over the edge of the examining table. The patient is instructed to actively extend the knee against resistance, which is applied through the examiner's grasp at the ankle. Active knee extension indicates quadriceps muscle and obturator nerve function.
2. Sartorius (L2, L3). This muscle's actions are very similar to the quadriceps femoris. It is activated during active knee extension. It cannot be readily differentiated from the quadriceps.

Sciatic Nerve in the Thigh (Fig. 9-12)

1. Semimembranosus (L5–S2). This muscle is one component of the hamstring group. To test it, the patient is positioned prone on the table and the knee is fully extended. The patient is instructed to flex the knee against resistance, which is applied

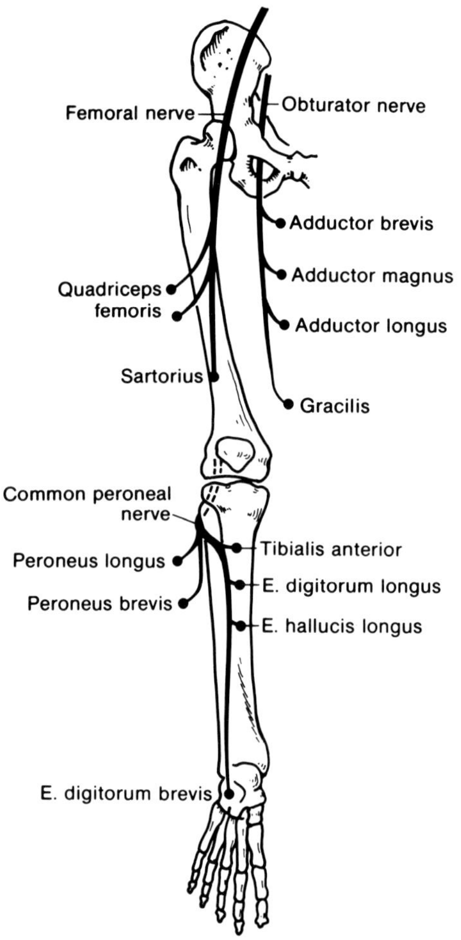

Figure 9–11. *Muscles innervated by the femoral, obturator, and common peroneal nerves, as viewed from the anterior aspect of the lower extremity. E, extensor.*

The sciatic nerve divides in the posterior thigh into the tibial and peroneal nerves. The tibial nerve continues down the posterior aspect of the upper extremity to innervate muscles in the posterior aspect of the leg. The peroneal nerve passes through the interval between the fibula and tibia to enter the anterior aspect of the leg. As it takes this course it supplies the muscles of both the lateral and anterior compartments of the leg.

Tibial Nerve (Fig. 9-12)

1. Gastrocnemius, medial and lateral heads (S1, S2). The patient is easily examined in the sitting position with the knees flexed and the feet over through the examiner's grasp at the ankle. Strong knee flexion indicates intact motor branches from the sciatic nerve. To better isolate the medial hamstrings from the lateral hamstrings, the leg is internally rotated while the test is repeated.
2. Semitendinosus (L5–S2). This is the second of the two medial hamstring muscles. It is tested in the same manner as the semimembranosus. It cannot be differentiated from that muscle on clinical examination.
3. Biceps femoris (L5–S2). This muscle is the lateral component of the hamstring group. It is tested in the same manner as the semimembranosus and semitendinosus muscles, except that it is better isolated by externally rotating the leg while performing the test.

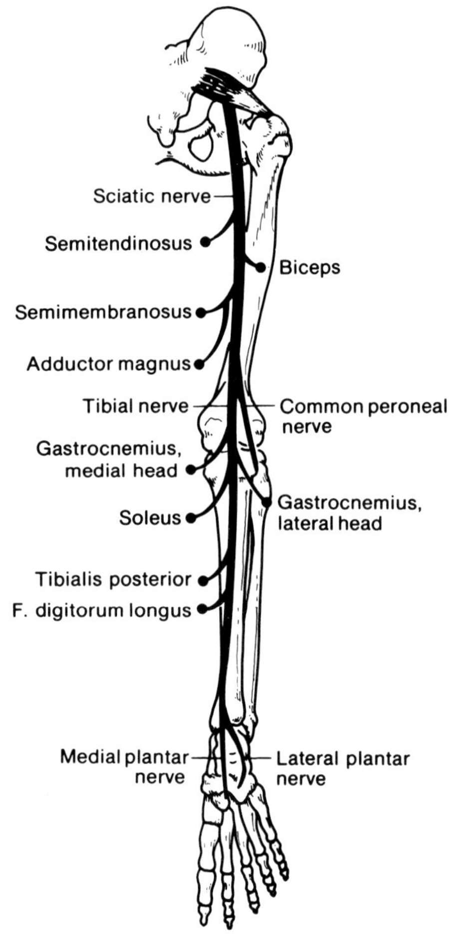

Figure 9–12. *Muscles innervated by the sciatic nerve and its major tibial nerve branch, as viewed from the posterior aspect of the lower extremity. F, flexor.*

the edge of the examining table. The feet are positioned plantigrade, and the examiner's hand is placed under the ball of the foot. The patient is instructed to flex the foot downward. Because this muscle is quite strong, it is difficult to grade strength using this maneuver. The patient should also be asked to walk on the toes.

2. Soleus (S1, S2). Because its anatomical location and function are very similar to the gastrocnemius, this muscle is tested in the same manner. The two muscles cannot be readily differentiated clinically. Changing knee position to include or exclude gastrocnemius activity is not reliable.
3. Tibialis posterior (L5, S1). The tendon is palpable as it comes around the medial malleolus and inserts into the tarsal navicular. It is tested with the patient in the sitting position. The examiner stabilizes the distal tibia with one hand and instructs the patient to flex and invert the foot against resistance. Simultaneous ankle flexion and foot inversion confirm tibialis posterior function.
4. Flexor digitorum longus (L5, S1). This muscle to the lateral four toes is tested by stabilizing the calcaneus with the ankle in a neutral position. The patient is then instructed to bend or curl the toes downward. The examiner assesses strength by attempting to straighten the toes with the opposite hand. Sustained toe flexion indicates good innervation.
5. Flexor hallucis longus (L5, S2). This muscle to the great toe is tested by stabilizing the calcaneus with the ankle in a neutral position. The patient is then instructed to bend or curl the great toe downward. The examiner assesses strength by attempting to straighten the great toe with the opposite hand.
6. Intrinsics on the plantar aspect of the foot (L5, S2). These muscles provide flexion of the toes through the MP joint without simultaneous flexion of the other joints and contribute to abduction and adduction of the toes. Testing does not isolate them well. The patient can be instructed to alternate spreading the toes apart and then squeezing them together.

Peroneal Nerve (Fig. 9-11)

The common peroneal nerve divides into superficial and deep nerves as it passes around the neck of the fibula. The superficial nerve continues down the leg to innervate the lateral compartment. The deep nerve travels distally and medially to enter and innervate the muscles of the anterior compartment of the leg.

1. Peroneus longus and brevis (L4–S1). These two tendons are just posterior to the lateral malleolus. They cannot be differentiated on clinical examination. The patient sits on the examining table with the knees bent 90°. The examiner stabilizes the distal tibia with one hand. The foot is placed in flexion and eversion. The patient is asked to maintain that position while the examiner applies resistance to the lateral border of the fifth metatarsal. A sustained position of flexion and eversion indicates good innervation of the peronei.
2. Tibialis anterior (L4–S1). This muscle is the primary extensor or dorsiflexor of the foot; it is also an invertor. During contraction it is visibly and palpably present on the anterior aspect of the ankle. To test it, the patient sits on the examining table with the knees flexed. The foot is placed in inversion and extension. The examiner stabilizes the distal tibia with one hand and grasps the patient's foot with the other. The examiner attempts to invert and flex the foot against the patient's resistance. Strong resistance confirms tibialis anterior integrity.
3. Extensor digitorum longus (L4–S1). This muscle is the primary extensor of the lateral four toes. To test it the patient assumes the sitting position with the knees flexed. The patient is instructed to extend or pull the toes upward. The examiner's index finger is placed transversely across the toes and attempts to flex the toes downward. Peroneal nerve function allows the patient's toes to resist the flexion force.
4. Extensor hallucis longus (L4–S1). This muscle is the primary extensor of the great toe. It is tested in the same manner as the extensor digitorum longus, except that the great toe is actively extended and the examiner attempts to flex it downward with only the tip of the index finger.
5. Extensor digitorum and extensor hallucis brevis (L5–S1). These muscles are secondary toe extensors. They are tested in the same manner as their long counterparts. They cannot be isolated for muscle testing.

Motor testing is easy to describe and comprehend, but it requires considerable retention of information and experience to translate these descriptions effectively into clinical practice. Optimum motor testing is not easily accomplished in every case. Associated muscle and tendon injury or decreased passive motion in joints across which each muscle acts confounds the interpretation of observations. Also, motor testing is predicated on the assumption that the patient is providing optimum effort. This may not always be the case, either because the patient does not understand the instructions, because the patient may be impaired from providing an optimum effort by systemic or psychological factors, or because the patient may have some interest in providing a suboptimum performance. These factors must be considered when interpreting the performance of each muscle test.

Despite these limitations, motor testing remains an invaluable method of systematically assessing the integrity of the peripheral nervous system.

REFERENCES

1. Evarts CM. Examination of the musculoskeletal patient. In: Evarts CM, ed. Surgery of the musculoskeletal system. New York: Churchill-Livingstone, 1983:9–17.
2. Hoppenfeld S. Physical examination of the spine and extremities. New York: Appleton-Century-Crofts, 1976:2–104, 153–235.
3. Lister G. The hand: Diagnosis and indications, ed 2. Edinburgh: Churchill-Livingstone, 1984:351–364.
4. Mannerfelt L. Motor function testing. In: Omer GE, Spinner M, eds. Management of peripheral nerve problems. Philadelphia: WB Saunders, 1980:16–29.

10

Electrophysiological Testing

Allen L. Van Beek
Philip Heyman

AUTHOR'S KEY POINTS

- Stimulus intensity, duration, and frequency are important variables for electrophysiological testing of the awake and the anesthetized patient.
- *Latency* is the delay between stimulus onset and electrical response. It is directly proportional to the distance between the electrode stimulating the response and the electrode recording that response.
- The motor unit potential (M-wave) is the potential created by a muscle fiber's contraction. It normally has a polyphasic wave form.
- *Fibrillation potential* is spontaneous electrical activity seen in denervated muscle caused by neuropathy or myopathy. It is produced by spontaneous depolarization of single muscle fiber units, creating miniature M-waves.
- The H-reflex and F-response are late response studies applicable to the assessment of long segments of peripheral nerve (eg, across the thoracic outlet or cervical spine foramen).

While the potential for clinical electrodiagnostic evaluations of peripheral nerve function started with the work of Helmholtz,[36] the work of Erlanger and Gasser[4] actually established the principles of modern electrodiagnosis. In the past two decades, significant changes in the operative management of peripheral nerve injuries have helped many injury victims and have decreased the incidence of late re-exploration and reconstruction of peripheral nerves. This chapter discusses the use of electrodiagnostic techniques as an adjunct to clinical examination in the objective evaluation of disorders of peripheral nerves. Electrodiagnostic studies also help isolate the segment of nerve that is injured.

Clinically, the most applicable of the electrodiagnostic studies is the electromyogram (EMG), which records the electrical activity produced by muscle units and detects changes in activity produced by disease. While it does not provide a specific diagnosis, it does detect changes in nerve or muscle that aid in establishing the diagnosis and determining its impact on the patient.[8,22,23] When the nerve is stimulated, it conducts in both antidrome and orthodrome directions. Because the nerve is conducting to the spinal cord, a reflex arc may be established.[3]

Electrical responses vary according to the electrical amplitude they elicit (Fig. 10-1). It is easy

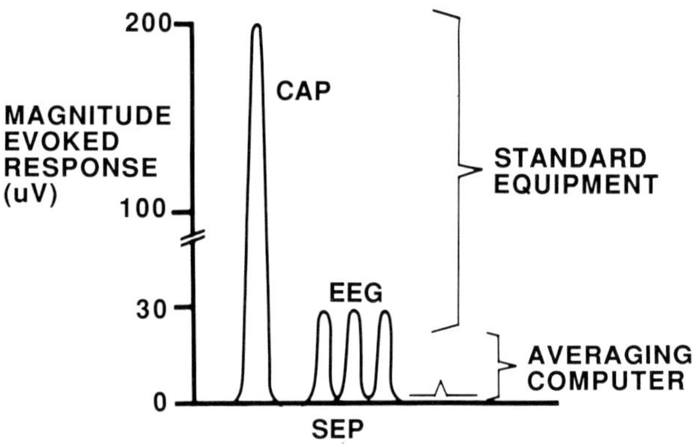

Figure 10–1. *A nerve action potential is usually 50 microvolts or greater when recording from the surface of large nerves. Recording an EEG from the scalp will usually produce 30 microvolt signals. Using transcutaneous recordings of the nerve action potential will usually produce an amplitude of 1 to 5 microvolts. Recording amplitudes less than 30 microvolts is easier when using a signal-averaging microprocessor.*

to record electrical responses with a magnitude over 50 microvolts (μV); amplitudes less than 50 μV are more difficult to record using standard EMG equipment because of electrical noise. Through the process of summation, signal-enhancing microprocessors diminish electrical noise while augmenting the biological response. This technique permits the recording of very small biological responses.[11,37]

Definitions

The surgeon should become familiar with the following commonly used terms and calculations.[8]

STIMULUS INTENSITY. The strength of the stimulus is variable; variation is provided by varying the volts or current. Because a stimulus creates a shock sensation, the patient should be told to prepare for it. The intensity level starts at zero and is slowly increased until the desired response is measured. This prevents surprises to the awake, unanesthetized patient and avoids overstimulating the anesthetized one.

STIMULUS DURATION. Duration is the period of time during which a potential difference occurs between the anode and the cathode of an electrode.

STIMULATION FREQUENCY. Stimulation frequency represents the depolarizing pulses per second (Hertz [Hz]) that are applied to the stimulating electrode. Usually, this parameter varies from 1 to 5 per second (1–5 Hz). This frequency induces a twitch response. To establish tetany, a 30- to 60-Hz stimulus is required.

LATENCY. The delay in time from the stimulus onset until an electrical response is measured is called latency. Latency is directly proportional to the distance between the electrode recording the response and the electrode inducing the response. Latency is measured by stimulating the nerve and recording an EMG response, or by stimulating the nerve and recording the nerve's action potential.

INSERTIONAL ACTIVITY. Motor unit potentials (M-waves) produced by mechanical stimulation and depolarization of muscle as the EMG needle is inserted are referred to as insertional activity. This is a normal response and is short in duration. An absent or diminished response occurs with severe muscle atrophy or fibrosis. An excessive response is seen with muscle irritability or inflammation.

MOTOR UNIT POTENTIAL. The M-wave is the recorded potential change created by a muscle fiber's contraction (Fig. 10-2). It is usually recorded as a polyphasic wave form. The amplitude and the frequency of this wave is related to fiber size, the distance the active motor unit is located from the needle, and other factors.[26]

RECRUITMENT PATTERN. When a patient volitionally contracts a muscle, multiple motor units fire simultaneously in the vicinity of the electrode, creating multiple M-waves. By asking the patient to progressively increase the strength of muscle contraction, additional motor units are progressively recruited, producing an increased frequency of M-waves (see Fig. 10-2). Failure of normal recruitment is seen with severe neuropathy, myopathy, or poor patient cooperation.

FIBRILLATION POTENTIAL. With muscle denervation, spontaneous electrical activity occurs even when the muscle is at rest. Normal muscle is electrically quiet. In denervated muscle, fibrillation potentials are produced by spontaneous depolar-

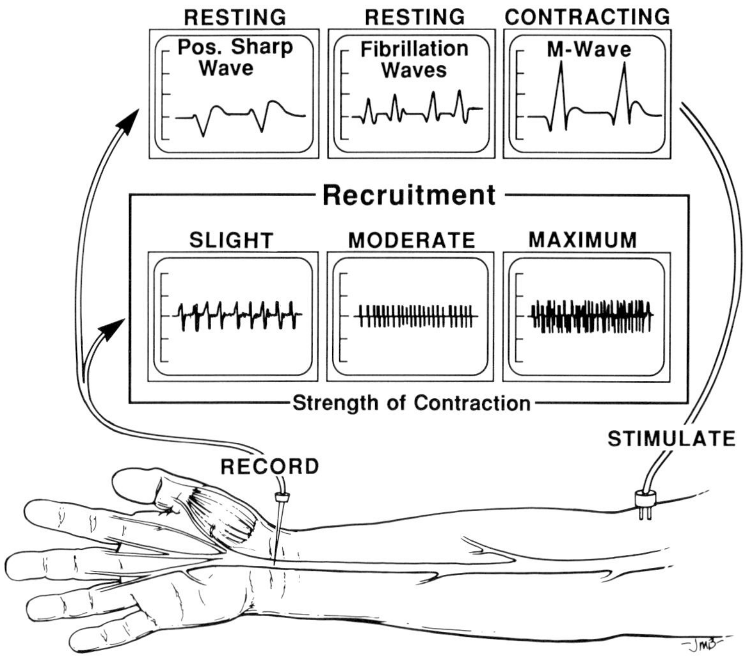

Figure 10–2. *When performing an EMG, nerve conduction studies are done by stimulating at the wrist and elbow and recording proximal and distal to the wrist. EMG recordings can be obtained from the thenar musculature. The M-wave is a large-amplitude, usually polyphasic, wave form. Positive sharp waves and fibrillation potentials are lower-amplitude waves with a fairly characteristic appearance. Recruitment is the volitional increase in active muscle fibers that occurs with progressively increasing contraction strength. For a detailed description of the wave forms and their implications, consult the text.*

ization of single muscle fiber units, creating miniature M-waves (see Fig. 10-2). In the absence of myopathy, fibrillation potentials imply muscle denervation and significant neuropathy.

POSITIVE SHARP WAVES. Like the fibrillation potential, this abnormal wave form is associated with muscle denervation or primary myopathy. The wave form has a very distinctive shape (see Fig. 10-2).

H-REFLEX AND F-RESPONSE. These late response studies, while more variable than the previous studies, assess long segments of peripheral nerve, detecting problems when conventional studies are normal. The H-reflex is the electrical equivalent of a tendon reflex. A submaximal stimulus is used to stimulate the nerve. The intensity is too low to trigger a direct orthodromic muscle response, but the simultaneous antidromic response does trigger a spinal cord reflex that produces a delayed muscle response. As the threshold of stimulation is incrementally increased, a direct response and reflex response are seen. With supramaximal stimulation, the direct response is much greater than the reflex response and may obscure it (Fig. 10-3).

This technique, which is more difficult to elicit and interpret, is used to calculate the nerve's conduction velocity along a long segment of nerve. This response is used to attempt evaluation across the thoracic outlet or through the spinal foramen. When testing elicits prolonged latency, fibrillation potentials, or positive sharp waves, it is necessary to identify the factors or problems causing the changes.

EVALUATION OF THE COMPRESSIVE NEUROPATHIES

Electrophysiological testing is of value in establishing the diagnosis and assessing the severity of a number of compressive neuropathies in both the upper and lower extremities.

Carpal Tunnel Syndrome

Nerve conduction and electromyographic studies are particularly useful in evaluating patients with carpal tunnel syndrome. Nerve conduction studies are more helpful in establishing the diagnosis; electromyographic studies are useful in determin-

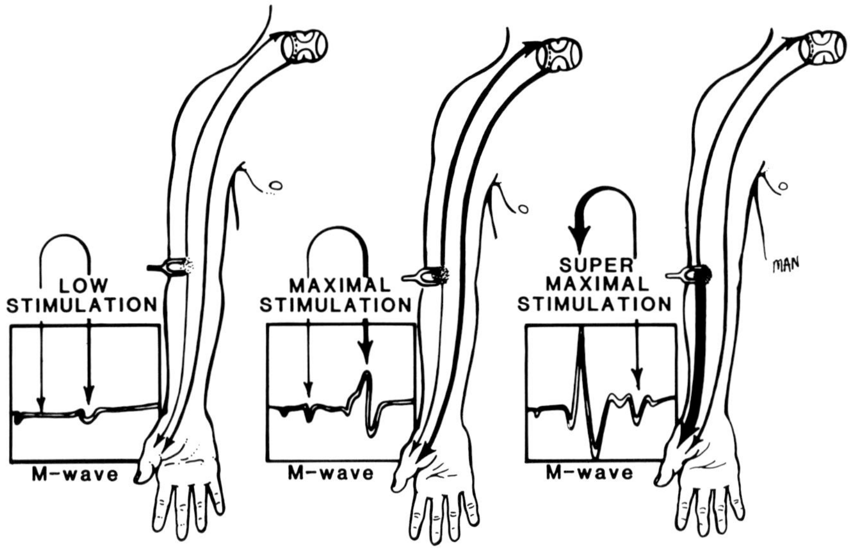

Figure 10–3. *The H-reflex allows recording over long segments of peripheral nerves and across the reflex arc of the spinal cord. The H-reflex is similar to a tendon reflex, but it is induced electrically. The advantage is that it permits one to look across the thoracic outlet and long segments of a nerve. The disadvantage is that short segment conduction delays may be unrecognized when included within a long segment study of peripheral nerve.*

ing the prognosis. Distal sensory latencies (DSL) and distal motor latencies (DML) are the most frequently ordered electrophysiological studies.

Distal Sensory Latency (DSL)

The DSL is generally more sensitive than the DML in studying patients with carpal tunnel syndrome. Standard methods position the stimulating electrode on the index finger and the receiving electrode at the wrist (Fig. 10-4). *A distal sensory latency of greater than 3.5 milliseconds is considered abnormal.* A .5 millisecond increase, compared to the opposite unaffected side, is also considered indicative of median nerve compression. Sensitivity of the DSL in establishing the diagnosis is approximately 85%. An alternate technique for measuring DSL involves placing the stimulating electrode in the palm and the receiving electrode at the wrist. This technique is theoretically more accurate, as only the diseased segment of the median nerve is examined. The technique is particularly useful in

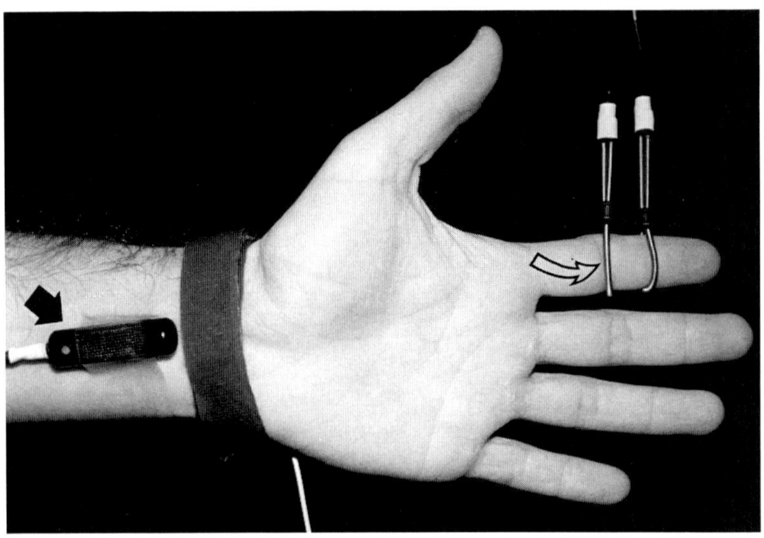

Figure 10–4. *Finger-to-wrist method of testing distal sensory latency in median nerve at the wrist. DSL > 3.5 milliseconds or 0.5 milliseconds > that of the unaffected side is considered abnormal.* Open arrow, *stimulating electrode;* closed arrow, *receiving electrode.*

cases involving peripheral polyneuropathy. Kimura reports a series of patients with clinically classic carpal tunnel syndrome in which 20% had a normal DSL over the finger-to-wrist segment and an abnormal DSL over the palm-to-wrist segment.[17]

Distal Motor Latency (DML)

The DML is usually obtained by measuring the response time of the abductor pollicis brevis muscle (APB) after stimulation at the wrist (Fig. 10-5). The upper limit of normal may be considered 4.5 milliseconds. A DML value on the affected side that is one millisecond greater than that of the unaffected side is considered abnormal. The sensitivity of the DML in establishing the diagnosis of carpal tunnel syndrome, according reports in the literature, ranges from 40% to 90%. On occasion, the DML value may be more markedly abnormal than the DSL. It has been postulated that this phenomenon is due to selective involvement of the motor fibers or to an anatomic variation in the arrangement of nerve fibers within the median nerve.[15] In severe cases of carpal tunnel syndrome, prolonged motor conduction in the forearm may also be seen. Electromyographic studies are useful in determining that the median nerve–innervated forearm muscles are normal, ruling out a more proximal compression site.

Not infrequently, clinical findings are consistent with carpal tunnel syndrome, but the distal motor and sensory latencies are normal.[30] When this is the case, some authors have suggested a role for provocative testing. It has been shown that, in normal wrists, wrist flexion for 2 minutes does not increase the DML or DSL more than 0.1 millisecond. In one study of 40 wrists with carpal tunnel syndrome, 16 had an increase of the distal motor latency or the distal sensory latency by 0.2 milliseconds or more.[28] The role of provocative testing has not yet been substantiated sufficiently to be recommended for routine use.

Axonotmesis, with denervation of the median nerve–innervated intrinsic muscles, occurs in more advanced cases of carpal tunnel syndrome. Electromyographic studies demonstrate denervation potentials (fibrillations, positive sharp waves, and complex potentials with minimal effort). These findings are significant for predicting the time and completeness of recovery.

Anterior Interosseous Nerve Compression Syndrome

The anterior interosseous nerve compression syndrome is characterized by motor weakness of the flexor pollicis longus, the flexor digitorum profundus of the index and long fingers, and the pronator quadratus muscles (see Chap. 70). Denervation patterns may be seen on electromyographic testing of these muscles. Nerve conduction studies have not been standardized for the evaluation of patients with this syndrome.

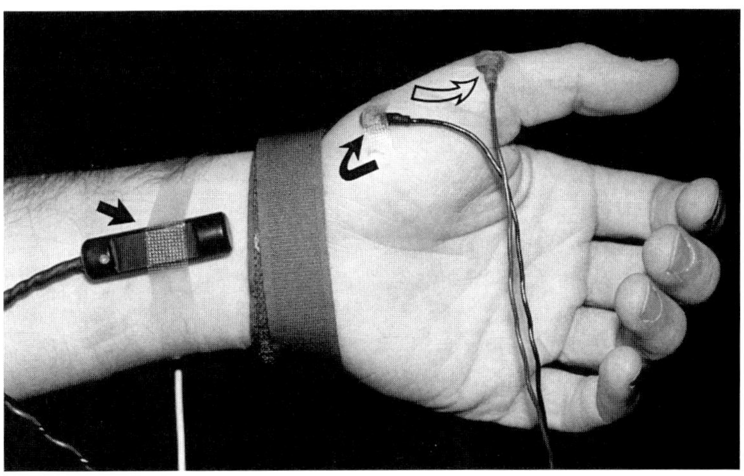

Figure 10–5. *Testing for distal motor latency in median nerve at the wrist. The upper limit of normal distal motor latency is 4.5 milliseconds, or 1 millisecond > that of the unaffected side.* Closed arrow, *stimulating electrode;* open arrow, *passive electrode. Receiving electrode is located distally over the metacarpophalangeal joint.*

Pronator Syndrome

Electromyographic studies have not been particularly helpful in establishing the diagnosis, or in determining the prognosis, of patients with pronator syndrome. Denervation patterns are infrequently seen in both the median nerve–innervated extrinsic and intrinsic muscles. It has been suggested that the magnitude of compression is generally insufficient to result in conduction values outside the normal range.[12] Hartz and Linscheid noted forearm muscle denervation in only 9 of their 40 patients with a diagnosis of pronator syndrome. They were able to document segmental compression of the sensory part of the median nerve in its course through the pronator teres in only 16% of patients.[12]

Ulnar Nerve Compression at Guyon's Canal

Isolated compression of the ulnar nerve at Guyon's canal is relatively infrequent (see Chap. 83). Three clinical syndromes exist. Mixed motor and sensory abnormalities correspond anatomically to a lesion in zone I[10]; this is the region of Guyon's canal in which both the sensory and motor components of the ulnar nerve travel together. Prolonged distal motor latency values to the first dorsal interosseous muscle and hypothenar muscles are expected with compression in this region. Distal sensory latency values from the wrist to the small finger are also prolonged. If an axonotmetic lesion is present, electromyographic studies show denervation patterns in these muscles.

In the presence of a pure motor syndrome, where the intrinsic muscles are involved but sensation is spared, the lesion is considered to be in zone II.[10] This is the portion of the canal where the motor branch courses under the pisohamate ligament. Compression here is demonstrated by an increase in distal motor latency values. Denervation potentials are seen in more severe cases.

The least common presentation involves the sensory branch to the ulnar side of the hand. The distal sensory latency is prolonged, while both the distal motor latency and electromyographic studies are normal. This corresponds to a lesion in zone 3.[10]

Cubital Tunnel Syndrome

The diagnosis of ulnar nerve compression at the elbow is based primarily on nerve conduction velocity (NCV). NCV is determined by the following equation:

$$\text{NCV} = \frac{\text{Distance between points of stimulation (mm)}}{\text{Proximal motor latency (msec)} - \text{distal motor latency (msec)}}$$

As motor latency includes transmission along the nerve as well as across the neuromuscular junction, it is necessary to subtract distal latency values from proximal latency values.

Nerve conduction velocity is altered by elbow position. *With elbow flexion, the normal range is 52 to 74 meters/second (average: 62.7 m/sec).*[2] The extended position reduces tension on the ulnar nerve resulting in a lower normal nerve conduction velocity value. In extension, the range of normal is 34 to 66 meters/second (average: 49.9 meters/second).[2] Standard NCV testing is done with the elbow in flexion. *Abnormal values are less than 45 meters/second (30% decrease relative to the normal side).* Alternatively, the NCV can be determined both above and below the elbow. A difference of 10 meters/second may be considered abnormal.

The prognosis for recovery after decompression depends largely on the degree of preoperative neural injury. Denervation patterns in the intrinsic muscles suggest an axonotmetic lesion with severe denervation, which is indicative of a reduced potential for full recovery. Electromyographic studies may also help localize the site of compression about the cubital tunnel by demonstrating denervation of the ulnar nerve–innervated forearm muscles. Occasionally, however, the flexor carpi ulnaris receives its innervation above the elbow. Thus, denervation of the flexor carpi ulnaris may be caused by more proximal compression (eg, Arcade of Struthers, medial intermuscular septum).

Thoracic Outlet Syndrome

Electrophysiological testing may be useful in the diagnosis of certain types of neurologic compression at the thoracic outlet (neurogenic compression). Four categories of neurogenic thoracic outlet syndrome (TOS) have been described[39]: classical, droopy shoulder, atypical, and disputed. In classical TOS, clinical wasting is present.[6] Electrophysiological studies characteristically show a decrease in the median compound motor action potential (CMAP) and a decrease in the ulnar sensory nerve action potential (SNAP). Median SNAP and ulnar CMAP may be normal or decreased.[7,38,39] This type of TOS is rare, however.

The droopy shoulder syndrome is a clinical entity associated with a characteristic body type and is characterized by vague sensory and motor complaints.[31] Electrical studies are generally negative in these patients. Atypical TOS is secondary to extrinsic compression, such as that seen from a shoulder strap or back pack. Electrophysiological studies of patients with this type of compression are usually normal. The majority of cases are of the disputed type. Symptoms are intermittent, and clinical and electrical evidence of denervation is frequently absent. Nerve conduction studies from Erb's point to the axilla may be prolonged.[1,33] Some feel that patients with reduced nerve conduction studies are more appropriate candidates for operative decompression.[1,33] Others feel that electrophysiological testing has little to offer in making the diagnosis of thoracic outlet syndrome (see Chap. 85).

Compressive Neuropathy in the Lower Extremity

Compressive neuropathies of each of the major motor and sensory nerves of the lower extremity have been described. Most important clinically are those affecting the peroneal nerve and the posterior tibial nerve (see Chap. 86).

The peroneal nerve is susceptible to stretch because it is fixed proximally as it exits the pelvis, as well as distally in the region of the fibular neck. Its superficial location at the neck of the fibula also makes it susceptible to compression in that location. Compression at the fibular neck may result in denervation of the muscles of the anterior and lateral compartments, as well as the extensor digitorum brevis muscle (Figs. 10-6, 10-7). While several standard textbooks on electromyography state that motor conduction studies are most reliable in assessing peroneal nerve entrapment, Singh and coworkers have reported that sensory studies may be significantly more helpful in making the diagnosis.[29] In this study, the diagnostic rate of motor conduction studies was 36%, while sensory studies had a diagnostic rate of 82%.

Injury to the peroneal nerve division of the sciatic nerve may occur after trauma (eg, dislocation or fracture/dislocation of the hip), and after reconstructive surgery of the hip (see Chap. 89). Denervation of the short head of the biceps femoris muscle suggests a more proximal compression lesion.

Posterior Tibial Nerve Compression

If the posterior tibial nerve is compressed in the tarsal tunnel, distal motor latency values along the medial and lateral plantar nerves may be prolonged. If the distal motor latency along the medial plantar nerve is determined, the muscle tested is the abductor hallucis. *Values greater than 6.5 msec are considered abnormal.* If the lateral plantar nerve is used, the muscle tested is the abductor digiti quinti. *Values greater than 7 msec are considered abnormal.* Oh and coworkers reported a 52% incidence of prolonged motor latencies in their series of patients with tarsal tunnel syndrome.[25] Distal sensory latencies of the medial and lateral plantar nerves have not been studies as thoroughly as distal motor latencies. Oh found that latency determination revealed an accuracy rate of 90% for compression of the posterior tibial nerve in the tarsal tunnel. Thus, as with carpal tunnel syndrome, distal sensory latency may prove to be more sensitive than distal motor latency.

Several reports have demonstrated denervation of the intrinsic muscles in the presence of normal nerve conduction. This suggests that the tarsal tunnel syndrome may be an axonal neuropathy and not a demyelinating compression neuropathy.[9,13,14,27] It may be appropriate to obtain EMGs of foot, back, and leg in patients with suspected tarsal tunnel syndrome.[21]

EQUIPMENT

While spontaneous peripheral nerve fiber electrical activity occurs constantly, the amplitude of the response is so low that it can be recorded only by microelectrodes and intracellular recording.[24] This

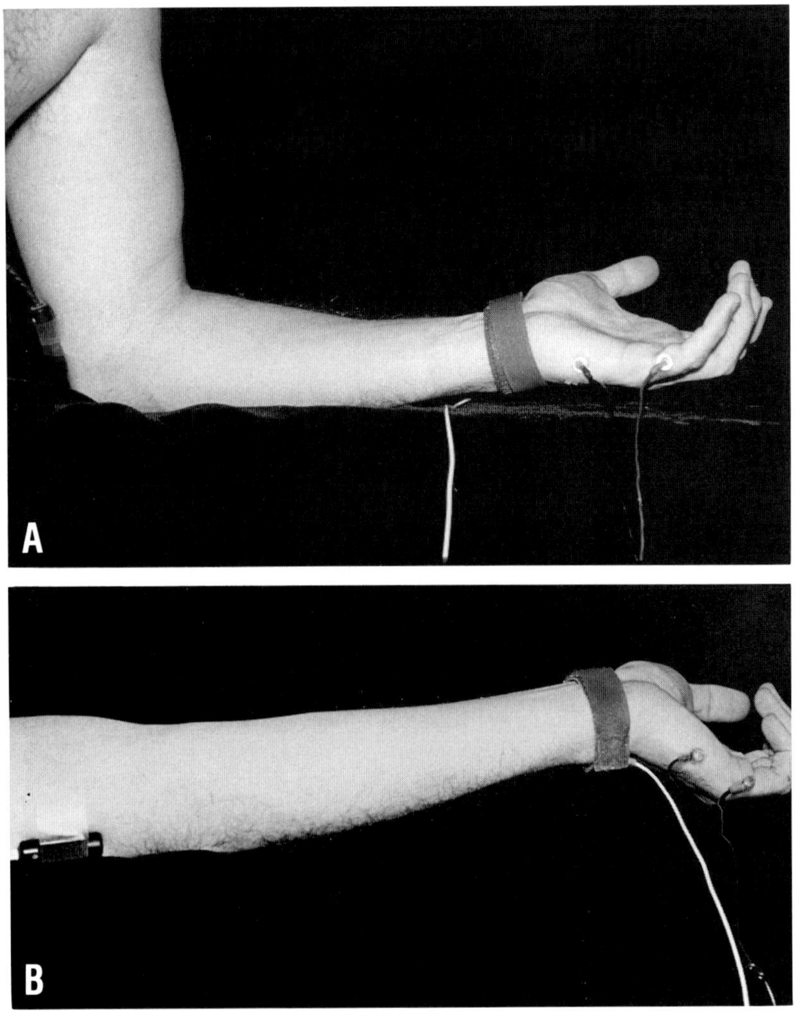

Figure 10–6. *Determining nerve conduction velocity (NCV) for ulnar nerve at the cubital tunnel with distal motor latency. The receiving electrode is over the hypothenar muscles. (**A**) The DML is determined with the stimulating electrode below the cubital tunnel. (**B**) Then the DML is determined with the stimulating electrode above the cubital tunnel. The distance between the two stimulation points is determined. NCV = distance between points of stimulation (in mm) (distal/proximal/DML (msec)) − distal DML (msec).*

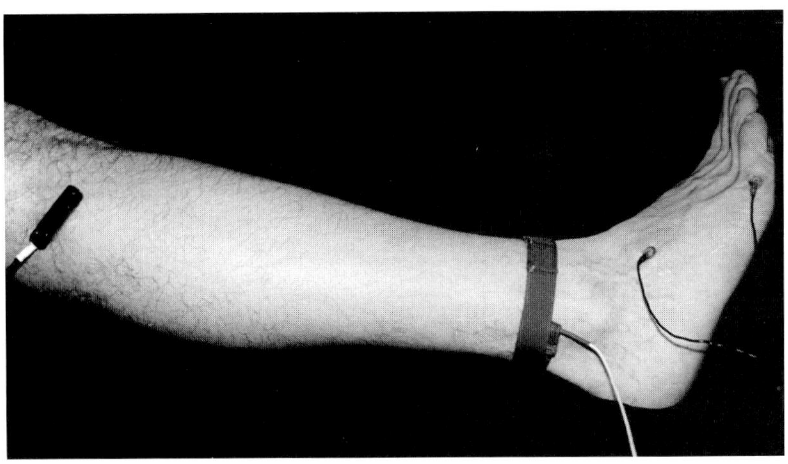

Figure 10–7. *NCV for the peroneal nerve at the fibular neck. DML may be used. The motor employed is the extensor digitorum brevis (not shown). The DML proximal to the fibular neck and distal to the fibular neck is determined; the NCV may be calculated from these. A drop in NCV across the fibular neck is indicative of compression at this level.*

system accurately assesses a few nerve fibers. However, if the peripheral nerve is stimulated mechanically or electrically, large numbers of nerve fibers discharge simultaneously. The result of a large number of axons depolarizing simultaneously is an electrical response large enough to be recorded by electrodes placed on the surface of the nerve, or even by using surface electrodes. Stimulators that produce a variable stimulus and a synchronization triggering impulses are essential for intraoperative assessment of nerves. The stimulator must have several variables: intensity, frequency, duration, stimulus delay, and triggering functions.

Stimulating and recording systems and electrodes for operative use are not readily available. In the past, silver or platinum wire electrodes were used because of their unique conduction and physical properties. Intraoperative equipment is the same equipment made for neurologists. Electrodes are custom-made using Grass electroencephalograph needle electrodes. The recording amplifier and display scope must have variable gain; high, low, and 60-cycle per second signal filters; digital oscilloscope; disk storage mechanism; and bipolar or unipolar recording capabilities. The recording system is linked to a signal-averaging microprocessor to permit transcutaneous nerve action potential (NAP) recordings.

NERVE STIMULATION TECHNIQUES

Sensory Identification

In nerve reconstruction for chronic nerve injury, appropriate alignment of nerve stumps is frequently impeded by size change, nerve trunk rotation, or loss of nerve trunk length. More accurate alignment of nerve stumps, especially in the distal forearm, can be accomplished using nerve stimulation (see Chap. 15).[5]

Author's Preferred Method

With intravenous regional anesthesia, the injured nerve is explored. When the nerve's status is established, the proximal neuroma is resected until normal-appearing fascicle patterns are identified. The operating microscope is then used to draw a schematic representation of the nerve's proximal stump. Local anesthetic agents should be injected into the skin before making the incision, to prevent incisional pain when the intravenous block is released and to prevent stray local anesthesia from blocking the resected nerve.

After reversing the block, it is necessary to wait at least 15 minutes before the patient can accurately interpret the stimulation. With twitch stimulation, the patient feels a tapping-type sensation in the distribution of the nerve. With higher-frequency stimulation (10–30/sec), the patient perceives a burning, painful feeling. Without small bipolar stimulating electrodes, excessive areas of depolarization may occur. Sensory-dominant fascicles have definite sensations associated with stimulation that are readily identified by patients. Motor-dominant fascicles are associated with weak or absent patient responses.

Once the nerve's topography has been studied and recorded, the patient is given a general anesthetic. The distal nerve stump is then traced across the wrist by microscopic dissection (Fig. 10-8). In the distal nerve, the anatomical components of the nerve are readily identified by group fascicular dissection. Using distal group fascicular dissection, the surgeon accurately identifies the fascicles innervating each finger; by using proximal nerve stimulation, he or she can determine which part of the nerve connects to the appropriate CNS location. The surgeon then connects the nerve stump to the correct location. By deduction, the quiet proximal fascicles are felt to be motor-fiber–dominant and are connected to what is anatomically identified as a motor fascicle in the distal stump.

Motor Fascicle Territory

The technique of composite tissue transfers using microneurovascular techniques has been an important addition to the reconstructive armamentarium of the surgeon. The success of reconstruction is frequently directly related to the success of nerve regeneration and the specificity of regeneration. Using stimulation to identify a motor fascicle's field offers the possibility of splitting a single muscle into two or more functional units (Fig. 10-9).

This is possible in the gracilis muscle.[35] The gracilis muscle's motor nerve has four fascicles. The large dominant fascicle supplies the anterior third of the muscle, and the remaining fascicles supply

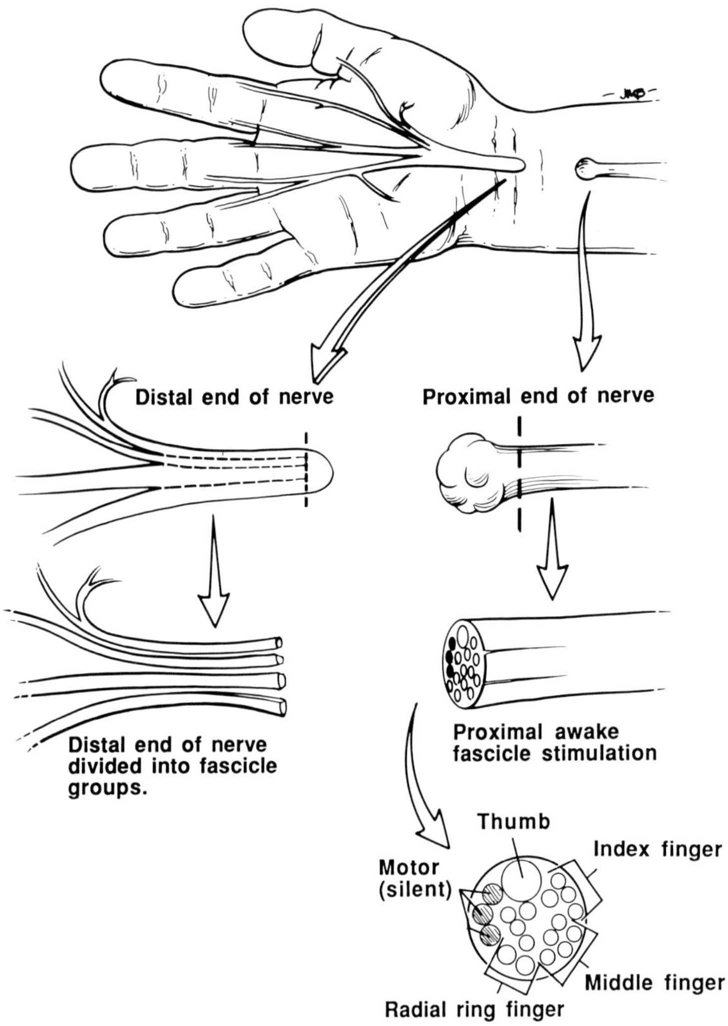

Figure 10–8. *In chronic nerve injuries, it is useful to stimulate the proximal nerve stump following its exposure and dissection with an intravenous regional block. This allows identification of proximal sensory dominant fascicle orientation. The distal fascicle orientation is determined by group fascicular dissection of the distal nerve. This is most reliable in the area of the wrist. If the injury is more proximal, mixing of motor and sensory components makes this technique less useful.*

the posterior two thirds of the muscle. If the muscle is split and the supplying nerve appropriately connected, the gracilis muscle can be used for two independent functions in its new location. Fascicles with two different functions must be available in the recipient bed. If these requirements are met, a single muscle unit can provide two almost completely independent functions.[35]

INTRAOPERATIVE STIMULATION AND RECORDING

Intraoperative stimulation and recording from peripheral nerves has been done for two decades. Several authors have described the use of intraoperative recording techniques directly on the surface of the nerve.[19,32] As computer technology has improved, equipment that helps eliminate noise problems and permits the recording of very small nerve action potentials (NAP) has become available. This has made stimulation and recording much easier, avoiding extra dissection of nerve away from the site of injury.

The intraoperative application of stimulation and recording of NAPs serves as an adjunct to the clinical and operative examination. While it does not substitute for a thorough clinical examination, it is helpful in the following situations:

- Early exploration of a segmental nerve injury where the nerve may be intact and early exploration is indicated

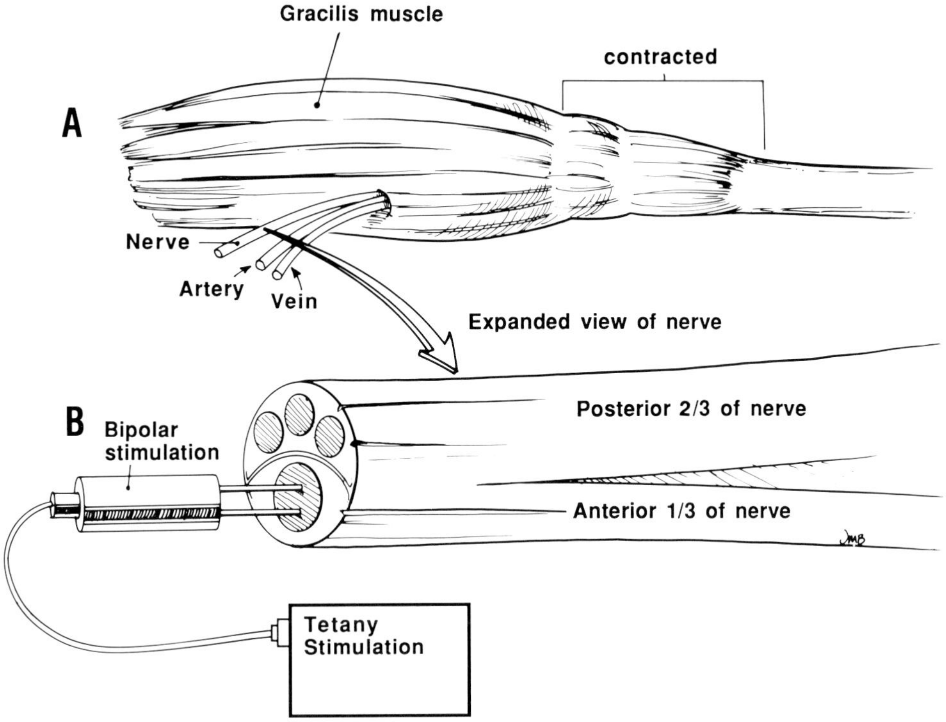

Figure 10–9. *Single fascicle stimulation is also useful in the identification of motor fascicle distribution. By careful stimulation of individual fascicles, the fascicle's motor territory within a muscle can be determined. The muscle can be divided into two components in an attempt to provide two functions with a single muscle. It is essential that in the recipient site, there are two separately identifiable motor fascicles available with discretely different functions. Division of the muscle is best accomplished using a tetany-inducing stimulus.*

- Exploration of a functioning neuroma-in-continuity (Fig. 10-10) (see Chap. 42)
- Exploration of a partially severed nerve (Fig. 10-11)
- Intraoperative evaluation of difficult brachial plexus injuries (see Chap. 92).[16,18,20,34]

Experience has shown that preoperative surgical plans have been changed intraoperatively in 20% of patients because of the findings of electrophysiological testing. When recording across a neuroma, the criteria used for determining favorable findings are as follows:

- The magnitude of the evoked response should be one third or more of the control.
- Conduction velocity calculated across a neuroma should be over 10 m/sec.

An illustrated methodology is shown in Figure 10-12. Recording needle electrodes are placed in the skin over the course of the nerve being studied, at mid-humerus, axilla, and Erb's point. The stimulating electrodes, which are hand-held, are made from Grass EEG needle electrodes. Stimulating and recording equipment is available from the Nicolet, Grass, or Techa instrument companies.

When performing nerve stimulation, several technical factors are important. Although the field is kept dry, desiccation must be avoided. The surface of the nerve is stimulated with the anode distally, to prevent anode block. When performing group fascicular or single fascicle stimulation, the operating microscope is used to enhance visualization of the nerve. A tetany-inducing stimulation frequency of 30 cycles/sec is used when identifying a motor fascicle field. The surgeon should begin below nerve threshold when performing fascicle stimulation with the patient awake and slowly increase the intensity until the patient recognizes the stimulus. This technique gains the patient's

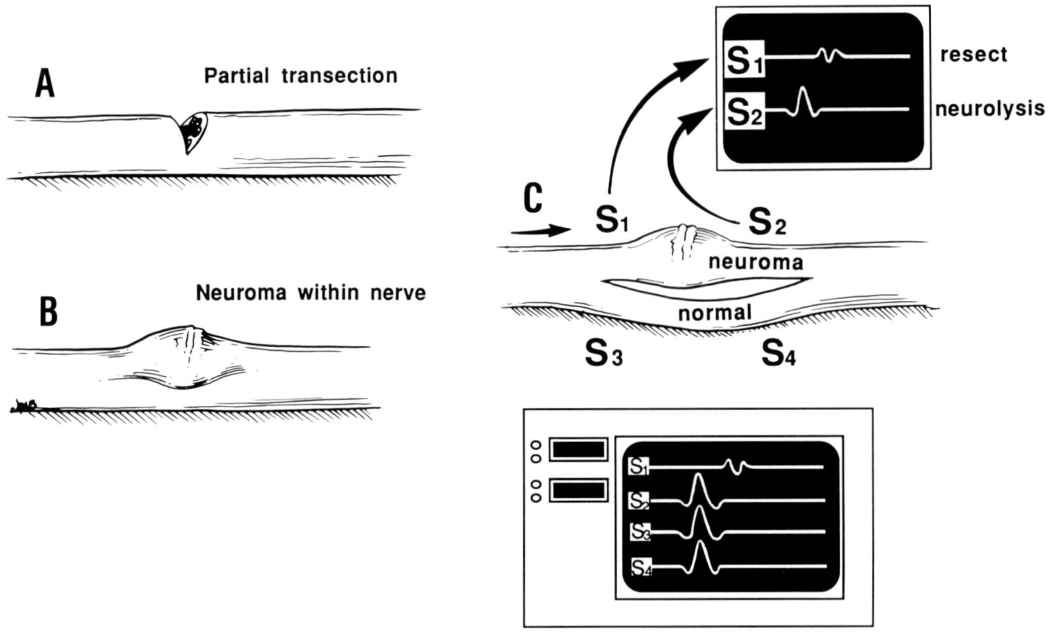

Figure 10–10. *In partial transections of nerves, a neuroma-in-continuity occurs with portions of the nerve being uninjured. In this instance, the surgeon needs to delineate whether the neuroma-in-continuity is a functional neuroma-in-continuity or a nonfunctional neuroma. This is best determined by intraoperative nerve stimulation. This is particularly important because of the function that will be going through the normal uninjured nerve, confusing the preoperative clinical picture. In this situation, the neuroma is stimulated on its proximal and distal ends, and an evoked response is measured proximally. The normal uninjured segment of nerve should conduct normally, whereas distal to the neuroma an increase in latency and a decrease in amplitude should be seen. If the amplitude and latency are excessively delayed, or the amplitude is diminished, a resection of neuroma is indicated.*

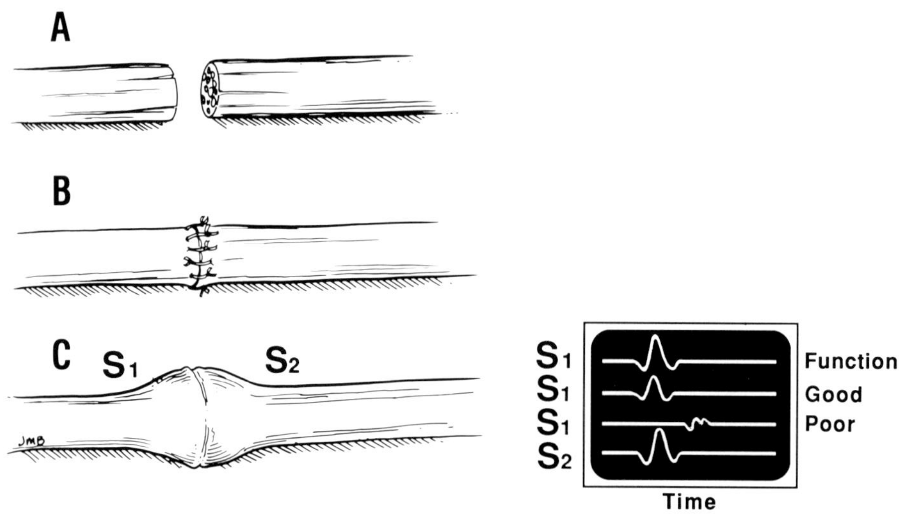

Figure 10–11. *When an entire nerve is transected, the neuroma may be functional or nonfunctional. Clinical and electrical assessment in the delayed setting determines whether the neuroma is functional. However, in the early phases of nerve regeneration, this may not be clinically possible; hence, early exploration of the nerve, along with intraoperative conduction, aids in assessment. If the neuroma shows function across it, then the nerve undergoes a neurolysis. If, however, the conduction characteristics of the nerve are untoward, the nerve is resected and the subsequent gap usually grafted.*

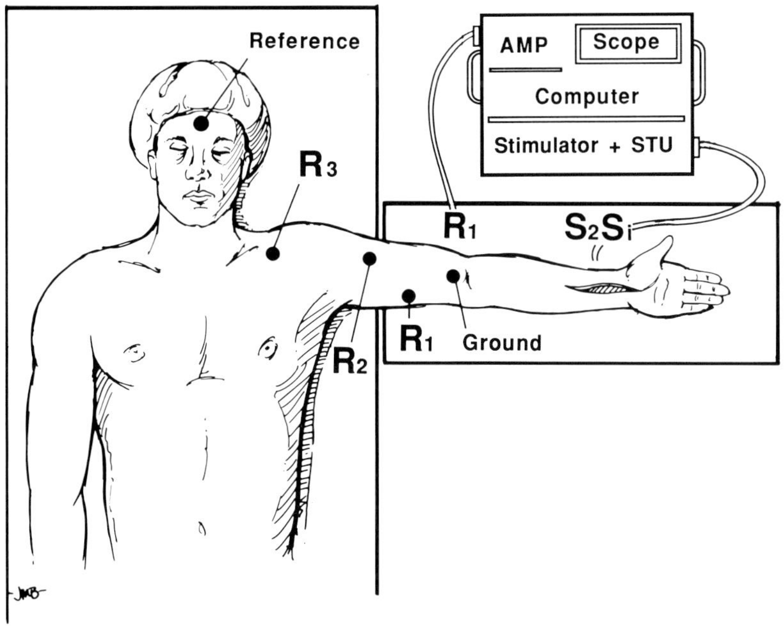

Figure 10–12. *The intraoperative mechanics for recording. With the patient in the supine position, and after anesthesia has been administered, needle electrodes are placed in the skin at the points indicated. In many instances, R1 cannot be used because of a tourniquet that is present. If a tourniquet is used, it must be deflated for at least 15 minutes before beginning recording studies. The stimulus is usually applied proximal and distal to the neuroma, and the recordings are most reliable when made from the axilla, or Erb's point.*

confidence, making it easier to identify the field of sensibility for the fascicle being stimulated.

It is our impression that peripheral nerves are more skillfully repaired using these methods, and that the number of severe peripheral nerve problems related to open nerve injuries is reduced.

REFERENCES

1. Caldwell JW, Crane CR, Krusen EM: Nerve conduction studies: An aid in the diagnosis of thoracic outlet syndrome. South Med J 1971; 64:210–212.
2. Checkles NS, Russakov AD, Piero DL: Ulnar nerve conduction velocity—effect of elbow position on measurement. Arch Phys Med Rehabil 1971; 52: 362.
3. DeLisa JA, Kraft GH, Gans BM. Clinical electromyography and nerve conduction studies. Ortho Rev 1978; 7:
4. Erlanger J, Gasser HS. Electrical signs of nervous activity. Philadelphia: University of Pennsylvania Press, 1937.
5. Gaul JS. Electrical fascicle identification as an adjunct to nerve repair. J Hand Surg 1983; 8:289–296.
6. Gilliatt RW, LeQuesne PM, Logue V, Sumner AJ: Wasting of the hand associated with cervical rib or band. J Neurol Neurosurg Psychiatry 1970; 33:615.
7. Gilliatt RW, Willison RG, Dietz V, Williams IR: Peripheral nerve conduction in patients with cervical rib and band. Ann Neurol 1978; 4:124.
8. Goodgold J, Eberstein A. Electrodiagnosis of neuromuscle diseases, ed 3. Baltimore: Williams & Wilkins, 1983:112–115.
9. Goodgold J, Kopell HP, Spielholz NI: The tarsal tunnel syndrome: Objective diagnostic criteria. N Engl J Med 1965; 273:742.
10. Gross MS, Gelberman RH: The anatomy of the distal ulnar tunnel. Clin Orthop 1985; 196:238.
11. Happel LT, LeBlanc HJ, Kline DG. Spinal cord potentials evoked by peripheral nerve stimulation. Electroencephalogr Clin Neurophysiol 1975; 38: 349–354.
12. Hartz CR, Linscheid RL, Gramse RR, Daube JR: The pronator teres syndrome: compressive neuropathy of the median nerve. J Bone Joint Surg [Am] 1981; 63:6.
13. Irani KD, Grabois M, Harvey SC: Standardized technique for diagnosis of tarsal tunnel syndrome. Am J Phys Med 1982; 61:26.
14. Johnson EW, Ortiz PR: Electrodiagnosis of tarsal tunnel syndrome. Arch Phys Med Rehabil 1966; 47: 776.
15. Johnson RK, Shrewsbury MM: Anatomical course of the thenar branch of the median nerve - usually

in a separate tunnel through the transverse carpal ligament. J Bone Joint Surg [Am] 1970; 52:269.
16. Jones SJ. Investigation of brachial plexus traction lesions by peripheral and spinal somatosensory evoked potentials. J Neurol Neurosurg Psychiatry 1979; 42:107–116.
17. Kimura J: A method of determining median nerve conduction velocity across the carpal tunnel. J Neurol Sci 1978; 38:1.
18. Kimura J, Davis FA. Electrodiagnosis in diseases of nerve and muscle. Philadelphia: FA Davis, 1983: 83–141.
19. Kline DG, Hackett ER. Value of electrophysiologic tests for peripheral nerve neuromas. J Surg Oncol 1970; 2:299–310.
20. Kline DG, Judice J. Operative management of selected brachial plexus lesions. J Neurosurg 1983; 58:631–649.
21. Kraft GH: Continuing Education Course E. American Association of Electromyography and Electrodiagnosis 1986:13.
22. Lambert E. Electromyography. In Youmans JR, ed. Neurological surgery, vol 1. Philadelphia: WB Saunders, 1973:358–367.
23. Lambert E. Electromyography and electrical stimulation of peripheral nerves and muscle. In: Mayo Clinic. Clinical examinations in neurology, ed 4. Philadelphia: WB Saunders, 1976:298–326.
24. Li CL, Bak A. Excitability characteristics of the A- and C-fibers in a peripheral nerve. Exp Neurol 1976; 50:67–79.
25. Oh SH, Sarala PK, Kuba T, Elmore RS: Tarsal tunnel syndrome: Electrophysiological study. Ann Neurol 1979; 5:327.
26. Peyronnard JM, Lamarre Y. Electrophysiological and anatomical estimation of the number of motor units in the monkey extensor digitorum brevis muscle. J Neurol Neurosurg Psychiatry 1977; 40:756–764.
27. Saeed MA, Gatens PF: Compound nerve action potentials of the medial and lateral plantar nerves through the tarsal tunnel. Ann Phys Med Rehabil 1982; 63:304.
28. Schwartz MS, Gordon JA, Swash M: Slowed nerve conduction with wrist flexion in carpal tunnel syndrome. Ann Neurol 1980; 8:69.
29. Singh N, Behse F, Buchthal F: Electrophysiological study of peroneal palsy. J Neurol Neurosurg Psychiatry 1974; 37:1202.
30. Stevens JL: AAEE minimonograph #26: The electrodiagnosis of carpal tunnel syndrome. Muscle Nerve 1987; 10:99.
31. Swift TR, Nichols FT: The droopy shoulder syndrome. Neurology 1984; 34:212.
32. Terzis JK, Dykes RW. Electrophysiological recording in peripheral nerve surgery: A review. J Hand Surg 1976; 1:52–66.
33. Urschel HC, Razuk MA, Wood RE, Parekh M, Paulson DL: Objective diagnosis (ulnar nerve conduction velocity) and current therapy of the thoracic outlet syndrome. Ann Thoracic Surg 1971; 12:608.
34. Van Beek AL. Electrodiagnostic evaluation of peripheral nerve injuries. Hand Clin 1986; 2:747–760.
35. Van Beek A, Hubble R, Kinkead L, Torros S, Suchy H. Clinical use of nerve stimulation and recording techniques. Plast Reconstr Surg 1983; 71:225–238.
36. Von Helmholtz G. Die Fortpflanzungsgeschwindigkeit der Nervenreizung. Archiv Fur Anatomie, Physiologie Und wissenschaft Liche Medicin. 199–216
37. Walsh JC. Somatosensory evoked responses in the diagnosis of thoracic outlet syndrome. J Neurol Neurosurg Psychiatry 1983; 46:234–240.
38. Wilbourn AJ: Case report #7: True neurogenic thoracic outlet syndrome. American Association of Electromyography and Electrodiagnosis, Rochester, Minnesota, 1982.
39. Wilbourn AJ: Thoracic outlet syndrome. Course D. Rochester, MN: American Association of Electromyography and Electrodiagnosis, 1984:28.

11

Pitfalls in Interpretation of Electrophysiological Testing

A. Lee Dellon

AUTHOR'S KEY POINTS

- The electrodiagnostic study is not a substitute for obtaining a careful history and physical examination.
- Normal values obtained with electrodiagnostic testing do not necessarily indicate absence of a neurologic abnormality.
- Conversely, an abnormal electrodiagnostic study does not mean that the patient requires operative treatment.
- Because an electrodiagnostic study may exceed the cost of surgery, sensibility testing (see Chap. 8) may be a more cost-effective means of assessment for most peripheral nerve problems.

Relying on the results of electrophysiological testing is a significant clinical problem, the basis for which is uncertainty in making a diagnosis and hesitancy in recommending treatment. The problem is the result of rapid history-taking and incomplete physical examination. As clinical uncertainty increases, electromyographers are consulted with increasing frequency (Fig. 11-1). At first localized to the physician's office, the problem spreads next to third-party payors and then to utilization reviewers who depend on electrophysiological studies to approve operative procedures. The expense of relying on the results of electrophysiological testing often exceeds the cost of the operative procedure itself. Cost containment has failed. Further, the problem is not confined to a single organ system: when the patient with upper extremity complaints, for example, is told that the results of electrophysiological testing are normal, the problem often will spread as the patient develops a compensation neurosis.

The pitfalls of electrophysiological testing can be avoided if the physician focuses on the patient's symptoms, the mechanism of injury, the regional anatomical peculiarities, and the associated anomalies. A meticulous sensorimotor evaluation is performed and the diagnosis is made. Electrophysiological testing is ordered *not* as a matter of course and *not* to confirm clinical suspicions, but only for assistance when a difficult diagnostic problem has been confronted (Table 11-1). Examples include the distinction of weakness due to primary myopathy, disorders of neuromuscular transmission, or axonopathies, or whether the numb thumb is

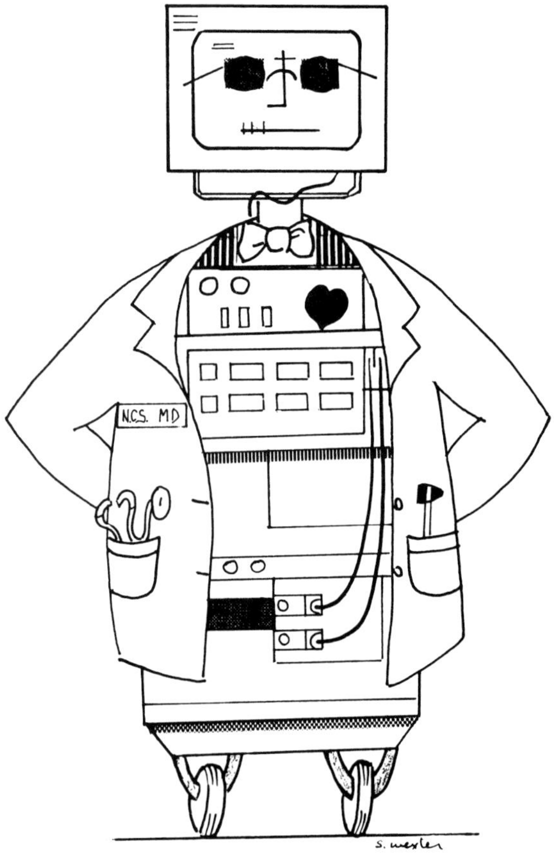

Figure 11–1. *Doctor Electrophysiology, NCS, EMG. This multichannel, oscilloscope-faced tyrant conceals his empire-building beneath a white lab coat. Reflex hammer and stethoscope are reminders of medicine's historic past, before the days of computer averaging, evoked potentials, and F&H waves. Put in your consult only when your careful history-taking and detailed sensorimotor testing indicate that electrophysiological testing is necessary to answer a particular question. Have sufficient confidence in your clinical skills that your judgment, not Doctor Electrophysiology's printout report, will be the final authority.*

due to either cervical radiculopathy or carpal tunnel syndrome, or both. Sufficient confidence in one's clinical skills (see Chaps. 8, 19, and 12) prevents overreliance on electrophysiological studies.

The theory and practical applications of electrophysiological testing have been well described (see Chap. 10).[4,21,25,29,30,43,45] This chapter focuses on areas in which the physician can easily reach the wrong clinical decision based on the interpretation of data derived from electrophysiological testing.

Table 11–1. *Indications for Electrophysiological Testing*

LOCALIZATION OF LESION
Radiculopathy vs compression or both
PROGRESSION OF LESION
Resolution of neurapraxia
Reinnervation following nerve repair[22]
Progression of inflammatory neuropathy[23]
Brachial plexopathy[20,24]
SYSTEMIC DISEASE
Peripheral neuropathy[25,26]
Drug toxicity[27]
Neuromuscular junction[28]
Myopathy[29,30]
VERIFICATION
Inability to communicate
Malingering
Martin-Gruber connection[31]

COMMON PITFALLS

The potential for a pitfall in electrophysiological testing is greatest in these areas:

1. The neurophysiology of electrical recording
2. The pathophysiology of chronic peripheral nerve compression
3. Anomalous innervation
4. Technical errors (Table 11-2)

The *neurophysiology of electrical recording* is such that the recording electrode will detect activity in the largest myelinated fibers first, since these fibers conduct at the fastest rates. Latency and conduction velocity, the commonly recorded parameters, depend on the time required from the electrical stimulus to the first recording. Electrically recordable events that occur thereafter, such as those related to activity in the slower-conducting, smaller, and more thinly myelinated fibers, are not reflected in routine electrodiagnostic reports. Further, if only a fraction of the large, thickly myelinated fibers remain and transmit impulses (that is, even if half of the fibers are *not* functioning), the recorded latency and conduction velocity re-

Table 11–2. *Pitfalls in Electrophysiological Testing*

NEUROPHYSIOLOGY
Large myelinated fibers preferentially recorded
PATHOPHYSIOLOGY
Sparing of central fascicles
Uneven fiber loss among fascicles
Incomplete remyelination
ANOMALOUS INNERVATION
Radial sensory nerve to thumb
Overlap of lateral antebrachial cutaneous nerve with radial sensory nerve
Lateral sural nerve entrapment
TECHNIQUE
Temperature
Patient age
Site along nerve
Temporal dispersion
Surface measurement of nerve length

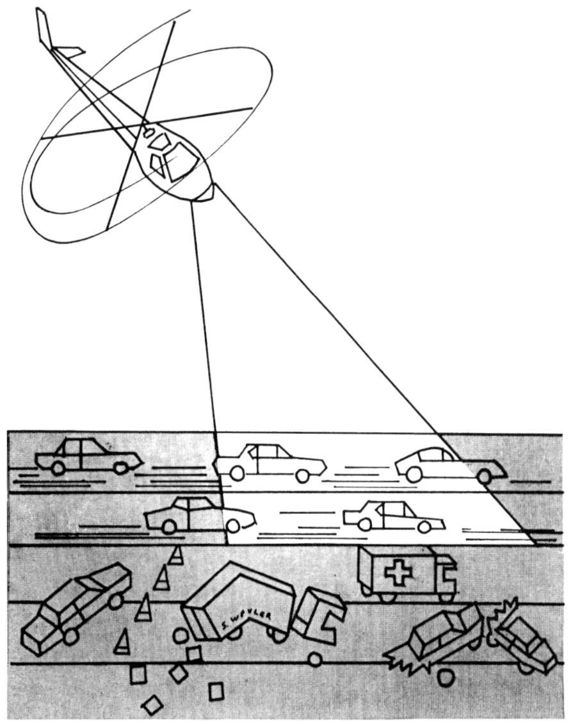

Figure 11–2. *"Reporter-in-the-sky" pitfall. The reported latency and conduction velocity of the electrodiagnostic report have the same inherent limitation as would the helicopter traffic reporter if he could report only the status of cars moving in the fastest lanes of the expressway. The thinly myelinated, smaller fiber nerves, analogous to the inner, slower lanes of the expressway, are simply ignored, or not reflected in the report of latency or conduction velocity, which depends on the first recorded impulse picked up from the large myelinated fibers. How different would be the report from the ambulance driver than from the helicopter pilot (ie, "complete block to traffic" versus "traffic moving normally")!*

mains normal because the pick-up electrode detects the fastest fibers as still functioning. This is analogous to hearing a morning traffic report based on the helicopter reporter's assessment of traffic moving in only the fastest lanes of the expressway (Fig. 11-2). There may be a total block to travel in the slow lanes due to an accident, and ambulances may be at the scene, but traffic may still be moving at 55 mph in the fast lane.

The pathophysiology of the pitfall in electrophysiological recordings is related to the consequences of chronic nerve compression and to the consequences of remyelination. The development of an experimental model of chronic nerve compression in the rat and in the primate[35,36,39] and the morphometric analysis of human examples of chronic nerve compression[32,37,38] have demonstrated that:

1. The periphery of a fascicle has a greater degree of injury than the center of the fascicle.
2. The fascicles within a nerve are not uniformly affected by compression.
3. Large myelinated and small unmyelinated fibers can be affected differently (Figs. 11-3, 11-4, Tables 11-3, 11-4).

This means that the patient's symptoms (ie, middle finger with persistent numbness or clumsiness) may be due to a severe degree of compression, with its attendant demyelination and axonal degeneration, while the "normal" findings on the electrodiagnostic testing are due to an adjacent, less severely affected fascicle.

During regeneration after operative decompression, despite restitution of neural blood flow[20,46–48] and distal axonal regeneration, remyelination is often incomplete.[19,33,40,41,49] Thus, although the patient may be without symptoms, fol-

(Text continued on p. 192)

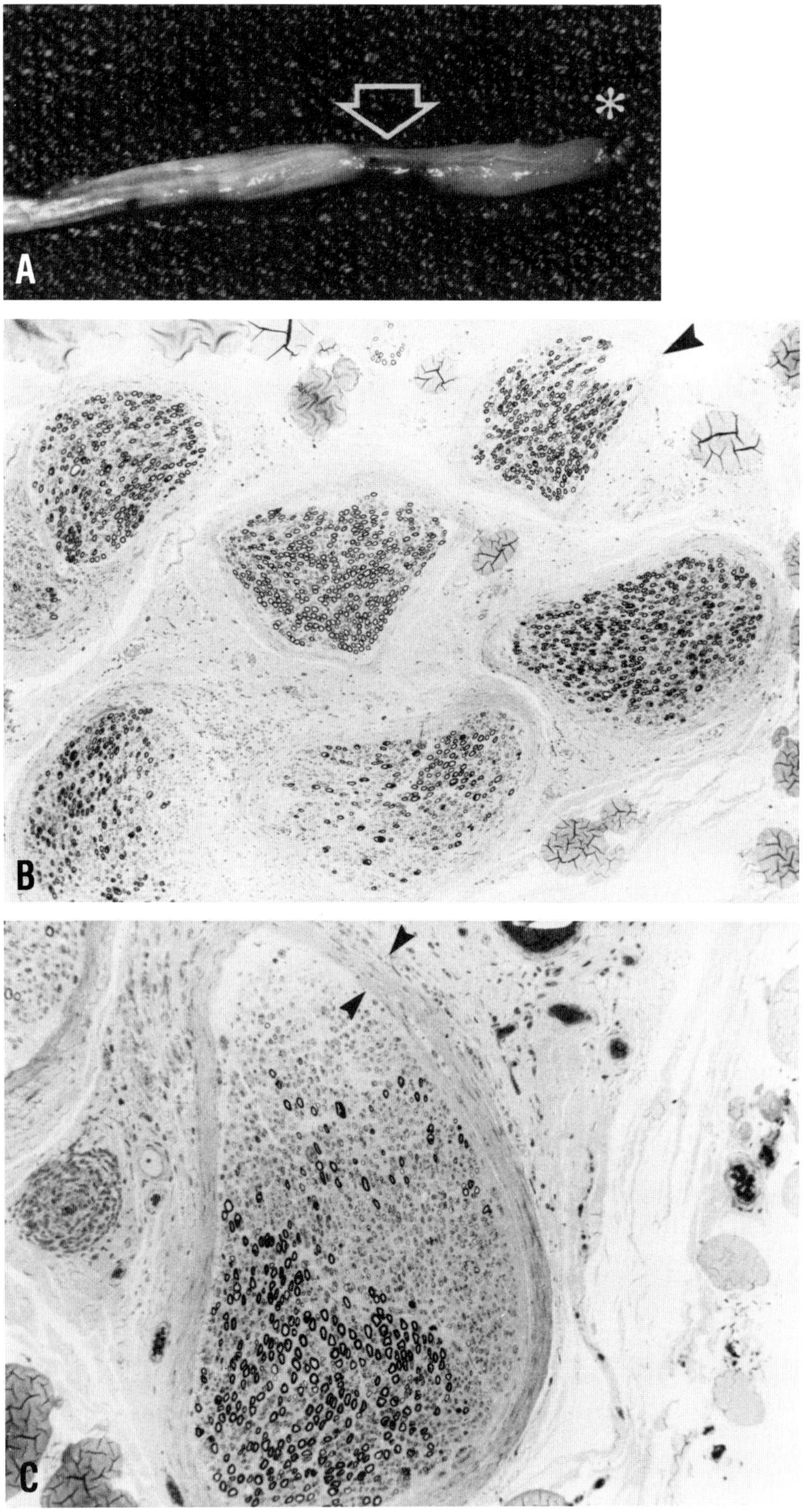

Figure 11–3. *Pathophysiology pitfall demonstrated with human radial sensory nerve. (**A**) Excised nerve. Asterisk denotes proximal end; arrow marks site of compression (see Case 2, Table 11–3). (**B**) Low-power (×78) photomicrograph from region of arrow in (A) demonstrates increased thickening in epineurium and perineurium of all six fascicles. Note Renaut body (arrow), which occurs with sheer plus compression forces. Note uneven distribution of fiber pathology within fascicle with spared central fascicle relative to peripheral fascicles, and (**C**) at higher magnification (×125) uneven fiber loss even within a fascicle. Arrows denote thickened perineurium.*

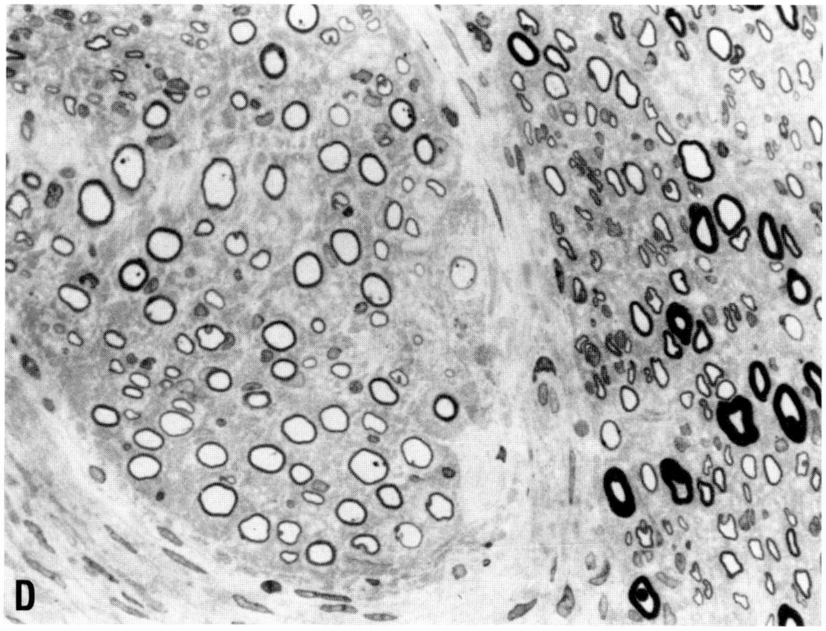

Figure 11–3. *(Continued) In (**D**) at higher magnification (×500), this variation within a fascicle is seen again (see Case 4, Table 11–3). Note thinning of myelin (increased axon/myelin ratio with nerve compression). This uneven fiber pathology seen with chronic human nerve compression is one of the pitfalls in electrophysiologic diagnosis. (Reprinted with permission from Mackinnon SE, Dellon AL, Hudson AR, Hunter DA. Chronic human nerve compression: A histologic assessment. Neuropathol Appl Neurobiol 1987;12:547.)*

Table 11–3. *Pathophysiology of a Pitfall: Radial Sensory Nerve*

	Case 1	***Case 2***	***Case 3***	***Case 4***
AGE (YEARS), SEX	32 F	24 F	44 M	62 M
PRECIPITATING FACTOR	Excessive writing	Crush injury	Crush injury	Forearm fracture
WCB	+	+	+	–
DURATION OF SYMPTOMS (YEARS)	7	1	3	15
PREVIOUS SURGERY	DQR	no	DQR	no
SENSORY EXAMINATION (SBR)				
M2PD (mm)				
Compressed SBR / Contralateral SBR	12/8	15/10	20/6	25/10
Tinel's sign	+	+	+	+
256 cps vibratory perception	↓	↓	↓	↓
Provocative test	+	+	+	+
NCS	NA	NA	N	AB

AB, abnormal; DQR, deQuervain's release; M2PD, moving two-point discrimination; N, normal; NA, not performed; NCS, nerve conduction studies; SBR, superficial branch of radial nerve; WCB, worker's compensation case.
(Data from Mackinnon SE, Dellon AL, Hunter DA. Histopathology of compression of the superficial radial nerve in the forearm. J Hand Surg [Am] 1986;11:206–209.)

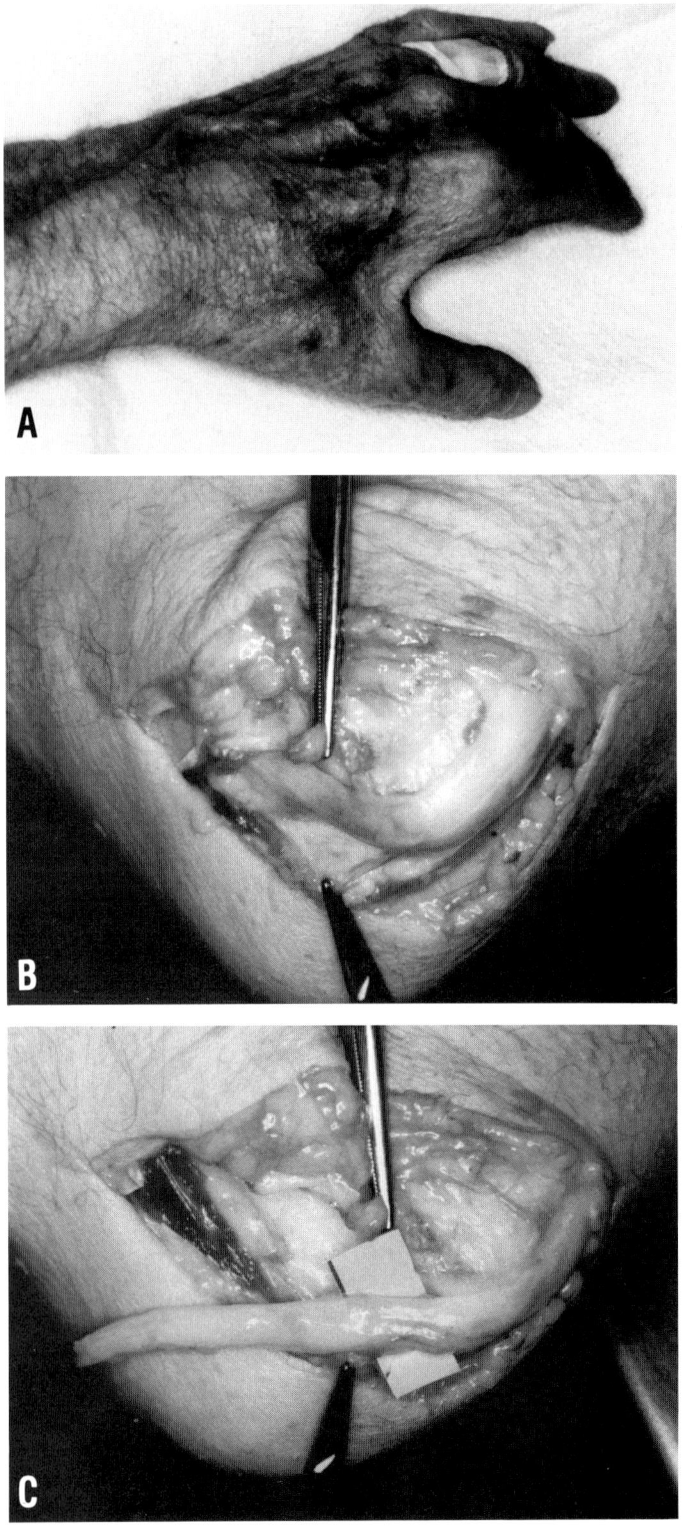

Figure 11–4. Pathophysiology pitfall demonstrated with human ulnar nerve at the elbow. (***A***) Severe intrinsic wasting related to unsuccessful intramuscular transposition of left ulnar nerve (see Table 11–4). (***B***) Fresh postmortem view of right cubital tunnel (see Table 11–4). Note area of narrowing at divided Osborne's band (between clamps). (***C***) Distal nerve has been divided. Note area of narrowing in nerve. Patient clinically had cubital tunnel syndrome.

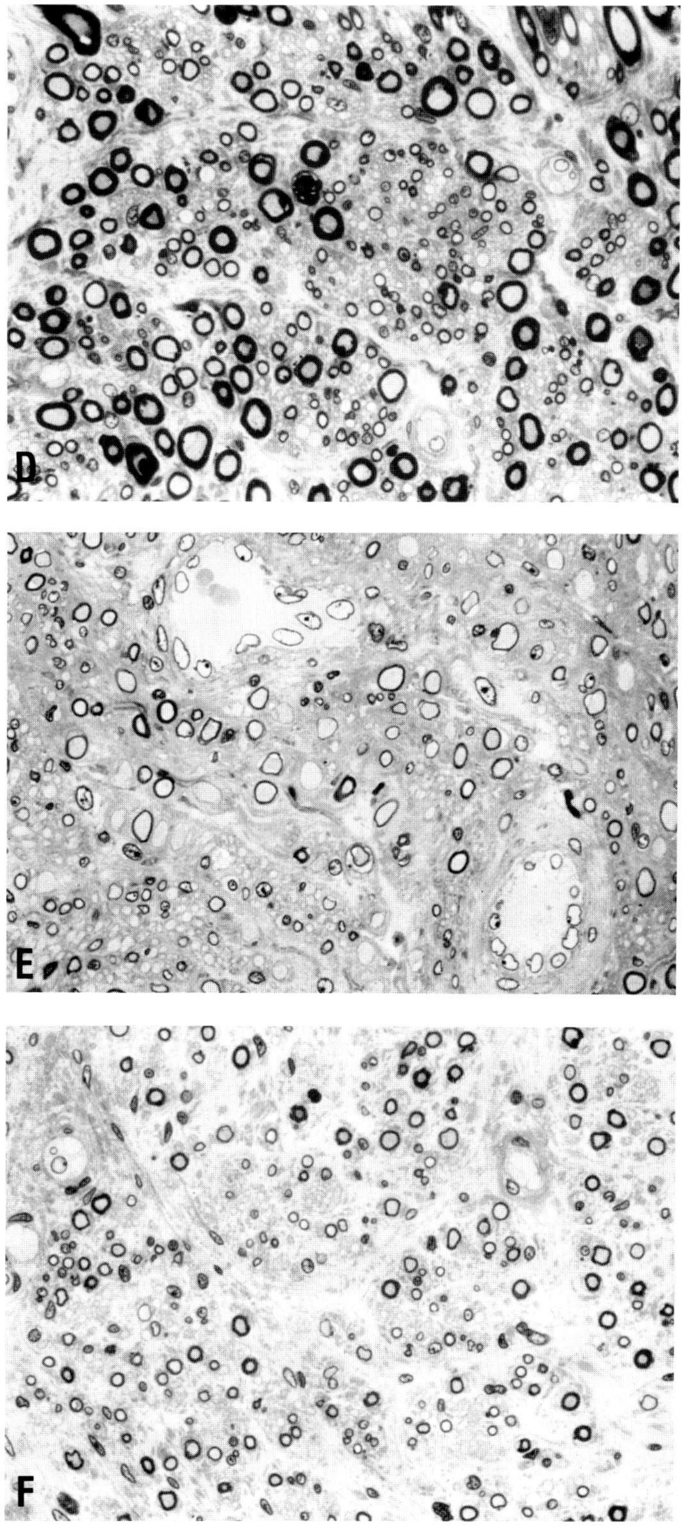

Figure 11–4. (Continued) *Histopathology that accompanies morphometry (Table 11–4) is noted (**D**) proximal to (**E**) at and (**F**) distal to Osborne's band (×588). (Reprinted with permission from Dellon AL, Mackinnon SE. Human ulnar neuropathy at the elbow: Clinical electrical and morphometric correlation. J Reconstr Microsurg 1988;4:179.)*

Table 11–4. *Pathophysiology Pitfall: Ulnar Nerve at Elbow*

Morphometric

	$\bar{x}$ Fiber Diameter (± SD)	% Neural Tissue	% Myelin	Axon/Myelin Ratio
RIGHT ULNAR NERVE				
Proximal	6.6 ± 2.38	31	66	0.5
Cubital tunnel	5.0 ± 2.37	29	49	1.0
Distal	6.6 ± 2.87	34	63	0.6
LEFT ULNAR NERVE				
Proximal				
Compressed	6.9 ± 3.1	34	64	0.5
region	5.2 ± 1.69	15	36	1.7
Distal	4.1 ± 1.28	10	52	0.5

Electrophysiology

	Latency (msec) Onset	Latency (msec) Peak	Distance (mm)	Velocity (m/sec)	Amplitude (uV)
RIGHT ULNAR					
Digit 5 to wrist	2.9	3.6	146	48	6
Wrist to ADM	3.3				5000
Below elbow to ADM	8.1		265	55	5000
Above elbow to ADM	10.3		110	50	2500
LEFT ULNAR					
Digit 5 to wrist	NR				
Wrist to ADM	2.7				5000
Below elbow to ADM	8.1		275	51	4500
Above elbow to ADM	12.8		125	27	3500

ADM, abductor digiti minimi; NR, no response.
(Data from Dellon AL, Mackinnon SE. Human ulnar neuropathy at the elbow: clinical, electrical and morphometric correlation. J Reconstr Microsurg 1988;4:179–184.)

low-up electrophysiological testing may suggest persistent or recurrent nerve compression.

While electrophysiological testing data may be crucial in identifying the presence of an anomaly, such as a Martin-Gruber communication[22] or innervation of the extensor digitorum brevis by the superficial peroneal nerve,[29] or sensory innervation of the thumb pulp by the radial sensory nerve,[12] the presence of an anomaly may also be a pitfall (see Chap. 12). For example, entrapment of the radial sensory nerve in the forearm is easily diagnosed by clinical criteria,[12,13] but it is difficult to diagnose by electrophysiological studies (see Table 11-3) due to the presence of an overlap in sensation by the lateral antebrachial cutaneous nerve in 75% of patients.[1,31] Normal conduction velocity may be found due to activity of the lateral antebrachial cutaneous nerve, which "shields" the abnormal conduction in the deeper radial sensory nerve (Fig. 11-5) (see Chap. 74).

Pitfalls due to the actual technique of recording the electrophysiological response have been summarized, but their description is beyond the scope of this chapter.[26] In general, these errors include temperature variability (velocity changes 5% for every degree Celsius),[17,23] variability along length of nerve (faster proximally than distally), variability due to age (half the adult value at birth, decrease 10 m/sec after age 60),[26] spread of stimulus current (inadvertent activation of neighboring nerves), temporal dispersion (action potential varies due to amplitude and area of subsets of fibers),[26] and error in surface measurement of nerve compared to actual length of nerve.[15,26]

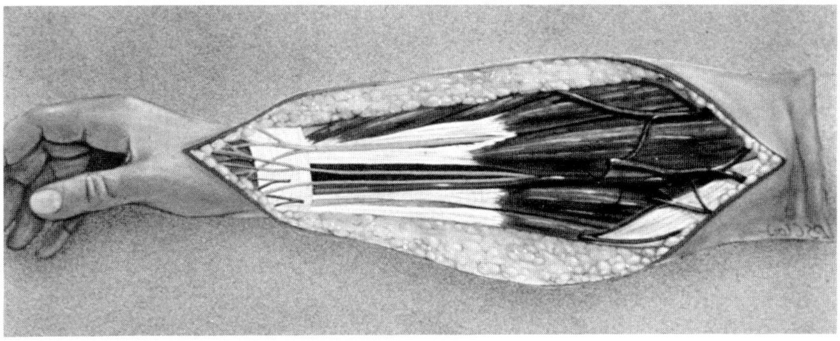

Figure 11–5. *Anatomic pitfall: Anomalous innervation. The radial sensory nerve and lateral antebrachial cutaneous nerve have great variability. Here the lateral antebrachial has a proximal split and distally partially overlaps the radial sensory nerve. Some overlap occurs in 75% of people. The site of radial sensory nerve entrapment is noted between the tendons of the brachioradialis and the extensor carpi radialis longus. (Reproduced with permission from Mackinnon SE, Dellon AL. Overlap of lateral antebrachial cutaneous nerve and superficial sensory branch of the radial nerve. J Hand Surg [Am] 1985; 10:522.*

COMMON PITFALLS

Thoracic Outlet Syndrome

Thoracic outlet syndrome is a clinical entity for which electrophysiological testing is not diagnostic (see Chap. 85). There is still some controversy over its existence.[6,8] The diagnosis is one of exclusion of other problems that give similar symptomatology, such as cervical disc disease, myofascial syndrome, shoulder impingement, or the cubital and carpal tunnel syndromes. Not only do accurate diagnostic criteria exist for these other problems, but specific therapy is available. The approach to diagnosis of thoracic outlet syndrome that I prefer considers each of these problems, rules them in or out, treats them, recognizes that several may coexist, and does not consider an operative approach until all other diagnostic possibilities have been pursued.[11,34]

Electrophysiological testing is helpful in diagnosis of the conditions that mimic brachial plexus compression (thoracic outlet compression), such as cervical radiculopathy and peripheral nerve entrapment. However, electrophysiological testing *cannot* make a diagnosis of brachial plexus compression. The sites of compression (eg, scalene anticus, scarring within the plexus itself, cervical rib, first rib and congenital bands) are widely distributed in three dimensions. The point for stimulus and for recording (eg, Erb's point) is poorly defined. The volume of tissue interposed between skin and any given trunk or cord of the brachial plexus is highly variable. The distance for measurement between stimulus and recording electrodes is inaccurate, since the relationship of skin to the brachial plexus is variable. Reflex tests such as the H wave can reflect abnormalities anywhere along the reflex arc and are not specific for brachial plexus compression.[7,44,50,51]

Multiple Compression Sites vs Distal Axonopathy

Traditionally, diffuse weakness or stocking and glove sensory loss has been attributed to peripheral neuropathy. Electrophysiological testing data is usually reported as indicating diffuse sensorimotor neuropathy. When terminal latencies and distal velocities are slower than proximal ones, which is usually the case, there is a neuropathy of the dying-back or distal axonopathy type. Diabetic neuropathy is the most common example.[2,18,24] If the neuropathy has not advanced to the point that "no response" is detectable to electrical stimulation, it may be possible, using the "inching" technique, to identify a superimposed entrapment neuropathy.[5,28,42] If this is identified, the report reads "diffuse peripheral neuropathy, distal axonopathy type with superimposed nerve compression" (of the posterior tibial nerve in the tarsal tunnel or the median nerve at the wrist). The surgeon's decision is clear if a site of superimposed compression is found: the nerve should be decompressed (see Chap. 68). But if diffuse neuropathy with no evidence of radiculopathy or nerve compression is detected, is surgery contraindicated? Could not a subclinical entrapment sufficient to produce symptoms still be present?

Recently, a clinical cause for optimism in diabetic neuropathy has been suggested, based on the theory that the diabetic nerve has increased susceptibility to compression.[9,16] Among other possibilities are the increased water content of the diabetic nerve and decreased axoplasmic transport observed in the diabetic patient.[34] The hypothesis is that symptoms of diabetic neuropathy may be due largely to multiple sites of compression along multiple peripheral nerves. The first clinical approach to this problem is encouraging, suggesting that up to 80% of diabetics can achieve good relief of symptoms by decompression of multiple peripheral nerves.[10] Just one third of patients in that study had nerve compression diagnosed by electrophysiological testing. This is not surprising: many diabetic patients are asymptomatic at times when their electrophysiological testing is abnormal, and there is a poor correlation between the diabetic patient's symptoms and severity as indicated by the electrophysiological test data.[3,52]

The answer to this paradox may lie in the following possibilities:

1. The observed electrophysiological changes may be related to metabolic events that do not correlate directly with symptoms.
2. Metabolic events increase neural water content and decrease axoplasmic flow, increasing the peripheral nerve's susceptibility to compression from the neuronal foramina at the spine (or base of skull) to the carpal and tarsal tunnels.
3. Multiple sites of compression along the course of a peripheral nerve may give the electrophysiological equivalent of a distal axonopathy.

In summary, if clinical criteria (positive Tinel's sign, positive provocative test) suggest there is nerve compression at a known anatomical site of narrowing along the course of a peripheral nerve, then even if the electrophysiological testing data are interpreted as diffuse neuropathy without sites of nerve compression, evidence is accumulating in support of accepting the clinical criteria that indicate compression and proceeding with operative decompression when indicated.

REFERENCES

1. Bourne MH, Wood MB, Carmichael SW. Locating the lateral antebrachial cutaneous nerve. J Hand Surg [Am] 1987;12:697–699.
2. Braddom RL, Hollis JB, Castell DO. Diabetic peripheral neuropathy: Correlation of nerve conduction studies and clinical findings. Arch Phys Med Rehabil 1977;58:308–313.
3. Brown MR, Dyck PJ, McLearn GE, Sima AAF, Powell HC, Porte D Jr. Central and peripheral nervous system complications. Diabet 1982;31[suppl]: 65–70.
4. Brown WF. The physiological and technical basis of electromyography. Boston: Butterworth, 1984.
5. Brown WF, Yates SK. Percutaneous localization of conduction abnormalities in human entrapment neuropathies. Canad J Neurol Sci 1982;9:391–400.
6. Carroll RE, Hurst LC. The relationship of thoracic outlet syndrome and carpal tunnel syndrome. Clin Orthop 1982;164:149–153.
7. Cherington M. Ulnar conduction velocity in thoracic outlet syndrome. N Engl J Med 1976;294:1185.
8. Cherington M. Surgery for thoracic outlet syndrome? N Engl J Med 1986;313:322.
9. Dellon AL. Optimism in diabetic neuropathy. Ann Plast Surg 1988;20:103–105.
10. Dellon AL. Treatment of symptoms of diabetic neuropathy by peripheral nerve decompression. Diabetes Care (submitted September 1990).
11. Dellon AL, Hendler N, Hopkins JET, Karas AC, Campbell JN. Team management of patients with diffuse upper extremity complaints. Maryland Med J 1986;35:849–852.
12. Dellon AL, Mackinnon SE. Radial sensory nerve entrapment. Arch Neurol 1986;43:833–837.
13. Dellon AL, Mackinnon SE. Radial sensory nerve entrapment in the forearm. J Hand Surg [Am] 1986;11: 199–205.
14. Dellon AL, Mackinnon SE. Human ulnar neuropathy at the elbow: Clinical, electrical and morphometric correlation. J Reconstr Microsurg 1988;4:179–184.
15. Dellon AL, Mackinnon SE, Schlegel R. Validity of

electrodiagnostic studies following anterior transposition of the ulnar nerve. J Hand Surg [Am] 1987;12:700–703.
16. Dellon AL, Mackinnon SE, Seiler WA IV. Susceptibility of the diabetic nerve to chronic compress. Ann Plast Surg 1988;20:117–119.
17. Denys EH. The role of temperature in electromyography. Rochester, Minn.: American Association for Electromyography and Electrodiagnosis, 1980, mini-monograph 14.
18. Dyck PJ, Thomas PK, Asbury AK, Winegard AF, Porte D Jr. Diabetic neuropathy. Philadelphia: WB Saunders, 1987.
19. Eversmann WW, Ritsick JA. Intraoperative changes in motor nerve conduction latency in carpal tunnel syndrome. J Hand Surg 1978;3:77–81.
20. Gelberman RH, Hergenroeder PT, Hargens AR, Lundborg GN, Akeson WH. The carpal tunnel syndrome. A study of carpal canal pressures. J Bone Joint Surg [Am] 1981;63:380–383.
21. Goodgold J, Eberstein A. Electrodiagnosis of neuromuscular diseases, ed 3. Baltimore: Williams & Wilkins, 1983.
22. Gutman L. Median–ulnar nerve communications and carpal tunnel syndrome. J Neurol Neurosurg Psychiatry 1977;40:982–986.
23. Halar EM, DeLisa JA, Soine TL. Nerve conduction studies in upper extremities: Skin temperature corrections. Arch Phys Med Rehabil 1983;64:412–416.
24. Halar EM, Graf RJ, Halter JB, Brozovich FV, Soine TL. Diabetic neuropathy: A clinical, laboratory and electrodiagnostic study. Arch Phys Med Rehabil 1982;63:298–303.
25. Johnson EW, ed. Practical electromyography. Baltimore: Williams & Wilkins, 1980.
26. Kimura J. Principles and pitfalls of nerve conduction studies. Ann Neurol 1984;16:415–429.
27. Kimura J. The carpal tunnel syndrome: Localization of conduction abnormalities within the distal segment of the median nerve. Brain 1979;102:619–635.
28. Lambert EH. The accessory deep peroneal nerve: A common variation in innervation of the extensor digitorum brevis. Neurol 1969;19:1169–1176.
29. Lang AH, Partanen VSJ. "Satellite potentials" and the duration of motor unit potentials in normal, neuropathic and myopathic muscles. J Neurol Sci 1976;27:513–524.
30. Lenman JAR, Ritchie AE. Clinical electromyograph. London: Pitman, 1983.
31. Mackinnon SE, Dellon AL. Overlap of lateral antebrachial cutaneous nerve and superficial sensory branch of the radial nerve. J Hand Surg [Am] 1985;10:522–526.
32. Mackinnon SE, Dellon AL. Experimental study of chronic nerve compression: Clinical implications. Hand Clinics 1986;2:639–650.
33. Mackinnon SE, Dellon AL. Evaluation of microsurgical internal neurolysis in a primate medial nerve model of chronic nerve compression. J Hand Surg [Am] 1988;13:345–351.
34. Mackinnon SE, Dellon AL. Surgery of the peripheral nerve. New York: Thieme, 1988: Ch 3, 14.
35. Mackinnon SE, Dellon AL, Hudson AR, Hunter D. Chronic nerve compression–experimental model in the rat. Ann Plast Surg 1984;13:112–120.
36. Mackinnon SE, Dellon AL, Hudson AR, Hunter DA. A primate model for chronic nerve compression. J Reconstr Microsurg 1985;1:185–194.
37. Mackinnon SE, Dellon AL, Hudson AR, Hunter DA. Chronic human nerve compression: A histologic assessment. Neuropathol Appl Neurobiol 1987;12: 547–565.
38. Mackinnon SE, Dellon AL, Hunter DA. Histopathology of compression of the superficial radial nerve in the forearm. J Hand Surg [Am] 1986;11: 206–209.
39. Mackinnon SE, O'Brien JP, Dellon AL, McLean AR, Hudson AR, Hunter DA. A model of chronic nerve compression in the rat model. Ann Plast Surg 1987;19:430–435.
40. Mackinnon SE, O'Brien JP, Dellon AL, MacLean AR, Hudson AR, Hunter DA. An assessment of different treatment strategies including internal neurolysis on a chronically compressed rat sciatic nerve. Plast Reconstr Surg 1988;81:251–256.
41. Melvin JL, Johnson EW, Duran R. Electrodiagnosis after surgery for the carpal tunnel syndrome. Arch Phys Med Rehabil 1968;49:502–507.
42. Miller RG. The cubital tunnel syndrome: Diagnosis and precise localization. Ann Neurol 1979;6:56–59.
43. Oh SJ. Clinical electromyography. Nerve conduction studies. Baltimore: University Park Press, 1984.
44. Relman AS. Responsibilities of authorship: Where does the buck stop? N Engl J Med 1984;310:1048–1049.
45. Robertson KB. Electrodiagnosis in neurological rehabilitation. In: Umphred DA, ed. Neurological rehabilitation. St. Louis: CV Mosby, 1985.
46. Rydevik B, Lundborg G. Permeability of intraneural microvessels and perineurium following acute, graded experimental nerve compression. Scand J Plast Reconstr Surg 1977;11:179–187.
47. Rydevik B, Lundborg G, Bagge U. Effects of graded

compression on intraneural blood flow. J Hand Surg 1981;6:3–12.

48. Seiler JG III, Milek MA, Carpenter GK, Swiontkowski MF. Intraoperative assessment of median nerve blood flow during carpal tunnel release with laser Doppler flowmetry. J Hand Surg [Am] 1989;14:986–991.
49. Stewart JD. Focal peripheral neuropathies. New York: Elsevier, 1987.
50. Urschel HC, Razzuk MA. Management of the thoracic outlet syndrome. N Engl J Med 1972;286: 1140–1143.
51. Wilbourn AJ, Lederman RJ. Evidence for conduction delay in thoracic outlet syndrome is challenged. N Engl J Med 1984;310:1052–1053.
52. Yagishashi S, Matsunago M. Ultrastructural pathology of peripheral nerves in patients with diabetic neuropathy. Tohoki J Exp Med 1979;129:356–366.

12

Anomalous Innervation of the Upper Extremity

Roy A. Meals
Edward R. Calkins

AUTHORS' KEY POINTS

- The types of peripheral nerve anomalies are neural loops, high neural origins, fibers temporarily coursing through different nerves, and fibers extending their entire courses within a different nerve.
- Communication from the median or anterior interosseous nerves to the ulnar nerve within the proximal forearm occurs in 10% to 30% of patients. The ramus (the Martin-Gruber communication), which causes varying degrees of anomalous innervation of the intrinsic muscles, is identified by correlation of physical findings before and after nerve blocks and electrophysiological findings.
- The Riche-Cannieu connection provides a mechanism for cross- or double-innervation of intrinsic muscles anywhere in the hand.
- A distal communicating sensory branch between median and ulnar nerves (communicating palmar branch of Berrettini) is a common finding. If injured during carpal tunnel release or palmar fasciectomy, a discrete area of digital numbness will occur.
- In 75% of cases, the radial sensory and lateral antebrachial cutaneous nerves share territories of innervation. Treatment of one or the other of these two nerves may not completely alleviate symptoms due to a neuroma.

At 24 days in human embryo development, the upper limb bud is only a slight swelling ventrolateral to the myotomes in the lower cervical region. By 33 days, the hand plate becomes recognizable, and spinal nerves extend into the root of the limb bud. As the myotomes fuse, contract, and lengthen to form a complex muscular system, the nerves distributed to the original parts of this system undergo similar rearrangements. Even by 37 days, the brachial plexus is evident, and radial, median, and ulnar nerves reach to the elbow. The musculature becomes stratified dorsally and ventrally by the central core of skeletal blastema, and the nerves are likewise stratified.[56]

Although the general arrangement is identical, no two individuals, excluding monozygous twins, have identical facial features, and the same is apparently true for nerves. Even side-to-side differences are noted in the same individual. Detailed anatomical dissections have delineated the usual peripheral nerve patterns and the incidence of major variations, and clinicians have related clinical findings to the recognized variations. The topic remains clouded, however, because a thorough functional examination and a thorough anatomical dissection cannot readily be done on the same limb. Thus the anatomist views nerve anomalies through one keyhole, finding a variation but remaining uncertain whether the branch carries motor or sensory fibers. The clinician views nerve anomalies through another keyhole, recognizing anomalous patterns on motor and sensory testing and perhaps glimpsing the anatomy through an operative approach, but remaining ignorant of the more proximal and distal arrangements of the nerves. Both the anatomist and the clinician are hampered by the inability to trace a single fiber back to its central origin.

Based on information gathered by these perspectives, however limited, a classification of nerve anomalies is proposed. In the primordial state, nerve fibers run directly from source to target end organ (Fig. 12-1*A*). With embryologic development, fusions and branchings occur to form the usually encountered pattern of plexus formation and distal branching with specific fibers still directed to specific target end organs (Fig. 12-1*B*). In the simplest variation fibers temporarily digress from their normal course and eventually rejoin the same trunk, forming a neural loop (Fig. 12-1*C*). Examples of Type 1 variations are short loops seen in the ulnar nerve around the pisiform and hamate. Long loops have been noted in the forearm.

Another type of variation (Type 2) is separation of a fiber from the parent trunk more proximally than usual. The fiber runs the remainder of its course to the target as a separate nerve (Fig. 12-1*D*). An example of the Type 2 variation is the bifid median nerve at the wrist level. A more complex arrangement, still in the Type 2 classification, is multiple median nerve branches to the thenar muscles.

The Type 3 variation is a nerve originating more proximally than usual and traveling temporarily with a different nerve (Fig. 12-1*E*). The Martin-Gruber communication between the median and ulnar nerves in the forearm is an example of a Type 3 variation.

In the final type of variation, Type 4, nerve fibers run their entire course in a different nerve trunk (Fig. 12-1*F*). Examples of this include variable innervation of the middle finger profundus belly and middle finger lumbrical from either the median or ulnar nerve.

Knowledge of nerve anomalies is important when deciding whether residual limb function is related to partial nerve injury or to complete nerve injury with function persisting via anomalous innervation. For the surgeon, knowledge of variations is also important in avoiding injury to nerves during operative procedures. What follows is a discussion of the more common upper limb nerve anomalies that have significant clinical implications for diagnosis and for planning surgical approaches. Although anomalies of the brachial plexus are common, most cannot be anticipated preoperatively, because nerve blocks and isolated conduction velocities at this level are difficult to perform and to interpret. Further, brachial plexus anomalies do not alter the operative approach to the region, although an awareness of the possibilities makes the surgeon more cautious and aware.

LATERAL PECTORAL NERVE

Case 1

An 18-year-old man sustained a closed injury to his left brachial plexus in a motorcycle accident. His left upper extremity is entirely flail and anesthetic from the cord level distally. However, the pectoralis major muscle is functioning well.

Is the lateral cord incompletely injured?

The medial and lateral pectoral nerves, arising respectively from the medial and lateral cords, usually innervate the pectoralis major muscle. The medial pectoral nerve also supplies the pectoralis minor, which is not functioning in this case. The lateral pectoral nerve often arises more proximally

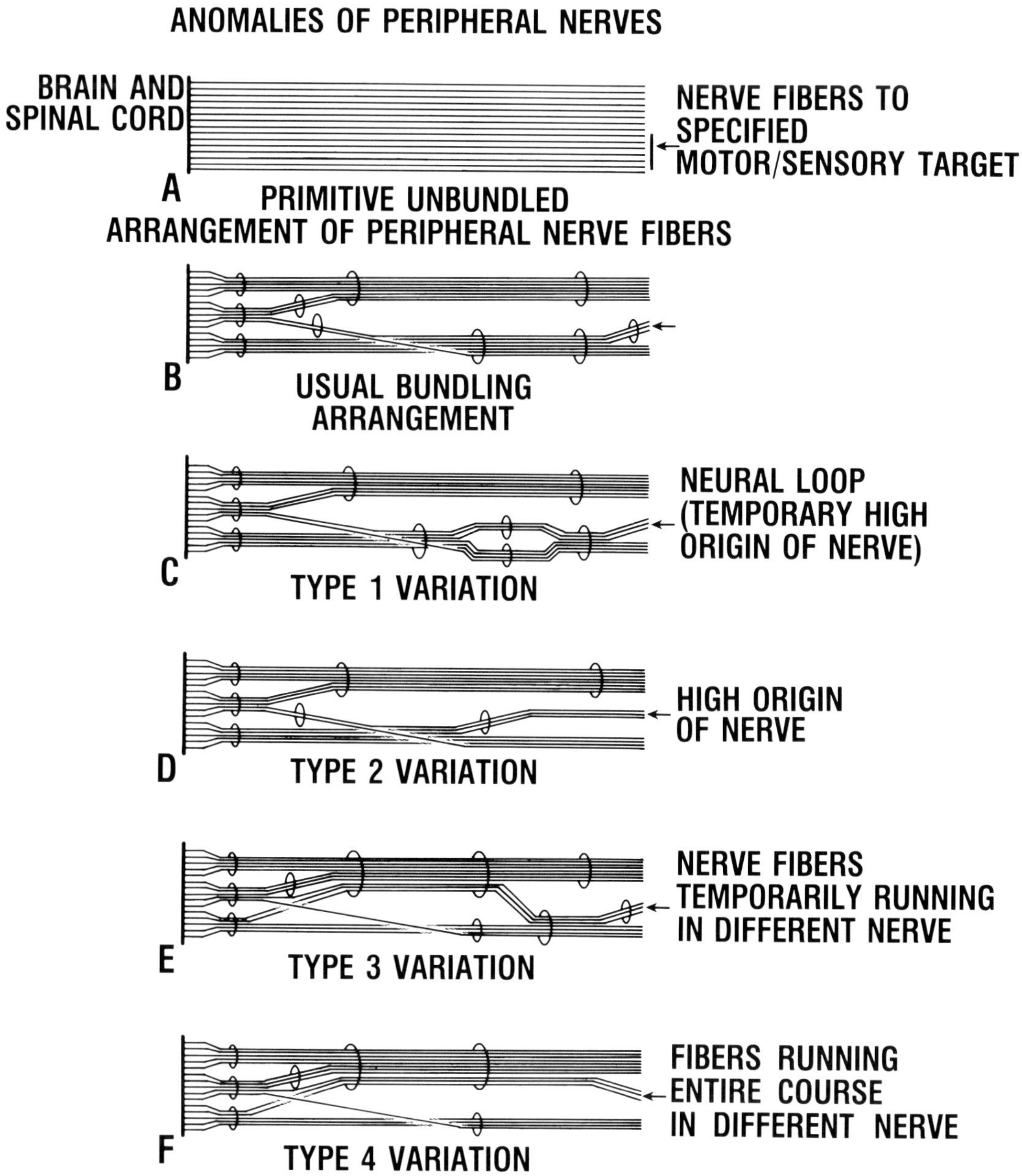

Figure 12–1. *Classification of nerve anomalies. See text for details.*

from the upper and middle trunk anterior divisions; the medial pectoral nerve occasionally arises from the lower trunk.[39] These are Type 2 variations in our classification of nerve anomalies. Thus, the lateral pectoral nerve originating proximal to the level of a brachial plexus cord injury is spared.

MUSCULOCUTANEOUS NERVE

Case 2

A 28-year-old man has been stabbed in the proximal, medial aspect of his arm with a small screwdriver. In addition to a complete motor and sensory median nerve deficit, he also cannot contract his biceps or brachialis muscles.

Is the damage more diffuse than anticipated by the mechanism of injury, since his musculocutaneous nerve is apparently not functioning?

Although fibers pass in both directions between the musculocutaneous and median nerves, anomalous sensory or motor innervation rarely results. Rather, fibers separated within the brachial plexus belatedly find their way to their respective nerves further down the arm. The musculocutaneous nerve is usually comprised of C5- and C6-derived fibers. In 24% of upper limbs, C7 fibers enter the musculocutaneous nerve and then pass to the median nerve through a Type 3 variation[38] (Fig. 12-2). Fibers pass from the median to the musculocutaneous nerve in only 2% of cases. An additional 2% have a combined musculocutaneous and median nerve. Thus, a small lesion disturbing both median and musculocutaneous nerve function could be anticipated in Case 2. Fibers coursing from the musculocutaneous to the median nerve have been traced to the pronator teres, the flexor carpi radialis, and the thenar muscles.[68]

In 89% of cases, the lateral cord divides into the musculocutaneous and median nerves. In 5% of cases, the median, ulnar, and musculocutaneous nerves arise from a common trunk. In another 5%, the musculocutaneous nerve is derived from the upper trunk anterior division.

MEDIAN–ULNAR NERVE COMMUNICATIONS

Case 3

A 20-year-old man received a severe penetrating injury to the forearm with considerable soft-tissue destruction. After hospital admission, he had complete function of the intrinsic muscles but anesthesia in the ulnar distribution. When the wound was debrided, the surgeons noted segmental loss of the ulnar nerve. Later physical and electrophysiological examinations confirmed initial physical findings.[13]

Did the surgeon confuse a disrupted tendon with the ulnar nerve?

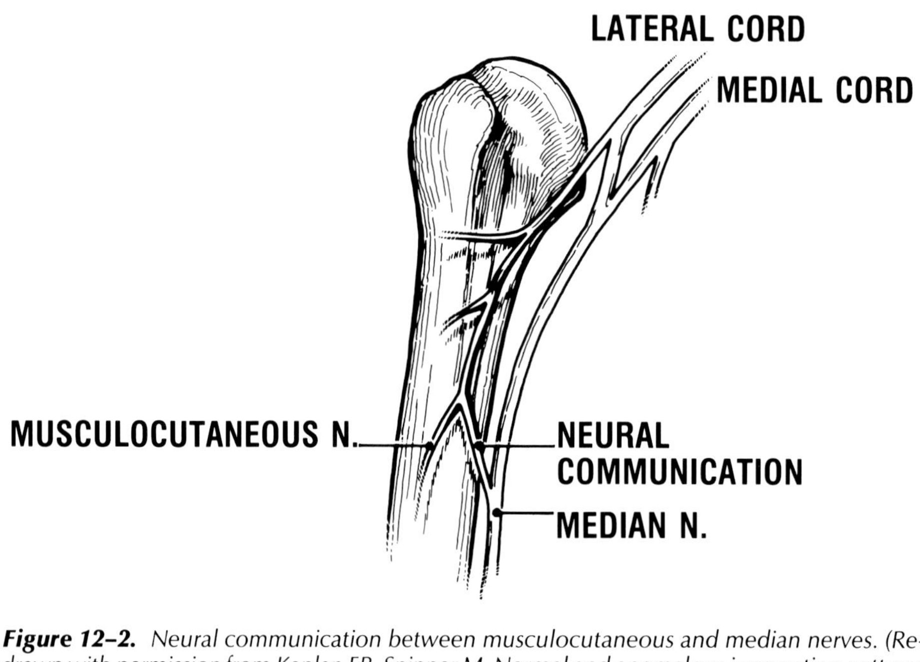

Figure 12–2. *Neural communication between musculocutaneous and median nerves. (Redrawn with permission from Kaplan EB, Spinner M. Normal and anomalous innervation patterns in the upper extremity. In: Omer GE, Spinner M, eds. Management of peripheral nerve problems. Philadelphia: WB Saunders, 1980:87.)*

Case 4

An 18-year-old man sustained a blast injury to the proximal, anterior forearm. He has extensive soft-tissue loss. At the time of debridement, segmental loss of his median nerve is noted. However, later physical and electrophysiological studies confirm normal function of all his forearm and hand muscles except the flexor digitorum profundus to the index finger and the flexor pollicis longus. He has no sensory deficit.[13]

Did the surgeons accurately identify the median nerve gap?

Case 5

A 69-year-old woman complains of numbness and tingling in the thumb, index, and middle fingers. She has no thenar wasting or weakness. She has a positive Phalen's test and a positive Tinel's sign over the median nerve. Two-point discrimination is diminished in the thumb, index, and middle fingers. Nerve conduction studies show delayed latency across the wrist, but normal latency from the elbow to thenar muscles.[34]

Should the nerve electrophysiological studies be repeated to resolve this discrepancy?

Case 6

A 72-year-old woman with lepromatous leprosy complains of severe dysfunction of her hands. The left hand is insensate. The left first dorsal interosseous muscle, abductor digiti minimi, and ulnar lumbricals are weak. The thenar muscles have normal strength. The ulnar three fingers of the right hand are shortened from multiple injuries. Sensation is markedly diminished over the hand except for the index finger. The abductor digiti minimi and flexor carpi ulnaris are paralyzed; the abductor pollicis brevis and opponens pollicis show marked wasting. The first dorsal interosseous and the flexor pollicis brevis are strong. There is no clawing.[8]

Are the findings related to atypically patchy involvement of leprosy?

General Patterns of Anomalous Median and Ulnar Innervation

In one fifth of 226 ulnar or median nerve-injured patients, Rowntree found evidence of anomalous innervation of hand muscles.[62] These cases ranged from median nerve innervating the first dorsal interosseous muscle or ulnar nerve innervating the abductor pollicis brevis, to complete median or complete ulnar innervation of the hand. The so-called all-ulnar or all-median hand explains cases in which one or the other nerve is cut without evident functional impairment of the hand.

The gradations between complete median and complete ulnar innervation of the hand reflect several anatomical arrangements. Fibers may pass between the ulnar and median nerves within the forearm and hand. Their terminal branches may send communicating fibers within the hand. The median nerve sometimes innervates the interosseous muscles, particularly the first dorsal interosseous, either alone or jointly with the ulnar nerve.[54,62] The ulnar nerve more commonly provides dual or replacement innervation to muscles usually innervated by the median nerve.[31,62,68] Less commonly, the median nerve innervates muscles that are usually ulnar-supplied.[68] The lumbricals sometimes receive double innervation.[10,46] Double innervation of the flexor pollicis brevis is common, and more extensive ulnar innervation of the thenar muscles occurs.[9,13,62] Several anatomical arrangements account for these observations.

Martin-Gruber Communication

There is communication between median and ulnar nerves within the proximal forearm in 10% to 30% of the population.[15,26,32,46] The communicating ramus often runs between the anterior interosseous nerve and the ulnar nerve.[70] Mannerfelt cites the earliest known description of the anomaly, by Martin in 1763.[46,49] Gruber made similar findings over a century later.[26] The Martin-Gruber communication is the crossover of motor fibers from the median or anterior interosseous to the ulnar nerve in the proximal forearm. Usually the connecting fibers travel in the plane between the flexor profundus and superficialis, dorsal to the ulnar artery; however, some examiners have traced fibers extending superficial to the flexor muscles.[70]

Electrophysiological studies, in addition to anatomical studies, have also identified Martin-Gruber communications carrying median nerve fibers to the hand via the ulnar nerve.[11,27,34,48,72] The connection carries fibers that result in varying degrees of anomalous innervation of the intrinsic muscles. Patients with carpal tunnel syndrome with median-to-ulnar nerve communication characteristically have normal latency from the elbow to thenar muscles and prolonged latency across the wrist, as in Case 5.[11,34]

The Martin-Gruber communication presents with several distinctly different types of anomalous motor innervation of the hand muscles. In one, motor fibers pass from the median to ulnar nerve, proceeding to innervate muscles usually innervated directly by median nerve branches.[13,46,68] In such cases, an additional crossover occurs within the palm for these fibers to reach the thenar muscles, a Type 4 variation. In another situation, fibers pass from the median to ulnar nerve, eventually terminating within muscles that usually are ulnar nerve targets.[13,46,48,64,65] Here the Martin-Gruber communication provides a pathway for redirecting nerve fibers that were not completely sorted within the brachial plexus, a Type 3 variation. Finally, ulnar nerve–derived fibers targeted for muscles normally innervated by the ulnar nerve sometimes cross over into the median nerve ulnar to median, a variation of the Martin-Gruber communication, and must therefore cross over again within the palm to reach their targets, another Type 4 variation.[62,65]

There is an increased incidence of the Martin-Gruber communication within some families, and an autosomal dominant inheritance pattern of median-ulnar nerve connections has been observed.[14] A communication between the median and ulnar nerves courses through the proximal forearm in all baboons, rhesus monkeys, and cynomolgus monkeys.[16,30]

Flexor Digitorum Profundus Innervation

While the flexor digitorum profundus belly of the index finger and first lumbrical muscle are nearly always supplied by branches of the median nerve, the innervation of the other flexor digitorum profundus bellies and their corresponding lumbricals are quite variable.[10,38,68] In general, the lumbrical is supplied by the same major nerve that supplies the corresponding belly of the flexor digitorum profundus. In 50% of cases, there are variations from the classic pattern of innervation (in which the median nerve motors the radial two bellies and the ulnar nerve motors the ulnar two bellies), with the median nerve usually encroaching on ulnar nerve distribution. However, the ulnar nerve can also encroach laterally to innervate the middle-finger belly partially or exclusively.

Riche-Cannieu Communication

Riche[60] and Cannieu[12] independently described a connection between the median nerve motor branch and the ulnar nerve deep branch. Each described a communication occurring between the fibers of the median motor branch traveling to the superficial head of the flexor pollicis brevis and the fibers of the deep ulnar branch going to the deep head of the flexor pollicis brevis (Fig. 12-3). The communicating fibers pass radially from the deep ulnar branch between the heads of the adductor

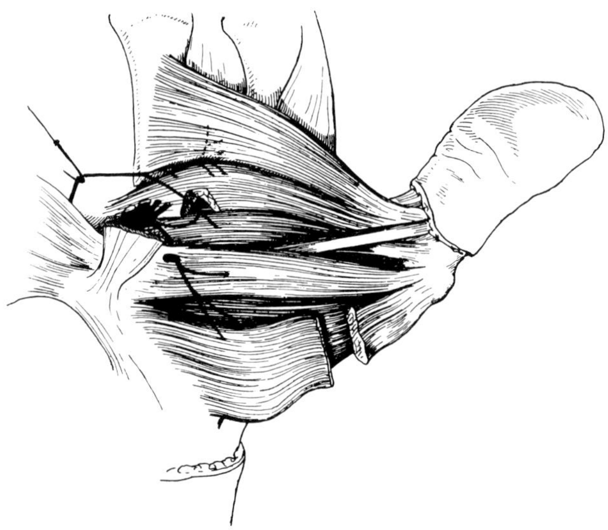

Figure 12–3. *Riche-Cannieu communication between the deep branch of the ulnar nerve and the motor branch of the median nerve. (Reproduced with permission from Hovelacque A. Anatomie des nerfs craniens and rachidiens et du système grand sympathique. Paris: Libraire Octave Doin, 1927.)*

pollicis, then deep to the flexor pollicis longus tendon. They continue proximally to the radial side of the tendon as they approach the median motor branch. Harness and Sekeles found such a communication in 77% of preserved cadaver hands and in virtually all fresh cadaver hands.[28]

Riche described two other anatomical situations.[60] In one, the communication occurs between a median-derived thumb digital nerve and fibers en route to the adductor pollicis from the deep ulnar nerve branch. The communicating fibers lie within the adductor muscle on the medial side of the flexor pollicis longus tendon. In another situation, the communicating fibers pass through the first lumbrical, which is innervated by the ulnar nerve.

The Riche-Cannieu connection probably carries motor fibers only.[28,46] Based on their data and that from clinical and electromyographic studies, Harness and Sekeles concluded that the Riche-Cannieu communication is the common and normal arrangement of thenar muscle innervation.[28] However, Mannerfelt noted that the nature (sensory, motor, or mixed), incidence, and direction of fiber passage (ulnar to median or opposite) remain unresolved.[46] At the very least, the communication provides a potential pathway for cross- or double-innervation of the intrinsic muscles anywhere in the hand. Spinner has reported a patient with a complete ulnar nerve laceration at the wrist with clawing occurring only after blocking the ulnar nerve at the elbow.[65] A Martin-Gruber communication in the forearm and a Riche-Cannieu communication distally may have been the pathway through which ulnar nerve–derived fibers reached the target muscles.

Palmar Ulnar-Median Communicating Branch of Berrettini

Case 7

A 32-year-old man sustained a 2-cm transverse laceration of the palm from a porcelain faucet handle that broke while he was forcefully turning it. The patient has no active flexion of the middle finger and no sensation along adjacent sides of the middle and ring fingers. He has subjectively diminished sensation along adjacent sides of the index and middle fingers and along adjacent sides of the ring and little fingers. Two-point discrimination is 8 mm in those areas. Circulation to the fingers is normal. A laceration of the superficial arterial arch is found during initial exploration.[61]

Should this be ligated before further exploration?

Case 8

Six months after right carpal tunnel release for median nerve compression, a 34-year-old woman complains of severe tingling over the radial aspect of the ring finger. Sudomotor activity and two-point discrimination over the radial side of the ring finger are absent; the other fingers are normal. The patient has a tender point in the proximal palm and a Tinel's sign that radiates only to the radial side of the ring finger.[50]

Can the findings best be explained by a slowly resolving axonotomesis from carpal tunnel syndrome?

Classically palmar sensation of the fingers is described as divided between ulnar and median nerves at the midline of the ring finger. However, a distal communicating branch between the ulnar and median nerves is the most common finding. Berrettini illustrated this branch in 1741.[5] In 40 of 50 dissected palms, Meals and Shaner found a branch coursing between the ulnar and median nerves.[52] Others have also noted a high incidence of the communication.[7,32,46,68] It usually passes immediately deep to the superficial palmar arch (Fig. 12-4); however, in some specimens it courses just distal to the transverse carpal ligament.[2,52] In this location, it could be injured during carpal tunnel release.[50] It is also vulnerable during flexor tendon surgery and during Dupuytren's contracture excision in the ring ray axis.

The palmar cutaneous branch of the median nerve consistently arises from the anterior, radial aspect of the median nerve well proximal to the wrist.[69] It then travels just below the ulnar edge of the flexor carpi radialis tendon to the transverse carpal ligament, where it passes through a short retinacular tunnel just ulnar to the flexor carpi radialis tendon, emerging to divide into radial and ulnar branches. However, in one case Amadio discovered the palmar cutaneous branch traveling with the median nerve into the distal flexor com-

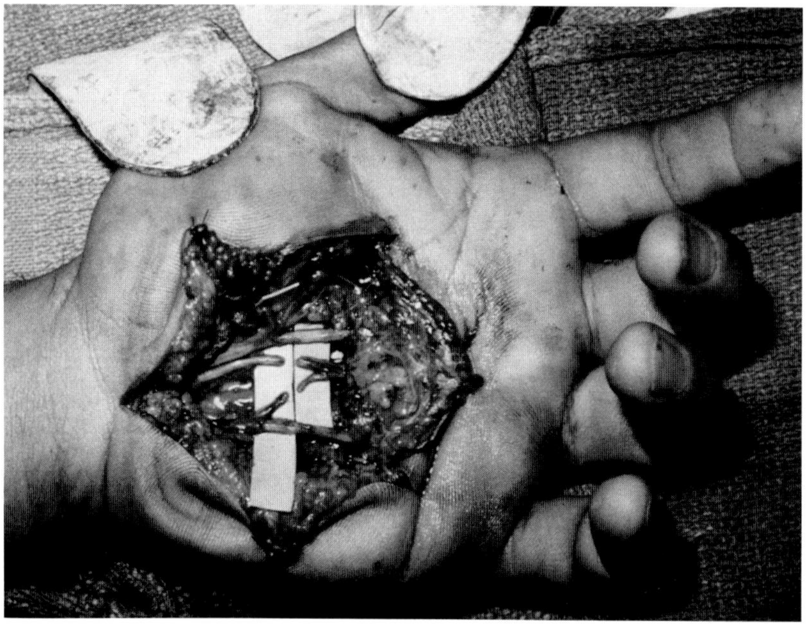

Figure 12–4. *Lacerated communicating branch of Berrettini (arrow). See Case 7. (Reproduced with permission from Rollins J, Meals RA. Recognition of acutely lacerated ulnar nerve–median nerve palmar communicating branch. Clin Orthop 1985;201:92.)*

partment before traversing the transverse carpal ligament.[2]

Other Median-Ulnar Nerve Variations

Other less common median and ulnar nerve variations occur. Rarely, the ulnar nerve sends fibers to the median nerve in the distal forearm.[38] This ramus carries mainly sensory fibers, but can transmit motor fibers as well. Large or small neural loops may leave the nerve, follow an aberrant course, and rejoin the main nerve.[29,38] Curtis found ulnar-derived sensory fibers traveling within a forearm connection to the median nerve.[15] Both motor and sensory fibers passed through the Martin-Gruber communication reported in Case 4.[13]

MEDIAN NERVE VARIATIONS AT THE WRIST AND HAND

Case 9

A 30-year-old woman underwent release of the left carpal tunnel one year ago. The procedure relieved preoperative symptoms of left hand numbness and tingling. However, she has had increasing difficulty using her left thumb. She has thenar atrophy and absent thumb abduction and opposition. Sensation is normal. Phalen's test and Tinel's sign are negative. An EMG shows normal sensory latencies but thenar motor denervation.[42]

Is it more likely that the motor branch remains compressed or that it was injured at the time of carpal tunnel release?

Since carpal tunnel release is commonly performed in treating carpal tunnel syndrome, many surgeons encounter variant median nerve anatomy within the carpal tunnel. Knowledge of these variations helps prevent iatrogenic injury to the branches of the nerve within or near the carpal canal. Amadio, after reviewing an earlier classification advanced by Lanz,[40] and basing his conclusions on his findings in 275 carpal tunnel releases, has recently proposed a classification for median nerve variations within the carpal tunnel (Table 12-1).[2]

Amadio found a 19% incidence of variations in the origin or course of the thenar motor branch. By far the most common variation was the motor branch penetrating the transverse carpal ligament rather than passing around its distal margin (Figs. 12-5, 12-6).[2] Others have confirmed the frequent transretinacular passage of the motor branch.[21,36,53,58,71] In these cases, the thenar branch traverses a tunnel 1.5 to 3.0 mm long within the ligament.[36] The motor branch sometimes emerges from the median nerve within the carpal canal (Fig.

Table 12–1. *Classification of Median Nerve Anomalies in the Carpal Tunnel*

HIGH DIVISION
Open branching
Closed loop
MOTOR BRANCH
Transretinacular
Multiple
Multiple and transretinacular
PALMAR CUTANEOUS BRANCH
Transretinacular
Multiple
Multiple and transretinacular
MEDIAN-ULNAR SENSORY RAMUS
(arising on median nerve proximal to superficial arch)
UNCLASSIFIED

(Adapted from Amadio PC. Anatomic variations of the median nerve within the carpal tunnel. Clin Anat 1988;1:23–31, with permission.)

12-5C).[58] Rarely, the entire median nerve passes superficial to the transverse carpal ligament.[68] One author has correlated palmar dermatoglyphic patterns with various courses of the motor branch.[63]

The clinical importance of transretinacular passage of the motor branch is shown in Case 9. Before surgical exploration, one could hypothesize that the findings are caused by iatrogenic injury to the nerve, or by unreleased, persistent impingement of the nerve as it passes through the transverse carpal ligament.[3,57,65] To protect the motor branch with an anomalous course, the surgeon dissects on the ulnar side of the median nerve in the carpal tunnel.

In 4% of cases, Amadio found multiple trunks of the thenar motor branch (Fig. 12-5D). Half of these passed through the retinaculum.[2] Mumford and coworkers reported two branches in one of ten dissections; one of the branches passed through the retinaculum.[53] Several others have reported this variation,[25,43,71] and two of these authors have reported transretinacular passage of nerve trunks.[25,43] Despite the potential for persistent entrapment of anomalous motor branches after carpal tunnel release, the greater potential for injuring an anomalous motor branch should discourage the surgeon from routinely exploring the motor branch.

Mumford and coworkers found an accessory thenar nerve arising from the first common digital nerve or the radial proper digital nerve in 15 of 20 dissected hands.[53] The accessory thenar nerve was the only median nerve supply to the flexor pollicis brevis in eight specimens. Harness and Sekeles[28] and Hovelacque[33] described a variation of the Riche-Cannieu communication in which a ramus from the deep ulnar nerve communicated with a thumb digital nerve. This presents the possibility that median motor fibers destined for the thenar muscles were traveling within the digital nerve.

Type 2 variations of the median nerve, branching proximal to the wrist, are also encountered. Gruber[26] described four cases in which the median nerve branch to the third web space originated in the proximal forearm (Fig. 12-5E), and there are two other reports of this anomaly.[29,73] Amadio found high branching of the median nerve in 3% of cases.[2] Other authors have reported a similar incidence.[17,40,71] In most of Amadio's cases, the two branches of the bifid median nerve remained independent of one another. However, two of nine cases had a loop communication in which one or the other median nerve branch received a communicating branch from the other within or just distal to the carpal canal, a Type 1 variation.[1,2] Amadio found that three of the 29 cases of bifid median nerve reported in the literature had a loop communication.[2] A high division of the median nerve is often seen in conjunction with the presence of a median artery (Fig. 12-5F). When this variation occurs, in addition to protecting the loop, the surgeon may need to release the median nerve branches from separate fascial channels within the transverse carpal ligament.[1]

Neither Amadio's nor Lanz's classifications consider the orientation of origin of the motor nerve trunk. The motor branch can arise from the ulnar side of the median nerve (Fig. 12-5G).[19,25,71] A motor branch may originate from the central, anterior surface of the median nerve, then pass ulnarly and distally until it clears the transverse carpal ligament, where it turns and passes radially and somewhat retrograde over the ligament into the thenar muscle mass (Fig. 12-5H).[47] The detailed intraneural topographic studies of Sunderland[67,68] and Jabaley and associates[35] suggest, but do not confirm, the orientation of the emerging motor branch.

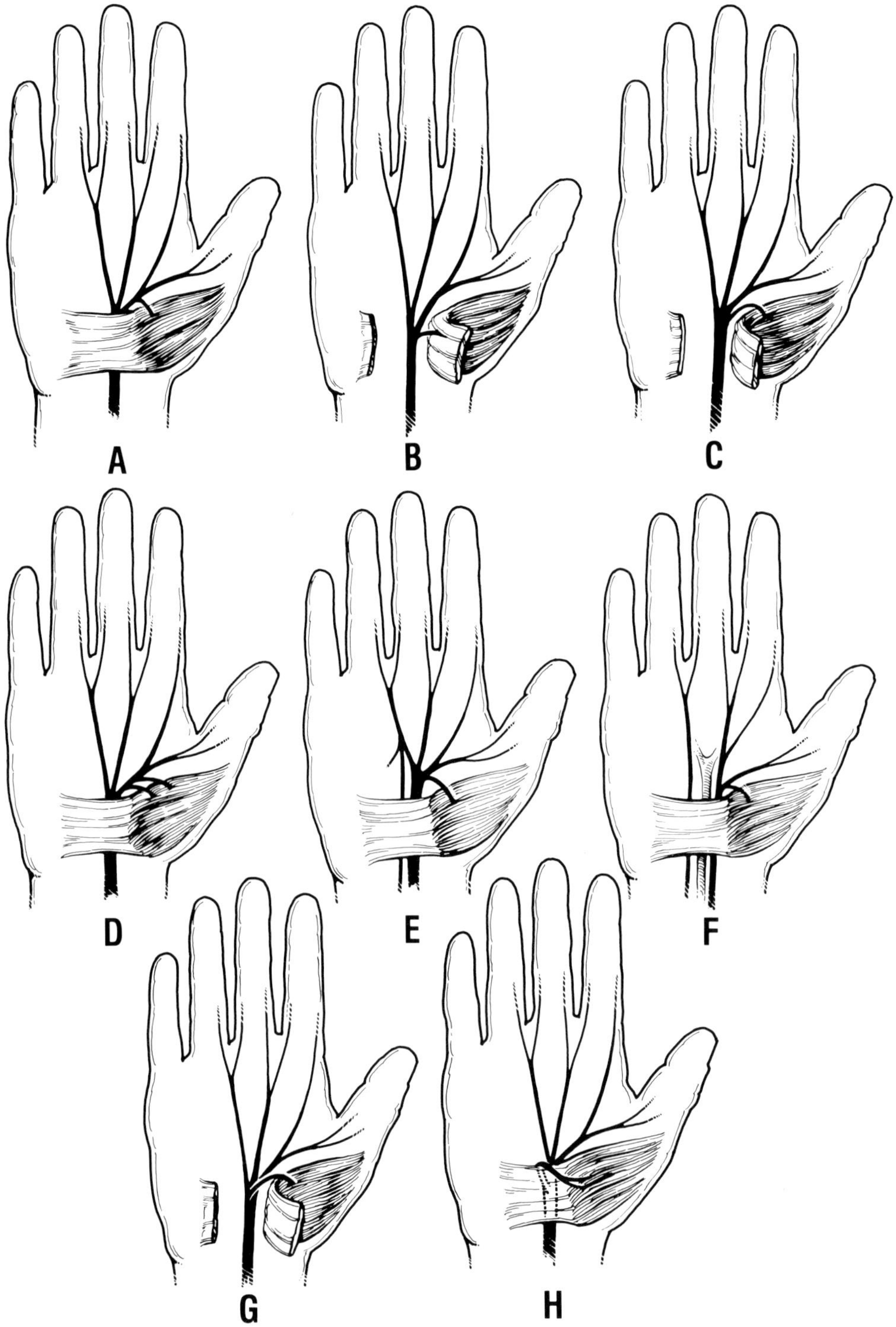

Figure 12–5. *Anatomy of the median nerve at the wrist. (**A**) Usual form and course of the median nerve and its motor branch. (**B**) Transretinacular passage of the motor branch. (**C**) Subligamentous origin of the motor branch. (**D**) Multiple motor branches. (**E**) High branching of the median nerve. (**F**) Bifid median nerve with median artery. (**G**) Motor branch arising from ulnar side of median nerve. (**H**) Motor branch arising anteriorly, then passing over surface of transverse carpal ligament. (Redrawn with permission from Lanz U. Anatomical variations of the median nerve in the carpal tunnel. J Hand Surg [Am] 1977;2:45–47.)*

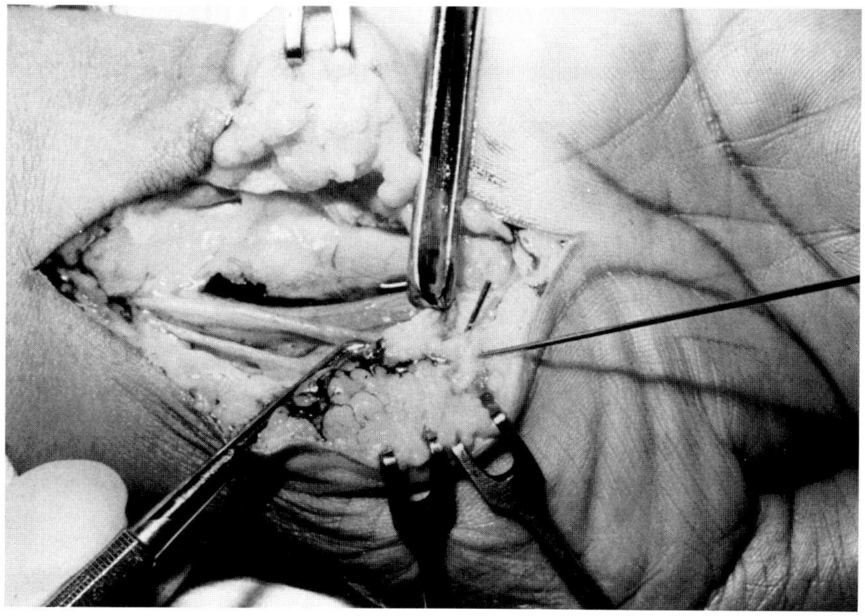

Figure 12–6. *A Type 2 variation of the median nerve motor branch with its origin proximal to the transverse carpal ligament. It then takes a transretinacular course (identified by probe) and emerges superficial to the ligament (identified by hook) before entering the thenar muscles.*

Mackinnon and Dellon dissected 50 hands to determine that the motor branch arises on the far radial aspect of the median nerve in 60% of cases, antero-centrally in 22% of cases, and from an anterior position one-third the distance between the radial and ulnar sides in 18% of hands.[45] Motor branches did not originate from the ulnar side of the median nerve. Mackinnon and Dellon believe that the motor branch emerges from the anterior, central aspect of the median nerve in most patients with carpal tunnel syndrome and thenar wasting. Papathanassiou described one clinical case and one dissection specimen in which the motor branch arose from the ulnar, anterior aspect of the radial division of the median nerve.[57] Mumford and coworkers found this arrangement in 16 of 20 dissected hands.[53] Lanz encountered it once.[40] (See Chap. 61 for more information.)

ULNAR NERVE VARIATIONS AT THE WRIST

Within Guyon's canal, the ulnar nerve usually divides into superficial sensory and deep motor branches. In about one fifth of cases the nerve terminates in three branches. A deep motor branch, the ulnar proper digital nerve of the little finger, and the common digital nerve of the fourth interosseous space enclose the pisiform on three sides.[7,37] This is no more than a high take-off of the superficial sensory branch, a Type 2 variation. In some cases, the deep motor branch divides as it passes the hook of the hamate. One ramus loops around the lateral side and the other ramus loops around the medial side of the hook of the hamate before rejoining distally or continuing to their destinations individually.[4,22,41,66] A loop arising from the ulnar nerve just proximal to the wrist and passing through the flexor carpi ulnaris tendon before reuniting with the main nerve has also been reported.[55,74] Awareness of these anomalous nerves prevents their injury during dissection around the ulnar head, hamate, and pisiform.

The ulnar palmar cutaneous nerve emerges from the epineurium of the ulnar nerve at the wrist and passes superficial to the transverse carpal ligament and ulnar to the axis of the ring finger to innervate the hypothenar eminence. However, Engber and Gmeiner in dissection of 21 specimens rarely found an ulnar cutaneous nerve.[18] Usually, the hypothenar region was innervated by multiple small branches from the superficial and dorsal branches of the ulnar nerve.

Case 10

A 17-year-old boy who has not been able to fully extend or adduct his left little finger since birth complains of extreme pain over the hypothenar region with grasping. He holds his little finger in abduction. He is exquisitely tender over the pisiform and with passive adduction of the little finger. When the wrist is flexed or the little finger adducted, the extensor digiti quinti and the extensor carpi ulnaris go into spasm.[51]

Does pisotriquetral arthritis account for the findings?

An anomalous neural branch, originating from the ulnar dorsal cutaneous nerve, courses under the flexor carpi ulnaris tendon and passes the pisiform on its ulnar side.[37,51] In Case 10, fibers of the flexor carpi ulnaris compress the anomalous nerve, which is stretched on little-finger extension or adduction.[51] It may also become encased in scar or callus after pisiform fracture.[37]

The ulnar dorsal cutaneous nerve usually perforates the fascia on the ulnar side of the flexor carpi ulnaris 3 to 5 cm proximal to the ulnar head. However, it often perforates the fascia more distally and may be placed at risk during ulnar head excision.[37]

COMMUNICATIONS BETWEEN PREAXIAL AND POSTAXIAL NERVES

Superficial Radial Nerve and Lateral Antebrachial Cutaneous Nerve Communication and Overlap

Case 11

A 26-year-old man sustained a laceration over the dorsal radial aspect of the wrist that was sutured one year ago. He has had severe pain in response to touch and movement in the area of the scar and dysesthesia over the dorsoradial aspect of the hand. A surgeon subsequently divided the radial sensory nerve proximally and buried the proximal end within the brachioradialis muscle. The patient's symptoms, although somewhat diminished in intensity, persist at the wrist.

Have the symptoms persisted because of incomplete division of the superficial radial nerve?

Mackinnon and Dellon emphasized that in 75% of cases, the radial sensory nerve and the lateral antebrachial cutaneous nerve share territories of innervation.[44] In some cases, the distribution of the two nerves overlaps (Fig. 12-7). In others, the branches of the two nerves form plexi. In their series, the radial sensory and antebrachial cutaneous nerves contributed to 23 of 30 dorsoradial neuromas. In another three patients, a neuroma of the lateral antebrachial cutaneous nerve persisted after proximal sectioning of the radial sensory nerve. In Case 11, a lidocaine block of the lateral antebrachial cutaneous nerve just lateral to the biceps tendon would have confirmed its involvement.

Froment-Rauber Communication

As would be anticipated from embryologic studies, communication between preaxial and postaxial nerves is quite rare. However, the posterior interosseous nerve can provide nerve fibers to the normally ulnar nerve–innervated first dorsal interosseous muscle.[24,59] Bichat described a communication between the posterior interosseous nerve and the deep branch of the ulnar nerve.[6] Although authors have documented passage of posterior interosseous nerve fibers through the interosseous membrane, passage of median or ulnar nerve fibers

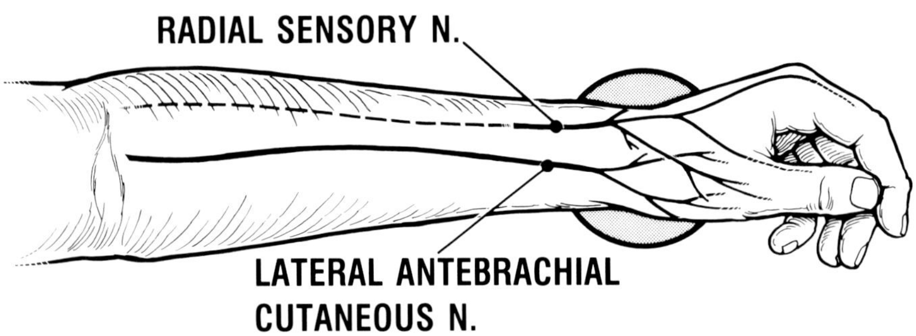

Figure 12–7. *Overlap of the lateral antebrachial cutaneous nerve and the radial cutaneous nerve. (Redrawn with permission from Mackinnon SE, Dellon AL. The overlap pattern of the lateral antebrachial cutaneous nerve and the superficial branch of the radial nerve. J Hand Surg [Am] 1985;10:523.)*

through the membrane has not been seen in humans. Probably, some C8–T1 fibers are sorted into the posterior cord rather than the medial cord within the brachial plexus, making their way to the interosseous muscles via the posterior interosseous nerve. Similarly, these fibers may reach the first dorsal interosseous muscle by way of the radial cutaneous nerve[20,33,68] or the lateral antebrachial cutaneous nerve.[23]

CONCLUSION

With a conceptual outline provided by the nerve variation classification, awareness of the most common and significant nerve anomalies, and careful physical examination, the astute clinician can correctly identify anomalous patterns of innervation in most patients with acute or chronic nerve injuries. Selective nerve blocks and electrodiagnostic studies confirm the suspected anomalous innervation. Awareness of variable nerve courses and branchings is of particular importance in the operating room.

REFERENCES

1. Amadio PC. Bifid median nerve with a double compartment within the transverse carpal canal. J Hand Surg [Am] 1987;12:366–368.
2. Amadio PC. Anatomic variations of the median nerve within the carpal tunnel. Clin Anat 1988;1: 23–31.
3. Bennett JB, Crouch CC. Compression syndrome of the recurrent motor branch of the median nerve. J Hand Surg [Am] 1982;7:407–409.
4. Bergfield TG, Aulicino PL. Variation of the deep motor branch of the ulnar nerve at the wrist. J Hand Surg [Am] 1988;13:368–369.
5. Berrettini P. Tabulae anatomicae. Rome: F Amidei, 1741.
6. Bichat XAV. Traité d'anatomie descriptive, tome troisième. Paris: Brosson and Gabon, 1802:269.
7. Bonnel F, Vila RM. Anatomical study of the ulnar nerve in the hand. J Hand Surg [Br] 1985;10:165–168.
8. Brandsma JW, Birke JA, Sims DS. The Martin-Gruber innervated hand. J Hand Surg [Am] 1986;11: 536–539.
9. Brooks HSJ. Variations in the nerve supply of the flexor brevis pollicis muscle. J Anat Physiol 1886;20: 641–644.
10. Brooks HSJ. Variations in the nerve supply of the lumbrical muscles in the hand and foot, with some observations on the innervation of the perforating flexors. J Anat Physiol 1887;21:575–585.
11. Buchthal F, Rosenfalck A, Trojaborg W. Electrophysiological findings in entrapment of the median nerve at the wrist and elbow. J Neurol Neurosurg Psych 1974;37:340–360.
12. Cannieu JMA. Note sur une anastomose entre la branche profunde du cubital et le médian. Bull Soc d'Anat Physiol Bordeaux 1897;18:339–340. [Cited by Hovelacque]
13. Cliffton EE. Unusual innervation of the intrinsic muscles of the hand by median and ulnar nerve. Surgery 1948;23:12–31.
14. Crutchfield CA, Gutmann L. Hereditary aspects of median-ulnar nerve communications. J Neurol Neurosurg Psych 1980;43:53–55.
15. Curtis F. Recherches anatomiques sur l'anatomoses et du médian et du cubital à l'avantbras. Intern Mschr Anat Physiol 1886;3:309–324. [Cited by Hovelacque]
16. Dellon AL, Mackinnon SE, Seiler WA. Peripheral nerve diseases. In: Adams RJ, Swindle MM, eds. Experimental surgery and physiology: Induced animal models of human disease. Baltimore: Williams & Wilkins, 1988:278–283.
17. Eiken O, Carstam N, Eddeland A. Anomalous distal branching of the median nerve. Scand J Plast Reconst Surg 1971;5:149–152.
18. Engber WD, Gmeiner JG. Palmar cutaneous branch of the ulnar nerve. J Hand Surg [Am] 1980;5:26–29.
19. Entin MA. Carpal tunnel syndrome and its variants. Surg Clin North Am 1968;48:1097–1112.
20. Fahrer M. Rare variations in a left radial nerve–case report. J Anat (London) 1968;103:208.
21. Falconer D, Spinner M. Anatomic variations in the motor and sensory supply of the thumb. Clin Orthop 1985;195:83–96.
22. Fenning JB. Deep ulnar nerve paralysis resulting from an anatomic abnormality. J Bone Joint Surg 1965;47A:1381–1382.
23. Foerster O. Spezielle anatomie und physiologie der peripheren nerven. In: Lewandowsky M, ed. Handbuch der neurologie, etgänzungsband. Berlin: Springer, 1929. [Cited by Sunderland]
24. Froment JBF. Traité d'anatomie humaine. Paris: Méquignon–Marvis, 1846:494.
25. Graham WP III. Variations of the motor branch of

the median nerve at the wrist. Plast Reconst Surg 1973;51:90–92.
26. Gruber W. Ueber die Verbindung des Nervus medianus mit dem Nervus ulnaris am Unterarme des Menschen und der Säugethiere. Arch Anat Physiol 1870;37:501–522.
27. Gutmann L. Median-ulnar nerve communications and carpal tunnel syndrome. J Neurol Neurosurg Psych 1977;40:982–986.
28. Harness D, Sekeles E. The double anastomotic innervation of the thenar muscles. J Anat 1971;109: 461–466.
29. Hartmann H. Étude de quelques anastomoses elliptiques des nerfs du membre supérieur. Bull Soc Anat Paris 1888;63:151–164.
30. Hepburn D. The comparative anatomy of the muscles and nerves of superior and inferior extremities of the anthropoid apes. J Anat Physiol 1892;26:149–186.
31. Highet WB. Innervation and function of the thenar muscles. Lancet 1943;1:227–230.
32. Hirasawa K. Plexus brachialis und die nerven der oberen extremität. Anatomischen Institutes der Kaiserlichen Universität Kyoto 1931; Serie A, Heft 2.
33. Hovelacque A. Anatomie des nerfs craniens et rachidiens et du système grand sympathique. Paris: Libraire Octave Doin, 1927.
34. Iyer V, Fenichel GM. Normal median nerve proximal latency in carpal tunnel syndrome: A clue to coexisting Martin-Gruber anastomosis. J Neurol Neurosurg Psych 1976;39:449–452.
35. Jabaley M, Wallace W, Heckler F. Internal topography of major nerves of the forearm and hand. J Hand Surg 1980;5:1–18.
36. Johnson RK, Shrewsbury MM. Anatomical course of the thenar branch of the median nerve–usually in a separate tunnel through the transverse carpal ligament. J Bone Joint Surg 1970;52A:269–273.
37. Kaplan EB. Variation of the ulnar nerve at the wrist. Bull Hosp Joint Dis 1963;24:85–88.
38. Kaplan EB, Spinner M. Normal and anomalous innervation patterns in the upper extremity. In: Omer GE, Spinner M, eds. Management of peripheral nerve problems. Philadelphia: W B Saunders, 1980: 75–99.
39. Kerr AT. The brachial plexus of nerves in man, the variations in its formation and branches. Am J Anat 1918;23:285–395.
40. Lanz U. Anatomical variations of the median nerve in the carpal tunnel. J Hand Surg [Am] 1977;2:44–53.
41. Lassa R, Shrewsbury MM. A variation in the path of the deep motor branch of the ulnar nerve at the wrist. J Bone Joint Surg 1975;57A:990–991.
42. Lilly CJ, Magnell TD. Severance of the thenar branch of the median nerve as a complication of carpal tunnel release. J Hand Surg [Am] 1985;10: 399–402.
43. Linburg RM, Albright JA. An anomalous branch of the median nerve. J Bone Joint Surg 1970;52A:182–183.
44. Mackinnon SE, Dellon AL. The overlap pattern of the lateral antebrachial cutaneous nerve and the superficial branch of the radial nerve. J Hand Surg [Am] 1985;10:522–526.
45. Mackinnon SE, Dellon AL. Anatomic investigations of nerves at the wrist: I. Orientation of the motor fascicle of the median nerve in the carpal tunnel. Ann Plast Surg 1988;21:32–35.
46. Mannerfelt L. Studies on the hand in ulnar nerve paralysis. Acta Orthop Scand Suppl 1966;87:1–176.
47. Mannerfelt L, Hybbeinette CH. Important anomaly of the thenar motor branch of the median nerve: A clinical and anatomical report. Bull Hosp Joint Dis 1972;33:15–21.
48. Marinacci AA, von Hagen KO. Misleading "all median hand." Arch Neurol 1965;12:80–83.
49. Martin R. Tal om nervus allmanna egenskaper 1 mannsikans kropp. Stockholm: Lars Salvius, 1763. [Cited by Kaplan and Spinner]
50. May JW Jr, Rosen H. Division of the sensory ramus communicans between the ulnar and median nerves: A complication following carpal tunnel release. J Bone Joint Surg 1981;63A:836–838.
51. McCarthy RE, Nalebuff EA. Anomalous volar branch of the dorsal cutaneous ulnar nerve: A case report. J Hand Surg [Am] 1980;5:19–20.
52. Meals RA, Shaner M. Variations in digital sensory patterns: A study of the ulnar nerve–median nerve palmar communicating branch. J Hand Surg [Am] 1983;8:411–414.
53. Mumford J, Morecraft R, Blair WF. Anatomy of the thenar branch of the median nerve. J Hand Surg [Am] 1987;12:361–365.
54. Murphey F, Kirklin JW, Finlayson AI. Anomalous innervation of intrinsic muscles of hand. Surg Gynecol Obstet 1946;83:15–23.
55. O'Hara JJ, Stone JH. Ulnar neuropathy at the wrist associated with aberrant flexor carpi ulnaris insertion. J Hand Surg [Am] 1988;13:370–371.
56. O'Rahilly R, Gardner E. The timing and sequence of events in the development of the limbs in the human embryo. Anatomy and Embryology 1975; 148:1–23.
57. Papathanassiou BT. A variant of the motor branch

of the median nerve in the hand. J Bone Joint Surg 1968;50B:156–157.

58. Poisel S. Ursprung und Verlauf des R muscularis des Nervus digitalis palmaris communis I (N medianus). Chir Praxis 1974;18:471–474. [Cited by Lanz]
59. Rauber A. Vater'sche körper der bänder und periostnerven. Inaug Diss. Münich, 1865. [Cited by Spinner (1978)]
60. Riche P. Le nerf cubitale et les muscle de l'éminence thenar. Bull Soc Anat Paris 1897;5:251–252.
61. Rollins J, Meals RA. Recognition of acutely lacerated ulnar nerve–median nerve palmar communicating branch. Clin Orthop 1985;201:91–93.
62. Rowntree T. Anomalous innervation of the hand muscles. J Bone Joint Surg 1949;31B:505–510.
63. Schwarz M. Kann die Hauttextur als Wegweiser für den Verlauf und die Variation des N medianus dienen? Handchirurgie 1988;20:344–346.
64. Spinner M. The anterior interosseous nerve syndrome with special attention to its variations. J Bone Joint Surg 1974;52A:84–94.
65. Spinner M. Injuries to the major branches of peripheral nerves of the forearm, ed 2. Philadelphia: W B Saunders, 1978.
66. Starke W, Rathay B, Hülsmann P. Anatomische Variante als seltene Ursache einer distalen Ulnariskompression. Handchirurgie 1988;20:347–348.
67. Sunderland S. The internal topography of the radial, median and ulnar nerves. Brain 1945;68:243–299.
68. Sunderland S. Nerves and nerve injuries, ed 2. New York: Churchill–Livingstone, 1978.
69. Taleisnik J. The palmar cutaneous branch of the median nerve and the approach to the carpal tunnel. J Bone Joint Surg 1973;55A:1212–1217.
70. Thomson A. Third annual report on the Committee of Collective Investigation of the Anatomical Society of Great Britain and Ireland for the year 1891–1892. J Anat Physiol 1893;27:183–194.
71. Tountas CP, Bihrle DM, MacDonald CJ, Bergman RA. Variations of the median nerve in the carpal canal. J Hand Surg [Am] 1987;12:708–712.
72. Uncini A, Lange DJ, Lovelace RE. Anomalous intrinsic hand muscle innervation in median and ulnar nerve lesions: An electrophysiological study. Ital J Neurol Sci 1988;9:497–503.
73. Winkelman NZ, Spinner M. A variant high sensory branch of the median nerve to the third web space. Bull Hosp Joint Dis 1973;34:161–166.
74. Zook EG, Kucan JO, Guy RJ. Palmar wrist pain caused by ulnar nerve entrapment in the flexor carpi ulnaris tendon. J Hand Surg [Am] 1988;13:732–735.

IV

ALIGNMENT

13 The Mechanical and Humoral Control of Specificity in Nerve Repair

14 Internal Topography of Peripheral Nerves as Related to Repair

15 Electrical Nerve Stimulation in the Awake Patient

16 Histochemical and Biochemical Aids to Nerve Repair

13

The Mechanical and Humoral Control of Specificity in Nerve Repair

Thomas M. E. Brushart

AUTHOR'S KEY POINTS

- Specificity of mammalian axon regeneration is viewed in a hierarchical framework, from gross through progressively finer distinctions. Specificity has been demonstrated at the tissue, nerve trunk, and sensory/motor levels; within both sensory and motor systems, topographic and end organ specificity are also possible.
- Neurotropism is the directional guidance of an axon or group of axons up a concentration gradient of a diffusible substance. It influences tissue and perhaps nerve trunk specificity in the "Y" tube model.
- Neurotrophic factors provide nutritive support to regenerating axons. Sensory/motor specificity is probably generated through neurotrophic support of motor axon collaterals that reinnervate motor Schwann cell tubes at the expense of those that enter sensory tubes.
- Operative alignment of fascicles may generate specificity at the nerve trunk and topographic levels in both sensory and motor systems.
- There is only limited evidence for humoral control of regeneration specificity after nerve repair by direct suture or entubation. Mechanical alignment of axons thus remains a primary determinant of mammalian regeneration specificity.

The results of peripheral nerve repair depend on several factors. Enough axons must reach the periphery to provide useful reinnervation, and this must occur before end organs atrophy beyond repair. In addition, axons must be specifically matched with appropriate end organs to restore motor function or provide meaningful sensory information to the central nervous system. This chapter reviews the types of regeneration specificity intrinsic to the peripheral nervous system (ie, independent of operative technique). Potential mechanisms for specificity generation are then discussed and placed in the context of operative repair.

In 1917, Langley and Hashimoto observed,

> Some fibers of the central end though they grow into the peripheral end are unable to make functional nerve endings. This occurs when efferent fibers grow into afferent, or afferent into efferent. It almost certainly occurs to some extent also in cross-union of afferent fibers of cutaneous sensation and afferent fibers of deep sensation, and may also occur in cross-union of the fibers serving the various forms of each of these classes of sensation.[45]

For ideal function to be restored, each regenerating axon should be matched with the same type of end organ it served previously. There is currently no evidence that changes occur in the central connections of individual axons in response to incorrect peripheral reconnection, so one must assume that incorrect peripheral reconnection results in permanently compromised function.[40,51] With smaller degrees of mismatch, as with similar sensory end organs, information continues to be generated and transmitted to the central nervous system.[40] However, with more significant mismatches, as between sensory and motor axons, the consequences are more severe. Regenerating motor axons are led to sensory end organs, and sensory axons to motor end plates. Not only do these axons fail to establish functional contacts, they also exclude appropriate axons from the pathways they occupy.[31,44,80]

The types of regeneration specificity possible within the mammalian peripheral nervous system are best viewed in a hierarchical framework, progressing from gross through progressively finer distinctions[12] (Fig. 13-1). Specificity at the tissue level is characterized by the preferential growth

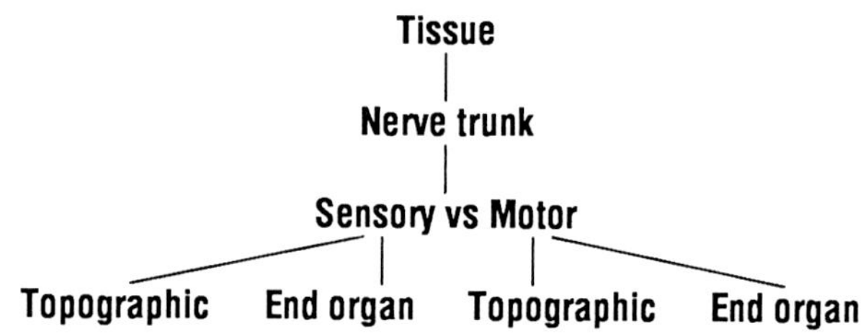

Figure 13–1. *The specificity hierarchy.*

of axons into nerve as opposed to other tissues, such as tendon, muscle, or visceral organ. At the nerve trunk level, sensory and motor axons are directed into the appropriate major nerve trunk, such as the tibial or peroneal division of the sciatic nerve. Within mixed nerve trunks (or at more proximal levels), sensory/motor specificity separates afferent and efferent fibers, and thus determines the makeup of individual distal sensory and motor branches. Finally, within both sensory and motor systems, axons are subject to topographic and end organ specificity. *Topographic specificity* describes reinnervation of the correct muscle within the motor system or correct patch of skin within the sensory system; *end organ specificity* involves reinnervation of the correct type of sensory end organ within the sensory system, and the correct fiber type (fast versus slow, motor end plate versus muscle spindle) in the motor system.

Several mechanisms are available for the generation of specificity in peripheral axon regeneration (Fig. 13-2). The peripheral nerve surgeon has been concerned traditionally with the mechanical control of specificity, the direction of regenerating axons to appropriate end organs by operative alignment of the proximal and distal nerve stumps. However, humoral mechanisms may be available as well. These rely on the capabilities of the axonal growth cone to explore the distal nerve stump (Fig. 13-3). *Contact recognition* would permit a regenerating axon to sample a variety of Schwann cell tubes in the distal stump, recognize one with an appropriate molecular signature, and selectively propagate through that tube to the correct end organ. *Neurotropism* refers to diffusion of factors from the distal nerve stump, guiding axons up a concentration gradient to an appropriate target. *Neurotrophic generation* of specificity would be less direct. Axons would randomly enter

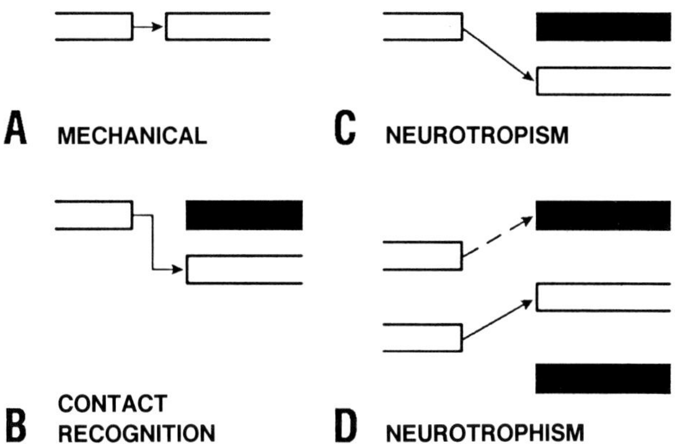

Figure 13–2. *Potential mechanisms of specificity generation. (**A**) Mechanical. The regenerating axon is guided to an appropriate distal Schwann cell tube by alignment of proximal and distal nerve stumps. (**B**) Contact recognition. The regenerating axon samples the molecular "footprints" of distal Schwann cell tubes, recognizing and selectively reinnervating an appropriate tube. (**C**) Neurotropism. The regenerating axon is guided directly to an appropriate Schwann cell tube by ascending a gradient of a diffusible substance. (**D**) Neurotrophism. Schwann cell tube reinnervation is initially random. Axons entering appropriate Schwann cell tubes receive trophic support, which leads to their maturation, while axons in inappropriate pathways do not receive this support and are resorbed.*

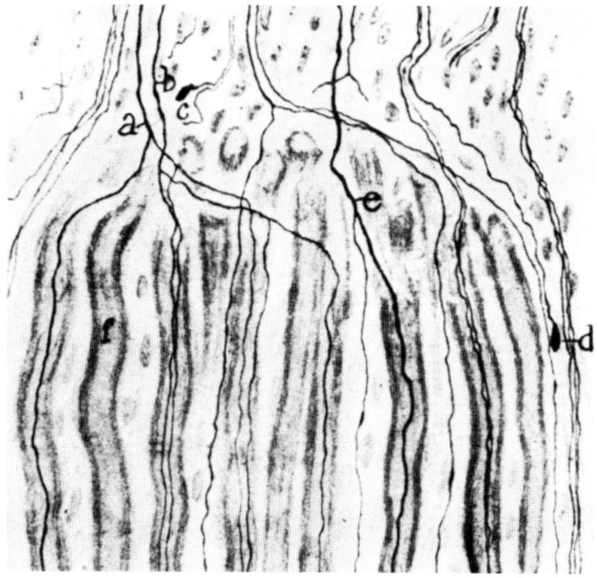

Figure 13–3. *This illustration demonstrates the behavior of regenerating axons as they reinnervate the distal nerve stump. The multiple collateral sprouts that are formed often move laterally across the mouths of several Schwann cell tubes before one is entered. A parent axon thus has access to a variety of Schwann cell tubes in the distal nerve stump.* a and b, *nerve fibers of the scar whose branches penetrate into various sheaths of the distal segment;* c, *fiber that bifurcates into a thick and a thin fiber, the latter being interstitial;* d, *club of growth;* e, *empty sheath. (Reprinted with permission from Ramon y Cajal S. Degeneration and regeneration of the nervous system. London: Oxford University Press, 1928, 233.)*

Schwann cell tubes of the distal stump; those entering a "correct" pathway or contacting a "correct" end organ would receive trophic, or nutritive, support in the form of chemical substances transported back to the parent neuron. These axons would increase in size and become myelinated, while those in inappropriate environments, with no trophic support, would be resorbed. This mechanism could be potentiated by the formation of multiple sprouts from each regenerating axon; if one sprout reached the correct target, it would survive at the expense of the others. This mechanism would give each neuron a chance of forming a correct peripheral connection.

THE SPECIFICITY HIERARCHY

Tissue

The earliest experiments on tissue specificity were performed by Forssman, who demonstrated that regenerating rat sciatic axons grow toward pieces of brain, but away from pieces of liver.[60] He attributed this selective attraction to elaboration of a neurotropic substance by degenerating myelin. In subsequent attempts to discredit the theory of neurotropism, Weiss and Taylor gave regenerating rat sciatic axons a choice of distal environment, this time in a conduit of allograft rat aorta in the shape of an inverted "Y."[77] They did not find evidence of specificity and argued against the possibility of neurotropism. Regeneration specificity at the tissue level was confirmed, however, when these experiments were repeated in an inert silicone "Y" chamber (Fig. 13-4).[49,50] Peripheral axons regenerated toward nerve and ignored tendon or granulation tissue. In retrospect, the allograft aortic tubes had provided a generalized stimulus to regeneration, mechanical or humoral, that had overpowered any target effect and masked the potential

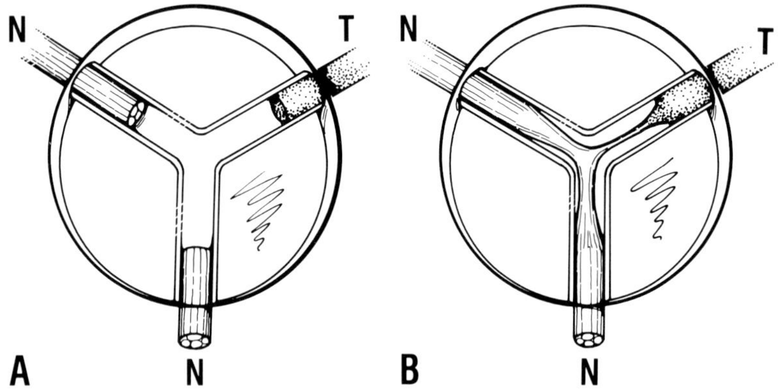

Figure 13–4. *A silicone "Y" chamber experiment. The regenerating rat sciatic nerve is given equal access to the distal nerve stump and a piece of tendon within the silicone "Y" (**A**). Preferential growth toward the nerve stump (**B**) results from tissue specificity in the regeneration process. N, nerve; T, tendon. (Redrawn, with permission from Lundborg GL, Dahlin L, Danielsen N, Nachemson AK. Tissue specificity in nerve regeneration. Scand J Plast Reconstr Surg Hand Surg 1986;20: 280.)*

for specificity. There have been no direct observations on the mechanism of tissue specificity, although either tropic or trophic mechanisms seem likely.

Nerve Trunk

Weiss also used the allograft aortic model to investigate specificity at the nerve trunk level, obtaining similarly negative results.[77] However, more recent work with inert silicone "Y tubes" confirmed the presence of specificity at the nerve trunk level and suggested a neurotropic mechanism.[57,58] Proximal stumps of transected peroneal or tibial nerves were used as the axon source in the proximal limb of the inverted "Y", with peroneal and tibial grafts serving as equally accessible targets in the distal limbs of the "Y". After 3.5 weeks, the majority of preparations showed preferential peroneal-to-peroneal or tibial-to-tibial growth of myelinated axons.[57] Specific regeneration at the nerve trunk level has been confirmed by other workers using axon count analysis of distal regenerates after 6 weeks.[65]

Sensory/Motor Reinnervation

Early observers believed sensory/motor reinnervation to be a selective process. Studies on cross-union of different peripheral nerves[44] and on the reinnervation of muscle spindles[60] demonstrated escape of motor axons from sensory pathways to innervate their original targets. These observations were followed by a series of experiments crossing sensory and motor nerves to evaluate end organ reinnervation.[31] Motor axons were seen to regenerate over long distances in sensory pathways and to remain stable in this foreign environment for over one year.[39] Sensory axons regenerated through motor pathways to muscle, where they formed persisting arborizations, but did not provide trophic support to the muscle.[77,80] These findings were taken as strong evidence against the sensory/motor specificity suggested by earlier workers. However, in this group of experiments *axons were forced into specific distal pathways*; they were not provided equal access to sensory and motor environments. When regenerating motor axons are given equal access to distal sensory and motor nerve stumps in the silicone inverted "Y tube," they reinnervate preferentially the motor nerve.[15]

The possibility of preferential motor reinnervation after routine nerve repair was investigated in a rat femoral nerve model.[12] This model is ideal for study of sensory/motor specificity because it is characterized by terminal sensory and motor branches of equal caliber that serve as equal "targets" for regeneration and dispersion of motor axons throughout the nerve at proximal levels. Axons regenerating after proximal nerve section thus have access to both sensory and motor Schwann cell tubes in the distal nerve stump. When the femoral nerve was severed and repaired, motor neurons preferentially reinnervated the femoral motor branch distally. This occurred not only after well-aligned end-to-end suture, but also when the repair was intentionally misaligned, or a 0.5-mm gap was imposed between proximal and distal stumps (Fig.

13-5). A specific interaction that was independent of mechanical axon alignment thus occurred between regenerating motor axons and the motor pathway and/or end organ. The mechanism of preferential motor reinnervation was then investigated by examining the development of specificity over time.[11] Motor axon regeneration was random at 2 weeks, with equal numbers of motor neurons projecting into the femoral sensory and motor branches (Fig. 13-6). However, the number of correct projections to the motor branch increased dramatically at subsequent time periods.

The possibility of sprouts from a single axon entering both sensory and motor branches was also investigated. At the end of the initial 2-week time period, 26% of femoral motor neurons had collateral sprouts projecting into both branches. This number decreased significantly at each time period, indicating that motor axon collaterals were "pruned" from the sensory pathway, increasing the number of correct projections at the expense of doubly projecting neurons (Fig. 13-7). These findings suggest *initial random reinnervation of the distal stumps by multiple axon sprouts, with the generation of specificity through trophic interaction between axons and the motor pathway or end organ.*

Topographic—Sensory

Currently, there is no evidence for topographic specificity in sensory axon regeneration. Only 53% of Type I fibers were associated with the correct distal fascicle after transection and repair of the cat femoral nerve.[36] Similarly, the narrow dorsal horn projection of the rat peroneal muscles uniformly expands to encompass the entire peroneal sensory territory after severance and repair of the peroneal nerve.[13] Sensory axons within the peroneal fascicle that previously served cutaneous re-

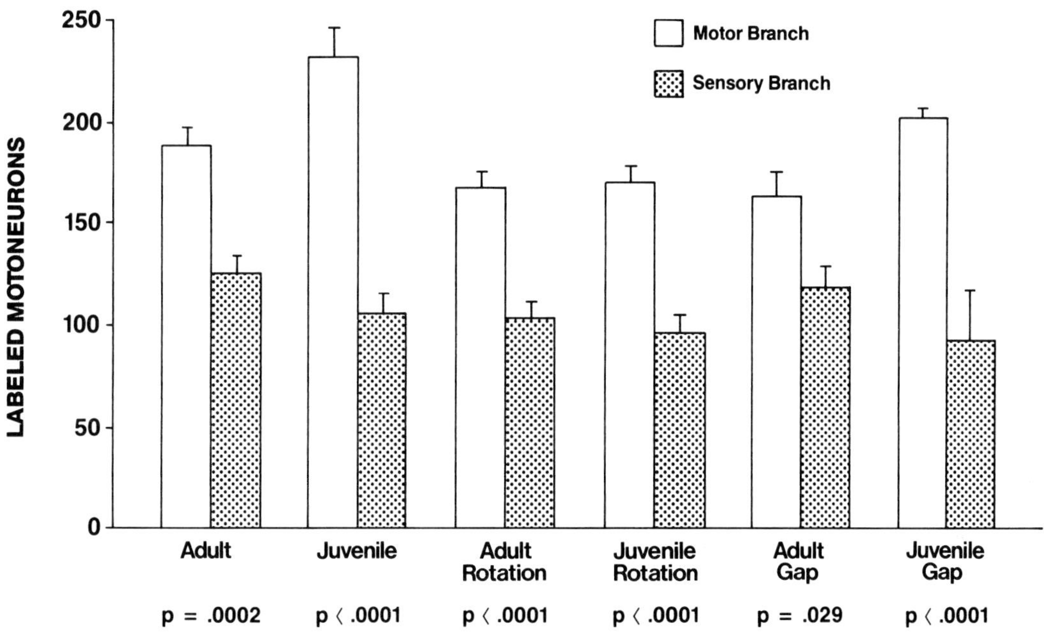

Figure 13–5. *Motor neuron counts resulting from application of horseradish peroxidase to the femoral motor (open bars) and sensory (stippled bars) branches after repair of the proximal femoral nerve. Adult and juvenile groups received well-aligned epineural repair, adult rotation and juvenile rotation groups had the distal stump rotated 180° before repair, and adult and juvenile gap groups had proximal and distal stumps separated by 0.5 mm in a silicone tube. Each bar represents the mean motor neuron count from a group of 20 sensory or motor branches. More motor neurons were labeled from the motor branch in all groups. (From Brushart TM. Preferential reinnervation of motor nerves by regenerating motor axons. J Neuroscience 1988;8:1028.)*

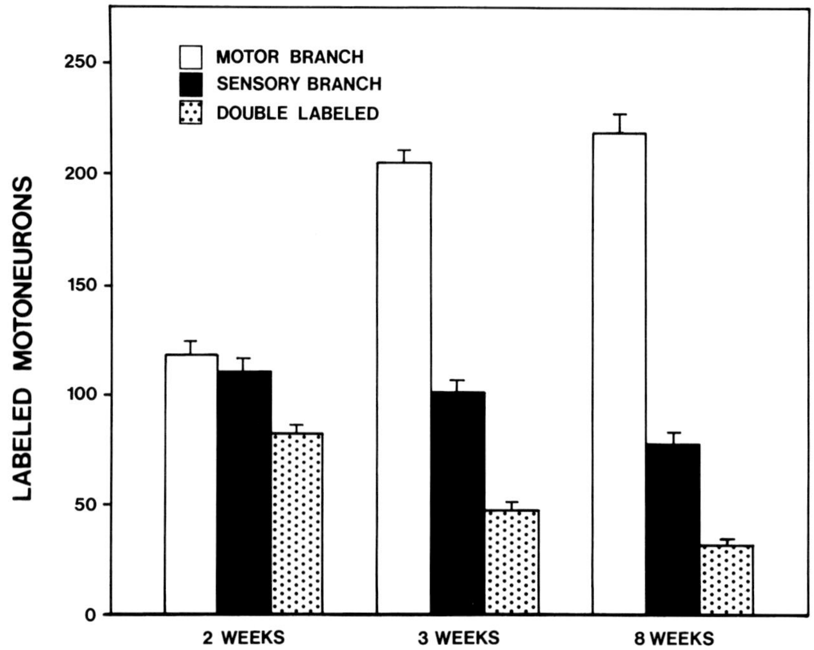

Figure 13–6. *Mean motor neuron counts resulting from simultaneous labeling of the femoral sensory and motor branches with separate tracers after proximal femoral nerve repair. Twenty nerves were evaluated at each time period. Motor neurons were scored as projecting correctly to the motor branch (light bar); incorrectly to the sensory branch (dark bar); or simultaneously to both branches, or double-labeled (stippled bar). Motor axon regeneration is random at two weeks, with equal numbers of motor neurons projecting to sensory and motor branches. However, at 3 and 8 weeks significantly more motor neurons project correctly to the motor branch than incorrectly to the sensory branch (P value < 0.0001). The number of double-labeled neurons, those with collateral projections to both branches, decreases significantly at each time period (P value < 0.0001). Axon collaterals are thus "pruned" from the sensory branch, increasing the number of correct projections at the expense of double-labeled neurons. (From Brushart TM. Preferential motor reinnervation: A sequential double-labeling study. Restorative Neurology and Neuroscience 1990;1:281–287.)*

ceptors regenerate inappropriately to peroneal muscles (Fig. 13-8).[8] Reinnervation of the rat vibrissa after trigeminal nerve section is also characterized by topographic disorganization.[61]

End Organ—Sensory

Conclusions regarding specific reinnervation of sensory end organs vary according to the model used. Cutaneous receptors are specifically reinnervated by axons with conduction velocities and dorsal column projections similar to their normal supply after sural nerve regeneration.[17] However, the sural nerve supplies a fairly limited receptor population, making appropriate reinnervation likely. In a larger mixed nerve where more receptor types are available, reinnervation is much less specific. A recent study elegantly combined anatomical and electrophysiological techniques to address this issue.[40] Individual regenerated axons were characterized electrophysiologically as to the receptor type they had reinnervated. The spinal cord projections of these axons were then defined anatomically with intracellular injections of horseradish peroxidase. Each receptor type has a characteristic central projection, making it possible to determine whether the "central wiring" was appropriate for the peripheral end organ. Fifty-one percent of the fibers studied reinnervated inappropriate recep-

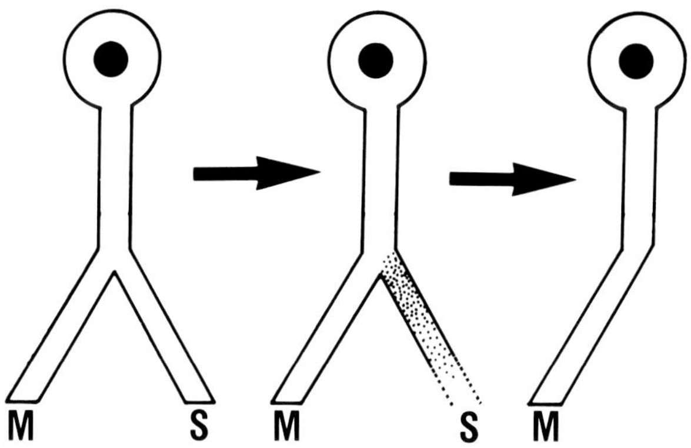

Figure 13–7. *Pruning of incorrect collateral projection. The neuron on the left has regenerated after transection of its axon. Collateral sprouts have formed, with one entering the motor branch and the other the sensory branch. Subsequently, the axon collateral in the motor branch matures while its counterpart in the sensory branch is resorbed. This could reflect trophic support to the collateral within the motor branch that is not available to its partner in the sensory branch. At the end of this process, on the right, the only projection remaining is that to the correct pathway, the femoral motor branch.*

tors. Mismatches included reinnervation of muscle receptors by cutaneous afferents and vice versa, reinnervation of low threshold cutaneous receptors by nociceptive afferents, and reinnervation of slowly adapting receptors by fibers previously supplying rapidly adapting receptors.

Structural and functional abnormalities of both muscle spindles and tendon organs persist long after sensory reinnervation of muscle.[4] Muscle spindles are randomly reinnervated by Group IA and Group II spindle afferents (their normal innervation), as well as by Group IB fibers (normally innervating tendon organs) after regeneration of the transected rat medial gastrocnemius muscle.[19] When cutaneous axons regenerate into muscle, muscle spindles are reinnervated with fine axon terminals, some of which respond to stretch; this observation confirms a potential for nonspecific muscle spindle reinnervation.[3] Reinnervation of tendon organs, in contrast, appears to be more specific.[54] This specificity is attributed to the ability of axons that previously innervated tendon organs to reenter appropriate Schwann tubes selectively at the operative site, although no direct evidence is presented.

Topographic—Motor

The topography of motor innervation is not restored in adult animals after lesions of the lumbar roots,[74] sciatic nerve,[6,14] hypoglossal nerve,[53] facial nerve,[2] or intercostal nerve.[33] However, reinnervation of the diaphragm and serratus anterior, muscles innervated by multiple spinal levels, is topographically specific in the adult rat.[46] This specificity is attributed to placement of the nerve lesion close to the muscles where contributions of the pathway are minimized, and to the presence of positional cues on the muscle fibers themselves that favor reinnervation by axons from correct spinal levels.[78] Such cues would be less useful during reinnervation of muscles innervated by only one or two spinal roots. In contrast to the adult situation, topography of motor innervation is restored after lesions of the neonatal rat facial and intercostal nerves.[1,33] This specificity may reflect the persistence into the early neonatal period of developmental path-finding cues.[33]

End Organ—Motor

Muscle fibers may be classified by speed of contraction (fast versus slow) or by motor neuron innervation (alpha motor neurons innervate skeletal muscle, beta and gamma motor neurons innervate skeletofusomotor and fusomotor fibers within muscle spindles). In the adult, there does not appear to be specific reinnervation of fast or slow muscles by axons that previously served either muscle type.[26,27,52] In neonatal rats, in contrast, soleus motor neurons selectively reinnervate slow muscle fibers, again producing evidence for a developmental cue present on neonatal muscle that is lost (or to which axons become insensitive) with later development.[68] Gamma motor neuron regeneration lags behind that of alpha and beta motor neurons, and the total number of gamma motor neurons contacting the periphery after nerve repair is significantly reduced from normal levels.[14,70,73] The spindle intrafusal fibers may also be incorrectly reinnervated by branches of alpha motor neurons.[9] These and other more subtle alterations of muscle spindle reinnervation result in profound functional alterations and give evidence for little specificity in the reinnervation process.[4,29]

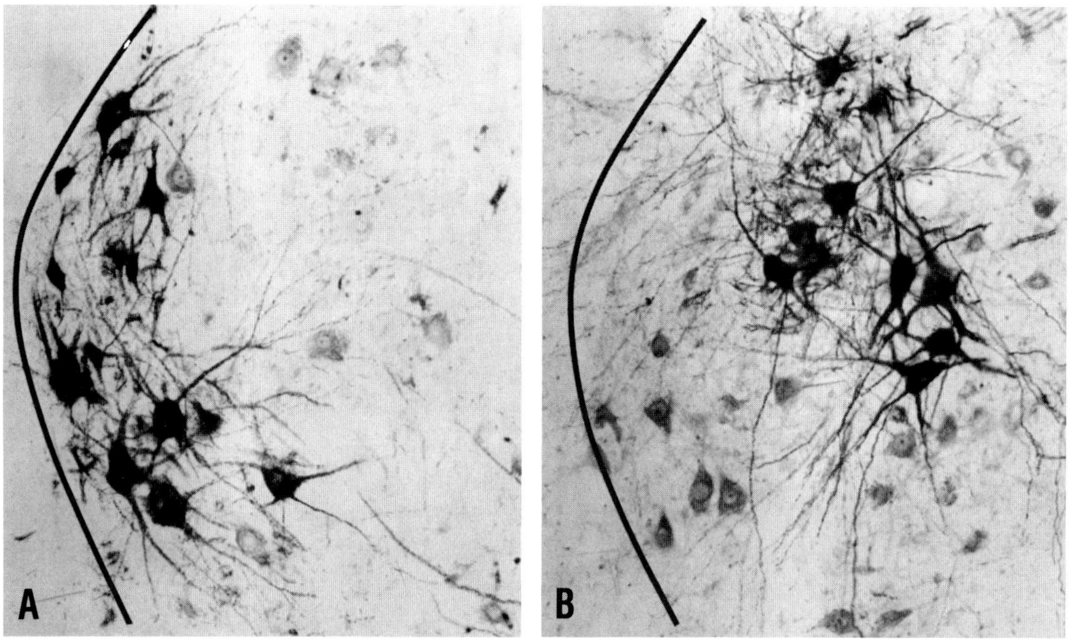

Figure 13–8. *Horseradish peroxidase–labeled motor neurons in the anterior horn of the rat spinal cord. (**A**) Normal peroneal motor neuron pool. HRP-labeled motor neurons are grouped in a crescentic pool at the lateral margin of the gray matter (solid line). Unlabeled motor neurons, those with light gray cell bodies and ill-defined dendrites, occupy locations centrally (to the right) and inferiorly. (**B**) Normal tibial motor neuron pool. HRP-labeled motor neurons are grouped centrally and superiorly to those of the peroneal pool. Unlabeled peroneal motor neurons are present, but do not occupy the entire peroneal pool location; this discrepancy results from variable spacing of neurons along the longitudinal axis of the spinal cord, so that some coronal sections contain fewer neurons. (**C**) The peroneal-innervated muscles are supplied by their original motor neurons after individual fascicular sciatic suture. Labeled motor neurons are confined to, but do not fill, the normal peroneal pool. Whether this discrepancy reflects incomplete reinnervation or simply the spacing of neurons cannot be judged from a single section. (**D**) After epineural suture, the peroneal-innervated muscles are supplied by some correct motor neurons as well as by those in the normal tibial pool location. Motor neurons in both pools remain unlabeled; they have either reinnervated muscle not exposed to HRP or have failed to make peripheral connections entirely. (Reproduced with permission from Brushart TM, Tarlov E, Mesulam MM. Specificity of muscle reinnervation after epineurial and individual fascicular suture of the rat sciatic nerve. J Hand Surg 1983;8:248–253.)*

POTENTIAL MECHANISMS OF SPECIFICITY GENERATION

Contact Recognition

Recognition of molecular "footprints" by advancing growth cones can serve as a basis for pathway selection in invertebrates.[5] Although Munson and coworkers have attributed specific reinnervation of tendon organs in the cat to a similar process, no direct evidence exists currently for specific recognition of Schwann cell tubes by regenerating mammalian axons.[54,64] However, Schwann cells or Schwann cell basal lamina of the distal stump contain molecular cues to their previous axonal associations, as suggested by the observation that sensory and motor axons differ in their surface glycoconjugates.[8,38,49] Similarly, motor axons selectively reinnervate synaptic basal lamina by preferential adherence to the glycoprotein S-laminin, and muscle fibers display positional cues that favor reinnervation by axons from correct spinal levels.[28,37,62,78]

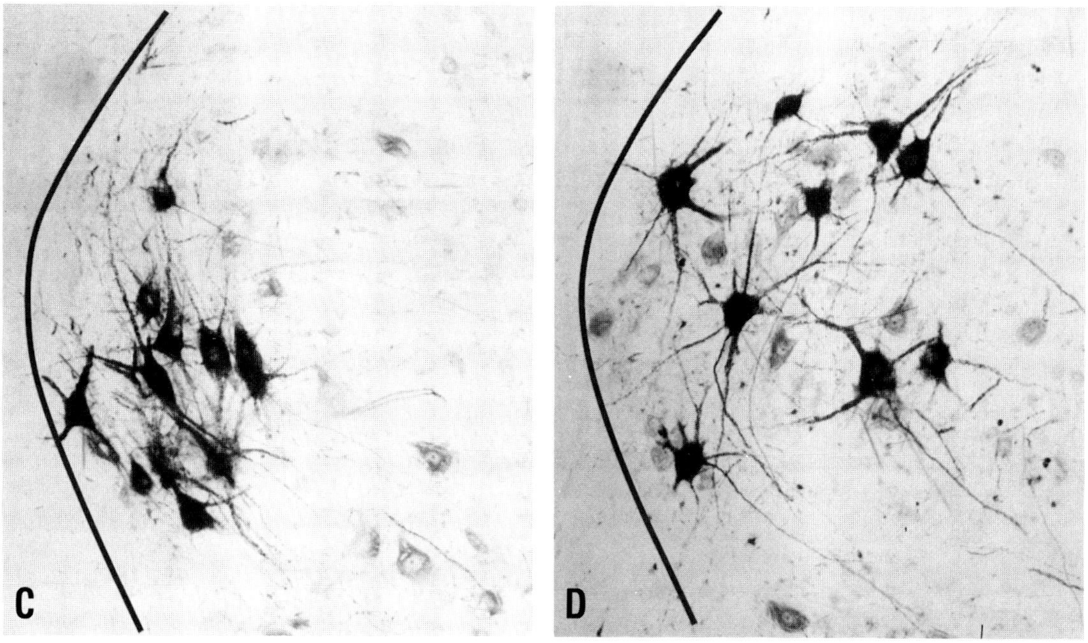

Figure 13–8. (Continued)

Neurotropism

Ramon y Cajal postulated the existence of both generalized and specific forms of neurotropism:

> We believe . . . that the action exerted by the peripheral stump—the cells of Schwann, etc.—on the growth of the young fibers is not individual and specific, that is, from tube to tube, but is general and collective, similarly directing the new axons towards the periphery . . . Once the axons are near the terminal structures, no matter what their position in the distal segment, the terminal clubs are influenced by another neurotropic influence which now has an individual and specific character . . . Among the specific orienting substances, those which appear especially necessary are those elaborated by the spindles of Kuhne and the musculo-tendinous structures of Golgi, and those also which are produced by the various categories of sensory organs of the skin and mucous membranes.[60]

According to this theory, tissue specificity is generated at the site of nerve injury; end organ specificity, in contrast, is generated within the target tissue. Recent experimental work is consistent with, but does not actually demonstrate, a neurotropic action in the generation of tissue specificity.[49,50] Neurotropism can only be proven when axons are seen growing toward a target they have not yet reached. Once the target is contacted, as in the above experiments, it may exert a positive neurotrophic effect, supporting the axons that reach it at the expense of those that do not. This criterion for neurotropism is met by the experiments of Politis, which demonstrate preferential growth towards a normal versus a metabolically compromised distal stump, even when a 0.2-micron millipore filter obstructs the pathway.[58] The direction of axon growth in these experiments is thus controlled by a diffusible substance that requires living cells for its production. Such a factor may be the basis for tissue specificity seen in other experiments,[49,50] as originally postulated by Ramon y Cajal. Specificity at the nerve trunk level could also result from neurotropic influence, but a clear definition of mechanism is impossible because the experiments were evaluated after reinnervation of the distal nerve stump.[57,65] Ramon y Cajal's "individual and specific" neurotropic effect at the end organ level has not yet been confirmed.

Evidence for the action of neurotropism has also been obtained in lower vertebrates and in tissue culture experiments. Kuffler's elegant morphologic work has shown directed growth of frog motor axons before target contact is made.[41] Sensory neurites ascend gradients of nerve growth factor and are selectively attracted to appropriate targets in co-cultures with either central or peripheral nervous tissue.[20,30,48] In the chick embryo, reversal of spinal cord segments or moderate limb shifts do not prevent motor axons from reaching appropriate targets, even if unique pathways are created to do so.[42,43]

In the past decade neurotropism has again been acknowledged as a significant determinant of peripheral nerve regeneration. However, its effect on the generation of specificity appears to be limited to the tissue and perhaps nerve trunk levels. Further, it has been demonstrated only after the creation of special circumstances and is not known to affect the outcome of end-to-end nerve suture. If a gap is imposed between nerve stumps to allow freedom of axonal movement in response to neurotropic "lures," motor reinnervation is random without evidence of nerve trunk or topographic specificity.[10,59]

Neurotrophism

The importance of neurotrophic effects has been well established in the sensory and sympathetic systems. *Nerve growth factor* (NGF), the first neurotrophic factor to be described, is released by tissues innervated by sympathetic and sensory axons.[25,34] It binds to specific receptors on the nerve terminal membranes and is transported to the parent neuron, where it accelerates metabolism.[24,69,72] Injected NGF stimulates axon growth and prevents neuronal death in the early stages of development.[7,32] Only recently has neurotrophism been identified as a potential mechanism of specificity generation in the motor system.[11] The evidence is derived from work on the regenerating rat femoral nerve (see above, Sensory/Motor). Initial reinnervation of distal sensory and motor branches by regenerating motor axons is random, with equal numbers of motor neurons projecting axons to correct (motor) and incorrect (sensory) pathways. This lack of initial specificity suggests the absence of neurotropic or contact mechanisms. Early in reinnervation many motor neurons project collateral sprouts into both pathways, permitting the neuron to sample neurotrophic influences from both sensory and motor environments. The subsequent generation of specificity coincides with the "pruning" of incorrect collateral projections from the sensory branch. This pruning most likely reflects the absence of trophic support for motor axons within the sensory branch.

These experiments produce only indirect evidence of a neurotrophic effect, but the inference is supported by evidence for a "motor nerve growth factor" similar to NGF. Muscle extracts, or media conditioned by them, significantly alter motor neuron behavior in tissue culture. Neuron survival is increased, neurite elongation is enhanced, and transmitter systems are potentiated.[18,23,65] Extracts are more potent when obtained from developing or recently denervated muscle, suggesting a role for this factor in development and regeneration.[35,55,67] Motor nerve growth factor may also be present in peripheral nerve, as fluid collected from enclosed peripheral nerve gaps contains separate growth factors for sympathetic, sensory, and spinal cord neurons.[47] In the living animal, target-derived neurotrophic factors reduce naturally occurring motor neuron death.[56]

In addition to influencing sensory/motor specificity, neurotrophism could also aid in the determination of specificity at the tissue, nerve trunk, and end organ levels. Positive confirmation will require identification of a substance that can itself support the population of axons in question, and antibodies that block the generation of specificity in the living animal.

MECHANICAL

Operative control of regeneration specificity has been studied extensively in the rat sciatic nerve model. Initial work compared the specificity of topographic motor and sensory reinnervation after epineural and individual fascicular nerve repair.[13,16] Topographic motor and sensory reinnervation are not subject to intrinsic humoral control in the extremities (see Topographic—Motor, Topographic—Sensory) and are thus an ideal substrate for these experiments. Normally, the motor neurons serving the peroneal and tibial sciatic fascicles are located in separate anatomical compartments or "pools" within the spinal cord (Fig. 13-8). After nerve repair and regeneration, the motor neurons reinnervating the peroneal fascicle were identified with a horseradish peroxidase (HRP) technique of axon tracing. They were counted and scored as "in" or "out" of the normal peroneal pool location; those scored as "out" had previously served the antagonistic tibial muscles. Their axons, regenerating from the proximal tibial fascicle, had entered the distal peroneal fascicle at the repair site, where they picked up HRP and transported it back to tibial motor neurons within the spinal cord. These motor neurons compromise function by incorrectly stimulating the peroneal muscles when plantar flexion is desired. The type of nerve repair did not significantly affect the number of motor neurons regenerating. However, reinnervation was significantly more accurate after individual fascicular suture (Fig. 13-8). *Individual alignment of nerve fascicles thus improved the specificity of topographic motor reinnervation.* These conclusions have been questioned, but on the basis of a limited study in which every third spinal cord section was evaluated in only four animals.[1] The large variability seen after epineural suture in our study mandates a larger sample to obtain meaningful results.[16]

A similar evaluation of mechanical contributions to topographic specificity in the sensory system is based on the topography of sensory axon projections to the dorsal horn of the spinal cord (Fig. 13-9).[13] The normal sensory territory corresponding to the peroneal muscles is quite limited, as muscle receives much less sensory innervation than does skin. Individual fascicular suture more closely restores this limited projection than does epineural suture, again demonstrating mechanical control of topographic specificity at the fascicular level (Fig. 13-9). However, the projection is still much wider than normal, and this abnormality persists even when only the peroneal fascicle is cut and repaired; it must thus reflect lack of specificity within the peroneal fascicle itself rather than axon ingrowth from other fascicles. On further examination, this persistently widened projection corresponds to that of skin served by the peroneal fascicle; axons normally serving skin have reinnervated the peroneal muscles. Topographic reinnervation within the fascicle thus proceeds on a random basis in spite of individual fascicular suture, defining the limits of suture technique.

The importance of mechanical factors in the generation of topographic specificity has been further emphasized by study of the "nerve reconnection" technique of deMedinaceli.[21,22,71,79,81] This technique involves gentle freezing of the nerve in solutions that limit metabolic axonal damage, transection of the nerve with a vibrating blade, and reapproximation of proximal and distal stumps without tension or sutures at the juncture. This technique has been applied to the rat sciatic nerve and the results analyzed by determination of the sciatic functional index (SFI), a numeric expression of muscle function derived from measurement of the rat's footprints. The functional results of "nerve reconnection" have been reproducibly superior to those of epineural suture (Fig. 13-10).[21,22,71,79,81] The success of the technique appears to reflect its excellent alignment of proximal and distal stump axons. The number of axons reinnervating the distal stump is not increased after "reconnection," suggesting that survival of axons or neurons is not improved.[71] One study showed an increase in the number of motor neurons reinnervating the peroneal nerve after "reconnection."[79] However, this finding is difficult to interpret, as it could result merely from increased overlap of the peroneal fascicle with sensory portions of the tibial fascicle after epineural suture, falsely decreasing the availability of motor axons in these repairs. Comparison of motor neuron pool topography, as described above, provides the most striking morphologic difference between epineural and "nerve reconnection" groups.[79] Only 66% of motor neurons labeled from the peroneal nerve after epineural suture had made correct peripheral connections, while 87% had reached the correct peripheral target after "reconnection." These differences correlated well with functional results as expressed by the SFI.

The "reconnection" technique produces optimal results in a laboratory setting where there is no tissue loss and proximal and distal stumps can be precisely realigned. However, experimental attempts to use the "reconnection" technique to im-

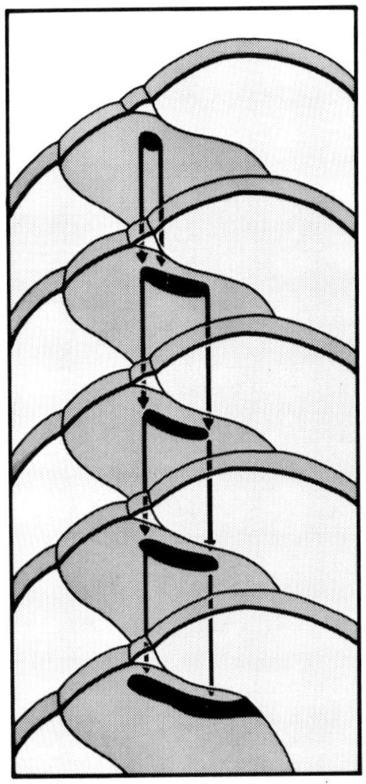

Figure 13–9. *Dorsal horn projections. The central processes of primary sensory neurons project topographically to the dorsal horn of the spinal cord. The normal projection from peroneal-innervated muscle is quite narrow. This projection is much wider after epineural repair of the sciatic nerve, reflecting reinnervation of peroneal muscle by axons from the tibial and sural fascicles. Individual fascicular sciatic suture narrows this projection significantly by providing mechanical control of topographic specificity at the fascicular level. However, the projection is still much wider than that of normal peroneal-innervated muscle. This widening persists even if only the peroneal fascicle itself is transected and repaired. The widened projection overlaps with that of peroneal-innervated skin, demonstrating lack of control of topographic specificity within the fascicle itself.*

prove on poor results after primary nerve suture have been unsuccessful.[21] This failure is attributed to mismatch of proximal and distal stumps after neuroma excision. Whatever its clinical applications may prove to be, this technique is important because it has reemphasized the role of mechanical factors in nerve repair at a time when surgeons, reaching the limits of suture technique, are looking progressively to humoral mechanisms to improve the results of nerve repair.

DISCUSSION

At our current level of knowledge, there is only limited evidence for humoral control of mammalian regeneration specificity. Contact recognition aids pathway selection in insects, but no mammalian examples are known.[5] Neurotropism contributes to generation of tissue specificity and may also influence specificity at the nerve trunk level.[57,58] Neurotrophic influences are strongly implicated in the generation of sensory/motor specificity.[11] Preferential motor reinnervation is of particular significance because it shapes the outcome of routine peripheral nerve suture, requiring no special circumstances for its demonstration. The factors responsible for this phenomenon are of sufficient magnitude to partially overcome the axonal disorganization imposed by stump malalignment or an interstump gap. Furthermore, preferential motor reinnervation can influence the population of axons that enter tributary nerves; progressively finer distinctions are meaningless if appropriate

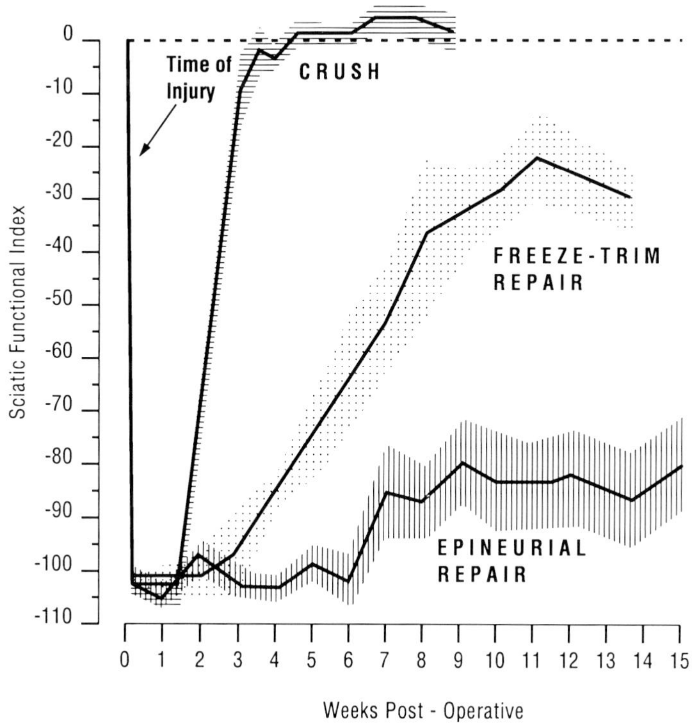

Figure 13–10. *Recovery of motor function (SFI) over time after nerve injury. The solid line in each curve represents the mean recovery for each group; the shaded zones represent one standard error of the mean. An SFI of 0 ± 5 is normal, while −100 shows no recovery. Crush injuries recovered rapidly to normal within 4 weeks. Epineurial repairs rarely improved beyond 20%, even after 12 weeks, whereas "reconnection" repairs reached about 70% recovery by 10 weeks (Wikholm R, Swett J, Torigoe Y, Blanks R. Repair of severed peripheral nerve: A superior anatomic and functional recovery with a new "reconnection" technique. Otol Head & Neck Surg 1988;99:357.)*

end organs are unavailable. These factors operate without our aid and until recently without our awareness. Our active role as surgeons is currently limited to the generation of specificity at the nerve trunk and topographic levels through mechanical restoration of fascicular alignment.

In the near future, improvement in the specificity of axon regeneration is likely to result from limited clinical use of the deMedinaceli technique. Sharp, clean lacerations without substance loss might benefit from a rapid, convenient "reconnection" technique applied at the fascicular or group fascicular level. (This would obviously be inappropriate for treatment of most injuries, in which exact correspondence of proximal and distal stumps has been lost.) In the years ahead, improvement in nerve regeneration specificity will result from analysis of axonal path-finding in development. Initial connections between the central nervous system and peripheral end organs are made with amazing accuracy, requiring only slight fine-tuning. The contact, neurotropic, or neurotrophic mechanisms underlying this specificity must be defined, and the structural components of these mechanisms sought in the regenerating adult system. Parallel research must define the comparative capabilities of developing and adult growth cones, as a well-marked path may be useless to a "blind" axon. Our increasing competence with molecular probes and genetic manipulation should ultimately allow us to reactivate expression of developmentally silenced genes, returning the regenerating neuron and perhaps even the supporting cells of the pathway to their original capabilities. If the messages that trigger wallerian degeneration can be identified and blocked, axon fusion with preservation of specificity could become a reality, restoring normal function within weeks of nerve transection.

REFERENCES

1. Aldskogius H, Molander C, Persson J, Thomander L. Specific and nonspecific regeneration of motor axons after sciatic nerve injury and repair in the rat. J Neurol Sci 1987;80:249–257.
2. Aldskogius H, Thomander L. Selective reinnerva-

tion of somatotopically appropriate muscles after facial nerve transection and regeneration in the neonatal rat. Brain Res 1986;375:126–134.

3. Banks RW, Barker D, Stacey MJ. Reinnervation of cat muscle spindles by foreign afferents after nerve section. J Physiol (Lond) 1984;357:21P.
4. Banks RW, Barker D, Brown HG. Sensory reinnervation of muscles following nerve section and suture in cats. J Hand Surg [Br] 1985;10:340–344.
5. Bastiani MJ, duLac S, Goodman CS. Guidance of neuronal growth cones in the grasshopper embryo. I. Recognition of a specific axonal pathway by the pCC neuron. J Neurosci 1986;6:3518–3531.
6. Bernstein JJ, Guth L. Nonselectivity in establishment of neuromuscular connections following nerve regeneration in the rat. Exp Neurol 1961;4:262–275.
7. Bjerre B, Bjorklund A, Mobley W, Rosengrene E. Short- and long-term effects of nerve growth factor on the sympathetic nervous system in the adult mouse. Brain Res 1975;94:263–277.
8. Borges LF, Sidman RL. Axonal transport of lectins in the peripheral nervous system. J Neurosci 1982;2:647–653.
9. Brown MC, Butler RG. Evidence for innervation of muscle spindle intrafusal fibers by branches of alpha motoneurons following nerve injury. J Physiol (Lond) 1974;238:41–42.
10. Brushart TM. Motor reinnervation across an 8-mm gap in the rat is non-specific. Topographic specificity of peripheral axon regeneration across enclosed gaps. Neurosci Abst 1990;16:806.
11. Brushart TM. Preferential motor reinnervation: A sequential double-labeling study. Restorative Neurology and Neuroscience 1990;1:281–287.
12. Brushart TM. Preferential reinnervation of motor nerves by regenerating motor axons. J Neuroscience 1988;8:1026–1031.
13. Brushart TM, Henry EW, Mesulam MM. Reorganization of muscle afferent projections accompanies peripheral nerve regeneration. Neuroscience 1981;6:2053–2061.
14. Brushart TM, Mesulam MM. Alteration in connections between muscle and anterior horn motoneurons after peripheral nerve repair. Science 1980;208:603–605.
15. Brushart TM, Seiler WA. Selective reinnervation of distal motor stumps by peripheral motor axons. Exp Neurol 1987;97:280–300.
16. Brushart TM, Tarlov E, Mesulam MM. Specificity of muscle reinnervation after epineurial and individual fascicular suture of the rat sciatic nerve. J Hand Surg 1983;8:248–253.
17. Burgess PR, Horch KW. Specific regeneration of cutaneous fibers in the cat. J Neurophysiol 1973;36: 101–114.
18. Calof AL, Reichardt LF. Response of purified chick motoneurons to myotube conditioned medium: Laminin is essential for the substratum-binding, neurite outgrowth-promoting activity. Neurosci Lett 1985;59:183–189.
19. Collins WF, Mendell LM, Munson JB. On the specificity of sensory reinnervation of cat skeletal muscle. J Physiol 1986;375:587–609.
20. Crain SM, Peterson ER. Selective innervation of target regions within fetal mouse spinal cord and medulla explants by isolated dorsal root ganglia in organotypic co-cultures. Developmental Brain Research 1982;2:341–362.
21. deMedinaceli L, Freed W, Wyatt R. Peripheral nerve reconnection: Improvement of long-term functional effects under simulated clinical conditions in the rat. Exp Neurol 1983;81:488–496.
22. deMedinaceli L, Seaber A. Experimental nerve reconnection: Importance of initial repair. Microsurgery 1989;10:56–70.
23. Dohrmann U, Edgar D, Sendtner M, Thoenen H. Muscle-derived factors that support survival and promote fiber outgrowth from embryonic chick spinal motor neurons in culture. Dev Biol 1986;118: 209–221.
24. Dumas M, Schwab M, Thoenen H. Retrograde axonal transport of specific macromolecules as a tool for characterizing nerve terminal membranes. J Neurobiol 1979;10:179–197.
25. Ebendal T, Olson L, Seiger A, Hedlund K-O. Nerve growth factors in the rat iris. Nature 1980;286:25–27.
26. Foehring RC, Sypert GW, Munson JB. Properties of self-reinnervated motor units of medial gastrocnemius of cat. I. Long-term reinnervation. J Neurophysiol 1986;55:931–965.
27. Gillespie MJ, Gordon T, Murphy PR. Reinnervation of the lateral gastrocnemius and soleus muscles in the rat by their common nerve. J Physiol (Lond) 1986;372:485–500.
28. Glicksman MA, Sanes JR. Differentiation of motor nerve terminals formed in the absence of muscle fibers. J Neurocytol 1983;12:661–671.
29. Gregory JE, Luff AR, Proske U. Muscle receptors in the cross-reinnervated soleus muscle of the cat. J Physiol 1982;331:367–383.
30. Gunderson RW, Barrett JN. Neuronal chemotaxis: Chick dorsal root axons turn toward high concentrations of nerve growth factor. Science 1979;206: 1079–1080.

31. Gutmann E. The reinnervation of muscle by sensory nerve fibers. J Anat 1945;79:1–8.
32. Hamburger V, Brunso-Beld J, Yip J. Neuronal death in the spinal ganglia of the chick embryo and its reduction by nerve growth factor. J Neuroscience 1981;1:60–71.
33. Hardman VJ, Brown MC. Accuracy of reinnervation of rat intercostal muscles by their own segmental nerves. J Neurosci 1987;7:1031–1036.
34. Harper G, Al-Saffar A, Pearce F, Vernon C. The production of nerve growth factor in vitro by tissues of the mouse, rat and embryonic chick. Dev Biol 1980;77:379–390.
35. Hill AM, Bennett MR. Motoneuron survival in extracts of denervated muscle is reduced by prior stimulation of the muscle. Developmental Brain Research 1986;24:305–308.
36. Horch K. Guidance of regrowing sensory axons after cutaneous nerve lesions in the cat. J Neurophysiol 1979;42:1437–1449.
37. Hunter DD, Shah V, Merlie JP, Sanes JR. A laminin-like adhesive protein concentrated in the synaptic cleft of the neuromuscular junction. Nature 1989;338:229–233.
38. Keynes RJ. Schwann cells during neural development and regeneration: Leaders or followers? Trends Neuroscience 1987;10:137–139.
39. Kilvington B. Some experiments on nerve regeneration. Aust N Z J Surg 1941;10:266–272.
40. Koerber HR, Seymour AW, Mendell LM. Mismatches between peripheral receptor type and central projections after peripheral nerve regeneration. Neurosci Lett 1989;99:67–72.
41. Kuffler DP. Isolated satellite cells of a peripheral nerve direct the growth of regenerating frog axons. J Comp Neurol 1986;249:57–64.
42. Lance-Jones C, Landmesser L. Motoneurone projection patterns in the chick hind limb following early partial reversals of the spinal cord. J Physiol (Lond) 1980;302:581–602.
43. Lance-Jones C, Landmesser L. Pathway selection by embryonic chick motoneurones in an experimentally altered environment. Proc R Soc Lond [Biol] 1981;214:19–52.
44. Langley JN, Anderson HK. The union of different kinds of nerve fibers. J Physiol (Lond) 1904;31:365–391.
45. Langley JN, Hashimoto M. On the suture of separate nerve bundles in a nerve trunk and on internal nerve plexuses. J Physiol (Lond) 1917;51:318–345.
46. Laskowski MB, Sanes JR. Topographically selective reinnervation of adult mammalian skeletal muscles. J Neurosci 1988;8:3094–3099.
47. Longo FM, Skaper SD, Manthorpe M, Williams LR, Lundborg G, Varon S. Temporal changes in neuronotrophic activities accumulating in vivo within nerve regeneration chambers. Exp Neurol 1983;81:756–769.
48. Lumsden AG, Davies AM. Earliest sensory nerve fibers are guided to peripheral targets by attractants other than nerve growth factor. Nature 1983;306:786–788.
49. Lundborg GL, Dahlin L, Danielsen N, Nachemson AK. Tissue specificity in nerve regeneration. Scand J Plast Reconstr Surg Hand Surg 1986;20:279–283.
50. Mackinnon SE, Dellon AL, Lundborg G, Hudson AR, Hunter DA. A study of neurotrophism in a primate model. J Hand Surg [Am] 1986;11:888–894.
51. Mendell LM, Scott JG. The effect of peripheral nerve cross-union on connections of single Ia fibers to motoneurons. Exp Brain Res 1975;22:221–234.
52. Miledi R, Stefani E. Non-selective re-innervation of slow and fast muscle fibers in the rat. Nature 1969;222:569–571.
53. Mizuno N, Uemura-Sumi M, Matsuda K, Takeuchi Y, Kume M, Matushima R. Non-selective distribution of hypoglossal nerve fibers after section and resuture: A horseradish peroxidase study in the cat. Neurosci Lett 1980;19:33–37.
54. Munson JB, Collins WF, Mendell LM. Reinnervation of muscle spindles by groups Ia and Ib fibers is consistent with specificity in the reinnervation process. In: Liss A. The current status of peripheral nerve regeneration. New York: Alan R Liss, 1988:259–268.
55. Nurcombe V, Hill MA, Eagleson KL, Bennett MR. Motor neuron survival and neuritic extension from spinal cord explants induced by factors released from denervated muscle. Brain Res 1984;291:19–28.
56. Oppenheim RW, Haverkamp LJ, Prevette D, McManaman JL, Appel SH. Reduction of naturally occurring motoneuron death in vivo by a target-derived neurotrophic factor. Science 1988;240:919–922.
57. Politis MJ. Specificity in mammalian peripheral nerve regeneration at the level of the trunk. Brain Res 1985;328:271–276.
58. Politis MJ, Ederle K, Spencer PS. Tropism in nerve regeneration in vivo. Attraction of regenerating axons by diffusible factors derived from cells in distal nerve stumps of transected peripheral nerves. Brain Res 1982;253:1–12.
59. Politis MJ, Steiss JE. Electromyographic evaluation of a novel surgical preparation to enhance nerve-muscle specificity that follows mammalian periph-

eral nerve trunk transection. Exp Neurol 1985;87: 326–333.

60. Ramon y Cajal S. Degeneration and regeneration of the nervous system, Vol 1. London: Oxford University Press, 1928:305–396.
61. Renehan WE, Munger BL. Degeneration and regeneration of peripheral nerve in the rat trigeminal system. II. Response to nerve lesions. J Comp Neurol 1986;249:429–459.
62. Sanes JR, Marshall M, McMahan UJ. Reinnervation of muscle fiber basal lamina after removal of myofibers. J Cell Biol 1978;78:176–198.
63. Sanes JR. More nerve growth factors? Nature 1984;307:500.
64. Scherer SS, Easter SS. Degenerative and regenerative changes in the trochlear nerve of goldfish. J Neurocytol 1984;13:519–565.
65. Seckel BR, Ryan SE, Gagne RG, Ho Chiu T, Watkins E. Target-specific nerve regeneration through a nerve guide in the rat. Plast Reconstr Surg 1986;78: 793–798.
66. Slack JR, Hopkins WG, Pockett S. Evidence for a motor nerve growth factor. Muscle Nerve 1983;6: 243–252.
67. Smith RG, Appel SH. Extracts of skeletal muscle increase neurite outgrowth and cholinergic activity of fetal rat spinal motor neurons. Science 1983;219: 1079–1081.
68. Soileau LC, Silberstein L, Blau HM, Thompson WJ. Reinnervation of muscle fiber types in the newborn rat soleus. J Neurosci 1987;7:4176–4194.
69. Stockel K, Paravicini U, Thoenen H. Specificity of the retrograde axonal transport of nerve growth factor. Brain Res 1974;76:413–421.
70. Takano K. Absence of gamma-spindle loop in the reinnervated hind leg muscles of the cat: "alpha muscle." Exp Brain Res 1976;26:343–354.
71. Terzis J, Smith K. Repair of severed peripheral nerves: Comparison of the "deMedinaceli" and standard microsuture methods. Exp Neurol 1987; 96:672–680.
72. Thoenen H, Angeletti P, Levi-Montalcini R, Kettler R. Selective induction of tyrosine hydroxylase and dopamine B-hydroxylase in rat superior cervical ganglion by nerve growth factor. Proc Natl Acad Sci USA 1971;68:1598–1602.
73. Thulin CA. Electrophysiological studies of peripheral nerve regeneration with special reference to the small diameter (gamma) fibers. Exp Neurol 1960;2:598–612.
74. Ungar-Sargon J, Goldberger ME. Maintenance of specificity by sprouting and regenerating peripheral nerves. II. Variability after lesions. Brain Res 1987;407:124–136.
75. Weiss P, Edds MV. Sensory-motor nerve crosses in the rat. J Neurophysiol 1945;30:173–193.
76. Weiss P, Hoag A. Competitive reinnervation of rat muscles by their own and foreign nerves. J Neurophysiol 1946;9:413–418.
77. Weiss P, Taylor AC. Further experimental evidence against neurotropism in nerve regeneration. J Exp Zool 1944;95:233–257.
78. Wigston DJ, Sanes JR. Selective reinnervation of adult mammalian muscle by axons from different segmental levels. Nature 1982;299:464–467.
79. Wikholm R, Swett J, Torigoe Y, Blanks R. Repair of severed peripheral nerve: A superior anatomic and functional recovery with a new "reconnection" technique. Otolaryngol Head Neck Surg 1988;99: 353–361.
80. Zalewski AA. Effects of reinnervation on denervated skeletal muscle by axons of motor, sensory, and sympathetic neurons. Am J Physiol 1970;219:1675–1679.
81. Zellem R, Miller D, Kenning J, Hoenig E, Buchheit W. Experimental peripheral nerve repair: Environmental control directed at the cellular level. Microsurgery 1989;10:290–301.

14

Internal Topography of Peripheral Nerves as Related to Repair

Michael E. Jabaley

AUTHOR'S KEY POINTS

- Specific sensory and motor function can be assigned to individual fascicles or fascicular groups.
- Although the cross-sectional appearance of the major nerves varies with the level, the path of functional units is less changeable and can be predicted over reasonably long lengths of nerve.
- Epineurium, whether internal or external, is the correct plane of dissection. Dissection within a nerve is accomplished with appropriate magnification and instrumentation and careful technique.
- The focus of nerve repair has shifted to the accurate alignment of functional components (fascicles). This is accomplished, where possible, by sutures placed in either the internal or external epineurium.
- Current repair techniques require the surgeon to understand internal topography and to be capable of internal dissection of nerves where necessary.

HISTORY

The internal topography of peripheral nerves was the subject of debate among anatomists long before it became a subject of investigation by surgeons.[3,6,8] Early in the 20th century, there was controversy in the literature as to whether plexuses existed within nerves or whether there were specific tracts, as had been described in the spinal cord. There was less debate as to what the functional significance of plexuses might be, and few publications considered this aspect.[5] Sunderland's now-classic studies defined the controversy and described the definitive investigations that addressed the questions clearly and laid the debate to rest. In his studies of the peripheral nerves of the upper and lower extremities of humans, Sunderland used the technique of serial sectioning and histologic examination to follow the distal-to-proximal course of specific branches as they entered and traversed a nerve trunk. He followed each fascicle until it was no longer identifiable, observing its position relative to other fascicles in the nerve trunk and the level where it eventually merged with adjacent fascicles.

From these studies, Sunderland concluded that the individual fascicles within a nerve were constantly branching and joining other fascicles, changing location, and generally contributing to the formation of a plexus or network of fascicles. Since Sunderland was interested primarily in changes in cross-sectional appearance, he stressed this aspect of his examinations, but he also appreciated the fact that the fibers of each branch were identifiable for considerable distances and that there was a general orderliness to nerve makeup. Moreover, proceeding distally in each nerve, the location of specific branches became more predictable and they became easier to identify.

In the second half of the 20th century, after World War II, interest in nerve injury and repair increased. Many surgeons who studied Sunderland's work concluded from it that accurate fascicular alignment was impossible during repair because of the constantly changing cross-sectional picture. This assumption was partly due to a misunderstanding on the part of some readers. Although Sunderland's tome contains few illustrations, a prominent one is a three-dimensional reconstruction of the musculocutaneous nerve (Fig. 14-1). The musculocutaneous nerve is a mixed motor and sensory nerve and, at least for a major extremity nerve, a relatively short one. It originates from C5, C6, and sometimes C7. In a relatively short space it must deliver branches to the coracobrachialis, biceps, and brachialis, then continue distally as the lateral antebrachial cutaneous nerve (a pure sensory trunk). Thus, it is not surprising that there is a complex fascicular arrangement with frequent branching and merging. These changes in appearance at each level are necessary to separate motor and sensory fibers arising from several cord levels over this relatively short distance.

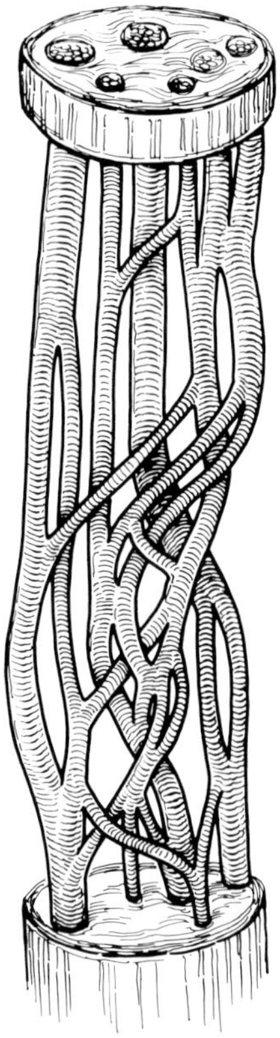

Figure 14–1. *A three-dimensional reconstruction of a human musculocutaneous nerve, prepared from histologic examination of serial sections. It demonstrates the natural plexus formation of fascicles as they branch and recombine within the nerve trunk. This process gathers fibers destined for a common destination and groups them into specific branches prior to exiting the main trunk.*

On the other hand, the major nerves to the most distal portions of the extremities travel a greater distance, and individual branches are well defined. In the more distal portions of the median and ulnar nerves, there are relatively few interconnections over greater distances. This point is of considerable clinical significance, since most nerve transections occur at the distal extremities (Fig. 14-2).

With the advent of optical magnification devices, fine suture material, and precision instruments, and an increased awareness of the potential for recovery following nerve grafting procedures, knowledge of internal topography took on more practical significance, and more precise information about internal anatomy became mandatory. For this reason, dissection of peripheral nerves was again investigated, but this time in the context of its surgical significance.

In the early 1970s, the general pessimism that pervaded the field of nerve repair was directly challenged.[4,11] The basis for this challenge was the inconsistency between what was generally assumed and what surgeons were observing in everyday practice. As early as the 1930s, Boyes had advised rerouting the motor branch of the ulnar nerve to permit a tension-free nerve suture following in-

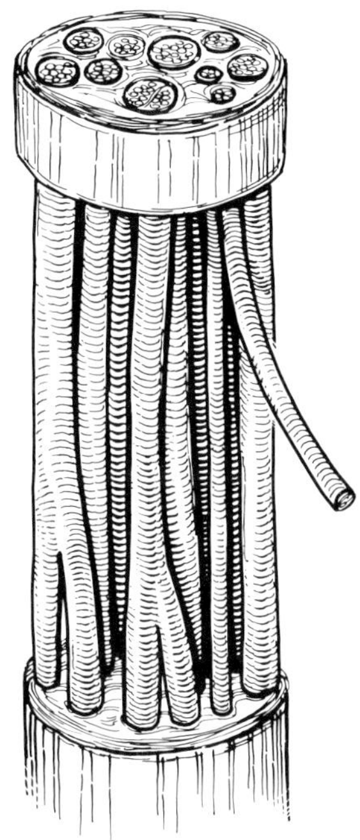

Figure 14–2. *Reconstruction of the human median nerve in the distal forearm. In contrast to the musculocutaneous nerve, the fascicular arrangement is more orderly and there are fewer interconnections in the terminal nerve because the branches are already defined. Surgical dissection for identification and alignment of fascicles is possible at this level, because fibers travel proximally in the same general quadrantic relationship for a considerable distance.*

juries at Guyon's canal. In addition, surgeons were also learning that they could, when indicated, incise the epineurium of intact nerves without harm to perform internal neurolysis. Finally, in managing transected nerves, they could excise epineurium where necessary for purposes of interfascicular nerve grafting. The notion of group fascicular repairs was accepted; some even advocated interfascicular suture. Thus, as a practical matter, contemporary nerve repair required a reinterpretation of available data in the light of everyday experience.

APPLIED ANATOMY

The terms used in this chapter are those recommended by the Committee on Nomenclature of the International Society of Reconstructive Microsurgery.[7]

A peripheral nerve consists of both conducting and nonconducting tissue. The conducting nervous tissue (axons and their Schwann cells) is ectodermal in origin; the nonconducting tissue is derived from mesoderm. The role of mesodermal tissue is structural, supportive, and nutritional. Each part of the nerve plays a different, highly specialized role in the repair process. Those tissues derived from mesoderm heal by formation of scar tissue (ie, they form a collagen bond between the ends of the nerve).[1] Axons, on the other hand, "heal" by regeneration and must subsequently bridge the bond of scar that has formed.

Mesodermal healing is similar to classical soft-tissue healing, beginning with inflammation and proceeding to a cellular phase dominated by fibroblasts. The epineurium, which is the main source of such fibroblasts, participates actively in the healing process (this active participation is the basis for Millesi's recommendation that the epineurium should be excised in nerve grafting procedures).

Transected axons do not "heal" in the usual sense of that word. Instead, they regenerate, a process that combines intense cellular activity at the cell body level, positive axonal flow, and a vigorous sprouting and elongation of axons at the zone of injury. The effect is an extension of the axon sprouts across a repair site (if one exists) or into a neuroma if no repair has been performed.

A peripheral nerve can be subdivided into bundles and individual fascicles (Fig. 14-3). A bundle consists of two or more fascicles. Each fascicle is bounded by the perineurium. This is a strong, well-organized, and tightly regimented structure of several layers or lamellae. They are oriented diagonally, transversely, or longitudinally. Perineurium provides the supporting framework for the structures contained within and also serves as a barrier separating the internal milieu from that without. Within the perineurium are located the endoneurium, the nerve fibers (myelinated or unmyelinated), and their Schwann cells. Myelinated fibers are each ensheathed by a Schwann cell, while several unmyelinated fibers may be associated with a single Schwann cell. In each case, the Schwann cells are the source of myelin. Pressure within the perineurium is slightly higher than that outside, and there is an ionic gradient.

The bundles are bounded by epineurium of two

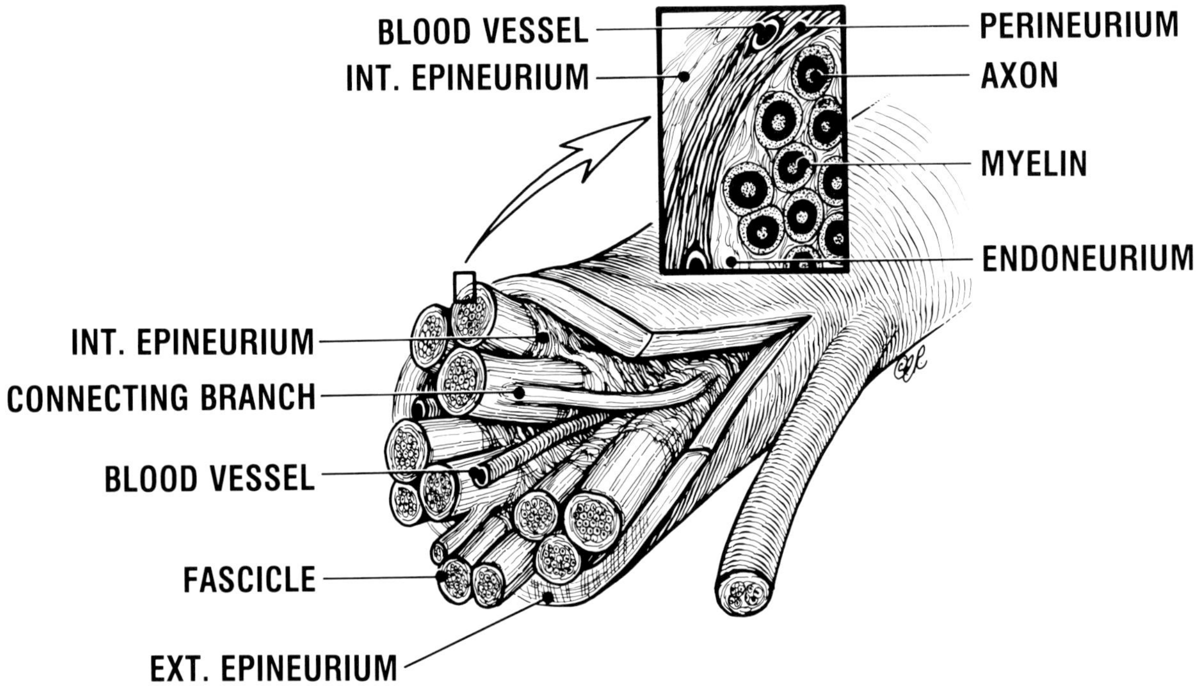

Figure 14–3. *Internal anatomy of a peripheral nerve. Epineurium, both internal and external, is the correct plane of dissection. The smallest unit of surgical significance is the fascicle, bounded by its perineurium. Groups of fascicles can be dissected, sutured, and joined by grafts, as indicated, as long as the perineurium is not damaged. (From Jabaley ME. Peripheral nerve repair. In: May JW Jr, Littler JW, eds. Plastic surgery: The hand. Philadelphia: WB Saunders, 1990:4760, with permission.)*

types: internal and external (or epifascicular). Epineurium is also primarily collagen, but it is looser and more areolar in nature than perineurium and it contains larger blood vessels. It also contains many fibroblasts. Epineurium both ensheathes the entire nerve and lies between the fascicles, where it blends with their perineurium. Epineurium is the preferred layer for suture placement in nerve repair.

From a practical standpoint, the significance of these nerve components is that the epifascicular and internal epineurium can be incised or excised as necessary without impairing nerve conduction. The epineurium contains many of the larger blood vessels that nourish the nerve and also provides the fibroblasts that produce much of the collagen in neuroma formation. Epineurium, when it is used in repair, holds suture well.

In contrast to the epineurium, the perineurium is a critical boundary and should be protected, both in dissection and in suturing. Injury to the perineurium results in a localized conduction block, at the very least. For example, sutures passed through the perineurium are likely to jeopardize conduction by those fibers in the immediate vicinity of the suture track. Presumably, surgical injury produces the same effect. For these reasons, perineural suturing should be carefully considered, if not avoided altogether. (Perineural sutures may be necessary if a single fascicle is being sutured, but they are unnecessary in group fascicular repair.) Thus, in both dissection and suturing, the principal reason for avoiding perineural injury is to avoid injury to the internal milieu, the conducting portion of the nerve.

At present, it is unlikely that surgeons will directly manipulate those structures that lie within the perineurium. Thus, the smallest identifiable unit for operative repair is the fascicle and its surrounding perineurium (Fig. 14-4). This is the structure that is correctly aligned in nerve repair. Once accurate alignment is achieved, it is main-

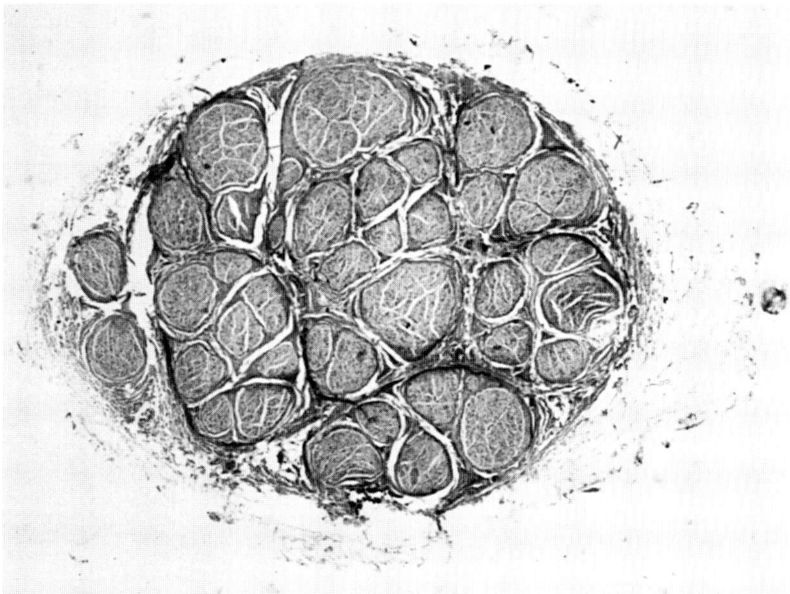

Figure 14–4. *Cross section of a peripheral nerve. The fascicles can be seen both individually and in bundles. Each fascicle is bounded by perineurium, the structure that defines it and that contains the conducting portion of the nerve. Epineurium, both internal and external, can be seen around and between the groups of fascicles. A well-formed branch consisting of two fascicles can be seen at the periphery in the 9 o'clock position.*

tained in the simplest way with the fewest number of sutures and the least amount of additional trauma. By extrapolating from a graph of the number of sutures and thread diameters used in recent years, it becomes apparent that nerve repair will soon use no sutures. Since 1950, suture material has diminished in size from 4-0 and 5-0 to 10-0 and 11-0 on 50- to 75-μm needles, and correspondingly fewer sutures are placed. In fact, suturing may well be disappearing, as the interest in tubulation suggests. The question that remains is whether tubulation will find a role in complex human nerves. In nerve repairs of the future, it may turn out that a certain number of sutures for alignment purposes will always be necessary.

NERVE FUNCTION

The function of nerve fibers, both afferent and efferent, is to conduct impulses. Conduction is primarily a chemical process that can be measured electrically; its velocity increases directly with increases in nerve fiber diameter and myelin thickness. Thus, myelinated nerves conduct impulses faster than unmyelinated ones. These differences serve as the basis for measurable action potentials and for sensory conduction times and motor latency measurements. Such measurements are useful in evaluating injury in intact nerves as well as in compression syndromes.

Conduction in individual fibers and fascicles may be impaired or slowed by a variety of processes. Chief among these (and best studied) are compression and segmental demyelination, but increasing degrees of physical disruption and complete transection produce changes as well. The variation in these degrees of injury is the basis for the schemes of classification developed by Seddon, Sunderland, and others. Each classification is based on an understanding of internal anatomy and the injury that different structures sustain. It is important to consider that not all fibers suffer the same degree of injury in stretch or avulsion injuries. In missile wounds, fractures, and other similar injury mechanisms, the clinical picture of recovery may be a very mixed (and sometimes confusing) one. The reader is referred to Chapter 7 for details on classification of nerve injury.

RECENT STUDIES

Sunderland's studies, culminating in his publications in the mid-1940s, describe each individual nerve in the extremities and its branches.[8] In these studies, cross sections were examined and the changes in fascicular arrangement documented. Sunderland concluded that the longest section of any nerve with a constant pattern was only 15 mm. He noted, however, that specific bundles or groups of bundles often traversed longer distances with minimal or no change in their positions relative to the overall nerve.

To determine what the practical importance of this information might be, laboratory investigation of internal topography was performed in the late 1970s.[4] Using techniques similar to Sunderland's, we harvested the major peripheral nerves from the upper extremities of fresh autopsy specimens, placed a labeling suture on the superficial surface, identified and labeled all branches, and divided the nerve into blocks 1.0 cm long. These blocks were then serially sectioned, stained, and examined microscopically. The path and location of individual branches were noted as they entered the main trunk, and each branch was followed as far proximally as it could be identified. In this way, we determined exactly when and where branches merged with other fascicles and, equally importantly, what their position was relative to the rest of the nerve trunk.

We obtained further information from fresh autopsy material in which in situ identification of branches was followed by microdissection of each branch. In these dissections, the epineurium was incised and the bundles separated at magnifications of 5× to 15×, noting the point where fusion with adjacent fascicles occurred. Merging of fascicles is easy to see, even with relatively low magnification, but small filamentous connections (the function of which is unknown) are difficult to see. The distance between the original entry point of a branch and its fusion with other fascicles is termed the *dissection distance,* the distance within a nerve that a fascicle can be dissected without transecting identifiable interconnections, large or small (Fig. 14-5).

Dissection distances, important when a major branch is being separated for identification and possible suture, have been defined by many authors. They vary from patient to patient and even between sides in the same individual. Dissection distances should serve only as guides, not as absolute values. Similar studies by other authors have confirmed these observations.[2,10–12]

Using these techniques, the three major forearm

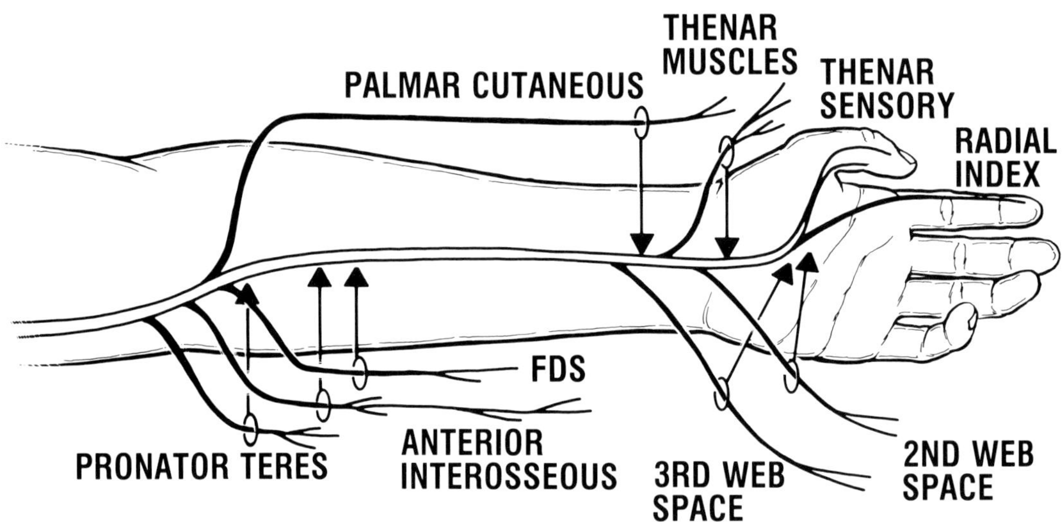

Figure 14–5. *Dissection distances in a human median nerve. The ring encircling each branch indicates the point of its original exit from the nerve trunk. The darkened area is the distance that each branch can be separated from the rest of the nerve trunk without division of interconnections. This is called the* dissection distance. *This distance varies with each branch and ranges from a few millimeters to several centimeters, a point of surgical significance in the repair of transected nerves. (From Jabaley ME, Wallace WH, Heckler FR. Internal topography of major nerves of the forearm and hand: A current view. J Hand Surg 1980;5:18, with permission.)*

nerves (median, ulnar, and radial) were dissected proximally from midpalm to above the elbow. Observations are described as they occurred in each major nerve.

Median Nerve

The sensory branches from the thumb, index and long fingers, and half of the ring finger were noted to fuse and form the terminal portion of the median nerve at the level of the distal edge of the transverse carpal ligament. Just proximal to this location, the motor branch also joins the main trunk. It usually enters from the radial side and assumes a palmar position, from which it gradually enters the substance of the nerve. The dissection distance for the motor branch (the distance over which it could be identified and freed without transecting any crossing branches) was about 70 mm, or about 30 mm proximal to the radial styloid. Individual sensory branches could be separated from one another over shorter, more variable distances. This means that a median nerve divided at the wrist level can be positively identified and separated distally into motor and sensory components, allowing separate repair of these units.

Proceeding proximally, the palmar cutaneous branch (PCN) of the median nerve sometimes arises singly and sometimes as two separate branches of one fascicle each. These always originate from the radial side of the median nerve, usually 2 to 3 cm proximal to the radial styloid. The serial sections showed clearly that the palmar cutaneous branches remained discrete and well localized proximal to this location for an additional 3 cm before they began to merge with other fascicles in the median nerve. The PCN can be separated when injured and repaired separately. This is not difficult in the distal forearm.

Proximal to the PCN was a long segment of the median nerve from which no branches were seen in most cases. The cross-sectional diameter of the nerve decreased as the connective tissue portion diminished; it became more circular and consisted mostly of fascicles over this region. This zone is characterized by a changing cross-sectional pattern; presumably the main purpose of these changes is to sort fibers into quadrants from which they will exit ultimately as the specific named terminal branches. Although the cross-sectional appearance is variable, there is reason to expect that functional units do not change their relative positions very much.

The next zone of significance in the median nerve is in the upper forearm, below the elbow. Here, the anterior interosseous nerve arises and branches to other extrinsic flexors originate. This occurred in the proximal third of the forearm in all cases studied, and the anterior interosseous nerve remained discrete and identifiable all the way to the level of the elbow, a distance of over 6 cm. In addition, branches to the flexor digitorum profundus, flexor digitorum superficialis, and pronator teres could be identified. They usually could be traced only for short distances within the nerve before intermingling with other fascicles. Above the elbow, no significant branches from the median nerve were noted, and dissections were terminated at this level. With median nerve transections in the proximal forearm, the anterior interosseous nerve is identified and repaired separately.

Ulnar Nerve

The anatomical simplicity of the ulnar nerve in the upper arm and forearm belies its complex function in the distal limb. Primarily a motor nerve, it provides branches to muscles at both the elbow and hand levels and is the major innervator of both power grip and pinch strength. Its two sensory branches take leave in the distal forearm and wrist. The main trunk terminates at Guyon's canal, where it divides into deep motor branch and sensory portions. From an operative standpoint, there are several anatomical points of interest.

The sensory portion of the ulnar nerve supplies the ulnar borders of the palm and small finger and the ring–little finger web space, where the common digital nerve branches proceed as proper digital nerves to the adjacent sides of the ring and little fingers. The two common digital nerves join in the proximal palm but remain clearly separable for an average of 26 mm within the main sensory trunk, reaching proximal to Guyon's canal. The sensory trunk, in turn, joins the deep motor component in Guyon's canal, and both proceed proximally as a single nerve. *The motor portion quickly comes to occupy a dorsoulnar position and remains clearly separable from the sensory component for about 80 mm.* This is one of the clearest and most distinct separations seen in a major nerve trunk, a particularly significant point since this zone is a common site of injury. This means that in ulnar nerve transections, motor and sensory components can clearly and easily be identified in the distal forearm and wrist, and they can and should be sutured individually.

The next branch of significance to join the ulnar nerve is the dorsal cutaneous branch. This branch is sensory to a variable territory over the dorsum of the ring and little metacarpals and their proximal phalanges. This branch is not considered a true branch, but rather a separate nerve traveling with the trunk of the ulnar nerve proper: investigators have consistently found this nerve to be clearly separable without interconnections for 170 mm to over 200 mm, a distance reaching nearly to the elbow.

There are several ramifications of this observation. First, the dorsal cutaneous nerve can be dissected away from the branches to the hand and repaired separately, minimizing chances for a mismatch. This maneuver, in turn, simplifies the anatomy of the remaining portion of the ulnar nerve and increases the likelihood of correct connection. Finally, under certain circumstances, a separation of the dorsal cutaneous branch makes it available as an excellent source for donor nerve grafts. If the ulnar nerve is irreparably damaged proximally or if many donor nerves are required, this maneuver is considered.

At elbow level, several motor branches to the flexor carpi ulnaris and a portion of the flexor digitorum profundus muscles are encountered. These may arise individually or as separate branches from a common trunk. Significantly, they can be separated from the main nerve for distances ranging from 75 mm to 100 mm, well above the elbow joint. Knowledge of these motor branches is important in repairs at the elbow level or in transposition operations for tardy ulnar palsy (cubital tunnel syndrome). With acute transections, branches to the forearm muscles can sometimes be identified for separate repair, although this is virtually impossible if they are small and multiple. Although unusual, such repairs can be valuable because the distance from injury to target muscles is relatively short and the likelihood of recovery is high. Repair at this level is well worth attempting whenever branches can be located. Finally, understanding motor branch anatomy is also useful in ulnar nerve transposition operations, where motor branches can be separated if necessary from the main trunk of the nerve without fear of injury.

Radial Nerve

Unlike the median and ulnar nerves (which continue to the hand), the radial nerve terminates in the proximal forearm as two main branches: the posterior interosseous and superficial radial nerves. The former is predominantly a motor nerve; the latter is a sensory nerve supplying a variable portion of the dorsum of the thumb, thenar web, and index and long rays. Along with the dorsal cutaneous branch of the ulnar nerve, it supplies the entire dorsum of the hand.

In the region of the lateral elbow, the terminal radial nerve is separated proximally into its two important branches for a distance of 70 to 90 mm, reaching a level at the junction of the middle and lower thirds of the upper arm. The significance of this observation in nerve repair is clear, where appropriate connections of motor and sensory components is mandatory. In nerve grafting situations, an understanding of the topographic composition of the radial nerve is also critical, because its distal portion can be easily separated into motor and sensory portions and connected by interfascicular grafts. Proceeding proximally in the nerve, the distinctions are less clear, but even here specific functional units have been shown to lie in the same quadrant for considerable distances. At upper arm levels, awake stimulation (see Chap. 15) can sometimes be valuable in determining functional capability. Without this technique, the surgeon must rely on Sunderland's topographic maps and make his or her best clinical guess. Functional recovery after radial nerve repair is often quite good, due in part to the smaller number of fascicles and their correspondingly larger size.

Lower Extremities

In our studies,[4] and those of other hand surgeons, the topographic anatomy of lower extremity nerves has not been defined, but Sunderland's complete works include such a study.[9] In his works, the lower extremity nerves were found to behave in a similar fashion to those in the upper extremity. The interested reader is directed to this and other publications for more specific information.

DISCUSSION

Most peripheral nerves, whether motor or sensory, arise from more than one level of the spinal cord. As they exit the spinal cord and enter the major plexuses, fibers bound for a specific muscle or sensory territories are initially distributed widely within many bundles. A sorting process then begins in which fibers from multiple origins are progressively gathered into specific bundles and named branches destined for specific muscles or sensory territories. As this convergence occurs, fibers first migrate toward specific nerves, then into fascicular bundles within nerves, and finally into branches. In this process of segregation, fibers move from one fascicle to another as they progress distally toward their destination. This movement of fibers from one fascicle to another is through well-recognized interconnections. Other than their obvious importance in the sorting process, the significance of these interconnections is unknown and has not been studied in detail.

Dissection of branches within and proximal to their points of exit from the main trunk of a nerve is feasible and practical. Such dissection is always within the epifascicular and internal epineurium. As long as interconnections are not divided, injury is avoided. The exact distance over which a branch may be separated (its dissection distance) varies considerably. Depending on the nerve and level in question, it may be as short as a few millimeters and as long as 200 mm. An appreciation of this fact allows the surgeon to make such identification and separation as is necessary in a specific clinical situation. This can be very valuable in planning repair or grafting procedures.

To dissect within a nerve, the surgeon acquires both the anatomical knowledge of that particular nerve's composition and the technical skill to perform the procedure. This latter requires optical magnification and microinstruments. With practice, dissection is performed speedily with relatively low magnification (4–6×) and with commonly available instruments. I prefer to dissect within the epineurium with a surgical knife, using a #15 blade and a "feathering" technique. With slight traction, the epineurium is easily separated without damaging the perineurium. The side of the blade actually lies against perineurium while the edge cuts the epineurium. Very little force is required, often little more than that provided by the weight of the knife. This technique seems less traumatic than the spreading of scissors (although I sometimes do this too), which always produces some stretching of fascicles. Scissors, by their nature, must either spread (stretch) tissue or shear it, and both of these maneuvers can be dangerous within a nerve.

Several investigations over many years confirm the observation that the natural state of peripheral nerves is to contain fascicles and bundles located in plexuses. These are more obvious in the proximal nerves where fiber segregation and localization occur than in the distal portions, where branches are more or less formed and ready for exit from the main trunk. Fibers pursue a localized course in a nerve for even longer than can be appreciated by the dissection distances described. In other words, although the cross-sectional pattern and the fascicular makeup changes from level to level, fibers continue onward in approximately the same quadrantic location within the nerve. This is a functional, not an anatomical, observation. Thus, in nerve grafting operations, gaps can be bridged between appropriate quadrants of a nerve over considerable distances with the expectation that some degree of recovery is still possible. As Sunderland noted, fibers "scatter gradually" and, even with some intermingling of fibers, "remain in the same quadrant over long distances."

It is unknown how many fibers must successfully regenerate, bridge a gap, and enter a distal nerve for useful function to occur. We know that axon sprouting after injury provides a large number of potential fibers; it appears that the number of correct connections is more important than the overall number of anatomical connections. Because we cannot say with certainty to what degree neurotrophic and neuronotrophic factors are at work in human nerves, for the present our greatest hope lies in using our knowledge of topographic anatomy to produce the most nearly correct anatomical alignment possible while inflicting the least amount of additional trauma by operative dissection and suturing.

REFERENCES

1. Bunge MB, Wood PM, Tynan LB, Bates ML, Sanes JR. Perineurium originates from fibroblasts: Demonstration in vitro with a retroviral marker. Science 1989; 243:229–231.
2. Chow JA, Van Beek AL, Meyer DL, Johnson MC. Surgical significance of the motor fascicular group of the ulnar nerve in the forearm. J Hand Surg [Am] 1985; 10:867–872.
3. Compton AT. The intrinsic anatomy of the large nerve trunks of limbs. J Anat 1917; 51:103.
4. Jabaley ME, Wallace WH, Heckler FR. Internal topography of major nerves of the forearm and hand: A current view. J Hand Surg 1980; 5:1–18.
5. Langley JN, Hashimoto M. On the suture of separate bundles in a nerve trunk and on internal nerve plexuses. J Physiol 1917; 51:318–345.
6. McKinley JC. The intraneural plexus of fasciculi and fibers in the sciatic nerve. Arch Neurol Psych 1921; 6:377–399.
7. Millesi H, Terzis JK. Problems of terminology in peripheral nerve surgery. Microsurgery 1983; 4: 51–56.
8. Sunderland S. The interneural topography of the radial, median, and ulnar nerves. Brain 1945; 68: 243–298.
9. Sunderland S. Nerves and nerve injuries, ed 2. Edinburgh: Churchill-Livingstone, 1971:925–1010.
10. Tamura K. The funicular pattern of Japanese peripheral nerves. Nippon Geka Hokan 1969; 38:35–58.
11. Williams HB. Peripheral nerve injuries in children. In: Kernahan D, Thompson HG, Bauer B, eds. Pediatric plastic surgery. St. Louis: CV Mosby, 1982: 266.
12. Williams HB, Jabaley ME. The importance of internal anatomy of the peripheral nerves to nerve repair in the forearm and hand. Hand Clin 1986; 2:689–707.

15

Electrical Nerve Stimulation in the Awake Patient

Michael E. Jabaley

AUTHOR'S KEY POINTS

- Current techniques of sedation and an intravenous lidocaine block permit adequate anesthesia for the dissection and mobilization of a peripheral nerve while still allowing immediate and complete dissolution of the anesthetic when desired.
- After a brief period to recover from ischemia, a peripheral nerve in an awake patient can be electrically stimulated and the patient's response noted.
- Using commonly available equipment, nerve stimulation in the awake patient is used to distinguish between motor and sensory fascicles and to further separate sensory fascicles on the basis of their cutaneous territories.
- In the distal forearm and wrist, the area where injuries to mixed nerves most commonly occur, electrical stimulation permits identification of specific nerve components and increases the likelihood of correct alignment of fascicles.

The relative position of the two ends of a nerve that is being repaired is critical if there is to be any hope of correct axonal regrowth. Because the focus of peripheral nerve surgery has shifted from whole nerve repair to group fascicular (or sometimes individual fascicular) suture, the challenge to determine the correct rotational orientation is greater than ever before.

During and immediately after World War II, the acceptable practice of nerve repair was *whole nerve suture*, in which epineural sutures were used to join the ends. During that period, immediate repair of sharply transected nerves, where possible, came to be the practice; external markings, such as blood vessels in the epineurium, were the basis for orientation. In preparation for nerve suture, the surgeon selected a prominent vessel or other landmark in the epineurium of each segment and placed a key stitch at this point to align the ends. The technique was, in effect, a whole nerve repair. Because the internal components of the nerve remained undisturbed, this approach more or less committed the surgeon to a specified rotational arrangement for the remainder of the repair. Unfortunately, we now know that this method does not always provide accurate alignment or prevent malrotation, particularly in mixed motor and sensory nerves.

In succeeding years, when surgeons' interest shifted to the smaller bundles and fascicles of nerves for both repair and grafting, the need arose for more specific identification of each fascicular group. At least two forces appear to have been responsible for the reassessment of internal identification. First, interest in *fascicular nerve repair* was heightened in the 1950s, even though it had been suggested before then. Second, *interfascicular nerve grafting* became popular in the 1970s, and correct fascicular identification took on more practical importance.

Both techniques had important differences from previous methods of external epineural suture. Unlike external epineural suture, where the first stitch determines the alignment for the entire nerve, fascicular dissection specifically allows for identification and reattachment of each individual fascicle or group of fascicles within a nerve segment. Because of this internal separation, more choices are presented and more potential sources for error exist. Thus, precise information is necessary if correct coaptation is to follow.

There are at least four specific techniques for fascicular identification, each with advantages and disadvantages. To date, no one technique has been generally accepted; indeed, it is probable that many surgeons perform nerve suture intuitively, without relying specifically on any of the four methods to be described. Nevertheless, it is generally agreed that accurate fascicular alignment is mandatory in the repair of a transected human nerve if there is to be any hope of restoring function, and correct fascicular identification remains a goal.

Direct Inspection

The simplest method for determining correct fascicular alignment is by *direct inspection*. In the immediate repair of a sharply transected nerve, the surgeon often sees the nerve ends as mirror images of each other and has only to reapproximate them in what appears to be the obvious position. This technique usually works, especially in relatively simple nerves (ie, those with few fascicles). Other methods are required only in untidy wounds where nerve ends must be trimmed, in injuries requiring secondary repairs, or in situations where there has been significant loss of nerve tissue and large gaps exist.

Cross-Sectional Mapping

If any of the above conditions is present, the next simplest approach used for topographic orientation is based on information available from Sunderland's classic *cross-sectional maps*.[12] By using serial transverse sections, Sunderland and other authors who have repeated his work produced cross-sectional drawings of the major nerves of both the upper and lower extremity, identifying specific functional units and noting their locations. To produce these maps, histologic sections of nerves were examined and drawings made of the cross section at specific locations relative to a fixed anatomical landmark, such as the radial styloid at the wrist.

In these serial mappings, individual branches are noted as they enter the main nerve trunk and are followed as far as they can be identified. By examining a cross section of a nerve at a specific level, the surgeon can then relate a specific branch to other fascicles, to a quadrant of the nerve, and to an external surface of the nerve, such as palmar or dorsal, radial or ulnar. Using these drawings, the surgeon can make a reasonable guess as to what quadrant the fibers that make up a particular branch are likely to occupy at some other level. This allows a reasonably correct anatomical connection and, theoretically, better results than could be obtained simply by guessing.

Sunderland emphasized three points in his works:

1. Branches can be identified and dissected for varying distances within a nerve, and individual fascicles can be separated for even greater distances.

2. Function-specific fascicles remain identifiable within the nerve trunk for distances of a few millimeters.
3. Even though the cross-sectional pattern changes constantly and a gradual diffusion of fibers among other fascicles occurs as one proceeds proximally in a nerve, function is likely to remain localized in specific quadrants for even greater distances.

In other words, even though the fascicular makeup may vary in number, location, and orientation, functional elements follow a reasonably consistent course. Although relatively imprecise, cross-sectional maps may be helpful when other techniques cannot provide specific information about functional location.

Histologic Staining

Histologic staining of individual fascicles has been available for some time and continues to have its proponents (see Chap. 16). In principle, the technique is quite attractive: a transverse slice of a nerve is obtained and stained differentially for its motor or sensory elements. Stains usually are specific for a particular enzyme. With staining, the composition of a specific fascicle can be determined and the appropriate connection made between it and a similar one in the opposite nerve end.

Earlier techniques stained whole sections of nerve for acetylcholinesterase activity.[5] In the earlier method, the essential difference is the staining of myelinated fibers. In motor fascicles, about half of the myelinated fibers stain and thus can be identified; in sensory fascicles, almost all the myelinated fibers remain unstained. The disadvantage of this technique is that is takes 2 to 3 days to prepare the sections, thus requiring the attendant risk, expense, and inconvenience of a two-stage nerve repair.

Efforts to find more rapid techniques led to the use of the enzyme choline acetylase as a marker.[1,2] Choline acetylase is normally synthesized in the nerve cell body and transported by axoplasmic flow to the nerve terminals. Radioactive acetyl-CoA activity is a measure of its presence. The test can be performed in 1 to 2 hours. The disadvantage of this technique is that individual fascicles or groups of fascicles must be separated and studied. Further, the activity of choline acetylase declines rapidly after injury, and identification in the distal stump is impossible after 3 to 4 days.

Another enzyme, carbonic anhydrase, has also been used as a marker.[11] It distinguishes dorsal sensory root axons from ventral motor root axons and has been proposed as another enzymatic method. Again, this method requires separation of individual fascicles for analysis and takes 3 to 4 hours for tissue processing.

In all of these staining methods, a cross section or part of a cross section of a nerve is analyzed for a marker, and the information gained is used for identification purposes. Thus, a portion of the nerve ends must be removed for study. This requires the assistance of personnel outside the operating room and means, at best, a delay for analysis of data and, at worst, two separate operations.

As noted, there are attractive features to this approach, but in practice the technique of histologic staining has proven more difficult to use. In the earlier techniques, the staining process took several hours to complete, requiring two operations. In the first operation, the nerve ends were dissected out, labeled, and cross-sectional slices obtained. The wound was then closed while the laboratory investigation was completed. A second operation was then necessary to join the identified nerve ends. In addition to the time consumed and the duplication of effort and expense of anesthesia and operating room time, the method also posed technical problems. Cutting and recutting the nerve ends shortened the trunks, magnifying the problems associated with tension.

Newer techniques have shortened the working time, minimizing many of the problems, but histologic staining still cannot distinguish between specific sensory territories and gives no insight into functional importance. As more is learned about the use of stains, the technique undoubtedly will continue to improve. Its role and value remain to be determined.

Electrical Stimulation and Recording

Perhaps the greatest innovations in functional evaluation of nerves have occurred with the development of computers, microprocessors, and improved nerve stimulators.[13] These devices have offered new possibilities and made *electrical stimulation and recording* a reality. In this approach (and the technique to be described), low-voltage electrical current is applied to various locations of a cut nerve end. Positive identifications are made that are, in turn, used for anatomical suturing. In the child, a sleeping patient, or an otherwise uncooperative candidate, stimulation and recording can give valuable information available by no other method. Similarly, conduction is measured and quantified in the intact or partially damaged nerve, and decisions can be made as to whether to resect a neuroma or perform a neurolysis.

But such sophisticated equipment, and the expertise necessary to use it, is unavailable in most operating rooms; when such stimulations are performed and recorded, interpreting them remains problematic. The technique seems most valuable in examining the in-continuity neuroma or in stimulating a specific branch of an intact nerve (see Chap. 42). It is less valuable in matching the ends of a divided nerve. For these reasons, sophisticated electrical stimulation is still not widely used.

Of all the techniques available, only *electrical stimulation in the awake patient* allows positive identification of motor and sensory fascicles in a proximal nerve end and associates them with specific distal territories.[8] In this method, the human brain is used as a computer to encode, sort, and collate data, rather than relying on external (and relatively crude) hardware. The potential advantages in terms of expense, time, and reliability are enormous. Information has been accumulated as surgeons have attempted to use variations of this technique for the past 20 to 30 years.

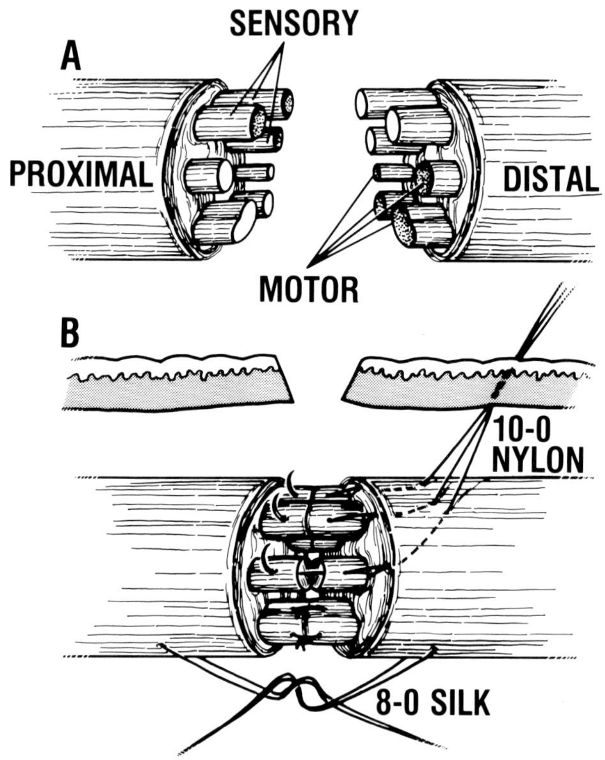

Figure 15–1. *Stimulation in an early repair of a transected mixed nerve. Proximal nerve end is to the reader's left. The upper figure shows a drawing of the proximal end in which the sensory endings (dark shading) have been positively identified. Stimulation of the lighter areas elicits no response. In the distal end, stimulation of the presumed motor bundles (dark shading) produces muscle contraction, while stimulation of the presumed sensory bundles is silent.*

In the lower figure, fascicular repair is performed by pull-out sutures of 10-0 nylon passed successively through skin and subcutaneous tissue, epineurium, and individual fascicles. The repair is splinted by 8-0 silk sutures in the external epineurium. (From Harris R. J Bone Joint Surg [Am] 1968;50:1178, with permission.)

TECHNIQUE OF NERVE STIMULATION IN THE AWAKE PATIENT

History

The literature describing awake stimulation is not extensive. Much of the early credit for this technique goes to Harris, who also is known as Hakstian (Fig. 15-1).[6] Later proponents, such as Gaul[3,4]; Vandeput, Tanner, and Huypens[14]; Nakatsuchi, Matsui, and Handa[10]; and Jabaley,[8] varied the technical details without altering the principle. Thus, the technique to be described has been in practice for over 20 years.

The method that I use takes advantage of modern techniques of sedation and anesthesia. Since the success of awake stimulation depends on its careful application, the technique will be described in detail; Table 15-1 presents a quick overview. The reader should appreciate that this is an evolving technique and that specific drugs and details

Table 15–1. *Outline for Awake Stimulation*

I. Preoperative counseling
 A. Outline anesthetic procedure
 B. Explain sedation
 C. Agree on nomenclature
II. Sedation, preoperative and intraoperative
 A. All medications are administered intravenously
  1. Versed, 5 mm IM preop, then 1.0-mg increments IV
  2. Sublimaze, analgesic of choice, 0.25 mL IV as necessary
III. IV lidocaine (Bier block) anesthetic
 A. Lidocaine 0.5%, without epinephrine
 B. 50–60 mL IV
IV. Tourniquet (two cuffs preferred)
 A. Setting at 80–100 mm Hg above systolic pressure
 B. Alternate cuffs as necessary
V. Timing
 A. 8–10 min required before beginning dissection
 B. 25–30 min tourniquet time with first cuff
 C. 30–45 min with second cuff
VI. Surgical dissection
 A. Identify transected nerve ends
 B. Trim nerve ends if necessary
 C. Draw maps of cut nerve ends
 D. Insert marking sutures for orientation
 E. Infiltrate subdermal plexus with bupivacaine 15 min before tourniquet deflation
VII. Deflate tourniquets
 A. Elevate and apply pressure for 8–10 min
 B. Cauterize remaining bleeding vessels
VIII. Nerve stimulation
 A. Start at low setting (0.3 mA)
 B. Increase voltage until patient perceives tingling
 C. Label proximal end fascicles as sensory or motor
 D. Stimulate distal ends where possible (3–4 days postinjury)
 E. Select bundles and fascicles for coaptation
IX. Completion of procedure
 A. Locally anesthetize nerve or switch to general anesthesia
 B. Proceed with repair or graft

will vary, not only with surgeon and geographic location but also with time and experience.

Preoperative Counseling

Preoperative counseling is extremely important and is carried out by either the surgeon or someone else who will be present at the operation. Ideally, the counseling session takes place 1 or more days before surgery, and more than once if possible. The procedure does not work as well when the subject is broached for the first time in the preoperative area, as the patient may be injured, sedated, or frightened (or all three).

First, the patient is reassured that the surgery can be performed comfortably and that he or she will have no pain. For many patients, this will be their first experience with both anesthesia and sedatives. The technique of intravenous lidocaine anesthesia (Bier block) is described in detail, since it may also be new to the patient. The patient is told that he or she will lose not only sensation but also proprioception. Sensation will return to sensory territories upon tourniquet deflation, but there will be no pain in the field of dissection.

The technique of stimulation is also described. The patient is assured that the procedure will not be painful and is told that he or she may feel nothing at some times or a light shock or tingling at others. The sensation will seem to arise from a specific area of the hand or a finger, and the purpose of the test is to determine which part of the nerve the patient associates with each area of the hand.

Finally, the surgeon and patient agree on a common terminology. It is important to know what the patient calls each digit and specific areas in the palm, as well as the radial and ulnar side of each digit. Often, the patient has no specific name for an area, such as the thenar or hypothenar eminences, and the surgeon should be prepared to suggest something. Three identifiable levels are necessary: the fingertips, the remainder of the finger, and the palm and muscle eminences.

Premedication and Sedation

There are two goals of the medications. First, the patient must be comfortable. Unfortunately, most operating rooms and operating tables are not designed with patient comfort in mind, and room temperature, the hardness of the operating table, extraneous noises, and the general atmosphere all detract from the success of the technique. These can be partly, but not completely, overcome by the careful use of sedation. Second, the well-medicated patient is better able to tolerate tourniquet ischemia and the high level of anxiety associated with awake surgery.

Our current drug choices are a short-acting narcotic such as Sublimaze and a sedative such as Versed. The surgeon may administer these, but we prefer to have an anesthetist or an anesthesiologist do so. This provides an experienced person who is concerned primarily with carefully monitoring the patient for signs of respiratory depression. More importantly, this person titrates the patient's medication to the appropriate level and anticipates the time of tourniquet deflation so that the patient is awake and ready to respond at the appropriate time. We routinely follow blood pressure, pulse, electrocardiogram, and tissue oxygenation. Most importantly, the level of wakefulness is carefully observed.

A single dose of Versed (5 mg in healthy young patients) given 30 minutes before the procedure gives a reliable estimate of the amount of sedative that will be necessary subsequently. If the patient arrives in the operating room placid and drowsy, small additional increments are usually adequate. If the patient is still fully awake, larger doses are necessary. In either event, Versed is best given in 1-mg increments, and the patient's response is carefully observed.

Use of the Tourniquet

The initial dissection with tourniquet ischemia is always a race against the clock. Every effort is made to ensure as long a period of comfortable tourniquet ischemia as possible. Several factors prolong tourniquet time:

1. An unpadded tourniquet or one lightly padded with cast padding is inadequate and should be avoided. I have found that a foam-rubber padding 1.0 to 1.5 cm thick increases patient comfort and prolongs tourniquet time.[7] Although we have not injected local anesthesia into the subcutaneous tissue beneath the cuff when applying a Bier block, we have done this with axillary blocks, and it is also an effective way to increase tourniquet tolerance. This technique blocks the axillary and intercostobrachial as well as other skin nerves.
2. So-called "double cuff" tourniquets, in which two inflatable bands are contained within a single tourniquet, are unsatisfactory. The balloon portion of each band is relatively narrow when both are contained within a single tourniquet, and a correspondingly higher pressure is required to produce arterial occlusion. This greatly reduces tourniquet tolerance and probably increases the possibility of nerve injury, since nerve compression is a function of cuff width and pressure. I use two 4-inch-wide cuffs, applied one above the other and attached to separate monitors.
3. The practice of arbitrarily setting the cuff pressure at the same level for every patient (eg, 300 mm Hg) and leaving it there is anachronistic and dangerous. Modern equipment makes it unnecessary. We find that 80 to 100 mm Hg above the patient's resting systolic pressure is generally adequate for circulatory arrest, although this varies with the shape of the upper arm and other factors. Generally, a thin, cylindrical arm requires a much lower pressure setting than an obese, conical one. Common adult settings are 200 to 225 mm Hg; children require less pressure.

By these measures, we routinely obtain 1.25 to 1.5 hours of comfortable tourniquet time. By alternate inflation of the two cuffs or by using a forearm tourniquet (in appropriate cases), tourniquet time can be extended even longer.

Anesthetic Technique

The patient is brought to a quiet, comfortably warm operating room and placed on the operating table. The back of the table is raised slightly and a pillow placed beneath the knees for comfort. The effect of premedication is carefully estimated, as it serves as a useful clue for judging subsequent doses. All medications are given intravenously, and the patient is monitored for pulse, blood pressure, tissue oxygenation (pulse oximetry), and electrocardiographic tracings.

Careful and complete exsanguination of the limb is accomplished. The effectiveness of the block is greatly enhanced by as tight a wrapping as can be accomplished during exsanguination. To fully empty the venous system, we routinely augment the wrapping with manual compression of the forearm prior to inflation of the cuff. The distal cuff is always inflated first to exsanguinate the area beneath it, and injection is carried out with both cuffs inflated. If there is no evidence of tourniquet leak, the distal cuff is then deflated, allowing the anesthetic to enter the area beneath it, and the procedure is begun with the upper cuff inflated. In this way, the anesthetic agent fills the veins beneath the distal cuff and anesthesia is more profound when this cuff is eventually inflated.

Anesthetic Agents

The drug of choice for intravenous anesthesia is 0.5% plain lidocaine. Although bupivacaine has been used for Bier blocks, in my opinion it is contraindicated for this technique. There is no particular advantage, and there is a potential risk associated with tourniquet leaks. Fifty to sixty milliliters (depending on limb size), well below the toxic level for lidocaine, is administered intravenously. It is important to administer enough volume to dilate the veins. If the surgeon is concerned about the amount of lidocaine required, a 0.4% solution appears to work equally well.

Operative Procedure

As many details as possible are attended to before inflating the tourniquet; for example, incisions are marked in advance, and someone stands ready to prep the extremity. Once the injection is completed and the surgeon has examined the extremity for a brief period to ensure that there is no tourniquet leak, skin preparation proceeds. A plane of surgical anesthesia is obtained in 8 to 10 minutes, more than enough time for prepping and draping the extremity. After administration of the drug, the skin remains blanched and mottled for a period of time, suggesting that the block is taking effect. The upper cuff is usually inflated for 30 or 35 minutes. It is deflated *after* the lower cuff is inflated. This latter is left inflated for 40 to 45 minutes if necessary.

Dissection is performed as quickly as possible. In cases of transection, both nerve ends are located and mobilized and either cleansed or recut. In an immediate repair of a tidy transection, it may be unnecessary to excise the nerve ends; simply washing away any hematoma may be sufficient. If the injury is a crushing or contusing type, the nerve ends are freshened, even though immediate repair is not planned. In secondary cases, of course, this step is mandatory.

While the tourniquet is still inflated, each nerve end is examined, preferably with a microscope, and the surgeon draws a simple cross section, showing the location of major bundles and fascicles and selecting those to be joined. If the external epineurium is to be excised or trimmed back, this is also done at this time. It is wise to place a small marking stitch in the epineurium for later orientation, since nerve ends swell after tourniquet deflation.

Tourniquet Deflation

In preparation for deflation of the tourniquet, the skin and superficial subcutaneous tissue *only* are infiltrated with 0.25% bupivacaine. This is done with a 25-gauge, 1½-inch needle 10 to 15 minutes before deflation. The anesthetic is injected through the wound edges, parallel to and just beneath the deep level of the dermis. In this way, the subdermal plexus is anesthetized, and the patient feels virtually no pain when the pneumatic cuff is deflated. Care is taken not to inject beneath the fascia or into the deeper muscles. *No anesthetic is placed about the nerve to be stimulated.*

After deflation, the extremity is elevated and pressure applied to the wound for several minutes. It takes about 15 minutes after deflation to completely reverse the effects of tourniquet ischemia.[15] By this time, most of the bleeding has stopped and the few remaining vessels of consequence are cauterized. Surprisingly, even cauterization at low settings produces little or no pain. Special care is taken not to cauterize or otherwise traumatize the unanesthetized nerve end, even with the bipolar coagulator. To do so is exquisitely painful and may even result in premature termination of the procedure.

The stimulator is the classical Hilgar nerve stimulator (Fig. 15-2). It has separate autoclavable handles and tips and a variable setting for milliamperage (mA) and frequency as well as separate settings for nerve and muscle. It is chosen because it is readily available in most operating rooms. A hand-held disposable stimulator has also been used,

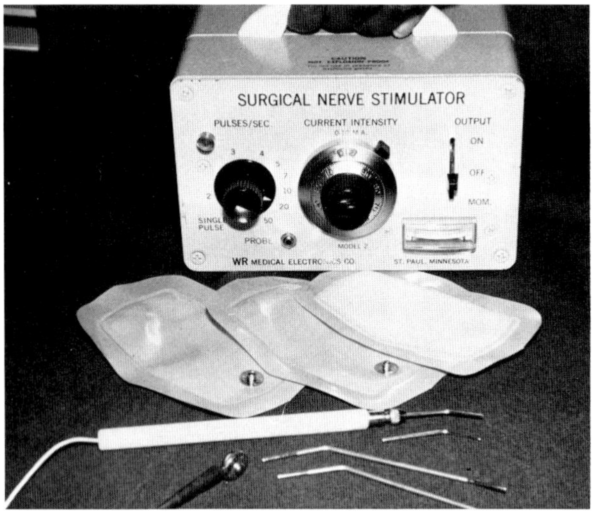

Figure 15–2. *Hilgar nerve stimulator. This instrument is present in most operating rooms and is adequate for nerve stimulation in the awake patient. It allows a variable strength of stimulus intensity and frequency of stimulation. Tips are interchangeable and different sizes and lengths are available. The instrument is relatively inexpensive and simple to use. It is more versatile than disposable stimulators and is adequate for analyzing most peripheral nerve injuries.*

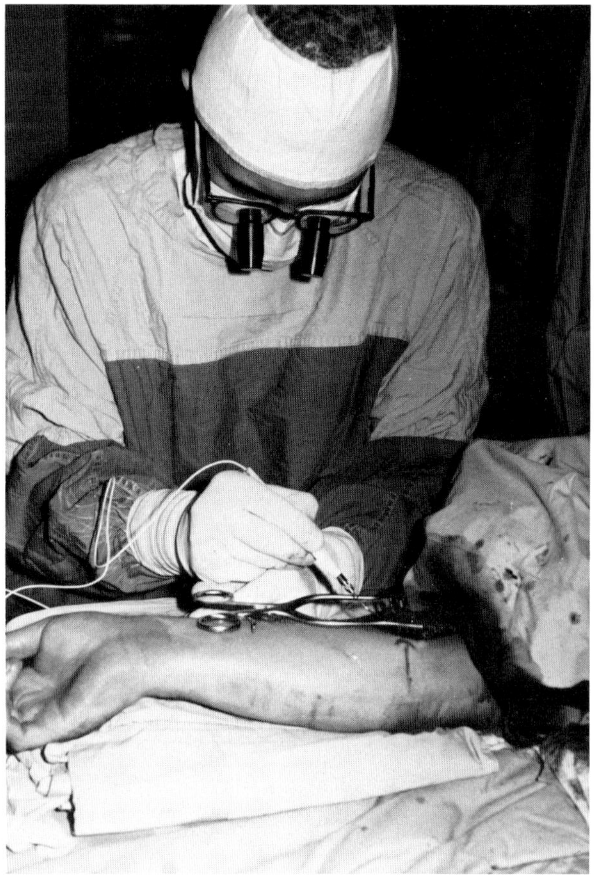

Figure 15–3. *An awake patient undergoing simulated stimulation of a median nerve in the forearm. The surgeon usually performs the stimulation and labels the drawing of the cut end. A nurse or other member of the operating team can vary the settings of the stimulator as necessary. No other technical assistance is required, for either stimulation or analysis.*

but it is limited in range and is not recommended for this purpose.

Stimulation of the nerve ends is carried out in an orderly fashion, beginning at some arbitrary location (such as the marking suture) on the map that has been prepared and proceeding until each bundle or fascicle has been tested (Fig. 15-3). The mA setting on the stimulator is intentionally started low and progressively increased until the patient first detects a tingling sensation. In practice, I usually begin at 0.3 mA, and some patients detect even this low setting. The level is increased to 0.5 to 0.6 mA without discomfort: practically all patients perceive sensation at this level. Even higher settings are used if necessary and are still tolerable.

In the beginning, the patient is asked, "Do you feel anything?" The procedure is repeated at increased settings until the patient answers "yes." The patient is informed that this is the sensation the surgeon is seeking and is then asked to localize it. For example, if the patient says, "That is my index finger," the surgeon might then ask, "Do you feel it at the tip or at the base?" and then, "Is it on the thumb side or the small finger side?" In this fashion, the surgeon systematically notes which bundles produce a motor response and which ones are sensory. This information is recorded on the drawings. Ordinarily, a proximal nerve's sensory fascicles are assigned to specific locations of the palm and digits; some patients can even subdivide these areas.

In acute transections, stimulation of the distal stump is performed as well, since motor responses can be seen for at least 3 to 4 days. More often, nerve reconstructions are secondary procedures, and distal stump stimulation is ineffective. In the acute case, patient cooperation is unnecessary for distal stump stimulation. If a motor response is obtained, the muscle twitch is obvious. If no twitch is seen, the surgeon can presume that the bundle in question is sensory.

If distal nerve stimulation is impossible, as is most often the case, the surgeon resorts to identifying specific named branches (such as the motor branch of the median nerve) and dissecting them proximally. (The information in Chapter 14 on internal topography and dissection distances of branches is helpful in this regard.) Specific named branches are then connected to bundles previously identified in the proximal stump. If this procedure cannot be accomplished, the surgeon must turn to Sunderland's topographic maps, making an appropriate connection by his or her "best clinical guess," as Sunderland recommended. As noted earlier, if dissection of distal branches is part of the operative plan, this is accomplished before the tourniquet is deflated.

A final note of caution: since the nerve, by necessity, is not anesthetized during awake stimulation, it is exquisitely sensitive, and all precautions are taken not to induce pain while handling it. Specifically, rubbing the nerve end with a gauze sponge is extremely painful; a small microsurgical cellulose wipe is preferred. Cautery near the nerve in any form, even with the bipolar coagulator, is painful and is avoided. Topical thrombin can be applied to the nerve end to stop bleeding, but we have found this unnecessary in most cases. When the nerve is picked up or otherwise handled, it is best done with jeweler's forceps applied to the external epineurium.

The entire process of deflation, equilibration time, stimulation, and mapping requires 30 to 45 minutes. Thereafter, the operation is completed using whatever anesthetic the surgeon chooses. General anesthesia is often chosen if a nerve graft is indicated, but a proximal nerve block with a local agent provides adequate anesthesia for direct nerve suture. Upon completion of the nerve stimulation, patients are usually fatigued, so my usual practice is to undertake general anesthesia at this point, a decision they usually welcome.

CLINICAL EXAMPLES

Case 1

Mr. N was injured when a circular saw lacerated his left forearm at the junction of the middle and distal thirds (Fig. 15-4). He was treated in an emergency room by wound cleansing and skin suture and admitted to the hospital. Definitive repair was performed 24 hours later. He suffered complete transection of the median nerve, four flexor tendons (brachioradialis, flexor pollicis longus, palmaris longus, and flexor carpi ulnaris) and the radial artery. All tendons and the artery were repaired at the time of nerve suture.

Initial dissection was performed with a Bier block anesthetic. The median nerve was found to have a high bifurcation (Fig. 15-4*B*, arrows). Stimulation of all fascicles in the radial portion of the distal end resulted in thenar muscle contraction, and they were presumed to be motor fascicles. No fascicles in the ulnar component responded to stimulation, and they were presumed to be sensory. In the proximal nerve stump, specific sensory territories corresponding to the thumb and index and long fingers were identified, as could the palmar cutaneous branch. No specific fascicles were found that were pure motor (ie, there were some sensory fibers in all fascicles). Thus, stimulation was not as beneficial as is sometimes the case.

Nerve repair was performed with three sutures of 6-0 Prolene to create an epineural bridge on the posterior surface, and individual fascicular alignment was obtained with 10-0 nylon on a 50-μm needle.

Three years later, all wounds were healed and tendon function had returned to normal. Sensation was present but impaired; specifically, vibration was present but two-point discrimination was 20 mm. Recovery to the thenar muscles had occurred and was graded as M4, and there was slight wasting. Tinel's sign was still positive at the site of nerve repair. A neurolysis of the repair site was recommended in an attempt to improve sensation, and this was performed about 2 months later. The repair site was examined and a large neuroma noted. It was cautiously trimmed but not divided. The wound healed without incident, and the patient was given a silicone Elastomere pad to wear over his scar in the postoperative period in an effort to further minimize scar formation.

When last seen in follow-up, 2 years and 4 months after neurolysis and 5.5 years after the initial repair, the patient was working at his old job and stated that he had no disability (Fig. 15-5). He had strong recovery of the thenar muscles

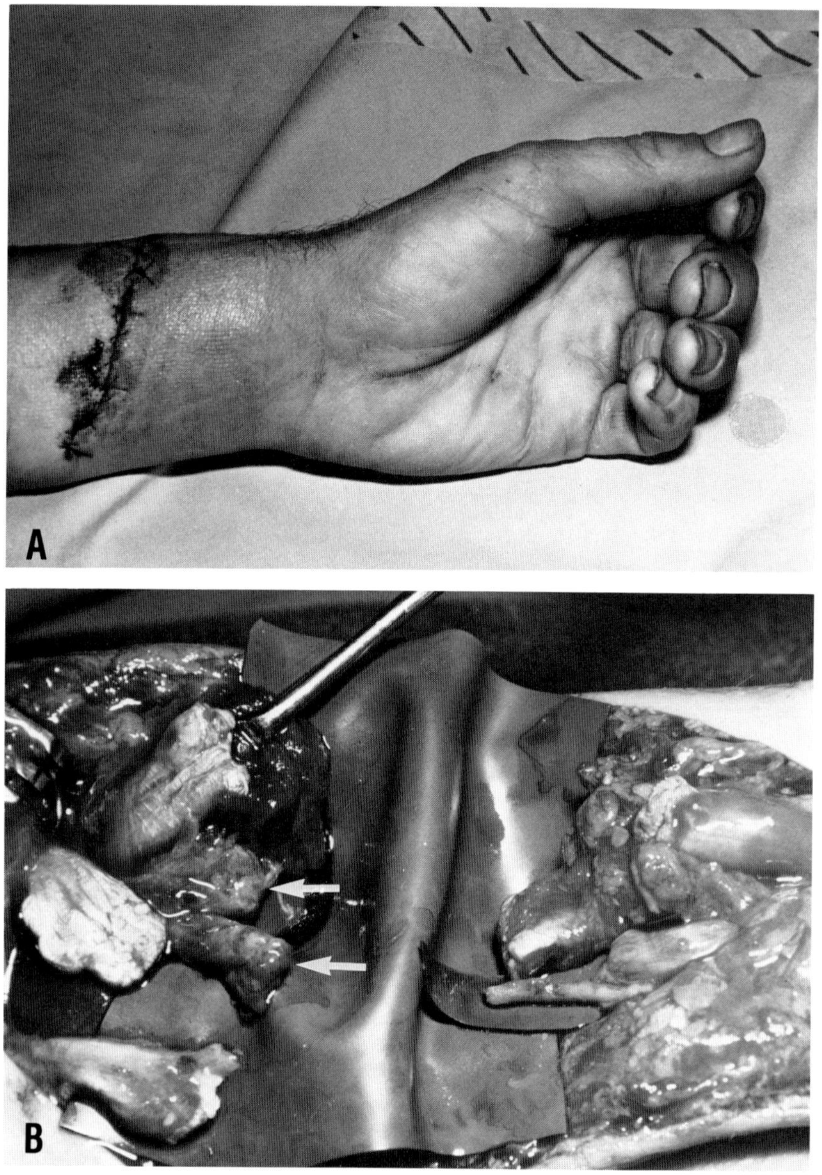

Figure 15-4. *(**A**) Mr. N, age 34, suffered transections of the radial artery, four tendons, and the median nerve 24 hours previously. Awake stimulation was performed. (**B**) Open wound at surgery. High division of proximal end of median nerve (arrows) can be seen.*

and good opposition of the thumb tip. His muscle strength was graded M5. Although he used his thumb and fingers to manipulate small objects and felt that sensation was "very good," he tested poorly. Two-point discrimination remained greater than 20 mm, and his ability to perceive von Frey monofilaments was reduced.

In this case, an anatomical variant of the median nerve was noted at the initial repair whose motor contribution was significantly greater than usual. With awake stimulation, confirmation of this finding allowed appropriate connections of the motor portion of the nerve to be made. Stimulation of the sensory section was not as specific as is usually the case at this level of the forearm, but an anatomical suture was accomplished by visually matching fascicles.

The long-term follow-up confirmed excellent motor recovery, as evidenced by bulk strength and function. The subjective quality of sensation could not be confirmed with clinical testing; the reason for this remains unclear. Although his "academic" test results were poor, he demonstrated excellent performance on the

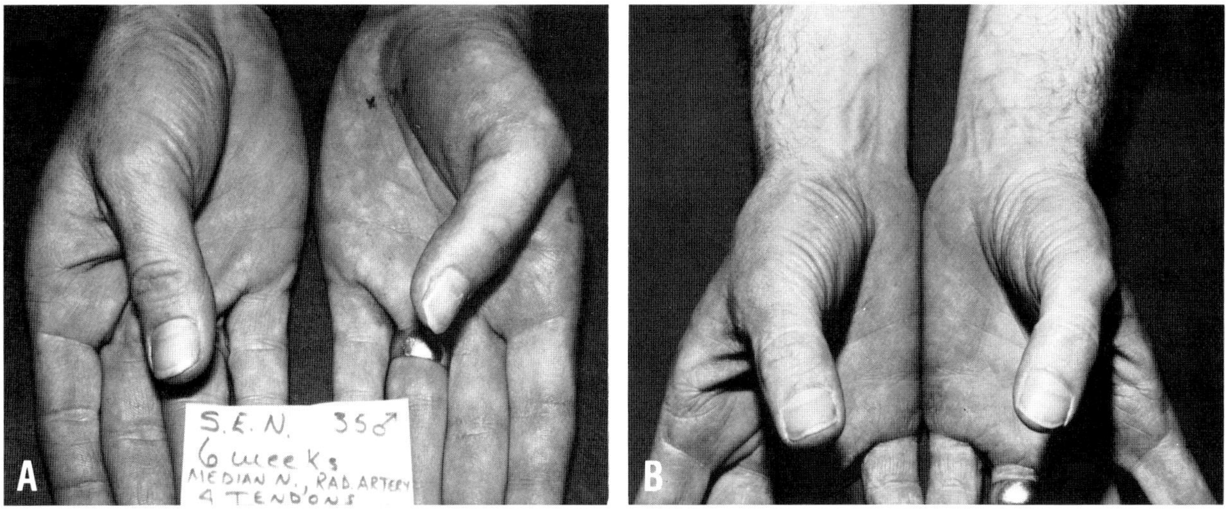

Figure 15-5. *(**A**) 6 weeks postoperative. Left thumb does not rotate for opposition. Note X on palm, designating level of paresthesias. (**B**) 5.5 years after repair, 2.5 years after neurolysis. Thenar muscles have recovered to M5. Sensory result is functionally good, but two-point discrimination is over 20 mm.*

pickup test, and his use pattern showed clearly his reliance on the median-innervated segment of the hand.

Case 2

Mr. J, a 29-year-old firefighter, was injured while breaking a window to enter a burning house. He suffered a laceration of his right wrist on the ulnar–volar surface, about 5 cm proximal to the proximal wrist crease. The wound was sutured, and 5 weeks later he was seen in consultation (Fig. 15-6). He was found to have absent sensation in the hypothenar eminence and the ulnar side of the small finger. Feeling in the ring finger web space and the small and ring fingers was normal. Significantly, there was a total motor paralysis of all muscles innervated by the ulnar nerve. The small and ring fingers were clawed, the intrinsic muscles were beginning to atrophy, and Froment's sign was positive. Tinel's sign was present at the level of the skin wound.

The patient underwent surgery 6 weeks after the injury. He was found to have an incomplete transection of the ulnar nerve with a neuroma-in-continuity. Awake stimulation proximal and distal to the neuroma indicated absence of transmission across the scarred area. Because of the lack of function, the intact portions of the nerve were surgically separated and the scar between the nerve ends excised. Drawings were made of the transected fascicles, and the tourniquet was deflated so that further stimulation could be performed. The intact portion of the nerve was found to consist of sensory fibers to the radial side of the small finger and the ulnar side of the ring finger. A single large bundle in the dorsal position of the proximal end was found to be electrically "silent" and was presumed to be motor in nature. Stimulation of the other bundles of the proximal stump produced sensation localized to the ulnar aspect of the small finger and hypothenar eminence.

Because grafting did not appear to be indicated, a perineural block was performed with bupivacaine, and group fascicular repair was performed with 10-0 nylon on a 75-μm needle. Sutures were placed in the internal epineurium and perineurium.

The patient was followed for 7 years. At 18 months, the claw deformity had disappeared and there was recovering function in the intrinsic muscles (Fig. 15-7). Lateral pinch was 22 pounds, compared to 26 pounds on the uninjured side. Two-point discrimination was 5 mm on the ulnar side of the small fingertip and moving two-point discrimination was 4 mm. The patient had returned to his job as a firefighter and noted only that he did not trust the hand completely when sliding down a pole.

When last seen, 7 years after his injury, he was found to have two-point discrimination of 4 mm in the small fingertip and 3 mm in all the other digits. In the hypothenar eminence, two-

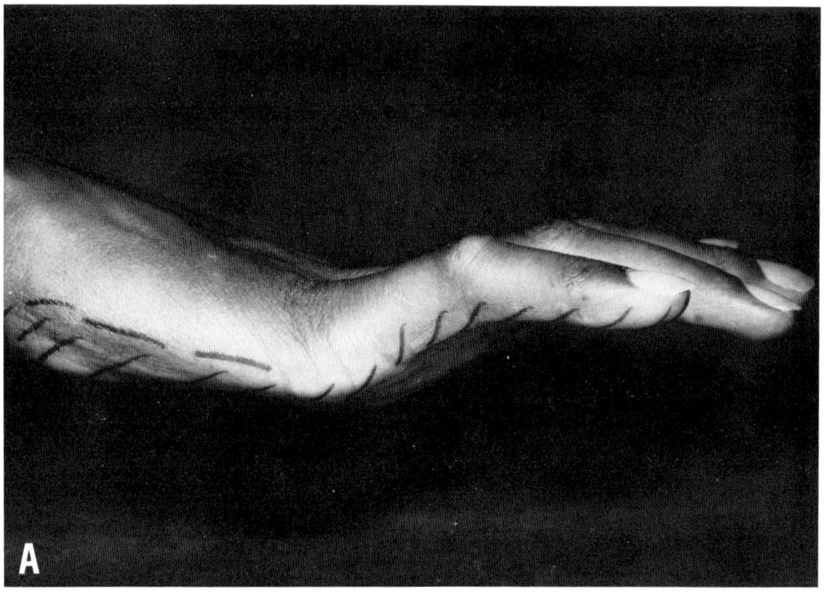

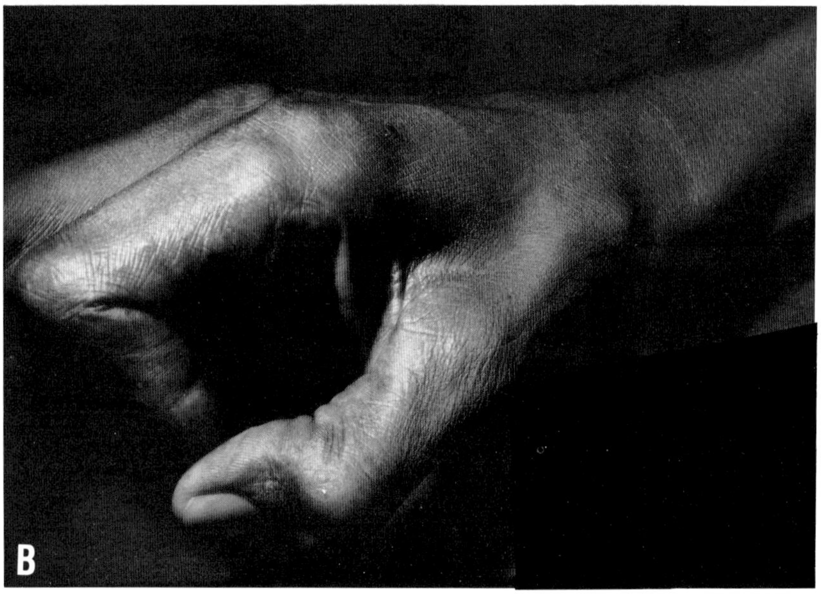

Figure 15–6. *(**A**) Mr. J, age 29, 5 weeks after ulnar nerve transection. Clawing of the small and ring fingers is present and numbness (striped skin) is noted in hypothenar eminence and ulnar side of small finger. (**B**) Atrophy of the first dorsal interosseous muscle can be seen and Froment's sign is present.*

point discrimination was 5 mm. Bulk in all the intrinsic muscles had improved, and the hand appeared normal. Wear marks were present, and grip strength was unchanged (Fig. 15-8).

This case illustrates the problems associated with a partially transected nerve and a secondary neuroma-in-continuity. When the nerve had been mobilized, stimulation proximally demonstrated a sensory response in the conscious patient but no motor response in the hand. Conversely, stimulation distal to the neuroma resulted in no conscious response by the patient, indicating that there was no transmission in either direction across the neuroma. Stimulation of the intact portions of the nerves showed normal sensory transmission from the ring–little finger web space and adjacent digits. Armed with this information, the neuroma was excised with confidence that no harm was being done. The distal motor portion of the ulnar nerve was identified by direct dissection and the proximal portion was

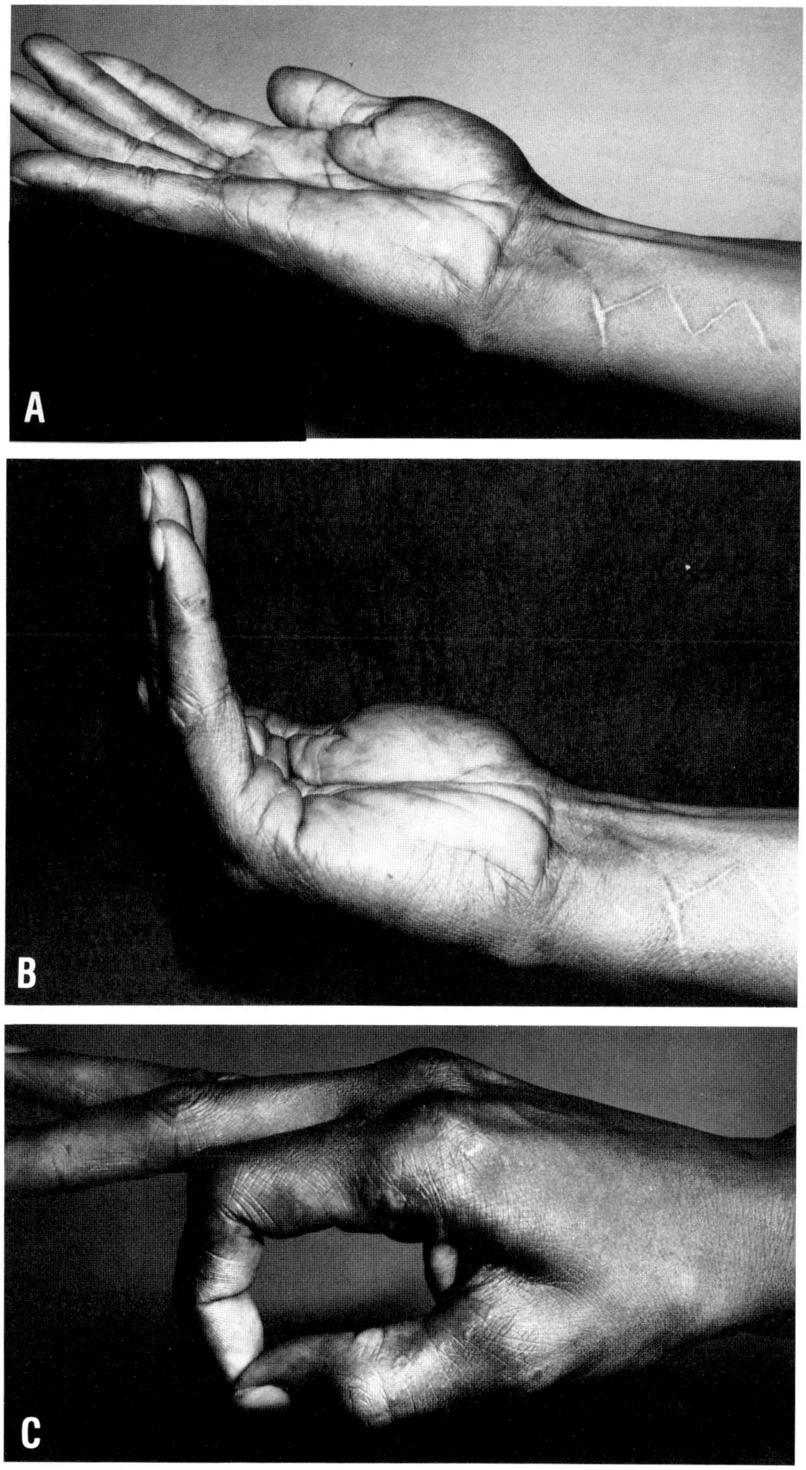

Figure 15–7. *1.5 years postoperative. (**A**) The claw deformity has disappeared. (**B**) Flexion is instituted at the metacarpophalangeal joints and the fingertips describe a wide arc. (**C**) Good, but not normal, bulk has returned to the first dorsal interosseous muscle. No Froment's sign is present.*

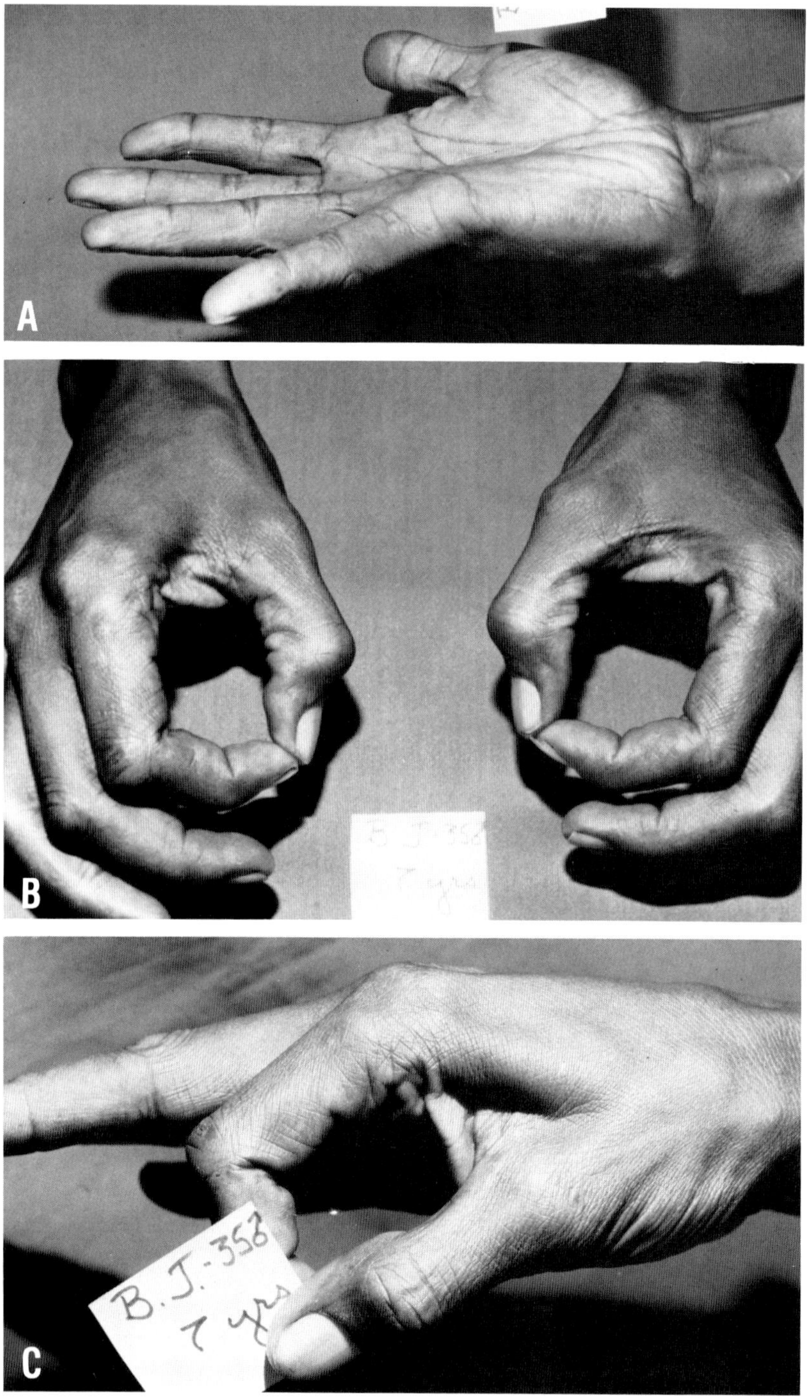

Figure 15–8. *7 years postoperative. The patient continues employment as a firefighter. (**A**) The fingers spread well and there is no clawing. (**B**) Forceful thumb adduction and index finger abduction is symmetrical. (**C**) Bulk and strength in the first dorsal interosseous is good.*

identified by stimulation. The remaining sensory portions were identified similarly, permitting accurate alignment and suturing.

Finally, the gradual improvement up to final follow-up underscores the importance of long-term follow-up. In many such cases, progressive improvement has been seen for up to 5 years.

DISCUSSION

Awake stimulation offers advantages that are unavailable either by stimulation in the anesthetized patient or by histologic or radioisotope techniques. Most importantly, it provides the opportunity for direct correlation between the results of electrical stimulation and the perception of sensation at the conscious level, a consideration that may be more valuable than it first appears. For example, anatomical variations in fascicular arrangement are certain to appear in some patients, and the degree of difference will increase with lengthening gaps between nerve ends. Despite these anatomical changes, however, the surgeon should still be able to identify dominant bundles or fascicles in the proximal end. When combined with stimulation or direct dissection of the distal end, positive identification and reasonably accurate functional alignment is still possible, regardless of differences in cross-sectional appearance between the nerve ends. In other words, the technique favors functional alignment while minimizing anatomical change.

The ideal way to determine the value of awake stimulation would be to compare the results of nerve repair in a group of patients in whom awake stimulation was carried out with those in a group of patients in whom this technique was not used. Unfortunately, this is impossible, and for several reasons it is not likely to become possible. First, there is a great deal of individual variation—compounded by age, sex, race, and biological variation—among patients. Second, wounds and wounding agents vary tremendously, not only from the standpoint of the structures injured, but also in the general degree of crush and stretch. Further, the time interval from injury to surgery may vary from a few hours to several days or even several months. Finally, operative technique and rehabilitation are also quite variable and further compound differences in results. For all these reasons, it is impossible to say with certainty that awake stimulation has a decided advantage in nerve reconstruction.

Fortunately, a few studies in the literature offer some help in assessing awake stimulation. In one, a group of patients treated by one surgeon with epineural suture without "electrical fascicle identification" was compared to a group in whom this technique was used.[3] The results suggest that nerve repairs as much as 100 to 150 mm proximal to the radial styloid are improved by such a technique. Gaul noted that he successfully mapped the proximal stump in 26 of 28 median and ulnar nerve injuries in the forearm, a success rate of 92.5%. In the distal stump, he was successful in 15 of 19 attempts (79%). The combined success rate of 87% underscores the applicability of the technique. The technique was not used in many distal stumps because of the time interval from injury to repair, and others were questionable because of probable wallerian degeneration. Finally, for reasons that he could not explain, he found median nerve results to be better than those in the ulnar nerve.

In a study by Nakatsuchi, Matsui, and Handa, 10 patients underwent repair of 11 nerves, by either fascicular suture or nerve graft.[10] The authors concluded that identification by electrical stimulation was possible in all instances and that satisfactory results could be achieved in cases of direct suture, but that the results with nerve grafting were not improved as much as with nerve suture.

Finally, Harris reported on nine patients treated between 1965 and 1967 with injuries to one or both major nerves at the level of the wrist and distal forearm.[6] All wounds were tidy and there was no tissue loss; as a consequence, little or no nerve tissue was resected. The results of ulnar nerve repair were generally better, with three of eight ulnar nerve repairs reaching a level of S3 within 6 months and five of eight recovering voluntary movement of the hypothenar muscles. Four of five patients with median repairs regained thenar function by 6 months, but sensation reached the fingertips in only one of five by this time. Because of the relatively short follow-up, specific statements could not be made about final outcome.

Kato and associates recently reported on 26 patients with 29 nerve injuries (13 median and 16 ulnar) at 0 to 7 cm above the wrist crease.[9] Successful stimulation was performed in 26 of 29 nerves. Sixteen nerve repairs (8 median and 8 ulnar) were followed for a minimum of 2 years. Fourteen (87%) recovered to a level of S3 and M3 or better. In contrast, only 50% of a comparable series treated by traditional epineural suture reached the S3 or M3 level.

I have used awake stimulation in 19 nerves (7 median, 10 ulnar, and 2 radial) in 17 patients. Both combined injuries were in the upper arm, one of the median and ulnar nerves, the other of the radial and ulnar nerves. The stimulation technique was successful in all cases attempted. Fascicular or group fascicular repairs or nerve grafts were performed in all cases using generally accepted microsurgical techniques. Appropriate magnification and suture with 10-0 or 11-0 nylon was used. Follow-up has been variable—3 patients were dropped because of insufficient follow-up—and percentages would be meaningless because of the small number of cases.

Sensory results with von Frey monofilaments are shown in Table 15-2. Motor results were also tested. One patient had previous transfers and was deleted, as were two patients with partial nerve injuries. Those with lesions above the elbow were scored separately for return to forearm muscles and intrinsic muscles of the hand; none of the latter group had recovery (Table 15-3).

Based on this small series, one conclusion seems reasonable: in nearly all cases, awake stimulation permitted the separate isolation of motor bundles and functionally identifiable sensory units. This held true even in injuries above the elbow, where successful recovery to forearm flexors and extensors was achieved but not to intrinsic muscles of the hand.

Table 15-2. *von Frey Monofilament Sensory Results*

Filament	Interpretation	No. of Patients
1.65–2.83 g	Excellent	5
3.22–3.61 g	Good	3
3.84–4.31 g	Fair	2
465 g	Poor	4

Table 15-3. *Motor Results*

Muscle Grade	No. of Patients
M5	8
M4	2
M3	1
M2	0
M1	0
M0	4

There seems little doubt that fascicular alignment, both anatomical and functional, is important and bears directly on the outcome in the complex human nerve (ie, one containing both motor and sensory elements). The more distal an injury and the more specifically function is defined, the more important correct alignment becomes. It seems likely that electrical stimulation techniques can aid in identification and correct matching, resulting in improved results.

REFERENCES

1. Engel J, Ganel A, Melamed R, Rimon S, Farine I. Choline acetyl-transferase for differentiation between human motor and sensory nerve fibers. Ann Plast Surg 1980; 4:376–380.
2. Ganel A, Engel J, Rimon S. Intraoperative identification of peripheral nerve fascicle: Use of a new rapid biochemical assay technique. Orthop Rev 1986; 15:85–88.
3. Gaul JS Jr. Electrical fascicle identification as an adjunct to nerve repair. J Hand Surg 1983; 8:289–296.
4. Gaul JS Jr. Electrical fascicle identification as an adjunct to nerve repair. Hand Clin 1986; 2:709–722.
5. Gruber H. Identification of motor and sensory funiculi in cut nerves and their selective reunion. Br J Plast Surg 1976; 29:70–73.
6. Hakstian RW. Funicular orientation by direct stimulation. J Bone Joint Surg [Am] 1968; 50:1178–1186.
7. Hansen FC. Personal communication.
8. Jabaley ME. Electrical nerve stimulation in the awake patient. Bull Hosp Jt Dis Orthop Inst 1984; 44:248–259.

9. Kato H. Torn median and ulnar nerve repair with electrical funicular orientation. J Hand Surg [Am] (in press).
10. Nakatsuchi Y, Matsui T, Handa Y. Funicular orientation by electrical stimulation and internal neurolysis in peripheral nerve suture. Hand 1980; 12: 65–74.
11. Riley DA, Lang DH. Carbonic anhydrase activity of human peripheral nerves: A possible histochemical aid to nerve repair. J Hand Surg [Am] 1984; 9:112–120.
12. Sunderland S. Nerves and nerve injuries, ed 2. Edinburgh: Churchill-Livingstone, 1978.
13. Van Beek AL. Electrodiagnostic evaluation of peripheral nerve injuries. Hand Clin 1986; 2:747–760.
14. Vandeput J, Tanner JC, Huypens L. Electrophysiological orientation of the cut ends in primary peripheral nerve repair. Plast Reconstr Surg 1969; 44: 378–382.
15. Wilgis EFS. Observations on the effects of tourniquet ischemia. J Bone Joint Surg [Am] 1971; 53: 1343–1346.

16

Histochemical and Biochemical Aids to Nerve Repair

David H. Lang
Graham D. Lister
Anthony W. Jevans

AUTHORS' KEY POINTS

- The transport of proteins present in one nerve fiber type but not in the other is the basis for the differentiation between sensory and motor axons by histochemical and biochemical methods.
- *Acetylcholinesterase* histochemistry provides a marker for motor axons; *carbonic anhydrase* histochemistry identifies sensory axons.
- Histochemical stains provide a significant improvement in resolution of sensory and motor axon topology within a peripheral nerve.
- The quickest histochemical techniques available require about an hour to complete.
- Distal nerve stump histochemical staining is effective for *7 to 10 days* following acute nerve injuries. Proximal stump staining is effective for prolonged periods.
- The use of histochemical techniques is probably not warranted in tidy injuries where fascicle size and distribution is clear and little or no nerve gap exists.

The outcome following repair of a major mixed peripheral nerve is influenced by many factors, including the patient's age, the presence of associated injuries to remote and local tissue, the extent and location of injury to the nerve, and the amount of scar tissue formed at the repair site.

The internal topology of mixed peripheral nerves affects both surgical technique and functional outcome. The plexiform nature of fascicular anatomy is well known.[15,31] The distribution of sensory and motor nerve fibers within a peripheral nerve is complex, becoming more organized as the distal end of the nerve is approached. While proximally, little identifiable functional organization of sensory and motor fibers is present,[31] distally, nerve fibers are organized into discrete fascicles and branches destined to innervate specific sensory and motor end organs. The anatomical organization of nerve fiber distribution is complicated by frequent intraneural branches between fascicles and complex intermingling of sensory and motor fibers within fascicles (see Chap. 14).

Several techniques have been developed in the past 30 years that differentiate between major motor and sensory components of a mixed peripheral nerve at the level of a traumatic or surgical lesion. These include electrical stimulation of the proximal and distal nerve stumps,[9,13,34] histochemical staining of nerve sections,[10,28] and biochemical assays of nerve fiber enzymes.[6] This chapter discusses the history, current clinical status, and methods of histochemical and biochemical aids to nerve repair.

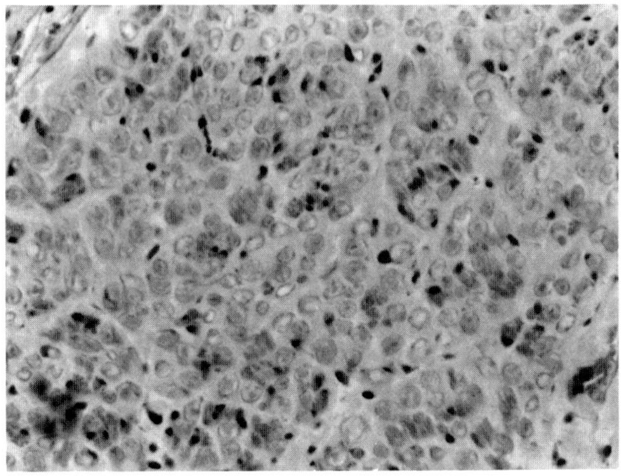

Figure 16-1. *An H&E-stained section of human ulnar nerve. Note that there is no differential staining between various axons. Compare to Figs. 16-5 through 16-8.*

BASIS FOR HISTOCHEMICAL AIDS

Unstained sections of nerve tissue are colorless. Peripheral nerve tissue stained with routine vital stains fails to demonstrate differential staining of motor and sensory fibers because routine stains label tissue components present in both types of nerve fibers. Most stains used in routine study of tissue function biochemically as acidic or basic compounds. These compounds form nonspecific salt complexes with nerve tissue, which provides contrast to the tissue section but fails to give specific information as to the chemical composition of the tissue. Examples of this type of stain include hematoxylin and eosin, orange G, and methylene blue (Fig. 16-1).

Numerous stains are available for specifically labeling tissues, cellular elements, and biochemical substances of interest. Stains are available for lipid, DNA, proteins, enzymes, and many other cellular constituents. Carbonic anhydrase and acetylcholinesterase histochemical techniques fall in this category of stain. Both of these techniques indirectly identify the location of an enzyme by marking a byproduct of its action. An alternate approach to enzyme location is the analysis of individual nerve fascicles for specific enzymes. Detection of choline acetyltransferase using a radiolabel is the basis of a biochemical method.

NERVE FIBER PHYSIOLOGY AND HISTOCHEMISTRY

Cellular proteins in neurons are produced in the cell body. Newly synthesized proteins are transported via *axoplasmic transport* (fast and slow) in an anterograde direction within the axon. This allows for replacement of axoplasmic proteins, which is necessary because the axon lacks the ribosomal machinery needed for protein synthesis.

Sensory and motor nerve fibers each synthesize distinct proteins. Axoplasmic transport of proteins present in one nerve fiber type but not in the other provides the basis for the differentiation between sensory and motor axons by histochemical and biochemical methods. If a sensory nerve cell body synthesizes and transports along its axon a protein that a motor neuron does not produce, identifying the protein in a mixed peripheral nerve axon means that the axon originated from a sensory cell body. The same would be true of a protein produced by motor fibers and not by sensory fibers.

Acetylcholinesterase, carbonic anhydrase, and *choline acetyltransferase* are enzymes synthesized differentially by sensory and motor axons. Histochemical and biochemical techniques currently used in clinical peripheral nerve research detect these enzymes.

CHOLINESTERASE HISTOCHEMISTRY

History

Several histochemical techniques have been used to label cholinesterases.[19,33] The techniques currently used in the clinical study of human peripheral nerves use modifications of the technique of Karnovsky and Roots.[16] Prior to the introduction of their method, cholinesterase histochemistry was felt to give unpredictable results, but a number of investigators have recently used their technique successfully in the study of nerve tissue in humans and other mammals.[1,2,10,11,18,21,37] The demonstration of differential staining in dorsal spinal roots has been demonstrated by many authors.[12,30] Gruber and Zenker demonstrated that the histochemical method of Karnovsky and Roots reliably stained 80% of motor and less than 10% of sensory fibers of the rat spinal root (Fig. 16-2).[11] Gruber later demonstrated similar findings in human peripheral nerves and applied them to clinical nerve repair.[10]

Gruber identified one of the major shortcomings of the use of acetylcholinesterase histochemistry in nerve repair: completing the histochemical process took 24 to 36 hours. This necessitated a two-stage approach to nerve repair. An initial procedure needed to obtain debridement specimens used the processing methods of Karnovsky and Roots. Two or three days later, the results of the histochemical staining were used in a second procedure to repair the nerve. Fascicles containing 50% or more stained axons in the proximal and distal nerve stumps were considered "motor."

Very little has been published on the clinical application of acetylcholinesterase histochemistry to human peripheral nerve repair. Yunshao and Shizhen recently supported Gruber's conclusions, demonstrating that motor axons stain but sensory axons do not.[37] Further, they defined the cholinesterase staining characteristics of human peripheral nerves in greater detail. Studying cryostat sections of major upper limb peripheral nerves and cervical ganglia taken from fresh cadavers, they found that both large ventral root myelinated fibers

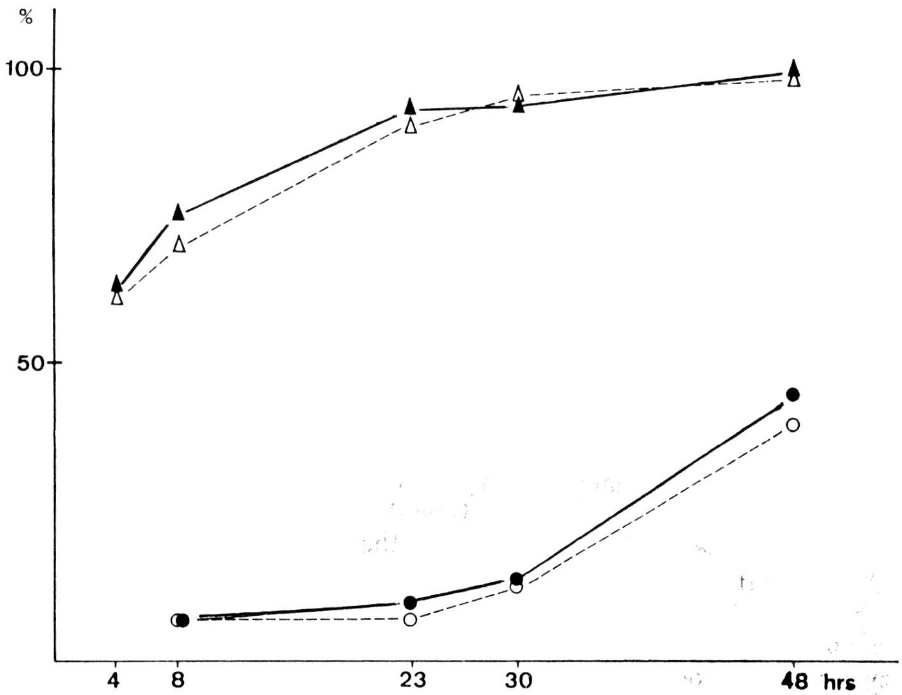

Figure 16-2. Cholinesterase staining results obtained by Gruber and colleagues. This graph demonstrates that a large percentage of motor axons (triangles) stain using Karnovsky and Roots histochemical stain, whereas sensory axons (circles) stain to a lesser degree. Open and closed circles represent left and right spinal ganglia, respectively. (From Gruber H, Zenker W. Acetylcholinesterase: Histochemical differentiation between motor and sensory fibers. Brain Res 1973; 51: 207–214, with permission.)

and small unmyelinated dorsal root fibers stained positive with acetylcholinesterase histochemistry. Dorsal root myelinated large fibers and ventral root unmyelinated fibers did not stain. They also described a modification of the staining technique designed to reduce the time required for incubation to less than 1 hour by altering the pH and the temperature of the reaction medium.

Basis for Acetylcholinesterase Histochemistry

Acetylcholinesterase histochemistry marks motor axons. Sectioned nerve tissue is incubated in a solution of acetylthiocholine, copper sulphate, and potassium ferricyanide. Intra-axonal acetylcholinesterase hydrolyzes the acetylthiocholine ester to thiocholine. Thiocholine reduces ferricyanide to ferrocyanide. The ferrocyanide then combines with the copper ions and forms the dark-brown precipitate copper ferrocyanide. The histochemical basis for the Karnovsky and Koelle stains has recently been clarified.[33] This staining process colors all axons that contain a significant amount of acetylcholinesterase dark brown in cross section. All axons that stain using this technique are motor axons. Further information on the chemistry of the reactions can be found in most histopathology texts.[20]

It appears that acetylcholinesterase synthesized in the perikaryon is transported as soluble and membrane-bound enzyme. The enzyme, which is modified slightly during its transport, is found bound to the axolemma and to cellular organelles.

CARBONIC ANHYDRASE HISTOCHEMISTRY

History

The enzyme carbonic anhydrase is present in numerous mammalian tissues. Its role is best understood in the kidney, the ciliary body of the eye, and the gastric mucosa. It maintains fluid and acid–base balance in these tissues. Carbonic anhydrase, one of the best-understood and most-studied enzymes, was first detected by Meldrum and Roughton in blood.[22] It catalyzes the reversible reaction:

$$H_2CO_3 \leftrightarrow H_2O + CO_2$$

Water and carbon dioxide are liberated as a result, with a subsequent elevation in pH in the region of the enzyme. Carbonic anhydrase, demonstrated by histochemical and immunohistochemical methods by numerous investigators,[32] exists in three isoenzymes: types I, II, and III.

Riley, Ellis, and Bain (and later, Wong and associates) demonstrated that carbonic anhydrase histochemistry could be used to differentiate between large myelinated dorsal root and ventral root axons in the rat.[25,35] They concluded that most large-diameter dorsal root sensory axons and few large-diameter ventral root motor axons stained with carbonic anhydrase histochemistry. Riley and Lang showed that carbonic anhydrase histochemistry could be used to differentiate sensory and motor components of mixed peripheral nerves in humans[28] and several different mammals.[27]

While the potential application of carbonic anhydrase histochemistry as an aid in human peripheral nerve repair has been recognized by several authors,[5,10] none has published a significant series of nerve repairs using this topographical aid.

Basis for Carbonic Anhydrase Histochemistry

Carbonic anhydrase is present in many large myelinated sensory axons, but only a few large myelinated motor axons (Fig. 16-3). It is unclear why more sensory axons than motor axons contain carbonic anhydrase, but there is evidence for increased tonic activity and need for increased clearance of CO_2 in sensory nerve pathways.[36] Perhaps the increased metabolic load secondary to tonic activity and the resulting metabolic need for improved pH balance explains the disparity between motor and sensory nerve staining.

Histochemical staining for carbonic anhydrase depends on the loss of CO_2 from the surface of peripheral nerve cryostat cut sections. Without the liberation of CO_2, the reaction will not proceed. The reactions relevant to carbonic anhydrase histochemistry are as follows:

$$HCO_3 + H_2O \leftrightarrow H_2CO_3 + OH \quad (1)$$

$$H_2CO_3 \leftrightarrow H_2O + CO_2 \quad (2)$$

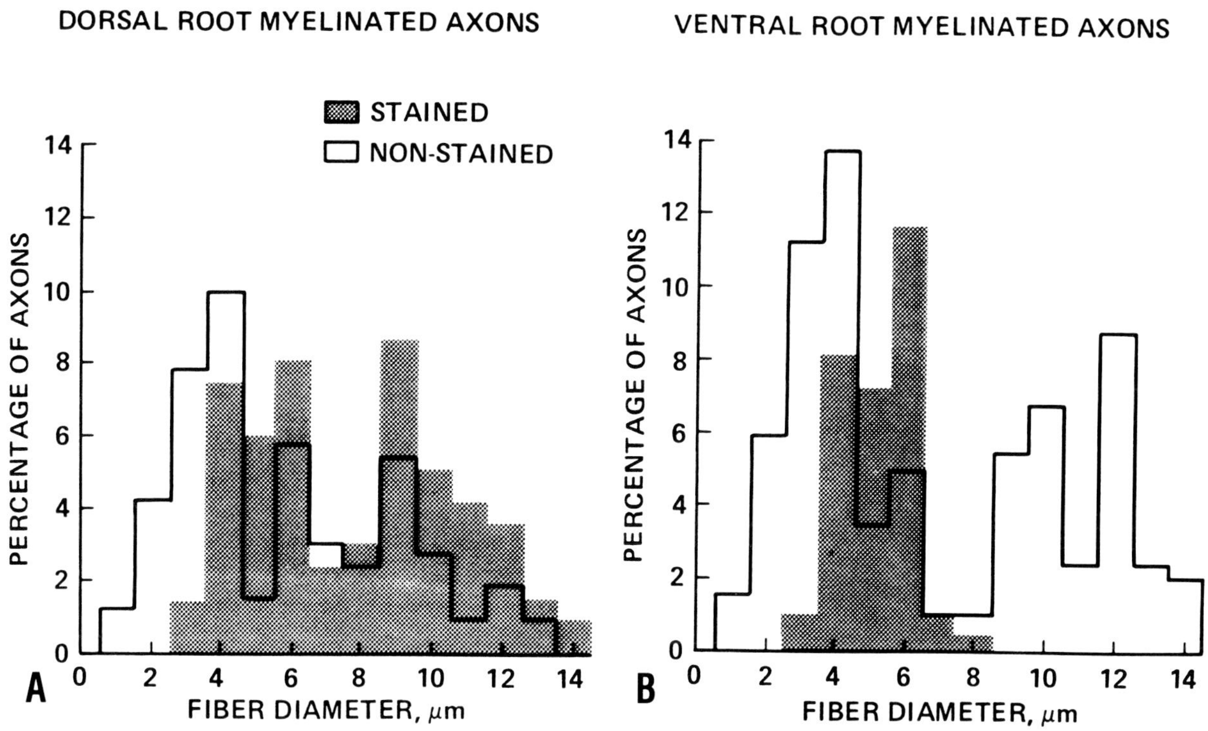

Figure 16-3. *These graphs demonstrate the percentage of stained axons vs nerve fiber diameter in dorsal and ventral root myelinated axons. Note that the dorsal root (**A**) contains a significantly higher percentage of large-diameter stained axons than the ventral root (**B**). (Used by permission of the Histochemical Society, Inc. and Danny A. Riley, PhD.)*

The loss of CO_2 in equation (2) forces the above reactions to the right by mass action. This results in local production of hydroxyl ions and increased pH. The basic environment of the reaction media in the region of the enzyme causes the deposition of a cobalt–phosphate complex. Exposing the white cobalt–phosphate precipitate to ammonium sulfide results in the deposition of the black precipitate cobalt sulfide (CoS). The net result is the precipitation of black CoS in the region of the carbonic anhydrase molecules present in sensory axons. Under the light microscope, this precipitate is visible as darkly stained axoplasm. The most commonly used technique uses a modified Hanson's medium, as described by Riddestrale.[24]

The ultrastructural localization of carbonic anhydrase has been demonstrated by Riley and coworkers.[26] Presence of the enzyme in both soluble axoplasmic and membrane-bound forms has been confirmed by biochemical assays.

CHOLINE ACETYLTRANSFERASE RADIOASSAY

History

The enzyme choline acetyltransferase (ChAC) was discovered in 1943 by Nachmansohn and Machado[23] and is found in all cholinergic neurons. It catalyzes the production of the neurotransmitter acetyl choline as follows:

$$\text{Choline} + \text{acetyl CoA} \xrightarrow{\text{ChAC}} \text{acetylcholine} + \text{CoA}$$

Choline acetyltransferase, synthesized in the cell body, is transported by axoplasmic flow to nerve terminals. Demonstration of higher choline acetyltransferase activity in ventral spinal roots compared to that in dorsal spinal roots, in several species, indicated a viable approach to nerve differentiation for human peripheral nerve repair.[14]

Although localization of choline acetyltransferase in tissues has been accomplished histochemically,[4,17] radiochemical assays have proved easier to use. In 1980, Engel and associates demonstrated rapid and precise nerve fascicle identification of homogenized fresh cadaveric nerve samples.[6] The radiochemical assay used showed that motor nerve fascicles had four to ten times the activity of sensory nerve fascicles. Subsequent studies of transected rat sciatic nerves indicated rapid decrease of choline acetyltransferase activity in the distal stump with time and that optimal results were obtained by performing the assay within 96 hours of injury.[7] However, demonstrable enzyme activity has been found in the distal nerve stumps of patients injured more than 5 months earlier.[8]*

The radiochemical assay time of 2 to 4 hours, depending on the age of injury and number of fascicles involved, allows interoperative nerve fascicle differentiation.

Basis for Choline Acetyltransferase Radioassay

Choline acetyltransferase activity is greater in motor axons than in sensory axons.

Sectioned nerve tissue is weighed and then incubated with acetyl-CoA (labeled with either ^{3}H or ^{14}C), choline chloride, and eserine. The labeled metabolite is selectively extracted into organic supernatant as its tetraphenylborate salt, and the activity of aliquots is determined by scintillation counting. To minimize the influence of tissue scarring on enzyme activity, fascicles can be screened by frozen section before analysis.

ADVANTAGES OF HISTOCHEMICAL AND BIOCHEMICAL TECHNIQUES

The peripheral nerve surgeon uses macroscopic and low-power microscopic anatomical guides for orientation of proximal and distal nerve stumps. Epineural vessels, the mesoneurium, fascicle size and arrangement, and groups of fascicles are often used to determine proper proximal and distal stump orientation. These anatomical guides work particularly well in peripheral nerves with relatively few fascicles and in cases of clean nerve transections where no significant gaps between nerve ends exists.

Electrical stimulation of nerve stumps has been used to aid in the identification of distal stump motor and proximal stump sensory fascicles. Several problems exist with electrical stimulation of nerve ends, however. A distal motor response to fascicle stimulation does not necessarily demonstrate that the stimulated fascicle is predominantly motor; it only indicates that motor fibers sufficient to cause a motor response have been stimulated. The same is true of positive proximal sensory responses. Further, negative responses can also be overinterpreted. Despite this shortcoming, nerve stimulation provides topographic information that is useful in nerve alignment.

Histochemical stains and biochemical assays provide a significant improvement in resolution of sensory and motor components of peripheral nerves. Not only do these techniques identify predominantly sensory and motor fascicles, but they can also locate fascicles with mixed sensory and motor components. Histochemical techniques provide additional spatial and quantitative information in those fascicles. These techniques demonstrate that motor or sensory fibers are present in a fascicle and also indicate the percentage and distribution of motor and sensory fibers within that fascicle. This represents a significant improvement in resolution of peripheral nerve functional topology.

Despite the apparent advantages of histochemical techniques, significant disadvantages have been identified. First, the time needed to complete the repair is increased due to the delay needed to process tissue. Even with the most rapid carbonic anhydrase or acetylcholinesterase histochemical techniques, 50 to 60 minutes is required to complete the staining and interpret the results. The most reliable results of histochemistry are obtained with longer processing times; in general, less reliable results are obtained when the processing time for tissue staining is shortened. Further, accurate interpretation of results requires special training. Similar time constraints are inherent in the biochemical technique used to identify choline

* *Jevans AW. Unpublished observations, 1987.*

acetyltransferase. Both techniques require the availability of a histochemical or biochemical laboratory, and most hospital pathology laboratories are not equipped to do these procedures routinely.

A more serious problem with histochemical and biochemical techniques is that staining in the distal stump diminishes with time. This is due to diffusion of soluble enzyme, metabolic degradation of cellular constituents, and dissolution of the distal stump axons. The reliability of these techniques is probably limited to the first 7 to 10 days post-injury.* After that time, one would not expect to obtain histochemical or biochemical information from the distal nerve stump. However, our experience has shown that *proximal* nerve stump staining persists and may actually increase with time.

These constraints are compounded by the time required to separate and label individual fascicles at both proximal and distal nerve stumps. Also, larger nerve sections may be required to provide adequate tissue mass for maintaining assay sensitivity for fascicles with small cross-sectional area.

CLINICAL USE OF HISTOCHEMICAL AND BIOCHEMICAL METHODS

Authors' Preferred Method

Use of these histochemical and biochemical methods does not significantly complicate the technical aspects of nerve repair, although additional time is needed to process tissue and construct a topographic map. The only significant change in the operative procedure is that tissue specimens must be obtained. Debridement trimmings 2 to 4 mm in length must be harvested from healthy-appearing portions of both the proximal and distal nerve stumps.

Before obtaining debridement trimmings, the orientation of the proximal and distal nerve stumps is labeled (Fig. 16-4). This is most easily done by placing sutures anteriorly on proximal and distal nerve stump epineurium. A similarly placed suture is placed on each debridement trimming, noting which trimming is from the proximal and distal stumps. An optional suture is placed 90° from the anterior suture to further clarify orientation of the nerve stumps and debridement trimmings. The labeled trimmings are then sent to the histochemical laboratory for processing. About 60 minutes later the surgeon receives a schematic drawing of the sensory and motor fascicle distributions of the proximal and distal stumps. The surgeon, guided by the maps constructed with staining results, proceeds with the repair using the most appropriate epineural, group fascicular, or fascicular repair methods.

* *Riley DA, Lang DH. Unpublished observation, 1984.*

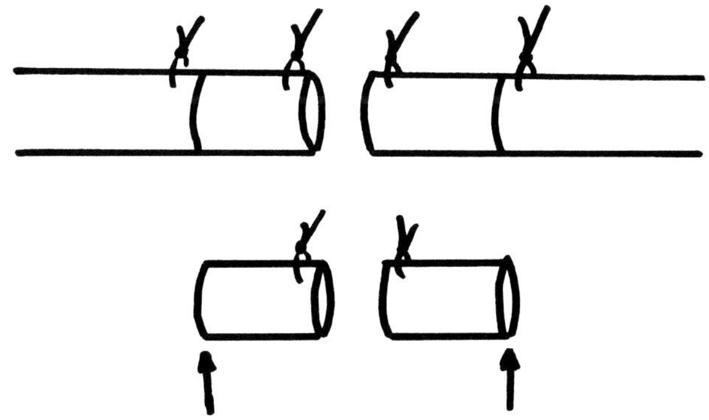

Figure 16-4. *The preferrred method of labeling proximal and distal nerve stumps and debridement trimmings to maintain spatial orientation during histochemical staining. Arrows indicate the correct starting point on the debridement trimming for tissue sections.*

Since the choline acetyltransferase radioassay usually involves many specimens from both proximal and distal stumps, a more complex identification system is required for the samples. Segments can be transported in a microtiter plate to the laboratory for analysis. Two to four hours later, depending on the number of segments and age of the injury, a report containing sample identification and relative choline acetyltransferase activity in cpm/mg tissue is delivered to the surgeon.

Specific Applications

At this time, peripheral nerve histochemical and biochemical techniques are not widely used and should be considered clinical research tools. Insufficient information from clinical trials has been available to establish the efficacy of these techniques compared to traditional alignment methods. However, since the techniques have been shown to identify sensory and motor components of peripheral nerves reliably, it follows that the use of the results of nerve staining to guide nerve repair should improve the results of nerve repair, provided that the other factors mentioned at the beginning of this chapter can be controlled.

The ability to identify predominantly sensory, motor, and mixed fascicles at the location of proximal nerve lesions could be used to improve the results of repaired distal brachial plexus injuries, innervated free muscle transfers,[29] segmental nerve injuries, and repairs involving long nerve grafts. These applications have been tried at our institutions and deserve further investigation. The use of these techniques is probably not justified in tidy injuries where the fascicle size and distribution is clear and little or no nerve gap exists.

TECHNIQUES OF CARBONIC ANHYDRASE AND ACETYLCHOLINESTERASE HISTOCHEMISTRY

Most clinical investigators do not have the training in histochemistry to run or interpret the results of carbonic anhydrase or acetylcholinesterase histochemistry. The techniques involved are not difficult, but complete understanding of the histochemistry and biochemistry involved entail significant study and practice. Fortunately, all of the methods described have been well worked out and are amenable to a cookbook-type approach. Accordingly, we describe the histochemical protocols for those interested in experimenting with the histochemical methods.

Those interested should practice using animal material first. The laboratory rat is an inexpensive, readily available source of nerve tissue for experimentation. The sciatic nerve is easiest to use. Several of the reagents are toxic, highly irritating to tissues, and potentially carcinogenic. Appropriate precautions should be taken, and all procedures should be done in an appropriately equipped laboratory. Only when the methods have been perfected and are repeatable should the techniques be applied to humans. (Most institutions require approval of clinical protocols by their human research committees.)

Carbonic Anhydrase Histochemical Materials and Methods

The following reagents are needed for carbonic anhydrase histochemistry:[24]

2.5% glutaraldehyde in 0.1 M phosphate buffer, pH 7.4
Sucrose cryoprotectant in 0.1 phosphate buffer, pH 7.4 (10%, 20%, and 30% sucrose solutions)
Solution A (100 mL of 0.067 M KH_2PO_4, 60 mL of 0.5 M H_2SO_4, 10 mL of 0.2 M $CoSO_4$)
Solution B (200 mL of 0.223 M $NaHCO_3$)
Acetazolamide
0.67×10^{-4} M NaK phosphate buffer, pH 5.9
0.5% NH_4S in distilled H_2O (this is highly toxic)
Ethanol dehydration series 70%, 80%, 90%, 95%, 100%
Xylene
Permount tissue mounting gel

The following materials are needed for carbonic anhydrase histochemistry:

2% gelatin-coated clean glass slides and cover slips
Coplin jars for dipping slides
Cryostat and supplies
Tissue-tek to adhere debridement trimmings to cryostat chucks

Carbonic anhydrase histochemistry is performed as follows:

1. Carbonic anhydrase is highly soluble in nerve tissue. In order to retain the enzyme in nerve trimmings, the nerve is fixed before starting the histochemical procedure. After the nerve stumps and debridement trimmings are labeled for orientation, the debridement trimmings are placed in separate, clearly labeled glass jars containing the 2.5% glutaraldehyde 0.1 M phosphate buffer, pH 7.4 at room temperature. Thirty minutes of immersion is sufficient to fix the tissue, provided the samples are 2 or 3 mm thick. The 0.1 M NaK phosphate buffer is made by mixing 0.1 M $K_2H_2PO_4$ (monobasic) and 0.1 M Na_2HPO_4 (dibasic) in a ratio of one to four by volume.
2. The fixed trimmings are then serially immersed in increasing concentrations of sucrose used as a cryoprotectant. This prevents most of the freezing artifact that occurs when nerve trimmings are frozen quickly in liquid nitrogen. The trimmings

should be allowed to sit in each serial sucrose solution (10%, 20%, 30%) until they sink.

3. The trimmings are then mounted to the cryostat chuck using Tissue-tek, and 8-μm sections are cut. The trimmings must be oriented properly, and the technician must keep track of the section orientation. Cut sections should be taken from the portion of the trimmings closest to the residual nerve stump.
4. The cryostat cut sections are picked up with room temperature 2% gelatin–coated glass slides. The section is allowed to sit at room temperature for 5 minutes. The tissue section will adhere to the slide.
5. The slide is placed on ice and the section covered with several drops of 2.5% glutaraldehyde in 0.1 M NaK phosphate buffer, pH 7.4, that has been chilled on ice.
6. The section is rinsed in a Coplin jar filled with 0.1 M NaK phosphate buffer, pH 7.4, at room temperature for 3 minutes.
7. Solutions A and B are added to a well-cleaned Coplin jar, and the effervescent pink solution is allowed to sit for 3 minutes. The slide is dipped into the solution every 15 to 30 seconds, just enough to cover the section. Between dippings, the slide is leaned vertically against the Coplin jar to allow excess solution to run off the section. *This is extremely important.* The liberation of CO_2 from the section is vital to the staining process. The slide is dipped for 10 to 12 minutes.
8. The sections are then rinsed in two serial Coplin jars containing .67 × 10^{-4} M NaK phosphate buffer, pH 5.9. The slide is left in each solution for 2 minutes.
9. The slide is then immersed for 3 minutes in 0.5% NH_4S diluted in distilled water. The section should turn black. This step must be done in a fume hood with a covered Coplin jar.
10. The slide is then again rinsed twice in 0.67 × 10^{-4} M phosphate buffer and dehydrated by serially dipping the slide in a graded series of ethanol. It is then immersed in xylene twice and mounted in Permount.

Visualizing the Stained Sections

Sections are then visualized under light microscopy. Nerve fascicles that contain a majority of myelinated large-diameter stained axons are considered sensory. Sections containing a majority of large myelinated unstained axons are considered motor. Hand-drawn maps of the distribution of sensory and motor fascicles in the proper orientation are then provided to the surgeon; this information is used to guide the nerve repair. Figures 16-5 and 16-6 show representative fascicles of a carbonic anhydrase–stained human ulnar nerve.

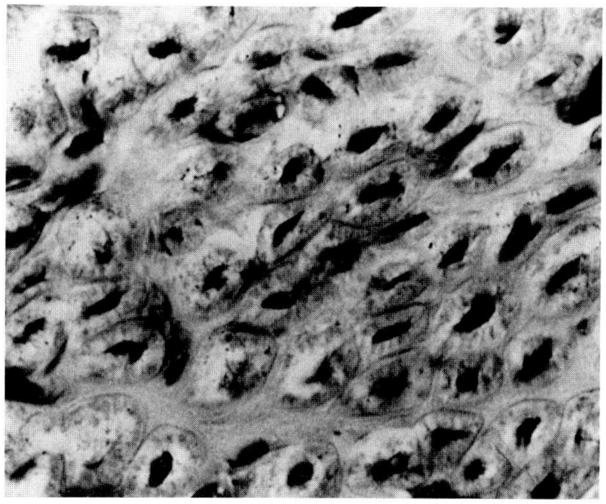

Figure 16-5. *A section of a carbonic anhydrase "positive" fascicle (magnification ×9) indicates a predominance of sensory fibers in this fascicle. Note that the axoplasm is darkly stained in this section. (From Riley DA, Lang DH. Carbonic anhydrase activity of human peripheral nerves: A possible histochemical aid to nerve repair. J Hand Surg [Am] 1984; 9:112–120, with permission.)*

Acetylcholinesterase Histochemical Materials and Methods

The following reagents are needed for acetylcholinesterase histochemistry:[37]*

Sodium citrate
Copper sulfate pentahydrate
Potassium ferricyanide (made fresh)
Acetyl-thiocholine iodide
0.1 M phosphate buffer, pH 6.5
2.5% glutaraldehyde, 0.1 M phosphate buffer, pH 7.4
Meserine (inhibitor)

In general, the tissue cryoprotection, tissue fixation, and sectioning procedures are the same for

* *Riley DA. Personal communication, 1988.*

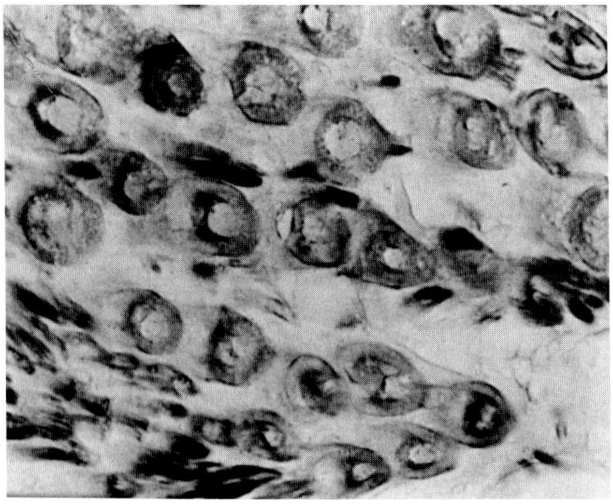

Figure 16-6. *A section of a carbonic anhydrase "negative" fascicle (magnified ×8) indicates a predominance of motor fibers in this fascicle. Note that the axoplasm is not stained in this section. (From Riley DA, Lang DH. Carbonic anhydrase activity of human peripheral nerves: A possible histochemical aid to nerve repair. J Hand Surg [Am] 1984; 9: 112–120.)*

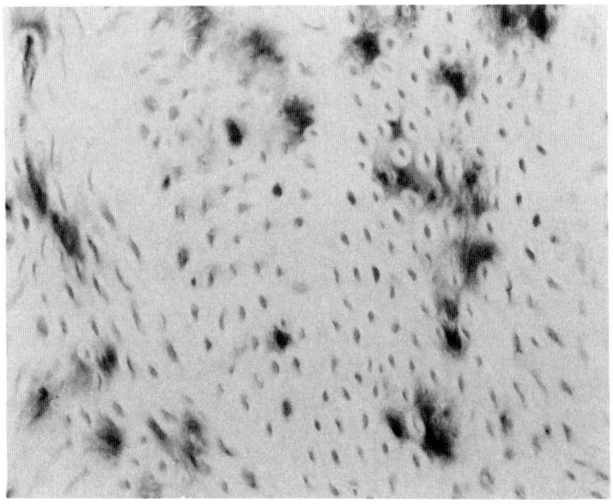

Figure 16-7. *A magnified section of a fascicle containing acetylcholinesterase "positive" axons. A predominance of axoplasmic staining indicates that the fascicle is probably a motor fascicle.*

acetylcholinesterase histochemistry as for carbonic anhydrase histochemistry. The steps that follow those are different.

1. The nerve ends are labeled as described previously and the debridement trimmings are cut.
2. The trimmings are immersed in the fixative at room temperature for 45 minutes.
3. The debridement trimmings are protected in serial sucrose solutions.
4. Sections 15 to 20 μm thick are frozen and cryostat-cut.
5. The sections are incubated for 24 hours at 4°C in Karnovsky and Roots medium. (This is the original protocol. Several authors have tried rapid tissue processing, which reduces the incubation time to under 1 hour,[37] but I have no experience with these methods.)*
6. The sections are mounted using water-soluble mounting medium, and the stained sections are visualized. Figures 16-7 and 16-8 show representative fascicles from a human ulnar nerve stained with acetylcholinesterase stain.

Choline Acetyltransferase Radioassay Materials and Methods

The following reagents are needed for the choline acetyltransferase radioassay.[6]*

50 mM sodium phosphate buffer, pH 7.4, containing 300 mM sodium chloride and 20 mM EDTA.
1.6 M choline chloride in deionized water (DIW)
0.005 M eserine in DIW (Note: highly toxic)
20 mM sodium s-acetyl coenzyme A in 0.1 M phosphate citrate buffer pH 6.0.
Working buffer solution (prepare fresh immediately before use):
  930 μL 50 mM phosphate buffer, pH 7.4
  10 μL choline chloride solution (1.6 M)
  50 μL eserine solution (0.005 M)
  13 μL sodium s-acetyl coenzyme A (20 mM) solution.
Substrate reagent (prepare immediately before use):
  220 μL working buffer solution
  20 μL acetyl coenzyme A (acetyl-^{3}H)
1.5% sodium tetraphenylborate in di-isobutylketone solution (Note: toxic).
Pico-fluor 30
Ringer buffer

* *Rimon S. Personal communication, 1981.*

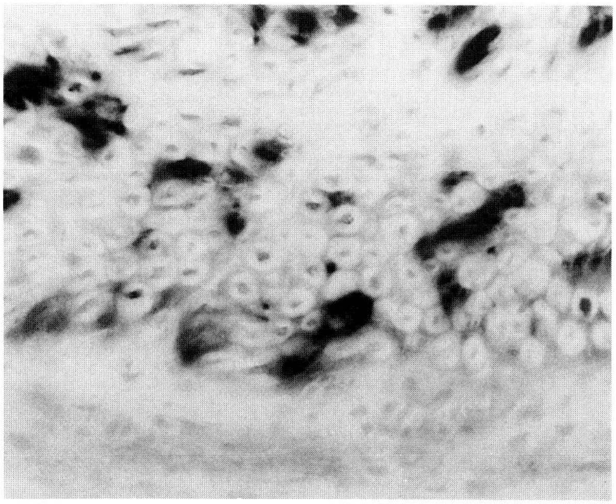

Figure 16-8. *A magnified section of a fascicle containing acetylcholinesterase "negative" axons. A predominance of unstained axons and slightly stained Schwann cells indicates that the fascicle is probably a sensory fascicle.*

The following materials are needed for the choline acetyltransferase radioassay:

1-mL polystyrene centrifuge tubes with caps
glassine weighing paper
filter paper
7-mL minivials (scintillation)
37°C incubator
reciprocal shaker
vortex mixer
10-, 20-, 50-, and 200-μL fixed volume pipets
10–100-μL adjustable pipet
50-μL repeater pipet
scintillation counter
microtiter plate

Nerve fascicles are transferred to separate wells of a microtiter plate and kept moist with Ringer buffer or an equivalent solution.

Each fascicle is dried on filter paper before being cut into 3.5- to 5-mg slices. It is preferable to assay each fascicle in duplicate if sufficient tissue is available. However, weights of less than 2 mg can give varying results. Each nerve slice is weighed to 0.1 mg and transferred to the bottom of a labeled 1-mL polystyrene centrifuge tube using tweezers. After the weight is recorded, 10 μL of phosphate buffer pH 7.4 is pipetted to the bottom of the tube, which is then capped. After all the specimens have been processed, two blank assay tubes are prepared using buffer only.

The working buffer solution and substrate reagent are then prepared; 10-μL aliquots of the radioactive substrate reagent are pipetted to the bottom of each polystyrene tube. The tubes are capped and vortexed, and then incubated at 37°C for 60 minutes with constant shaking.

Fifteen minutes before the incubation is complete the sodium tetraphenylborate solution is prepared. Termination of the reaction is achieved by adding 50 μL of sodium tetraphenylborate solution to each assay tube and vortexing vigorously for 30 seconds. Tritiated acetylcholine is isolated as its tetraphenylborate salt, which is soluble in the organic phase of the reaction mixture. The reaction tubes are then centrifuged, four at a time, at 10–12,000 rpm for 2 minutes to produce a clear organic supernatant. Ten microliters of each clear supernatant, followed by 5 mL of Pico-fluor 30, is transferred to individually labeled minivials. Each vial is capped and mixed well before being placed in the scintillation counter. The vials are allowed to stand for 10 minutes before being counted for 1 minute each.

The average cpm (counts per minute) of the assay blanks are then subtracted from each specimen's cpm, and the corrected cpm divided by fascicle weight. Where appropriate, replicate values for each nerve fascicle are averaged.

The report, consisting of each specimen's ID number, cpm, corrected cpm, fascicle slice weight and corrected cpm per mg nerve, is then provided to the surgeon.

The technique described above differs in several respects from the original work of Ganel and associates[6,7] (doubling the incubation time as well as the volume of tracer used) and reflects experience with patients whose nerve repair was undertaken 6 to 36 months after injury, requiring a more sensitive assay to detect lower levels of choline acetyltransferase in both distal and proximal specimens. In these patients motor nerve fascicle activity was usually greater than 350 cpm/mg nerve, while the sensory nerve fascicle activity was usually less than 80 cpm/mg nerve.

CONCLUSION

Histochemical techniques have become practical for operative nerve repair. Numerous investigators have demonstrated the reliability of the staining procedures with human peripheral nerve tissue. However, the efficacy of histochemically guided nerve repair over traditional nerve repair techniques has not yet been established. With the completion of large series of patients in whom histochemical aids to nerve repair were used, this challenging question should soon be answered.

REFERENCES

1. Adams CW, Grant RT, Bayliss B. Cholinesterases in nervous system. I. Mixed, motor and sensory trunks. Brain Res 1967; 5:366–376.
2. Baljet B, Drukker J. An acetylcholinesterase method for in toto staining of peripheral nerves. Stain Technol 1975; 50:1.
3. Bancroft JD. Histochemical techniques, ed 2. London: Butterworth & Co, 1975.
4. Burt AM. A histochemical procedure for the localization of choline acetyltransferase activity. J Histochem Cytochem 1970; 18:408–415.
5. Carson KA, Terzis JK. Carbonic anhydrase histochemistry: A potential diagnostic method for peripheral nerve repair. Clinics Plast Surg 1985; 12: 227–229.
6. Engel J, Ganel A, Melamed S, Rimon S, Farine I. Choline acetyltransferase for differentiation between human motor and sensory nerve fibers. Ann Plast Surg 1980; 4:5.
7. Ganel A, Engel J, Luboshitz S, Melamed R, Rimon S. Choline acetyltransferase nerve identification method in early and late nerve repair. Ann Plast Surg 1980; 4:228–230.
8. Ganel A, Farine I, Aharonson Z, Horoszowski H, Melamed R, Rimon S. Intraoperative nerve fascicle identification using choline acetyltransferase: A preliminary report. Clin Orthop 1982; 165:228–232.
9. Gaul JS. Electrical fascicle identification as an adjunct to nerve repair. Hand Clin 1986; 2:4.
10. Gruber H, Freilinger G, Holle J, Mandl H. Identification of motor and sensory funiculi in cut nerves and their selective reunion. Br J Plast Surg 1976; 29:70.
11. Gruber H, Zenker W. Acetylcholinesterase: Histochemical differentiation between motor and sensory fibers. Brain Res 1973; 51:207–214.
12. Gruber H, Zenker W, Hohberg E. Untersuchungen über die spezifitat der cholinesterin im perpherin nervensystem der ratte. Histochemie 1971; 27:78–86.
13. Hakstian RW. Funicular orientation by direct stimulation: An aid to peripheral nerve repair. J Bone Joint Surg [Am] 1968; 50:6.
14. Hebb C. Formation, storage and liberation of acetylcholine. In: Handbuch der Experimentellen Pharmakologie. Berlin: Springer, 1963: 56–88.
15. Jabaley ME, Wallace WH, Heckler FR. Internal topology of major nerves of the forearm and hand: A current view. J Hand Surg 1980; 5:1–18.
16. Karnovsky MJ, Roots CA. A "direct coloring" thiocholine method for cholinesterases. J Histochem Cytochem 1964; 12:219–221.
17. Kasa P, Mann SP, Hebb C. Localization of choline acetyltransferase. Nature 1970; 226:812–814.
18. Kasa P, Rakonczay Z. Histochemical and biochemical demonstration of the molecular forms of acetylcholinesterase in peripheral nerve of rat. Acta Histochem 1982; 70:244–257.
19. Koelle GB, Freidenweld JS. A histochemical method for localizing cholinesterase activity. Proc Soc Exp Biol Med 1949; 70:617–622.
20. Lojda Z, Gossrau R, Schrieber TH. Enzyme histochemistry: A laboratory manual. New York: Springer-Verlag, 1979.
21. Lubinska L, Niemierko S, Oderfeld B, Szwarc L. The distribution of cholinesterase in peripheral nerves. J Neurochem 1963; 10:25–41.
22. Meldrum NV, Roughton FJ. Carbonic anhydrase: Its preparation and properties. J Physiol 1933; 80: 113–142.
23. Nachmansohn D, Machado AL. The formation of acetylcholine. A new enzyme "choline acetylase." J Neurophysiol 1943; 6:397–404.
24. Riddestrale Y. Intracellular localization of carbonic anhydrase in the frog nephron. Acta Physiol Scand 1976; 98:465–469.
25. Riley DA, Ellis S, Bain J. Carbonic anhydrase activity in skeletal muscle fiber types, axons, spindles, and capillaries of rat soleus and extensor digitorum longus muscles. J Histochem Cytochem 1982; 30: 1275–1288.
26. Riley DA, Ellis S, Bain J. Ultrastructural cytochemical localization of carbonic anhydrase activity in peripheral sensory, motor nerves, dorsal root ganglia and dorsal column nuclei. Neuroscience 1984; 13:189–206.
27. Riley DA, Ellis S, Lang DH, Bain J. Examination of

carbonic anhydrase activities in the peripheral nervous system of humans, rhesus monkeys, cats, and rats. Ann NY Acad Sci 1984; 429:408–411.

28. Riley DA, Lang DH. Carbonic anhydrase activity of human peripheral nerves: A possible histochemical aid to nerve repair. J Hand Surg [Am] 1984; 9:112–120.
29. Sanger JR, Riley DA, Yousif NJ, Matlaub HS. Histochemical staining of nerve endings as an aid to free muscle transplant (submitted for publication).
30. Schlaepfer W. Acetylcholinesterase activity of motor and sensory nerve fibers in the spinal nerve roots of the cat. Z Zellforsh 1968; 88:441–456.
31. Sunderland S. The anatomic basis of nerve repair. In: Jewett DL, McCarroll HR, eds. Nerve repair and regeneration. St Louis: CV Mosby, 1980.
32. Tashian RE, Hewett-Emmett D. Biology and chemistry of the carbonic anhydrases. Ann NY Acad Sci 1984; 429.
33. Tsuji S. Histochemical demonstration of membrane-bound acetylcholinesterase: A methodological consideration on Koelle's copper thiocholine reaction and on Karnovsky's copper ferrocyanide reaction. Acta Histochem 1986 (supp); 33:147–156.
34. Vandeput MD, Tanner JC, Huypens L. Electrophysiological orientation of the cut ends on primary nerve repair. Plast Reconstr Surg 1969; 44:4.
35. Wong V, Barrett CP, Donati EJ, Eng LF, Guth L. Carbonic anhydrase activity in first-order sensory neurons of the rat. J Histochem Cytochem 1983; 31:293–300.
36. Wong V, Barrett CP, Donati EJ, Guth L. Distribution of carbonic anhydrase activity in neurons of the rat. J Comp Neurobiol 1987; 257:122–129.
37. Yunshao H, Shizhen Z. Acetylcholinesterase: A histochemical identification of motor and sensory fascicles in human peripheral nerves and its use during operation. Plast Reconstr Surg 1988; 82:125–32.

V

OPERATIVE TECHNIQUE

17 Instrumentation for Nerve Repair

18 Techniques of Epineural and Group Fascicular Repair

19 Fascicular Repair

20 Sutureless Methods of Nerve Repair

21 Modified Techniques of Nerve Repair: Epineurial Splint

22 New Approaches in Nerve Suture

23 Partial Nerve Injuries

17

Instrumentation for Nerve Repair

Paul W. Gorman
Paul C. Dell

AUTHORS' KEY POINTS

- Instruments are kept in a storage case lined with rubber dowels to protect delicate tips.
- The microsurgical set is steam-autoclaved, rather than gas-autoclaved, to prevent wear.
- Loupes of 2.5× to 4.5× are the most versatile since the depth of field and field of view are inversely proportional to magnification power.
- Operating microscope features important in peripheral nerve suture include automatic, motorized foot controls with constant focusing up to 40×; high-intensity fiber-optic lighting; microscope mounting on a movable base; an x-y feature for horizontal and vertical excursion; and a beam splitter.
- The most commonly used instruments for microneurosurgery are bipolar cautery; No. 2, 3, 4, and 5 jeweler's forceps; spring-handled needle holders with straight or curved tips; spring-handled scissors; circular nerve-holding forceps; and a nerve approximator.
- Demagnetization of microinstruments is performed with a demagnetizer that generates a von Graefe electric field.
- Most commonly indicated for microneural repair are 70- to 100-μm, 3/8-circle needles on 8-0 to 10-0 nylon suture. Epineural suture is carried out with 8-0 or 9-0 nylon suture, perineural suture with 9-0 or 10-0 nylon.

Advances in metallurgy, optics, and electronics have greatly contributed to the field of peripheral microsurgery. Microneurosurgery instrumentation and techniques have evolved in parallel with those used in microvascular surgery over the last four decades. Wartime injuries, the industrialization of society, and civilian violence have provided increasing numbers of patients requiring nerve reconstruction.

The purpose of this chapter is to review the instrumentation used clinically and experimentally in peripheral nerve reconstruction. Specific methods of nerve repair are addressed in other chapters.

OPERATING ROOM CONSIDERATIONS

Adherence to standard microsurgical principles is as important in microneural as in microvascular surgery.[3,5,9,10]

Microinstruments are finely machined, with precision points that provide accurate tip approximation. Instruments are kept in a storage case lined with rubber dowels to protect the delicate tips (Fig. 17-1). The microsurgical set is steam-autoclaved, rather than gas-autoclaved, to prevent wear. Periodic examination and replacement of defective instruments ensures atraumatic handling of nerves and facility of suture manipulation. Replacements for frequently used items are maintained in stock in case of breakage.

A large operating room is extremely helpful in reducing operating time and providing the surgeon and assistants ample room for variable positioning of the operating microscope. Careful handling of the mobile microscope and other bulky items, such as anesthesia and electrodiagnostic equipment, is also facilitated. Background electrical "noise" is kept to a minimum, and the room is well grounded when using intraoperative electrodiagnostic techniques. Most often, the end or corner room in an operating suite is conducive to achieving the appropriate environment.

LOUPES AND MICROSCOPES

Magnifying loupes, or operating telescopes, in powers of 2.5× to 6.0× are used to perform initial dissection of nerves and surrounding structures. Loupes have become lighter in recent years and are now constructed with improved optics and a variety of fields with interchangeable optical powers. For versatility and cost containment, some loupes have adjustable interpupillary distances so they can be used by different surgeons, although considerable preoperative time is necessary for accurate adjustment. For individual use, telescopes are mounted with the surgeon's own corrective lenses or a plain glass frame (Fig. 17-2). The choice of loupe depends on the clinical requirements for magnification, focal length, field of vision, comfort, and cost. Loupes of 2.5× to 4.5× are most versatile, since the depth of field and field of view are inversely proportional to magnification power.

Numerous types of operating microscopes are commercially available from a variety of manufacturers. Well-maintained or reconditioned older models are affordable options for those facilities in which nerve repair is only occasionally performed or where a laboratory microscope is needed. Several features now available on these microscopes merit discussion, for they have made microsurgery less tedious and time-consuming.

Control of magnification by an automatic, motorized, foot-controlled device with constant focusing up to 40× magnification permits the surgeon to continue working at a fixed focal length while

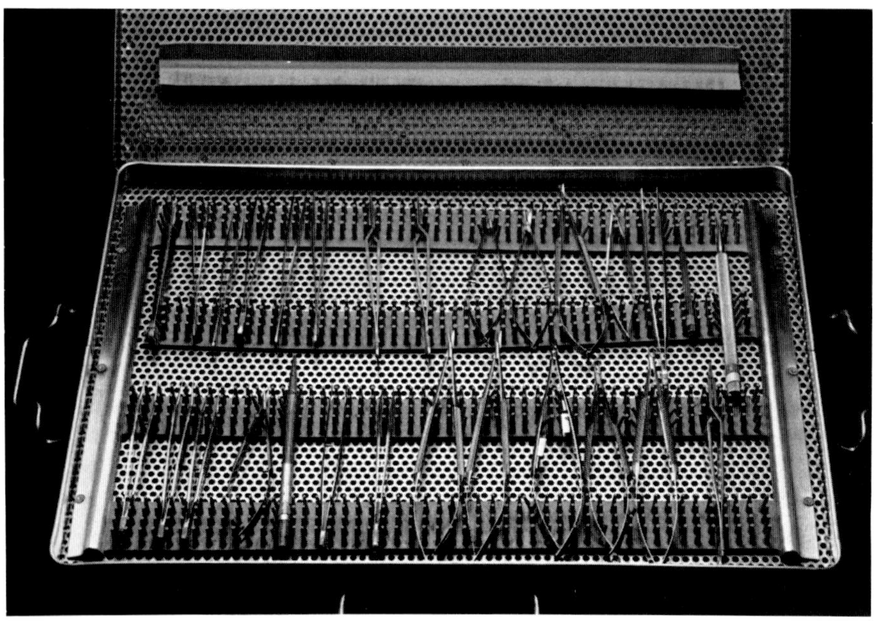

Figure 17–1. *Instruments are protected in a storage case lined with rubber dowels.*

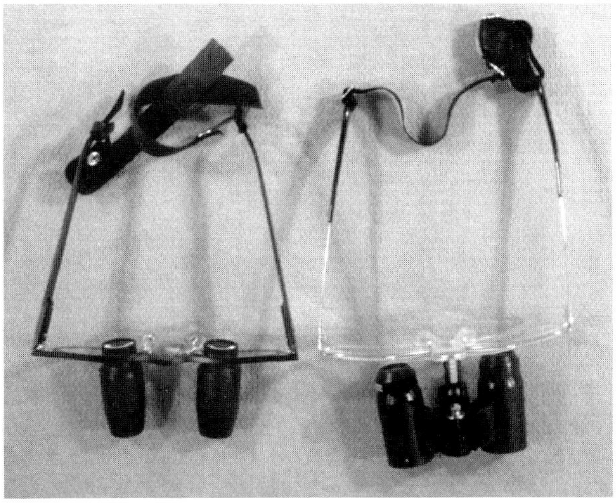

Figure 17–2. *Two types of loupes. The telescopes are mounted on the lenses or to a plain glass frame.*

changing magnification (Fig. 17-3). Improvements in illumination paralleled advances in magnification. Early operating microscopes relied on incandescent light bulbs that, by necessity, were close to the operating field and could desiccate tissue with the heat they generated. High-intensity fiberoptic light sources, located away from the surgical field, decreased heat generation and improved illumination.

Microscopes may be mounted on the ceiling or wall or on movable bases. Microscopes with floor stands allow the most versatility in positioning, particularly for operating on different areas of the body, and are the most widely used in peripheral microneurosurgery. Microscope heads have a variable horizontal and vertical excursion controlled by automated foot controls. When properly positioned at the time of nerve dissection, this *x-y feature* is set in the middle of both axes directly over the nerve ends to provide the greatest extent of field (see Fig. 17-3). Additionally, positioning the horizontal axis parallel to the extremity permits the surgeon to visualize proximally and distally by activating only one control pedal. A voice-activation control unit is an expensive accessory now being marketed, but we have no experience with this device.

Prisms, called *beam splitters*, have made it possible for cameras and stereoscopic observation tubes to be attached to the microscope (see Fig. 17-3). The problem of decreased illumination with their use has been largely eliminated with fiberoptic light sources. The development of the diploscope joined through a common network of prisms provides the assistant with separate binocular vision and zoom capabilities directly opposite the surgeon, while simultaneously ensuring the same field of view. When the surgical exposure requires focusing the microscope at an angle other than vertical, as in brachial plexus surgery, the microscope must tilt from its support column in order to place the objective perpendicular to the field of dissection. With the microscope in Figure 17-3, this is accomplished by adjusting a knob adjacent to the beam splitter. This allows the surgeon to bring the maximal amount of surgical field into focus. Further adjustments in the x-y axis may be needed, and the surgical assistant's positioning may be compromised.

Several studies have questioned whether the use of the operating microscope versus loupe magnification improves the results of peripheral nerve suture.[6,7] There are advantages and disadvantages to both methods, and larger clinical trials are needed to reach any definitive conclusions.

INSTRUMENTS

With the input of the Microsurgical Instrumentation Research Association (MICRA, est. 1952) and numerous surgeons and engineers, an array of highly specialized precision instruments has become available for use in peripheral neurosurgery. Many of the instruments are designed for use with or without microscopy and are equally applicable to microvascular surgery.

Bipolar electrocautery is preferred over unipolar systems for providing controlled thermonecrosis (Fig. 17-4). No. 5 jeweler's forceps are commonly attached to the insulated tip of the bipolar lead. When current is applied, it travels only between the two tips of the cautery, with no excessive burning. To prevent adherence of tissue to the bipolar tips, cauterization is done under saline irrigation.

Nos. 2, 3, 4, and 5 *jeweler's forceps* are indispensable for delicate tissue handling (Fig. 17-5). The narrow jaws and bit of the No. 5 forceps are

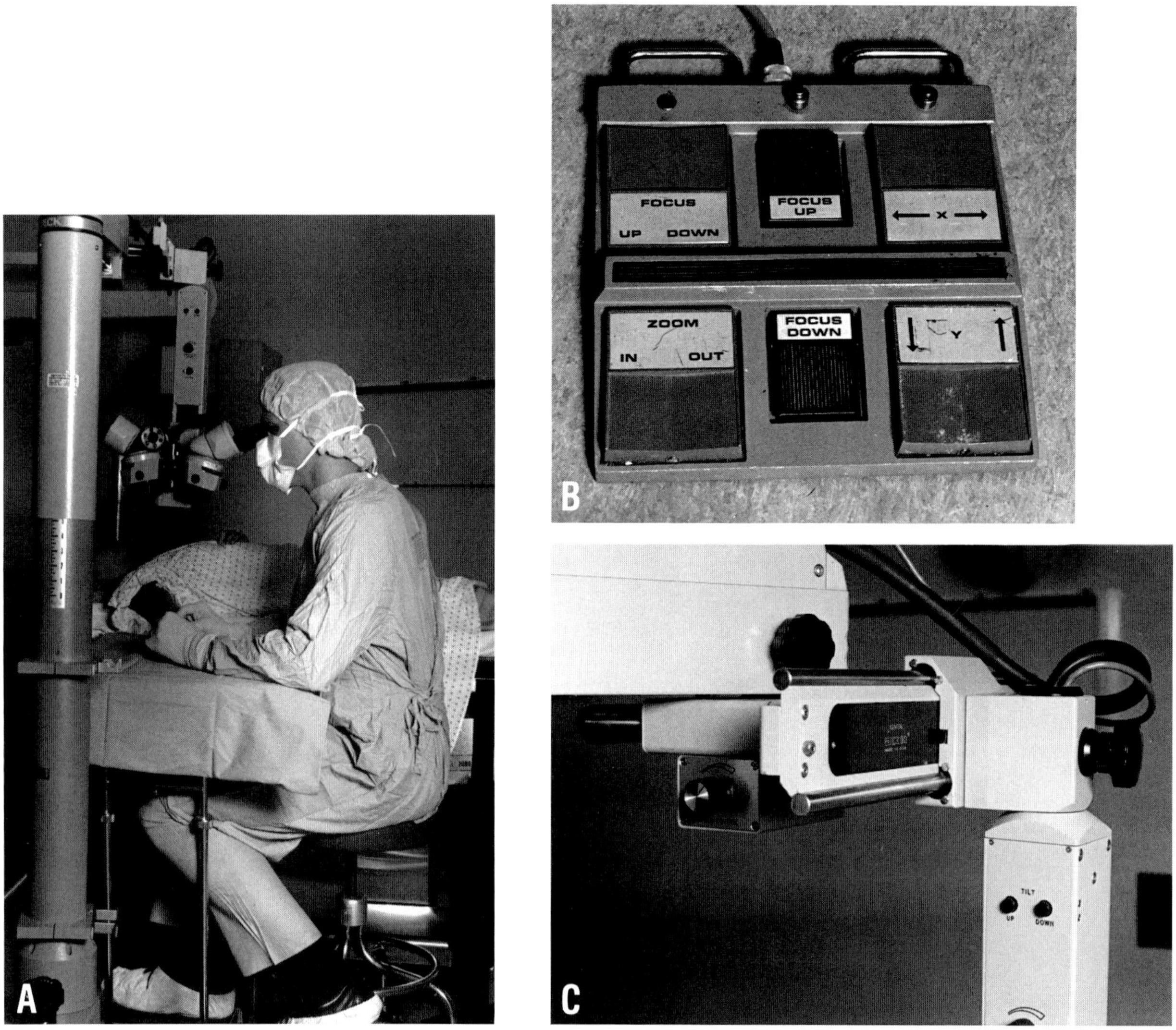

Figure 17–3. *An operating microscope. This floor stand diploscope provides an assistant with separate binocular vision and zoom capabilities. (**A**) The microscope is positioned for use, and the surgeon is seated comfortably with forearms supported. Note that the x track of the x-y movement attachment is parallel with the limb for easier longitudinal positioning in longer wounds. (**B**) The motorized foot control device for this scope allows adjustments in focusing, magnification (zoom), vertical control, and x-y movements. (**C**) The x-y portion of the microscope is shown in midposition for movement in the plane parallel to the floor. (**D, E**) The microscope is shown at the limits of two tilted positions for further variable positioning in a surgical field that is not horizontal. (**F**) The beam-splitter prisms are located in the head of the microscope.*

well suited for microscopic work. Toothed jeweler's forceps are helpful in manipulating the neuroma and glioma in preparation for neurorrhaphy. Frequent inspection of the tips and filing when needed with an emery board or Arkansas whetstone are helpful. Gentle handling and storing the tips in soft plastic scabbards help them last longer. Short segments of intravenous tubing or small rubber catheters make excellent, cost-effective tip protectors. To permit delicate balancing in the surgeon's

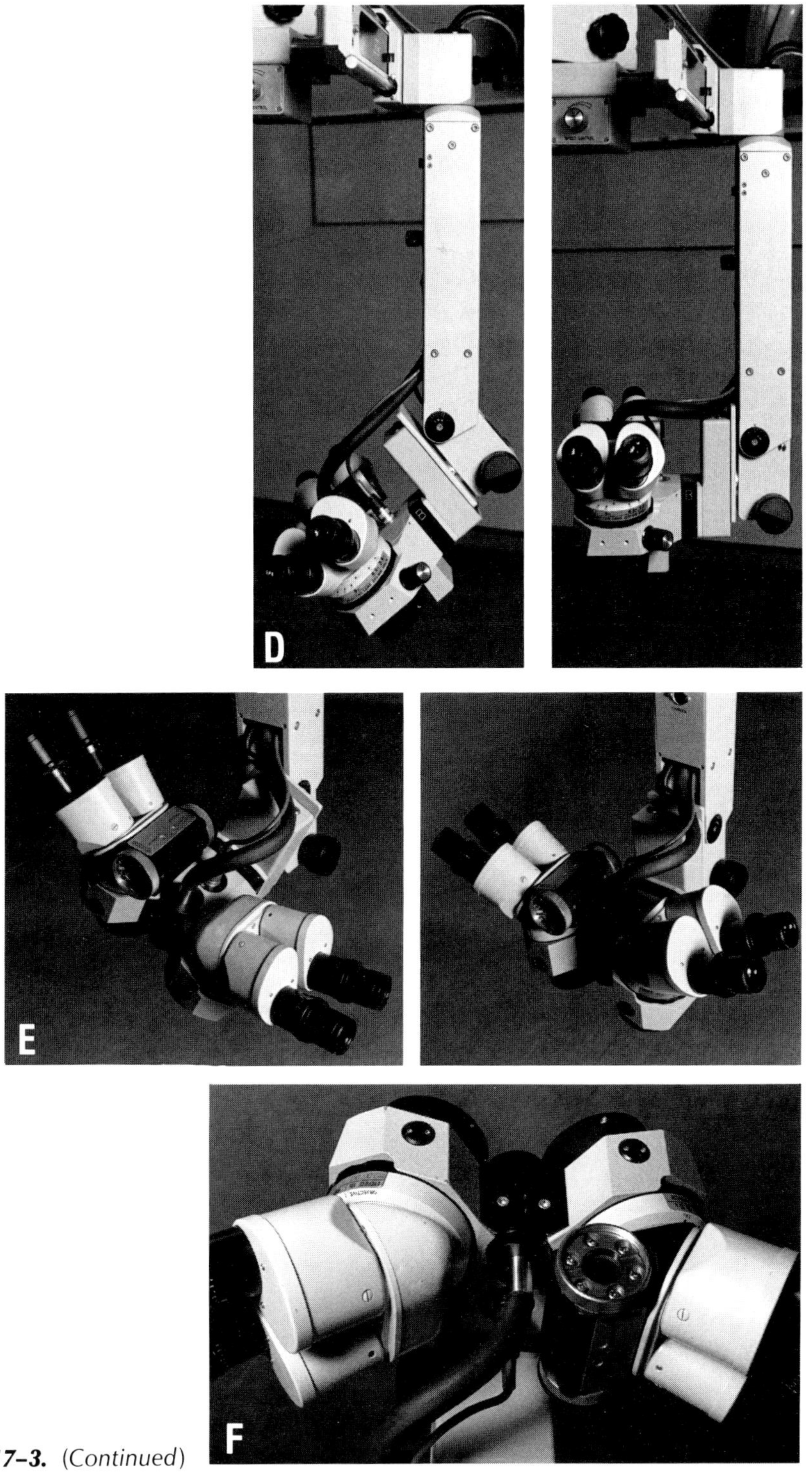

Figure 17–3. (Continued)

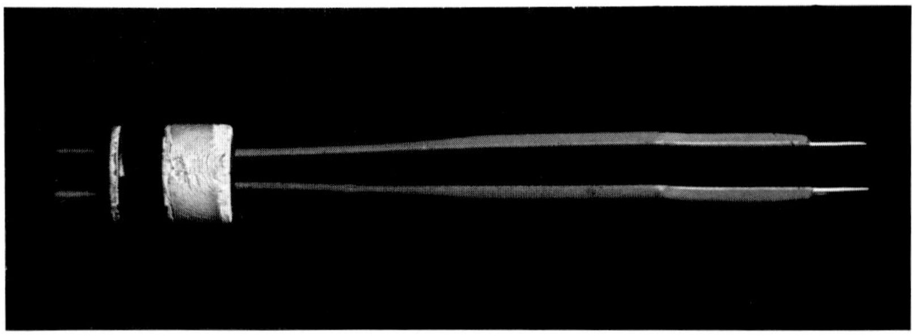

Figure 17–4. *Bipolar cautery forceps.*

first web space, forceps should be long enough to rest delicately on the first dorsal interosseous muscle (Fig. 17-6).

Demagnetization of microinstruments is easily done by putting them through one of the commercially available units that generate a von Graefe electric field.

Needle holders may be as simple as a No. 2 jeweler's forceps or as complex as ratcheted models for a fixed grasp. The ratcheted needle holder is unacceptable for microneurosurgery since the ratchet is too forceful to be manipulated delicately. Microneedles are most easily manipulated by a spring-handled needle holder to ensure control without undue force (Fig. 17-7). Jaws may be straight or curved, and newer shanks are available with better length and contouring for larger-handed surgeons or for work in deep wounds. Curved jaws provide less interference to viewing the suture. Other variations include dual-purpose holders that have a suture cutting surface at the base of the jaws and another specifically designed to hold the microneedle. The needle holder can grasp needles ranging from 30 to 130 μm as well

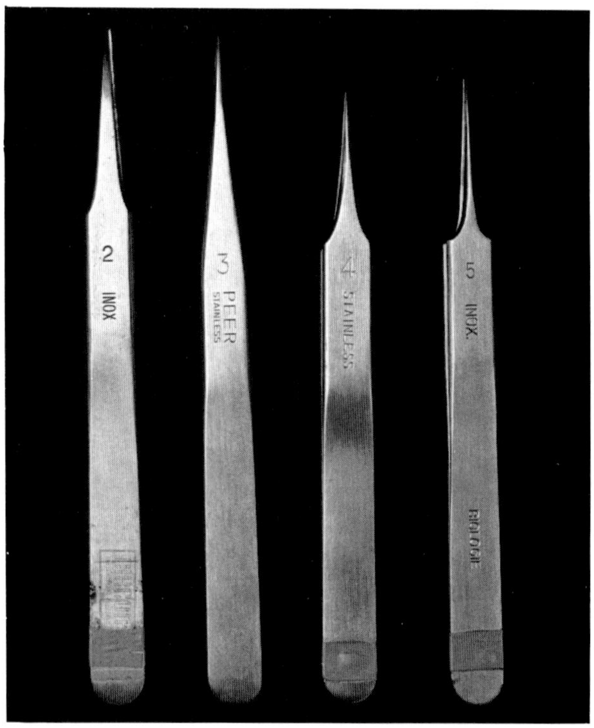

Figure 17–5. *No. 2, 3, 4, and 5 jeweler's forceps.*

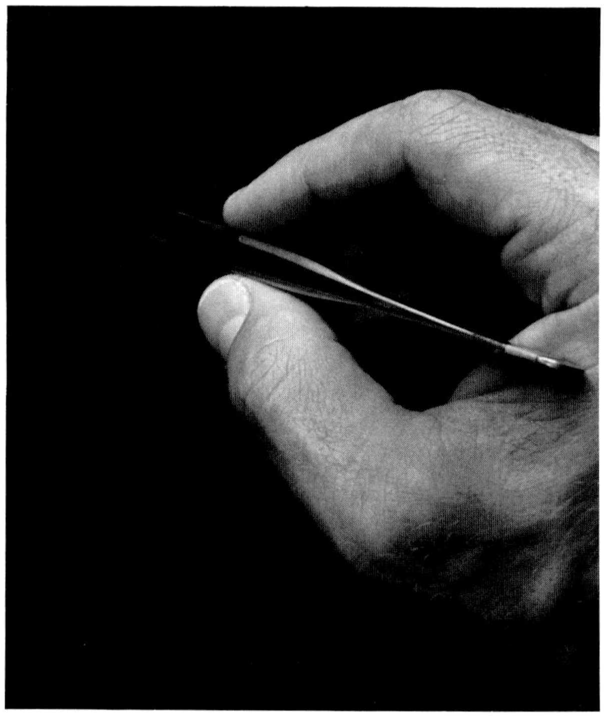

Figure 17–6. *An instrument should rest comfortably on the surgeon's first web space.*

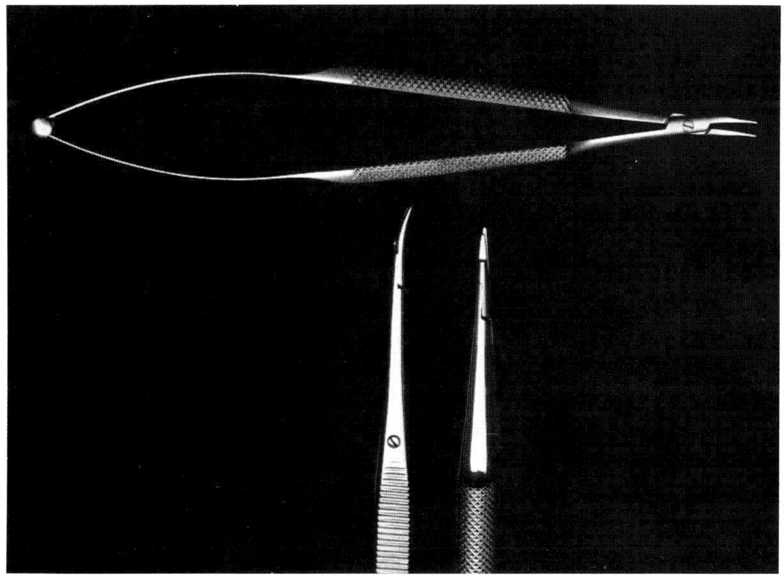

Figure 17–7. *A spring-handled needle holder, with straight or curved tips.*

as 22-μm suture material. The needle holder should rest comfortably in the surgeon's first web space.

Straight and angled spring-handled scissors are available in numerous sizes and shapes (Fig. 17-8). Angled scissors with blunt tips are especially helpful in intrafascicular nerve dissection and neurolysis. Scissors with serrated blades serve to secure the nerve better when sectioning but produce more focal damage than a knife blade. Microsurgical knives have evolved from razor-blade knives to diamond knives.[11] Although more expensive, *the diamond knife* never dulls if properly protected from chipping. The extremely sharp cutting edge greatly facilitates atraumatic nerve dissection and sectioning. While the razor-blade chip knife is less sturdy and dulls quickly, it is more versatile and is adequate for occasional use. It is much cheaper than a diamond knife. *Circular nerve-holding forceps* with apertures of 2 to 7 mm may also be helpful for nerve stabilization during sectioning (Fig.

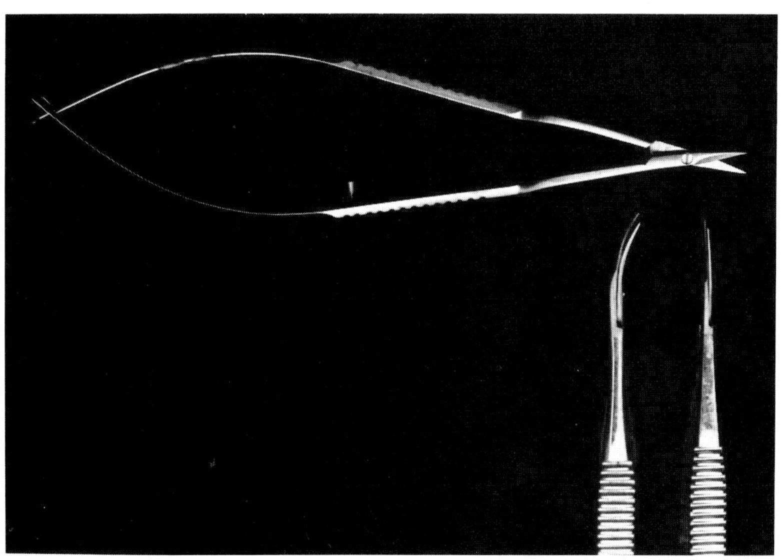

Figure 17–8. *Spring-handled scissors also come with straight or curved tips.*

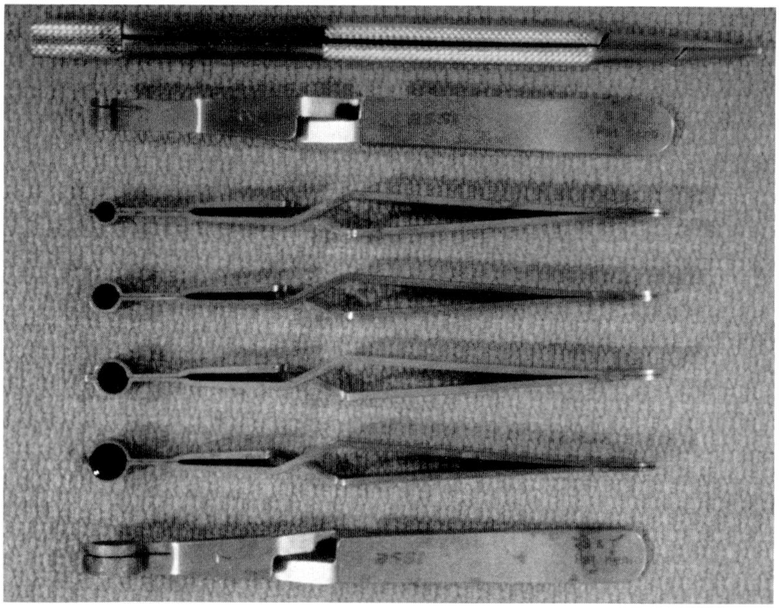

Figure 17–9. *Circular nerve-holding forceps for transecting nerves.*

17-9). A slot is oriented transverse to the nerve in the ring of the forceps for accurate perpendicular fascicular sectioning.

Topical thrombin is helpful in controlling bleeding from nerve ends, and the contrast provided by plastic background material is helpful in the microscopic field. We use a pneumatic tourniquet (sterile, if needed) on the operative extremity whenever possible.

We have used the *Van Beek nerve-approximating clamp* and have found it helpful during neurorrhaphy when there is adequate exposure (Fig. 17-10).[12] The device is placed after adequate mobilization of the nerve ends, and 28-gauge needles are inserted through the epineurium to stabilize the nerve. The clamps are then brought together on the connecting bar to approximate the nerve stumps. The more precise alignment and gentler handling of the nerve outweigh the negligible trauma caused by piercing the epineurium with the needle.

SUTURES

The development of *durable swaged-on microneedles* to suture structures that are finer than human hair has been a major advance in materials design and manufacturing. Although stainless steel sutures incite less fibroblastic response, monofilament nylon sutures of sizes 8-0 through 11-0 are easier to handle, pass well through tissue, are relatively nonreactive, and are sufficiently strong. The 70- to 100-μm 3/8-circle needles on 8-0 to 10-0 nylon suture are most commonly indicated. Suturing of

A

B

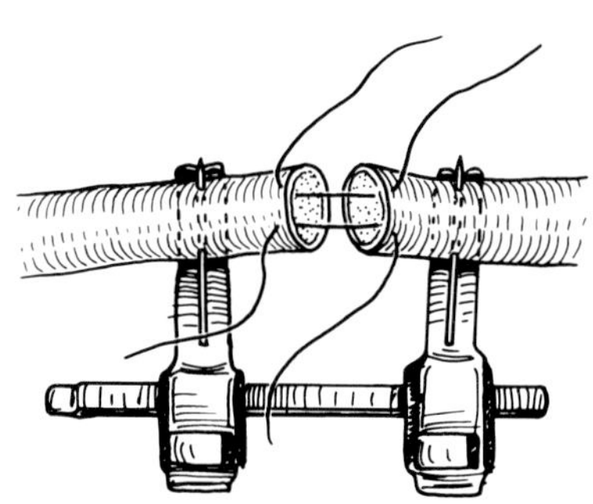

Figure 17–10. *The Van Beek nerve approximator with proper placement of the needle through the epineurium.*

epineurium with 8-0 or 9-0 nylon and perineurium with 9-0 or 10-0 nylon is recommended.

Many biological and synthetic nerve-wrapping materials have been clinically tested over the last half-century in an attempt to limit adhesions, promote longitudinal axonal growth, and provide mechanical support to the suture line.[10] No clear evidence has emerged beyond preliminary reports that wrapping improves recovery rates. One presterilized device is a silicone microprosthetic tube that encapsulates the nerve repair or graft junction (Fig. 17-11).

Protective wrappings do not impede the epi- and perineurial fibrosis that is deleterious to reconstruction of multifasciculated nerves. Further, cuffs can become too loose or too tight depending on the amount of postoperative neural edema that occurs. Thus, blood supply may be impaired at the repair site. Removal at a later date necessitates another operative procedure.

SUTURELESS NEURORRHAPHY

Concern about the reaction to sutures and the impediment their use poses to axonal regeneration has spurred the search for a technique for sutureless neurorrhaphy. Of the techniques and materials described below, only fibrin clot has significant clinical application with encouraging results (see Chaps. 20 and 22).[8] Autologous plasma and prepared fibrin clot are contraindicated when there is tension at the nerve ends. Fibrin glue, popularized in Europe, consists of a human fibrinogen solution and lyophilized bovine thrombin, the fibrinogen activator. Narakas has published an excellent review of his recent experience with its use in nerve repairs and grafts.[8] Micropore adhesive tape neurorrhaphy has not yet been widely applied on a clinical basis.[10] Tissue adhesives (cyanoacrylates) have also been largely experimental, and until problems with tissue reactivity are solved they will not gain wide clinical use.[10]

Tubulation

Sutureless tubulation using tubes and cuffs of various resorbable and non-resorbable materials to bridge segmental defects has generated much research interest as well, and investigators are searching for a material appropriate for clinical application. Akelman has reported on axonal growth across gaps up to 3 mm with resorbable isomeric alpha-hydrocarboxylic acid polymer tubes in rat and primate models.[1] Silicone tubes and cuffs have yet to earn a role in clinical practice. The objections to suture-line wrapping mentioned above apply as well to sutureless tubulation. More conclusive clinical trials based on sound laboratory models are needed before recommendations of methods other than suture neurorrhaphy are made.

Lasers

While the laser was introduced in 1950, it is only in the last decade that it has gained some acceptance in nerve repair (see Chaps. 20 through 22). Laser energy has three general effects on tissue. *Photostimulation*, which occurs from low energy, directs cellular reactions in the target tissue as in

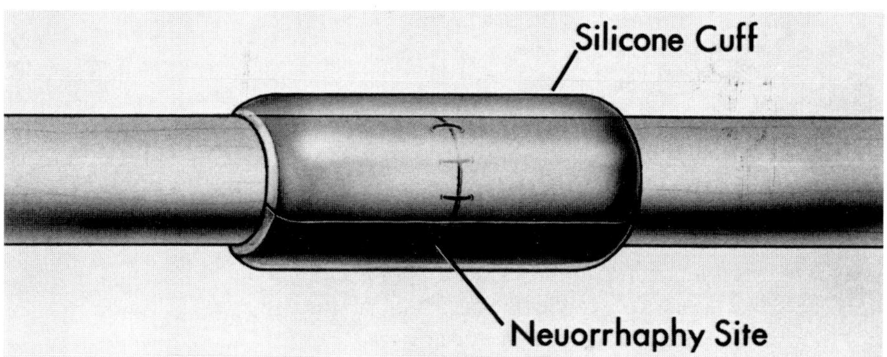

Figure 17-11. *A diagrammatic representation of a silicone nerve cuff in place over the repair.*

cancer therapy applications. *Vaporization* is the tissue effect that allows the laser to be used as a scalpel. *Coagulation*, the third and newest application of the laser to tissue, is based on the graded absorption of energy to heat the target to a specified temperature. Laser effects on tissue depend on three factors: the optical characteristics of the tissue, the absorption and scattering characteristics of the laser energy, and the dosage of the laser energy. Each tissue, in turn, has unique absorption properties.[2]

The argon laser, with its high-energy source, was first used in ophthalmologic procedures. Its use for nerve repairs in a rabbit model was recently reported by Campion.[4] He demonstrated an improved histologic appearance of laser-repaired nerves compared to controls with epineural suture. The *standard high-energy carbon dioxide (CO_2) laser*, designed for cutting, is less useful in nerve repair than the newly developed *milliwatt CO_2 laser*, with its surface-coagulating properties. The *neodymium:YAG laser* has wavelength energy properties that make it a coagulator that is conveniently transmissible through fiber-optic cables.

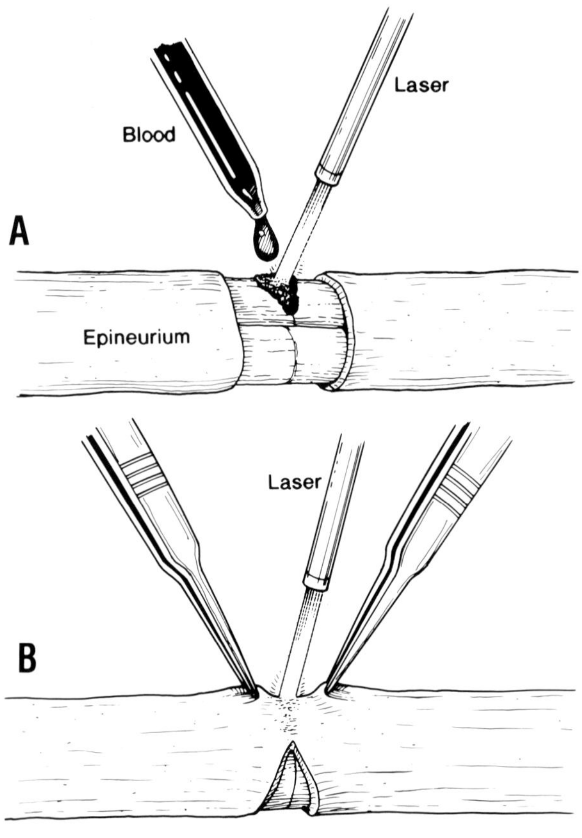

Figure 17–12. *The two techniques of experimental laser-guided neurorrhaphy. (**A**) Cauterization of a cuff of blood around a group of fascicles. (**B**) Epineurial welding.*

Coaptation of nerves by two methods—coagulation of a cuff of blood at the nerve or fascicular junction and thermal epineural fusion—is outlined in Figure 17-12. As with the fibrin clot, a theoretical advantage with laser-assisted repair is the speed with which the repair can be performed. The argon laser typifies the method of coagulating the minicuff of blood, and the CO_2 and YAG lasers operate on the principle of controlled surface depth thermal tissue welding (see Fig. 17-12). Although many of the practical aspects of laser use remain to be worked out, we feel that this method of nerve repair merits further study. The advantages over conventional techniques of less operative time, easier access to nerves in awkward locations, avoidance of foreign body reaction, decreased nerve tissue dissection, and more precise realignment of nerve fibers are compelling reasons for further investigation.

AUTHORS' PREFERRED METHOD

For initial dissection, 3.5× wide-angle loupes are used. The floor-mounted operating diploscope has foot-control zoom magnification, focus, and x-y excursion for nerve dissection and repair. We use electrical fascicular stimulation for acute repairs of mixed nerves in the appropriate patient (see Chap. 15); otherwise, we rely on surface topographical mapping (particularly for nerves repaired after extended delays or nerves with segmental defeats).

The following instruments are considered most important in the clinical practice of nerve repair: bipolar cautery, No. 3 and No. 5 jeweler's forceps, curved spring-loaded needle holder, nerve sectioning knife, and nylon suture with 50- to 100-μm needles. We do not use nerve-wrapping materials at the site of repair.

While the future of the technical aspects of nerve repair is undecided, instruments continue to develop, facilitating nerve coaptation and suture. Sutureless neurorrhaphy may become the standard as better adhesives and laser techniques are developed and as the biological basis for promoting nerve regrowth becomes more completely understood.

REFERENCES

1. Akelman E. Regeneration of peripheral nerves through bioresorbable nerve guides in primates. In: Proceedings from the 44th meeting of the Am Soc Surg Hand (abstract) 1989;3:17.
2. Almquist E. Nerve repair by laser. Orthop Clinic North Am 1988;19:201–208.
3. American Academy of Orthopaedic Surgeons. Microsurgical Skills Development Laboratory Manual. Chicago: AAOS, 1985:1–35.
4. Campion E. Peripheral nerve repair with the argon laser. In: Proceedings from the 35th meeting of the Orthop Res Soc (abstract) 1989;19.
5. Daniel R, ed. Reconstructive microsurgery. Boston: Little, Brown, 1977:9–41, 351–355.
6. Marsh D. Does the use of the operating microscope improve the results of peripheral nerve suture? J Bone Joint Surg [Br] 1987;69:625–630.
7. McManamny D. Comparison of microscope and loupe magnification: Assistance for the repair of median and ulnar nerves. Br J Plast Surg 1983;36: 367–371.
8. Narakas A. The use of fibrin glue in repair of peripheral nerves. Orthop Clin North Am 1988;19: 187–198.
9. Omer G, ed. Management of peripheral nerve problems. Philadelphia: WB Saunders, 1980:353–365.
10. Sunderland S. Nerves and nerve injuries. Baltimore: Williams & Wilkins, 1968:539–548.
11. Terzis J. A diamond knife for microsurgical repair of peripheral nerves. Plast Reconstr Surg 1974;54: 102–103.
12. Van Beek A. A nerve-approximating device. Plast Reconstr Surg 1980;66:143–146.

18

Techniques of Epineural and Group Fascicular Repair

E. F. Shaw Wilgis

AUTHOR'S KEY POINTS

- Nerves are subdivided into monofascicular, oligofascicular, and polyfascicular types. The method of nerve repair selected depends on both nerve type and nerve injury location.
- When considering repair of a divided peripheral nerve, in addition to the internal elastic tension of nerve, the necessity for longitudinal excursion during limb movement must be considered. The median and ulnar nerves at the elbow have an excursion of 7.3 and 9.8 mm, respectively, with full motion.
- There are four overriding principles for coaptation of divided nerves: preparation of neural stumps with resection of damaged tissue, approximation of stumps with special reference to length of gap and tension, coaptation of nerve stumps, and nerve suture.
- In preparation for *epineural suture,* the surgeon divides nerve ends proximal and distal to the injury site until fascicles mushroom from the neural stumps and the epineurium retracts slightly. The goal of epineural repair, to accomplish suture without tension under appropriate rotational alignment, is then accomplished. For larger nerves 8-0 nylon is used, and for small nerves 10-0 nylon is used.
- If nerve stumps cannot be approximated with 8-0 nylon suture, tension is considered excessive. Either further mobilization or a secondary procedure is then performed.
- Depending on the specific area within the extremity in which a nerve is injured, a combination of fascicular, group fascicular, and epineural suture techniques are indicated. For the *ulnar* nerve at the wrist, fascicular repair of the motor branch and group fascicular repair of sensory branches, supported by an epineural suture of the sensory component of the nerve, is indicated. For the *median* nerve, a group fascicular repair of fascicles to the motor branch, combined with a loose epineural repair of the sensory components of the nerve, is most appropriate. It is preferable to match motor nerves to motor nerves, on a fascicular or group fascicular basis, and it is inappropriate to carry interneural dissection, as this causes considerable scarring, detracting from the results of neural suture.

Epineural and group fascicular repair are two accepted techniques for repair of a severed nerve. The purpose of all nerve repair techniques is to restore continuity of the nerve trunk, including all of its elements, in order to achieve optimal and useful reinnervation of the end-organs, both sensory and motor. This chapter provides the rationale for choosing these techniques and describes the actual techniques of repair.

No single repair method is appropriate for every instance of nerve injury. The choice of repair technique depends on several overriding anatomical factors.

Type of Nerve

Nerves are subdivided into three types:

- A *monofascicular* nerve is one containing one large fascicle with many axons. An example is one of the terminal branches of a digital nerve. Monofascicular nerves are usually either pure sensory or pure motor.
- An *oligofascicular* nerve is one in which the cross section consists of few fascicles. Examples are the digital nerves and the ulnar nerve at the elbow. The latter usually contains four fascicles. Oligofascicular nerves can be either single-purpose or mixed nerves with both sensory and motor components.
- *Polyfascicular* nerves are nerves in which the cross section consists of many small fascicles, such as the radial nerve in the upper arm.

In its course from the brachial plexus to the fingertips, the nerve may undergo changes (polyfascicular in the upper arm, oligofascicular in the elbow region, and monofascicular in the hand). The ulnar nerve, as it emerges from the brachial plexus, is classified as polyfascicular; at the elbow, as oligofascicular; and, after the division to the motor branch in the hand, as monofascicular. One selects the type of nerve repair according to both nerve type and location.

Excursion

A second anatomical feature to be considered when treating a transected nerve is longitudinal neural excursion. During limb movement, peripheral nerve accommodates changes in the length of its bed. The longitudinal excursion of nerve during motion has been studied recently in several ways.

McLellan and Swash recorded action potentials in the median nerve before and during active and passive motion of limbs.[5] They found that active and passive movement had equal effects. Greatest excursions were produced by extension of the wrist and fingers and by flexion of the elbow. Extension of the wrist and fingers caused 7.4 mm excursion, flexion of the elbow 4.3 mm. The authors estimated that hyperextension of the wrist caused the median nerve to glide 10 to 15 mm. They also found that displacement of the median nerve during flexion of the wrist and fingers was two to four times greater at the wrist than in the upper arm.

Dellon and coworkers postulated that the radial sensory nerve had a significant excursion on radial and ulnar deviation of the wrist.[1] Wilgis and Murphy, using 15 fresh intact adult cadaveric arms, dissected the entire peripheral nervous system, focusing on longitudinal nerve excursion.[10] They noted that the brachial plexus had an average excursion of 15 mm when ranged from the frontal plane with the arm in full abduction to full adduction. The median and ulnar nerves at the elbow moved an average of 7.3 and 9.8 mm, respectively, with full motion. The greatest excursion of peripheral nerves occurred at the wrist, proximal to the carpal tunnel. Here the median and ulnar nerves had 15.5 and 14.8 mm of longitudinal sliding respectively, with the wrist ranged through a full arc of flexion and extension in the sagittal plane (Fig. 18-1).

These studies are consistent with the studies of McLellan and Swash. In the palm and digits, the excursion was considerably less. To summarize the amount of motion of the median nerve and the digital nerves at the wrist and fingers, the excursion of these components approaches 2 cm.

When planning repair of a divided peripheral nerve, the surgeon must consider not only the internal elastic tension of nerve, but also the need for longitudinal excursion during limb movement. For example, the normal retraction of the median nerve at the level of the wrist is 1.5 cm after a clean division. By adding the 1.5 cm of longitudinal excursion needed when taking the wrist from full flexion to full extension, the immediate demand

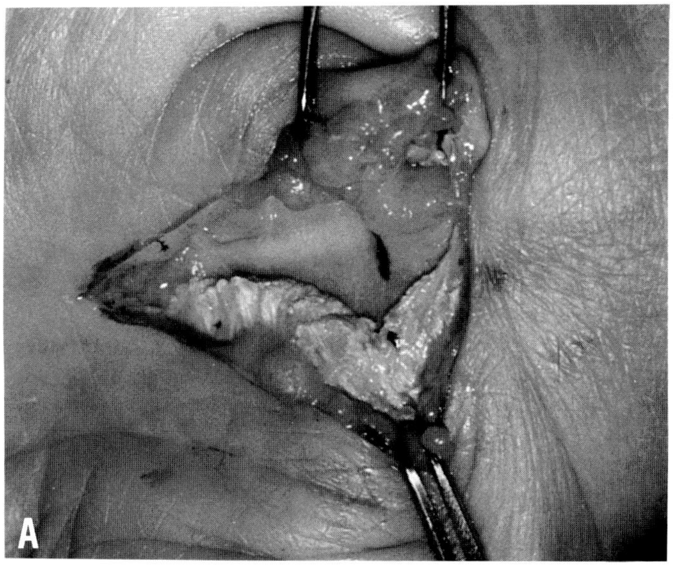

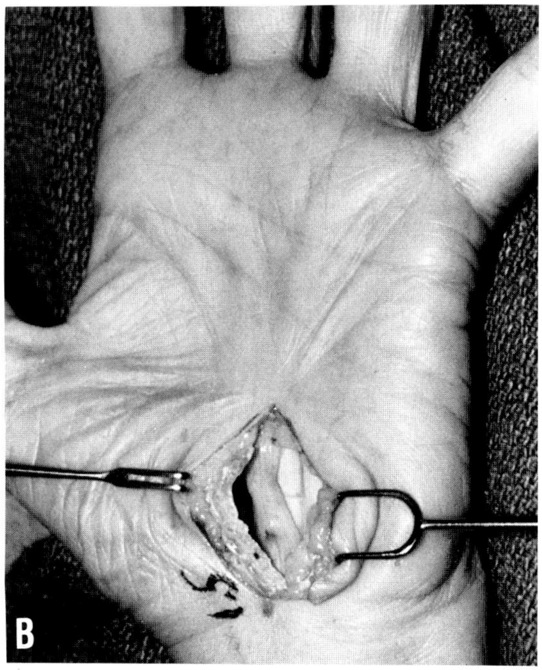

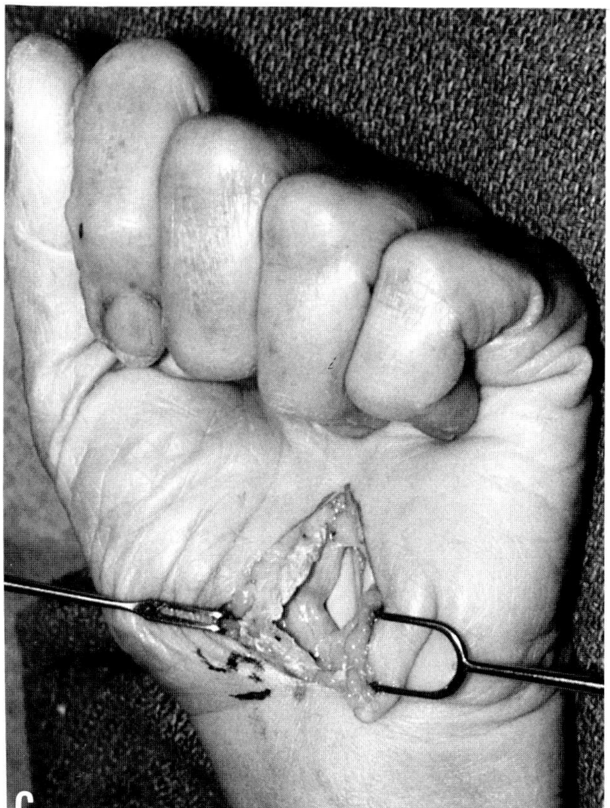

Figure 18–1. (***A***) The median nerve exposed at the wrist, with a marker on the median nerve in the transverse carpal ligament. (***B***) The median nerve dissected, with the fingers in full extension. (***C***) The median nerve dissected with the fingers in full flexion. A 1.5-mm excursion is noted.

for appropriate length of the nerve becomes apparent.

Acutely, when nerve can be approximated with minimal tension, one would expect normal longitudinal excursion to occur once local scarring factors have subsided. However, conditions are altered with the prolonged delays brought about by secondary nerve suture. Nerve loses elasticity as a result of the injury itself and subsequent scarring. Therefore the stumps cannot be approximated under normal tension with the anticipation of normal excursion, without acute flexion of an adjacent joint. In other words, nerve length is lost due to both the injury and the elapsed time interval. If nerve is sutured under tension with the wrist in acute flexion, the nerve becomes unable to slide adequately when the adjacent joint is moved into the position opposite the one in which it was placed for the repair. The existing gap between the two ends is increased because of the excursion factor.

For example, in a secondary repair of the median nerve at the wrist, when the existing gap after resection of a neuroma is 2 cm, the surgeon must consider the additional 1.5 cm that must be provided in order to accommodate the nerve's requirement for longitudinal excursion. This creates a physiological gap of 3.5 cm, a gap sufficient to influence the surgeon to choose an alternative method of repair, such as nerve grafting.

At the elbow, the need for excursion can be satisfied by transposing the ulnar nerve anteriorly, thereby reducing its need for longitudinal excursion and bridging the gap (see Chap. 78). This aspect of nerve anatomy, in its dynamic state, is of particular importance to the surgeon undertaking primary and secondary repair of peripheral nerve.

PRINCIPLES OF REPAIR

The four overriding principles for coaptation of divided nerve were outlined by Millesi and Terzis in 1984[6]:

1. Preparation of the stump, often involving resection or interfascicular dissection with separation of individual fascicles or groups of fascicles. In this step, the zone of injury is removed as completely as possible by microscopic dissection.
2. Approximation with special reference to the length of the gap between the stumps, as well as the amount of tension present.
3. Coaptation of the nerve stumps. Coaptation connotes the apposition of corresponding nerve ends with special attention to bringing fascicles into optimal contact. A direct neurorrhaphy apposes stump to stump, fascicle to fascicle, or fascicle group to fascicle group, in the corresponding ends. An indirect coaptation is performed by interposing a nerve graft. In this section we deal only with direct coaptation by epineural or group fascicular repair.
4. Maintenance of coaptation involving the use of sutures.

In performing any of the repair techniques, proper fascicular identification is mandatory. Hakstian,[3] Jabaley,[4] and Gaul[2] have proposed using electrical stimulation to aid in the identification of the fascicular structure (see Chap. 15). Intraoperative nerve stimulation is also helpful in identifying specific motor and sensory bundles.

A second aid in the proper identification of fascicles is the use of histochemical reaction and staining techniques, as described by Lister (see Chap. 16). It is particularly helpful to use the histochemical techniques in situations of late repair in which the fascicular structures are confusing. In the acute phase, the cleanly transected and divided nerve can usually be matched without the use of staining techniques.

EPINEURAL REPAIR

Epineural suture has been the traditional method of repair. Nerve repair is enhanced with the use of magnification, either magnifying loupes or the operating microscope (see Chap. 17). I use magnification in every nerve repair.

In accomplishing the epineural suture technique in the primary situation, the surgeon first divides nerve ends proximal and distal to the injury site until all visible signs of damage have been debrided. Fascicles then mushroom from the neural stumps, and the epineurium retracts slightly. The goals of epineural repair are to establish continuity without tension, with proper rotational alignment.

The nerve is inspected for longitudinal blood vessels that can be aligned in the epineurium. Also, fascicular arrangement is noted and fascicles from both stumps are matched. This ensures appropriate rotational alignment.

Neurorrhaphy is carried out using nonabsorbable suture. I recommend 8-0 nylon for larger nerves and 10-0 nylon for small nerves, such as digital nerves. The nylon is passed through the epineurium proximally and distally and tied (Fig. 18-2). The epineurium is not closed so tightly that the fascicular ends become mismatched and malaligned. It is preferable to leave a small gap in the epineurium held together by a suture, with the fascicular ends in more appropriate alignment. Therefore, the suture, which is not tied tightly, acts as a guiding suture rather than a retention suture.

The second suture is placed opposite the first, and then the epineurium is closed by halving the distance on the anterior and posterior aspects of the nerve. The number of sutures used is the minimal number required to ensure approximation of the nerve stumps. If the nerve cannot be approximated with 8-0 nylon suture, tension is considered excessive. Either further mobilization or a secondary procedure is then performed.

The nerve is inverted and the posterior aspect sutured in a similar fashion. No fascicles should protrude between the suture lines.

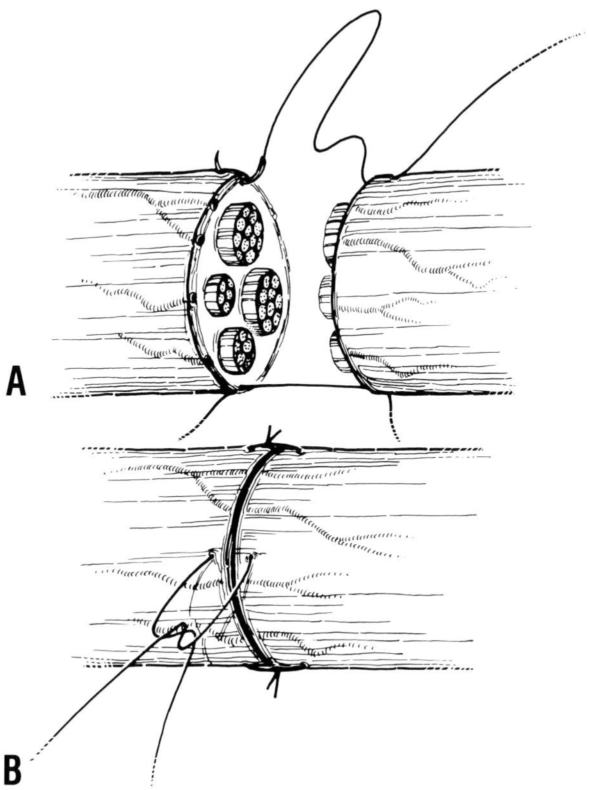

Figure 18-2. Epineural repair.

GROUP FASCICULAR REPAIR

A potentially more accurate technique is the group fascicular repair. In this method, I use Sunderland's anatomical dissections[7-9] and Millesi's concepts[6] in grouping a number of fascicles together for matching. Again, the nerve ends are matched by resecting damaged tissue, followed by a careful analysis of the anatomical cross-sectional appearance of the nerve stumps. Fascicular groups are drawn out and dissected and the groups of fascicles joined by interfascicular epineurial suture (Fig. 18-3). In the median nerve at the forearm level, it is possible to identify five groups of fascicles; in the ulnar nerve at the wrist, approximately four.

With this technique the margin of error is reduced considerably because axons remaining in the same groups of fascicles cross the juncture, reinnervating appropriate areas. The interfascicular anatomical arrangement of nerve is thus preserved more appropriately than with fascicular suture.

Author's Preferred Method

I prefer to use a combination of the above types of repairs, depending on the specific area within the

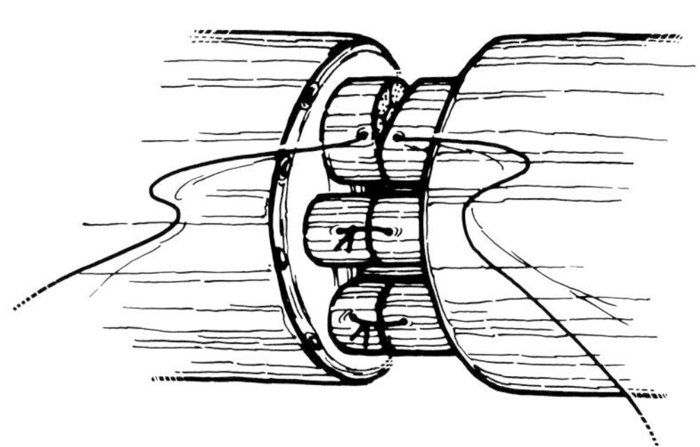

Figure 18-3. Group fascicular repair.

extremity. For instance, the ulnar nerve at the elbow is composed of four fascicles. A fascicular repair is the appropriate repair here. When faced with division of the ulnar nerve at the wrist, I would prefer to do a fascicular repair of the motor branch and then a group fascicular repair of sensory branches, supported by an epineural repair of the sensory component of the nerve. In the median nerve, I prefer to do a group fascicular repair of the fascicles to the motor branch and then a loose epineural repair of the remainder of the sensory nerve (Fig. 18-4).

Adhering strictly to one type of repair or another is not useful in peripheral nerve surgery. The surgeon should have all the techniques in his or her armamentarium and should use them in appropriate situations. The anatomical arrangement of nerve differs considerably throughout the extremity, and the surgeon should adjust the nerve repair depending on the anatomical arrangement he or she confronts.

In my opinion it is preferable to match motor nerves with motor nerves, on a fascicular or group fascicular basis, and it is inappropriate to proceed with intricate interneural dissection, as this causes sufficient scarring to detract ultimately from the results of nerve suture.

A fresh, cleanly transected nerve demonstrating complete correspondence between the fascicular patterns of both nerve ends is best treated by coaptation with the correct orientation by use of superficial epineural sutures. Epineurial sutures are inserted at levels where the fascicles are closely packed with minimal interfascicular epineurial tissue. On the other hand, when the transected areas are dominated by epineural tissue, group fascicular sutures are advisable, since misalignment of fascicular structures creates a high risk of axonal misdirection into epineurial tissues. Proximal in the arm, where separate fascicles contain a mixture of fibers belonging to several peripheral branches, separate fascicular units cannot be created, and thus group fascicular repair is not advisable. However, at distal levels where branches representing unique functions are well-formed and confined to separate fascicles within nerve trunks, the group fascicular technique is superior. This is especially true for the median and ulnar nerves, at or just above the wrist, where motor and sensory components are separated and well-defined. This is also true for the radial nerve at the elbow and the sciatic nerve in the distal thigh.

Epineural and group fascicular techniques can be combined, as I suggest. It may be useful to preserve a sector of the epineurium in the dorsal portion of the repair site to improve strength and maintain orientation of interneural structures, while the group fascicular technique is used in the central portion of the nerve. This is particularly useful when suturing the median nerve at the wrist.

A

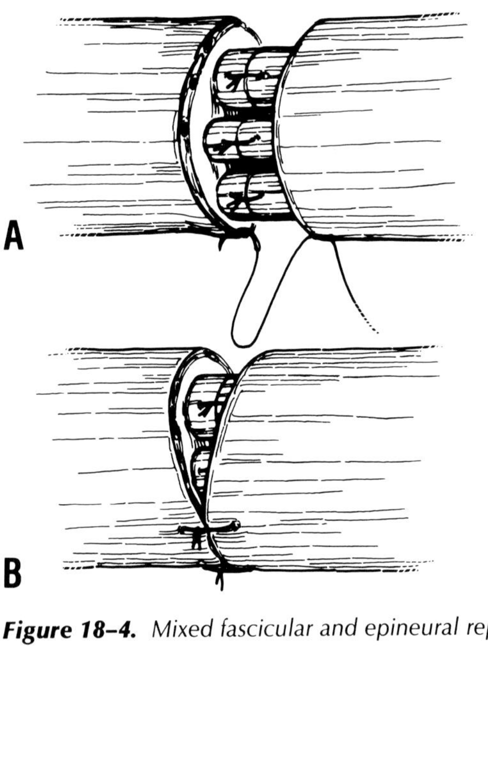

B

Figure 18-4. *Mixed fascicular and epineural repair.*

REFERENCES

1. Dellon AL, Mackinnon S, Pestronk A. Implantation of sensory nerve into muscle: Preliminary clinical and experimental observations on neuroma formation. Ann Plast Surg 1984; 12:30–40.
2. Gaul S. Electrical fascicle identification as an adjunct to nerve repair. J Hand Surg 1983; 8:289.
3. Hakstian RW. Funicular orientation by direct stimulation. J Bone Joint Surg [Am] 1968; 50:1178.
4. Jabaley ME. Electrical nerve stimulation in the awake patient. Bulletin of the Hospital for Joint Disease Ortho Inst 1984; 4:248–259.
5. McLellan DL, Swash M. Longitudinal sliding of the median nerve during movements of the upper limb. J Neurol Neurosurg Psychiatry 1976; 39:566.

6. Millesi H, Terzis JK. Nomenclature in peripheral nerve surgery. Clin Plast Surg 1984; 11:3.
7. Sunderland S. The intraneural topography of the radial, median and ulnar nerves. Brain 1945; 68: 243.
8. Sunderland S. The adipose tissue of peripheral nerves. Brain 1945; 68:118.
9. Sunderland S. The pros and cons of funicular nerve repair. Founder's Lecture, the American Society for Surgery of the Hand. J Hand Surg 1979; 4:201.
10. Wilgis EFSW, Murphy R. The significance of longitudinal excursion in peripheral nerves. Clin Hand Surg 1986; 2:761–776.

19

Fascicular Repair

Jack W. Tupper

AUTHOR'S KEY POINTS

- The fascicle, the outer layer of which is the perineurium, is the smallest suturable component of peripheral nerve.
- In 1969, it became possible to repair small fascicles (0.2–1 mm) when a 70-μm stainless steel needle was swaged onto a 25-μm nylon filament suture.
- Pure motor and sensory fascicles, repaired by fascicular suture, provide optimal functional return.
- With partial nerve severance, a technically superior repair is accomplished by dissecting individual fascicles from intact ones and suturing them directly. While reports on the results of fascicular suture do not conclusively demonstrate its superiority over other techniques, this method is preferred in well-defined situations.

HISTORY

The possibility for repair of individual intraneural elements was described initially in 1917 by Langley and Hashimoto.[8] Sir Sydney Sunderland provided the basic information necessary for clinical fascicular repair: in 1945 he described upper-extremity intraneural anatomy and, from a theoretical standpoint, described fascicular suture.[10] In 1953 he stated, "An ideal suturing method will achieve full restoration of the funicular pattern of the divided nerve."[11]

The clinical attempts I have made since 1960 have been limited, because of limited suture availability, to groups of fascicles. The needles that could be successfully joined to suture at that time were too large, injuring the perineurium of 1-mm fascicles. Although 11-0 steel was an adequate suture material, static charges under low depth of microscopic fields made its use impractical. Attempts to temper the end of stainless steel suture to form its own needle were unsuccessful. The practical application of perineural suturing was impossible until an adequate needle–thread ratio was provided. Buncke and Schultz* attempted to electroplate a chromium needle onto the tip of a nylon suture in 1962, but the method did not prove practical. O'Brien,† in similar fashion, plated stainless steel onto a nylon thread, but this method also was clinically impractical.

In 1964 Edshage showed experimentally that epineural suture often resulted in poor fascicle ap-

* *Buncke H, Schultz W. Personal communication, 1990.*

† *O'Brien B. Personal communication, 1972.*

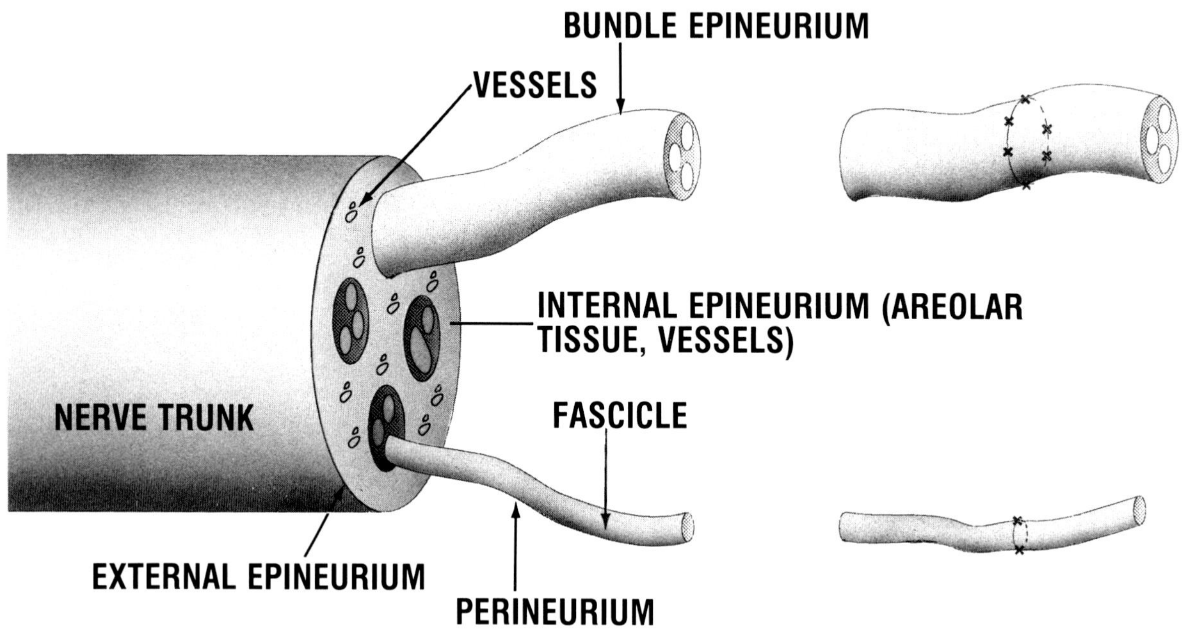

Figure 19–1. *Anatomy of peripheral nerve.*

position.[4] In 1968 Hakstian discussed orientation of fascicles in the process of nerve repair, but only alluded to the possibility of fascicular repair.[5] Bora, in 1967, reported on and showed diagrams of true epineural repair in the large fascicles of cat sciatic nerve.[1] In 1976 Cabaud, Rodkey, McCarroll, Mutz, and Niebauer compared results of epineural and perineural repairs and found little difference.[3]

The repair of small fascicles (0.2–1 mm) in humans was impossible until suitably small needles were swaged on to sufficiently fine threads. In 1969, Werner Spingler and Eugen Tritt (S&T Co.) in West Germany, working with Robert Acland‡ from Scotland, swaged a 70-μm stainless steel needle onto a 25-μm nylon filament suture. The needles were hand-sharpened and polished. Portions of each batch were tested with the expectation that they would be able to penetrate shoe leather. Quality control was so stringent (up to 50% rejects at the factory) that the product, although in short supply, was extremely reliable. These handmade sutures supplied the world's microsurgery needs until 1977, when Ethicon, and later other manufacturers, were able to fabricate them on automated machinery.

Sunderland said, "The most serious factors which complicate the regeneration and adversely affect the quality of the recovery after nerve repair are those which foster the wasteful regeneration of axons outside funiculi and their entry into functionally unrelated endoneural tubes."[12] While many factors influence recovery after nerve disruption (ie, age, local tissue condition, nerve growth factors, basal laminin, phosphorylation and ion transport; see Chap. 24), the major effect the surgeon has had, to date, is on the quality of the actual repair. On theoretical grounds, it appears that the more accurate the alignment of the smallest nerve elements, the greater the likelihood that tropic influences will encourage regrowth of axons into appropriate channels.

ANATOMY

Each peripheral nerve is surrounded by an external epineural sheath. Blood vessels are located just inside looser surrounding areolar paraneurium (see Chap. 1). The contents of the external epineurium

‡ *Tritt E. Personal communication, 1990.*

are a matrix of internal epineurium, composed of connective tissue and areolar tissue through which blood vessels and lymph vessels pass; fascicles surrounded by a perineural sheath; and bundles of fascicles surrounded by their own sheath of condensed internal epineurium (Fig. 19-1).

The perineurium surrounding each fascicle forms a physiological barrier, interruption of which leads to demyelinization (see Chap. 1).[13] From a physiological standpoint it is the smallest suturable structure in peripheral nerve.

Fascicles comprise 25% to 75% of nerve volume, depending on the nerve involved and its location.[14] Nerves commonly used for grafting purposes (ie, the sural and lateral antebrachial cutaneous nerves) are approximately 75% non-neural tissue. Fascicles vary in size from just over 1 mm to less than 0.1 mm. Using the microscope and microinstruments, sutures may be placed easily in fascicles as small as 0.2 mm (see Chap. 17).

INDICATIONS FOR FASCICULAR REPAIR

Completely severed pure motor or sensory nerves repaired in epineural fashion provide results equal to those undergoing the more painstaking perineural repair.[2,3,6,9,15–17] Terminal branches are the size of individual fascicles. These terminal fascicles, which not only are pure, but also are in close proximity to their receptors, are appropriately sutured as soon as possible after sharp transections. Thus, sensory branches beyond the distal flexion crease of the fingers and motor divisions of the median nerve beneath the abductor pollicis brevis may be sutured directly. The abductor pollicis brevis may be detached at its insertion and reflected proximally toward its blood and nerve supply, exposing the terminal motor elements to the flexor pollicis brevis and opponens pollicis. The abductor pollicis brevis is then re-attached to its insertion with no loss of function.[19] Similar branches to specific intrinsic muscles, emerging from the deep motor branch of the ulnar nerve as it crosses the depths of the palm, are also repaired by fascicular suture.

Case 1

A 15-year-old girl, stabbed through the dorsal apex of the thumb–index metacarpal angle, presented 1 week later complaining of inability to extend the index finger at the middle and distal interphalangeal joints. Ulnar nerve damage alone would not account for the functional loss, as not only were the motor branches of the ulnar nerve to the first dorsal and first palmar interossei damaged, but also the median motor branch to the index finger lumbrical muscle. The patient had a positive Froment's sign, indicating that the adductor pollicis was also involved.

At surgery, the ulnar motor branches to the adductor pollicis, first dorsal interosseous, and first volar interosseous muscles, which were found to have been transected, were repaired individually. The motor branch to the index finger lumbrical muscle was repaired where it had been severed, 0.5 cm from its entry into muscle. This latter nerve had the shortest distance to regenerate.

The first indication of functional return was the loss of the index claw posture. The return of function of the other muscles followed with a loss of the Froment's sign.

Case 2

A 14-year-old boy was stabbed in the dorsal forearm. Loss of function of the extensor pollicis longus and extensor indicis proprius, assumed to be the result of muscle–tendon severance, was noted. Exploration revealed severance of the fascicle motor branch that passed to these two muscles after exiting the supinator. Operative repair resulted in full return of function.

Repair of Mixed Nerves Where Motor and Sensory Elements are Identifiable (Median and Ulnar Nerves at the Wrist)

This larger type of nerve provides more opportunity for axons to grow into functionally unrelated fascicles or to be lost in interfascicular tissue. The motor branch distally is identified where small fascicles emerge from beneath the abductor pollicis brevis, condensing more proximally into one large fascicle or occasionally into a bundle of small fascicles in the carpal tunnel area where it branches from the median nerve. This branch is traced as a separate unit for approximately 5 cm proximal to the flexion crease of the wrist.[7] As the branch joins the median nerve at one of a number of sites, it can be identified by tracing it from its point of entry into the thenar muscles. Following acute sharp injury, the identified distal stump is visually aligned with its proximal counterpart. Even if the injury is a crush injury and a decision is made to carry out secondary repair later, this proximal fasciculus is identified and tagged.

The motor bundle of the ulnar nerve at the wrist, because of its consistent posterior location, is also readily identifiable (Fig. 19-2*A*). Repair of the remaining sensory elements of either nerve is then accomplished by simple bundle repair, after part of the external epineurium has been excised. This method gives results equal to the very time-consuming total fascicular repair of this nerve (Fig. 19-2*B*). Misdirected sensory-to-sensory axons can result in useful function due to cortical recognition of new signals, but motor axons misdirected into

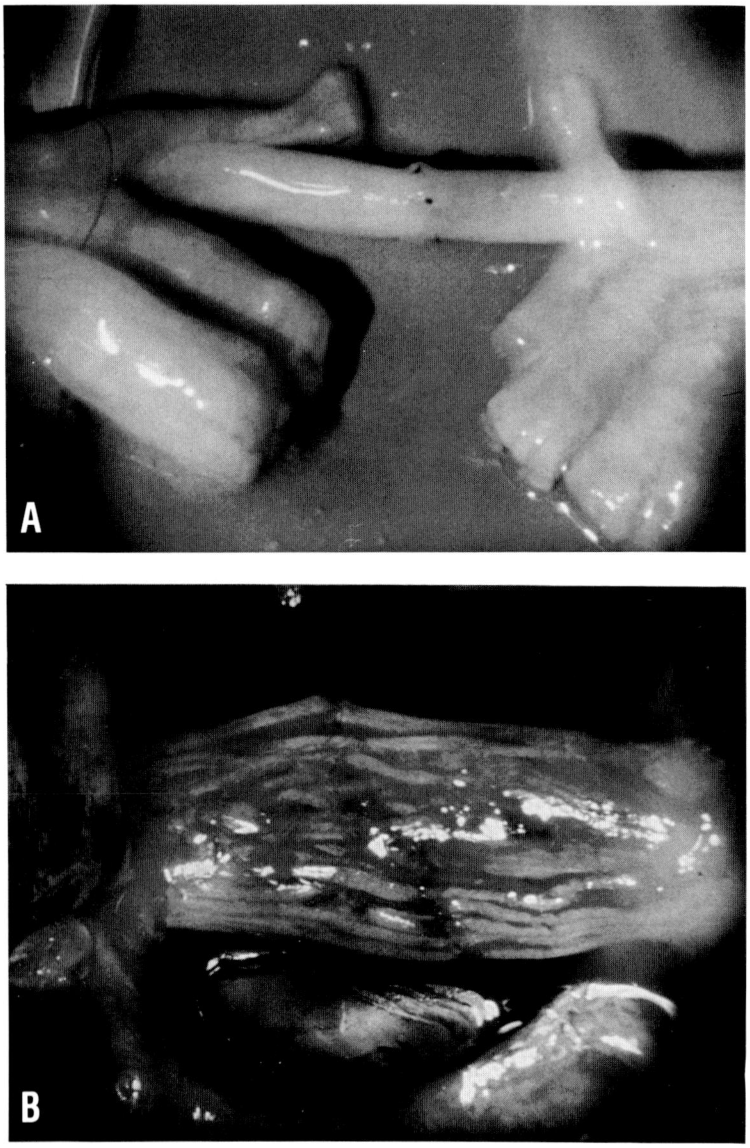

Figure 19–2. *(**A**) Ulnar nerve at wrist with motor fascicle repaired. The remaining fascicles may be repaired as fascicle groups. (**B**) Total fascicular repair.*

sensory pathways or into the interfascicular epineurium do not become functional.

PARTIALLY SEVERED NERVES

If a nerve has been partially severed, a neater repair is accomplished by individually dissecting the divided segment from the intact one, followed by individual fascicular or small bundle repair. An example is the partially severed digital nerve that continues to provide some sensation but also has developed a tender neuroma (Fig. 19-3). Most digital nerves have five fascicles. If two have been severed, forming a neuroma-in-continuity, they can be dissected free from undamaged fascicles, trimmed, and repaired by perineural suture. Thus, the sensibility present preoperatively is preserved and the tenderness due to the neuroma is alleviated. In addition, there is hope of some sensory return, depending on the delay from the original injury. In the case of an old, scarred hemisection of a large nerve, the dissection is tedious and fascicular grafts may be required.

Nerves severed at the site of branching are more easily dissected into fascicular or bundle elements for individual repair. There are no contraindications for this type of dissection, except where there is so much intraneural scarring that the terminal elements cannot be identified (ie, in the fingertip or muscle insertional area).

Author's Preferred Method

General or adequate axillary block anesthesia is given. The extremity is maintained in a stationary position during the procedure. Tourniquet control facilitates dissection and the placement of sutures.

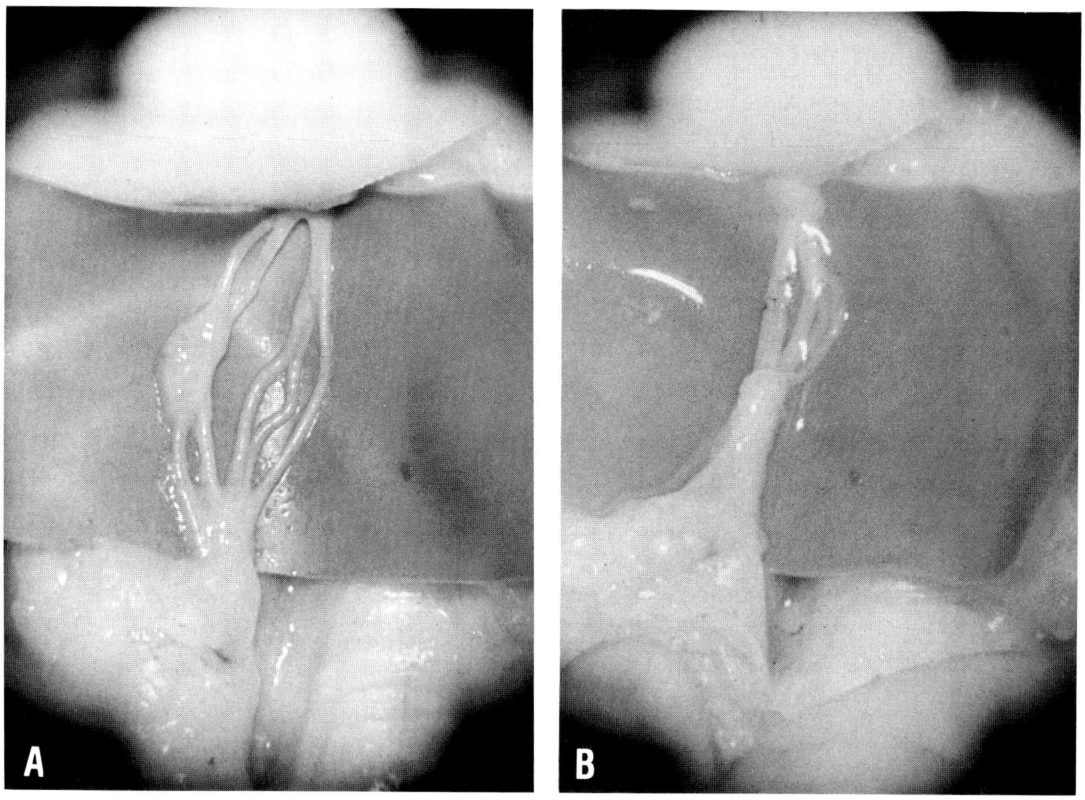

Figure 19–3. *Digital nerve (**A**) with three fascicles intact and tender neuroma from two fascicles; (**B**) after excisional repair of damaged fascicles.*

If tourniquet control is lost, or is interrupted because of time involved, the portion of the nerve being dissected is placed on an elevated bolster, allowing blood to drain. Irrigation is used liberally. It is best to work rapidly so that the the repair can be carried out within the confines of tourniquet time.

After repair, the part is splinted so that tension on the suture line is eliminated. In the case of the median nerve at the wrist, a 1-cm portion of the transverse carpal ligament is preserved so that when the wrist is splinted in flexion postoperatively, the flexor tendons do not bowstring, pushing the nerve into the subcutaneous wound scar.

Dissection is done with 2.5× to 3.5× loupes. Adjacent paraneurium, which carries the blood supply, is preserved as a layer for later closure over the repair site. A bipolar coagulator with very small tips (ie, No. 5 jeweler's forceps) for use on the intraneural vessels of larger nerves is used for hemostasis. The external epineurium is discarded for a length equal to twice the diameter of the nerve on each side. The general alignment of fascicles and bundles is assessed visually and matched with corresponding groups on the opposite side. If additional nerve must be resected to arrive at unscarred bundles, or if the delay to repair has allowed atrophy of distal fascicles, matching is more difficult. Two or three 10-0 sutures placed in groups that appear to match help maintain alignment.

With the help of repeated saline flushes, the loose intraneural epineurium and vessels between the fascicles or bundles are excised with microscissors. Individual fascicles are identified by the spiral bands of Fontana located in the perineurium. If longitudinal tension is applied to the perineurium, these bands disappear, indicating that they are tension wrinkles probably affording some protection from stretch deformation (Fig. 19-4). Beyond the perineural brim on the end of a

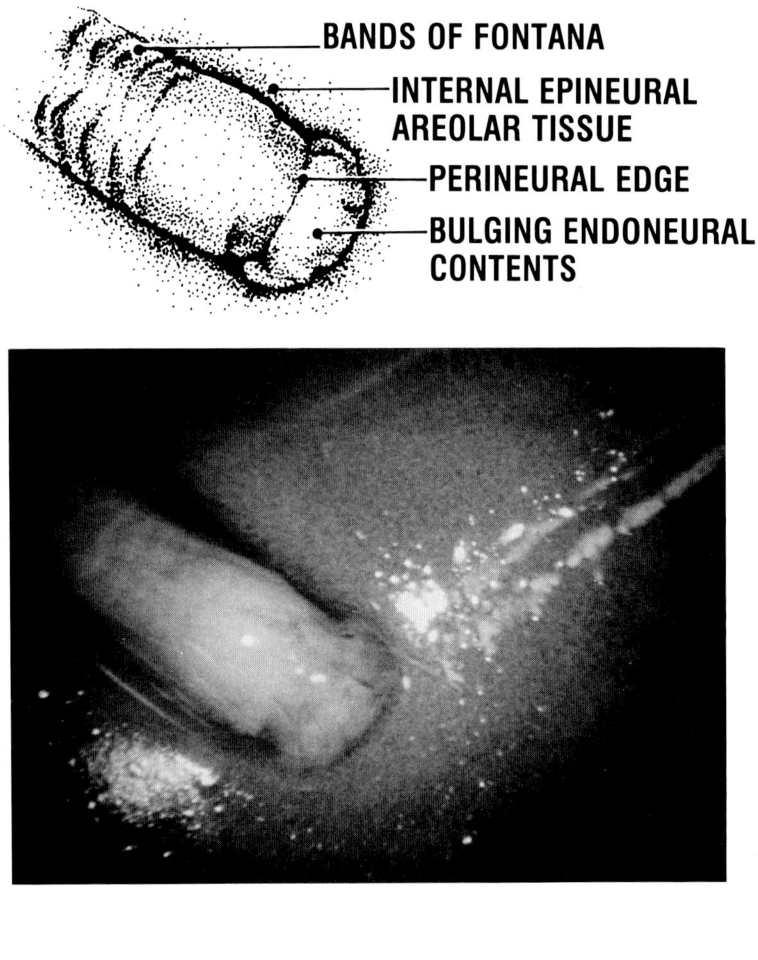

Figure 19–4. *Fascicle bands of Fontana. Note endoneural bulge beyond the edge of the perineurium.*

fascicle, a bulge of intrafascicular contents is noted that looks like the end of an ice-cream cone. This is trimmed prior to suture placement; it rapidly recurs unless sutures are placed promptly. Two sutures placed through the perineurium 180° from each other are usually adequate for each fascicle. Depending on fascicle size, either a 70-μm or 50-μm needle on a 10-0 nylon suture is preferred. Placement of sutures is done under high power, taking care to include only perineurium. The power may then be zoomed down to the low end of the spectrum for the purpose of tying knots rapidly. The cleaner the initial fascicular preparation, the easier the final repair.

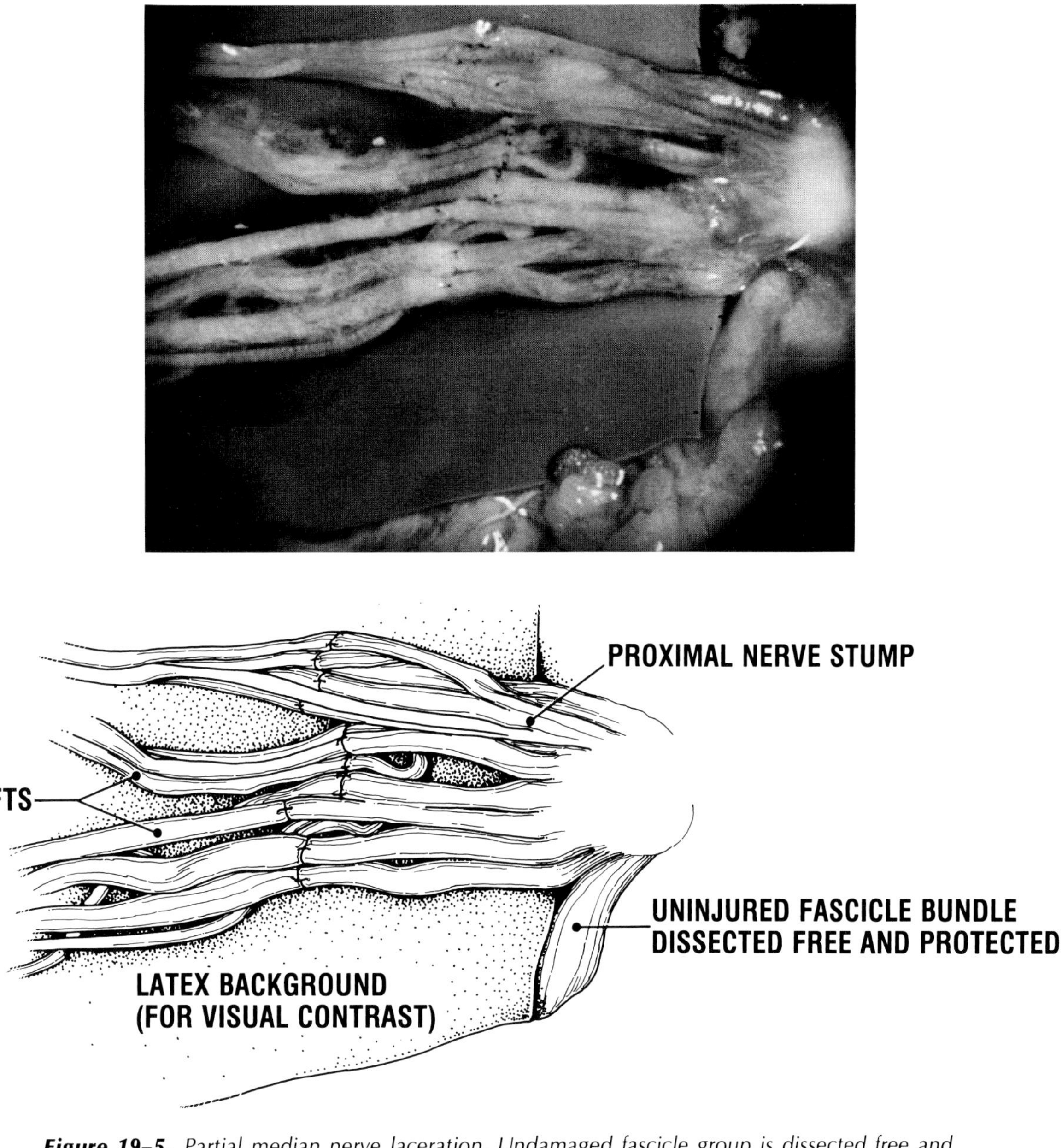

Figure 19–5. *Partial median nerve laceration. Undamaged fascicle group is dissected free and placed beneath latex sheet. (Left) Distal junctures out of the field. (Right) Free fascicles from sural nerve sutured one-to-one to proximal nerve trunk fascicles.*

At the end of the procedure, closure should provide at least a subcutaneous layer of fat overlying the repair. A free fat graft from the forearm or the medial brachium, including the deep fascia, may be used if necessary. This is secured with four percutaneous corner sutures.

Postoperatively, a splint is applied for 3 weeks, followed by exercises to regain joint motion. In the case of repair of nerves in the hand, although the fingers and wrist are prevented from extending, passive flexion of the fingers is carried out in the early postoperative interval to reduce stiffness.

NERVE GRAFTING

There is some evidence that a better result may be obtained if a graft has a fascicular volume equal to that of the proximal and distal stumps (Fig. 19-5). In a limited series of six epineural and ten fascicular (perineural) grafts, the epineural repairs achieved Von Frey hair values averaging 3.24, compared to 1.92 achieved with fascicular grafts. Epineural repair provided two-point discrimination averaging 11.5 mm, compared to 8.2 mm in the fascicular repair group. As donor nerves have as much as 75% nonfascicular tissue, it is advantageous to seek equal fascicular graft volume both proximally and distally. To accomplish this, the fascicles are removed from the donor sural nerve, using loupe magnification on a moist plastic background. The fascicles are sized by length and diameter, individually paired, and sutured. Initially the distal stumps and grafts are sutured, followed by the proximal stumps. The distal suture sites junctures are protected by a plastic sheet in order to prevent damage while working on the final proximal suture line. Two sutures are sufficient in most fascicles, but more may be required for a bundle. Depending on the size of the fascicle, a 70-μm or 50-μm needle on a 10-0 nylon suture is indicated.

RESULTS

The ability to accomplish fascicular repair using the microscope seems to be the only way, mechanically, to repair small near-terminal branches of peripheral nerves. This technique provides a better visual result in cases of hemisection or section at a point of branching. It also appears most appropriate for specific repair of motor-to-motor fascicles and sensory-to-sensory fascicles. However, varied results have been reported in the literature, some indicating improved, others poorer results.[2,3,6,9,15,17] My results indicate little discernible difference. It has not been possible to prove clinically that an accurate suture of individual fascicles provides better results than those achieved with epineural suture.[16]

There may be a problem with the assessment of return of function. Mechanical repair of nerves is not analogous to the repair of other tissues where mere accurate coaptation of structures offers reasonable correlation with function (ie, bowels, skin, bone). Success with nerve repair depends on complex intercellular physiological processes resulting in new growth of axons reaching end-organs appropriately and then maturing. Success is relative, never total, and methods of assessment are crude.

Based on the data available, the indications for fascicular nerve repair are limited to specific situations. Group fascicular repair is optimal, where possible, and in some cases epineural methods suffice. Improved assessment methods may provide greater insight into the efficacy of the specific types of nerve suture.

REFERENCES

1. Bora FW. Peripheral nerve repair in cats—the fascicular stitch. J Bone Joint Surg [Am] 1967; 49:659–666.
2. Cabaud HE, Rodkey WG, McCarroll HR Jr. Peripheral nerve injuries: Studies in higher non-human primates. J Hand Surg [Am] 1980; 5:201–206.
3. Cabaud HE, Rodkey WG, McCarroll HR Jr, Mutz SB, Niebauer JJ. Epineurial and perineurial fascicular nerve repairs: A critical comparison. J Hand Surg [Am] 1976; 1:131–137.
4. Edshage S. Peripheral nerve suture technique for improved intraneural topography evaluation of some suture materials. Acta Chir Scand [Supp] 1964: 331.
5. Hakstian RW. Funicular orientation by direct stimulation: An aid to peripheral nerve repair. J Bone Joint Surg [Am] 1968; 50:1178.
6. Hudson AR, Hunter D, Kline DG, Bratton BR. Histological studies of experimental interfascicular graft repairs. J Neurosurg 1979; 51:333–340.

7. Jabaley ME, Wallacke WN, Heckler FR. Internal topography of major nerves of the forearm and hand: A current view. J Hand Surg [Am] 1980; 5:1–18.
8. Langley JN, Hashimoto M. On the suture of separate nerve bundles in a nerve trunk and on internal nerve plexuses. J Physiol [London] 1917; 51:318.
9. Orgel MG. Epineurial vs perineurial repair of peripheral nerves. Clin Plast Surg 1984; 11:101–104.
10. Sunderland S. The intraneural topography of the radial, median and ulnar nerves. Brain 1945; 68: 243.
11. Sunderland S. Funicular suture and funicular exclusion in the repair of severed nerves. Brit J Surg 1953; 40:580.
12. Sunderland S. Nerves and nerve injury, ed 2. Edinburgh: Churchill-Livingstone, 1978:593.
13. Sunderland S. Nerves and nerve injury, ed 2. Edinburgh: Churchill-Livingstone, 1978:42.
14. Sunderland S. Nerves and nerve injury, ed 2. Edinburgh: Churchill-Livingstone, 1978:37.
15. Tupper JW. Surgical exposure of terminal median motor nerve branches in the thenar muscles. Sunderland Society, Vienna 1986.
16. Tupper JW, Crick JC, Matteck LR. Fascicular nerve repairs, a comparative study of epineurial and fascicular (perineurial) techniques. Orthop Clin North Am 1988; 19:57–69.
17. Young L, Wray RC, Weeks PM. A randomized prospective comparison of fascicular and epineurial digital nerve repairs. Plast Reconstr Surg 1981; 68: 89–93.

20

Sutureless Methods of Nerve Repair

Edward Diao
Clayton A. Peimer

AUTHORS' KEY POINTS

- Nerve repair using fibrin glue has been a generally successful technique for experimental repair of a variety of intracranial, facial, and peripheral nerves in animals.
- Clinical experience with fibrin glue nerve repair has been limited to commercially available preparations in Europe, with good results. Successful fibrin glue neurorrhaphy depends on elimination of tension and may be most appropriate for reconstruction by nerve grafting.
- Conduits of a variety of materials, biodegradable and non-biodegradable, synthetic and biological, have been used successfully in experimental animals and a limited number of clinical trials to bridge nerve gaps.
- Laser nerve repair remains in its infancy, but it has shown promise in several experimental studies.
- In the future, reconstructive neurorrhaphy may employ a combination of established and experimental techniques to improve results.

With modern optics and microsurgical techniques, instrumentation, and sutures, the approximation of divided nerves has been refined to minimize the operative trauma and improve alignment accuracy. Despite successes with such techniques, researchers continue to seek further improvements in methods, to improve anatomical accuracy in repair, and to avoid the deleterious effects of suture placement. Late fibrosis may be related to excessive manipulation of nerve with forceps and suture, traumatic placement of sutures, foreign body reaction from suture materials, and inclusion of nerve tissue into sutures, as well as fascicular misalignment and "buckling" associated with the tying of sutures.[1,2,4,5,8] This chapter examines the alternatives to current clinical microsuture techniques for acute and reconstructive neurorrhaphy.

FIBRIN GLUE

Historical Perspective

In 1940 Young and Medawar first described a method of sciatic nerve repair using concentrated blood plasma that was allowed to coagulate in rabbits and dogs.[80] They used cockerel plasma "fortified" by centrifugation with six to 10 times its normal content of fibrinogen to improve the tensile strength of the resulting plasma clot. Using autologous plasma, they applied this method clinically to reapproximate the median nerve in the wrist of one patient.[68] At that time, accepted macrosuture materials included linen, silk, and human hair.

Tarlov and Benjamin, attempting to repeat the original experiments, found histologic evidence of significant inflammation and fibrosis.[76] Their experiments with other types of plasma clots identified unmodified autologous plasma as an acceptable alternative, yielding stronger clots and less inflammation. However, nerve dehiscence remained a problem. Like Seddon and Medawar, they emphasized that the presence of tension at the repair site was a contraindication to the use of "plasma clot suture" because of the high risk of nerve separation.[68] Tarlov used a rubber mold to maintain alignment and a tantalum wire suture 1 cm from each end to hold nerves in approximation until the autologous clot formed. Seven of 14 cases had sufficient follow-up and demonstrated "nerve recovery" by clinical evidence of motor reinnervation.[75]

Singer used a thin fibrin film prepared from human plasma fractionation, impregnated with thrombin and surfaced with fibrinogen. Human nerves were apposed after in vitro tests with rabbit sciatic nerves had demonstrated steadily increasing tissue strength from the 5th to 10th postoperative days.[71] Nerve histologic features were regular when telescoping or flanging of fibers was avoided, and best when 1- to 4-mm gaps were created. These findings supported Weiss's findings in his studies of tubular splicing of rat nerves.[78] Singer also noted that the sequence of cellular changes at the juncture began as invasion of polymorphonuclear leukocytes, rapidly followed by lymphocytes and giant cells, which disappeared after the 5th to 6th postoperative day.

Despite these positive early experimental and clinical reports with plasma clot and fibrin gluing, these methods were still considered less reliable and considerably more complicated than macroscopic epineural suture repair.

Recent Experience

Interest in the use of fibrin glue as an alternative to suture occurred was revived in Europe in the 1970s.[17,37,50–53,77] An animal model for the use of fibrinogen cryoprecipitate was described by Matras and coworkers. Homologous adhesive materials (rabbit plasma-cryoprecipitate) and heterologous clotting substance were coagulated by adding human fibrinogen with factor XIII to bovine thrombin solution.[52,53] The authors compared glued nerve grafts to sutured nerve grafts across a 1.5-cm gap in rabbit sciatic nerves: electrophysiological and histologic evaluation confirmed satisfactory nerve regeneration in both.

In another study, Matras and associates demonstrated that clot strength increased with increasing fibrinogen concentrations. Adding factor XIII produced a statistically significant improvement in tensile strength at low fibrinogen concentrations.[51] Adding fibrinolysis inhibitor retarded clot lysis and prevented early dehiscences.[37,52] Pooled homologous plasma concentrates were subsequently used to concentrate the quantity of clottable substances and to improve the tensile strength of the sealant.[38]

In the late 1970s, a highly concentrated human fibrinogen solution with an enriched factor XIII content was introduced in Europe as a two-compound fibrin seal and was marketed by Immuno AG of Vienna. The first component consisted of fibrinogen and plasma proteins, including cold insoluble globulin, albumin, and factor XIII. Thrombin and calcium chloride were contained in the second component. Mixing these components resulted in thrombin-mediated conversion of fibrinogen into fibrin, which initiates clotting and solidification. Thrombin also activates factor XIII to factor XIIIA in the presence of ionized calcium, which then catalyzes the cross-linkage of fibrin and cold insoluble globulin.

Experimental and clinical work have been facilitated by the advent of this commercial fibrin glue system. Several experimental studies comparing fibrin glue to microsuture have reported largely similar results in animals by biochemical, muscle weight, histologic, and electrophysiological data.[4,5,7,15,21,54,72] Rat sciatic nerve regeneration after fibrin gluing has been demonstrated by ^{32}P radiolabeling after delayed primary repairs.[4] When Becker and associates used morphologic and metabolic data to study divided rat nerves coapted with fibrin glue and suture, the two methods achieved comparable results, but the results were inferior to recovery outcomes after nerve crush.[5] Studies of rat and mouse facial nerves comparing suture alone with suture plus fibrin glue demonstrated no difference in axon counts distal to the repair. Neither repair site itself nor function post-repair was examined in this study.[54] Intracranial cat facial nerve gluing gave evidence of excellent histologic and functional recovery, as did electromyography results in another study.[61,62] One 1985 study described good results with sutureless neurorrhaphies in 29 humans.[15]

Reports of fibrin glue failures have focused on the common problem of nerve dehiscence with the use of fibrin glue alone. Several reports compared rat sciatic nerve repair by suture, suture plus glue, and glue alone, finding that two sutures plus glue produced more inflammatory infiltrates, but glue alone produced 100% dehiscence.[12,27,28] However, fibrin glue performed admirably when used to maintain apposition of nerve grafts without tension. Accidental glue interposition inhibited neural regeneration histologically.[28]

Nishihira and McCaffrey reported no difference in nerve–muscle twitch strength between suture and glue groups, but compound action potentials were much better in the sutured nerves.[58] More significantly, two of 12 glued nerve grafts failed and, in fact, actually resorbed.

Moy, Peimer, and colleagues compared fibrin seal to nonabsorbable microsuture repairs in rat tibial nerves.[56] To achieve fibrin seal repair it was necessary first to place two epineural sutures to maintain nerve approximation while gluing (Fig. 20-1). While glue reduced operative time by 40%, mean conduction velocity was similar for both. However, mean amplitude in the fibrin-treated nerves was 40%, compared to 53% in the sutured nerves. An increase in inflammatory cells was found after fibrin seal that persisted until 18 weeks postoperatively (Figs. 20-2 through 20-5). Herder and others noted no significant difference in collagen content or in cumulative action potentials between glued and sutured nerves in rat experiments.[30,32] In some studies homologous plasma seemed to stimulate rat sciatic nerve regeneration in silicone chamber models.[79] Based on these experimental studies, any significant fibrosis from fibrin glues may, in fact, be secondary to nerve dehiscence rather than neurotoxicity.[22,31]

Clinical Experience

Clinical experience with fibrin glue nerve repairs has been reported in Europe.[15,20,50,55,57,73] Merle and associates, describing the clinical applications in 53 post-traumatic brachial plexus reconstruc-

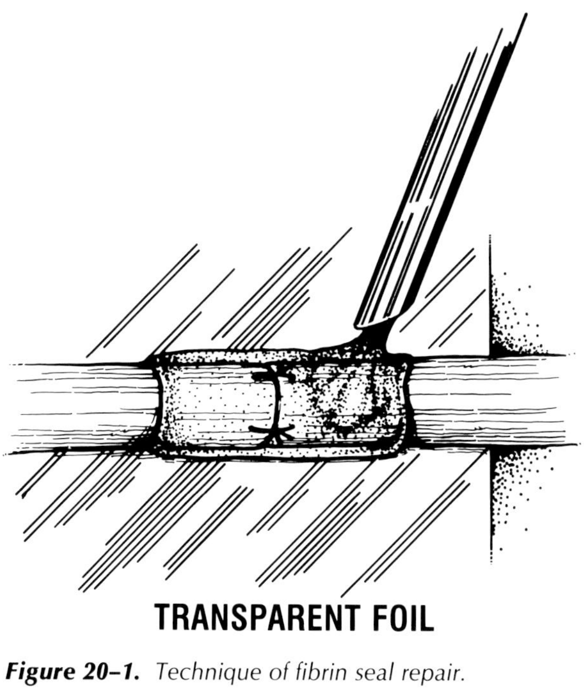

Figure 20–1. *Technique of fibrin seal repair.*

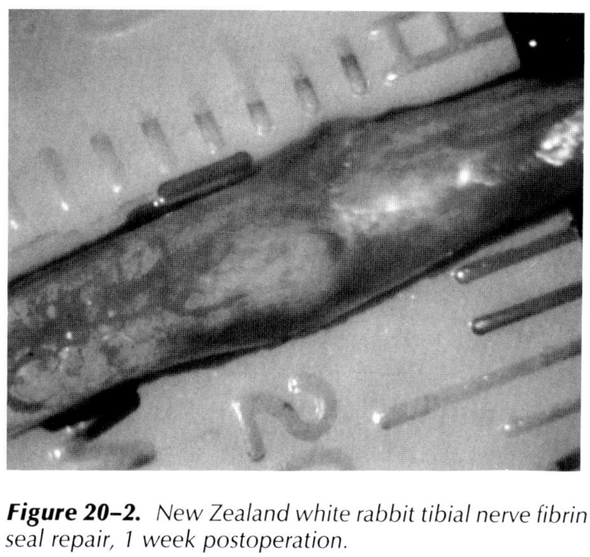

Figure 20–2. *New Zealand white rabbit tibial nerve fibrin seal repair, 1 week postoperation.*

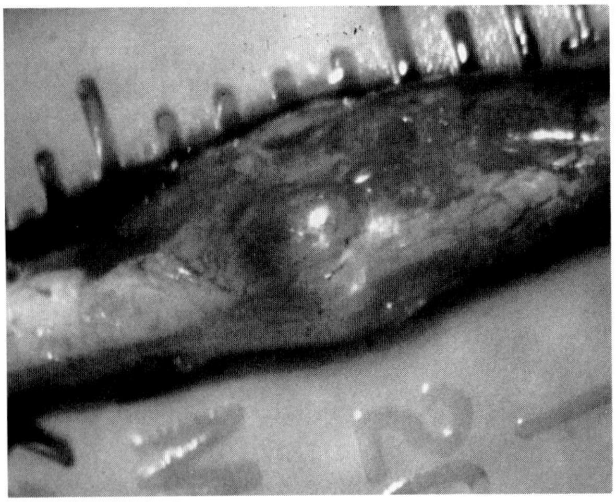

Figure 20–3. *New Zealand white rabbit tibial nerve conventional suture repair, 1 week postoperation.*

tions, had results equivalent to conventional suturing with a considerable saving in operative time.[56] Narakas and Egloff compared fibrin glue primary repairs and nerve grafting to microsuture in 244 patients.[20,57] A 15% improvement in results with glue use was reported based on *subjective* criteria without electrophysiological or quantitative assessment. They also noted a 30% reduction in operative time without loss of technical precision in nerve alignment. Successful fibrin glue suture of the facial nerve in humans has also been reported.[15,73]

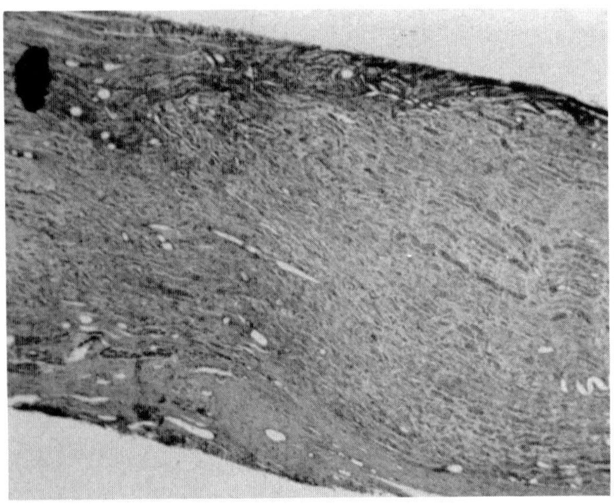

Figure 20–4. *Fibrin seal, 6 weeks postoperation (20×).*

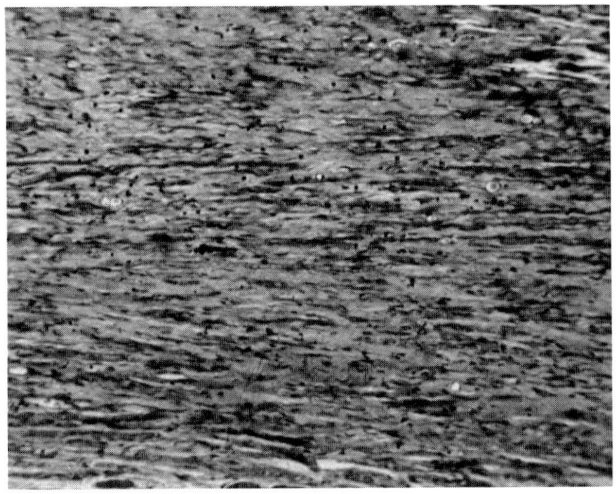

Figure 20–5. *Fibrin seal, 18 weeks postoperation (45×).*

Autologous Preparation

Because of concern about transmitting hepatitis, acquired immunodeficiency syndrome (AIDS), and other diseases, the United States Food and Drug Administration has *not* approved commercial (pooled-source) tissue adhesives for human use. To circumvent this problem, techniques for preparing autologous fibrin glue have been developed.[19,23,25,70] However, one study of autologous fibrin tissue adhesive reported that the bonding strength was lower than that of pooled commercial preparations.[70]

Technique of Nerve Repair Using Fibrin Glue

The nerve stumps are prepared in the conventional manner. Fibrotic nerve is resected sharply until normal fascicles are noted. Neurorrhaphy without tension is performed using fibrin alone. If the repair is subjected to any tension, one to three epineural stay sutures are added. Nerve stumps are isolated from blood with a thin transparent foil placed beneath the repair site. Fibrin glue is then applied as a thin layer four times longer than the diameter of the nerve in order to create a cylinder sufficient to resist shear. The glue hardens in about 3 minutes. Foil or a piece of surgical glove wrapped around the nerve repair site for 30 seconds ensures even distribution of the fibrin glue and separation from surrounding tissues. Postoperative immobilization for at least 2 weeks is required, as fibrin glue may start to break down after only 3 days. Long-term stability is maintained by nerve callus formation as Schwann cells rebuild the bridge between the stumps.

TUBULATION AND CONDUITS

Experimental Data

Tubulation is a method of sutureless repair that requires insertion of proximal and distal portions of a divided nerve into a hollow tube (see Chap. 41). Nerve regeneration proceeds through contact guidance and containment of neural tissue by the tube itself, and the creation of a microenvironment in which neuronotrophic factors may stimulate and direct neural regeneration.

In 1943, Weiss used a closely fitting sleeve of artery to repair rat sciatic nerves.[78] He concluded that nerve regeneration occurred across gaps up to 3 mm between the nerve stumps using this technique; in fact, a slight gap was found, on histologic examination, to be preferred over having divided ends of nerve in direct physical contact.

Lundborg and associates in a series of studies examined nerve regeneration through preformed pseudosynovial sheaths.[41,42,44] A mesothelial tube was created by using a 2-mm diameter silicone rod and a thin metal spiral. They obtained good axon density and diameter when compared to sutured nerves. Mean conduction velocities were also comparable. Non-repair controls with a 10-mm nerve gap showed only rare axons and no action potentials.[41] In another study with a control using only a proximal nerve introduced into a synovial tube, the authors found that regeneration ceased after a few weeks, supporting the concept that local factors elaborated from, or related to, the distal nerve stump or nerve-target tissue positively influenced regeneration.[42]

Mackinnon, Dellon, and coworkers evaluated application of pseudosynovial tube–stimulated nerve regeneration across a 3-cm gap in baboon ulnar nerves and reported that histologic evaluation confirmed both regeneration and fiber maturation of the regenerated nerves over 3 to 9 months.[47]

Seckel and associates successfully obtained histologically well-defined nerve regeneration distal to the repair site, with secondary biodegradation of polylactic acid tubes within 3 months.[66] The absence of a distal nerve stump resulted in failure of regeneration of the proximal nerve, again supporting the concept of a positive trophic effect on nerve regeneration from target tissues. They studied several gap sizes and concluded that a gap distance of *less than 10 mm* was required for successful tubulized regeneration of rat sciatic nerve. The presence of specific target-derived neuronotrophic factors was considered when follow-up studies using Y-shaped conduits as guides showed that the proximal peroneal nerve grew preferentially, by a two-to-one ratio, to the appropriate distal fascicle.[67]

Biodegradable polyester tubes of different compositions were studied to evaluate the effect of the rate of biodegradation on nerve regeneration, revealing that the more biodegradable the tube, the greater the incidence and degree of distortion and luminal narrowing.[14,29] Madison and coworkers compared biodegradable polylactate tubes to a nondegradable polyethylene and found no difference in mouse sciatic nerve regeneration after 2, 4, and 6 weeks.[48] This model also demonstrated a stimulative effect by placing laminin-containing gel in the nerve tubes.

Synthetic bioabsorbable tubes have been successfully used in the primate model to achieve regeneration across a 3-cm ulnar nerve gap.[16] The polyglycolic acid tube concept has been extended by some investigators who have designed a nerve-coupling device consisting of two tubules that hold the nerve ends and slide into a hollow cylinder to achieve nerve coaptation.[49]

Silicone tubes used experimentally to support nerve regeneration and for testing neuronotrophic factors have been evaluated.[13,25,32,34–36,39,40,43,63,69] However, some studies have noted that silicone tubes have deleterious effects on nerve regeneration. Le Beau and Ellisman described failure of occurrence of late maturation in rats with 10-mm sciatic nerve gaps bridged by silicone tubes, noting axonal degeneration and secondary demyelination at 56 days post-repair.[39] Gibson and Daniloff found silicone tube mediated nerve regeneration inferior to nerve allograft.[26] Jenq and Coggeshall studied regeneration through silicone tubes with microscopic holes pierced in the walls and found improved axon numbers when compared to regeneration through solid silicone tubes.[34,36] The regenerating axons successfully crossed larger gaps when tubes with holes were used. A similar study by Hurtado and associates used semipermeable tubes of acrylic and noted that a fibrin-containing matrix formed, which was then invaded by fibroblasts and blood vessels and finally colonized by nerve fibers.[32] Their results approached those reported for impermeable tubes, but were inferior to those obtained for fully permeable tubes.

Autogenous vein graft has been used for rat sciatic nerve regeneration.[9,10] Nerve conduction studies, obtained 4 months postoperatively, demonstrated restoration of conduction with muscle reinnervation.[9] Electrophysiological evaluation of nerve grafts and autogenous vein grafts was performed in another study.[10] While nerve conduction velocities compared well in the two groups, the nerve action potentials of vein-grafted nerves were about 50% of that in conventionally grafted nerves.

Clinical Data

Mackinnon and Dellon used bioabsorbable polyglycolic acid tubes in clinical nerve reconstruction, primarily for short nerve gaps in the digital nerves and revision surgery of failed primary repairs of major nerves at the wrist level.[45,46] They reported excellent results, comparable to classic techniques of nerve grafting. They reported their "impression" that nerve regeneration appeared accelerated in some patients compared to those treated with nerve grafting or repair.

The medial brachial cutaneous nerve of the forearm was used as an empty perineural tube graft for a digital nerve defect in one patient treated for a sensory deficit in the index finger.[60] Clinical and electromyographic data confirmed successful regeneration, which the authors said was superior to what would have been expected from conventional nerve grafting.

Chiu and Strauch analyzed 22 patients with small peripheral sensory nerve gaps, comparing autogenous vein nerve conduits to conventional nerve grafts and direct nerve repair. They selected patients with painful neuromas and segmental nerve injuries of 3 cm. Results demonstrated that the autogenous vein conduit was successful in obtaining sufficient nerve regeneration to provide protective sensibility and 256-cps and 30-cps vibration sensibility in all operated parts, with no cases of neuroma formation. Static two-point discrimination was 7.4 mm in controls (direct repair group), 9.0 mm in the sural nerve graft group, and 11.1 mm in the autogenous vein nerve conduit group.[11]

LASER: EXPERIMENTAL AND CLINICAL DATA

Laser is an acronym for **L**ight **A**mplication by **S**timulated **E**mission of **R**adiation. In contrast to ordinary light, which consists of photons of many random wavelengths scattered in all directions, laser light has uniform wavelength, color (if any), and direction. The light may be the ultraviolet (UV, 150 to 400 nM), visible (390 to 700 nM), or infrared (IR, >700 nM) portions of the electromagnetic spectrum.[2,18,64] Effective transfer of laser energy depends on multiple factors, including the type of laser used, the particular wavelength of the laser (as it relates to the absorptive capacity of the tissue at that particular wavelength), and the duration and energy output of the laser.

Laser energy must be absorbed by the target tissue to have an effect. *Photostimulation* occurs when low energy is absorbed and causes cellular reactions. *Vaporization*, in which high energy absorption occurs, leads to heat; when the heat exceeds 100°C (212°F), cellular water is converted to steam, resulting in an "explosion," with cell debris emitted as steam and smoke. *Tissue coagulation*, a third type of laser action, is the most useful in terms of nerve repairs. Graded absorption of energy results in moderate heat, which causes protein denaturing and a welding effect without vaporizing surrounding tissue.

The types of lasers in current experimental and clinical use include the CO_2 laser, neodymium-doped yttrium-aluminum-garnet (neodymium-YAG laser), and the argon laser (see Chap. 22).

The CO_2 laser–water interaction is absorption-dominated; tissue penetration is minimal and independent of pigment. Fisher, Beggs, and coworkers used the CO_2 laser to spot-weld rat sciatic nerves and connective tissue to create microepineural repairs.[6,24] Action potentials were recorded across the repair in 85% of laser-treated nerves compared to 78% of sutured ones. Morphologic studies showed greater scar formation and more constriction at sutured nerves than at laser-treated nerves.[24] Morphometric analysis of myelinated nerve fibers revealed that the laser had no deleterious effects on nerve histologically as determined by the degree of retrograde axonal degeneration and regeneration, as compared to traditional suture techniques.[6]

The neodymium-YAG laser is delivered through a flexible quartz fiber-optic system designed for use in microsurgical tissue welding. It has been used to repair rat carotid artery and sciatic nerve lesions.[65] Collagen homogenization and tumefaction of the supporting neural structures, predominantly of the epineurium, was observed histologically, with minimal reactive changes compared to the foreign body granulomas observed around silk stay sutures. The authors also noted a reduction in laser-induced carbonaceous deposits compared to studies using CO_2 lasers. Over time, vascularization and neuromatous neurotization of the supportive nerve structures were seen histologically.[33]

Argon laser produces a blue-green light with a wavelength of 488 to 521 μm, which is almost completely absorbed by red-colored materials and reflected by white surfaces and enables it to coagulate blood on the surface of nerve tissue while being reflected by underlying nerve. This is the theoretical basis for use of the argon laser in the construction of a mini-tubule of coagulated blood in repairing nerves.[2,3] Transmission and scanning electron microscopic studies demonstrated that argon laser repairs performed in rat sciatic and baboon median nerves were superior to conventionally sutured nerves. Laser repairs had mild fibrosis and a well-developed pattern of regeneration. Scarring was not excessive, and escapement of axon sprouts was minimal.

There have been interesting recent reports on the use of a fibrin film fastened to rat nerve using a CO_2 70-mW laser.[59] Satisfactory tensile strength was noted with nerve counts of myelinated fibers and mean nerve diameters indicative of successful nerve recovery.

THE FUTURE

The sutureless methods of nerve repair described in this chapter represent primarily experimental techniques; quantifiable clinical studies have yet to be done. The future of alternative methods to suture repairs may lie in the application and refinement of one or, possibly, a combination of several of these techniques.[74] The concept of creating "mini-tubules" of coagulated blood using a laser or of using fibrin glue in combination with a nerve conduit or tubule[3,7] is intriguing. But until further work is done, sutured nerve repair using the refinements of microsurgical techniques, although imperfect, remains the standard for clinical care.

REFERENCES

1. Akoweb TH, Kokuh C, Ymacob EH. Petehepallh. Zhurnal Voprosy Neirokhirurgii Imeni N-N-Burdenko 1988; 6:32–36.
2. Almquist EE. Nerve repair by laser. Orthop Clin N Am 1988; 19:201–208.
3. Almquist EE, Nachemson A, Auth D, Almquist B, Hall S. Evaluation of the use of argon laser in repairing rat and primate nerve. J Hand Surg [Am] 1984; 9:792–799.
4. Becker C, Gueuning C, Graff G. Réparation du nerf périphérique: Intérêt des colles biologiques et de la suture épipérineurale dans les interventions tardives. Ann Chir Main 1985; 4:259–262.
5. Becker CM, Gueuning CO, Graff GL. Sutures or fibrin glue for divided rat nerves: Schwann cell and muscle metabolism. Microsurg 1985; 6:1–10.
6. Beggs JL, Fischer DW, Shetter AG. Comparative study of rat sciatic nerve. Microepineural anastomosis made with carbon dioxide laser and suture techniques: Part 2. Neurosurg 1986; 18:266–269.
7. Boedts D. A comparative experimental study on nerve repair. Arch Otorhinolaryngol 1987; 244:1–6.
8. Cham RB, Peimer CA, Howard C, Walsh WP, Eckert BS. Absorbable vs. non-absorbable suture for microneurorrhaphy. J Hand Surg [Am] 1984; 9:434–440.

9. Chiu DTW, Janecka I, Krizek TJ, Wolff M, Lovelace RE. Autogenous vein graft as a conduit for nerve regeneration. Surgery 1982; 91:226–233.
10. Chiu DTW, Lovelace RE, Yu LT, Wolff M, Stengel S, Middleton L, Janecka IP, Krizek TJ. Comparative electrophysiologic evaluation of nerve grafts and autogenous vein grafts as nerve conduits: An experimental study. J Reconstr Microsurg 1988; 4: 303–312.
11. Chiu DTW, Strauch B. A prospective clinical evaluation of autogenous vein graft used as a nerve conduit for distal sensory nerve defect of 3 cm or less. Submitted for publication.
12. Cruz NI, Debs N, Fiol RE. Evaluation of fibrin glue in rat sciatic nerve repairs. Plast Reconstr Surg 1986; 78:369–373.
13. Cuadros CL, Granatir CE. Nerve regeneration through a synthetic microporous tube (expanded polytetrafluoroethylene): Experimental study in the sciatic nerve of the rat. Microsurgery 1987; 8:41–46.
14. Da Silva CF, Madison R, Dikkes P, Chiu TH, Sidman RL. An in vivo model to quantify motor and sensory peripheral nerve regeneration using bioresorbable nerve guide tubes. Brain Res 1985; 342:307–315.
15. Daverio PJ. Facial nerve repair. Facial Plastic Surgery 1985; 2:351–356.
16. Dellon AL, Mackinnon SE. An alternative to the classical nerve graft for the management of the short nerve gap. Plast Reconstr Surg 1988; 82:849–856.
17. Duspiva W. Nerve erkenntnisse zur anastomosierung durchtrennter peripherer nerven. Fortschr Med 1978; 96:2214–2218.
18. Edwards MSB, Boggan JE, Fuller TA. The laser in neurological surgery. J Neurosurg 1983; 59:555–566.
19. Egloff DV, Narakas A. Nerve anastomoses with human fibrin. Ann Chir Main 1983; 2:101–115.
20. Epstein GH, Weisman RA, Zwillenberg S, Schreiber AD. A new autologous fibrinogen-based adhesive for otologic surgery. Ann Otol Rhinol Laryngol 1986; 95:40–45.
21. Faldini A, Puntoni P, Magherini PC, Lisanti M, Carlucci F, Risaliti R. Comparative neurophysiological assessments of nerve sutures performed by microsurgical methods and with fibrin glue: Experimental study. Ital J Orthop Traumatol 1984; 10:527–532.
22. Feldman MD, Sataloff RT, Ballas SK. Autologous fibrin tissue adhesive for cerebrospinal fluid leaks: A controlled study of neurotoxicity. Am J Otol 1988; 9:302–305.
23. Feldman MD, Sataloff RT, Epstein G, Ballas SK. Autologous fibrin tissue adhesive for peripheral nerve anastomosis. Arch Otolaryngol Head Neck Surg 1987; 113:963–967.
24. Fischer DW, Beggs JL, Kenshalo DL Jr, Shetter AG. Comparative study of microepineurial anastomoses with the use of CO_2 laser and suture techniques in rat sciatic nerves. Part 1. Neurosurg 1985; 17:300–308.
25. Gestring GF, Lerner R. Autologous fibrinogen for tissue adhesion, hemostasis and embolization. Vasc Surg 1983; 17:294–304.
26. Gibson KL, Daniloff JK. Comparison of sciatic nerve regeneration through silicone tubes and nerve allografts. Microsurgery 1989; 10:126–129.
27. Hamm KD, Steube D, Beer R, Pothe H. Mikrochirurgische naht und fibrinklebung von nervenanastomosen. Zent bl Neurochir 1987; 48:206–218.
28. Hamm KD, Steube D, Pothe H, Beer R. Experimental studies in animals on the use of fibrin glue from the human plasma fraction Cohn I in nerve reconstruction. Folia Haematol 1988; 115:208–212.
29. Henry EW, Chiu TH, Nyilas E, Brushart TM, Dikkes P, Sidman RL. Nerve regeneration through biodegradable polyester tubes. Exp Neurol 1985; 90: 652–676.
30. Herter T. Problems of fibrin adhesion of the nerves. Neurosurg Rev 1988; 11:249–258.
31. Herter T, Schleep J, Windman D. Führen fibrinklebermanschetten zur fibrosierung von nerventransplantaten? Neurochirurgia 1989; 32:16–20.
32. Hurtado H, Knoops B, Aguilar P. Research note: Rat sciatic nerve regeneration in semipermeable artificial tubes. Exp Neurol 1987; 97:751–757.
33. Jain KK. Repair of small blood vessels with neodymium-YAG laser: A preliminary report. Surgery 1979; 85:684–688.
34. Jenq C, Coggeshall RE. Nerve regeneration through holey silicone tubes. Brain Res 1985; 361:233–241.
35. Jenq C, Coggeshall RE. Regeneration of transected rat sciatic nerves after using isolated nerve fragments as distal inserts in silicone tubes. Exp Neurol 1986; 91:154–162.
36. Jenq C, Coggeshall RE. Permeable tubes increase the length of the gap that regenerating axons can span. Brain Res 1987; 408:239–242.
37. Kuderna H. Klinische anwendung der klebung von nervenanastomosen mit fibrinogen. Fortschr der Kiefer und Gesichts Chirurgie 1976; 21:135.
38. Kuderna H, Matras H. Die klinische anwendung der klebung von nervenanastomosen bei der rekonstruktion verletzter peripherer nerven. Wien Klin Wochenschr 1975; 87:495.
39. Le Beau JM, Ellisman MH, Powell HC. Ultrastruc-

tural and morphometric analysis of long-term peripheral nerve regeneration through silicone tubes. J Neurocytology 1988; 17:161–172.
40. Lundborg G, Dahlin LB, Danielsen N, Gelberman RH, Longo FM, Powell HC, Varon S. Nerve regeneration in silicone chambers: Influence of gap length and of distal stump components. Exp Neurol 1982; 76:361–375.
41. Lundborg G, Dahlin L, Danielsen N, Hansson HA, Johannesson A, Longo FM, Varon S. Nerve regeneration across an extended gap: A neurobiological view of nerve repair and the possible involvement of neuronotrophic factors. J Hand Surg 1982; 7: 580–587.
42. Lundborg G, Dahlin LB, Danielsen NP, Hansson HA, Larsson K. Reorganization and orientation of regenerating nerve fibres, perineurium, and epineurium in preformed mesothelial tubes: An experimental study on the sciatic nerve of rats. J Neurosci Res 1981; 6:265–281.
43. Lundborg G, Gelberman RH, Longo FM, Powell HC, Varon S. In vivo regeneration of cut nerves encased in silicone tubes. Growth across a 6-mm gap. J Neuropath Exp Neurol 1982; 41:412–422.
44. Lundborg G, Hansson H. Nerve regeneration through preformed pseudosynovial tubes. J Hand Surg 1980; 5:35–38.
45. Mackinnon SE. Surgical management of the peripheral nerve gap. Clin Plast Surg 1989; 16:587–603.
46. Mackinnon SE, Dellon AL. Surgery of the peripheral nerve. New York: Thieme, 1988:562–571.
47. Mackinnon SE, Dellon AL, Hudson AR, Hunter DA. Nerve regeneration through a pseudosynovial sheath in a primate model. Plast Reconstr Surg 1985; 75:833–839.
48. Madison RD, da Silva C, Dikkes P, Sidman RL, Chiu TH. Peripheral nerve regeneration with entubulation repair: Comparison of biodegradable nerve guides versus polyethylene tubes and the effects of a laminin-containing gel. Exp Neurol 1987; 95:378–390.
49. Marshall DM, Grosser M, Stephanides MC, Keeley RD, Rosen JM. Sutureless nerve repair at the fascicular level using a nerve coupler. J Rehabil Res Dev 1989; 26:63–76.
50. Matras H. Fibrin seal: The state of the art. J Oral Maxillofac Surg 1985; 43:605–611.
51. Matras H, Braun F, Lassman H, Ammerer HP, Mamoli B. Plasma clot welding of nerves (experimental report). J Maxillofac Surg 1973; 1:236–247.
52. Matras H, Dinges HF, Lassman H, Mamoli B. Zur nahtlosen interfaszikulären nerventransplantation im tierexperiment. Wien Med Wschr 1972; 122: 517–523.
53. Matras H, Dinges HP, Mamoli B, Lassman H. Nonsutured nerve transplantation (a report on animal experiments). J Maxillofac Surg 1973; 1:37–40.
54. Medders G, Mattox DE, Lyles A. Effects of fibrin glue on rat facial nerve regeneration. Otolaryngol Head Neck Surg 1989; 100:106–109.
55. Merle M, Becker C, Pankovic C, Bagot d'Arc M. La réparation microchirurgicale des nerfs périphériques et des vaisseaux par le Tissucol: Étude clinique et expérimentale. Revue de Laryngologie 1987; 108:13–14.
56. Moy OJ, Peimer CA, Koniuch MP, Howard C, Zielezny M, Katikaneni PR. Fibrin seal adhesive versus nonabsorbable microsuture in peripheral nerve repair. J Hand Surg [Am] 1988; 13:273–278.
57. Narakas A. The use of fibrin glue in repair of peripheral nerves. Orthop Clin North Am 1988; 19: 187–199.
58. Nishihira S, McCaffrey TV. Repair of motor nerve defects: Comparison of suture and fibrin adhesive techniques. Otolaryngol Head Neck Surg 1989; 100:17–21.
59. Osedo M. An experimental study on nerve repair using carbon dioxide laser. J Jpn Orthop Assoc 1988; 62:653–663.
60. Restrepo Y, Merle M, Petry D, Michon J. Empty perineurial tube graft used to repair a digital nerve: A first case report. Microsurg 1985; 6:73–77.
61. Sandvoss G, Cervos-Navarro J, Yasargil MG. Intracranial repair of the oculomotor nerve in cats. Neurochirurgia 1986; 29:1–8.
62. Sandvoss G, Stoltenburg-Didinger G, Yasargil MG. Experimental transclival exposure and repair of the abducens nerve in cats. Neurochirurgia 1987; 30: 65–68.
63. Satou T, Nishida S, Hiruma S, Tanji K, Takahashi M, Fujita S, Mizuhara Y, Akai F, Hashimoto S. A morphological study on the effects of collagen gel matrix on regeneration of severed rat sciatic nerve in silicone tubes. Acta Pathol Jpn 1986; 36:199–208.
64. Saunders ML, Young HF, Becker DP, Greenberg RP, Newlon PG, Corales RL, Ham WT, Povlishock JT. The use of the laser in neurological surgery. Surg Neurol 1980; 14:1–10.
65. Schrober R, Ulrich F, Sander T, Durselen H, Hessel S. Laser-induced alteration of collagen substructure allows microsurgical tissue welding. Science 1986; 232:1421–1422.
66. Seckel BR, Chiu TH, Nyilas E, Sidman RL. Nerve regeneration through synthetic biodegradable nerve

guides: Regulation by the target organ. Plast Reconstr Surg 1984; 74:173–181.

67. Seckel BR, Ryan SE, Gagne RG, Chiu TH, Watkins E. Target-specific nerve regeneration through a nerve guide in the rat. Plast Reconstr Surg 1986; 78:793–798.
68. Seddon HJ, Medawar PB. Fibrin suture of human nerves. Lancet 1942; 2:87–88.
69. Shine HD, Harcourt PG, Sidman RL. Cultured peripheral nervous system cells support peripheral nerve regeneration through tubes in the absence of distal nerve stump. J Neurosci Res 1985; 14:393–401.
70. Siedentop KH, Harris DM, Sanchez B. Autologous fibrin tissue adhesive. Laryngoscope 1985; 95:1074–1076.
71. Singer M. The combined use of fibrin film and clot in end-to-end union of nerves. J Neurosurg 1945; 2:102–115.
72. Smahel J, Meyer VE, Bachem U. Gluing of peripheral nerves with fibrin: Experimental studies. J Reconstr Microsurg 1987; 3:211–218.
73. Sterkers O, Becherel P, Sterkers JM. Réparation du nerf facial par colle de fibrine exclusive. Ann Oto-Laryngol 1989; 106:176–181.
74. Sugiura K, Nakatsuchi Y, Yagi R, Sugimoto Y. New method for venous interposition grafts using fibrin glue. Microsurgery 1985; 6:125–128.
75. Tarlov IM. Autologous plasma clot suture of nerves. JAMA 1944; 12:741–748.
76. Tarlov IM, Benjamin B. Plasma clot and silk suture of nerves: An experimental study of comparative tissue reaction. Surg Gynecol Obstet 1943; 76:366–374.
77. Ventura R, Torri G, Campari A, Giandomenico A, Peretti G. Experimental suture of the peripheral nerves with fibrin glue. Ital J Orthop Traumatol 1980; 6:407–414.
78. Weiss P. Nerve regeneration in the rat following tubular splicing of severed nerves. Arch Surg 1943; 46:525–547.
79. Williams LR. Exogenous fibrin matrix precursors stimulate the temporal progress of nerve regeneration within a silicone chamber. Neurochemical Res 1987; 12:851–860.
80. Young JZ, Medawar PB. Fibrin suture of peripheral nerves. Lancet 1940; 2:126–128.

21

Modified Techniques of Nerve Repair: Epineurial Splint

Michael E. Jabaley

AUTHOR'S KEY POINTS

- The goal of nerve repair is accurate fascicular alignment with minimal tension.
- In using an epineurial bridge to splint a nerve repair, a strip of epineurium is left attached to the deep surface *only* of each nerve end and the strips are sutured to each other, forming a bridge that serves as a tension-relieving device. The bridge permits coaptation of fascicles with a minimum number of sutures.
- A few small stitches, placed in the internal epineurium rather than the perineurium, align individual fascicles or groups of fascicles, completing the repair.

Functional recovery after nerve suture is influenced by many factors. These are operative at all levels of the extremity, from the nerve cell body to the peripheral organs, including the point of nerve coaptation. The process is initiated at the time of injury. The surgeon's ability to influence events is quite limited; he or she cannot influence events at the cell body or at the periphery and can control only the timing and techniques of repair. Many of us have believed and have taught for years (while ignoring central or peripheral factors) that results improve as technique improves. But in light of current information, it seems clear that the technique of nerve suture is only one (and often not the dominant) factor in determining the functional outcome of nerve suture.[10] Nevertheless, the emphasis on operative technique has led to significant advances in instrument manufacture, reduction of needle and suture diameter, and the availability of magnifying devices that are comfortable to use, provide a wide field of vision, and are accurately lighted.

Despite these advances, the outcome of nerve suture remains unpredictable, and many patients who suffer nerve transections are left with major functional losses. Because there is room for improvement, new approaches are warranted.[5,12,13,17,20,25]

Over the past 20 to 25 years, surgeons have come to appreciate the importance of a tension-free suture line and minimal scar formation. The technique of interfascicular nerve grafting, as practiced and studied in many centers, has given considerable credence to these two points. Investigators and surgeons now agree that *a major advantage of nerve grafting is that it permits nerve coaptation without tension.*[9,15] Further, the conscious removal of external epineurium seems to limit the amount of scar formation about the nerve juncture. Ideally, nerve grafting results in a thin scar interface between recipient nerve and graft, allowing the rapid and orderly advance of regenerating axons into the graft and ultimately into the distal nerve. Providing an abundance of axon sprouts beyond the zone of injury is one of the most beneficial aspects of nerve grafting.[19]

In an effort to mimic as closely as possible the conditions that prevail in nerve grafting procedures, a technique has been devised and practiced for the past 10 years in which the external epineurium is trimmed back from the cut nerve end, except for a strip left attached to the deep surface of each nerve end. Proximal and distal strips then are sewn together, coapting the fascicle ends and creating an epineurial bridge or splint, thereby relieving tension on those sutures that are placed to join the fascicles themselves. While the interfascicular sutures themselves are few in number and are quite small (10-0 or 11-0), they are critical in aligning individual fascicles. This technique leaves less foreign body, permits a tension-free nerve junction, and results in a thinner scar and less neuroma, with eventually better axonal regeneration.

INDICATIONS

Epineurial splinting can be used in both primary and secondary nerve repairs (ie, in any situation where tension is not excessive and where otherwise ends would be joined by direct suture). Such conditions usually exist in tidy wounds. Classifying wounds as "tidy" and "untidy" dates at least to the writings of Rank and Wakefield and is still a useful concept.[24] Tidy wounds result from knives, glass, choppers, and cutters of various types where primary or delayed primary repair is indicated. The technique can also be used in untidy wounds when an early secondary repair might be performed. In secondary repairs, use of the epineurial splint is limited to those situations where there has been no significant loss of nerve substance and where major retraction of the nerve ends is not a factor.

A contraindication to the use of the epineurial splint is a nerve division that requires secondary repair and in which there is a long length of neuroma formation or retraction of the nerve ends. Similarly, if there has been significant loss of nerve substance or if extreme joint flexion is necessary to join the nerve ends, this technique is not used.

The epineurial bridge technique is *not* a method for overcoming otherwise excessive tension, but is rather an approach that mimics the favorable aspects of nerve grafting. The bridge itself takes up the tension, allowing fascicular ends to fall toward each other without tension. This, in turn, permits accurate coaptation of bundles while using a minimum of sutures.

APPLIED ANATOMY

Nerve suture by epineurial bridging requires intraneural dissection within both the proximal and distal nerve ends. Successful preparation of a nerve requires the surgeon to understand the details of topographic anatomy and to be familiar with the necessary techniques of dissection (Fig. 21-1). Specifically, he or she must be able to incise and manipulate the external epineurium and separate fascicles or bundles, as well as identify and map these structures for subsequent coaptation. This is done with appropriate magnification. Useful adjuncts in the performance of this technique are described in the chapters on electrical stimulation in the awake patient (see Chap. 15) and topographic anatomy (see Chap. 14). A summary of the important details of anatomy follows.

A peripheral nerve consists of structures of both ectodermal and mesodermal origin.[22] Tissue of mesodermal origin heals by cellular proliferation and collagen formation (scar); structures of ectodermal origin do not. The mesodermal tissue includes the epineurium, both internal and external, and the perineurium. The ectodermal derivatives include the axon and the endoneurium. An injury to these structure is actually an injury to part of the nerve cell itself, and it "heals" by regeneration,

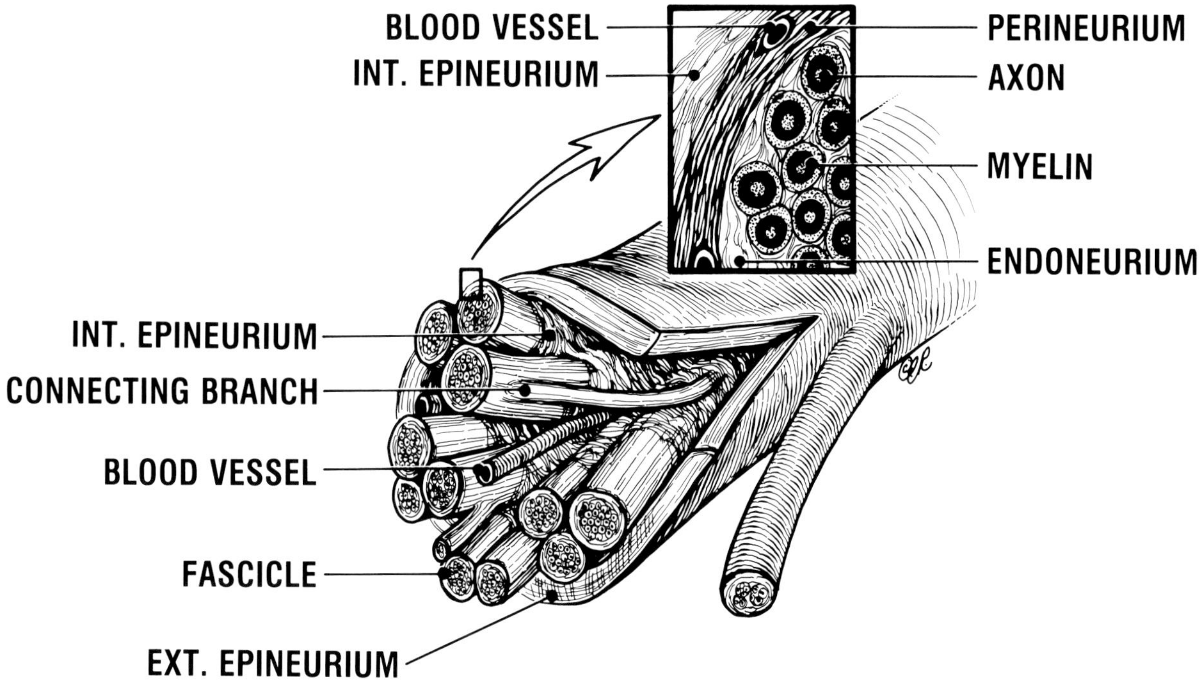

Figure 21–1. *Anatomy of a peripheral nerve. The conducting units are the fascicles, which may be either single or in bundles. Each fascicle is bounded by its perineurium, which delineates its internal environment. Within the perineurium, both pressure and ionic content differ from the area outside the perineurium. Internal epineurium separates the fascicles from one another, and the entire nerve is bounded by the epifascicular (external) epineurium. Epineurium can be incised and dissected or excised where necessary. In the epineural bridge repair, a strip of external epineurium is retained for suture to the opposite nerve end, and fascicles are coapted by sutures placed in the internal epineurium.*

not division. Thus, nerve "healing" is a unique phenomenon. The ends of a cut nerve are bonded by scar tissue that must, in turn, be bridged by regenerating axons.

Perineurium defines each nerve fascicle; two or more fascicles in close proximity are called a bundle. The perineurium is a strong, well-organized structure, 3 to 15 lamellae thick, made up of a flattened layer of cells on its inner surface and separated by longitudinally, transversely, or obliquely oriented collagen fibers and an external layer of transition to epineurium. This structure is of great strength and also has an important barrier function: it defines and preserves the fascicle's internal milieu. When perineurium is damaged, conduction and axon regeneration are impaired or made impossible. For this reason, dissection of the perineurium is done carefully. Although perineurium can be sutured, it need not be in most instances. It apparently heals by scar formation, and will do so if properly aligned.

The cross-sectional appearance of a nerve changes constantly from level to level, but functional axons appear to travel in a more orderly fashion and may occupy the same quadrant for a considerable distance. For this reason, nerve ends are joined with some hope of useful return, even when a short gap exists and even though the cut surfaces are not mirror images of each other. There is every reason to assume that axons will cross a nerve juncture to the distal end, given otherwise favorable circumstances. In the case of nerve repair by direct suture, "favorable circumstances" means the elimination of tension at the suture line, coaptation of viable nerve ends, and a well-vascularized bed containing minimal foreign body.

ALTERNATIVE PROCEDURES

Because transected nerves are common, most hand and extremity surgeons are familiar with nerve repairs. Over the past several generations, a great deal of experience has accrued with *epineurial nerve suture*, and this technique remains the standard against which others are measured. More recently, several reports have described *interfascicular repair*, both in animals and humans.[2,8,14] To date, there does not appear to be enough improvement in results with this technique to justify its routine use.[3,23,26,29] Finally, *nerve grafting* has increased in popularity as a way to deal with excessive gaps.[27] While separate chapters describes each of these techniques, their specific advantages and disadvantages are briefly described here.

Epineurial Repair

Epineurial repair, the oldest technique, remains popular among nerve surgeons. It has a number of advantages: it is quick and relatively simple to perform, and it requires no special surgical skills. It can be performed without magnification. It often requires little additional nerve dissection and consequently inflicts little surgical trauma on the nerve end. In practice, epineurial repair probably includes a range of techniques instead of only one, including those performed with no magnification, those performed with loupes only, and those done with microscopes.

The main disadvantage of epineurial suture is that it is a whole nerve suture. As such, it does not necessarily permit precise alignment (except by chance) of individual fascicles or bundles of fascicles within a nerve end. In other words, the technique does not incorporate individual fascicular control and is not function-specific. This may be of little consequence in relatively simple nerves with only a few fascicles or bundles, but may be more critical in complex or mixed nerves.

In epineurial repair, an external landmark on the epineurium, such as a blood vessel, is selected and a key suture is placed there. This commits the surgeon to a rotational alignment based on that suture, and the remaining stitches are placed in more or less random fashion. It has been shown that an epineurial suture that looks adequate from the outside may, in fact, contain major problems within the nerve.[7] For example, if the sutures are tied loosely, the normal elasticity of the perineurium may cause the fascicle ends to retract from each other, leaving a wide space between them. This space will be filled with blood, fibroblasts, fibrin, and ultimately scar tissue. A widened band of such scar at a nerve juncture may serve as a major barrier to regenerating axons. Some axon sprouts may be deflected off this scar and proceed no further. Some of those that penetrate it may do so in a more or less random fashion, and there is little control over which fascicles they enter in the distal end. Although regenerating axons apparently will follow any physical substrate (including scar), they do not do so in a purposeful fashion, and they may enter vessels or collagen fibers as well as endoneural tubes. In any event, when fascicle ends are distracted, the yield of functional axons bridging the gap is low, and their paths are random.

Alternately, if there is a deficiency of nerve tissue, sutures placed in the epineurium necessarily take larger bites and are tied more tightly. This may result in a telescoping or overlapping of fascicles and bundles. As a result, the regenerating axons may reach no fascicles at all but may enter only the internal epineurium.

In either event, the effect of the above-described conditions is that a fewer-than-ideal number of axons may enter the distal segment, and they may or may not end up in the appropriate fascicles.

Despite these drawbacks, a carefully performed epineurial repair can often produce a satisfactory outcome when it is performed in the most proximal portion of the nerve, where fibers destined for a specific muscle or sensory territory are present in a number of fascicles and may be more or less represented in all of the areas. Epineurial suture is also useful in the most distal portion of nerves, such as a common or proper digital nerve. Here, alignment is less of a problem because nerve composition is relatively homogeneous and fascicles are few in number.

Interfascicular Repair

As the name suggests, interfascicular repair is based on individual suturing of each fascicle, usually by stitches placed in the perineurium (see Chap. 19). This means that one or two sutures may be required in as many as 30 to 40 fascicles of a major nerve such as the median or ulnar nerve. The cost of the additional surgical trauma may more than offset any advantage gained in fascicular alignment. However, if a single fascicle or bundle is associated with a specific function (such as a motor bundle), individual alignment and suture is justified. Further, if rotation of the proximal or distal end occurs in an interfascicular repair, the effect might be a malalignment of all the fascicles, since they are joined individually.

Although this technique has been reported on, it is not likely to gain wide favor as a routine way of treating transection of a major forearm nerve. It requires considerable additional effort and operative manipulation, and available data to date do not justify it.

Interfascicular Nerve Grafting

Since its introduction around 1970, interfascicular nerve grafting has increased in popularity. Its major features are described in detail in Chapter 37. Perhaps its major advantage is that by inserting autografts between transected ends, the surgeon can completely eliminate tension at the nerve junctures, assuming that the grafts are long enough to allow the proximal and distal ends to lie naturally in their bed with the extremity in full extension. A second consideration in nerve grafting is that the external epineurium is removed from nerve ends, a technique thought to minimize suture line scarring and neuroma formation. With these two maneuvers, a thinner scar is likely to be produced at the graft–nerve interface, a scar that offers less resistance to regenerating axons.

Nerve grafting probably will never be practiced as the primary technique for dealing with nerve transection; instead, it will be reserved for cases in which nerve substance has been lost and tension is deemed excessive. This probably will limit its use to secondary cases and gaps of more than 3 cm.

Theoretically, there are significant disadvantages to nerve grafting. There are two suture lines, and a donor defect is produced. The operation takes longer and requires specific microsurgical skills and equipment. Because a graft is used, and grafts must vascularize to survive, the quality of the bed becomes all-important. Most importantly, the technique requires the surgeon to be skilled in microsurgery and dissection of the internal components of nerves.

Tubulation

Although the concept of tubulation has been familiar and has been practiced in laboratory animals for nearly 50 years, it is only in the last 10 years that it has been researched with modern techniques.[16] Its potential use in patients has opened new doors and modified the thinking of surgeons. There is hope that an acceptable conduit for tubulation soon may become available and that chemical substances that enhance regeneration may be perfected and used to fill such tubes (see Chap. 41).

Finally, there is keen interest in neurotrophic and neuronotrophic factors that might influence regenerating axons and guide them to appropriate targets in the distal nerve ends. Although early reports describe the result of this technique in humans, at this time it is not recommended for general use and is considered primarily a research technique, albeit one with considerable potential.[18]

EPINEURIAL SPLINT REPAIR

Author's Preferred Method

Because no technique currently in use reliably provides satisfactory results, it appears that some modification of suture technique might be warranted to deal with the problems of nerve tension and the inability to align fascicles accurately.[11] The technique and the underlying principle to be described are not new, and I claim no credit for either. The technique of the epineurial bridge was inspired by Tsuge's anchoring funicular suture (Fig. 21-2)[28] and was born out of the frustration of trying to overcome the normal elasticity of peripheral nerves with 10-0 suture. It was some years before the underlying principle was explained by deMedinaceli and Seaber.[6] In 1956, de Saint-Venant described a principle dealing with the distribution of tensile forces in elastic bodies, noting that "only near the loaded ends does the stress distribution depend on the manner of applying the tensile force; in cross-sections at a distance from the end, the stresses are uniformly distributed. For practical purposes, a distance equal to 1.5 or 2 diameters of the structure is sufficient to obtain the effect."[6] deMedinaceli and Seaber reversed this principle: "In order to manipulate and displace an elastic body without inflicting stress at the tip of the structure, it suffices to apply mechanical traction at a distance from the tip equal to at least one-and-a-half times the diameter of the structure" (Fig. 21-3).[6]

This approach is neither necessary nor ideal for all nerve transections. It is probably unnecessary in acute severance of the proper and common digital nerves, where a simple epineurial suture can be satisfactory. Similarly, if injuries involve the motor and sensory branches of the ulnar or median nerves, these again might be sutured individually. The technique is most commonly used in transections of the major forearm nerves, beginning at the wrist and going at least to the midportion of the upper arm. Thus, it can be used for the median, ulnar, and radial nerves in those portions that contain both motor and sensory elements.[4] It has also been used and is equally applicable in the lower extremity.

Epineurial splint repairs can be complemented by awake stimulation or dissection of individual branches in the distal stump to identify specific motor or sensory units. It can be applied in either acute situations or in early secondary repairs. If

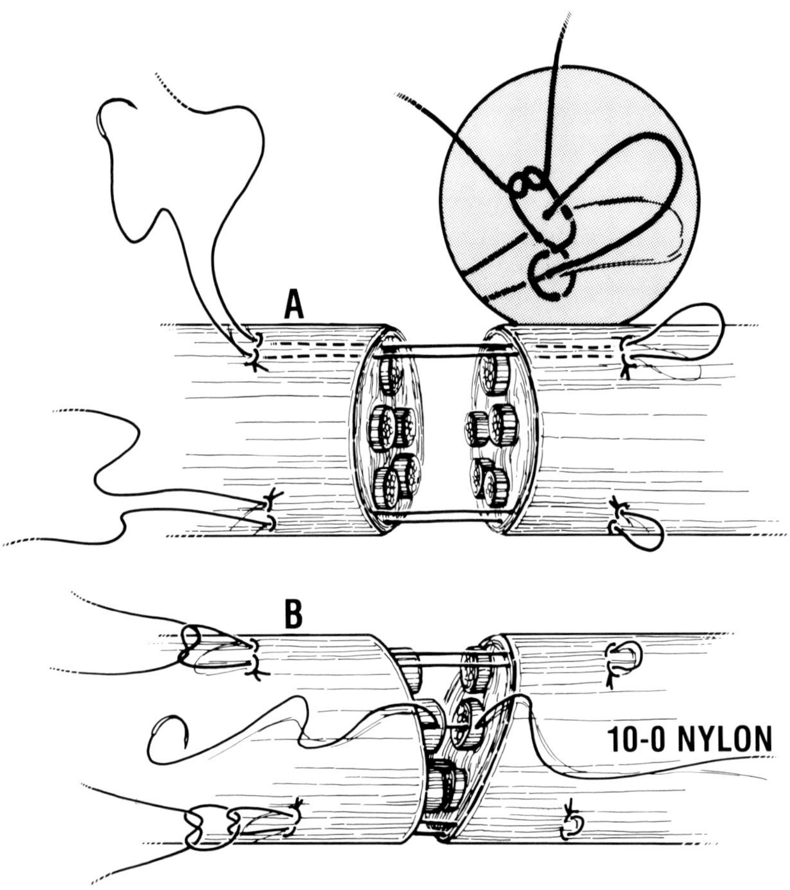

Figure 21–2. *The anchoring funicular suture of Tsuge, Ikuta, and Sakaue. The upper figure shows details of the anchoring suture, passed through external epineurium only at a distance from the cut end of the nerve. Its purpose is to grasp a remote site of external epineurium so that the transected nerve ends can be coapted without tension. In the lower figure, 10-0 nylon sutures are placed in the perineurium if there are areas of inadequate coaptation. (From Tsuge K, Ikuta Y, Sakaue M. A new technique for nerve suture: The anchoring funicular suture. Plast Reconstr Surg 1975;56:497, with permission.)*

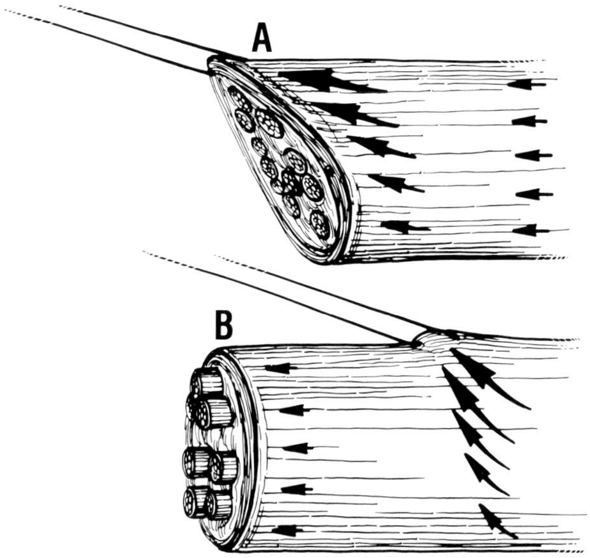

Figure 21–3. The principle of Saint-Venant. In the upper drawing, tension (large arrow) on the edge of an elastic cylinder loads that side asymmetrically. At some distance from the edge (small arrows), tension is equally distributed. In the lower drawing, the reverse situation can be seen. Asymmetrical tension at a distance (large arrow) from the edge absorbs the elastic force of the nerve and shields the cut surface from tension (small arrows). Fascicular coaptation can be accomplished with a minimum of foreign body and very few stitches.

there is loss of nerve substance or if neuroma excision produces an excessively long gap that would require extremes of joint flexion, a grafting procedure is indicated and the epineurial splint is not useful. This is *not* a procedure to overcome otherwise unacceptable tension, but is primarily a technique for minimizing tension and allowing careful approximation of individual components in a mixed nerve, one where direct suture might be performed anyway.

Technique

In the acute case, both nerve ends are identified and mobilized for a short distance. In tidy wounds, this need not be very far. If hematoma is present on the ends of the nerve, it is cleansed away manually and by irrigation. If the transection results from a sharp instrument, whether glass or steel, the nerve ends need not be recut. Such injuries usually produce satisfactory cuts and inflict no damage on adjacent nerve tissue. Because the ends are mirror images, they are ideal for repair. If the transection is slightly diagonal, as is often the case, recutting is also unnecessary and is not recommended.[21] Retaining the original cuts makes rotational alignment easier to interpret, wastes no length, and slightly offsets each stitch so that a circular scar is avoided. Recutting the nerve ends is recommended *only* if the newly cut ends are likely to produce a more tidy edge for repair than the original injury. There appear to be both advantages and disadvantages to trimming the "endoneural bulge" from a transected end.[1]

If the ends are to be recut, it is wise to make whatever positive identifications are possible before beginning and to cut the bundles individually, rather than all at once. To further aid in bundle identification, an awake stimulation can be done but is unnecessary. In the delayed primary repair and in secondary cases where a neuroma is forming or has formed, recutting the ends is mandatory. The normal reaction about cut nerve ends (whether a neuroma or glioma) results in a random arrangement of fibers, and the ends are unfit for repair. Recutting (and consequent shortening) is mandatory in such cases.

Once the nerves are mobilized and the ends prepared, a map is drawn of each end showing the configuration and location of bundles and major fascicles, and a marking stitch is placed for orientation. The two ends are then compared, and specific bundles or individual fascicles are identified for subsequent coaptation. In practice, the number of units selected may vary from as few as three to as many as eight. The number is likely to be greater in primary cases, where there has been no shrinkage of the fascicles in the distal end, than in secondary cases.

A longitudinal incision is made through the external epineurium on the superficial surface of the nerve end (Fig. 21-4A). Using appropriate magnification, the epineurium is then trimmed off the underlying fascicles for about 1 to 1.5 cm. A certain amount of judgment is necessary to decide how much trimming is required. This maneuver serves two purposes: it preserves the epineurium for construction of the bridge, and it trims the external epineurium back away from the fascicle ends, a step thought to be important from the standpoint of subsequent scarring. When this step has been completed, both ends are ready for coaptation.

A few sutures, perhaps as few as two or three of

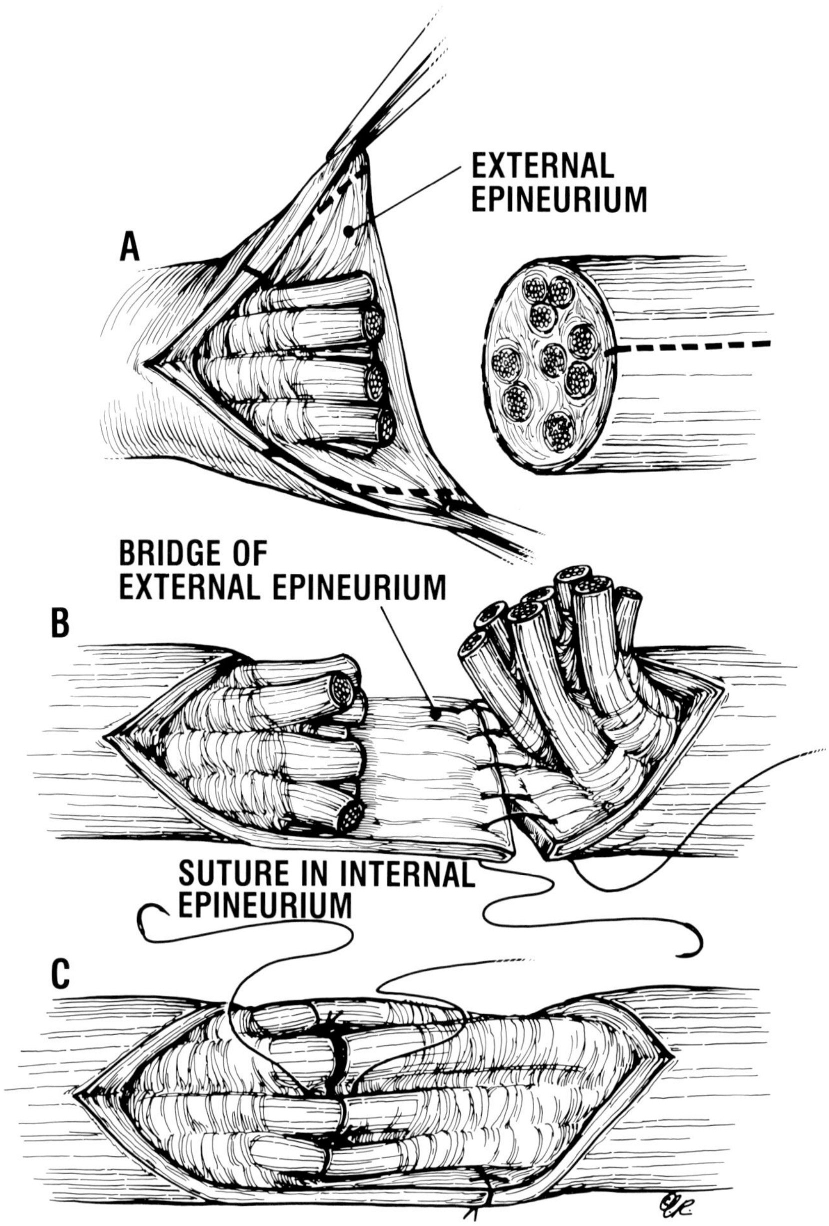

Figure 21-4. *Epineural bridge technique of nerve repair. (**A**) The epifascicular epineurium is incised longitudinally on the superficial surface of the nerve and dissected away from the underlying fascicles. A strip is retained on the posterior surface. (**B**) The epineural strip from each end is sutured with 8-0 nylon, usually two or three sutures, constructing the epineural bridge. This bridge uses the principal of Saint-Venant to absorb the tension and allow coaptation of the fascicles in a tension-free state. One of the epineural strips may be shortened slightly so as to offset the suture line away from the fascicular coaptation. (**C**) A few sutures of 10-0 nylon are placed in the internal epineurium to join individual fascicles or bundles of fascicles and complete the repair. External epineurium is not sutured on the superficial surface.*

8-0 nylon, are used to construct the bridge (Fig. 21-4*B*). A few millimeters of epineurium may be excised from one end of the bridge while the other end is left at its original length. The effect of this step is to offset the epineurial suture line in one direction or the other, so that it lies beneath intact fascicles rather than at the point of fascicular coaptation. As the epineurial sutures are tied, the fascicular ends are drawn toward each other and will be seen to naturally abut as the tension is taken up by the epineurium.

Once the epineurial splint is constructed, fascicular coaptation becomes relatively simple. Sutures of 10-0 or 11-0 nylon (my current choice is the Sharpoint MET needle) are placed *in the internal epineurium*, not in the perineurium. Two (sometimes only one) sutures are required to join a bundle. The fascicle ends naturally stick together and are held by a fibrin seal (Fig. 21-4C).

Any further external epineurial closure is contraindicated. By leaving the superficial surface open, minimal epineurium is left in the region of the nerve juncture, and this may well limit the number of fibroblasts available for neuroma formation. It may also relieve any constriction resulting from a circular suture (Fig. 21-5).

Figure 21-6 illustrates a patient in whom the epineurium was used in an acute repair.

Postoperative Care

Prior to wound closure, the repair site is visually inspected while adjacent joints are moved through a range of motion. The surgeon then selects a position of slightly more flexion so as to relieve any tension on the repair site. It is advisable, where possible, to measure the correct position with a goniometer. When wound closure is complete, the limb is splinted in that position for 3 weeks.

Even though the splint prohibits excessive flexion and disruption of the repair site, patients are

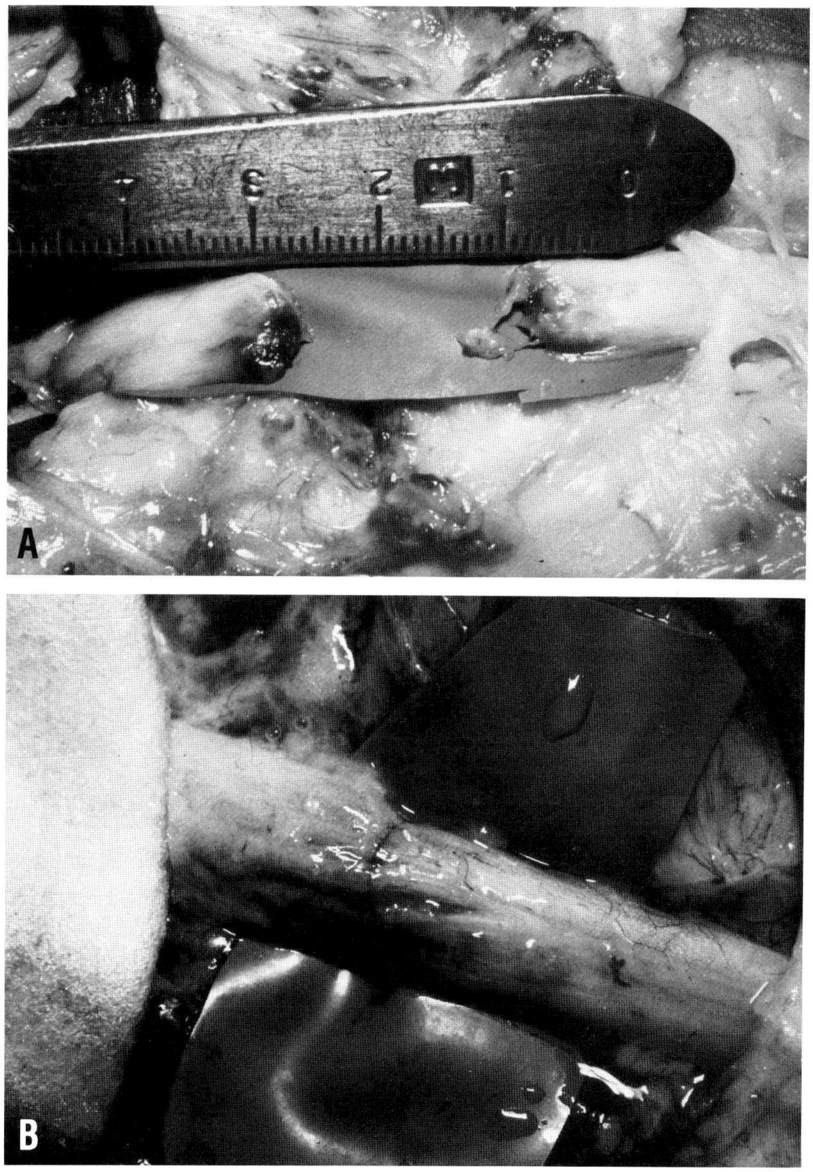

Figure 21–5. (**A**) Delayed primary repair of common peroneal nerve 1 week after sharp transection. No nerve tissue has been removed and the 2-cm distance between the nerve ends is the result of natural elasticity of the nerve ends. Once the ends have been trimmed, a 3-cm gap and a 1-cm nerve deficit are present. (**B**) An epineural bridge has been constructed (and cannot be seen) on the deep surface of the nerve, and individual fascicles have been aligned and sutured with 10-0 nylon. The external epineurium is not sutured on the superficial surface.

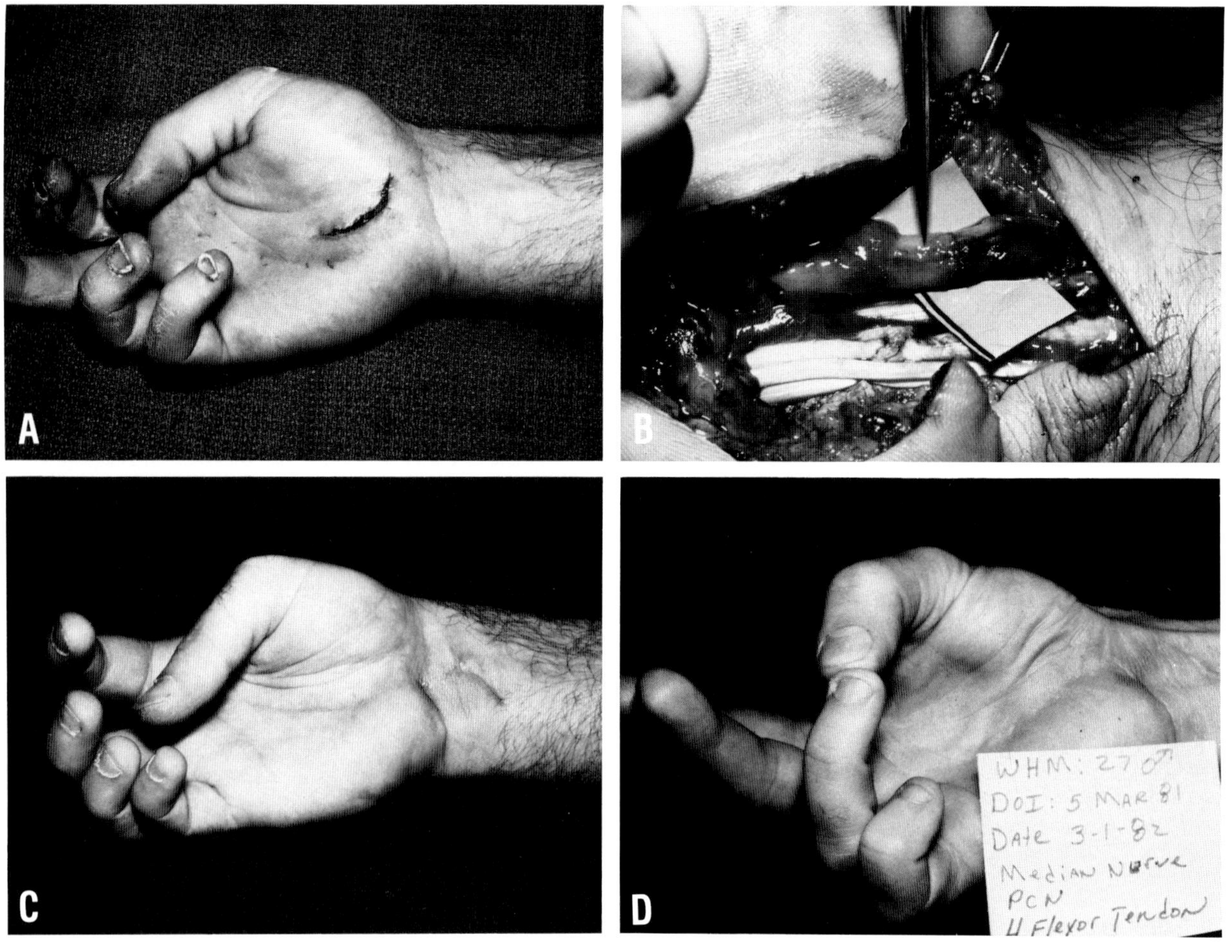

Figure 21–6. *A 26-year-old right-handed printer suffered a wine-glass laceration at the transverse carpal ligament area. (**A**) He divided the median nerve and flexor tendons to the thumb, index, and both long fingers. An immediate repair was performed. (**B**) Awake electrical stimulation and epineural bridge repair of the median nerve (pointer) was performed. (Fingers to the left.) The pointer is on the median nerve, just distal to the repair. Epineurium just distal to the pointer will be excised. The repaired tendon is visible beneath the nerve. (**C**) 6 weeks postoperative. Sensation is absent and opposition of the thumb is impossible. Note drying of thumb tip, scar crossing wrist. (**D**) 1 year postoperative. Sensation has returned and opposition of the thumb is now present and forceful. Patient returned to his job as a printer and had virtually normal sensation, pinch strength, and opposition 4 years after repair.*

allowed (and even encouraged) to actively flex their joints and move the digits passively. The intent is to minimize the likelihood of adherence of the repair site to surrounding tissue.[30]

At 3 weeks, joints are allowed to extend to neutral, but a protective dorsal splint on joints such as the wrist is worn for another 3 weeks. This can be a removable one; its purpose is to prevent hyperextension without restricting flexion.

At 6 weeks, baseline sensory and motor tests are performed and a full active range of motion is permitted. The patient then proceeds to strengthening and endurance-building, sensory re-education, and whatever other rehabilitative techniques are indicated.

The specific indications for this technique may be apparent and have been outlined previously. Whenever group fascicular nerve suture is indicated, it appears that the use of an epineurial bridge may assist in the technique.

In recent years, primary nerve repair has generally been advocated and more and more primary repairs have been performed. The experience of the major wars and civilian practice thereafter suggest (and I agree) that primary repair of peripheral nerves should be limited to tidy wounds. In wounds where there has been a significant stretch or crush component, the basic dilemma is that we have no way to determine in the period immediately after injury what portion of a nerve is viable. As a consequence, repair is sometimes carried out between nerve ends that are less than satisfactory (ie, that may be irreparably damaged), reducing the capability for functional recovery. In such instances, the surgeon is better advised to close the soft tissues, allow primary healing, and then return for an early secondary repair.

If this practice is to be followed, it is advisable to place one or two sutures between the nerve ends to prevent retraction and to be prepared to excise a neuroma at the time of early secondary surgery. At that time, the surgeon makes a judgment as to whether the gap is an acceptable one or whether it is excessive, in which case grafts must be inserted. As a rule, gaps of 2.5 to 3 cm or less are acceptable for direct suture; longer gaps are grafted.

Summary

Epineurial splint repair is not a method for overcoming otherwise unacceptable tension, nor is it a way to avoid an excessive gap. It is a method to relieve tension so that accurate fascicular coaptation is achieved without having to resort to an excessive number of heavier-than-desired and tightly tied sutures.

COMPLICATIONS

Few complications are associated specifically with this technique; the problems common to peripheral nerve surgery in general can be expected. Specifically, the bed in which the nerve lies plays a major role in the outcome. If there is excessive fibrosis and scarring as a result of major soft-tissue injury, scar formation about the repair can be expected. A scar adhesion of the repair site to the surrounding tissue may produce a traction phenomenon on the repair site (see Chap. 18). At best, this results in local symptoms and slow progress in recovery; at worst, the nerve repair fails. In such instances, an external neurolysis of the nerve repair is indicated and can be helpful. Neurolysis is best deferred for 4 to 6 months, after reasonable tissue equilibrium has occurred. If neurolysis of a repaired nerve is performed, *it is an external neurolysis only*. Rarely, if ever, can bundles of fascicles be separated at the repair site. Surgeons who do so run the risk of losing whatever regeneration has occurred up to that point.

Tinel's sign is the best way to monitor progress in a recently repaired nerve. I perform the test by simple digital percussion rather than with a hammer. Percussion is begun distally and proceeds proximally toward the area of the repair. Two specific points are usually apparent: the most distal location at which paresthesias can be elicited, and the point at which the sensation of tingling is maximal (the major Tinel's sign). If paresthesias radiate to a specific area or digit, this is also noted. As progress occurs, the more distal point will move further and will spread out over a longer length of nerve. The maximal point of paresthesia gradually lessens and progresses distally as well. If the major Tinel's sign does not advance, the surgeon should be prepared to re-explore the wound and perform a neurolysis, resection and resuture, or graft, as is indicated.

In addition to Tinel's sign, the only other ways to follow the progress of nerve repair are with clinical muscle and sensory testing. Careful baseline observations are made shortly after the operation. In the postoperative period, we rarely see progress within the first 6 weeks, but we test frequently thereafter and have found such testing to be a useful monitor of progress.

Although electrodiagnostic studies can be used, we have not found them particularly helpful in following the progress of a repaired nerve. They are expensive and uncomfortable, and interpretation is open to question and requires an informed examiner (see Chaps. 10 and 11).

In injuries to major nerves containing motor fibers, such as the radial and ulnar nerves, protective splinting is important to prevent secondary joint deformity. Clawing of the small and ring fingers has been the most common deformity and should be watched for; it may result in permanent proximal interphalangeal (PIP) joint contracture, which is extremely difficult to treat. If splinting is done, it is best to keep it simple. Patients will not wear hot, bulky, or cumbersome splints. In addition, splints that mask sensory stimuli are useless. Sensory input can be very helpful in sensory recovery and should be encouraged. Finally, sensory reeducation has been shown to be valuable in patients who are recovering sensation, and should be used where possible (see Chap. 58).

REFERENCES

1. Archibald SJ, Fisher TR. Microsurgical fascicular nerve repair: A morphological study of the endoneurial bulge. J Hand Surg [Br] 1987; 12:5–10.
2. Bora FW, Pleasure DE, Didizian NA. A study of nerve regeneration and neuroma formation after nerve suture by various techniques. J Hand Surg 1976; 1:138–143.
3. Cabaud HE, Rodkey WG, McCarroll HR, Mutz SB, Niebauer JJ. Epineurial and perineurial fascicular nerve repairs: A critical comparison. J Hand Surg 1976; 1:131–137.
4. Chow JA, Van Beek AL, Bilos ZJ, et al. Anatomical basis for repair of ulnar and median nerves in the distal part of the forearm by group fascicular suture and nerve grafting. J Bone Joint Surg [Am] 1986; 68:273–280.
5. deMedinaceli LD, Freed WJ. Peripheral nerve reconnection: Immediate histologic consequences of distributed mechanical support. Exp Neurol 1983; 81:459–468.
6. deMedinaceli LD, Seaber AV. Experimental nerve reconnection: Importance of initial repair. Microsurgery 1989; 10:56–70.
7. Edshage S. Peripheral nerve suture: A technique for improved intraneural topography. Acta Chir Scand 1964; 331:1–104.
8. Hakstian RW. Perineural neurorrhaphy. Orthop Clin North Am 1973; 4:945–956.
9. Highet WB, Sanders FK. The effects of stretching nerves after suture. Br J Surg 1943; 30:355–369.
10. Hubbard JH. The quality of nerve regeneration. Surg Clin North Am 1972; 52:1099–1108.
11. Jabaley ME. Technical aspects of peripheral nerve repair. J Hand Surg 1984; 9:14–19.
12. Jabaley ME. Peripheral nerve repair. In May JW Jr, Littler JW, eds. Plastic surgery: The hand. Philadelphia: WB Saunders, 1990:4757–4775.
13. Kline DG, Hudson AR. Selected recent advances in peripheral nerve injury research. Surg Neurol 1985; 24:371–376.
14. Kutz JE, Shealy G, Lubbers L. Interfascicular nerve repair. Orthop Clin North Am 1981; 12:277–286.
15: Lundborg G. The intrinsic vascularization of human peripheral nerves: Structural and functional aspects. J Hand Surg 1979; 4:34–41.
16. Lundborg G. Nerve injury and repair. Edinburgh: Churchill-Livingstone, 1988:196.
17. Mackinnon SE. New directions in peripheral nerve surgery. Ann Plast Surg 1989; 22:257–273.
18. Mackinnon SE, Dellon AL. Clinical nerve reconstruction with a bioabsorbable polyglycolic acid tube. Plast Reconstr Surg 1990; 85:419–424.
19. Millesi H. Healing of nerves. Clin Plast Surg 1977; 4:459–472.
20. Millesi H. Reappraisal of nerve repair. Surg Clin North Am 1981; 61:321–340.
21. Millesi H. The nerve gap: Theory and clinical practice. Hand Clin 1986; 2:651–663.
22. Millesi H, Terzis JK. Problems of terminology in peripheral nerve surgery: Committee report of the International Society of Reconstructive Microsurgery. Microsurgery 1983; 4:51–56.
23. Orgel MG. Epineurial vs perineurial repair of peripheral nerves. Clin Plast Surg 1984; 11:101–104.
24. Rank BK, Wakefield AR. Surgery of repair as applied to hand injuries, ed 2, Chapter 5. Edinburgh & London: E & S Livingstone Ltd, 1960:62–64.
25. Rosen JM. Concepts of peripheral nerve repair. Ann Plast Surg 1981; 7:165–171.
26. Sunderland S. The pros and cons of funicular nerve repair. J Hand Surg 1979; 4:201–211.
27. Sunderland S. Nerve repair. J Hand Surg [Am] 1984; 9:1–3.
28. Tsuge K, Ikuta Y, Sakaue M. A new technique for nerve suture: The anchoring funicular suture. Plast Reconstr Surg 1975; 56:496–500.
29. Tupper JW, Crick JC, Matteck LR. Fascicular nerve repairs: A comparative study of perineurial and fascicular (perineurial) techniques. Orthop Clin North Am 1988; 19:57–69.
30. Wilgis EFS, Murphy R. The significance of longitudinal excursion in peripheral nerves. Hand Clin 1986; 2:761–766.

22

New Approaches in Nerve Suture

Kenya Tsuge
Takaya Mizuseki

AUTHORS' KEY POINTS

- The most important technical aspects of nerve suture are atraumatic technique with avoidance of suture site tension and placement of the repair or graft in an unscarred environment.
- Use of the anchoring funicular suture greatly reduces tension at the suture site. Moderate-sized gaps are overcome safely without sacrificing neural capillary circulation.

BASIC CONSIDERATIONS

Surgeons should keep in mind several basic points when performing peripheral nerve suture, regardless of the specific technique and suture material used.

Topological Coaptation

In performing nerve suture, it is ideal to match proximal fibers to distal fibers. This is technically difficult, as the only method in common use is ocular identification of the topology of fascicles under magnification. Several studies have reported on the differentiation of sensory and motor nerve components by histochemical staining (see Chap. 16),[3,6] but these methods are experimental and are not practiced on a routine basis. It has been acceptable to use topograms of peripheral nerves as presented in the literature.[17] The emphasis has been on suturing or grafting nerves to corresponding fascicles so that better alignment is obtained (see Chap. 14). This is not an easy task. Generally speaking, the more proximal the lesion, and the larger the gap, the more difficult the fascicle identification and alignment.

Suture Site Tension

Tension on the site of nerve suture is undesirable. Experimentally it has been found that if the initial tension of sutured nerve is greater than 25 g, axonal regeneration is inhibited.[13] Clinically, there is little agreement regarding the units of tension that are tolerated at the suture site.[12,15] In our experience, after freshly preparing and mobilizing nerve stumps, a 3-cm gap can be overcome for the median and ulnar nerves in the forearm, whereas 2 cm is the limit that can be overcome in the upper arm. Nerve grafting is indicated when the defect exceeds these limits.

Leakage of Axonal Flow

It is postulated that neuronotropic factors play an important role in the regenerative process.[2,5,9,10] In order to keep factor concentration as high as possible, the elapsed time prior to surgery is minimized and leakage of axonal fluid from the suture site is prevented. Trials to limit axonal leakage as much as possible have been accomplished with a variety of adaptics or films, both artificial and biological.

Sound Soft-Tissue Environment

If the nerve bed is severely scarred and lacking in ample extrinsic blood supply, nerve regeneration after neurorrhaphy is disappointing.[8] In such cases, conventional nerve suture or grafting techniques are not used. Vascularized nerve grafts may be indicated in order to overcome the avascularity of a scarred bed (see Chap. 40).[18]

SPECIAL TECHNIQUES

Adhesive Repair

Nerve repair without suture is ideal for avoidance of trauma. For this reason, a number of procedures have been devised, including the use of plasma glue,[11] fibrin film,[16] Micropore tape,[4] and fibrin sealant.[7,21] Their advantages are that they are atraumatic and prevent leakage of axonal flow. However, they have failed to gain popularity because they do not provide sufficient suture site adhesiveness to resist tension and subsequent deformation, and because these adaptic materials often cause local tissue reactions. Some surgeons use fibrin film and fibrin sealant in combination with conventional suture techniques.

Fibrin Sealant

The technique of nerve repair with each of the available adhesives is similar. The nerve ends are approximated with fine jeweler's forceps, and an adhesive agent, such as fibrin sealant, is applied topically. Fibrin sealant is highly concentrated and has greater adhesive strength now than it had in the past. It is commercially available, prepared in two separate syringes, one containing fibrinogen and the other containing thrombin. At the time of injection, they are mixed to form adhesive fibrin. Afterwards, the fibrin film is wrapped around the repair site (Fig. 22-1).

With either technique, tension at the suture site is minimized because the nerve stumps are easily separated. If a gap occurs, the fibrin product will enter the repair site between the nerve stumps, possibly creating a barrier to axonal regeneration.

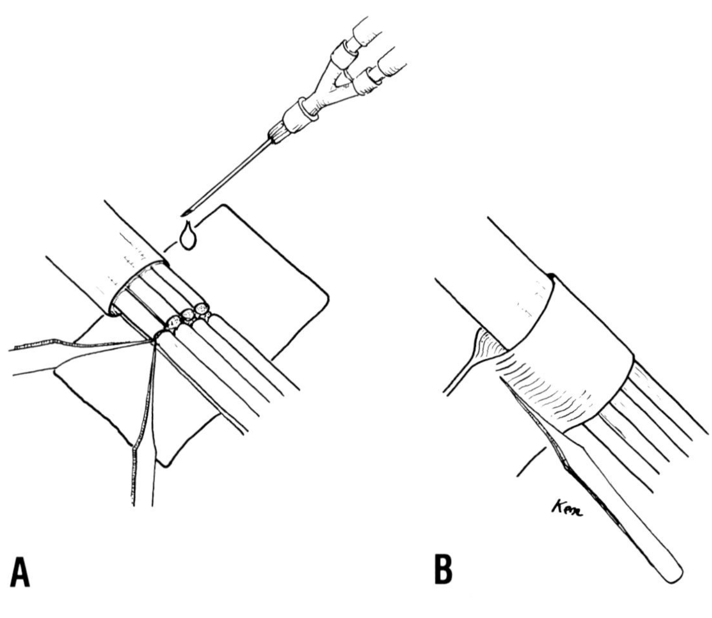

Figure 22-1. *Nerve repair technique using fibrin sealant. (**A**) With forceps, the nerve end and the nerve graft are approximated. A drop or two of the fibrin sealant is topically applied. The nerve should be held by the forceps until the seal is stable. (**B**) Toward the end, fibrin film may be used to wrap the entire anastomosis.*

Current indications for this technique include cases in which cable nerve grafts are being applied because of repair site gap; as a result, tension at the suture site is nonexistent.

Laser-Assisted Repair

The laser, originally invented for industrial use, has been modified for various surgical purposes. One of its applications is for nerve suture. Two types of laser beams are used experimentally, argon[1] and low-output carbon dioxide.[14] Neither can bond transected nerve stumps by itself. By converting nonadherent into adherent material, however, laser-assisted repair becomes possible. Argon laser energy, selectively absorbed by porphyrine derivatives, converts blood erythrocytes into an adhesive coagulant. Low-output carbon dioxide laser energy is absorbed primarily in superficial tissue layers, creating fibrin film adhesive.

With these methods, scar formation around the suture site is reduced. Axonal regeneration after laser-assisted neurorrhaphy is significantly superior to that of conventional neurorrhaphy.

The Osedo technique of laser-assisted nerve repair uses the low-output carbon dioxide laser, which is specially prepared for microscopic operative use.[14] Its output is 60 to 70 mW, and the diameter of the beam is less than 0.2 mm. The He-Ne laser beam is used as a guide beam because the carbon dioxide laser wave, which is ultra-red, cannot be monitored without a guide.

Prior to laser use, two stay sutures are inserted, approximating the nerve ends. Then several sheets of thin fibrin film are wrapped around the suture site, and the entire surface of the film irradiated with the laser beam (Fig. 22-2). Total laser irradiation time averages 2.5 minutes. As most of the energy of the carbon dioxide laser is absorbed in the surface of the fibrin film, it does not affect the deeper layers, including the nerve fibers. The fibrin film is then adhesive enough to withstand some tension at the suture site. The stay sutures are removed at the end of the procedure.

The advantages of laser repair are significantly improved regeneration of nerve fibers, diminished axonal sprouting, and reduced scarring around the suture site (Fig. 22-3). Although laser repair is still in the experimental stages, its ability to seal the nerve, preventing axonal sprouting, is very attractive. Further experiments should clarify its effectiveness for earlier revascularization and nerve regeneration and will identify any adverse effects.

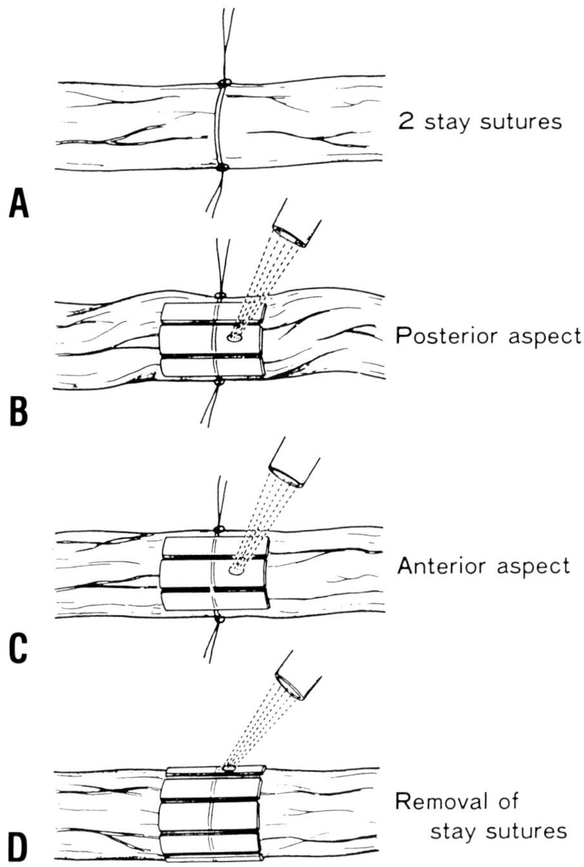

Figure 22-2. *CO_2 laser-assisted nerve anastomosis. (**A**) Two stay sutures are applied. (**B**) Several sheets of thin fibrin film are wrapped around the suture site and irradiated with CO_2 laser beam. It is usually easier to start with the posterior aspect and then proceed to the anterior aspect (**C**). (**D**) The stay sutures are removed at the end of the procedure. (Reproduced with permission from Osedo M. An experimental study on nerve repair using carbon dioxide laser. J Jpn Orthop Assoc 1988;62:655.)*

Anchoring Funicular Suture

Authors' Preferred Method

Surgeons often are confronted with a nerve defect at or just beyond the critical limit for direct approximation (eg, 3 cm for the median nerve in the forearm) in which the gap is too large for primary repair. In an effort to reduce the morbidity

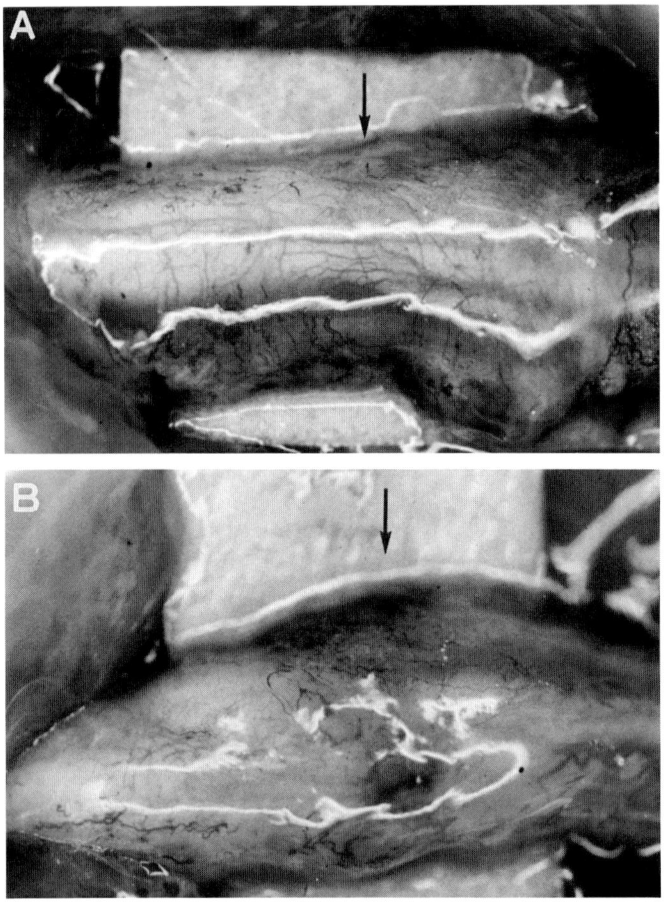

Figure 22–3. *Comparison of the results of laser-assisted nerve suture and conventional suture.* ***A*** *shows microscopic findings 8 weeks after* CO_2 *laser-assisted anastomosis.* ***B*** *shows the results of conventional technique. Arrows indicate suture site. Note that less neuroma is formed in the laser-assisted anastomosis. (Reproduced with permission from Osedo M. An experimental study on nerve repair using carbon dioxide laser. J Jpn Orthop Assoc 1988;62:657.)*

and time associated with nerve grafting, and to reduce the repair site tension created by conventional techniques, the anchoring funicular suture is used.[20]

The nerve repair is performed in a bloodless field with prior exsanguination. The severed nerve ends are exposed under magnification. In chronic cases, the neuroma of the proximal end and the glioma of the distal end are identified. (When the severed nerves have been neglected for an extended time, the cut ends will have retracted and will be difficult to approximate.) The nerve ends are palpated and transected with a sharp knife at the site where the funicular arrangements are intact (Figs. 22-4, 22-5). The other side of the epineurium is maintained in continuity so that the funicular pattern can be studied by holding the neuroma or glioma.

A decision is made as to whether nerve grafting or primary repair is indicated. If the decision is made to suture the nerve primarily, the following steps are taken.

A 5-0 or 6-0 nylon looped suture is used for nerves larger than 4 mm in diameter. It is similar in configuration to the looped suture commonly used for tendon repair.[19] The suture is specially designed with the needle fitted on the end of the looped suture. Two types of suture material are commercially available: nylon monofilament suture and braided polyester suture. For nerve repair, monofilament nylon is preferred, because it causes less friction as it extends through tissue and allows easier approximation of nerve ends at the desired tension. The technique is illustrated in Figure 22-6.

The superficial loop stay is made at a point 1 cm from the nerve end (point A). The radius of the needle is enlarged after making the loop so that it more easily passes through the epineurium. The needle is passed through the epineurium along the longitudinal axis of the nerve. Then, taking the funicular pattern into consideration, the stay suture is inserted at the corresponding point of the opposite nerve end (point B) and drawn out at a point 1 cm from the cut end (point C). One of the

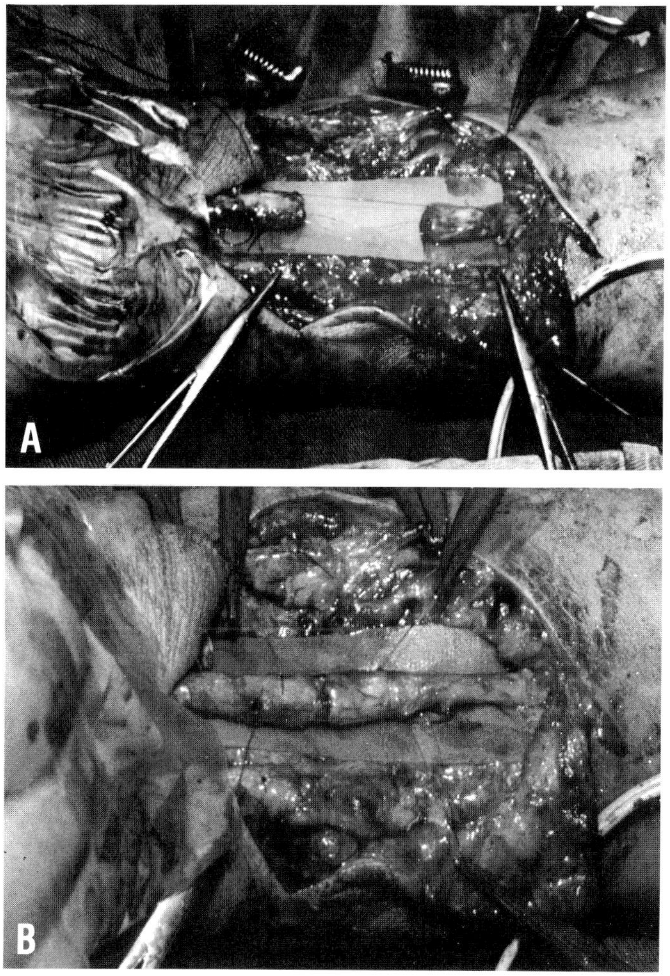

Figure 22–4. *Anchoring funicular suture. (**A**) There is a gap of about 2.5 cm in the median nerve of a 41-year-old male. (**B**) The anchoring funicular suture with two looped nylon sutures is completed. (Reproduced with permission from Tsuge K, Ikuta Y, Sakaue M. A new technique for nerve suture: The anchoring funicular suture. Plast Reconstr Surg 1975;56:500.)*

two sutures is cut, after which the needle is once again drawn into and out of the epineurium in order to allow a knot to be tied. When tying the knot, the nerve ends are approximated carefully, neither too tightly nor too loosely. While slight gapping or unevenness is tolerable, buckling of the fasciculi is avoided. When necessary, a second anchoring suture is inserted 180° from the first, after the neuroma and glioma have been resected.

Group fascicular suture then follows. This is accomplished with 8-0 or 9-0 nylon suture. As this technique is applied only when there is a moderate gap between the nerve ends, special care is taken in managing nerve stumps. If the nerve is stretched, further damage to the nerve end will occur. Therefore, when suturing, the neighboring joints are flexed or extended in an effort to reduce tension and minimize nerve stump damage.

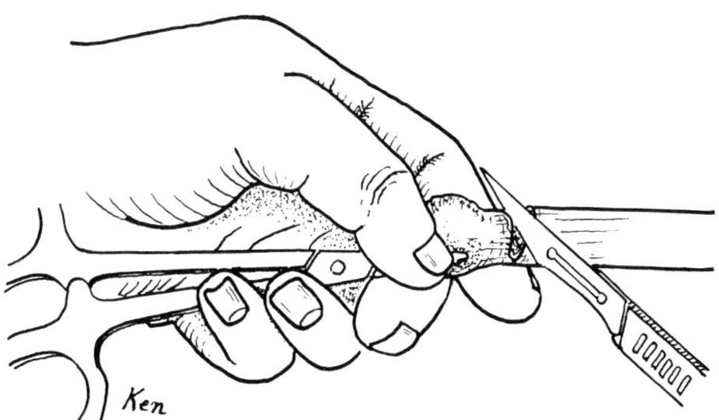

Figure 22–5. *The nerve end is prepared. The neuroma or glioma can be removed with a single stroke of the sharp scalpel. The edge of the nerve is held by mosquito forceps, and the nerve is pushed up with the other index finger, keeping it immobile.*

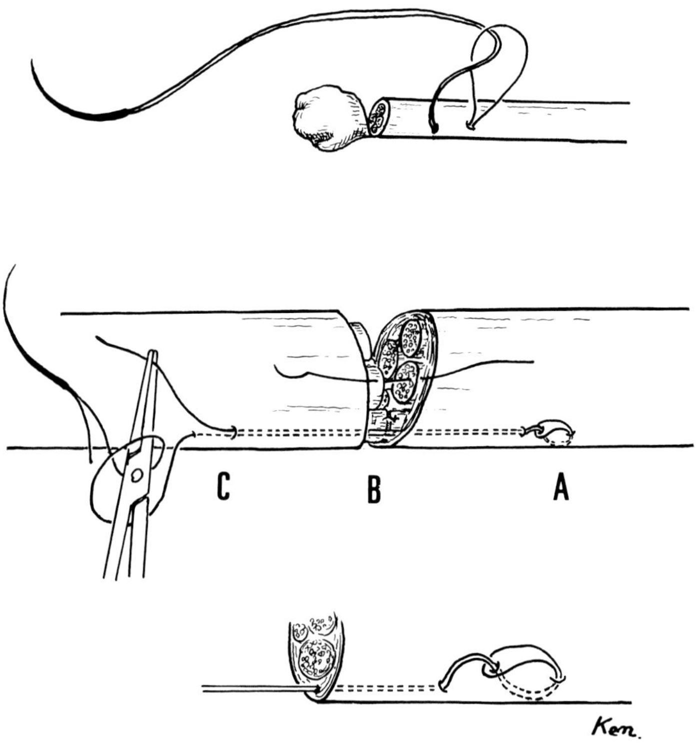

Figure 22–6. *Anchoring funicular suture. A stay loop is made about 1 cm from the suture site (**A**). The suture is passed through the epineurium to the other side of the nerve (**B**). The knot suture is made about 1 cm from the suture site after accommodating the gap (**C**). (Modified with permission from Tsuge K, Ikuta Y, Sakaue M. A new technique for nerve suture: The anchoring funicular suture. Plast Reconstr Surg 1975;56: 497.)*

Postoperative management is similar to that for conventional suture methods. The suture site and neighboring joints are immobilized postoperatively for 3 weeks, after which controlled mobilization is carried out for 3 additional weeks.

With this method, tension of the suture site is maintained in the epineurium where the stay sutures are anchored, reducing tension at the suture site and maintaining nerve stump vascularity. Figure 22-7 shows the differences in vascularity at the suture site between the conventional and anchoring funicular suture technique. Significantly increased capillary anastomoses have been observed in the latter group.

The advantages of this technique are that it easily approximates nerve ends with moderate gaps,

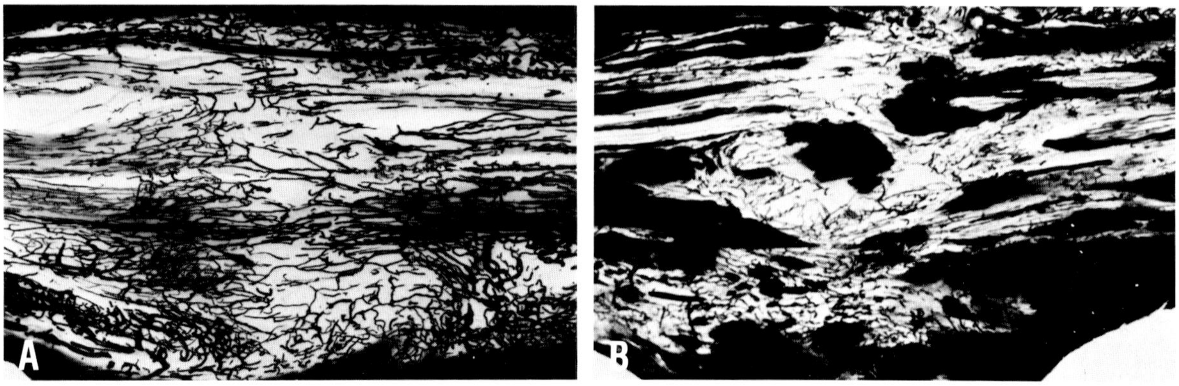

Figure 22–7. *Microcirculation demonstrated by injection of india ink at the suture site 3 weeks after nerve suture. Abundant anastomosis of capillary vessels is demonstrated on the anchoring funicular suture (**A**) as compared to the conventional suture (**B**). (Reproduced with permission from Tsuge K, Ikuta Y, Sakaue M. A new technique for nerve suture: The anchoring funicular suture. Plast Reconstr Surg 1975;56:498.)*

does not sacrifice the circulation of the repair site, requires less time than conventional repair, and does not need special instrumentation.

This technique is indicated in situations where tension is too great for direct epi-perineural (group fascicular), end-to-end suture but not great enough to require interfascicular nerve grafting. However, this technique should not be used in situations where the gap is excessive or mobilization of the nerve will impair neural blood supply. Undue tension and reduced circulation predictably compromise results.

FUTURE PERSPECTIVE

With the advent of microsurgical techniques, the technical aspects of nerve repair have been investigated thoroughly. However, recovery of nerve function after nerve repair is not uniformly satisfactory, regardless of the refined suture technique used, especially when the injury is well proximal to the end organ or when it has occurred in an older individual. In the future, experimental studies will be directed toward the elucidation of the biochemical properties of nerve regeneration, both locally and systemically, including activating factors, biological sealing, and differences between motor and sensory nerves. The success of these experiments will open the door to a new era of nerve repair.

REFERENCES

1. Almquist EE, Nachemson A, Auth D, Almquist B, Hall S. Evaluation of the use of the argon laser in repairing rat and primate nerves. J Hand Surg [Am] 1984; 9:792–799.
2. Bueker ED, Bane JL. The problem of distribution of a nerve growth factor specific for spinal and sympathetic ganglia. Cancer Res 1960; 20:1220–1228.
3. Cruger H, Freilinger G, Holle J, Mandl H. Identification of motor and sensory funiculi in cut nerves and their selective reunion. Br J Plast Surg 1976; 29:70–73.
4. Freeman BS. Adhesive anastomosis techniques for fine nerves: Experimental and clinical techniques. Am J Surg 1964; 108:529–532.
5. Gundersen, Barrett JN. Neuronal chemotaxis: Chick dorsal root axons turn toward high concentrations of nerve growth factor. Science 1979; 206:1079–1080.
6. Karnovsky MJ. A "direct-coloring" thiocholine method for cholinesterases. Journal of Biochemistry Cytochemistry 1964; 12:219–221.
7. Koshima I, Matsunaga Y, Harii K. Experimental study on nerve union using fibrin seal. Rinsho Seikei Geka (Clin Orthop Surg) 1983; 18:735–741.
8. Lundborg G. Structure and function of the intraneural microvessels as related to trauma, edema formation, and nerve function. J Bone Joint Surg [Am] 1975; 57:938–948.
9. Lundborg G, Dahlin LB, Danielsen N, et al. Nerve regeneration across an extended gap: A neurobiological view of nerve repair and the possible involvement of neuronotrophic factors. J Hand Surg 1982; 7:580–587.
10. Mackinnon SE, Dellon AL, Lundborg G, Hudson AR, Hunter DA. A study of neurotrophism in a primate model. J Hand Surg [Am] 1986; 11:888–894.
11. Matras H, Braun F, Lassmann H, Ammerer HP, Mamoli B. Plasma cloth welding of nerves (experimental report). Journal of Maxillofacial Surgery 1973; 1:236–247.
12. Millesi H, Meissl G, Berger A. The interfascicular nerve-grafting of the median and ulnar nerves. J Bone Joint Surg [Am] 1972; 54:727–750.
13. Miyamoto Y. Experimental study of results of nerve suture under tension vs. nerve grafting. Plast Reconstr Surg 1979; 64:540–549.
14. Osedo M. An experimental study on nerve repair using carbon dioxide laser. J Jpn Orthop Assoc 1988; 62:653–663.
15. Schultz RJ. Management of nerve gaps. In: Omer GE, Spinner M, eds. Management of peripheral nerve problems. Philadelphia: WB Saunders, 1980: 388–409.
16. Singer M. The combined use of fibrin film and cloth in end-to-end union of nerves. J Neurosurg 1945; 2:102–125.
17. Sunderland S. Funicular suture and funicular exclusion in the repair of severed nerves. Br J Surg 1953; 40:580–587.
18. Taylor GI, Ham FJ. The free vascularized nerve graft: A further experimental and clinical application of microvascular techniques. Plast Reconstr Surg 1975; 56:166–170.
19. Tsuge K, Ikuta Y, Matusishi Y. Repair of flexor tendons by intratendinous tendon suture. J Hand Surg 1977; 2:436–440.
20. Tsuge K, Ikuta Y, Sakaue M. A new technique for nerve suture: The anchoring funicular suture. Plast Reconstr Surg 1975; 56:496–500.
21. Young JZ, Medawar PB: Fibrin suture of peripheral nerves. Lancet 1940; 239:126–128.

23

Partial Nerve Injuries

Lawrence C. Hurst
Andrew Dowd

AUTHORS' KEY POINTS

- Partial nerve lacerations are a unique problem for the peripheral nerve surgeon. Their repair demands precise microsurgical techniques, as potential operative complications include damage to intact fascicular groups.
- Partial nerve lacerations are rare in civilian practice but common in war-related injuries.
- Partial nerve repairs are technically easier immediately after injury. End-to-end repair of the lacerated fascicular groups is usually possible in sharp, clean civilian lacerations.
- Dissection within the internal epineural plane allows end-to-end repair of the lacerated fascicular groups.
- True defects and their resultant tension, not simply the presence of a gap secondary to elastic recoil, should be the indication for grafting.

Partial nerve injury is defined as any nerve damage that causes incomplete functional loss. A classic example of partial nerve injury occurs in the patient who presents with a sharp laceration of the median nerve at the wrist but has sensation in the thumb and radial aspect of the index finger (Fig. 23-1).

Sunderland defines five types of partial nerve injuries.[29] The first type has a positive correlation between the partial neurologic defect and the operative dissection, which reveals incomplete transection of the median nerve. Lundborg calls this type "subtotal nerve transection."[19] The second type of partial nerve injury causes complete functional loss in the distribution of a particular nerve, but operative dissection shows transection of some fascicular groups and a neurapraxia of the remaining fascicular groups. While the third type of partial nerve injury presents with no functional loss, at surgery an isolated epineural laceration or even partial damage of a few fascicles is found. The third type occurs when a proximal laceration partially damages a fascicular group that contains numerous fascicles. The resultant damage is slight and the functional defect so diffuse that it is clinically undetectable.

The fourth type of partial nerve injury is a traumatic compression neuropathy, a tractional injury, or blunt trauma. The fifth type is demonstrated by the incomplete recovery after repair of a completely lacerated nerve. Incomplete nerve regen-

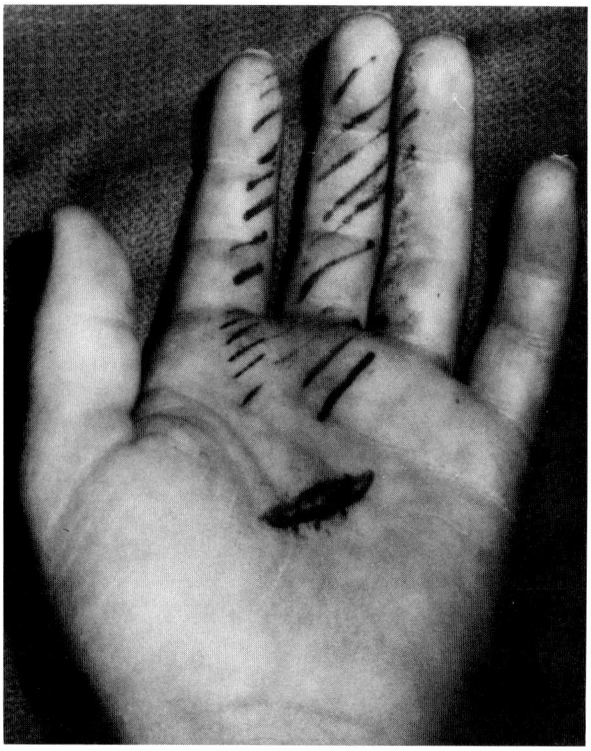

Figure 23–1. *Midpalm laceration that went proximally into the middle of the carpal tunnel. Patient had intact median motor function and intact sensation in the thumb and radial side of the index. Sensation in the areas marked by parallel lines was completely absent.*

eration and compression neuropathies are discussed in Chapters 42 and 60 through 88.

The incidence of partial nerve injury is difficult to assess. In our practice, 12 partial nerve lacerations occurred between 1981 and 1987. During this same period, 75 complete nerve lacerations were treated by surgical neurorrhaphy, 1975 other hand operations were performed, and 6564 new patients were seen in the hand center. This means the incidence of partial nerve lacerations was 6.6 per 1000 new patient visits, or 0.18%. Of procedures performed, partial nerve repairs represented 0.6% of all operations and only 16% of the nerve repairs. This shows that in our civilian practice partial nerve injuries are uncommon, in direct contrast to the wartime experience reported by Kline and others where 60% of injuries to peripheral nerves lacerated only part of the nerve.[15,16]

PERTINENT ANATOMY

To deal appropriately with the operative repair of partial nerve lacerations, the surgeon must have a thorough understanding of the internal topography of the peripheral nerves. As Sunderland has emphasized, the surgeon who attempts repair of a partial nerve injury must understand how the level of the injury affects the funicular (fascicular) pattern, funicular distribution, and funicular redistribution.[29] Jabaley and Williams emphasize that surgeons' review of this work must be comprehensive and include Sunderland's microdissections or their interpretation of his work will leave them with an overly pessimistic view of the operability of peripheral nerve fascicular groups.[14,31,34] The connections between fascicles within a given fascicular group are considerable, particularly at the level of the brachial plexus. However, in the forearm and hand the connections between fascicular groups are minimal.[3,31] Gunther, DiPasquale, and Martin have recently confirmed this with dissections at the elbow. Except for the flexor digitorum superficialis, the branches of the median nerve could easily be dissected proximally in the nerve for 2 to 9 cm.[10] Jabaley has shown that the lack of connections between fascicular groups allows intraneural neurolysis, fascicular nerve repair, and fascicular level nerve grafting.[13,14,21,34] The microsurgical plane of these dissections is between the fascicular groups within the internal epineurium. Our recent study of the repair of partial lacerations of the median and ulnar nerves has shown that this plane can also be used to dissect the transected fascicular groups, allowing direct repair of these groups (Fig. 23-2).[12]

TIMING OF REPAIR

At present, the consensus on the timing of repair for a completely lacerated nerve appears to be that early repair is ideal.[13] Nerve repairs are not done as acute emergencies or in the face of untidy wounds, however. We agree with Braun that whole nerve repairs should be done as urgent but elective cases.[2] The surgical team should be well rested, with experienced support personnel available, ap-

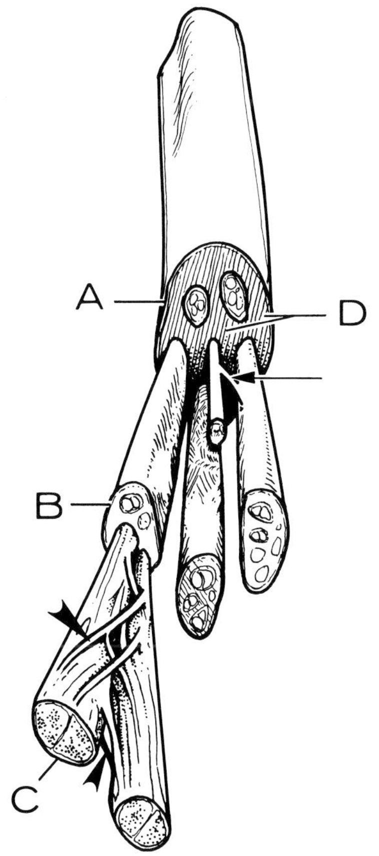

Figure 23–2. *Schematic drawing of a peripheral forearm nerve showing (**A**) the whole nerve, (**B**) the fascicular groups, (**C**) the fascicles, and (**D**) the external and internal epineurium. The thin arrow indicates the minimal connections between the fascicular groups, and the wide arrow shows the more numerous connections between the fascicles within each fascicular group.*

propriate microsurgical instruments ready, and the surgical microscope on hand.[20] In the case of a partial nerve laceration, early repair is perhaps even more important than in nerve repair following a complete laceration. Primary repair facilitates the dissection of the transected fascicular groups and their separation from intact groups.[7] In secondary repair, Edshage recommends nerve grafting.[7] Lovett also has emphasized the technical difficulty of partial nerve repair and the increased difficulty associated with delay. He recommends repair within 6 hours.[17]

In our study of partial nerve injuries, we obtained good results when repairs were done *within 2 months*. However, the data also suggest that increased intervals between injury and repair may negatively influence the result. The data revealed a trend toward better results in those nerves repaired early.[12] We agree with Edshage and Lovett that early repairs are technically easier. Unfortunately, some of our patients did not present at the time of injury. In the ideal situation we recommend repair within 7 days and prefer to do these repairs within 72 hours.

PREOPERATIVE EXAMINATION

The preoperative evaluation of the patient with a potential partial nerve laceration is important. Appropriate discussion of operative risks, prognosis, and surgical planning are definitely different when the surgeon expects a partial nerve injury. Therefore, a detailed preoperative history and examination are *mandatory* in all potential nerve injury cases. Historical factors such as patient age, occupation, hand dominance, type of trauma, and general medical condition are recorded. Proximal injury is distinguished from distal injury.

If the injury is acute and associated with tendon lacerations, then the preoperative motor examination may seem difficult, but a gentle, calm approach will usually allow the surgeon to decide which motors are functioning, which are transected, and which are denervated. For potential partial median nerve lacerations, an opponens muscle strength test is done. For potential partial ulnar lacerations, the first dorsal interosseous and the hypothenar muscles are tested. For the radial nerve, the digital extensors are examined. A light touch examination of the radial and ulnar side of each digit will provide an accurate assessment of the sensory losses.

If the patient's reporting appears uncertain, a more detailed examination of two-point discrimination on each side of each digit will help establish the true functional deficit. However, it is noted that, even distally, some partial nerve injuries leave gradations of sensory function. One finger may have normal two-point discrimination, one finger or side of a finger may have absent sensation, and one finger or side may have partial sensation.

INTRAOPERATIVE ELECTRODIAGNOSTIC EVALUATION

Acute partial nerve laceration is usually accurately assessed by preoperative physical examination, intraoperative palpation in secondary repairs, a knowledge of the internal topography of the nerve at the level of the laceration, and intraoperative microsurgical observation. We share Lundborg's view that the surgeon can use these skills to determine successfully which fascicular groups need neuroma excision and repair and which groups are intact.[19] In our recent study none of the preoperative clinically detectable functioning fascicular groups were damaged by this method of assessing the fascicular functional integrity.[12]

In late cases with an established lateral neuroma or a neuroma-in-continuity, intraoperative nerve conduction studies may be useful (see Chap. 42) (Fig. 23-3).[19,28,30,33,35] To use these techniques fully, appropriate equipment and technical support personnel must be available so that single fascicle recording and signal averaging techniques can be used.[28,33]

Even with this sophisticated approach, there is a potential disparity between the operative and clinical realities and the electrodiagnostic results.[1,5,6,8,9] When electrodiagnostic studies demonstrate function, a reliable operative decision to retain and neurolyse a particular fascicular group is made. However, the decision to resect and graft based on no detectable or measurable electrical response has a greater potential for error. Electro-

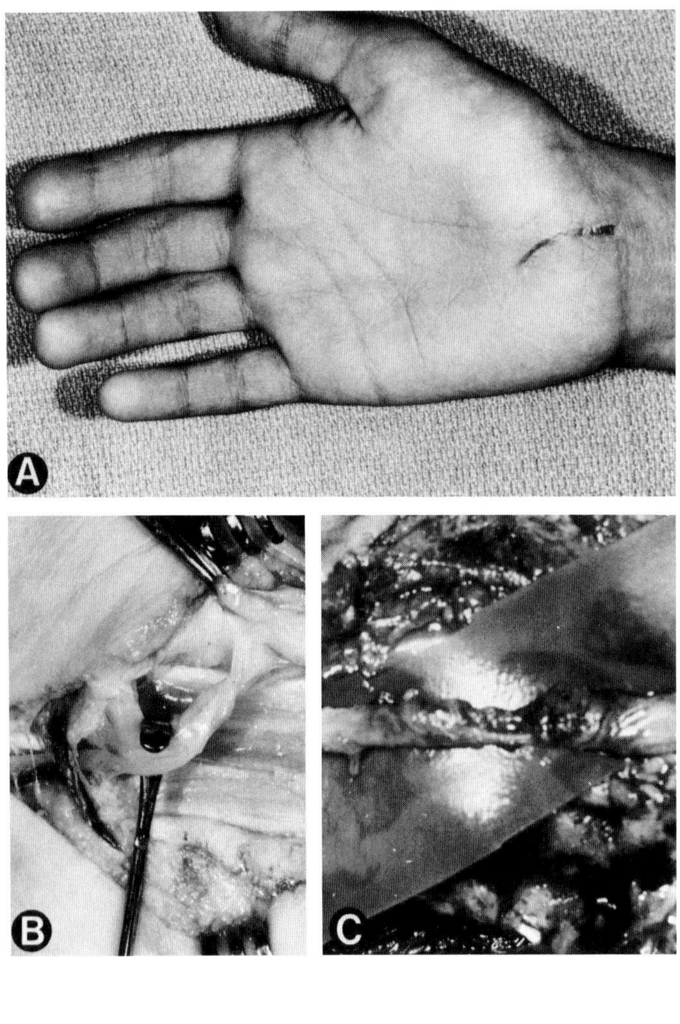

Figure 23–3. *(**A**) This patient presented 3 months after injury with a laceration of the median nerve. The preoperative sensory and motor examination was consistent with a complete laceration. (**B**) The distal nerve in loop retractor was found adherent to the transverse carpal ligament, and part of the proximal nerve in the hemostat was severely scarred into the wound. (**C**) After dissection, an epineural bridge and a few scarred fascicles were left intact. This is the ideal time for an operative electrodiagnostic study to confirm the nonfunctioning status of these fascicles and to support the decision to resect the neuroma-in-continuity and repair the whole nerve.*

diagnostic studies are more likely to produce false-positive results (no conduction in a nerve that can regain conductivity) than false-negative results (electrical conduction without impulse conduction). Nerve conduction studies cannot distinguish neurapraxia from axontomesis. Intraoperative electrodiagnostic tests also add operative time and often mandate an extended surgical dissection (see Chap. 10).[28,33]

TENSION AND REPAIR OF PARTIALLY TRANSECTED NERVES

Before explaining the individual technical options for repairing partial nerve lacerations, we will review the management of the more generic problem of tension (see Chap. 36). Tension on a nerve repair or partial nerve repair is poorly tolerated.[7,13,23,27,30] If a nerve is acutely elongated more than 15% of its resting length, intraneural blood flow is impeded.[18] However, extensive nerve dissection is tolerated if longitudinal vessels remain intact.[27] If a nerve or collection of fascicular groups is severely and suddenly stretched to overcome a significant defect, functional recovery is poor. Achieving end-to-end fibrous connection by excessive tension with large-diameter sutures to overcome gaps is not enough.[23,30]

Before deciding how to deal with a gap, it is appropriate to remember Steven's definition of gap.[27] As he points out, a *gap* occurs when a nerve is cut and the natural elasticity separates the ends. A *defect* occurs when a portion of the nerve is actually removed. The separate concepts of the physiological gap and the traumatic defect are important when managing partial nerve injuries. In many civilian, nonurban partial nerve injuries, the injury is a true sharp laceration with a gap and no defect (Fig. 23-4). This has an important implication for the potential success of the primary direct group fascicular repair of the isolated transected groups.

While opinion is unanimous that tension is to be avoided, there is little agreement regarding the management options for overcoming defects. In partial nerve injury, tension may be controlled completely by the intact fascicular groups adjacent to transected ones.[7] If tension is not overcome in this manner, then adjacent joints are flexed. Loop sutures temporarily control gaps or permanently control small defects without harming the functional result of repaired or intact fascicular groups.

How large should a gap or defect be before grafting is indicated? In the partial nerve injury there is no clinical or laboratory research data to form a scientific basis for an answer. In complete nerve transections in rats, Terzis showed poor results with acute stretch greater than 4 mm and in grafts longer than 6 mm.[30] In complete nerve lacerations Millesi recommended direct repair for defects of 1.5 to 2.0 cm and definite grafting for defects of 5.0 to 6.0 cm or greater. Further, Millesi states that grafting is debatably appropriate for defects in the 3- to 4-cm range (for more detail, see Chap. 36).[21]

TYPES OF OPERATIONS

Observation Alone

Seddon, Kline, and Sunderland have recommended observation alone when a late secondary repair was needed, when the laceration was very proximal, or when the laceration represented a very small portion of the nerve.[15,25,29] Without modern operating microscopes, Seddon concluded that separating normal fascicular groups from cut ones was difficult and potentially detrimental.[11,25,26] Today, this nonoperative approach may be indicated occasionally in patients who are not operative candidates for other medical reasons, or who have such small partial nerve injuries that symptoms are absent. The possibility of increased neuroma pain should be kept in mind whenever observation alone is the therapeutic choice.

Nerve Wrapping

The advantage of this approach, advocated by Hooper and Kuczynski, is that suture material is not required.[11] These surgeons hypothesize that suture and scar produce entrapment in intact fascicular groups. Although there is no clinical evidence to support this hypothesis, Kline has shown experimentally that scar in unrepaired fascicular groups damages intact fascicular groups in a mon-

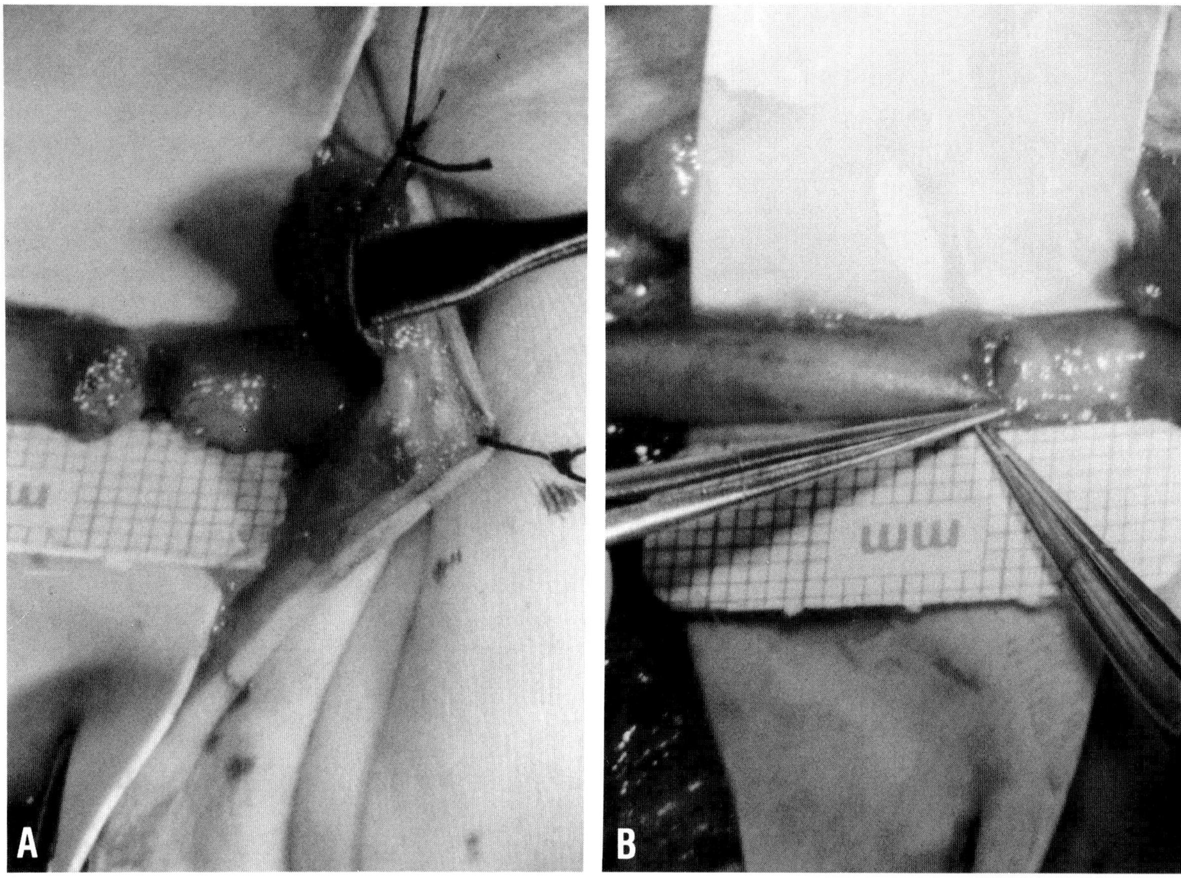

Figure 23–4. *(**A**) Note the 4-mm gap in this recent sharp partial laceration. This is a physiological gap but there is no traumatic defect in the nerve. (**B**) Note how easily the ends can be approximated.*

key model.[15,16] The clear disadvantage to nerve-wrapping technique is that it does not allow precise coaptation of transected fascicular groups and does not allow excision of individual traumatic fascicular neuromas. We have no experience with this technique, but Hooper and Kuczynski recommend Silastic sheath wrapping because they observed several nerves that were not repaired and resulted in no apparent deficits. However, they also add that late neurolysis and resection of neuroma may be needed.

Completion of Partial Nerve Injury Followed by Complete Nerve Repair

Seddon, Sunderland, and Kline have recommended resection of the entire injured area and whole nerve repair if more than 50% of the nerve is cut or if the intact portion was "functionally unimportant."[15,26,29] The advantage is that this technique does not require interfascicular dissection.

There are two obvious disadvantages to this approach. First, the intact fascicles are an important guide to the fascicular matching that is discarded when the laceration is completed. Second, what might seem functionally unimportant to the surgeon may be quite important to the patient. This is particularly true with distal lesions. Functional recovery after repair of complete nerve lacerations is not total. In our opinion, this approach to partial nerve injury is now rarely indicated, particularly if the patient demonstrates, on preoperative examination, only partial function of the damaged nerve. An exception may be the patient in whom preoperative examination shows no significant function but operative exploration shows some part of the nerve intact (see Fig. 23-3). In this situation transection and total nerve repair is indicated. In our opinion this approach is justified only if operative microscopy reveals that the intact part of the nerve is only epineurium or a few severely scarred fascicles or a hard fusiform neuroma-in-continuity involving the whole diameter of the nerve. Operative electrodiagnostic studies are helpful in this situation (see Chaps. 18, 19).

Repair of Transected Fascicular Groups

Direct end-to-end repair of the transected fascicular groups alone is usually possible following acute clean civilian partial nerve lacerations. Direct repair has the advantage that it involves only one repair site (as opposed to two with a nerve graft). Further, retained normal function in the intact fascicular groups is useful to the patient. Direct repair is most appropriate following acute injuries with minimal secondary scarring and with minimal retraction of the transected fascicular groups due to their natural elastic recoil. Another advantage of direct repair in early injuries is the ease of fascicular matching by using both the fascicular pattern and the internal and external epineural blood vessels.

One disadvantage is the theoretical consideration that the normal neuroma of repair may injure the intact portion of the lacerated nerve.[15,16] However, this has been shown not to be the case in our recent studies.[12] Another disadvantage is the fact that fascicular repairs of the transected portion require precise microsurgical techniques that often include gentle interfascicular dissection in both the proximal and distal stumps in order to separate the damaged from undamaged portions. Successful separation and precise identification require microsurgical experience, an operative microscope, and microsurgical instruments. The surgeon must be aware of the fascicular topography of the involved nerve at the level of the laceration.

The indication for a direct end-to-end repair is a partially lacerated nerve in a clean wound. The damaged fascicular groups involve a narrow, well-defined injury zone in which the proximal and distal portions are approximated without excessive tension. The gap tension is controllable by a single 10-0 suture connecting the damaged fascicular groups after appropriate control of tension by flexion of the adjacent joints and, if necessary, a temporary loop suture in the intact fascicular groups.[27]

The repair of transected fascicular groups is begun with the aid of loupe magnification. The traumatic wounds are extended proximally and distally. Once the nerve laceration is identified, the dissection is continued with the operative microscope and microsurgical instruments. In cases done within a week, the junction between transected fascicular groups and intact fascicular groups is easily determined at the level of laceration (Fig. 23-5*A*). The proximal lacerated fascicular groups should be separated as a unit from the intact groups by dissecting the internal epineural planes (Fig. 23-5*B*). An identical dissection is then done distally. The vessels on the external and internal epineurium are preserved and used to guide the dissection. For injuries seen after 1 week, the dissection is begun 1 to 2 cm proximal to the laceration. The external epineurium is opened, and the interval between the lacerated and intact fascicular groups is enlarged. The fascicular groups are then dissected as a unit into the early neuroma. The distal fascicular groups are similarly dissected in a distal-to-proximal direction into the glioma. These dissections also define the intact distal fascicular groups. In some very early cases with only a few fascicular groups cut (80% intact) or with only a few fascicular groups uncut (80% transected), wide separation of the cut from the intact groups is unnecessary.

Next, tension between the cut ends of the fascicular groups is assessed. In some cases wrist flexion overcomes all or part of the tension. If needed, the remaining tension is controlled by a loop in the intact fascicular groups, which is held with a single strand of 8-0 nylon in the external epineurium (see Fig. 23-5*B*). This makes approximation of the cut fascicular groups easy. Prior to repair, the proximal 2- to 5-mm neuroma and the distal 2- to 5-mm glioma are resected. The resultant true defect is usually less than 1 cm, although the functional gap may appear slightly larger due to fascicular elasticity.[7] In some immediate sharp partial lacerations, no resection of nerve tissue is required.

Next, fascicular matching is done by comparing distal and proximal fascicular size and orientation and by observing the epineural vessels. The rotational alignment is determined by examining the connections between the lacerated fascicular groups and the intact fascicular groups. The repair is done using 10-0 nylon external epineural sutures and an occasional internal 10-0 epineural suture (see Fig. 23-5*B*,*C*). In most cases the 8-0 loop suture is removed after repair (see Fig. 23-5*C*).[12,36] Occasionally, partial nerve injury is represented by a very small clean epineural laceration (Fig. 23-6). In this case, insertion of one or two 10-0 nylon sutures in the epineurium is all that is needed.

Postoperative management includes flexion of adjacent joints for 4 weeks in a long arm cast. From

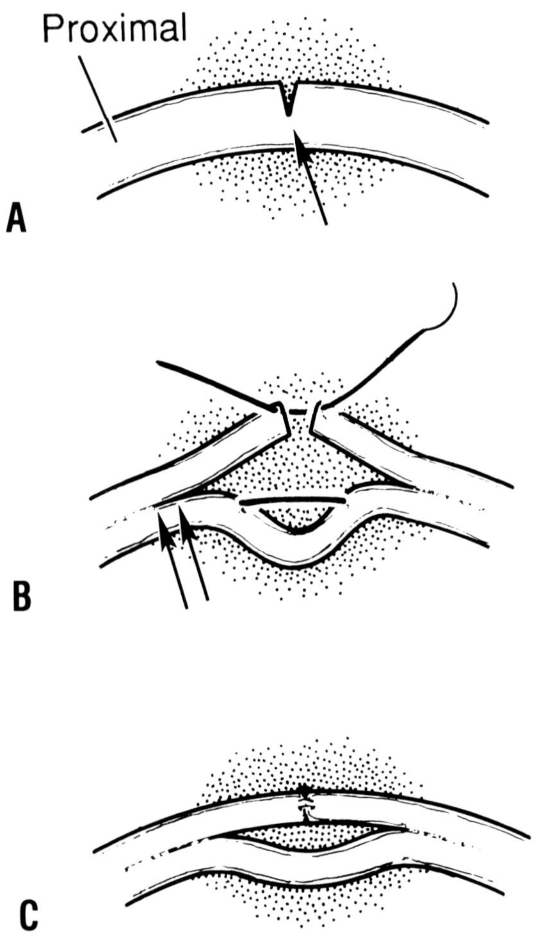

Figure 23–5. (***A***) *A 50% laceration is shown. In early cases the dissection begins at the arrow.* (***B***) *Once the proximal and distal fascicular groups are dissected, a temporary loop suture is placed to control tension and 10-0 nylon is used to repair the nerve. In late cases dissection starts at the double arrow.* (***C***) *After repair the loop is removed.*

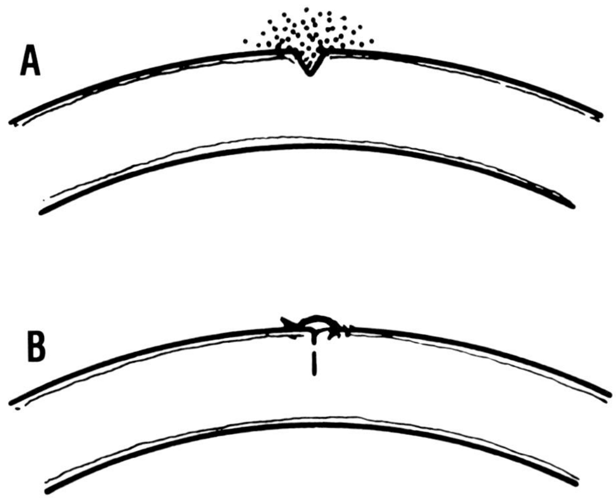

Figure 23–6. (***A***) *Small epineural injury.* (***B***) *Injury repaired with single simple 10-0 suture.*

4 to 6 weeks the wrist and fingers are held in neutral position with no passive or active wrist extension exercises, but splints are designed that allow wrist flexion and free finger motion. The postoperative management is altered depending on the nature and extent of associated injuries and the reliability of the patient.

Nerve Grafting of Transected Fascicular Groups

Most civilian partial nerve lacerations are managed by direct fascicular repair with or without tension-relieving temporary loop sutures. However, those injuries complicated by extensive partial nerve defects, such as those associated with gunshot wounds, require nerve grafting. In addition, some chronic or late partial nerve transections repaired secondarily have excessive scarring and fascicular retraction. These too require nerve grafting. The obvious advantage of nerve grafting is that it allows spanning of larger defects and placement of regenerating axonal graft conduits in nonscarred, well-vascularized beds.

Opinions vary on the size of defects requiring nerve grafts following complete nerve injuries. Millesi uses a nerve graft for a complete lesion with a defect of 4 cm or greater and sometimes for a defect as small as 2 cm.[21,22] He does not use joint flexion to approximate the ends and uses only limited nerve mobilization. For most surgeons, the critical defect to manage with nerve graft is *4 cm or larger.*[23,27,30] Nerve grafting of larger defects has the advantage of leaving the undamaged fascicular groups intact, hence preserving their maximum function. Despite this, several animal experiments have demonstrated inferior results with grafting when the results of grafting are compared to end-to-end repair without tension.[27,30] In the laboratory, Miyamoto has shown that nerve repair under tension of more than 25 g disrupts blood flow and gives a result inferior to grafting.[23] With grafting under ideal conditions, Millesi and others had clinical results that approximated results seen after end-to-end repair.[21]

The disadvantages of nerve grafting include difficulty with nerve regeneration across two suture sites and need for a donor site with its associated morbidity. In animal studies, Stevens showed that repairs using nerve grafts have significantly slower conduction velocities than those performed without grafts.[27] Miyamoto demonstrated delay in axon regeneration with use of nerve grafts, although at 10 months following repair, the number of regenerating axons was comparable to those with end-to-end repair.

The operative technique for grafting of nerves partially injured is similar to that used for direct repair.[4] First, the zone of injury is defined with the operative microscope (Fig. 23-7*A*). The dissection is begun at the corners of the rectangle outlined by the dotted line. The damaged tissues are debrided. The transected but usable fascicular groups are separated from the intact fascicular groups, both proximal and distally (Fig. 23-7*B*). The defect size is measured and a suitable nerve graft or grafts are obtained (see Fig. 23-7*B*). The sural nerve is used (see Chap. 38). The graft or grafts are sutured in place with a minimal number of 10-0 nylon sutures. A separation between each of the grafts and between the grafts and intact fascicular groups is maintained (Fig. 23-7*C*).

Postoperative management following nerve grafting of partial nerve injuries is identical to that used for direct repair except for appropriate additional care of the donor site.

For additional information on nerve grafting, the reader is referred to the works of Millesi and Wood,[21,22,36] and to Chapters 36 through 41.

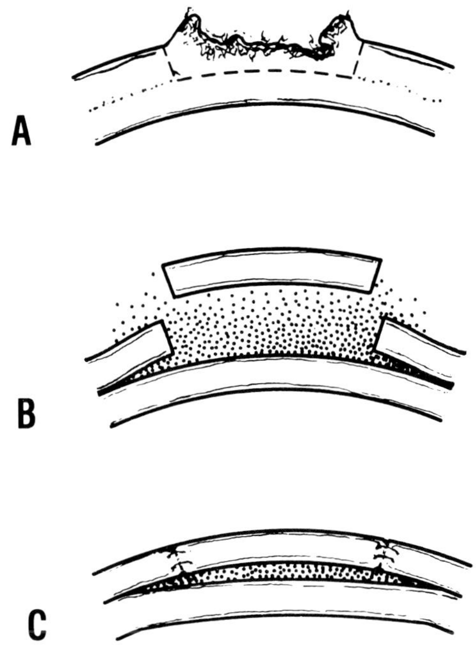

Figure 23–7. *(**A**) First the damaged section is removed (dotted line). (**B**) The true defect is measured, and an appropriate-sized graft is harvested. (**C**) The graft is sutured with a minimal number of 10-0 nylon sutures.*

Author's Preferred Method

Observation alone is appropriate only if the patient lacks symptoms or is nonoperable for other medical or psychiatric reasons. We do not use nerve-wrapping techniques. The work of De Medinacelli may add this to our armamentarium in the future, but his repair technique is still experimental.[5,32] We complete the laceration and repair the entire nerve only if the intact portion consists of epineurium alone or the remaining epineurium and fascicles are totally scarred and nonfunctional according to both the preoperative examination, operative microscopic examination, or intraoperative electrodiagnostic assessment.

Most partial nerve injuries present as acute partial lacerations secondary to glass or knife injuries. The true defect is usually tiny or nonexistent, and direct repair of the cut fascicular groups only, with or without a temporary loop suture, is accomplished directly. The microneural iris scissors are helpful for interfascicular dissections needed with this technique.

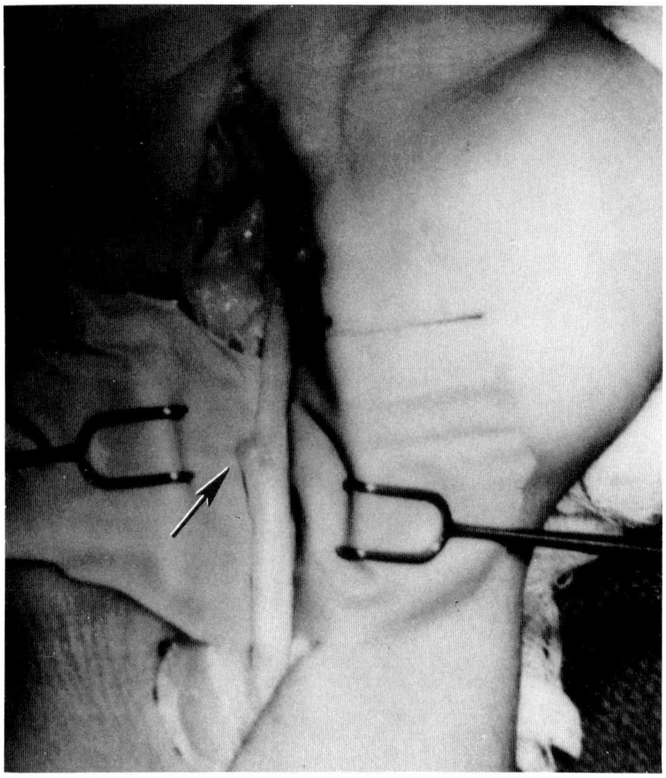

Figure 23–8. *Chronic painful lateral neuroma (arrow) from an unrepaired partial nerve laceration. Successfully treated by resection and end-to-end secondary repair of the lacerated fascicular groups.*

Nerve grafting is recommended in the repair of partial nerve lacerations only for large true defects (greater than 3 cm). These injuries usually result from severe trauma or from injuries seen late.

POSTOPERATIVE COMPLICATIONS

Potential complications after repair of partial nerve injury include infection, failure to recover adequate function, loss of function in the originally intact fascicular groups, and painful neuromas. In our recent study of 12 partial median and ulnar nerve transections, we had only one complication, when a patient removed the cast prematurely and disrupted the repair; resuture was partially successful. Our overall results were good, according to Moberg's rating system of excellent, good, fair, and poor. According to the British Medical Research Council rating, motor values averaged 4.0 (M = 5.0 [normal]) and sensory values 3.81 (S = 4.0 [normal]) (see Chap. 25).[24] Further, there was no sign of functional deterioration of originally intact fascicular groups.

While we have not experienced postoperative infection with this procedure, management includes wound culture and sensitivity studies, irrigation and debridement, and appropriate intravenous antibiotic therapy before further reconstructive nerve surgery is attempted.

Painful postoperative lateral neuromas (Fig. 23-8) are treated by reoperation with direct repair after resection, or by grafting of disrupted fascicular groups.

REFERENCES

1. Ballantyne J, Campbell M. Electrophysiological study after surgical repair of sectioned human peripheral nerves. J Neurol Neurosurg Psychiatry 1973; 36:797–805.
2. Braun R. Epineural nerve repair. In: Omer G, Spinner M, eds. Management of peripheral nerve problems. Philadelphia: WB Saunders, 1980:366–379.
3. Chow J, Sunderland S, Van Beek A, et al. Surgical significance of the motor fascicular group of the ul-

nar nerve in the forearm (abstract). J Hand Surg [Am] 1984; 9:605.
4. Daniel R, Terzis J. Reconstructive microsurgery. Boston: Little, Brown, 1977:387–429.
5. De Medinacelli L, Seaber A. Experimental nerve reconnection: Importance of initial repair. Microsurg 1989; 10:56–70.
6. Dennis M, Miledi R. Lack of correspondence between the amplitudes of spontaneous potentials and unit potentials evoked by nerve impulses at regenerating neuromuscular junctions. Nature 1971; 232: 126–128.
7. Edshage S. In: Jewett D, McCarroll H, eds. Nerve repair and regeneration: Its clinical and experimental basis. St. Louis: CV Mosby, 1980:279–283.
8. Goldberg N, Deshpande S, May C, et al. Disparity between neurophysiologic measurements and clinical reality following peripheral nerve transection and microneurorrhaphy. Surg Forum 1984; 35: 608–610.
9. Grace P, Augustine S, Lynch G. Immediate return of nerve function following microsurgical repair. Br J Plast Surg 1989; 42:212–215.
10. Gunther S, DiPasquale D, Martin R. Internal anatomy of the median nerve in the region of the elbow. Seattle: ASSH, 1989:3–16.
11. Hooper G, Kuczynski K. Nerve injuries. In: Lamb D, Hooper G, Kuczynski K, eds. The practice of hand surgery. Oxford: Blackwell, 1989:196–217.
12. Hurst L, Dowd A, Sampson S, Badalamente M. Partial lacerations of median and ulnar nerves. J Hand Surg [Am] 1990; 15:in press.
13. Jabaley M. Technical aspects of nerve repair. J Hand Surg [Br] 1984; 9:14–19.
14. Jabaley ME, Wallace W, Heckler F. Internal topography of major nerves of the forearm and hand: A current view. J Hand Surg 1980; 5:1–18.
15. Kline D. Evaluation of the neuroma-in-continuity. In: Omer G, Spinner M, eds. Management of peripheral nerve problems. Philadelphia: WB Saunders, 1980:451–461.
16. Kline D, Hackett E, May PR. Partial nerve laceration evaluated by evoked potentials. J Surg Res 1970; 10:81–90.
17. Lovett W, McCalla M. Nerve injuries: Management and rehabilitation. Orthop Clin North Am 1983; 14: 767–778.
18. Lundborg G. Structure and function of the intraneural microvessels as related to trauma, edema formation, and nerve function. J Bone Joint Surg [Am] 1975; 57:938.
19. Lundborg G. Nerve injury and repair. Edinburgh: Churchill-Livingstone, 1988:197–213.
20. Mackinnon S, Dellon A. Surgery of the peripheral nerve. New York: Thieme, 1988:115–129.
21. Millesi H. The current state of peripheral nerve surgery in the upper limb. Ann Chir Main 1984; 3: 18–34.
22. Millesi H. The nerve gap: Theory and clinical practice. Hand Clinics 1986; 2:651–664.
23. Miyamoto Y. Experimental study of results of nerve suture under tension vs. nerve grafting. Plast Reconstr Surg 1979; 64:540–549.
24. Omer G. The evaluation of clinical results following peripheral nerve suture. In: Omer G, Spinner M, eds. Management of peripheral nerve problems. Philadelphia: WB Saunders, 1980:431–442.
25. Seddon H. Surgical disorders of the peripheral nerves, ed 2. Edinburgh: Churchill-Livingstone, 1975:276–280.
26. Seddon H, Riddoch G. Peripheral nerve injuries: (i) Surgery of the peripheral nerves. In: History of the Second World War. London: Her Majesty's Stationery Office, 1953:517–533.
27. Stevens W, Hall J, Young V, Weeks P. When should nerve gaps be grafted? An experimental study in rats. Plast Reconstr Surg 1985; 75:707–713.
28. Stewart J. Electrodiagnostic techniques in the evaluation of nerve compression and injuries in the upper limb. Hand Clinics 1986; 2:677–688.
29. Sunderland S. Nerve and nerve injuries, ed 2. Edinburgh: Churchill-Livingstone, 1978:36, 140, 190, 206–208, 470, 489, 522–524, 629.
30. Terzis J, Faibisoff B, Williams H. The nerve gap: Suture under tension vs. graft. Plast Reconstr Surg 1975; 56:166–170.
31. Terzis J, Feeker B, Sismour E. A computerized study of the intraneural organization of the median nerve (abstract). J Hand Surg [Am] 1984; 9:605.
32. Terzis J, Smith K. Repair of severed peripheral nerves: Comparison of the "de Medinacelli" and standard microsuture methods. Exp Neurol 1987; 96:681–691.
33. Van Beek A. Electrodiagnostic evaluation of peripheral nerve injuries. Hand Clin 1986; 2:747–760.
34. Williams H, Jabaley M. The importance of internal anatomy of the peripheral nerves to nerve repair in the forearm and hand. Hand Clin 1986; 2:689–707.
35. Williams H, Terzis J. Single fascicular recordings: An intraoperative diagnostic tool for the management of peripheral nerve lesions. Plast Reconstr Surg 1976; 57:562–569.
36. Wood M. Nerve repair and reconstruction. In: Wood M, ed. Atlas of reconstructive microsurgery. Rockville, MD: Aspen, 1990:13–36.

VI

APPLIED ANATOMY, OPERATIVE EXPOSURE, RESULTS OF REPAIR

24 Factors Affecting the Results of Peripheral Nerve Repair

25 Median Nerve: Applied Anatomy and Operative Exposure

26 Median Nerve Repairs: The Results of Treatment

27 Radial Nerve: Applied Anatomy and Operative Exposure

28 Radial Nerve—Results

29 Ulnar Nerve: Applied Anatomy and Operative Exposure

30 Ulnar Nerve Repair

31 Axillary Nerve

32 Spinal Accessory Nerve

33 Digital Nerves

34 Facial Nerve Paralysis

35 Peripheral Nerve Injuries to the Lower Extremity

24

Factors Affecting the Results of Peripheral Nerve Repair

David R. Steinberg
L. Andrew Koman

AUTHORS' KEY POINTS

- Nerve repair has the best potential for achieving recovery in children less than 10 years of age.
- The functional results of neurorrhaphy become less satisfactory as the time between injury and repair increases . Clinically, 6 months represents a delay that significantly limits recovery.
- The level of injury has a significant effect on the results of nerve repair.
- In order to appreciate maximal nerve recovery, children are followed for at least 2 years and adults for 5 years after neurorrhaphy.

Despite advances in hand surgery and medical care, it remains difficult to predict functional recovery after peripheral nerve repair. The focus of this chapter is a description and analysis of factors that significantly affect the results of nerve repair. Those most often discussed are patient age, elapsed time interval from injury to repair, level of injury (proximal vs distal), mechanism of injury (crush/avulsion vs sharp), specific nerve injured (eg, median vs radial, tibial vs peroneal), type of nerve injured (pure motor vs pure sensory vs mixed), and time between injury and clinical evaluation. Other important factors have been described in other chapters, including pain (Chaps. 100 through 105), the effect of associated vascular injuries (Chap. 47), defect size (Chap. 36), nerve graft vs primary repair (Chaps. 26, 28, 30, 35, 39), repair site tension (Chap. 36), and technical factors, including magnification, suture size, and suture technique (Chaps. 17 through 22, 33), alignment techniques (Chaps. 14 through 16), and suture methods (Chaps. 18 through 20).

ANALYSIS OF EXISTING DATA

Presenting a concise, complete evaluation of the results of neurorrhaphy is difficult. In order to obtain a sufficient number of cases for analysis, results from many centers and surgeons, based on different objective and subjective criteria, must be pooled and analyzed retrospectively. Some of the largest series in the literature, on which many of our present perceptions are founded, deal with wartime injuries, repair techniques that by today's standards are suboptimal, and variable evaluation parameters. Conclusions based on these results therefore are primarily observational and represent documented information from suboptimal and technically imprecise studies.

Various authors have used different classification schemes for reporting "successful" results of neurorrhaphy. Those using Highet and Sanders' criteria have been inconsistent concerning the stage used to define functional recovery.[41] In this chapter we use Dellon's modification of this system to discuss sensory recovery because it incorporates static two-point discrimination (see Table 39-2).[23] For the purpose of the following analysis, functional recovery includes those patients rated S3 or better (two-point discrimination <20 mm). Functional motor return denotes values of M3 or greater in the upper extremity (see Table 39-1).

FACTORS INFLUENCING FUNCTIONAL RECOVERY

Factors affecting the quality of nerve recovery are evaluated in terms of the following:

1. Host anatomy and function
2. Pathophysiologic consequences of the injury
3. Operative repair process
4. Physiologic events associated with recovery.

Host Anatomy and Physiology

Age

The prognosis for functional nerve recovery after repair is best in the very young.[1,31,53,59,78,91,95,112] Teenagers and young adults obtain poorer results than children, but their prognosis for neural recovery is better than in the rest of the adult population.[59,75,78,81,84,91,102]

In the first large series of civilian nerve repairs published after World War II, children under age 10 were noted to have "sensory recovery . . . adequate in all, and in only one case was motor recovery defective."[73] This contrasted with the series' adult population, which exhibited functional motor and sensory recoveries in less than 70% of cases. Subsequent reports over the next 30 years have confirmed the excellent recovery potential in young children, with good to excellent results in more than 90% of cases.[31,53,59,78,91,95,112] In patients between the ages of 10 and 20 years, good to excellent motor and sensory recovery can be expected in over 75% of cases.[1,43,56,59,61,63,78,81,84,91,102,112]

In a classic paper, Lars Önne evaluated 91 distal nerve repairs followed for 4 to 5 years.[78] In this group, two-point discrimination in millimeters was approximately equal to the age of the patient in years up to 20 years and deteriorated thereafter, although digital nerve repairs recovered functional two-point discrimination (less than 21 mm) in patients up to age 50. A linear relationship between age and two-point discrimination in patients under 20 years has also been described more recently.[1,59]

In addition to achieving better results, children also appear to recover more quickly. These young patients achieve normal or near-normal motor and sensory function in distal nerve injuries by 2 years post-repair, whereas adults may take as long as 5 years to obtain their optimum results.[31,95]

Clinical results in the adult population show no significant correlation with age. While specific values vary for different nerves in various series, motor and sensory recovery to a functional level can be expected in 50% to 70% of adults between ages 20 and 50.[31,33,43,53,59,63,73,91] Prognosis for complete recovery in adults is more optimistic today than in the past: previous studies often reported residual sensory defects in almost all adults after nerve injury.[53,95] Recent series are more encouraging, with approximately 25% of adult patients attaining near-premorbid sensory and motor function.[16,59,96,105,112]

No conclusions can be drawn regarding recovery after neurorrhaphy in the population over 50, as the numbers are very small. Most reports indicate a poor prognosis, although anecdotal evidence of good results can be found in the literature.[23,58,60] Seddon noted that in 24 patients older than 50 years with upper extremity nerve repairs, 58% achieved fair and 21% poor results.[91] Mailander and coworkers described 60% patients over the age of 50 who had no measurable two-point discrimination at 2 years after distal nerve repair.[59]

There are a number of possible explanations for age-related neural recovery. It may be related to inherent physiologic factors (eg, increased neural regeneration rates), the length of extremities, or increased adaptability and capacity for re-education in the young.

Gutmann and associates sectioned and repaired sciatic nerves in rabbits and found that the young animals, compared with mature ones, exhibited decreased latencies at the suture line and a more rapid return of muscle function.[36,38,39] They could not demonstrate any differences in sensory return in the two age groups as measured by the pinch test. This would indicate either the presence of differential rates of motor and sensory axonal regeneration in the two age groups, or increased rates of recovery at the suture line and motor end-organs in the young, with no difference in axonal growth. In another experiment, young rats demonstrated more rapid axonal transport of radioactively labeled proteins in a regenerating crushed sciatic nerve model.[4]

A similar age difference in peripheral nerve regeneration, however, was not observed in a primate model.[2] The median nerves of adult and baby monkeys were transected and repaired and subsequently evaluated 3 years postoperatively. In both groups of animals, sensory conduction velocities were 25 m/sec in the repaired nerves and 39 m/sec in contralateral control nerves. Histologically, there was no difference in the total number of axons in either age group or in control vs repaired nerves. While the repaired nerves demonstrated decreased myelination compared with controls, there were no age-related myelin differences. These findings supported clinical observations in 19 repaired human median and ulnar nerves studied electrophysiologically more than 5 years postoperatively.[1] The repaired nerves had slower nerve conduction velocities and required a greater stimulus than uninjured nerves, yet there was no correlation with patients' ages (which ranged from 10 to 35 years at the time of the study). Those patients under 14 years at the time of neurorrhaphy demonstrated significantly improved two-point discrimination; however, no correlation between nerve conduction velocity or stimulus intensity and two-point discrimination could be found.

These observations indicate that age-related differences after nerve repair are due, at least in part, to changes occurring centrally rather than in the periphery. This capacity for cortical reorganization of the somatosensory homunculus has been described in primates and other mammals.[48,66–68] In a series of experiments, monkeys underwent median nerve sectioning, digital amputation, and restricted use of portions of the hand. Mapping of the somatosensory cortex immediately and at 2 to 9 months post-intervention revealed changes in the area originally receiving input from the altered peripheral receptors. For example, 9 months after median nerve transection, cortical regions previously representing median nerve responded to stimuli from ulnar- and radial-innervated skin. This phenomenon is age-dependent, with younger animals demonstrating enhanced capacities for cortical reorganization after spinal and peripheral nerve injury.[49,62]

Congenital/Genetic Factors

Scientific evidence is insufficient to make definitive statements regarding any genetic factors that affect nerve recovery following neurorrhaphy. However, the quality of functional nerve recovery may prove to be related to genetically controlled physiologic capabilities. Genetic control of neural degeneration distal to the injury or axonal regrowth is not understood but is theoretically important. "Physiologic adaptability" and vasomotor, thermoregulatory, and sudomotor control, all predetermined by genetic factors, may contribute to the quality of functional recovery.[78] Factors that may be controlled genetically in part include the regenerative power of neurons; central factors that may affect myelination, axonal budding, and branching; and potential myoneural end-plate recovery.[100]

Type of Nerve

The type of nerve injured (ie, pure motor, pure sensory, sudomotor, or mixed) has some bearing on outcome. Repair of a "pure" motor or sensory nerve will lead to better results than mixed nerves, due to a decreased chance of fascicular mismatching (sensory axons growing into motor endoneural tubes and vice versa). The specific prognosis for motor vs sensory recovery is more controversial. A number of studies report essentially equal motor and sensory recovery after neurorrhaphy.[73,75,91] Some of this may be artifactual, however, secondary to the methods of reporting results in these series, rather than a true reflection of equal recovery capabilities.

Another group of clinical reports indicates that sensory function recovers to a greater degree than motor function. Functional recovery to S3 in ulnar nerve repair was 10% to 25% higher than M3 recovery in distal lesions and 15% to 44% higher in proximal lesions.[53,56,59,61,63,73,84,113] Such a comparison is less remarkable in median nerve injuries, in which four series demonstrated approximately 10% better sensory than motor recovery in both distal and proximal lesions.[53,61,113]

A few reports recorded greater motor than sensory recovery.[44,56,105,111] One of these concerns the large United States World War II experience with median and ulnar nerve injuries; the discrepancy is so different from all other series that one questions the validity of the figures provided.[111]

Experimental data can be found to support any of the above clinical observations. Changes occurring in the neuron after axonal injury occur more rapidly, and to a greater degree, in sensory than in motor cells, and sensory fibers degenerate earlier and more rapidly than motor fibers.[100] Some of the differences seen between motor and sensory recovery may be related to reinnervation of respective end-organs. Muscle and motor end-plates undergo irreversible changes after 2 to 3 years, after which reinnervation will be ineffective.[10,99] Sensory receptors may be successfully reinnervated after denervation periods greater than 1 year, although the maximum time over which this may occur is unclear (see Timing of Repair, below).[85] That denervated mechanoreceptors can be reinnervated has been shown experimentally and clinically.[22,45] Denervated sensory nerve endings may be compensated by overlap of already present adjacent nerve fibers and by new ingrowth of neighboring fibers.[38,43,54,107] Cortical reorganization, as discussed previously, could also play a role in enhanced recovery of sensory compared to motor function.

Regeneration of sympathetic fibers after neurorrhaphy was thought to be important for vasomotor control and for optimal sensory recovery. Normal sweating patterns and ninhydrin tests have been observed after nerve repairs at 2 years in children and 5 years in adults.[95] Nevertheless, no correlation between the results of two-point discrimination and the pick-up test and sudomotor recovery has been demonstrated.[63,78,95]

Specific Nerve Involved

The specific peripheral nerve involved affects functional recovery. For example, radial nerve injuries are more likely to have functional motor return in the forearm than median or ulnar nerve lesions of similar levels.[76] As discussed above, if all other factors are comparable, a mixed motor-sensory nerve (eg, ulnar) demonstrates inferior recovery compared to a primarily motor (eg, radial) or sensory (eg, digital) nerve.

In the major nerves of the upper extremity, radial nerves have a reputation for the best recovery, followed by median and ulnar nerves. In a series of 917 wartime injuries, spontaneous recovery was observed in 73% of radial, 71% of median, 69% of ulnar, and 54% of musculocutaneous nerves.[75] While the exact numbers are not identical, similar patterns of recovery have been reported after neurorrhaphy.

A review of results in the literature on digital nerve repairs is gratifying; there are a large number of cases that use modern techniques and reporting methods. Such is not the case for radial, musculocutaneous, tibial, and peroneal nerves; there are few reports, and most of these are based on World War II experience. While there are more cases of median and ulnar nerve repairs, fewer have been reported in the recent literature, perhaps in part due to poor patient follow-up. In discussing general prognosis for recovery of digital, median, and ulnar nerves, only civilian studies published after 1972 will be evaluated. All of these use currently accepted operative techniques, and most present data in sufficient detail to allow meaningful discussion of functional results. Due to the paucity of information on the other major peripheral nerves, all reports since World War II will be used, although caution must be taken when applying these results to modern practice (Tables 24-1 through 24-4). Only results of distal medial and ulnar nerve lesions

Table 24–1. *Results of Digital Nerve Repair*

Author	Number in Study	Ages (yr)	Children (%)*	Avg F/U (mo)	S2 (%)	S2+ (%)	S3 (%)	S3+ (%)	S4 (%)
Buncke, 1972[16]	18	–	6	–	←	11	→	28	61
Ito et al, 1976[44]	16	2–68		48	←	12	→	88	→
Poppen et al, 1979[81]	26	6–19	100	106	0	4	0	58	38
	48	20–67	0	106	0	38	15	42	4
Young et al, 1981[112]	9	2–19	100	10	0	0	0	22	78
	23	20–67	0	10	0	0	34	44	22
Sullivan, 1985[96]	42	20–65	0	6–12	0	0	26	50	24
Tupper, 1988[105]	109	16–70	0	30	0	17	→	48	35
Mailander et al, 1989[59]	107		8	24	1	8	20	48	23
AVERAGE	401	2–70	11	40	0	8	16	48	27
Adults†	366	20–70	2		0	8	19	48	25
Children	35	2–19	100	58	0	3	0	40	58

* *Variously defined as <10–20 years old.*
† *A few children are unavoidably included as they were not differentiated from adults in the original reports.*

are included. Differences in distal and proximal lesions are discussed in Level of Injury, below.

Digital Nerve

Of 401 cases followed for an average of 2 years (6–48 months), 91% achieved functional sensory recovery (S3 or better). Seventy-five percent attained two-point discrimination of 15 mm or less. Patients under age 20 years recovered normal two-point discrimination (≤6 mm) in 58% of cases, compared with 26% of adults (Table 24-1).

Median Nerve

Of 58 civilian cases after 1972, 91% achieved functional motor recovery, with 27% having normal muscle function. Seventy-nine percent obtained functional sensory recovery; normal two-point discrimination was noted in 41% (Table

Table 24–2. *Results of Distal Median Nerve Repair*

Author	Number in Study	Ages (yr)	Children (%)	Avg F/U (mo)	S2+ (%)	S3 (%)	S3+ (%)	S4 (%)	M2 (%)	M3 (%)	M4 (%)	M5 (%)
Ito et al, 1976[44]	8	2–68	–	48	12	25	12	25	0	38	0	38
McManamny, 1983[63]	6	0–16	100	–	0	0	17	83	0	16	33	33
	14	17–50	0	–	14	→	57	29	7	21	57	14
Tupper, 1988[105]	13	18–53	0	45	54	→	36	10	23	0	77	→
Mailander et al, 1989[59]	10	–	–	24	20	10	10	40	0	10	60	30
Tajima, Imai, 1989[102]	7	1–13	100	56	0	0	43	57	–	–	–	–
AVERAGE	58	0–50	21	42	17	8	30	41	7	16	48	27
Adults	45	16–50	0	40	27	6	32	33	9	16	53	18
Children	13	0–16	100	56	0	0	30	70	0	16	33	33

Table 24–3. Results of Distal Ulnar Nerve Repair

Author	Number in Study	Ages (yr)	Children (%)	Avg F/U (mo)	S2+ (%)	S3 (%)	S3+ (%)	S4 (%)	M2 (%)	M3 (%)	M4 (%)	M5 (%)
Ito et al, 1976[44]	14	2–68	–	48	21	29	14	21	28	14	29	21
McManamny, 1983[63]	5	0–16	100	–	0	0	20	80	0	40	60	0
	10	17–50	0	–	20	→	70	10	20	40	0	10
Tupper, 1988[105]	9	16–62	0	50	67	→	22	22	22	11	44	→
Mailander et al, 1989[59]	10	–	–	24	0	20	0	60	10	30	40	10
AVERAGE	48	2–68	12	41	23	12	25	34	18	25	32	10

24-2). The high percentage of motor recovery may be misleading, as at least 38% of patients with distal median nerve injuries have sufficient ulnar innervation of the thenar muscles to have functional opposition of the thumb.[83]

Ulnar Nerve

Of 48 patients, 67% acquired functional motor recovery of M3 or better. Seventy-one percent registered S3 or better sensory return (Table 24-3). Evaluating intrinsic recovery, Gaul found that average key pinch in children reached 86% of normal by 2 years, whereas it required 5 years for adults to attain 82% of normal pinch.[31]

Radial Nerve

In 100 transections in the civilian population, 76% achieved useful motor function. Adding the British World War II experience,[113] functional results of 214 patients decreased to 68%. Mixed radial nerve injuries (proximal) resulted in 65% functional sensory recovery after repair, compared with a 72% return in pure radial sensory nerve repairs in civilians (Table 24-4).

Musculocutaneous Nerve

In a very small number of patients, 88% obtained M4 or better and 100% noted functional motor recovery.

Table 24–4. Results of Radial Nerve Repair

Author	Number in Study	Level	S2 (%)	S2+ (%)	S3 (%)	S3+ (%)	S4 (%)	M2 (%)	M3 (%)	M4 (%)	M5 (%)
Larsen, 1958[53]	17	high	←	35	→	59	0	6	←	76	→
	6	low*	←	17	→	83	0	–	–	–	–
Sakellarides, 1962[84]	13	all	–	–	–	–	–	23	39	15	0
Seddon, 1975[91]	63	high	–	–	–	–	–	8	24	54	0
Ito et al, 1976[44]	5	all	20	0	40	0	20	0	0	20	80
Mailander et al, 1989[59]	2	high	50	0	0	0	0	0	0	100	0
	5	low*	0	40	40	0	20	–	–	–	–
AVERAGE	111†	all	6	26	11	43	11	9	21	52	4
	11	low*	0	40	40	0	20	–	–	–	–

* N = 100, motor evaluation; N = 35, sensory evaluation
† Dorsal radial sensory nerve

Lower Extremity Nerves

The incidence of significant injury to the nerves of the lower extremity is extremely low when compared to that of the upper extremity (see Chap. 35). The definition of useful recovery is slightly different in the lower extremity: a sensory level of S2 (autonomous sensibility) and motor level of M1(4) (proximal muscle contractions against some resistance) result in a functional leg.[20] Functional motor recovery in the tibial nerve averaged 64% in two large wartime series, with 37% useful sensory recovery.[20,113] Peroneal nerves regained useful motor function in only 15% of repairs, although 69% resulted in useful sensory return. Ito reported satisfactory sensory function in seven repairs of lower extremity nerves, with only 28% achieving "good" motor return.[44] A good functional result after lower extremity nerve repair has been defined as the ability to walk 1 mile, with or without an orthosis, with minimal pain and no evidence of trophic ulcers.[21,113] Little correlation has been found when relating good function with objective ratings. Clawson and Seddon noted that 70% of sciatic nerve injuries with good motor/sensory recovery had a "good" functional result, compared with 45% of patients with poor motor/sensory return who had good function. Results after peroneal repair were even more confusing, with 94% of good recoveries and 82% of poor recoveries achieving satisfactory function.[21] Zachary found that 28% of patients with absolutely no motor recovery fell into the "good functional result" category.[113]

Authors' Perspective

There appear to be specific patient, autonomic, or physiologic factors that affect neural recovery. How can these factors help in clinical decision making? First, a physiologic age assignment is more pertinent than one of chronologic age. An active, healthy 60-year-old patient may have a far better prognosis than an overweight 40-year-old patient with diabetes mellitus. Second, assuming that the magnitude of the extremity injury and the mechanism of injury are favorable, good results (M3, S3+) can be expected in physiologic 10- to 20-year olds and excellent results (M4, S4) in children. Third, all neural injuries should be approached in a patient-oriented manner (ie, long nerve grafts to restore intrinsic muscle function are not likely to be successful in an 80-year-old patient, but are an appropriate technique in a 10-year-old patient).

Injury

Mechanism

The mechanism of injury is of considerable importance. Omer evaluated 917 upper-extremity injuries with particular emphasis on mechanism and prognosis.[75] Of the 143 injuries that required neurorrhaphy, acceptable clinical recovery occurred in 44% of lacerations, 31% of low-velocity gunshot wounds, and 21% of high-velocity gunshot wounds. These results were no different from those reported during World War II.

Many of the subsequent studies that have looked at mechanism of injury involve civilian nerve injuries associated with amputations. In one series of 64 thumb replantations, there was no correlation between sensory recovery and type of injury.[86] Half the patients followed for more than 6 months retained two-point discrimination of 10 mm or less. However, there was a 27% nonsurvival rate, most occurring in crushed or avulsed digits; therefore, most of the digits surviving were secondary to cleaner transections. A later report of thumb avulsions indicated two-point discrimination of greater than 10 mm in all patients in whom nerve repair was attempted.[3] Other studies have demonstrated superior sensory or motor recovery in clean/sharp transections, with poorer results in neurorrhaphies secondary to severe crushing or avulsion injuries.[33,47,93]

There are several explanations for the above observations. The more severe injuries are also associated with significant vascular and soft-tissue damage, which will affect nerve regeneration (see Chap. 47). This perineural environment has been shown to be highly significant. Nerve repair in high-energy, untidy war wounds is significantly inferior to nerve repair in civilian wounds.[73,98,111,113] The extent of soft-tissue damage may affect the results of neurorrhaphy directly, by physical or chemical factors at the repair site, or indirectly, by damage to the end-organs to be reinnervated. Extensive muscle and soft-tissue damage may result in a scarred hostile environment, which increases mechanical stresses at the suture line, decreases potential diffusional nutrition, interferes with axoplasmic flow, and slows neural recovery.[24] Nicholson and Seddon demonstrated the adverse effects of nerve mobilization, which is another indication that an altered soft-tissue environment/vascular bed may be deleterious to neural regeneration.[73] Avulsion/crushing injuries often result in segmental nerve damage, increasing the zone of injury (see Chap. 39). These injuries are also more difficult to deal with, as the full extent of involvement may not be recognized at the time of injury. The extremity may also be predisposed to infection, which would further impede neural recovery.

Experimental data have shown that more severe trauma is associated with an increased depression of protein synthesis and transport.[50] However, in comparing sharp and blunt nerve division in a primate model, Grabb observed no difference in recovery after repair.[35]

Unfortunately, many nerve transections are secondary to complex events, and classifying the mechanism of injury is difficult. In general, low-energy sharp transections have the best prognosis, and high-energy crush/avulsion injuries with segmental damage have a poorer outcome.

Level of Injury

The level of neural disruption has a significant bearing on the quality of nerve recovery following repair. Numerous clinical studies have demonstrated that distal injuries are associated with a better prognosis.[31,33,43,53,59,61,73,75,81,84,85,91,113] In repaired median nerve injuries, useful recovery (to M3/S3 or greater) has been reported in 50% of distal lesions, compared to 30% of proximal lesions.[53,73,75,84,91,111,113] Distal ulnar nerve repairs resulted in approximately 44% useful recovery, which decreased to 24% M3 and 32% S3 in proximal lesions.[31,53,75,84,91,111,113] In digital nerve repair, all studies note better sensibility with distal injuries, yet few break down the data by level.[33,53,81,85,112] Two reports indicate that sensory recovery of S3 or greater can be expected in 80% of proper digital nerve injuries and in about 45% of common digital nerve injuries.[43,59]

Less has been published on radial nerve repair, as many of these injuries are closed and proceed to spontaneous recovery.[75] Zachary noted motor recovery to M3 in 70% of distal, 65% of intermediate, and 44% of proximal repairs.[113] In one of the largest civilian series, Larsen and Posch observed sensory recovery of the radial nerve in 83% of distal and 59% of proximal lesions.[53] However, the results were reversed regarding complete or partial motor recovery (40% distal vs 82% proximal lesions). They attributed this to the fact that the distal lesions usually occurred at the level of branching, making accurate repair much more difficult. Similar differences have been noted in the tibial and peroneal nerves, although the exact levels of injury are not described.[113]

A faster functional recovery has also been demonstrated in the laboratory in more distal lesions.[38] This may be due to several factors. Greater retrograde degeneration, sometimes leading to neuronal death, takes place following lesions occurring close to the cell body.[100] Thus, there may be less regenerative potential following proximal injuries. Bowden and Sholl demonstrated clinically that the rates of neural regeneration decrease with time and, therefore, with distance traveled.[11] This is perhaps due to the greater strain placed on the synthetic capabilities of the cell.

The fascicles in the proximal nerves contain greater mixtures of motor and sensory fibers arranged in plexi that maintain constant patterns for only 1.5 cm, making fascicular alignment more difficult (see Chap. 14).[97] This differs from the internal topography of distal nerves, in which greater lengths of separate fascicles can be dissected out before forming interconnections.[46] Sensory fibers make up 94% of the median nerve at the wrist, while only 66% of the median nerve above the elbow consists of sensory fibers destined for the hand. For the ulnar nerve, 56% is sensory at the wrist, whereas 35% is made up of terminal sensory nerves above the elbow.[100] Thus, the chance of fascicular misalignment at proximal levels is increased. While mismatched motor neurons can reinnervate other muscles, sensory nerves cannot innervate motor end-plates.[37,115] Similarly, regenerating sensory nerves may sometimes innervate the "wrong" mechanoreceptors (see Chap. 6).

Authors' Perspective

Wounding itself has a profound effect on the prognosis for neural recovery. The events that disrupt nerve continuity, however, are not under the control of even the most dedicated and skilled surgeon—a fact that is often forgotten. Surgeons often fail to document the extent of injury and amount of energy involved, stating only the mechanism of injury. The details of the extent of soft-tissue injury and skeletal involvement are rarely addressed in the literature and are difficult to analyze retrospectively.

An assessment of the *magnitude of insult* to the extremity is crucial and is helpful in predicting potential outcome. High-energy wounds, often associated with more proximal injuries, have a poorer prognosis, a fact well substantiated by a comparison of war wounds to civilian injuries.

Repair Process

Timing of Repair

Outcome deteriorates with increasing delay between the time of injury and repair, but determining a specific time interval in which to repair the nerve is difficult by reviewing the available literature. *Primary neurorrhaphy* has been variously defined as either the immediate repair or suture within 5 to 7 days of a lacerated nerve from the time of injury (this latter period is sometimes referred to as delayed primary neurorrhaphy). *Secondary neurorrhaphy* is defined as repair done at a later date. In general, it assumes a new incision is necessary and involves operative resection of the scarred nerve ends (ie, removal of the proximal neuroma and distal glioma). Secondary neurorrhaphy allows optimization of the soft-tissue bed and other factors. Seddon also believes that the thicker epineurium observed 3 weeks after injury is more conducive to better repair.[91]

Based on results from the earliest series of both wartime and civilian nerve repairs, some authors actually advocated secondary repair,[73,84,114] while others found no difference in primary vs secondary neurorrhaphy.[43,60,78,81,91,106] Poppen and coworkers looked at 30 digital nerves repaired within 24 hours and 31 repaired between 6 weeks and 6 months, and found no difference in outcome.[81]

Most authors agree that nerve repairs have a better prognosis if performed before 6 months have elapsed.[29,75,81,85,113,114] Poppen and coworkers noted that all their patients repaired after 6 months had poor results.[81] Schaffer and Cleveland stated that the delay to repair was not significant in the "rapidity and completeness of nerve regeneration."[85] However, closer examination of their data reveals that 50% of those repaired within 6 months recovered two-point discrimination, whereas 20% or less of those repaired after 6 months achieved return of two-point discrimination. Omer observed that 75% of his successful results were repaired prior to 6 months.[75]

The British World War II experience revealed significantly poorer outcomes in those nerves repaired later than 6 months. In the major nerves of the upper extremity, 43% to 71% functional recovery was found in repairs before 6 months, which decreased to 15% to 53% in repairs after 6 months.[113] In the lower extremity, functional tibial sensory recovery decreased from 45% to 0%, and useful peroneal motor function decreased from 32% to 14% in the pre- and post-6 months repairs, respectively.

Looking at the overall effect of delay and ultimate recovery, after a 2- to 3-week latency period, the potential for motor recovery decreases 1% every 6 days; no similar time correlation has been described for sensory recovery.[111] Zachary and Seddon also looked at the "critical delay" to repair, after which no functional recovery could be expected.[91,113] Proximal lesions had a two to three times shorter critical delay than distal ones. In all major peripheral motor nerves, no functional recoveries were noted after delays of 9 to 18 months. In distal median and ulnar nerves injuries, delays of 31 to 48 months were still compatible with functional sensory recovery. While both authors claimed to have seen median nerve recovery after 24 to 48 months, this should be viewed cautiously in light of the partial ulnar innervation of the thenar muscles previously discussed.[83]

As mentioned above, there are no clinical data to support the widespread belief and current teaching that the earlier neurorrhaphy is performed—other factors being equal—the better the prognosis for functional motor and sensory recovery. Experimental studies evaluating immediate vs delayed repair are controversial. In a rabbit sciatic nerve model, greater myelin content was found in nerves repaired immediately compared to those sutured at 3 weeks.[7] A comprehensive evaluation of transected nerves to extensor digitorum longus (EDL) in the rabbit suggest that muscular morphology and function is adversely affected by delays of 3 weeks to 6 months.[5] Immediate neurorrhaphies were associated with mild fibrosis and atrophy and force generation of 93% of controls. Delayed repair correlated with greater fibrosis and atrophy and force generation of 40% to 50% of controls. An electrophysiological evaluation of a primate model demonstrated significantly better results in immediate vs 3-week neurorrhaphies.[35]

Certain animal studies would appear to support delayed nerve repair. On the cellular level, the synthetic machinery of the neuron is disabled during the first week after injury. Over the following 2 weeks, there is reorganization within the cell bodies, including a two-fold increase in protein content and activity. This has led some authors to advocate nerve repair at 2 to 3 weeks to take advantage of the "turned-on" neurons.[25,26,91] Conditioning lesions applied 2 days to 2 weeks prior to a second lesion in various animal models were associated with increased rates of axonal growth from the proximal stumps.[13,28,57,65] It is unclear, however, how such conditioning lesions might relate to functional return in the clinical setting.

The maximal delay acceptable for successful neurorrhaphy has not been determined experimentally. Axons in the proximal stump have the ability to regenerate at least 1 year after injury.[42] Based on clinical observations of more measurable deterioration in motor recovery, investigators have focused on time factors related to changes in motor neurons/axons and the neuromuscular end-organ. Variable effects of denervation on muscle have been reported. While Bolesta and colleagues described changes occurring as early as 3 weeks, an opossum model demonstrated decreasing weight but no fibrosis or other changes in muscle; a mass loss of 1% per day, plateauing at 60% to 80%, was described.[101] The number and properties of motor end-plates appear to change 9 to 12 months after denervation in animals.[40,82] Denervated human muscle has also exhibited changes as early as 6 weeks, with abnormal motor end-plates after 1 year.[9] Irreversible changes were not found until 3 years after denervation.[10] Despite these changes, human muscle can still be functional after 1 year of denervation.[98,100]

Type of Repair

End-to-end neurorrhaphy may be achieved by four basic methods: epineural, fascicular, group fascicular, or a combination involving one or more of these techniques. Traditional neurorrhaphies are variations of epineural repairs and are performed after resection of the neuroma proximally and the glioma distally. Appropriate alignment is based on external landmarks, but this is often difficult and no longer definitive after resecting large portions of nerve. Fascicular and group fascicular repairs are potentially more accurate but require a critical alignment of motor and sensory fascicles and more sutures.[104,105,110] A combination repair (epineural plus group fascicular) may be used to improve alignment of one segment of the nerve while decreasing the number of sutures or the operating time. An example is repair of the median nerve at the wrist with group fascicular repair of the motor portion and epineural repair of the remainder of the nerve. The theoretical merits of group fascicular alignment of motor or sensory components of the median nerve in the distal forearm and the ulnar nerve are well reported, but superiority of one technique is not well validated.[88,110] Treatment of the ulnar nerve motor component and sensory portion as two separate nerves has been demonstrated to be superior.[76,77] There is no evidence that fascicular repair is superior to epineural repair in the experimental model[7,17,18,52,80] or the clinical situation.[55,104,105]

Nerve grafting may decrease excessive tension at the site of a repair. Graft techniques include various autogenous nerve grafts or other material (see Chap. 37). Autogenous neural tissue includes the following:

1. Intrafascicular nerve grafts[70,71]
2. Trunk cable[89]
3. Pedicle grafts[94]
4. Free vascularized nerve grafts[34,92,103]
5. True fascicular grafts.[104,105,109]

Other materials, such as veins and muscle autografts,[30,74] may be used as interposition conduits to promote neural reattachment, and experimental studies suggest that synthetic material may also be effective.[6,58] To date, however, autologous nerve grafts remain the structures of choice for interposition grafting.

While nerve grafting results are discussed in detail in Chapter 39, several pertinent points deserve emphasis:

1. Small-caliber intrafascicular nerve grafts using autogenous noncritical sensory or motor nerve (eg, sural, medial antebrachial cutaneous) give results superior to those with trunk grafts or cable grafts.[87,90,108] These small grafts do not undergo central fibrosis or necrosis as readily as trunk or cable grafts in supple well-vascularized wounds.
2. Vascularized pedicle grafts are currently experimental, and, except in very large defects in poor soft-tissue beds, they have not been shown to be superior to other types of grafting (see Chaps. 37 and 40).[34]
3. Pedicle nerve grafts are rarely indicated, because they require severe injury to multiple nerves, one of which must be nonsalvageable.[94,110]
4. The shorter the graft (assuming adequate resection of damaged nerve and elimination of tension), the more likely it is that there will be a good functional recovery. The best results are seen in grafts less than 50 mm long; grafts 10 cm or longer have a poorer prognosis for motor and sensory recovery (see Chaps. 37 and 39).[69]
5. Peripheral nerve repair using muscle autografts is a new technique with promising results in a small series and deserves additional evaluation.[30,74]

Grafting vs Repair

Primary neurorrhaphy is considered the optimal approach and provides the best clinical prognosis for complete recovery.[18] The advantages of end-to-end repair include a single suture line and delivery of equal or more proximal axons to the distal stump. Potential neural damage or hindrance of neural transfer secondary to mobilization, manipulation, and tension affects recovery. Nerve grafting diminishes manipulation and tension but adds an additional suture line, and the available nerve graft may not provide access of all the proximal axons to the distal stump.

Although nonprimate experimental data suggest that ultimate sensory and muscular function with primary neurorrhaphy or nerve grafting is equal,[64] there are no data that justify nerve grafting if primary or delayed end-to-end suture may be performed without extensive mobilization (<2–4 cm) or tension. In large nerves (eg, median, sciatic) there are insufficient fascicles available from autogenous neural tissue to allow transmission of a majority of proximal axons. Although functional recovery will still be acceptable, potential repair processes will be compromised to a certain extent.

Authors' Perspective

The physiologic variables in which time affects functional recovery include the following:

1. Regenerative potential of the proximal nerve
2. Ability of the distal segment to accept regenerating axons
3. The restorative capacity of the myoneural junction
4. The degree of responsiveness after deterioration of the denervated muscles and sensory mechanoreceptors.

Neurorrhaphy is performed as early as is justified by the condition of the neural elements and the status of the wound. A delay in repair of longer than 6 months diminishes the likelihood of functional recovery. However, there is little clinical documentation that immediate repair is significantly superior to delayed primary or early secondary repair. In primary repair, end-to-end tension-free apposition is more likely to be possible, and electrodiagnosis of the distal stump allows definitive recognition of motor vs sensory fascicles, which is impossible in a secondary procedure (see Chap. 15).[32] In general, it is inadvisable to perform primary nerve grafts, since an established and proven well-nourished and infection-free environment is necessary for graft survival (see Chap. 37).

Recovery Process

The recovery process itself is crucial and is a factor generally overlooked in the analysis of nerve repair. It is important to protect the extremity in the recovery period, especially if the primary or secondary repair has been performed after extensive nerve mobilization. Joint motion proximal and distal to the repair site is performed in a protected and controlled manner, and appropriate sensory or motor re-education is provided.

Post-Recovery Protection

Following peripheral neurorrhaphy with or without tension, it is important that the anastomotic site be protected from disruption. Since excessive graft lengths are potentially deleterious to functional recovery, extremes of motion may provide tension at the suture line; such tension should be avoided.[12,19,27,29]

Time to Evaluation

Many of the reports in the literature examining the results of nerve repair suffer from inadequate follow-up of 1 to 2 years.[8,14,15,59,85,86,96,112] When dealing with nerve regeneration, longer periods are required before recovery plateaus. While Nicholson and Seddon observed maximal changes 2 to 3 years after repair, a slower but continued improvement in function was noted up to 5 years.[73] Adult patients after ulnar nerve repair demonstrated 7% intrinsic motor recovery at 14 months, which improved to an average of 82% after 26 to 51 months.[31] In another demonstration of the superior regenerative abilities of youth, recovery in children in this study plateaued at 86% after only 2 years. Others have also recognized the need to follow young patients for at least 2 years and adults for 5 years.[72,95]

Re-Education

Sensory and motor re-education can improve functional recovery.[22,58] Sensibility may be improved by techniques that reduce hyperesthesia or pain and stress early sensibility training in the extremity (see Chap. 58).

SUMMARY

The factors influencing the success of operative repair of peripheral nerves are poorly understood, with experimental and clinical data often supporting opposing views. It has been difficult to isolate prognostic factors, as many are interrelated (eg, proximal lesions are often associated with extensive soft-tissue damage and delayed repairs).

Many of the important factors that affect potential functional recovery after neurorrhaphy have been predetermined by the mechanism of injury, the type of nerve injured, the level of injury, and the age of the patient (Table 24-5). Of these, age is the most important variable, with significantly superior recovery observed in children and teenagers. Sharp transections favor a better outcome than crushing/avulsion injuries. Distal lesions generally recover better than proximal ones, in part due to the decreased synthesis/regeneration required of the cell body.

Sensory nerves appear to have a better prognosis for functional recovery than motor nerves. No functional significance has been attributed to sudomotor return. This improved prognosis after repair does not appear related to axonal regenerative potentials, which are inferior to those of motor neurons. This may be due to the longevity of sensory end-organs (see Chap. 6), overlap and ingrowth from neighboring sensory fibers, or the brain's ability for cortical reorganization.

Distal median and digital nerves attain significant functional return, most likely due to the high per-

Table 24–5. *Factors Affecting Nerve Recovery**

1. Patient age
2. Level of injury
3. Specific nerve injured
4. Mechanism/nerve defect
5. Rehabilitation/time to evaluation
6. Repair techniques
7. Associated injuries
8. Delay to repair

* *Factors 1–3 are listed in order of probable significance, substantiated by data in the literature. While factors 4–8 are all important, it is difficult to place them in any meaningful order.*

centage of sensory nerve fibers. Ulnar nerves may have a poorer prognosis, as their recovery depends on reinnervation of small, distal muscles that are responsible for very fine movement. Poor peroneal recovery has been attributed to numerous factors.[51] In the thigh, the peroneal portion of the sciatic nerve is situated laterally and is therefore more susceptible to injury. Distally it is tethered at the fibular head. This nerve innervates muscles more distally in the lower extremity, thus requiring greater distances for axonal regeneration.

No significant differences in epineural vs fascicular repair,[52,79,80] loupe vs microscopic magnification,[63] and defects less than 5 cm have been observed.[88–91,110,113,114] While experimental evidence advocates immediate or delayed primary repair, clinical results argue strongly for nerve repair within 6 months of injury. At least 2 years for children and 5 years for adults must be allowed for follow-up before meaningful conclusions can be discussed.

The timing of the repair process and the technical details that influence the quality of the repair bed are under the control of the operating surgeon. Which mechanism to use to decrease tension while overcoming the nerve gap is the single most important decision required of the surgeon. His or her decisions as to the appropriate degree of mobilization, the handling of neural tissue, and the best type of repair are the factors that will most significantly influence functional recovery.

REFERENCES

1. Almquist EE, Eeg-Olafsson O. Sensory-nerve conduction velocity and two-point discrimination in sutured nerves. J Bone Joint Surg [Am] 1970; 52: 791–796.
2. Almquist EE, Smith OA, Fry L. Nerve conduction velocity, microscopic, and electron microscopy studies comparing repaired adult and baby monkey median nerves. J Hand Surg 1983; 8:406–410.
3. Bieber EJ, Wood MB, Cooney WP, Amadio PC. Thumb avulsion: Results of replantation/revascularization. J Hand Surg [Am] 1987; 12:786–789.
4. Black MM, Laseck RJ. Slowing of the rate of axonal regeneration during growth and maturation. Exp Neurol 1979; 68:108–119.
5. Bolesta MJ, Garrett WE Jr, Ribbeck BM, Glisson RR, Seaber AV, Goldner JL. Immediate and delayed neurorrhaphy in a rabbit model: A functional, histologic, and biochemical comparison. J Hand Surg [Am] 1988; 13:352–357.
6. Bora FW Jr, Bednar JM, Osterman AL, Brown MJ, Summer AJ. Prosthetic nerve grafts: A resorbable tube as an alternative to autogenous nerve grafting. J Hand Surg [Am] 1987; 12:685–692.
7. Bora FW Jr, Pleasurable DE, Didizian NA. A study of nerve regeneration and neuroma formation after nerve suture by various techniques. J Hand Surg 1976; 1:138–143.
8. Boswick JA Jr, Schneewind J, Stromberg J Jr. Evaluation of peripheral nerve repairs below elbow. Arch Surg 1965; 90:50–51.
9. Bowden REM. Factors influencing functional recovery. In: Seddon HJ, ed. Peripheral nerve injuries. Medical Research Council Special Report No. 282. London: Her Majesty's Stationery Office, 1954; 326–353.
10. Bowden REM, Gutmann E. Denervation and reinnervation of human voluntary muscle. Brain 1944; 67:273–313.
11. Bowden REM, Sholl DA. Rates of regeneration of peripheral nerve injuries. In: Seddon HJ, ed. Peripheral nerve injuries. Medical Research Council Special Report No. 282. London: Her Majesty's Stationery Office, 1954:16–24.
12. Braun RM. Epineurial nerve suture. Clin Orthop 1982; 163:50–56.
13. Brisby MA, Keen P. The effect of a conditioning lesion on the regeneration rate of peripheral nerve axons containing substance P. Brain Res 1985; 336: 201–206.
14. Brown PW. The time factor in surgery of upper extremity peripheral nerve injury. Clin Orthop 1970; 68:14–21.
15. Brown PW. Factors influencing the success of the surgical repair of peripheral nerves. Surg Clin North Am 1972; 52:1137–1155.
16. Buncke HJ Jr. Digital nerve repairs. Surg Clin North Am 1972; 52:1267–1286.
17. Cabaud HE, Rodkey WG, McCarroll HR Jr, Mutz SB, Niebauer JJ. Epineurial and perineurial fascicular nerve repairs: A critical comparison. J Hand Surg 1976; 1:131–137.
18. Cabaud HE, Rodkey WG, McCarroll HR Jr. Peripheral nerve injuries: Studies in higher nonhuman primates. J Hand Surg 1980; 5:201–206.
19. Chiu DTW, Ishii C. Management of peripheral nerve injuries. Orthop Clin North Am 1986; 17: 365–373.
20. Clawson DK, Seddon HJ. The results of repair of

the sciatic nerve. J Bone Joint Surg [Br] 1960; 42: 205–212.

21. Clawson DK, Seddon HJ. The late consequences of sciatic nerve injury. J Bone Joint Surg [Br] 1960; 42:213–225.
22. Dellon AL. Re-innervation of denervated Meissner corpuscles: A sequential histologic study in primates following interfascicular nerve repair. J Hand Surg 1976; 1:98–109.
23. Dellon AL. Evaluation of sensibility and re-education of sensation in the hand. Baltimore: Williams & Wilkins, 1981:117–118.
24. De Medinaceli L, Wyatt RJ, Freed WJ. Peripheral nerve reconnection: Mechanical, thermal and ionic conditions that promote the return of function. Exp Neurol 1983; 81:469–487.
25. Ducker TB. Metabolic factors in surgery of peripheral nerves. Surg Clin North Am 1972; 52: 1109–1122.
26. Ducker TB, Kempe LG, Hayes GJ. The metabolic background for peripheral nerve surgery. J Neurosurg 1969; 30:270–280.
27. Fess EE. Rehabilitation of the patient with peripheral nerve injury. Hand Clin 1986; 2:207–215.
28. Forman DS, McQuarrie IG, Labore FW, et al. Time course of the conditioning lesion effect on axonal regeneration. Brain Res 1980; 182:180–185.
29. Frykman GK, Waylett J. Rehabilitation of peripheral nerve injuries. Orthop Clin North Am 1981; 12:361–379.
30. Gattuso JM, Davies AH, Glasby MA, Gschmeissner SE, Huang CLH. Peripheral nerve repair using muscle autografts: Recovery of transmission in primates. J Bone Joint Surg [Br] 1988; 70:524–529.
31. Gaul JS Jr. Intrinsic motor recovery: A long-term study of ulnar nerve repair. J Hand Surg 1982; 7: 502–508.
32. Gaul JS Jr. Electrical fascicle identification as an adjunct to nerve repair. J Hand Surg 1983; 8:289–296.
33. Gelberman RH, Urbaniak JR, Bright DS, Levin LS. Digital sensibility following replantation. J Hand Surg 1978; 3:313–319.
34. Gilbert A. Vascularized sural nerve graft. Clin Plast Surg 1974; 2:73–77.
35. Grabb WC. Median and ulnar nerve suture: An experimental study comparing primary and secondary repair in monkeys. J Bone Joint Surg [Am] 1968; 50:964–972.
36. Gutmann E. Factors affecting recovery of motor function after nerve lesions. J Neurol Neurosurg Psychiatry 1942; 5:81–95.
37. Gutmann E. The re-innervation of muscle by sensory nerve fibres. J Anat 1945; 79:1.
38. Gutmann E, Guttmann L. Factors affecting recovery of sensory function after nerve lesions. J Neurol Neurosurg Psychiatry 1942; 5:117.
39. Gutmann E, Guttmann L, Medawar PB, Young JZ. The rate of regeneration of the nerve. J Exp Biol 1942; 19:14–44.
40. Gutmann E, Young JZ. The re-innervation of muscle after various periods of atrophy. J Anat 1944; 78:15.
41. Highet WB, Sanders FK. The effects of stretching nerves after suture. Br J Surg 1943; 30:355.
42. Holmes W, Young JZ. Nerve regeneration after immediate and delayed suture. J Anat 1942; 77: 63.
43. Honner R. Fragiadakis EG, Lamb DW. An investigation of the factors affecting the results of digital nerve division. Hand 1970; 2:21–30.
44. Ito T, Hirotani H, Yamamoto K. Peripheral nerve repairs by the funicular suture technique. Acta Orthop Scand 1976; 47:283–289.
45. Jabaley ME, Burns JE, Orcutt BS, Bryant WM. Comparison of histologic and functional recovery after peripheral nerve repair. J Hand Surg 1976; 1:119–130.
46. Jabaley ME, Wallace WH, Heckler FR. Internal topography of major nerves of the forearm and hand: A current view. J Hand Surg 1980; 5:1–18.
47. Jaeger SH, Tsai T, Kleinert HE. Upper extremity replantation in children. Orthop Clin North Am 1981; 12:897–907.
48. Jenkins WM, Merzenich MM, Ocho MT. Behaviorally controlled diferential use of restricted hand surfaces induce changes in the cortical representation of the hand in area 3b of adult owl monkeys. Soc Neurosci Abstr 1984; 10:665.
49. Kaleska J, Pomeranz B. Chronic paw denervation causes an age-dependent appearance of novel responses from forearm in "paw cortex" of kittens and adult cats. J Neurophysiol 1979; 42:618–633.
50. Karlström L, Dahlström A. The effect of different types of axonal trauma on the synthesis and transport of amine storage granules in rat sciatic nerves. J Neurobiol 1973; 4:191–200.
51. Kline DG. Operative experience with major lower extremity nerve lesions including lumbosacral plexus and the sciatic nerve. In: Omer GE Jr, Spinner M, eds. Management of peripheral nerve problems. Philadelphia: WB Saunders, 1980:607–625.

52. Kline DG, Hudson AR, Bratton BR. Experimental study of fascicular nerve repair with and without epineurial closure. J Neurosurg 1981; 54:513–520.
53. Larsen RD, Posch JL. Nerve injuries in the upper extremity. Arch Surg 1958; 77:469–482.
54. Leonard MH. Return of skin sensation in children after repair of nerves. Clin Orthop 1973; 273–277.
55. Levinthal R, Brown WJ, Rand RW. Comparison of fascicular, interfascicular, and epineural suture techniques in the repair of simple lacerations. J Neurosurg 1977; 47:744–750.
56. Lindsay WK, Walker FG, Farmer AW. Traumatic peripheral nerve injuries in children: Results of repair. Plast Reconstr Surg 1962; 30:462–468.
57. Lundborg G, Dahlin LB, Hansson H, Kanje M, Necking L. Vibration exposure and peripheral nerve fiber damage. J Hand Surg [Am] 1990; 15: 346–351.
58. Mackinnon SE, Dellon AL. Surgery of the peripheral nerve. New York: Thieme, 1988:89–130.
59. Mailänder P, Berger A, Schaller E, Ruhe K. Results of primary nerve repair in the upper extremity. Microsurg 1989; 10:147–150.
60. Marble EH, Hamlin JR, Watkins AL. Regeneration in ulnar, median, and radial nerves. Am J Surg 1942; 55:274–294.
61. McEwan LE. Median and ulnar nerve injuries. Aust NZ J Surg 1962; 32:89–104.
62. McKinley PA, Jenkins WM, Smith JL, Merzenich MM. Age-dependent capacity for somatosensory cortex reorganization in chronic spinal cats. Brain Res 1987; 428:136–139.
63. McManamny DS. Comparison of microscope and loupe magnification: Assistance for the repair of median and ulnar nerves. Br J Plast Surg 1983; 36: 367–372.
64. McNamara MJ, Garrett WE Jr, Seaber AV, Goldner JL. Neurorrhaphy, nerve grafting, and neurotization; a functional comparison of nerve reconstruction techniques. J Hand Surg [Am] 1987; 12: 354–360.
65. McQuarrie IG, Grafstein B. Axon outgrowth enhanced by a previous nerve injury. Arch Neurol 1973; 29:53–55.
66. Merzenich MM, Kaas JH, Wall JT, Nelson RJ, Sur M, Felleman DJ. Topographic reorganization of somatosensory cortical area 3b and 1 in adult monkeys following restricted deafferentation. Neurosci 1983; 8:33–55.
67. Merzenich MM, Kaas JH, Wall JT, Sur M, Nelson RJ, Felleman DJ. Progression of changes following median nerve section in the cortical representation of the hand in areas 3b and 1 in adult owl and squirrel monkeys. Neurosci 1983; 10:639–665.
68. Merzenich MM, Nelson RJ, Stryker MP, Cynacker MS, Schoppmann A, Zook JM. Somatosensory cortical map changes following digital amputation in adult monkeys. J Comp Neurol 1984; 224:591–605.
69. Millesi H. Interfascicular nerve grafting. Orthop Clin North Am 1981; 12:287–301.
70. Millesi H. Nerve grafting. Clin Plast Surg 1984; 11:105–113.
71. Millesi H, Meissl G, Berger A. The interfascicular nerve-grafting of the median and ulnar nerves. J Bone Joint Surg [Am] 1972; 54:727–750.
72. Moberg E. Nerve repair in hand surgery: An analysis. Surg Clin North Am 1968; 48:985–991.
73. Nicholson OR, Seddon HJ. Nerve repair in civil practice: Results of treatment of median and ulnar nerve lesions. Br Med J 1957; 11:1065–1071.
74. Norris RW, Glasby MA, Gattuso JM, Bowden REM. Peripheral nerve repair in humans using muscle autografts: A new technique. J Bone Joint Surg [Br] 1988; 70:530–533.
75. Omer GE Jr. Injuries to nerves of the upper extremity. J Bone Joint Surg [Am] 1974; 56:1615–1624.
76. Omer GE Jr. The evaluation of clinical results following peripheral nerve suture. In: Omer GE Jr, Spinner M, eds. Management of peripheral nerve problems. Philadelphia: WB Saunders, 1980:431–442.
77. Omer GE Jr. Acute management of peripheral nerve injuries. Hand Clin 1986; 2:193–206.
78. Önne L. Recovery of sensibility and sudomotor activity in the hand after nerve suture. Acta Chir Scand Suppl 1962; 300:1–69.
79. Orgel MG. Epineurial versus perineurial repair of peripheral nerves. Clin Plast Surg 1984; 11:101–104.
80. Orgel MG, Terzis JK. Epineurial versus perineurial repair: An ultrastructural and electrophysiological study of nerve regeneration. Plast Reconstr Surg 1977; 60:80–91.
81. Poppen NK, McCarroll HR Jr, Doyle JR, Niebauer JJ. Recovery of sensibility after suture of digital nerves. J Hand Surg 1979; 4:212–226.
82. Richter HP, Frosch D, Ketalsen VP. Functional and morphological motor regeneration after different periods of denervation and following microsurgical suture of the peroneal nerve. Acta Neurochir Suppl 1979; 28:605–607.
83. Rowntree T. Anomalous innervation of the hand

and muscles. J Bone Joint Surg [Br] 1949; 31:505–510.

84. Sakellarides H. A follow-up study of 172 peripheral nerve injuries in the upper extremity in civilians. J Bone Joint Surg [Am] 1962; 44:140–148.
85. Schaffer JM, Cleveland F. Delayed suture of sensory nerves of the hand. Ann Surg 1950; 131:556–563.
86. Schlenker JD, Kleinert HE, Tsai T. Methods and results of replantation following traumatic amputation of the thumb in 64 patients. J Hand Surg 1980; 5:63–70.
87. Seddon HJ. The use of autogenous grafts for the repair of large gaps in peripheral nerves. Br J Surg 1947; 35:151–167.
88. Seddon HJ. Peripheral nerve repair in man. In: Seddon HJ, ed. Peripheral nerve injuries. Medical Research Council Special Report No. 282. London: Her Majesty's Stationery Office, 1954:110–134.
89. Seddon HJ. Nerve grafting and other unusual forms of nerve repair. In: Seddon HJ, ed. Peripheral nerve injuries. Medical Research Council Special Report No. 282. London: Her Majesty's Stationery Office, 1954:389–417.
90. Seddon HJ. Nerve grafting. J Bone Joint Surg [Br] 1963; 45:447–461.
91. Seddon HJ. Surgical disorders of the peripheral nerves, ed 2. Edinburgh: Churchill-Livingstone, 1975; 242–249, 303–314.
92. Shibata M, Tsai T, Firrell J, Breidenbach WC. Experimental comparison of vascularized and nonvascularized nerve grafting. J Hand Surg [Am] 1988; 13:358–365.
93. Stevenson JH, Zuker RM. Upper limb motor and sensory recovery after multiple proximal nerve injury in children: A long-term review of 5 patients. Br J Plast Surg 1986; 39:109–113.
94. Strange FG. An operation for nerve pedicle grafting: Preliminary communication. Br J Surg 1946; 34:423–425.
95. Stromberg WB Jr, McFarlane RM, Bell JL, Koch SL, Mason ML. Injury of the median and ulnar nerves: 150 cases with an evaluation of Moberg's ninhydrin test. J Bone Joint Surg [Am] 1961; 43: 717–730.
96. Sullivan DJ. Results of digital neurorrhaphy in adults. J Hand Surg [Br] 1985; 10:41–44.
97. Sunderland S. The intraneural topography of the radial, median, and ulnar nerves. Brain 1945; 68: 243–298.
98. Sunderland S. Observations on the course of recovery and late end results in a series of cases of peripheral nerve suture. Aust NZ Surg 1949; 18: 264–341.
99. Sunderland S. Capacity of reinnervated muscles to function efficiently after prolonged denervation. Arch Neurol Psychiat 1950; 64:755–771.
100. Sunderland S. Nerves and nerve injuries, ed 2. Edinburgh: Churchill-Livingstone, 1978:18, 87–96, 116–124, 232–246.
101. Sunderland S, Ray LJ. Denervation changes in mammalian striated muscle. J Neurol Neurosurg Psychiatry 1950; 13:159.
102. Tajima T, Imai H. Results of median nerve repair in children. Microsurg 1989; 10:145–146.
103. Taylor GI. Nerve grafting with simultaneous microvascular reconstruction. Clin Orthop 1978; 133:56–70.
104. Tupper JW. Fascicular nerve repair. In: American Academy of Orthopaedic Surgeons. Symposium on microsurgery. St. Louis: CV Mosby, 1979:215–226.
105. Tupper JW, Crick JC, Matteck LR. Fascicular nerve repairs: A comparative study of epineural and fascicular (perineural) techniques. Orthop Clin North Am 1988; 19:57–69.
106. Weckesser EC. The repair of nerves in the palm and the fingers. Clin Orthop 1961; 119:200–207.
107. Wedell G, Guttmann L, Gutmann E. The local extension of nerve fibers into denervated areas of skin. J Neurol Neurosurg Psychiatry 1941; 4:206.
108. Wilgis EFS. Nerve repair and grafting. In: Green DP, ed. Operative hand surgery. New York: Churchill-Livingstone, 1982:1373–1403.
109. Wilgis EFS, Maxwell GP. Distal digital nerve grafts: Clinical and anatomical studies. J Hand Surg 1979; 4:439–443.
110. Wilgis EFS, Murphy R. The significance of longitudinal excursion in peripheral nerves. Hand Clin 1986; 2:761–766.
111. Woodhall B, Beebe GW eds. Peripheral nerve regeneration: A follow-up study of 3,656 World War II injuries. Veterans Administration monograph. Washington DC: US Government Printing Office, 1956:71–201, 241–310.
112. Young L, Wray RC, Weeks PM. A randomized prospective comparison of fascicular and epineural digital nerve repairs. Plast Reconstr Surg 1981; 68:89–92.
113. Zachary RB. Results of nerve suture. In: Seddon HJ, ed. Peripheral nerve injuries. Medical Research Council Special Report No. 282. London: Her Majesty's Stationery Office, 1954; 354–388.
114. Zachary RB, Holmes W. Primary suture of nerves. Surg Gynecol Obstet 1946; 82:632–651.
115. Zalewski AA. Effects of neuromuscular reinnervation on denervated skeletal muscle by axons of motor, sensory, and sympathetic neurons. Am J Physiol 970; 219:1675–1679.

25

Median Nerve: Applied Anatomy and Operative Exposure

David B. Siegel
Richard H. Gelberman

AUTHORS' KEY POINTS

- The ligament of Struthers attaches to the supracondyloid process, which projects anteromedially from the medial supracondylar ridge of the humerus, 3 to 5 cm above the medial epicondyle. The ligament attaches to the medial epicondyle, forming a fibro-osseous tunnel that is a site for median nerve compression in the arm.
- The median nerve enters the forearm between the humeral and ulnar heads of the pronator teres; it passes deep to the humeral head when there is congenital absence of the ulnar head (6% of cases). The pronator teres is the most common site of nerve compression in the forearm.
- The anterior interosseous nerve arises from the dorsoradial surface of the median nerve immediately distal to the flexor digitorum superficialis arch, 5 cm distal to the medial epicondyle. The nerve is compressed most frequently near its origin, where it is least mobile, by a tendinous arch along the ulnar head of the pronator teres.
- The most common variation for the median nerve in the hand and wrist is high separation of the motor branch (subligamentous pattern), seen in 31% of limbs.
- The anterior branch of the medial cutaneous nerve of the forearm crosses the elbow in the subcutaneous tissue between the medial epicondyle and biceps tendon, and is at risk when the median nerve is explored in the proximal forearm.

ANATOMY

Median Nerve in the Arm

The median nerve, which arises from the lateral and medial cords of the brachial plexus, contains fibers from the fifth cervical through first thoracic nerve roots and is formed anterior or anterolateral to the third portion of the axillary artery (Fig. 25-1). Rarely, cords join to form the median nerve posterior to the axillary artery, or more distal than normal, in the upper third of the arm.[8] The nerve descends in the arm, posterior to the pectoralis major muscle, lateral to the brachial artery. It lies

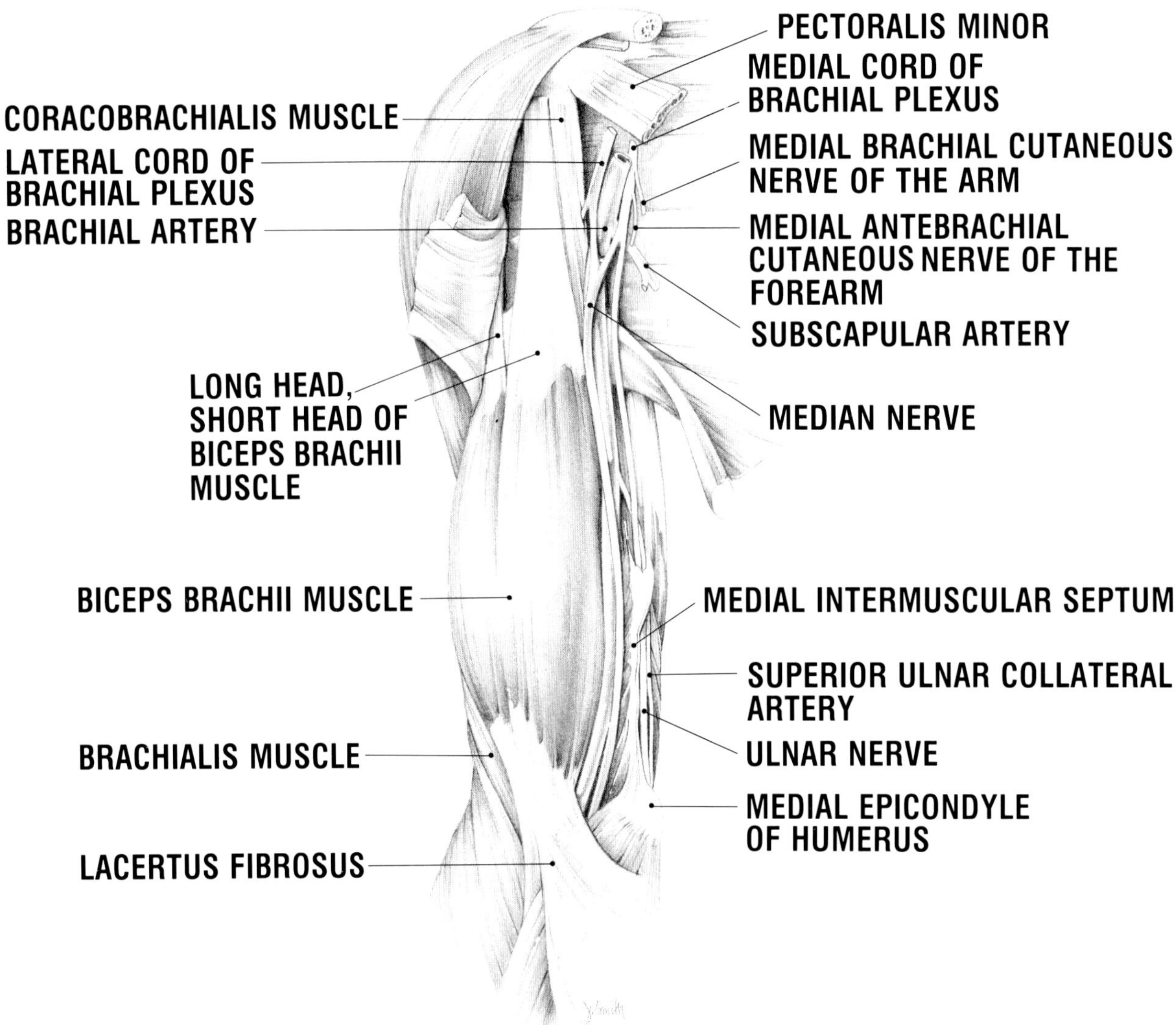

Figure 25–1. *The median nerve crosses from medial to lateral anterior to the brachial artery at the level of the insertion of the coracobrachialis muscle. It then runs distally along the medial side of the biceps brachii muscle.*

anteromedial to the brachialis muscle and posteromedial to the biceps brachii throughout its course in the arm. In the midportion of the arm, at the point of insertion of the coracobrachialis, the nerve crosses anterior to the brachial artery to lie on its medial side. It descends to the cubital fossa, medial to the artery. The median nerve typically gives off several vascular branches, but does not provide innervation to muscles in the arm.[20]

Potential Points of Neural Compression in the Arm

Six points of potential compression of the median nerve along its course in the arm have been described:

1. As the nerve descends medial to the coracoid process, it may be compressed by the pectoralis minor muscle, which lies on the anterior surface of the nerve. This is noted most often when the arm is hyperabducted.[13]
2. Several anomalous muscles have been reported to cause infraclavicular median nerve entrapment.[7] Langer's muscle, for example, arises from the latissimus dorsi tendon, crosses the axillary neurovascular bundle, and inserts on the pectoralis major.
3. Anomalous vascular arches, or perforations of the nerve by anomalous vessels, may be found in the axilla. The vascular anomalies may be arterial or venous in origin. An 8% incidence of abnormal relationships between the vascular and neural elements in the axilla has been reported.[14]
4. Occasionally the deltopectoral fascia, when thickened and fibrotic, may compress the median nerve at it distal edge. This has been reported following blunt trauma to the shoulder.[16]
5. The supracondyloid process may project anteromedially from the medial supracondylar ridge of the distal humerus, 3 to 5 cm above the medial epicondyle (Fig. 25-2). It is the origin of the ligament of Struthers, which attaches to the supracondyloid process and the medial epicondyle, forming a fibro-osseous tunnel. This anomaly, present in 1% of limbs, may represent an accessory origin of the pronator teres muscle. The nerve passes through the tunnel with either the ulnar or brachial artery and veins, medial to the vessels. Neural compression may be caused by either the supracondyloid process itself or the ligament.[2]

SUMMARY OF ANATOMICAL COMPRESSION POINTS OF THE MEDIAN NERVE

ARM

1. Pectoralis minor muscle
2. Anomalous axillary arch muscles
3. Anomalous vascular arches in the axilla
4. Deltopectoral fascia
5. A supracondyloid process
6. Ligament of Struthers

FOREARM

1. Lacertus fibrosus
2. Pronator teres muscle
3. Flexor digitorum superficialis arch
4. Anomalous muscles
5. Ulnar collateral or radial artery branches

HAND/WRIST

1. Carpal tunnel
2. Palmar cutaneous branch within the transverse retinacular ligament

Variations

A branch from the musculocutaneous nerve occasionally joins the median nerve after the former pierces the coracobrachialis muscle. This variation has been reported in 8% to 36% of dissected specimens.[9] Fibers enter the musculocutaneous nerve from the lateral cord rather than passing into the lateral root of the median nerve. The communicating branch leaves the musculocutaneous nerve, descends from lateral to medial between the brachialis and biceps muscles, and joins the median nerve in the midportion of the arm. When this anomaly occurs, the branch (or branches) of the lateral cord that joins the medial cord is smaller than normal. Fibers from the median to musculocutaneous nerve are rare. A nerve to the pronator teres muscle may leave the main median nerve trunk in the arm as high as 7 cm above the epicondyles.[5]

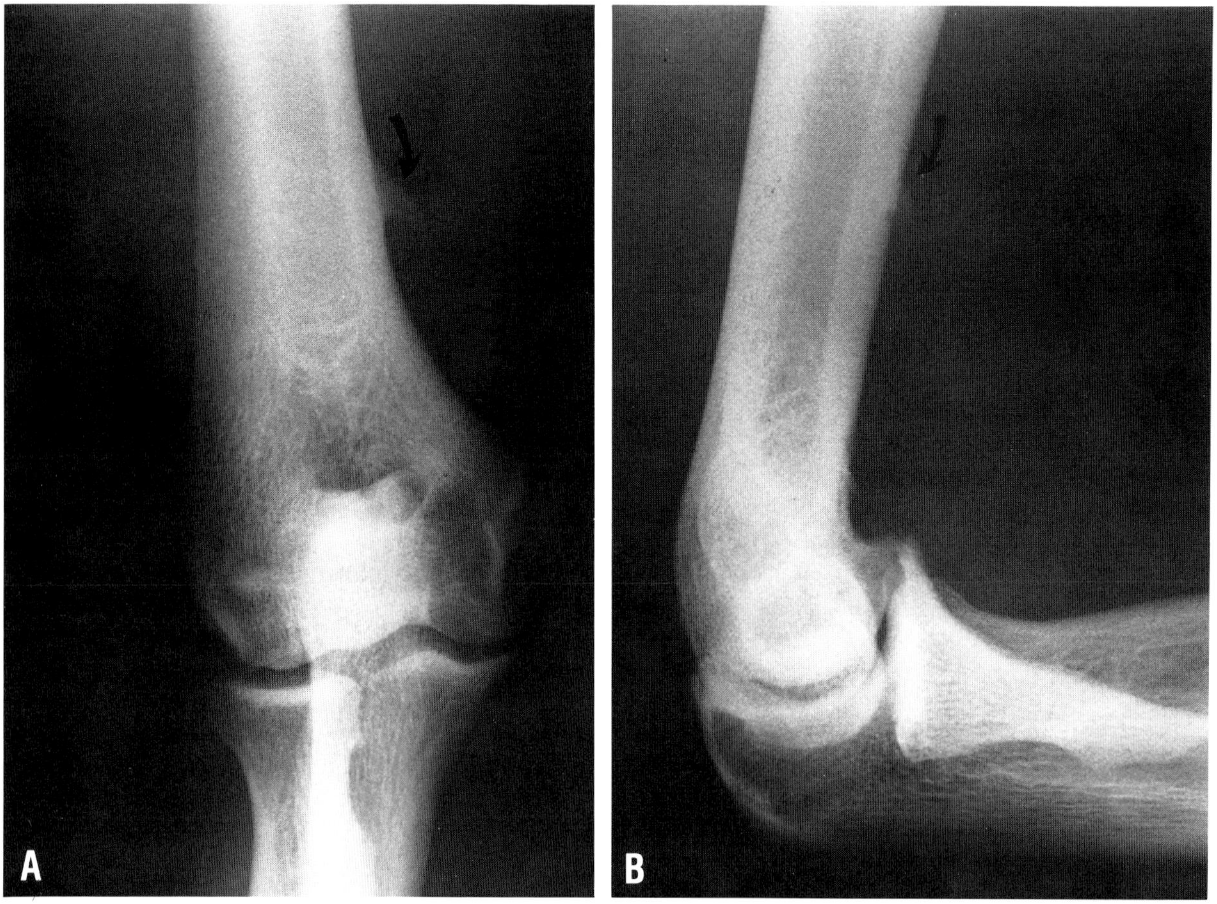

Figure 25–2. *(**A**) Anteroposterior and (**B**) lateral radiographs demonstrating a supracondyloid process. The process projects anteromedially toward the elbow joint, in contrast to the pattern seen with characteristic osteocartilaginous exostoses.*

Median Nerve in the Forearm

As the median nerve enters the cubital fossa, it lies posterior to the lacertus fibrosus, anterior to the brachialis muscle, and medial to the brachial artery (Fig. 25-3). Articular branches supply the elbow and proximal radioulnar joints as the nerve crosses the elbow. The nerve enters the forearm between the superficial (humeral) and deep (ulnar) heads of the pronator teres muscle. It passes deep to the humeral head even when there is congenital absence of the ulnar head (in 6% of cases).[1] As it passes through the muscle bellies, it crosses the ulnar artery anteriorly, from medial to lateral, separated from the artery by the deep head of the pronator teres. After emerging from the pronator teres, the nerve passes deep to an arch created by the two heads of the flexor digitorum superficialis. It descends in the forearm between the flexor digitorum superficialis and flexor digitorum profundus, occasionally within the substance of the flexor digitorum superficialis.[6] It becomes superficial 5 cm above the wrist, emerging between the flexor digitorum superficialis and flexor carpi radialis, dorsal and slightly radial to the tendon of the palmaris longus.[3]

The median nerve supplies the pronator teres, flexor carpi radialis, palmaris longus, and flexor

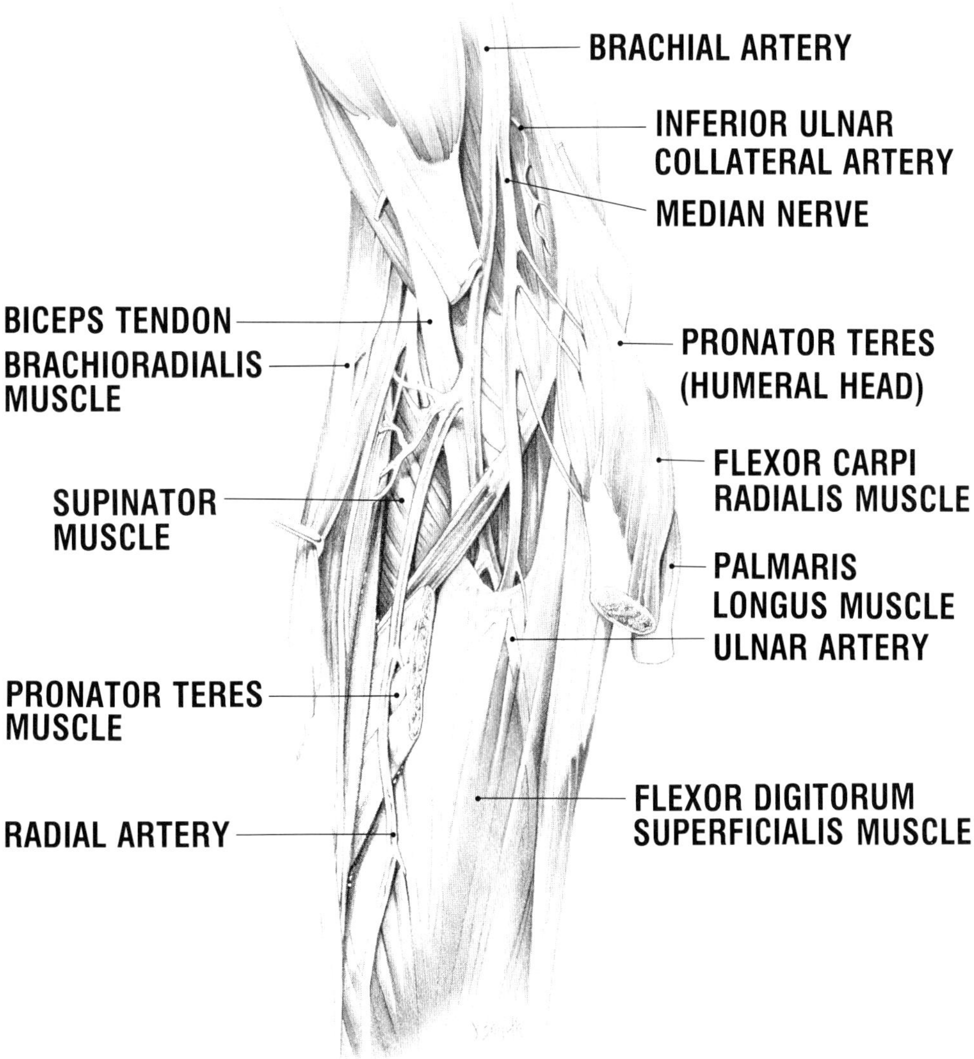

Figure 25–3. *The median nerve has been exposed under the lacertus fibrosus. After supplying the pronator teres muscle and flexor carpi radialis muscle, the nerve passes volar to the deep head of the pronator teres muscle and dorsal to the fibrous arch of origin of the flexor digitorum superficialis muscle. Note that the ulnar artery passes dorsal to the deep head of the pronator teres muscle.*

digitorum superficialis in the proximal forearm (Table 25-1). The branch to the pronator teres arises from 7 cm above to 2.3 cm below the medial epicondyle.[5] In 45% of arms dissected, Sunderland found two branches to the pronator teres, in 30% one branch, and in 25% three or four branches.[18] Proximal to the anterior interosseous branch, the nerve supplies the flexor carpi radialis, palmaris longus, and flexor digitorum superficialis. There is usually a single nerve to the flexor carpi radialis and one to the palmaris longus, but there are from two to seven branches to the flexor digitorum superficialis. The branch to the index finger portion of the flexor digitorum superficialis arises in the midportion of the forearm, up to 20 cm distal to the medial epicondyle. The muscular branches of

Table 25–1. *Level and Order of Innervation of Muscles Supplied by Median Nerve*

Muscle	cm From Medial Epicondyle (Shortest to Longest)
Pronator teres	12.9–16.1
Flexor digitorum superficialis	15.4–23.0
Flexor carpi radialis	15.9–16.6
Palmaris longus	
Flexor digitorum profundus	19.3–22.6
Flexor pollicis longus	20.0–24.3
Pronator quadratus	29.8–30.2
	cm From Radial Styloid
Flexor pollicis brevis	6.0–6.8
Abductor pollicis brevis	6.5–6.9
Opponens pollicis	6.9–7.0
First lumbrical	6.9–7.0
Second lumbrical	7.4–7.4

(Data from Sunderland S, Ray LJ. Metrical and non-metrical features of the muscular branches of the median nerve. J Comp Neurol 1946;85:191.)

the median nerve arise primarily from its medial surface.[4]

The anterior interosseous nerve branches typically from the dorsoradial surface of the median nerve. It arises immediately distal to the flexor digitorum superficialis arch, 5 cm distal to the medial epicondyle. Characteristically, it innervates the portion of flexor digitorum profundus to the index and long fingers, the flexor pollicis longus, and the pronator quadratus.[15] The largest muscular branch of the median nerve, the anterior interosseous nerve, lies initially between the flexor digitorum superficialis and profundus. It passes dorsally, in the interval between the flexor pollicis longus and the flexor digitorum profundus, providing two to six branches to each of these muscles.[17] Accompanied by the anterior interosseous artery, the nerve descends in the forearm on the surface of the interosseous membrane. It passes deep to and supplies the pronator quadratus muscle. The nerve contains sensory afferent fibers for the intercarpal, radiocarpal, and distal radioulnar joints.

The palmar cutaneous branch of the median nerve arises 5 to 7 cm above the wrist. It travels with the epineurium of the median nerve for 16 to 25 mm before exiting along the palmar–radial surface, at the point of its emergence from the radial margin of the flexor digitorum superficialis (5–7 cm above the proximal wrist crease).[19] This purely sensory nerve courses distally along the ulnar side of the flexor carpi radialis, adherent to the undersurface of the antebrachial fascia. At the proximal edge of the transverse carpal ligament, it deviates ulnarly and enters its own tunnel within the ligament. It pierces the transverse carpal ligament in line with the ring finger and enters the subcutaneous tissue. The nerve divides within the ligament into medial and lateral branches, which supply the skin of the proximal two fifths of the palm on the radial side and the thenar eminence.[2]

Potential Points of Neural Compression in the Forearm

The median nerve and its branches may be compressed at several levels in the forearm. The most proximal is at the point where the main median nerve trunk passes under the lacertus fibrosus. Hypertrophy of the brachialis may compress the nerve between the muscle and the aponeurosis. Compression may occur as the nerve passes through the humeral and ulnar heads of the pronator teres. Fibrous bands between the two heads, fibrous origins of the deep head, fibrous arches beneath the superficial head, and hypertrophic pronator teres muscles have been reported.[16]

The third potential point of compression lies under the fibrous aponeurotic arch formed by the ulnohumeral and radial heads of the flexor digitorum superficialis. In the distal third of the forearm the median nerve may be compressed by one of two anomalous muscles. The palmaris profundus originates from the radius at the proximal origin of the flexor pollicis longus and inserts on the transverse carpal ligament. The flexor carpi radialis brevis originates near the proximal origin of the flexor pollicis longus and joins the flexor carpi radialis.[16]

The anterior interosseous nerve may be compressed near its origin, where it is least mobile. A tendinous origin of the ulnar head of the pronator teres or a distinct flexor digitorum superficialis arch is commonly found in compressive neuropathies of the anterior interosseous nerve.[2] Ulnar collateral and aberrant branches of the radial artery may cross the anterior interosseous nerve under the arch of the flexor digitorum superficialis. Gantzer's muscle is an anomalous muscle that originates from the medial humeral condyle and inserts into the flexor pollicis longus muscle. It arises posterior to the deep palmar compartment muscles and passes dorsal to the anterior interosseous nerve. The muscle, present in 45% of dissected limbs, has been implicated in compression neuropathy of the anterior interosseous nerve.[1]

Variations

Connections between the median and ulnar nerves are the most common variations in neural anatomy in the forearm (see Chap. 12). A connection often exists between the anterior interosseous and ulnar nerves within the substance of the flexor digitorum profundus. This intramuscular communication leads to multiple variations in patterns of innervation of the muscle. Dual innervation is most common in the long finger flexor, but may occur in all the digits. The median nerve, or rarely the ulnar nerve, may innervate the entire flexor digitorum profundus.[12]

The Martin-Gruber connection is an anomalous communication containing motor, sensory, or mixed fibers from the median or anterior interosseous nerve to the ulnar nerve in the proximal forearm (Fig. 25-4). It has been found in 15% (range 10%–44%) of dissected forearms.[12] The connection passes ulnarly and distally, adjacent to the ulnar artery, between the flexor digitorum superficialis and profundus muscles, occasionally innervating the latter. A looped communication, with its convexity distally, typically contains motor fibers. Straight connections are usually sensory. Some of the fibers from the median to ulnar nerves may innervate the thenar muscles via a second connection in the hand, the Riche-Cannieu connection, which is discussed later in this chapter. Preservation of intrinsic muscle function after high injury of the ulnar nerve, coupled with absence of function of the flexor carpi ulnaris and flexor digitorum profundus to the little finger, suggests a Martin-Gruber connection distal to the area of nerve injury. Connections from ulnar to median nerves are rare; when present, they occur in the distal forearm, palmar to the flexor digitorum profundus muscle.[9]

Other variations occur when the ulnar head of the pronator teres is absent (in 8% of cases), in which case the nerve passes either deep to (6%) or through (2%) the humeral head.[1]

Median Nerve in the Wrist and Hand

After emerging 5 cm above the wrist, the median nerve lies immediately palmar to the flexor digitorum superficialis tendons and dorsal to the transverse carpal ligament (Fig. 25-4). The boundaries of the carpal tunnel are the palmar radiocarpal ligaments dorsally, the scaphoid and trapezium radially, the transverse carpal ligament palmarly, and the hook of the hamate and pisiform ulnarly. After passing through the carpal tunnel, the motor branch to the thenar muscles arises from the radial surface of the median nerve. Variations occur in branching of the motor nerve (see Chap. 58).[11] Most commonly, an extraligamentous recurrent branch exits the main trunk at the distal margin of the transverse carpal ligament. It curves proximally and radially, entering the thenar musculature. This pattern has been noted in 46% of dissected specimens. The first branch is to the flexor pollicis brevis, followed by a branch to the abductor pollicis brevis. The nerve then passes deeply to innervate the opponens pollicis from its ulnar border. Variations in the nerve supply of the thenar muscles are discussed further in Chapter 12. Rarely, the motor branch innervates the first dorsal interosseous muscle.

After exiting the carpal tunnel, the median nerve splits into two divisions, radial and ulnar. The radial division further divides into the common digital nerve to the thumb, and the proper digital nerve to the radial side of the index finger. The proper palmar digital nerve supplies the first lumbrical muscle.[3] The common digital nerve to the thumb immediately divides into two proper digital nerves to supply the radial and ulnar sides of the thumb. The ulnar division of the median nerve branches into the common digital nerves of the second and

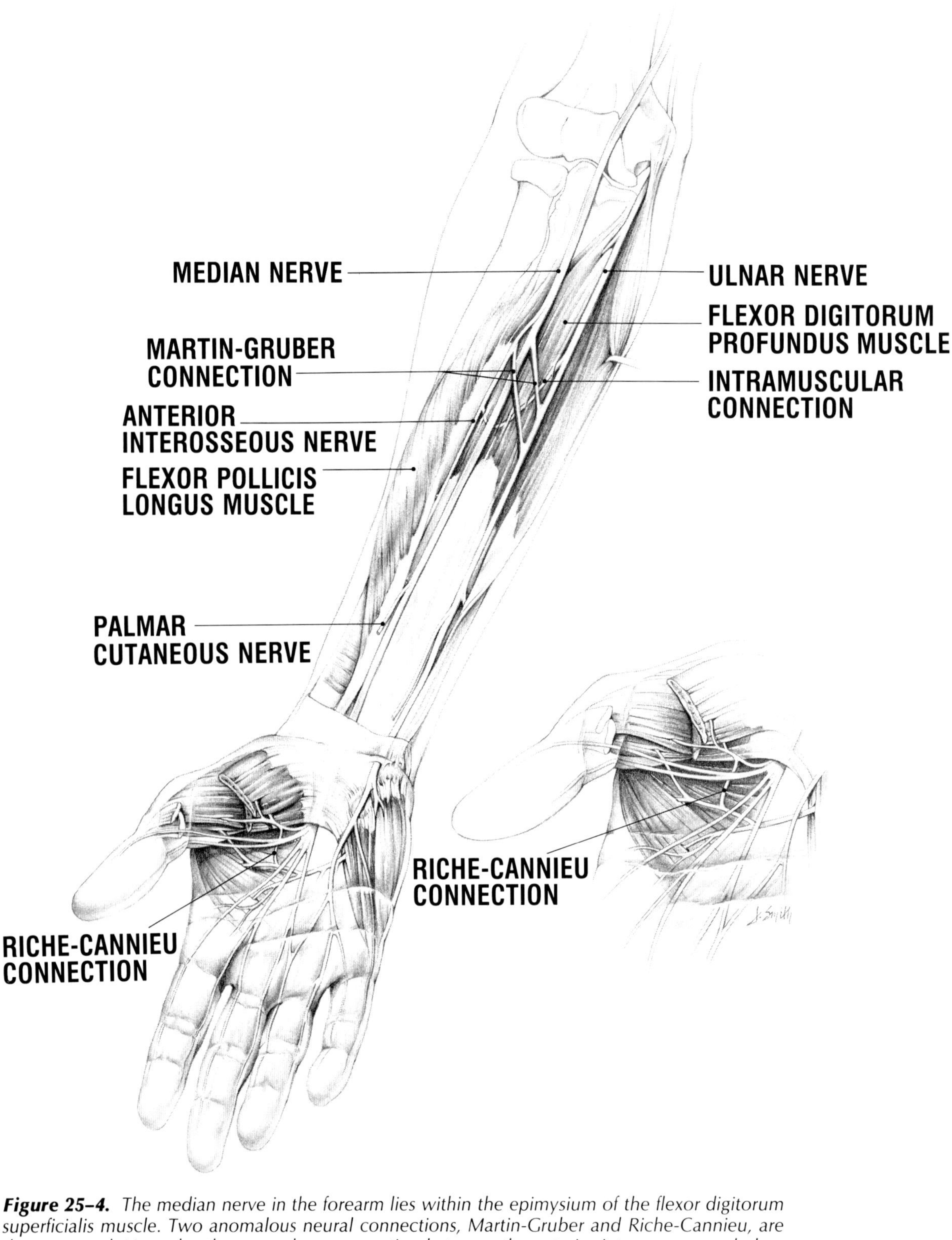

Figure 25–4. *The median nerve in the forearm lies within the epimysium of the flexor digitorum superficialis muscle. Two anomalous neural connections, Martin-Gruber and Riche-Cannieu, are demonstrated. Note also the anomalous connection between the anterior interosseous and ulnar nerves.*

third web spaces. The common digital nerve to the index and long fingers innervates the second lumbrical muscle. The common digital nerves divide at the junction of the middle and distal thirds of the metacarpal shafts, about 1 cm distal to the superficial palmar arch. In the palm the nerves are dorsal to the superficial palmar arch and palmar to the flexor tendons. Immediately after the division of the common digital nerves, at the level of the metacarpal necks, the proper digital nerves come to lie palmar (superficial) to the digital arteries. The nerves enter the fingers between the deep and superficial transverse metacarpal ligaments, maintaining their palmar relationship to the digital arteries.

Points of Neural Compression in the Wrist and Hand

Compression of the median nerve in the carpal tunnel is the most common compressive neuropathy of the upper limb.[2] The nerve is compressed within the canal beneath the transverse retinacular ligament. The palmar cutaneous branch of the median nerve may be compressed within its tunnel within the transverse retinacular ligament.

Variations

There are five major patterns of variability involving the median nerve in the hand and wrist. The most common involves the motor (thenar) branch, which may divide from the main trunk of the median nerve within the carpal canal and pass through the canal before curving proximally toward the thenar muscles. This pattern, the subligamentous pattern, is found in 31% of upper limbs.[10] The motor branch may perforate the transverse retinacular ligament at any point within its substance, where it may be compressed. This transligamentous pattern occurs in 23% of upper extremities. Rarely, the motor branch may exit the ulnar surface of the median nerve, or may become recurrent on top of the transverse carpal ligament before innervating the thenar muscles.

The second common pattern of variability, occurring in 7% of hands, concerns the branching of the motor nerve itself. Thin accessory branches leave the median nerve directly to innervate thenar muscles. True double motor branches are rare.

High divisions of the median nerve in the distal forearm occur in about 3% of upper limbs. This pattern is commonly associated with the presence of a median artery. An accessory lumbrical muscle to the index finger has been reported to divide the median nerve. The calibers of the ulnar and radial divisions determine the patterns of innervation. When the radial division is large, it may innervate the thenar muscles and the skin on the palmar aspect of the thumb, index, and long fingers. Large ulnar divisions may innervate the index, long, and ring fingers. The radial division always supplies the thumb and thenar muscles. Accessory branches may leave the radial or ulnar surface of the median nerve in the distal forearm, rejoining the nerve, or any of its branches, distally. These accessory branches, occurring in fewer than 1% of upper extremities, may pierce or pass under the transverse retinacular ligament.

Anomalous communications between the median and ulnar nerves in the hand may involve sensory or motor fibers. The most common communication is between the ulnar sensory branch in the palm and the common digital nerve to the third web space. This communication leads to dual innervation of the adjacent sides of the long and ring fingers.[8] The Riche-Cannieu communication, noted above, is a motor nerve connection between the terminal portion of the deep ulnar nerve and the recurrent thenar branch of the median nerve (Fig. 25-3). It occurs most commonly within the substance of the thenar eminence, but may occur in midpalm. Through this communication, which occurs in 50% of hands, the median nerve may innervate the third lumbrical muscle or rarely all of the lumbricals. In the former case, a low ulnar nerve lesion leads to clawing of the little finger only, while in the latter case a low ulnar nerve lesion does not lead to clawing at all.

Alternately, if a Martin-Gruber connection exists in the forearm, median nerve fibers are carried within the substance of the ulnar nerve. These fibers may then innervate the thenar muscles via the Riche-Cannieu connection, and a low median nerve lesion will not cause thenar palsy.[12]

OPERATIVE EXPOSURE

Median Nerve in the Arm

The medial approach provides the most extensile exposure of the median nerve in the arm. In the proximal third of the arm the nerve lies medially, in the sulcus between the coracobrachialis anteriorly and the long head of the triceps posteriorly. In the middle third, the nerve lies between the biceps brachii anteriorly and the medial intermuscular septum and the long head of the triceps posteriorly. The nerve courses laterally in the distal third of the arm and lies between the biceps brachii anteriorly and the brachialis muscle posteriorly.

Exposure of the median nerve throughout the upper extremity is accomplished with the patient positioned supine, with the arm on a hand table. The shoulder is abducted 90° and externally rotated. The forearm is positioned in supination and slight flexion. The coracoid process is palpated beneath the anterior fibers of the deltoid muscle and its position marked. The sulcus between the biceps brachii and the triceps is palpated and traced proximally to the anterior axillary fold (Fig. 25-5). A straight incision is made from this point distally toward the medial epicondyle, curving gently laterally, 4 cm above the epicondyle. The dissection is continued deeply to the brachial fascia, which is incised in line with the skin incision. Proximally, the median nerve lies lateral to the brachial artery (see Fig. 25-1). At the level of the insertion of the coracobrachialis (10–12 cm proximal to the medial epicondyle) it passes anterior to the artery and lies on its medial side. There are no branches of the median nerve in the arm (except the rare proximal branch to the pronator teres), and it is easily mobilized.[6]

Proximal extension of the exposure may be achieved by continuing the incision over the pectoralis major tendon, into the deltopectoral interval, toward the coracoid process. The pectoralis major is retracted medially and the deltoid laterally. Coracoid osteotomy and release of the pectoralis major U-shaped tendon from the humerus provide wider exposure.

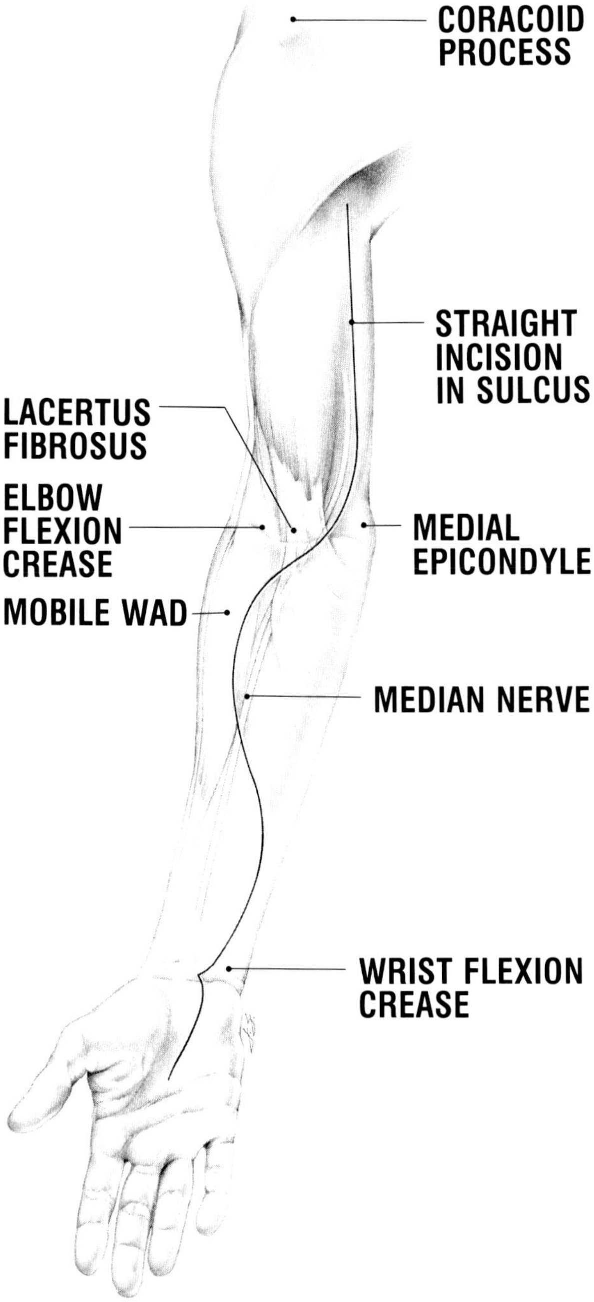

Figure 25–5. *Incision for operative exposure of the median nerve (see text).*

Median Nerve at the Elbow and in the Forearm

At the elbow the median nerve is covered by the lacertus fibrosus and antebrachial fascia. It lies on the surface of the brachialis, medial and posterior to the biceps and medial to the brachial artery. Two fingerbreadths above and lateral to the medial epicondyle, the nerve may be palpated in the sulcus between the biceps and the brachialis. After it passes beneath the bicipital aponeurosis, it is no longer palpable. The brachial artery is a useful landmark to palpate proximally and can be traced distally to the elbow flexion crease. The mobile wad (brachioradialis, extensor carpi radialis longus and brevis) should be palpated, and its ulnar border marked. Henry's mnemonic provides useful topographical anatomy.[4] The opposite hand is placed on the palmar surface of the supinated forearm, with the thenar eminence covering the medial epicondyle and the fingers pointing distally. The ring finger rests on the ulnar border of the forearm and the little finger is free. In this position, the thumb covers the pronator teres, the index finger covers the flexor carpi radialis, the long finger covers the palmaris longus, and the ring finger covers the flexor carpi ulnaris.

Elbow and Proximal Forearm (Extensile to Arm and Hand)

A variety of skin incisions has been proposed for exposure of the median nerve at the elbow and in the proximal forearm. The choice is determined best by the extent of exposure required, the pathologic process for which the nerve is being explored, and the associated structures requiring exposure. The surgeon should avoid making skin incisions that cross the elbow flexion crease at right angles. If the crease is crossed perpendicularly, 45° to 60° Z-plasty flaps should be created and transposed to prevent longitudinal scarring.

Authors' Preferred Method

The incision begins 2 cm above the medial epicondyle, over the medial intermuscular septum. At the elbow flexion crease the skin incision curves obliquely, laterally, and distally, over the bicipital aponeurosis. At the ulnar border of the mobile wad, the incision curves distally, continuing over the interval between the superficial flexor–pronator mass and the brachioradialis muscle (Fig. 25-5). In the midforearm, the incision curves obliquely medially and continues along the ulnar border of the distal third of the forearm toward the radial border of the pisiform. The incision ends at the proximal wrist crease but may be extended into the hand (see Chap. 61). Proximally, the extensile approach is continuous with the medial approach to the median nerve in the arm (see above). This approach is similar to the volar fasciotomy incision used for decompression of forearm compartment syndrome.[3] An alternative approach uses a zigzag incision in the proximal forearm, providing similar exposure.[2]

Proximal Forearm Combined with Exposure of the Radius

The anterior approach is most useful for median nerve decompression in the proximal forearm, particularly when exposure of the radius is necessary. The median cubital vein may be ligated. After identifying the median nerve and the brachial artery and veins proximally, the lacertus fibrosus and its aponeurotic expansion are incised to provide wide exposure of the median nerve proximal to the flexor–pronator muscles. Antebrachial fascia is incised throughout the length of the incision, the brachioradialis muscle is retracted laterally, and the radial artery is followed distally to the conjoined tendinous insertion of the pronator teres (see Fig. 25-3). The radial artery begins at the medial side of the biceps tendon and follows the humeral head of the pronator teres to the radial shaft. The artery is superficial to the muscle and is bound to it by fascial attachments. Ligation of the radial recurrent leash of vessels permits further radial retraction of the mobile wad and is necessary for exposure of the radial shaft. The insertion of the pronator teres is identified clearly on the radial shaft, the humeral head is isolated, and its tendon is divided distally. Retraction of the humeral head ulnarly exposes the median nerve distally to the level of the flexor digitorum superficialis arch. The anterior interosseous nerve may then be visualized

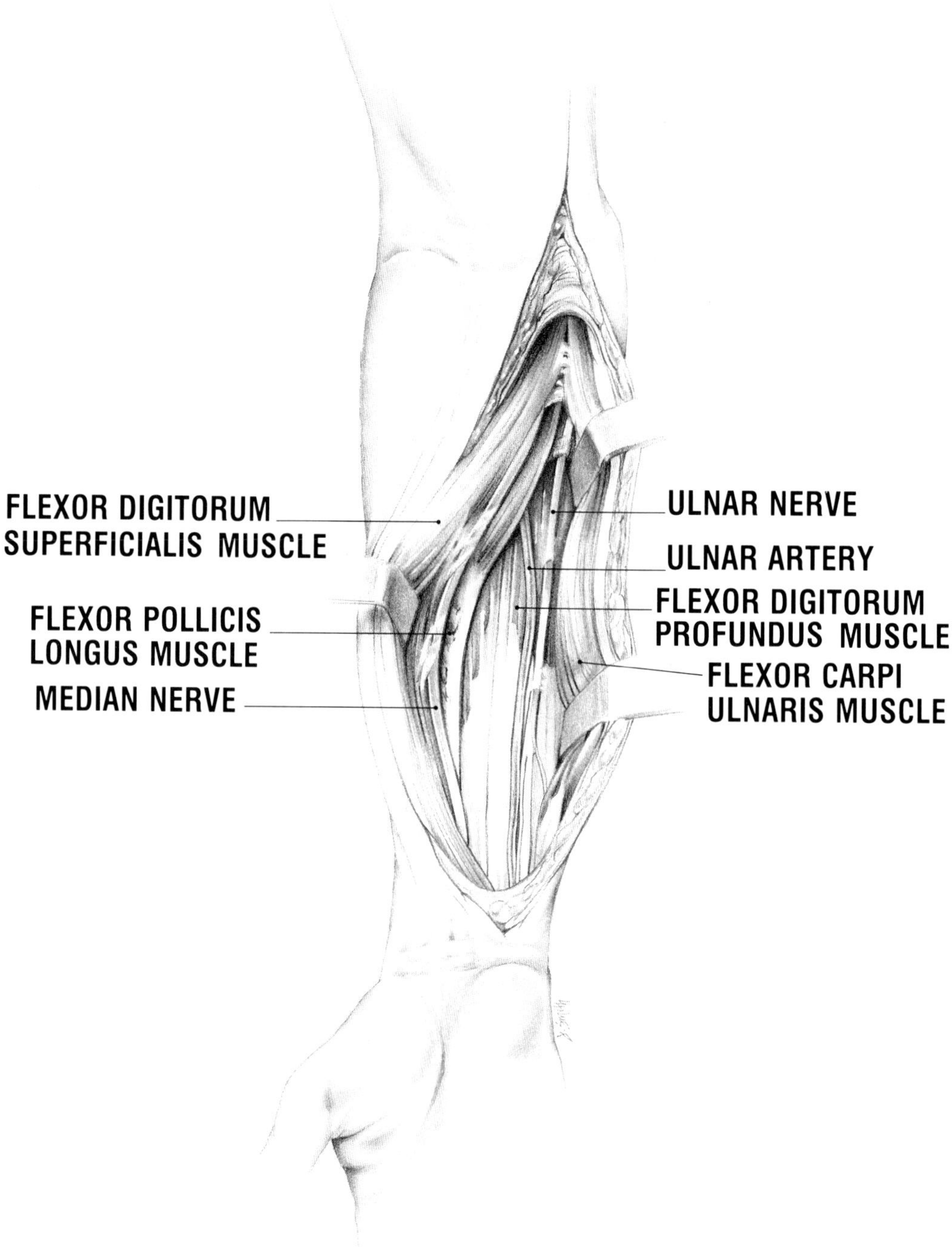

Figure 25–6. *Deep operative exposure of the median nerve in the forearm. Note that the median nerve lies within the epimysium of the flexor digitorum superficialis muscle.*

by gently retracting the ulnar head of the pronator teres.[2]

Anterior Interosseous Nerve and Median Nerve in the Middle to Distal Forearm

To expose further the median and anterior interosseous nerves, the flexor digitorum superficialis origin is divided.[6] The radial head of the flexor superficialis is identified and its origin is visualized by retracting the deep head of the pronator teres muscle radially. The radial origin, on the anterior oblique line of the radius, is incised sharply and elevated from the radius subperiosteally. The superficialis arch and proximal muscle belly are retracted ulnarly to expose the anterior interosseous and median nerves. Through this incision the median nerve may be traced distally to the wrist, where it lies between the flexor carpi radialis and the flexor digitorum superficialis. The nerve often lies within the epimysium of the flexor digitorum superficialis, and the epimysium must be incised to free the nerve. The ulnar nerve may be exposed by retracting the flexor carpi ulnaris medially. The ulnar neurovascular bundle is found on the epimysium of the flexor digitorum profundus.

Authors' Preferred Method

McConnell's approach, as described by Henry, is the preferred approach to both the median nerve and ulnar neurovascular bundle (Fig. 25-6).[4] Superficially, this medial approach uses the interval between the palmaris longus and the flexor carpi ulnaris. Deeply, the interval is between the flexors digitorum superficialis and profundus. The ulnar nerve is found between the two heads of origin of the flexor carpi ulnaris proximally and between the flexor digitorum profundus and flexor carpi ulnaris in the middle and distal forearm. Alternatively, the ulnar nerve may be found at the distal end of the incision, along the radial border of the flexor carpi ulnaris tendon. It is traced proximally into the interval between the flexors digitorum superficialis and profundus. The flexor carpi ulnaris is retracted medially and the flexor digitorum superficialis laterally. The median nerve is found within the epimysium of the flexor digitorum superficialis.

REFERENCES

1. Dellon AL, Mackinnon SE. Musculoaponeurotic variations along the course of the median nerve in the proximal forearm. J Hand Surg [Br] 1987; 12: 359–363.
2. Eversmann WW Jr. Entrapment and compression neuropathies. In: Green DP, ed. Operative hand surgery, ed. 2. New York: Churchill-Livingstone, 1988:1424–1432.
3. Gelberman RH, Zakaib GS, Mubarak SJ, et al. Decompression of foreman compartment syndromes. Clin Orthop 1978; 134:225–229.
4. Henry AK: Extensile exposure, ed. 2. New York: Churchill-Livingstone, 1973:94–99.
5. Hollingshead WH. Anatomy for surgeons: The back and limbs, vol. 3. Philadelphia: JB Lippincott, 1982: 341–529.
6. Inglis AE. Surgical exposure of peripheral nerves. In: Omer GE, Spinner M, eds. Management of peripheral nerve problems. Philadelphia: WB Saunders, 1980: 317–331.
7. Kameda Y. An anomalous muscle (accessory scapularis-teres latissimus) in the axilla penetrating the brachial plexus in man. Acta Anat 1976; 96:513.
8. Kaplan EB, Spinner M. Normal and anomalous innervation patterns in the upper extremity. In: Omer GE, Spinner M, eds. Management of peripheral nerve problems. Philadelphia: WB Saunders, 1980: 75–99.
9. Kerr AT. The brachial plexus of nerves in man, the variations in its formation and branches. Amer J Anat 1918; 23:285–288.
10. Lanz U. Anatomical variations of the median nerve in the carpal tunnel. J Hand Surg [Am] 1977; 2:44–53.
11. Linell EA. The distribution of nerves in the upper limb with reference to variabilities and their clinical significance. J Anat 1920–21; 55:79.
12. Mannerfelt L. Studies of anastomoses between the median and ulnar nerves in the forearm. Acta Universitatis Lundensis Sectio II, No. 6, 1964.
13. Mayfield FH. Compression syndromes of the shoulder girdle and arms. In: Vinken PJ, Bruyn GW, eds. Handbook of clinical neurology, vol 7: Diseases of nerves. New York: American Elsevier, 1970:441–444.
14. Miller R. Observations upon the arrangement of the axillary artery and brachial plexus. Amer J Anat 1939; 64:143.
15. Spinner M. Anterior interosseous nerve syndrome,

with special attention to its variations. J Bone Joint Surg [Am] 1970; 52:84–94.
16. Spinner M. Management of nerve compression lesions of the upper extremity. In: Omer GE, Spinner M, eds. Management of peripheral nerve problems. Philadelphia: WB Saunders, 1980:569–587.
17. Sunderland S. The innervation of the flexor digitorum profundus and lumbrical muscles. Anat Rec 1945; 93:317–321.
18. Sunderland S, Ray LJ. Metrical and non-metrical features of the muscular branches of the median nerve. J Comp Neurol 1946; 85:191.
19. Taleisnik J. The palmar cutaneous branch of the median nerve and the approach to the carpal tunnel. J Bone Joint Surg [Am] 1973; 55:1212–1217.
20. Warwick R, Williams PL, ed. Gray's anatomy, ed 35 [Br]. Philadelphia: WB Saunders, 1973:1041–1043.

26

Median Nerve Repairs: The Results of Treatment

William P. Cooney

AUTHOR'S KEY POINTS

- In considering results of median nerve repair, both patient-related factors (age, type of injury, interval from injury to repair) and operative repair–related factors (technique of repair, magnification, level of injury) are of prime importance.
- While sophisticated methods of clinical and electrophysiological assessment have been introduced, sensory and motor examination, following the British Medical Research Council's program, has become standard for assessing the results of nerve repair.
- The results of repair of the median nerve in adults have ranged from M3/S3 (fair) to M4/S3+ (good) in most clinical series. While thenar motor strength is regained in 50% of patients, recovery of two-point discrimination is not generally attained.
- While conclusive clinical reports demonstrating efficacy have not been provided, group fascicular repair under magnification is currently favored for the median nerve in the distal third of the forearm.
- Results with median nerve grafting, indicated for nerve gaps greater than 2.5 cm or failure of 8-O nylon suture to maintain nerve stump coaptation, have been comparable to those reported for primary epineural repair.

The treatment of peripheral nerve injuries has changed significantly since the substantive reports of Woodall and Beebe[49] following study of World War II injuries from the United States and Seddon's review regarding the British war experience.[38,39] Since their discouraging reports of incomplete or poor return of motor and sensory nerve function, a number of investigators have identified important factors that lead to more reliable nerve recovery and, as a result, improved function of the injured extremities. The effects of age,[14,26,33] type of injury,[29,39] length of time from injury to nerve repair,[4,7,21] and length of nerve gap[4,33,34] correlate directly with final results. The elapsed time from nerve repair to assessment is also considered a significant variable, since recovery measured at 1 year has not been as good as that measured at 3 to 4 years.[26] Studies that average only 1 to 2 years of follow-up are discounted in comparison to longitudinal studies of similar patients.[46]

Despite widespread recognition of the importance of these factors, there have been few well-controlled, prospective studies comparing results in a meaningful way.[16,19,26,28] Thus, definite conclusions regarding the optimal factors for median nerve repair have not been presented previously. Results from war-related injuries[36,40] are considerably different from civilian nerve injuries[24,41] because of the intensity and extent of the injuries. Cooperative studies involving a number of medical centers should provide the numbers of cases needed to achieve statistical significance as long as operative and patient-related factors are controlled.

In the assessment of results of repair of injuries to the median nerve, both patient-related factors (age, type of injury, time since injury) and operative repair–related factors (method of repair, magnification, location of the injury, topographical anatomy, nature of the vascular bed, and the skill and experience of the surgeon) are of considerable importance. Grading of sensory and motor recovery with a scheme of universal application, combined with a controlled group of patient and injury-related factors, is required in order to compare functional results. Animal studies provide new concepts and guidelines for clinical use, but direct extrapolation to the clinical setting is not justified without careful interchange with the eventual outcome.

UNIFORM ASSESSMENT OF CLINICAL RESULTS

The Medical Research Council (MRC) (London, 1943) provided a reliable and reproducible means of assessing function following peripheral nerve surgery (Tables 26-1, 26-2).[29] Some have objected that the definition of specific end points is unclear and that more detailed subclassification (Table 26-3) is needed to define sensibility[35] and motor function.[23,27] Young and coworkers[50] argued, for example, that the category S3+ lacks precision and

Table 26-1. *Median Nerve: Motor Recovery*

Level of Motor Recovery	*Classification**
No contraction	M0
Return of perceptible contraction in proximal muscles	M1
Return of perceptible contraction in distal muscles	M2
Return of contraction sufficient to act against resistance or gravity	M3
Return of muscle(s) to act against strong resistance and independent movement	M4
Return of full muscle strength	M5
Median Nerve Specific Test	
Abduction of thumb against force Full finger flexion without resistance	M3
Full abduction/opposition with 50% pinch Full finger flexion with 50% grip	M4
Normal grip and pinch strength (80% of uninjured side)	M5

* *Medical Research Council classification of functional recovery*

Table 26-2. Median Nerve: Recovery of Sensibility

Recovery of Sensibility	**Classification***
Absence of sensibility in the autonomous area†	S-0
Recovery of deep pain sensibility (response to pin prick)	S-1
Recovery of superficial sensibility (some response to touch and pain stimulus)	S-2
Full recovery of pain and touch (protective sensibility not localized, moving two-point discrimination is greater than 15 mm)	S-3
Localization of stimulus (pain and touch; moving and static two-point discrimination is 7–15 mm)	S-3+
Complete recovery of sensibility (moving and static two-point discrimination 3–6 mm)	S-4

** Medical Research Council classification of functional recovery*
† All testing is within the autonomous zone of the median nerve, the palmar surface of the index or long finger.

that the description "some two-point discrimination" is virtually meaningless. Dellon and Mackinnon stated that a major flaw exists in the classification of sensory recovery, since there is no separation of painful and painless sensations.[10] They also objected to quantitation of sensory recovery in some studies by measurement of static two-point discrimination, where research has demonstrated that *moving* two-point discrimination is the best predictor of hand function.[9] They noted that tactile gnosis and object identification correlate well with moving two-point discrimination.

The measurement of motor recovery, which dates back to the work of Highet and Sanders,[17] also is controversial. In Highet and Sanders' classification, the level of return of contraction for proximal and distal muscles is graded by clinical examination of the muscle. A level of M3 is the minimum accepted indication of some level of useful function. There is no clear definition, however, of M4, which requires that "all synergistic and independent movements are possible," in addition to the muscle being "sufficiently powerful to act against resistance." It is difficult to discern when muscle recovery advances from M3 to M4 since there is no gradient to full recovery (M5). A definition of specific tests to indicate the level of return is beneficial.[19]

To improve the rating criteria for peripheral nerve return, some authors have added factors of functional use, such as writing, button fastening, key turning, and handling of tools.[27,39] Moberg's pick-up test, a timed test of hand function, has been used in several studies.[2,4,39] In addition to use of the MRC criteria, disabling symptoms of pain from neuromas,[24,25] cold sensitivity,[25] and loss of sensation for pain, temperature, and touch[19,27] are noted in reports assessing the results of nerve repair.

To improve the grading of low vs high median nerve lesions, Moneim isolated proximal (extrinsic) from distal (intrinsic) muscles.[33] He defined functional motor recovery as a level of M3 or greater. To better determine functional strength after low median and ulnar nerve injuries, key pinch and extension of the fingers against resistance was required for M3; strong key pinch and ability to abduct and adduct the fingers was M4; and full strength of pinch and grasp was needed for M5. For low median nerve injuries alone (see Table 26-1), abduction and opposition of the thumb were assessed; for greater return, the level of pinch and grip strength were measured.

Clinical neurophysiologic studies and sensory detection threshold studies (Table 26-4) have also been suggested to quantitate the level of recovery following peripheral nerve repair.[1,3,13] Dyck studied median nerve repair by nerve conduction stud-

Table 26–3. *Functional Sensory Recovery Score*

Test	Partial Points for Each Test	Total Points for Each Test
1. Sharp vs dull discrimination		15
2. Temperature:		15
hot (approximately 100°)	7.5	
cold (approximately 32°)	7.5	
3. Vibration with tuning forks:		10
30 cps	5	
256 cps	5	
4. Moving touch:		10
single point	5	
two points between 10 mm and 20 mm	2.5	
two points < 10 mm	5	
5. Static two-point discrimination:		10
between 10 mm and 20 mm	5	
< 10 mm	10	
6. Thickness (distinguishing between blocks 1 cm, 2 cm, and 3 cm thick):		10
two blocks	5	
three blocks	10	
7. Texture (differentiating between textures of canvas cloth, lock component Velcro, and medium-grade sandpaper):		15
any two	10	
any three	15	
8. Sharp identification using four objects (two 5-mm diameter cylinders, one 1 mm deep and one 4 mm deep, and two 5-mm rectangles, one 1 mm deep and one 4 mm deep):		15
identification of any two	5	
identification of any three	10	
identification of any four	15	

(From Lewis RC, Tenny J, Irvine D. The restoration of sensibility by nerve translocation. Bull Hosp Jt Dis Orthop Inst 1984; 44:290, with permission)

ies, needle electromyography, maximal isometric twitch recordings of thenar muscle activity evoked by supramaximal stimulation, estimation of tactile and vibratory detection thresholds (a computer-assisted sensory examination), and tactile hemidigit localization tests.[12] A statistically significant increase in index pulp tactile detection threshold (TDT) and vibratory detection threshold (VDT) was present in the injured extremity after median nerve repair when compared to the contralateral side.

Kanakamedala and Hong used electrophysiological studies to evaluate median nerve regeneration after incomplete transection, reporting the value of nerve conduction studies and measurement of compound muscle and nerve action potentials.[20] They noted that "prolonged distal latencies and compound nerve action potential amplitudes correlated with the degree of regeneration . . . the decrease in amplitude of the evoked potential related to conduction block, axon loss or to the temporal dispersion of the compound potential resulting from differential slowing of conduction along different nerve fibers."[20]

More recent studies have combined clinical evaluation of muscle power, sensibility, and object identification with neurophysiologic testing of motor amplitude and distal latency and sensory action potentials to analyze end results.[6,16,27,41,44,45,50]

Table 26-4. *Detection Thresholds of Touch-Pressure and Vibratory Sensations of Pulp of Index Finger of Patients with Median Nerve Injury*

	Touch-Pressure*†		Vibration††	
Case	No. Sensitive	Threshold (in mg)	No. Sensitive	Threshold in μm
1	9 (9)	7.6 (6.3)	9 (8 super)	0.9 (−1.9)
2	9 (9)	6.8 (6.2)	9 (9)	3.5 (2.5)
3	9 (9)	6.9 (5.2)	9 (2 super)	3.6 (0.1)
4	9 (9)	6.9 (4.9)	9 (8 super)	2.9 (−1.5)
5	9 (9)	6.7 (5.8)	9 (1 super)	3.0 (−0.1)

* Pulp of index finger; results on contralateral finger are in parentheses; super = supersensitive.
† For difference between nerve-injured and contralateral fingers, $p = 0.004$ (Student's paired t test).
†† For difference between nerve-injured and contralateral fingers, $p = 0.003$ (Student's paired t test).
(With permission from Dyck PJ, Lambert EH, Wood MB, Linscheid RL: Assessment of nerve regeneration and adaptation after median nerve reconnection and digital neurovascular flap transfer. Neurology 1988; 38:1586.)

These findings, while providing a higher level of functional testing, are of little value standing alone, however, since they cannot easily be compared with other studies unless they use the same testing procedures.

From a practical viewpoint, clinical groups have had neither the technical capability to perform many of the exacting clinical studies[45] nor the ability to carry out in-depth neurophysiologic studies using sophisticated computer sampling.[12] We have been better served by comparative studies using the MRC program, modifying the broad classifications and criteria so that adaptations are made for specific nerve lesions (eg, separating low from high median, ulnar, and radial nerve injuries and dividing them into respective sensory and motor functional levels). If patient-related factors are controlled (particularly age, time from injury, type of trauma, and time of follow-up), comparative longitudinal studies can be obtained.

RESULTS OF PRIMARY REPAIR OF MEDIAN NERVE LESIONS

Primary repair connotes direct suture within 7 to 10 days of complete nerve transection. Nerve grafts are excluded. Either epineural, perineural, or combined epineural-perineural repairs have been recommended. Epineural repair includes group fascicular repairs involving inner epineural fibrous tissue. Using the functional criteria of motor and sensory return, most studies interpret useful recovery of median nerve function as M3 and S2+.[11,22,32,38] A motor level of M3 and sensory level of S2+ provides little more than superficial cutaneous pain and tactile sensation, however, and muscle return sufficient only to achieve mild resistance (antigravity).

To have good to excellent clinical results, most authors believe that sensory return of S3+ to S4 and motor return of M4 are needed. With primary nerve repair, one anticipates a return of function to these levels. Previous reports demonstrate, however, that predictably good function following median nerve repair in the wrist and forearm is unusual. Larsen and Posch, for example, reported that 35% of patients had motor return only to M2 and 65% to M4[22]; Sakallarides recorded 50% return to M2/M3 and 12% to M4[37]; Lijftogt and associates had 21 of 25 median injuries return to S3/S3+, and 8 of 25 (32%) had fair results (M3+); 14 of 25 (56%) had good results (S4/M4) (Fig. 26-1).[24] Jongen and Van Twisk reported on 22 primary repairs at the wrist with 2-year follow-up, 12 of which were of the median nerve.[19] Ten of 12 cases were in the M3/S3 (fair) to M4/S3+ (good) category, and they concluded that primary neurorrhaphy is the treatment of choice for serious median nerve injuries. The poor results were associated with neuromas and sympathetic dystrophy.

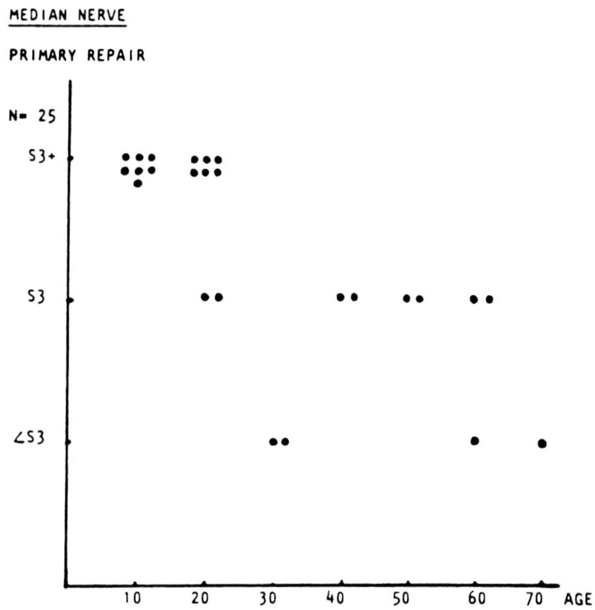

Figure 26–1. *Sensory recovery following primary repair of the median nerve according to patient age. S3–S3+ provides useful sensibility. (Reprinted with permission from Lijftogt HJA, Dykstra R, Storm R, Van Leeuwen B. Results of microsurgical treatment of nerve injuries of the wrist. Netherlands J Surg 1987;39:172.)*

Median Nerve Repair by Fascicular Alignment and Suture

A persistent controversy is the relative value of primary epineural median nerve repair vs primary fascicular repair. Tupper examined thirteen patients with median nerve repairs, eight with epineural repairs, and four with fascicular repairs.[45] The age of the patient, type of injury, tension, and other factors such as delay interval to repair were examined closely. He concluded that epineural and fascicular nerve repairs performed under the operating microscope produced almost identical results in adults (children were not included in his study). A potential for increased damage to nerve axonal transmission associated with removing the protective epineurium, part of the technique of fascicular repair, was noted. The potential for increased fibrosis appears to outweigh the possible advantages of improved alignment of nerve fascicles.

Magnification and Other Variables

Controversy surrounds the use of magnification for median nerve repair. Marsh and Barton questioned whether the operating microscope improved results.[26] In a controlled sequential study, they noted that primary epineural repair without the microscope produced results equal to combined epineural-perineural suture with microscopic augmentation (Table 26-5). Muscle power scores on the MRC scale and sensibility measured by moving two-point discrimination showed better values in the group that did *not* have microscopic assistance, despite a delay in treatment favoring the microscopic repair group. There was no statistically significant difference between the two groups ($p > 0.05$) when the follow-up period was equalized at 5 years.

The question of whether an operating microscope is necessary was also studied by McManamny.[27] For primary repair of ulnar and median nerves, he found that there was no significant difference between use of the operating microscope and magnification loupes. Other injuries and patient-related factors appeared more important. In his study, the only factor showing a significant difference was age, with children clearly showing a greater degree of recovery than adults.

Vahvanen, Gripenberg, and Nuutinen support the observation of improved results in children in a report of 38 cases of peripheral nerve injury in the hand and wrist.[49] Following twenty primary median neurorrhaphies with epineural suture, there were eight good (40%), ten fair (50%), and only two poor results. A fair to good result had a minimum of 6 to 15 mm two-point discrimination.

Suture Technique

If there is an operative technique associated with improved functional return following primary median nerve repair, our experience indicates that it is group fascicular suture, isolating motor from sensory fascicles. While a number of experimental studies have addressed this question, there are few studies in humans. Gaul reported experience with group fascicle identification in the repair of ten median and four ulnar nerves with minimum two years follow-up.[14] Using a patient "wake-up"

Table 26–5. *Microscopic-Assisted vs Loupe Magnification Repair of Peripheral Nerves*

	Mean Scores in 1982			Mean Scores in 1985	
	Microscope (n = 11)	No microscope (n = 13)	p	Microscope (n = 9)	No microscope (n = 9)
Muscle power	55	69	0.20	73	66
Moving 2PD	9	15	0.29	20	19
Localization	83	95	0.11	88	99
Shapes	32	48	0.02	50	43
Textures	36	55	0.07	40	47
Pick up	54	66	0.31	77	62
Motor amplitude	33	58	0.01	57	67
Motor velocity	99	92	0.39	97	86
Motor latency	72	84	0.07	75	81
SAP peak	15	32	0.03	20	31
SAP cumulative	25	42	0.13	27	41
SAP velocity	78	84	0.48	71	78
SAP dispersion	68	81	0.26	82	78

All scores are expressed as a percentage of the normal side. All are calculated in such a way that a higher score means better function. 2PD, two-point discrimination; SAP, sensory action potential; p, the probability value associated with a two-tailed t-test of differences of means in 1982; in 1985 there were no significant differences.

(From Marsh D, Barton N. Does the use of the operating microscope improve the results of peripheral nerve suture? J Bone Joint Surg [Br] 1987; 69:628, with permission.)

technique combined with proximal fascicular identification and distal motor nerve stimulation or dissection, Gaul was impressed with the level of motor recovery in the muscles of opposition. He noted that nine of ten patients regained normal function. Studies on the fascicular orientation of peripheral nerves have supported the concept of isolating major motor and sensory bundles.[8,18,48] Critical to this technique is a knowledge of the internal topography of the median nerve. Conclusive clinical reports demonstrating the value of group fascicular nerve repair have not been provided, however.

RESULTS FROM NERVE GRAFTING

Based on the belief that even under ideal conditions a small zone of scar tissue will develop at the site where an injured nerve has been repaired, peripheral nerve grafting has been promoted by Millesi and collaborators.[30–32] As a result of extensive clinical experience, they propose nerve resection and interposition grafting in all but sharp localized injuries. Nerve grafts, which are felt to minimize the effects of tension at the repair site, present "to the axon sprouts the same conditions as a distal stump."[32] Median nerve grafts are indicated for segmental injuries, nerve gaps of 2.5 cm or more, combined neurolysis and nerve repair, poor vascular bed, crush injury where the specific level or extent of injury is unknown, and open nerve injuries.[10]

In a summary of early results, Berger and Millesi reported on 38 cases of median nerve grafts.[4] They noted sensory return to S3+ or S4 in fifteen (40%), S3 in twenty-two (57.9%), and S2 in one. In a group of 28 patients, motor function in seventeen reached the M4 or M5 level (60.7%), six reached M3 (21.4%), and only five did not achieve a useful level of recovery. Shorter nerve grafts (2.5 to 5 cm) were superior to longer grafts.

Pluchino and Luccarelli argued that interfascicular nerve suture with autografts was the treatment of choice for all peripheral nerve injuries and reported on 30 patients followed for 2 to 7 years.[36] Using MRC criteria they evaluated 15 patients with median nerve lesions. Follow-up demonstrated that seven cases attained the M4-5 level (46.6%), while five cases had grade M3 (33.3%). A total of 80% acceptable results was achieved. Sensory recovery was good (S3–S3+) in 13 cases (86.6%). Poor results were related to either the proximal level of the lesion, length of graft (>12 cm), or delay from injury to repair. The authors agreed with Millesi that primary repair was indicated only when a gap of less than 1 to 2 cm existed and there was no tension at the repair site.

In another excellent study that considered the variables of age, length of graft, and level of injury, Haase, Bjerre, and Simesen reported results of interfascicular grafting for 37 median and 27 ulnar nerve injuries.[16] Useful motor recovery (M3 or higher) was achieved in 84%, and sensory return with measurable two-point discrimination was found in 63% of the low median nerve injuries (Fig. 26-2). The results were superior to other civilian and wartime studies that have included both primary and secondary nerve repairs (Tables 26-6, 26-7).[17,23,37,38,47] The authors emphasized careful clinical examination of moving two-point discrimination within one autonomous zone of digits without neurologic cross-over (index and little finger) as well as muscle testing of pure median-nerve innervated muscles.

In the United States, the results of peripheral nerve grafting have been less encouraging. Young, Wray, and Weeks reported on nerve grafts in 38 patients, 11 of whom had injuries to the median nerve.[50] They used group fascicular repair with magnification. While they noted sensory recovery of S3 or better in 63%, they found functional motor repair of M4 or better in only one patient. They compared these results with several other series on nerve grafts and found the results of poorer motor function difficult to explain.[4,31,40]

Moneim reported experience with 21 patients,

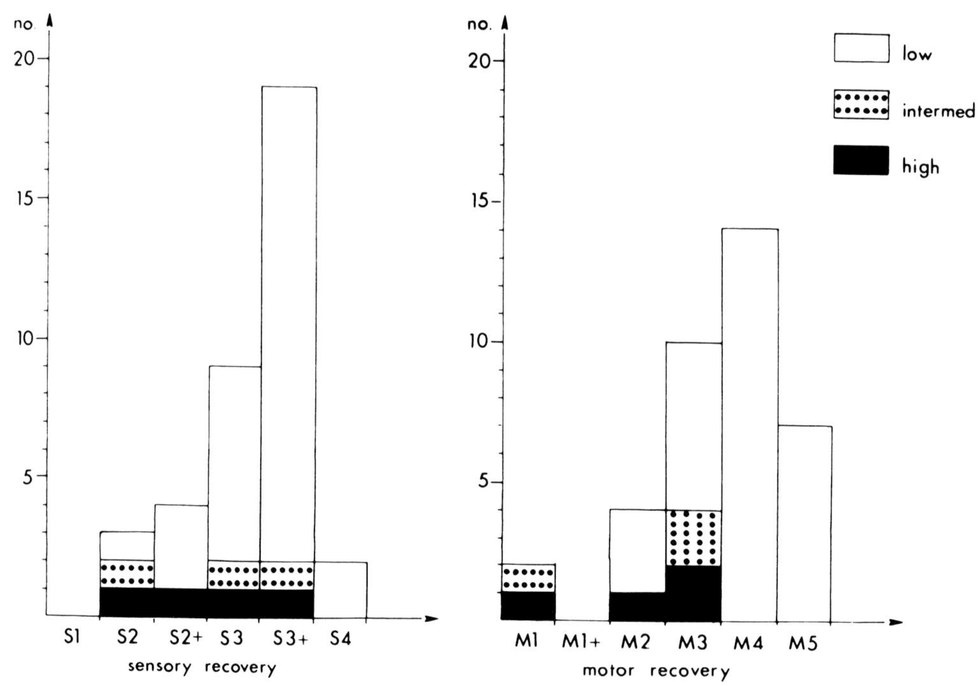

Figure 26–2. *Sensory (S1–S4) and motor (M1–M5) recovery following pain, intermediate and high median nerve transection, and repair by nerve grafts. (Reprinted with permission from Haase J, Bjerre P, Simesen K. Median and ulnar nerve transections treated with microsurgical interfascicular cable grafting with autogenous sural nerve. J Neurosurg 1980;53:73.)*

Table 26–6. *Functional Results Following Grafting of the Median Nerve*

Recovery Grade*	Sakellarides†	%	Nicholson & Seddon†	%	Zachary†	%	Millesi et al.‡	%	Haase et al.‡	%
M4	9	43%	20	65%	41	40%	13	81%	21	90%
M3	22		14		22		4		61	
M2	13		11		41		1		3	
M1+	0		7		54		0		0	
M1 & M0	28		0		0		3		0	
Total	72		52		158		21		30	
S4 & S3+	3		13		16		12		19	
S3	14	53%	21	79%	46	55%	19	100%	7	97%
S2+	23		8		18		0		3	
S2	17		11		65		0		1	
S1 & S0	19		0		0		0		0	
Total	76		53		145		31		30	

* *Grade according to Zachary.*
† *Studies of epineural suture.*
‡ *Study with interfascicular nerve grafting.*
(From Millesi H. Nerve grafting. Clin Plast Surg 1984; 11:108, with permission.)

Table 26–7. *Sensory (S1–S4) and Motor (M1–M5) Recovery Following Intermediate and High Median Nerve Transection and Repair by Nerve Grafts*

Recovery Grade*	Sakellarides†	%	Nicholson & Seddon†	%	Zachary†	%	Millesi et al.‡	%	Haase et al.‡	%
M4	0	11%	2	43%	13	24%	4	86%	0	57%
M3	1		1		19		2		4	
M2	4		2		48		1		1	
M1+	0		1		41		0		0	
M1 & M0	4		1		11		0		2	
Total	9		7		132		7		7	
S4 & S3+	0		1		8		4		2	
S3	1	11%	2	43%	36	51%	2	86%	2	71%
S2+	0		0		24		0		1	
S2	4		4		65		1		2	
S1 & S0	4		0		0		0		0	
Total	9		7		133		7		7	

* *Grade according to Zachary.*
† *Studies of epineural suture.*
‡ *Study with interfascicular nerve grafting.*
(From Haase J, Bjerre P, Simesen K. Median and ulnar nerve transections treated with microsurgical interfascicular cable grafting with autogenous sural nerve. J Neurosurg 1980: 53, 73, with permission.)

in whom interfascicular nerve grafting was used for the median nerve in 10.[33] Indications for nerve grafts were a nerve gap of over 2.5 cm or failure of 8-0 nylon to hold a nerve together when adjacent joints were placed in a range of motion from full extension to slight flexion. Moneim isolated high from low median nerve injuries in examining his results and found that four of seven nerve repairs within the distal forearm or wrist achieved M3 to M5 motor return. The remaining three did not have functional (M3 or better) motor recovery. With high median nerve grafts, M4 was obtained with testing of proximal muscles, but there was no recovery (M0–M2) noted in the intrinsic muscles. Sensory recovery, however, was S3 or above in four patients.

In a recent analysis of results by Millesi (Table 26-8), 39 patients undergoing interfascicular nerve grafts were assessed.[30] The degree of sensory return was good to very good (S3–S3+). Motor return was usually to M3+ or M4. Important associated factors of age, interval, and length of defect were included. Millesi believed that with the addition of the operating microscope, free nerve grafting has become as reliable a procedure as primary neurorrhaphy when it is performed under favorable conditions. Nerve grafting is felt to be superior if tension exists at the repair site.

Table 26–8. *Motor and Sensory Recovery*

	Mixed Innervation*			***M4–5***			***M3***			***M2***		
	Age (yrs)	*Interval (months)*	*Defect (cm)*	*Age (yrs)*	*Interval (months)*	*Defect (cm)*	*Age (yrs)*	*Interval (months)*	*Defect (cm)*	*Age (yrs)*	*Interval (months)*	*Defect (cm)*
S3+ −4	21	4	5.0	19	6	2.5				23	4	7.0
	20	1	2.0	22	8	8.0						
	25	2	3.5	18	7	7.0						
	40	2	2.0	21	2	6.0						
	27	2	3.5	10	9	5.0						
	49	1	6.5	9	2	5.0						
	44	8	5.0	20	3	5.0						
	7	2	2.0	46	5	3.5						
	13	4	4.0	50	2	2.0						
				10	4	4.0						
S3	21	4	4.5	35	6	2.0	43	8	5.0	41	28	15.0
	21	2	6.0	19	2	4.0	44	36	12.0			
	46	4	2.0	50	2	3.0	48	18	7.0			
	24	4	5.0				25	2	5.0			
	27	2	4.0				6	5	4.0			
	52	12	4.5									
	30	9	10.0									
	23	5	4.0									
	61	3	4.0									
S2	26	11	16.0									

(From Haase J, Bjerre P, Simesen I. Median and ulnar nerve transections treated with microsurgical interfascicular cable grafting with autogenous sural nerve. J Neurosurg 1980; 53:73, with permission.)

VASCULARIZED NERVE GRAFTS

When large nerve defects are present and when the neural bed is either scarred or relatively avascular as a result of associated trauma, the use of a vascularized nerve graft has been suggested (see Chap. 40).[43] While free vascularized grafts have been applied clinically,[10,11] the basic research question of whether a vascularized nerve graft increases nerve regeneration has not yet been answered.[40] With respect to median nerve injuries, in particular, our own experience has been limited to two patients with extensive forearm trauma in which free vascularized nerve grafts were used. Protective sensibility with M3 motor was acquired in one, but sensory only in the other. Further clinical experience is needed to evaluate the potential benefit in selected cases.

Another option for median nerve reconstruction that has been used for over 40 years is a vascularized nerve transfer. First described by St. Clair Strange in 1947,[42] the pedicle ulnar nerve transfer is a procedure that appears to work well. Usually performed in two stages, it consists of rotating the uninjured part of the ulnar nerve on a vascular pedicle, either proximally or distally, to replace the median nerve. Alpar and Brooks report experience with this technique in six children and three adults.[2] Good sensory return was present in the children, and thenar muscle return was noted if the procedure was done within 1 year of injury. Results in the adults were not as good.

Using a slightly different technique, Greenberg and coworkers reported on seven patients with the St. Clair Strange operation.[15] Five patients, followed for a mean of 10 years, achieved protective median nerve sensibility with accurate localization, stereognosis, and vibration responses in a majority of digits. Intrinsic hand muscle function was not regained, however. The level of sensory and motor return was similar to that reported in several previous papers.[5,40] In a report by Louis and Eckenrode, three patients undergoing this procedure were studied carefully.[21] These authors reported subjective improvement in sensibility, but objective testing was less convincing. While light touch and vibration were regained, there was poor localization of touch and no object or two-point discrimination.

Transfer of the ulnar nerve on a vascular pedicle based on the ulnar artery is another reported method of median nerve reconstruction, but preliminary results only are described in one patient.[7] The St. Clair Strange procedure remains limited to cases of severe forearm crush injuries or fractures resulting in Volkman's ischemia. In a well-vascularized soft-tissue bed, there are no current indications for a vascularized nerve graft. Until such evidence points to the superiority of vascular grafts over conventional techniques, nonvascularized nerve grafts remain the procedure of choice for cases where there are median nerve defects.

REFERENCES

1. Almquist E, Olofsson O. Sensory-nerve-conduction velocity and two-point discrimination in suture nerves. J Bone Joint Surg [Am] 1970; 52:791–796.
2. Alpar EK, Brooks DM. Long-term results of ulnar to median nerve pedicle grafts. Hand 1978; 10:61–64.
3. Ballantyne JP, Campbell MJ. Electrophysiologic study after surgical repair of sectioned human peripheral nerve. J Neurol Neurosurg Psychiatry 1973; 36:797–805.
4. Berger A, Millesi H. Nerve grafting. Clin Orthop 1978; 133:49–55.
5. Braun RM. Epineurial nerve suture. Clin Orthop 1981; 163:50–56.
6. Buchthal F, Kuhl V. Nerve conduction, tactile sensibility, and the electromyogram after suture or compression of peripheral nerve: A longitudinal study in man. J Neurol Neurosurg Psychiatry 1979; 42:436–451.
7. Chase RA. The severely injured upper limb—to amputate or reconstruct? Arch Surg 1970; 100: 382–392.
8. Chow JA, Van Beck AL, Belos ZJ, Meyer DL, Johnson MC. Anatomical basis for repair of ulnar and median nerves in the distal part of the forearm by group fascicular suture and grafting. J Bone Joint Surg [Am] 1986; 68:273–280.
9. Dellon AL, Kallman CM. Evaluation of functional sensation in the hand. J Hand Surg 1983; 8:865–870.
10. Dellon AL, Mackinnon SE. Surgery of the peripheral nerves, chapter 4. New York: Thieme Med Pub, 1988:89–129.
11. Doi K, Kuwata N, Kawakami F, Tamaru K, Kawai

S. The free vascularized sural nerve graft. Microsurgery 1984; 5:175–184.
12. Dyck PJ, Lambert EH, Wood MB, Linscheid RL. Assessment of nerve regeneration and adaptation after median nerve reconnection and digital neurovascular flap transfer. Neurology 1988; 38:1586–1591.
13. Dyck PJ, Stevens JC, Lambert EH, Linscheid RL, Cooney WP. Increased tactile detection threshold and perceptual territory after successful median nerve reconnection and the possible basis. In: Persson A, ed. Symposia, Sixth International Congress of Electromyography, Stockholm, Sweden, June 1979:93–101.
14. Gaul JS Jr. Electrical fascicle identification as an adjunct to nerve repair. J Hand Surg 1983; 8:289–296.
15. Greenberg BM, Cuadros CL, Panda M, May JW. St. Clair Strange procedure: Indications, technique, and long-term evaluation. J Hand Surg [Am] 1988; 13: 928–935.
16. Haase J, Bjerre P, Simesen K. Median and ulnar nerve transections treated by microsurgical interfascicular cable grafting with autogenous sural nerve. J Neurosurg 1980; 53:73–84.
17. Highet WB, Sanders FK. The effects of stretching nerves after suture. Br J Surg 1943; 30:355–369.
18. Jabaley MD, Wallace WH, Heckler FR. Internal topography of major nerves of the forearm and hand: A current review. J Hand Surg 1980; 5:1.
19. Jongen SJ, Van Twisk K. Results of primary repair of ulnar and median nerve injuries at the wrist: An evaluation of sensibility and motor recovery. Netherlands J Surg 1988; 40:86–89.
20. Kanakamedala RV, Hong CZ. Electrophysiologic studies of the median nerve and its palmar cutaneous branches after nerve grafting. Arch Phys Med Rehabil 1988; 69:344–347.
21. Kline DG, Hackett ER. Reappraisal of timing for exploration of civilian peripheral nerve injuries. Surgery 1975; 78:54–63.
22. Larsen RD, Posch, JL. Nerve injuries in the upper extremity. Arch Surg 1958; 77:469.
23. Lewis RC, Tenny J, Irvine D. The restoration of sensibility by nerve translocation. Bull Hosp Jt Dis Orthop Inst 1984; 44:288–296.
24. Lijftogt HJ, Dykstra E, Storm R, Van Leeuwen JB. Results of microsurgical treatment of nerve injuries of the wrist. Netherlands J Surgery 1987; 39:170–174.
25. Louis DS, Eckenrode JF. Autogenous nerve pedicle graft in the forearm. J Hand Surg [Am] 1986; 11: 703–706.
26. Marsh D, Barton N. Does the use of the operating microscope improve the results of peripheral nerve suture? J Bone Joint Surg [Br] 1987; 69:625–630.
27. McManamny DS. Comparison of microscope and loupe magnification: Assistance for the repair of median and ulnar nerves. Br J Plast Surg 1983; 36: 367–372.
28. McQuarrie IG. Peripheral nerve surgery—today and looking ahead. Clinical Plastic Surgery 1986; 13:255–268.
29. Medical Research Council. Aids to the investigation of peripheral nerve injuries. London: Her Majesty's Stationery Office, 1943.
30. Millesi H. Reappraisal of nerve repair. Surg Clin North Am 1981; 61:321–340.
31. Millesi H. Nerve grafting. Clin Plast Surg 1984; 11: 105–113.
32. Millesi H, Meissl G, Berger A. The interfascicular nerve grafting of the median and ulnar nerves. J Bone Joint Surg [Am] 1972; 54:727–750.
33. Moneim MS. Interfascicular nerve grafting. Clin Orthop 1982; 163:65–74.
34. Omer G. Injuries to nerves of the upper extremities. J Bone Joint Surg [Am] 1974; 56:1615–1624.
35. Parry CB. Peripheral nerve injuries, a symposium: Sensation. J Bone Joint Surg [Br] 1986; 68:15–29.
36. Pluchino F, Luccarelli G. Interfascicular suture with nerve autografts for median, ulnar, and radial nerve lesions. Italian J Neurol Sci 1981; 2:139–146.
37. Sakallarides H. A follow-up study of 172 peripheral nerve injuries in the upper extremity in civilians. J Bone Joint Surg [Am] 1962; 44:140–148.
38. Seddon HJ. Nerve grafting and other unusual forms of nerve repair. In: Seddon HJ, ed. Peripheral nerve injuries. Medical Research Council Special Report Series No. 282. London: Her Majesty's Stationery Office, 1954:389–417.
39. Seddon HJ. Surgical disorders of the peripheral nerves. London: Williams & Wilkins, 1972.
40. Settergren LK, Wood MB. Comparison of blood flow in free vascularized vs nonvascularized nerve grafts. J Reconstr Microsurgery 1984; 1:95.
41. Simesen K, Haase J, Bjerre P. Interfascicular transplantation in median nerve injuries. Acta Orthop Scand 1980; 51:243–248.
42. St. Clair Strange FG. An operation for nerve pedicle grafting (preliminary communication). Br J Surg 1947; 34:423–425.
43. Taylor EG, Ham FJ. The free vascularized nerve graft. Plast Reconstr Surg 1976; 57:413.
44. Thomas CK, Stein RB, Gordon T, Lee RG, Elleker MG. Patterns of reinnervation and motor unit re-

cruitment in human hand muscles after complete ulnar and median nerve section and resuture. J Neurol Neurosurg Psychiatry 1987; 50:259–268.

45. Tupper JW, Crick JC, Matteck LR. Fascicular nerve repairs: A comparative study of epineurial and fascicular (perineurial) techniques. Orthop Clin North Am 1988; 19:57–69.

46. Vahvanen V, Gripenberg L, Nuutinen P. Peripheral nerve injuries of the hand in children: A follow-up of 38 patients. Scand J Plast Reconstr Surg 1981; 15:49–51.

47. Waeton R, Finseth F. Nerve grafts in the repair of complicated peripheral nerve trauma. J Trauma 1977; 17:793.

48. Williams HB, Jabaley ME. The importance of internal anatomy of the peripheral nerves to nerve repair in the forearm and hand. Hand Clin 1986; 2:689–707.

49. Woodall B, Beebe WG. Peripheral nerve regeneration. A follow-up study of 3,656 World War II injuries. In: VA Medical Monograph. U.S. Government Printing Office, Washington DC, 1956.

50. Young VL, Wray RC, Weeks PM. The results of nerve grafting in the wrist and hand. Ann Plast Surg 1980; 5:212–215

27

Radial Nerve: Applied Anatomy and Operative Exposure

David B. Siegel
Richard H. Gelberman

AUTHORS' KEY POINTS

- The radial nerve crosses the posterior aspect of the arm obliquely, separated from the humeral shaft by the medial head of the triceps muscle, piercing the lateral intermuscular septum 10 cm above the lateral epicondyle. Injured most frequently following short oblique fractures at the junction of the middle and distal thirds of the humeral shaft, the nerve becomes entrapped within the proximal portion of the lateral intermuscular septum, proximal to the level at which it actually pierces the septum.
- The nerve along the anterior aspect of the elbow requires dissection deeply within the interval between the brachioradialis and brachialis muscles; the lateral cutaneous nerve of the forearm lies superficially within the interval between the brachialis and biceps muscles.
- The anterolateral exposure of the radial nerve, extensile to the arm and forearm, is the recommended approach to the nerve in the radial tunnel.
- The autonomous zone of cutaneous innervation of the radial nerve, the dorsum of the first web space, may be overlapped partially or completely by the lateral or posterior cutaneous nerves of the forearm.
- The posterior interosseous nerve passes from the flexor to the extensor surface of the forearm between the two heads of the supinator muscle; however, it may lie directly on the radius, a fact that should be kept in mind when exposing the proximal third of the radial shaft, either anteriorly or posteriorly.

ANATOMY

Radial Nerve in the Arm

The radial nerve arises from the posterior cord of the brachial plexus behind the third portion of the axillary artery. Containing neural elements from the fifth through eighth cervical nerve roots, it is the largest terminal branch of the brachial plexus. The lower trunk contributes fibers from the first thoracic nerve root to the radial nerve in 8% of upper limbs.[8] In the proximal third of the arm, the nerve descends behind the brachial artery, anterior to the subscapularis muscle, the teres major and latissimus dorsi muscle tendons, and the long head of the triceps muscle.[25] At the junction of the proximal and middle thirds of the humerus, the nerve deviates dorsolaterally and passes between the medial and long heads of the triceps muscle, accompanied by the profunda brachii artery. Continuing obliquely across the back of the humerus, the nerve and artery pass between the medial and lateral heads of the triceps muscle. The nerve reaches the lateral intermuscular septum separated from the humeral shaft by the medial head of the triceps muscle, lying adjacent to but not within the spiral groove of the humerus (Fig. 27-1).[26] At the lateral border of the medial head of the triceps muscle, the nerve leaves the extensor compartment and enters the flexor compartment of the arm. It pierces the lateral intermuscular septum 10 cm above the lateral humeral epicondyle, accompanied by the radial collateral artery, a terminal branch of the profunda brachii artery. Distally, the artery contributes to the collateral circulation about the elbow by joining the radial recurrent branch of the radial artery. Proximally, the nerve lies deeply within the intermuscular interval between the brachialis and brachioradialis muscles. Distally, it comes to lie between the brachialis and extensor carpi radialis longus muscles, often covered by the lateral portion of the brachialis muscle. The nerve leaves the arm anterior to the tip of the lateral epicondyle, dividing into superficial and deep terminal branches as it enters the forearm.

Arising from the radial nerve in the arm are three cutaneous nerves, several muscular branches, and articular fibers supplying the elbow joint. The posterior cutaneous nerve of the arm is the first branch arising from the main nerve trunk in the axilla. It pierces the axillary fascia and passes dorsally, medial to the long head of the triceps muscle, supplying the dorsomedial skin of the arm. It communicates with the intercostobrachial and medial cutaneous nerves of the arm. The second branch of the radial nerve, arising about 7 cm below the tip of the acromion (Table 27-1), supplies the long head of the triceps muscle.[13] It leaves the main trunk with the posterior cutaneous nerve of the arm in 30% of limbs.[8] The branch to the medial portion of the medial head arises just distal to the branch to the long head, 9 cm below the tip of the acromion. Known as the ulnar collateral nerve, this branch lies adjacent to the ulnar nerve as far distally as the lower third of the arm, and provides several branches to the medial head of the triceps muscle.[25] As the radial nerve passes deep to the long head, it may provide additional branches to this muscle. The posterior muscular branch arises from the main trunk as it lies between the lateral and medial heads, near the spiral groove of the humerus. This is the largest muscular branch of the radial nerve in the arm, innervating the medial and lateral heads of the triceps and anconeus muscles. The division to the lateral head arises about 1 cm proximal to the branch to the medial head.[13] The nerve to the anconeus muscle descends distally within the substance of the medial head of the triceps muscle, giving several branches to this muscle before innervating the anconeus muscle posterior to the elbow. The middle collateral artery, the second terminal branch of the profunda brachii artery, travels with the nerve posterior to the lateral epicondyle, and anastomoses with the interosseous recurrent branch of the posterior interosseous artery. At the level of the deltoid muscle insertion, the inferior lateral cutaneous nerve of the arm and the posterior cutaneous nerve of the forearm arise from a common trunk, traversing the lateral head of the triceps muscle before dividing. The inferior lateral cutaneous nerve pierces the fascia and supplies the lower half of the lateral surface of the arm. The posterior cutaneous nerve of the forearm travels within the lateral intermuscular septum, piercing the fascia in the lower third of the arm and passing distally on the dorsal surface of the brachioradialis muscle. It innervates the skin on the dorsum of the forearm, terminating near the wrist where it joins the dorsal branches of the lateral cutaneous nerve of the forearm.[8]

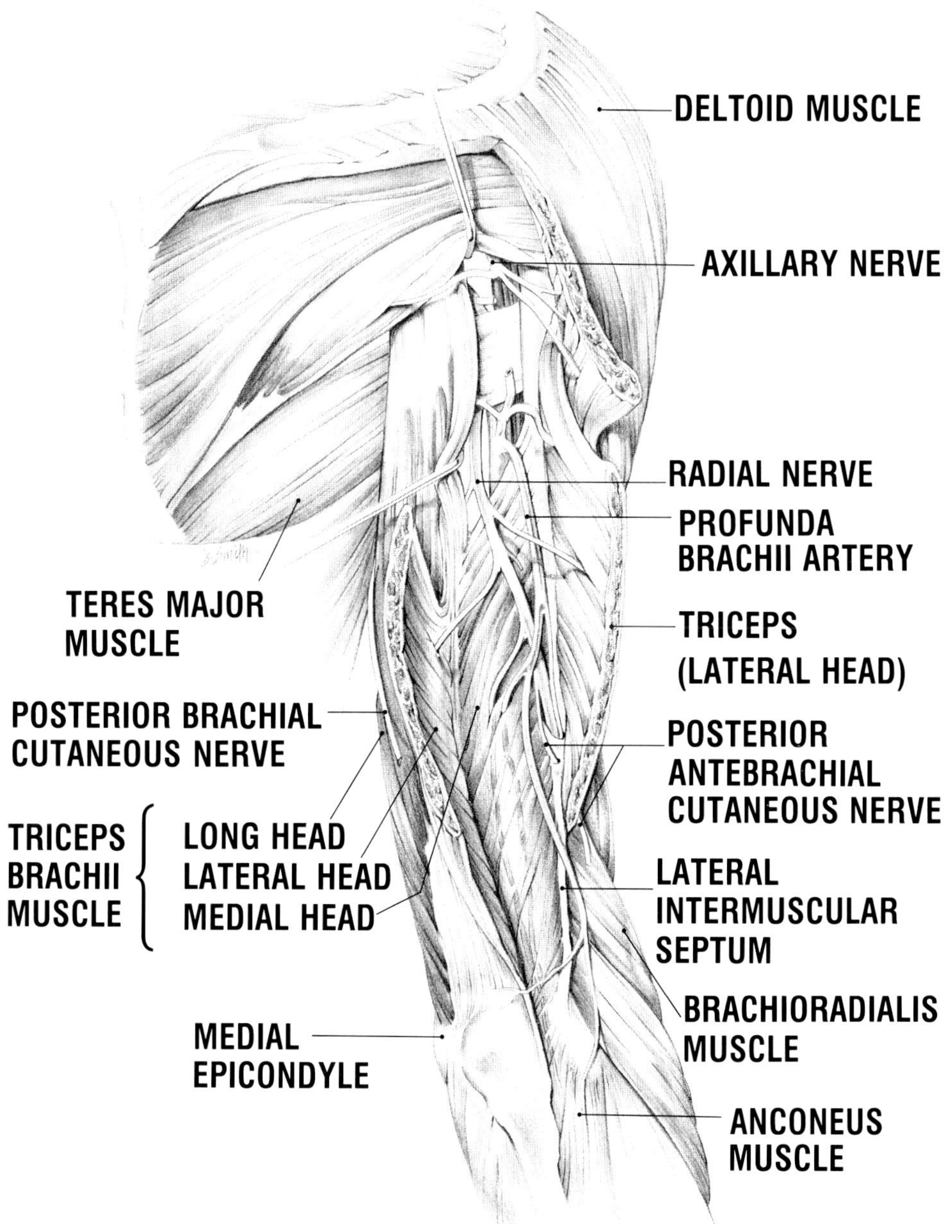

Figure 27–1. *The radial nerve enters the extensor surface of the arm in conjunction with the profunda brachii artery. It crosses the posterior surface of the arm obliquely on the surface of the fibers of the medial head of the triceps muscle.*

After piercing the lateral intermuscular septum, the radial nerve lies deeply within the interval between the brachialis and brachioradialis muscles. It is covered anteriorly by the lateral portion of the brachialis muscle and may lie on the humerus. One or more branches leave the main trunk at this level, innervate the lateral portion of the brachialis muscle, and course distally within the substance of this muscle to supply the elbow joint. Additional articular fibers leave the nerve as it passes in front

Table 27–1. *Level and Order of Innervation of Muscles Supplied by Radial Nerve*

Muscle	cm From Tip of Acromion (Shortest to Longest)
Triceps	–
long head	7.1
medial head	9.5–11.2
lateral head	10.1
Anconeus	–
	cm From Humerus (From 10 cm Above Lateral Epicondyle)
Brachioradialis	8.2–10.0
Extensor carpi radialis longus	10.5–12.3
Extensor carpi radialis brevis	14.7–16.5
	cm From Lateral Epicondyle
Extensor carpi ulnaris	10.2–10.6
Extensor digitorum communis	10.2–12.5
Extensor digiti minimi	11.7–12.0
Abductor pollicis longus	11.4–14.2
Extensor pollicis longus	13.9–17.6
Extensor pollicis brevis	15.9–16.4
Extensor indicis proprius	16.9–18.0

(From Linnell EA. The distribution of nerves in the upper limb, with reference to variabilities and their clinical significance. J Anat 1921;55:79, and Sunderland S. Metrical and non-metrical features of the muscular branches of the radial nerve. J Comp Neurol 1946;85:93–97, with permission.)

of the radiocapitellar joint, supplying the lateral epicondyle and orbicular ligament.[25] The brachioradialis and extensor carpi radialis longus muscles arise from the lateral supracondylar ridge and are each supplied by a branch of the radial nerve 2 to 3 cm above the lateral epicondyle as it lies under cover of these muscles.

Potential Points of Neural Compression in the Arm

Four potential points of compression of the radial nerve in the arm have been described:

1. Compression of the nerve at the level of the lateral head of the triceps muscle has been reported as a cause of high radial nerve palsy.[17] A fibrous band of origin of the lateral head of the triceps muscle attaches to the humerus above and below the nerve and is a potential site of compression.[15]
2. Radial palsy following fractures of the humerus may be caused by compression of the nerve within the lateral intermuscular septum.[26]
3. Anomalous vessels in the axilla, such as an aberrant subscapular artery, may penetrate and compress the radial nerve.[22]
4. An anomalous muscle, the accessory scapularis-teres-latissimus muscle, has been reported to cross the radial nerve, compressing it over the subscapularis muscle.[11]

SUMMARY OF ANATOMICAL COMPRESSION POINTS OF THE RADIAL NERVE

ARM

1. Accessory subscapularis-teres-latissimus muscle
2. Lateral head of the triceps muscle
3. Lateral intermuscular septum

FOREARM

1. Posterior interosseous nerve within the radial tunnel
   Fibrous bands attached to the radiocapitellar joint
   Extensor carpi radialis brevis muscle
   Arcade of Frohse
   Fibrous bands within the supinator muscle
2. Superficial radial nerve
   Between brachioradialis muscle and radial shaft
   Between brachioradialis and extensor carpi radialis longus tendons

HAND/WRIST

None

Variations

In about 20% of upper limbs, there are variant patterns of formation of the radial nerve.[13] The most common variation is the division of axillary and radial nerves proximal to the contribution of the lower trunk, in which case the posterior division of the lower trunk joins the radial nerve directly, distal to the posterior cord.[25] The radial nerve may be formed directly from the posterior division of the lower trunk and may receive fibers distally from the posterior division of the lateral trunk.[12] In that case, the posterior cord does not exist, and the axillary nerve is formed directly from the posterior division of the upper and middle trunks. As it courses through the axilla, the radial nerve may pierce the subscapularis muscle at various points before entering the arm.[8] Rarely, communicating fibers may exist between the ulnar collateral branch of the radial nerve and the ulnar nerve in the arm, above the level at which the ulnar nerve pierces the medial intermuscular septum.[12] The function of this neural communication is poorly described. Most commonly, there are four muscular branches to the triceps muscle; however, there may be as many as five to ten branches leaving the nerve in the upper arm.[24]

The final pattern of variation of the nerve in the arm concerns the innervation of the extensor carpi radialis brevis muscle. This muscle is most commonly innervated by the posterior interosseous nerve below the elbow; however, a branch may leave the main nerve trunk distal to the branch to the extensor carpi radialis longus muscle to supply the extensor carpi radialis brevis muscle.

Radial Nerve in the Forearm

As the main trunk of the radial nerve passes anterior to the lateral epicondyle, it divides into superficial and deep terminal branches, under cover of the brachioradialis and radial wrist extensor muscles. The superficial branch passes anterior (superficial) to the supinator muscle in the proximal third of the forearm and comes to lie on the deep surface of the brachioradialis muscle (Fig. 27-2). Initially, the nerve lies under the anterior third of the brachioradialis, but courses laterally as it descends in the forearm, under cover of this muscle. The radial artery passes palmar to the insertion of the pronator teres muscle and comes to lie on the ulnar border of the brachioradialis muscle in the middle third of the forearm. The superficial branch of the radial nerve is lateral to the radial artery, palmar to the origins of the radial head of the flexor digitorum superficialis and flexor pollicis longus muscles. The nerve crosses over the radius, deep to the brachioradialis tendon, and pierces the fascia on the ulnar side of this tendon, about 7 cm above the wrist. Descending on the dorsoradial side of the wrist, it divides into five dorsal digital nerves. The only branch of the nerve in the forearm innervates the extensor carpi radialis brevis muscle (in about 55% of upper limbs).[8]

The posterior interosseous nerve, the deep terminal branch of the radial nerve, innervates the extensor muscles of the forearm and contains afferent fibers to the wrist joint. The supinator muscle, arising from the lateral epicondyle, radial collateral ligament, orbicular ligament, and proximal ulna, is divided into deep and superficial laminae, through which the posterior interosseous nerve passes. The nerve courses obliquely through the supinator, crossing the proximal radius, to enter the extensor compartment of the forearm (Fig. 27-3). It is separated from the radius by the deep head of the supinator muscle, but may come into contact with the bone, especially when the fibers of the deep head parallel the course of the nerve.[3] After leaving the supinator muscle, the nerve lies between the abductor pollicis longus muscle deeply and the extensor carpi ulnaris, extensor digiti minimi, and extensor digitorum communis muscles superficially. It is joined on the extensor surface of the forearm by the posterior interosseous artery, a branch of the common interosseous artery. Coursing distally in the forearm, the nerve passes superficial to the extensor pollicis brevis and deep to the extensor pollicis longus muscles. It penetrates deeply, either over or through the extensor pollicis brevis muscle, and comes to lie on the interosseous membrane between the radius and the ulna. Continuing distally on the interosseous membrane, it divides into terminal branches that provide sensory innervation to the wrist.

The extensor carpi radialis brevis may be innervated by the radial nerve, its superficial branch, or the posterior interosseous nerve. Branches to this muscle most commonly originate 2 cm below the tip of the lateral epicondyle, but may arise between 2 and 5 cm below it.[24] The posterior interosseous nerve gives one or more branches to the supinator muscle before entering it; however, additional fibers may travel within the epineurium of the main trunk for several centimeters, supplying the muscle between its two heads. As the nerve leaves the supinator, it gives off three short and two long mus-

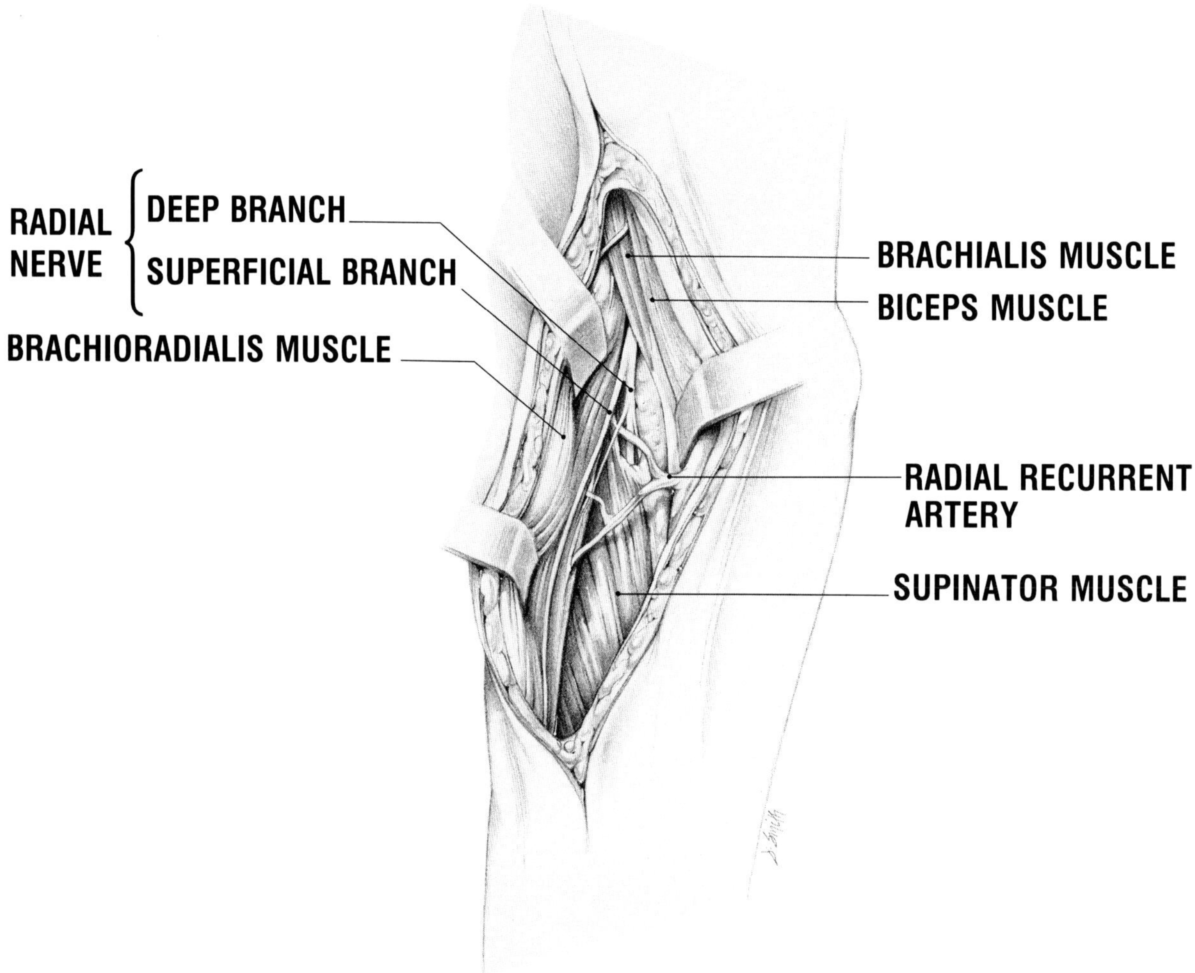

Figure 27–2. *Radial nerve in the anterior forearm. Note that the superficial branch of the radial nerve passes volar (superficial) to the supinator muscle and comes to lie adjacent to the radial artery on the undersurface of the brachioradialis muscle.*

cular branches, the order of which is highly variable. The short branches to the extensor digitorum communis, followed by the extensor digiti minimi and extensor carpi ulnaris muscles, arise in close succession and travel a variable distance before entering their respective muscles (see Table 27-1). The extensor carpi ulnaris muscle is innervated 1.25 cm, the extensor digitorum communis muscle 1.5 cm, and the extensor digiti quinti muscle 1.8 cm below the posterior interosseous nerve division.[19] A long medial muscular branch provides innervation to the extensor indicis proprius 6.8 cm below the nerve division and to the extensor pollicis longus 7.5 cm below the division. A long lateral branch supplies the abductor pollicis longus 5.6 cm below the division and ends in the extensor pollicis brevis, 6.8 cm below the division.[19] Multiple branches to these muscles are common.

Potential Points of Neural Compression in the Forearm

Compression neuropathy of the radial nerve most often occurs within the anatomical region known as the radial tunnel.[24] The tunnel, 10 cm long, begins after the nerve enters the flexor surface of the arm by piercing the lateral intermuscular septum

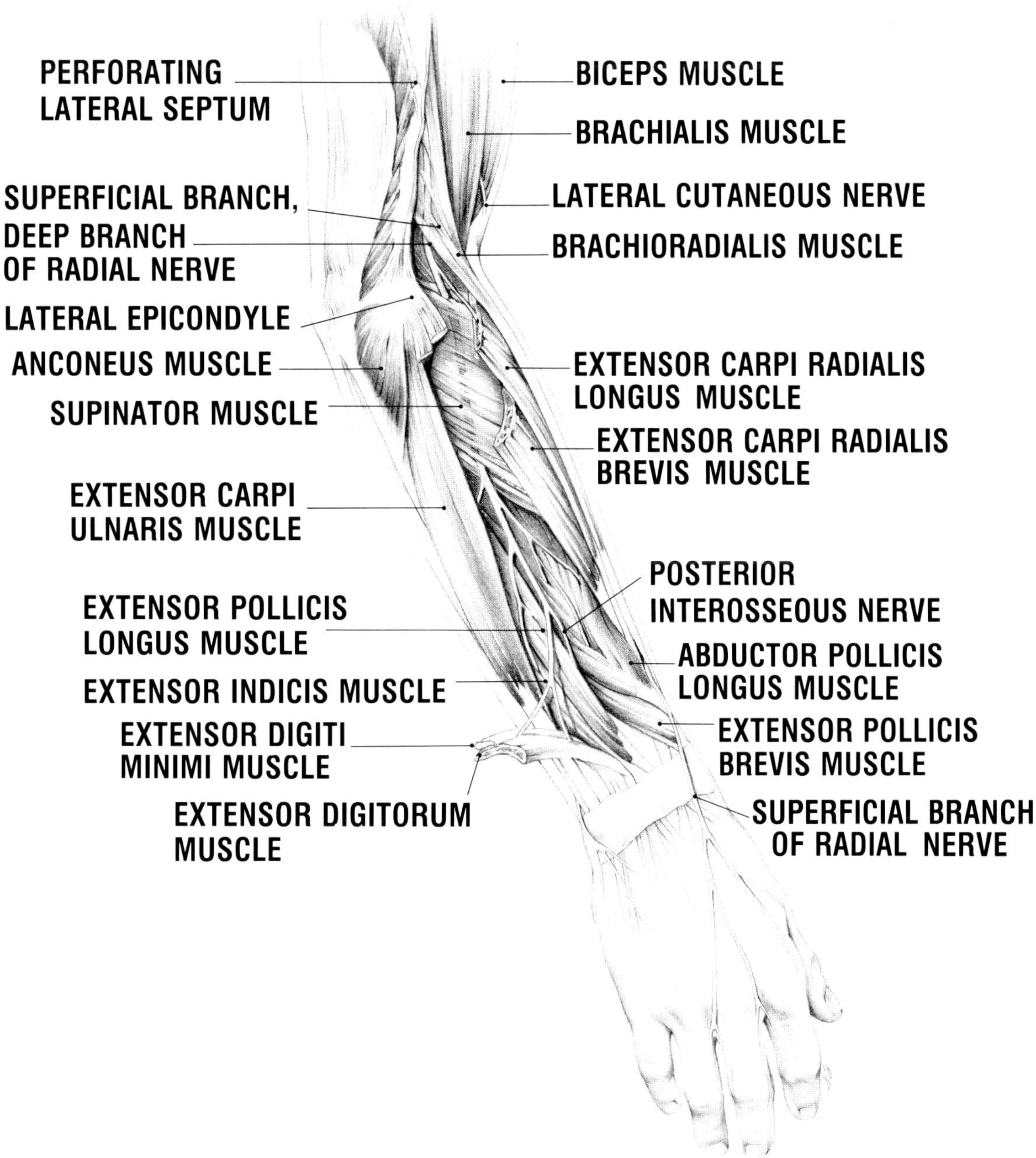

Figure 27–3. *The posterior interosseous nerve enters the extensor surface of the forearm between the two heads of the supinator muscle. Note that the extensor carpi radialis longus and brevis muscles receive their innervation prior to the entrance into the supinator muscle.*

and ends as the nerve enters the extensor surface of the forearm, leaving the supinator muscle. At the entrance to the tunnel, the nerve lies deeply in the interval between the brachialis muscle medially and the brachioradialis muscle laterally. At the elbow the tunnel is bordered posteriorly by the capitellum, medially by the biceps tendon and brachialis muscle, laterally by the extensor carpi radialis longus muscle, and anterolaterally by the brachioradialis muscle. At this level the nerve may be crossed by fibrous bands that attach it to the radiocapitellar joint.[14]

A fanlike leash of vessels extending from the radial recurrent artery and vein to the mobile wad muscles is the second potential site of nerve constriction.[14,20] This group of vessels, known as the radial recurrent leash of Henry, courses posterolaterally, crossing the radial or posterior interosseous nerve, before the nerve enters the supinator muscle.[7]

Fibrous bands may extend from the extensor carpi radialis brevis muscle to the antebrachial fascia and have been reported to compress the nerve with pronation of the forearm.[5] The nerve may be compressed by a fibrous band at the proximal edge of the supinator muscle. This band, known as the arcade of Frohse, is present in 30% to 90% of adult upper limbs. It compresses the nerve beneath the medial half of the superficial head of the supinator muscle.[1,21] At the distal edge of the supinator, the nerve may become constricted by fibrous bands within the supinator muscle.[23]

The superficial branch of the radial nerve may be compressed in the distal third of the forearm before it pierces the forearm fascia.[4] Emerging from under the brachioradialis tendon, the nerve is closely applied to the dorsolateral aspect of the radius. It may be tethered at this level by fascia blending with the periosteum of the radius. Further, with pronation of the forearm and ulnar deviation of the wrist, the nerve may be entrapped by a scissoring effect between the brachioradialis and extensor carpi radialis longus tendons.[4]

Variations

Three patterns of variability are recognized in the course of the radial nerve in the forearm. The first concerns the terminal branching pattern of the radial nerve trunk. Most commonly, the nerve bifurcates into superficial and deep branches at the level of the tip of the lateral epicondyle. The level of division may vary from 4.5 cm above to 4 cm below the epicondyle; distal division is more common.[13]

The second pattern of variability concerns the level of innervation of the forearm muscles. The extensor carpi radialis brevis muscle may be innervated directly from the radial nerve trunk, from its bifurcation, from the posterior interosseous, or from superficial branches. The supinator muscle usually receives a single branch from the posterior interosseous nerve before it enters the muscle and several short branches within the muscle. However, Sunderland found several branches dividing proximally to supply the supinator muscle.[22,24] As the posterior interosseous nerve leaves the supinator, several branches arise to supply the superficial and deep forearm extensor muscles. Although the level of innervation and branching described above is generally adhered to, great variation exists among individuals. All of the branches may arise from one common stem or may divide much like the cauda equina.

The third pattern of variability concerns the course of the terminal branches of the radial nerve. Rarely, the posterior interosseous nerve passes superficial to rather than through the supinator muscle. Distally the nerve may pass under, over, or through the extensor pollicis brevis muscle before coming in contact with the interosseous membrane. The superficial branch of the radial nerve may pass over the brachioradialis muscle in the proximal forearm and course distally on the dorsal surface of the muscle fascia or within the subcutaneous tissue on the dorsolateral surface of the forearm.[12]

Radial Nerve in the Hand

The superficial branch of the radial nerve pierces the dorsoradial fascia of the forearm 5 to 7 cm above the wrist.[8] It crosses over the abductor pollicis longus and extensor pollicis brevis muscles, bifurcating into radial and ulnar divisions on the dorsal surface of the extensor retinaculum between the first and second extensor compartments. Within the subcutaneous tissue it divides into four or five dorsal digital nerves and several small branches that communicate with the terminal fibers of the posterior cutaneous nerve of the forearm. The radial division supplies the skin on the dorsum of the radial side of the thumb and palmar–radial side of the thenar eminence, communicating with the terminal branches of the lateral cutaneous nerve of the forearm and the palmar cutaneous branch of the median nerve.[16] The first branch of the ulnar division supplies the dorsoulnar side of the thumb. The second branch innervates the radial side of the index finger, and the third supplies the second web space and the adjacent sides of the index and long fingers. The fourth branch supplies the third web space and adjacent sides of the long and ring fingers, communicating with the dorsal cutaneous branch of the ulnar nerve.[25] The dorsal digital nerves provide innervation as far distally as the base of the thumbnail, the middle phalanx of the index finger, and the proximal interphalangeal joints of the long and ring fingers. Fingertip innervation is supplied by the proper palmar digital nerves. The dorsal digital nerves also supply the metacarpophalangeal and proximal interphalangeal joints. The autonomous area of innervation of the radial nerve is the dorsum of the first web space; however, this may be overlapped partially or completely by branches of the posterior and lateral cutaneous nerves of the forearm.[16]

The posterior interosseous nerve ramifies on the dorsum of the wrist to supply the capsule, ligaments, and carpal bones. Occasionally it innervates an accessory finger extensor in the hand, the extensor brevis manus. It supplies no other muscles in the hand.[12]

Potential Points of Compression in the Hand and Wrist

Compression of the terminal branches of the radial nerve has not been described.

Variations

The level at which the superficial branch of the radial nerve divides often varies by 2 to 3 cm, and the pattern of division varies among individuals. The branch to the ulnar side of the thumb may arise from the radial division of the main nerve trunk. In as many as 70% of upper limbs, the dorsal cutaneous branch of the ulnar nerve supplies the third web space and adjacent sides of the long and ring fingers (Fig. 27-4).[13] Rarely, the radial nerve innervates the entire dorsum of the hand.

The posterior interosseous nerve may communicate with the deep branch of the ulnar nerve. Through this connection, the Froment-Ruber nerve, the posterior interosseous nerve may innervate the first dorsal interosseous muscle.[12]

OPERATIVE EXPOSURE

Radial Nerve in the Arm

The posterior or anterolateral approach may be used to expose the radial nerve in the arm. The choice of approach is determined by the extent of exposure necessary, the pathologic process for which the nerve is being explored, and associated structures requiring exposure. The nerve enters the arm inferior to the teres major muscle, between the long and medial heads of the triceps muscle. It courses obliquely across the extensor surface of the arm, between the medial and lateral heads of the triceps muscle, and pierces the lateral intermuscular septum 10 cm above the lateral epicondyle, where it enters the radial tunnel. It lies deeply in the intermuscular interval between the brachialis and brachioradialis muscles proximally and the extensor carpi radialis longus muscle distally. It is important to note that the lateral antebrachial cutaneous nerve of the forearm lies in the interval between the biceps and brachialis muscles, and exposure of the radial nerve requires deeper dissection in an adjacent interval between the brachioradialis and the brachialis muscles.

Exposure of the radial nerve in the arm is best accomplished with the patient in the lateral decubitus or prone position, with the entire upper extremity draped freely.

Posterior Approach to the Radial Nerve and Humerus (Extensile to Shoulder and Elbow Joints)

The cutaneous bony landmarks are the posterior border of the acromion and the tip of the olecranon. The long head of the triceps, palpated medially below the deltoid muscle, is relatively mobile, whereas the lateral head and deltoid muscles are more firmly held to bone. A straight incision along a line connecting the acromion and olecranon will expose the sulcus between the long and lateral heads of the triceps muscle. Beginning 5 cm below the acromion, the incision extends distally to the olecranon fossa. Proximally, the incision may be extended to expose the posterior aspect of the shoulder by curving medially across the scapular spine. Distally, the incision may continue over the

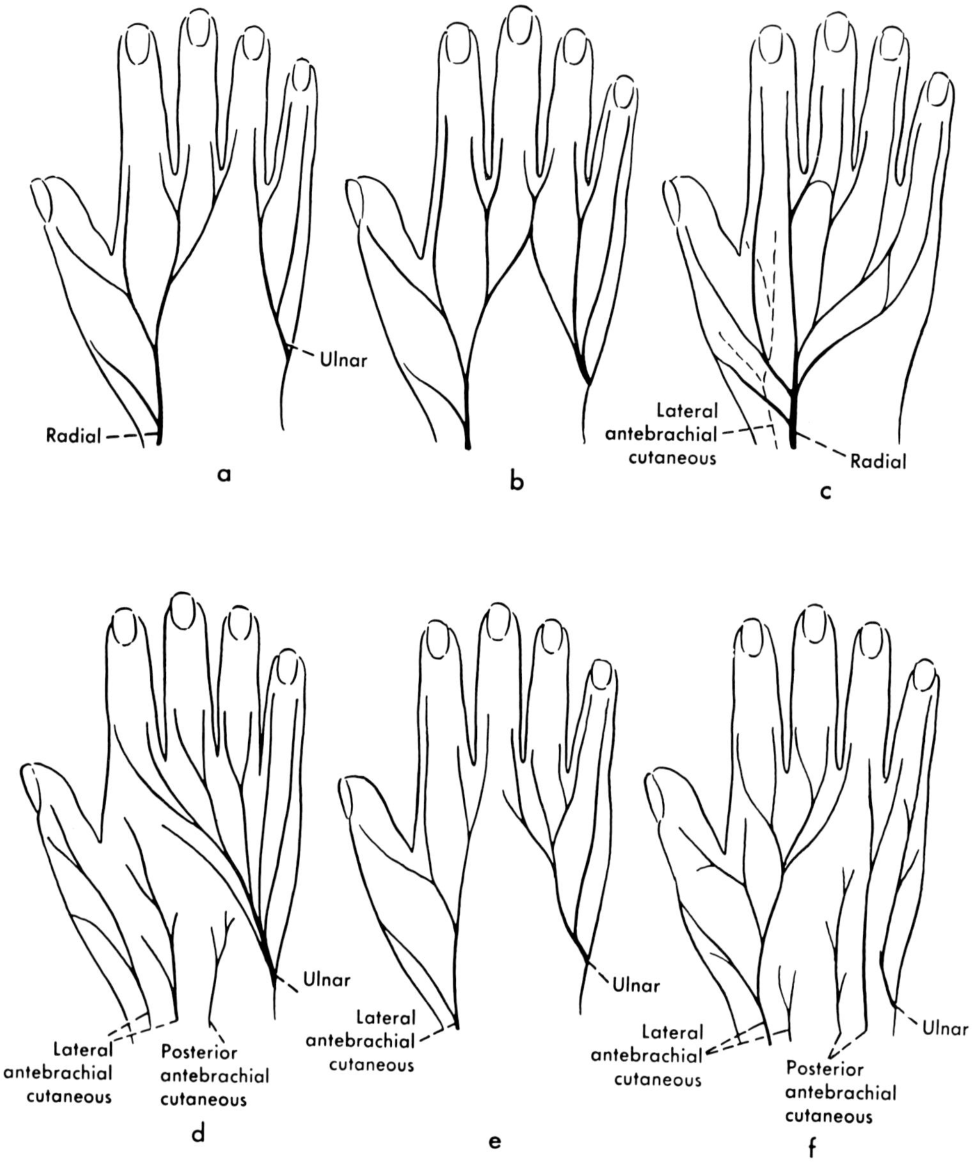

Figure 27–4. *Anatomical variations in the cutaneous nerve distribution to the dorsum of the hand. (From Hollingshead WH. The back and limbs, ed 3. Philadelphia: Harper and Row, 1982:532, with permission.)*

olecranon to facilitate exposure of the elbow. The fascia is incised along the lateral border of the long head of the triceps muscle proximally in line with the skin incision distally. The interval between the long and lateral heads is divided bluntly, from proximal to distal, to the level of the triceps tendon, which is incised sharply.[7] Retraction of the superficial muscle bellies exposes the radial nerve and profunda brachii artery proximally and the medial head of the triceps deeply. The nerve is identified as it pierces the lateral intermuscular septum and may be traced proximally, exposing the ulnar nerve and brachial artery.[10] Branches to the triceps muscle limit the mobility of the radial nerve in this area. However, to expose the posterior aspect of the humeral shaft, the nerve may be retracted gently, both proximally and laterally, allowing the medial head to be incised safely in the midline. Adduction of the arm relaxes the nerve, facilitating retraction.[9] The muscle is incised sharply to periosteum. The humerus is exposed by subperiosteal dissection, avoiding injury to the radial nerve as well as the ulnar nerve, which pierces the medial intermuscular septum 8 cm above the medial epicondyle. Further radial nerve exposure proximally requires release of the long head of the triceps muscle and the tendons of the teres major and latissimus dorsi.[10] The lateral intermuscular septum should be incised close to bone to facilitate distal exposure of the nerve.

Authors' Preferred Method

Thompson's anterolateral approach is recommended for exposure of the radial nerve in the distal half of the arm.[2] This approach may be extended proximally, joining the posterior approach in the upper arm, or distally, exposing the nerve in the radial tunnel and forearm. The incision begins posterolaterally in the interval between the deltoid and lateral head of the triceps muscles, about 8 cm below the posterior axillary crease (Fig. 27-5). It courses distally over the intermuscular sulcus between the biceps and lateral head of the triceps muscles, crossing the lateral intermuscular septum obliquely, 10 cm above the lateral epicondyle. Continuing distally between the biceps and brachioradialis muscles, this incision is contiguous with the anterolateral approach to the radial nerve at the elbow and forearm. The superficial fascia is incised, and the cephalic vein is either retracted or ligated. The lateral cutaneous nerve of the forearm, the terminal branch of the musculocutaneous nerve, should be identified and protected in the distal third of the incision. It emerges between the biceps and brachialis muscles, piercing the fascia anterior to the elbow, posterior to the cephalic vein, and lateral to the biceps tendon.[18] The deep fascia is incised in line with the skin incision, and the biceps muscle is retracted medially. The interval between the brachioradialis and brachialis muscles is developed just above the elbow. The radial nerve is found deeply within the intermuscular interval and traced proximally to the point at which it pierces the lateral intermuscular septum. The septum is divided and the nerve traced proximally under the lateral head of the triceps muscle. To gain further exposure, the interval between the long and lateral heads of the triceps muscle is divided, as described in the posterior approach to the radial nerve in the arm. The distal third of the humeral shaft is exposed in the interval between the brachioradialis muscles. If further proximal exposure of the humerus is needed, the plane between the brachialis and the lateral head of the triceps muscles may be developed.

Radial Nerve in the Forearm

The radial nerve enters the forearm anterior to the tip of the lateral epicondyle and divides into superficial and deep branches. The superficial branch courses distally under the brachioradialis muscle, where it is joined by the radial artery in the midforearm. It pierces the forearm fascia at the dorsoulnar margin of the brachioradialis tendon 7 cm above the wrist. The deep branch passes through the superficial and deep heads of the supinator muscle, coursing over the radius to supply the extensor muscles of the forearm. The lateral cutaneous nerve of the forearm divides into anterior and posterior branches at the elbow, supplying sensation to the radial half of the forearm.[18]

Modified Henry Anterior Approach Combined with Exposure of Radius

This approach uses the interval between the brachioradialis muscle and several adjacent muscles: the brachialis at the elbow, the pronator teres in the proximal forearm, and the flexor carpi radialis in the middle and distal forearm.[2] It may be used to expose the entire radial shaft.

The patient is positioned supine, with the upper limb on a hand table and the forearm supinated and slightly flexed. The incision begins 3 cm medial to the upper border of the lateral supracondylar ridge, about 6 cm above the lateral humeral epicondyle. Continuing distally in the sulcus between biceps and brachioradialis muscles, the incision crosses the elbow flexion crease obliquely, then crosses the proximal portion of the flexor–pronator muscle mass before turning distally and radially. The incision crosses the midforearm obliquely and turns distally at the ulnar border of the brachioradialis muscle. A modification of this incision uses

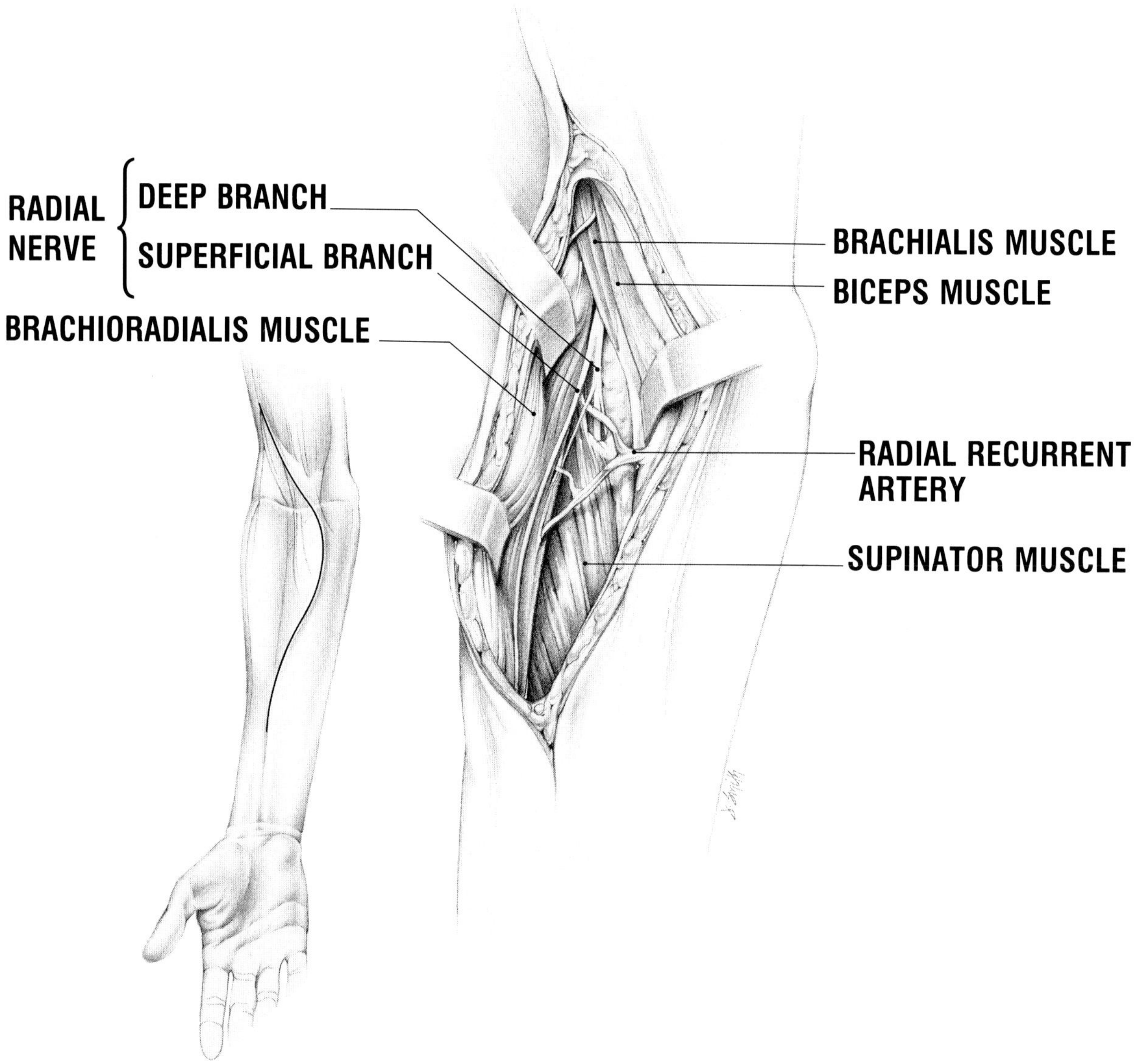

Figure 27–5. *The operative incision and deep surgical dissection to expose the posterior interosseous nerve in the proximal forearm. Note the relationship of the deep and superficial branches to the radial recurrent artery.*

the same starting point but turns laterally 2 cm above the elbow flexion crease, curving gently over the mobile wad and medially to the ulnar border of the brachioradialis muscle. Both incisions may be carried distally to the wrist along the ulnar border of the brachioradialis muscle. The cephalic vein is ligated, and the lateral cutaneous nerve of the forearm is identified and protected. The deep fascia and lacertus fibrosus are divided on the lateral side of the biceps tendon, along the medial side of the brachioradialis muscle.[6] Biceps and pronator teres muscles are retracted medially and brachioradialis muscle laterally.

In the proximal part of the incision, the radial nerve is found deeply between brachioradialis and brachialis muscles and is traced distally to its division. The superficial branch may be followed on the deep surface of the brachioradialis muscle to the point at which it courses dorsomedially under the brachioradialis tendon.

The radial recurrent leash of vessels is isolated and ligated, facilitating medial retraction of the radial artery. The posterior interosseous nerve is traced distally, isolating branches to the extensor carpi radialis brevis and supinator muscles, before entering the latter. The fibers of the superficial head are divided sharply as the nerve is traced through the supinator muscle. Thompson's approach is recommended for exposure of the nerve distal to the supinator muscle.

The entire radial shaft may be exposed through Henry's approach. With the forearm supinated fully and elbow flexed 90°, the biceps tendon is traced to its insertion on the radius. The bicipital bursa is incised on the lateral side of the tendon, exposing the broad insertion of the supinator. The insertion is incised sharply and the muscle elevated subperiosteally. Pronation of the forearm exposes the radial shaft.

Thompson's Approach to Posterior Interosseous Nerve and Upper Two Thirds of Radial Shaft

The mnemonic described by Henry provides a useful way to remember the topographic anatomy of the superficial extensor muscles of the forearm.[7] With the upper extremity fully pronated, the opposite hand is placed on the dorsal surface of the forearm so that the thenar eminence covers the lateral epicondyle and the fingers point distally. The index finger rests on the subcutaneous border of the ulna, the ring finger on the radial border of the forearm, and the little finger wraps around the radius, pointing toward the radial styloid. In this position the thumb covers the anconeus, the index finger covers the extensor carpi ulnaris, the long finger covers the extensor digiti minimi, the ring finger covers the extensor digitorum communis, and the little finger covers the mobile wad muscles.

Thompson's approach uses the interval between

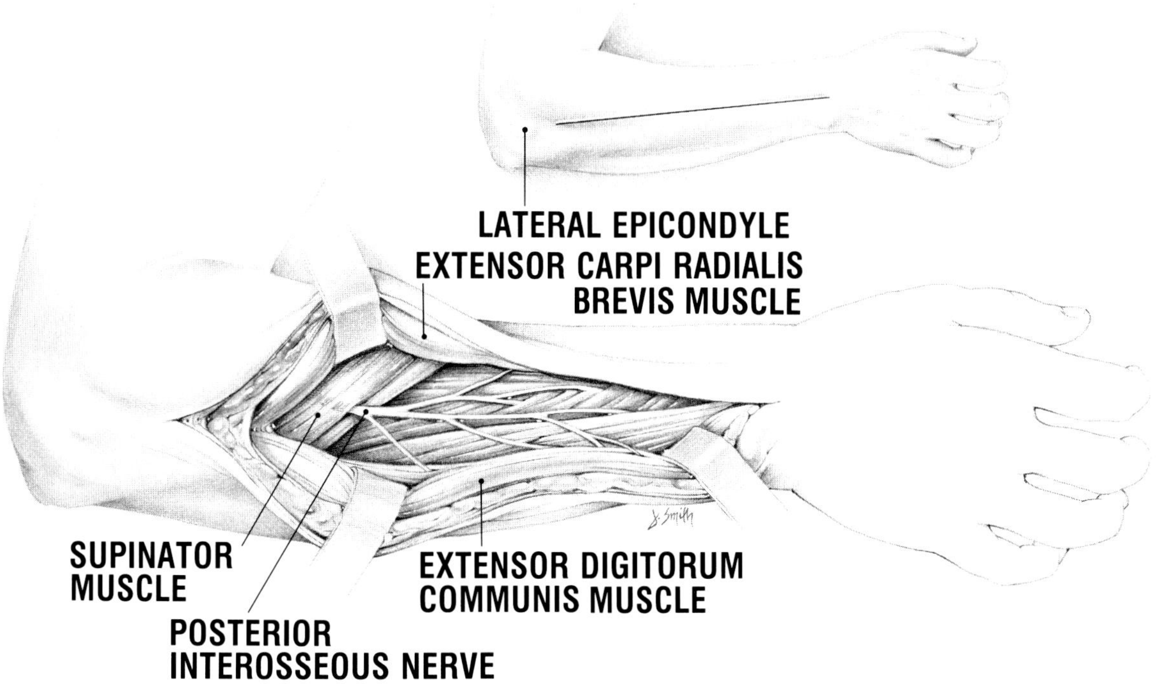

Figure 27–6. *A straight longitudinal incision is used to expose the posterior interosseous nerve in the forearm. The nerve is exposed in the interval between the extensor carpi radialis brevis and extensor digitorum communis muscles (See text).*

the extensor digitorum communis and extensor carpi radialis brevis muscles (Fig. 27-6). The forearm is supinated, and a point 2 cm anterior to the lateral epicondyle is marked. The forearm is then pronated and a straight line drawn from this point distally to the center of the dorsum of the wrist. The skin incision, along the upper two thirds of this line, is deepened through the subcutaneous tissue, protecting the posterior branch of the lateral cutaneous nerve of the forearm. The fascia is incised along the radial border of the extensor digitorum communis muscle, developing the interval from distal to proximal between it and the extensor carpi radialis brevis muscle. The interval may be developed as far proximally as the lateral epicondyle, where the extensor digitorum communis muscle may be detached from its origin if necessary. The supinator muscle is seen in the proximal third of the incision, deep to the superficial extensor muscles. Exposure of the nerve within the supinator muscle requires a muscle incision perpendicular to the direction of the fibers of the superficial head in its midportion.

The upper two thirds of the radial shaft may be exposed in the interval between the extensor carpi radialis brevis and extensor digitorum communis muscles. The supinator muscle is elevated from the radial shaft by subperiosteal dissection and retracted proximally with the posterior interosseous nerve. The abductor pollicis longus is retracted ulnarly, exposing the middle third of the radial shaft.

Superficial Branch of the Radial Nerve in the Distal Forearm

The superficial branch of the radial nerve may be found in the distal forearm two to three fingerbreadths proximal to the tip of the radial styloid process, along a line connecting the radial styloid and the lateral humeral epicondyle. A 6-cm longitudinal incision is made palmar to this line, beginning 2 cm proximal to the tip of the radial styloid.[4] The nerve is found distally in the subcutaneous tissue and may be traced proximally to the point where it emerges from under the brachioradialis tendon, in the axilla formed by this tendon and the extensor carpi radialis longus tendon.

REFERENCES

1. Capener N. The vulnerability of the posterior interosseous nerve of the forearm. J Bone Joint Surg [Br] 1966; 48:770–772.
2. Crenshaw AH. Surgical approaches. In: Crenshaw AH, ed. Campbell's operative orthopaedics, 7th ed. St. Louis: CV Mosby, 1987:94–99.
3. Davies F, Laird M. The supinator muscle in the deep radial (posterior interosseous) nerve. Anat Rec 1948; 101:243–250.
4. Dellon AL, Mackinnon SE. Radial sensory nerve entrapment in the forearm. J Hand Surg [Am] 1986; 11:199–205.
5. Eversmann WW Jr. Entrapment and compression neuropathies. In: Green DP, ed. Operative hand surgery, ed 2. New York: Churchill-Livingstone, 1988:1454–1460.
6. Hall HC, Mackinnon SE, Gilbert RW. An approach to the posterior interosseous nerve. Plast Reconstr Surg 1984; 74:435–438.
7. Henry AK. Extensile exposure, ed 2. New York: Churchill-Livingstone, 1973:91–115.
8. Hollingshead WH. Anatomy for surgeons: Vol. 3, The back and limbs, ed 3. New York: Harper & Row, 1982:341–529.
9. Hoppenfeld S, deBoer P. Surgical exposures in orthopaedics. Philadelphia: JB Lippincott, 1984:109–140.
10. Inglis AE. Surgical exposure of peripheral nerves. In: Omer GE, Spinner M, eds. Management of peripheral nerve problems. Philadelphia: WB Saunders, 1980:317–331.
11. Kameda Y. An anomalous muscle (accessory scapularis-teres-latissimus muscle) in the axilla penetrating the brachial plexus in man. Acta Anat 1976; 96:513–533.
12. Kaplan EB, Spinner M. Normal and anomalous innervation patterns in the upper extremity. In: Omer GE, Spinner M, eds. Management of peripheral nerve problems. Philadelphia: WB Saunders, 1980: 75–99.
13. Linell EA. The distribution of nerves in the upper limb, with reference to variabilities and their clinical significance. J Anat 1921; 55:79.
14. Lister GD, Belsole RB, Kleinert HE. The radial tunnel syndrome. J Hand Surg [Am] 1979; 4:52–59.
15. Lotem M, Fried A, Levy M, Solzi P, Najensoss T, Nathan H. Radial palsy following muscular effort: A nerve compression syndrome possibly related to a fibrous arch of the lateral head of the triceps. J Bone Joint Surg [Br] 1971; 53:500–506.

16. Mackinnon SE, Dellon AL. The overlap pattern of the lateral antebrachial cutaneous nerve and the superficial branch of the radial nerve. J Hand Surg [Am] 1985; 10:522–526.
17. Manske PR. Compression of the radial nerve by the triceps muscle. J Bone Joint Surg [Am] 1977; 59: 835–836.
18. McFarlane RM, Mayer JR. Digital nerve grafts with the lateral antebrachial cutaneous nerve. J Hand Surg [Am] 1976; 1:169–173.
19. Packer JW, Foster RR, Garcia A, Grantham BA. The humeral fracture with radial nerve palsy: Is exploration warranted? Clin Orthop 1972; 88:34–38.
20. Roles NC, Maudsley RH. Radial tunnel syndrome: Resistant tennis elbow as a nerve entrapment. J Bone Joint Surg [Br] 1972; 54:499–508.
21. Spinner M. The arcade of Frohse and its relationship to posterior interosseous nerve paralysis. J Bone Joint Surg [Br] 1968; 50:809–812.
22. Spinner M. Management of nerve compression lesions of the upper extremity. In: Omer GE, Spinner M, eds. Management of peripheral nerve problems. Philadelphia: WB Saunders, 1980:569–587.
23. Sponseller PD, Engber WD. Double entrapment of radial tunnel syndrome. J Hand Surg [Am] 1983; 8: 420–423.
24. Sunderland S. Metrical and non-metrical features of the muscular branches of the radial nerve. J Comp Neurol 1946; 85:93–97.
25. Warwick R, Williams PL, eds. Gray's anatomy. 35th ed [Br]. Philadelphia: WB Saunders, 1973:1045–1048.
26. Whitson RO. Relation of the radial nerve to the shaft of the humerus. J Bone Joint Surg [Am] 1954; 36: 85–88.

28

Radial Nerve—Results

Curtis M. Steyers

AUTHOR'S KEY POINTS

- Repair of radial nerve injuries provides better results than repair of comparable median and ulnar nerve injuries, irrespective of level or mechanism of injury.
- Repair of radial nerve injuries below the elbow (when technically possible) provides better results than repair of radial nerve injuries above the elbow.

The purpose of this chapter is to review the available data relating to outcomes following penetrating injury and direct repair of the radial nerve and to review those factors that appear to have a significant influence on outcomes following repair. Results of treatment for closed injuries, including blunt trauma, fractures, thermal injuries, and open injuries associated with gunshot wounds and complex soft-tissue trauma are reviewed in separate chapters and are not included here. Results following late reconstruction using nerve grafting techniques and tendon transfer are also discussed in separate sections of this book.

Most reviews of penetrating injuries of the peripheral nerves of the upper extremity have concluded that outcomes following radial nerve repair are generally better than those for other nerves.[18] However, many authors have cautioned that interpretation of these studies is extremely difficult for numerous reasons.[10,14,16] Objective, reproducible outcome measures are often missing or ambiguous, rarely include functional measures, and are inconsistent among studies, so that comparisons among these studies have little practical value. Sensory and motor recovery are usually weighted equally, despite significant differences in the relative importance of sensory recovery in median nerve lesions when compared to radial nerve injuries.[16] Little information is available relative to static measures of gross hand function such as grip and pinch strength in patients who have had a radial nerve repair, despite available documentation that these measures deteriorate in radial nerve palsy.[7]

In a series of 10 normal volunteers who had radial nerve blocks, Labosky and Waggy demonstrated a substantial loss of grip and key pinch strength.[7] Persistent strength decrements were observed in these patients even with use of a static wrist splint that stabilized the wrist in dorsiflexion. Most available studies of upper-extremity peripheral nerve lesions include multiple injury types and therefore are made up of heterogeneous patient groups. Final outcome assessments are often done prematurely, and evaluation of older series, collected prior to the introduction of microsurgical techniques, may be misleading because of the anticipated improvement in outcome directly related to the newer operative techniques.[18]

EARLY STUDIES—EXPERIENCES IN WORLD WARS I AND II

The radial nerve was the most commonly injured nerve in World Wars I and II.[18] However, most large series of upper-extremity peripheral nerve trauma indicate that most of these injuries are lesions in continuity and do not require exploration and repair as often as injuries to the median and ulnar nerves.[5,12,13,16,18,19] Based on wartime data, Sunderland estimates that fewer than 30% of radial nerve injuries require exploration and repair.[18]

In 1932, Pollock and Davis reviewed the literature up to that date that reported the results of treatment of radial nerve injuries in World War I.[14] Reported results varied drastically, with failure rates ranging from 3% to 87.5%. The cumulative experience of 397 cases cited by Pollock revealed a "success" rate of 72% for radial nerve repairs, compared to 69% and 57% "success" rates for median and ulnar nerves respectively. However, Pollock also cited the Surgeon General's Report of the Medical Department of the United States Army, which indicated that only 11% of the 99 cases reported achieved a good result. Several other series were also cited by Pollock and served to highlight the wide variations in outcome following peripheral nerve repair at that time.

In 1956, Woodhall and Beebe reported on the American experience with peripheral nerve injuries sustained in World War II. Of the 197 radial nerve injuries, 21.3% achieved a "good" result. "Good" indicated that all synergistic and independent movements were possible or recovery was normal (British Medical Research Council rating of M4 or M5).[19] Seddon reported on the British experience with a similar group of 114 radial nerve injuries; 36.9% of these patients achieved an M4 or M5 motor level.

In 1975, Seddon reported on his cumulative experience with peripheral nerve injury and repair.[16] This experience spanned 25 years and included both civilian and war-injured patients. Of 2229 patients, 82 had radial nerve injuries. Four patients underwent immediate primary repair and two achieved a "good" result (described as M4- or M5-level motor function). Of the 63 patients who underwent "secondary suture," 54% achieved a "good" result.

LATER EXPERIENCE—VIETNAM WAR

Most series of nerve injuries since World War II have included patients treated with newer microsurgical techniques, including the routine use of magnification. Omer reported the largest series of nerve-injured patients from the Vietnam War in 1974.[12] However, data relative to outcomes for injuries to specific nerves were not provided in that study. In 1970, Brown reported a similar series of patients from Vietnam in which 135 nerves were repaired and followed from 6 to 24 months postoperatively.[3] Five radial nerves were repaired, and 40% showed "some return" of function at last evaluation.

FACTORS INFLUENCING OUTCOME FOLLOWING REPAIR

Level of Injury

Several series provided sufficient data to compare the results of repair of injuries sustained above the elbow with those sustained below the elbow.[1,2,8,10,15,16] Marble and coworkers reviewed their experience with civilian peripheral nerve injuries during the 1930s.[10] Of the 11 radial nerves repaired, 37.5% achieved a "good" result; all of these injuries were above the elbow. Mayer and associates repaired 39 posterior interosseous nerves during this same era and reported 72% excellent results with full recovery.[11] Allbritten repaired eight posterior interosseous nerves.[1] Three patients with sufficient follow-up had excellent results, but follow-up information was unavailable for the other five patients. Larson and Posch, reporting on the results of five posterior interosseous nerve repairs and 17 above-elbow radial nerve repairs, found that 40% of the below-elbow repairs had partial or complete extensor return, while 82% of the above-elbow repairs had the same result.[8] Sakellarides repaired 13 radial nerves in a series of 172 peripheral nerve injuries; 17% of the above-elbow repairs achieved a "good" result, while 57% of the below-elbow repairs reached the same level.[15] Seddon recorded 71% "good" results following repair of the posterior interosseous nerve and 54% "good" results following repair of the radial nerve above the elbow.

In summary, the available literature from the past 60 years supports the conclusion that repair of radial nerve injuries below the elbow provides a more satisfactory outcome than repair above the elbow (Table 28-1).

Other Factors

Many other factors undoubtedly play a role in determining outcome following radial nerve injury and repair (see Chap. 24). Most of these factors, including mechanism of injury, associated soft-tissue and skeletal injuries, length of nerve injured, and time interval between injury and attempted repair, are interrelated and cannot be considered independently. However, despite these limitations several trends are apparent. Tidy wounds with a narrow zone of nerve injury are associated with better outcomes than injuries associated with segmental nerve and soft-tissue damage. Omer noted that 44% of the nerve injuries characterized as lacerations in his Vietnam series had a "successful" outcome, compared to 25% of the injuries associated with gunshot wounds from military weapons.[12]

Numerous studies have documented the detrimental effects of excessive tension on outcome following direct nerve repair.[18] However, there is very little agreement on the size of the gap that can be overcome safely by nerve mobilization and joint positioning (see Chap. 36). Level of injury, nerve injured, time since injury, and the condition of the surrounding soft tissues all determine the maximum gap that can be closed. Granthan has indicated that 6-cm gaps in the arm and 3.4-cm gaps about the elbow can be successfully closed,[6] while Brown and others have indicated that 8-cm gaps can be successfully managed by these techniques.[4] No data are available for direct comparison between these techniques and interfascicular nerve grafting.

Timing of nerve repair following injury appears to play some role in outcome. Prolonged delays beyond which repair is unlikely to provide useful recovery have been established.[18] Zachary has indicated that delays beyond 13 months for injuries above the spiral groove, 16 months for injuries below the spiral groove and above the terminal branches of the radial nerve, and 9 months for injuries of the posterior interosseous nerve predictably lead to poor results. Less clear are the roles

Table 28-1. *Radial Nerve—Results*

Author	**Injury Type**	**Location**			**% Recovery M4–M5**
		Above Elbow	*Below Elbow*	*Not Specified*	
Marble, 1942[10]	Civilian	11	–	–	37.5
Mayer, 1947[11]	Civilian	–	39	–	72
Albritten, 1946[1]	Civilian	–	8	–	100
Larsen, 1958[8]	Civilian	17	–	–	76
			11	–	40
Seddon, 1954[17]	Military	–	–	114	36.9
Woodhall, 1956[19]	Military	–	–	197	21.3
Brown, 1970[3]	Military	–	–	5	40.0 ("some return")
Sakellarides, 1962[15]	Civilian	6	–	–	17 (M3 or better)
		–	7	–	57 (M3 or better)
Seddon, 1975[16]	Military & Civilian	67	–	–	54
		–	7	–	72

of immediate primary, delayed primary, and early secondary repair. Results in World War II patients appeared to be best when repair was delayed 2 to 3 weeks, as noted by Brown.[4] Omer noted that 70% of the successful repairs done in his series were completed within 6 weeks of injury and all were done within 3 months.[12] These findings tend to support the theoretical advantage of delayed repair noted by Lundborg.[9]

COMPARISON OF RESULTS—MEDIAN AND ULNAR NERVES VS RADIAL

As indicated previously, these series are very difficult to evaluate and compare because they include heterogeneous patient groups with respect to injury mechanisms, level of injury, and other factors. Different outcome measures are used, repairs were done at different time intervals following injury, and different surgical techniques were used. However, comparison of the outcomes for radial, median, and ulnar nerve repairs within each series indicates that radial nerve injuries have more satisfactory outcomes than median and ulnar nerve injuries (see Chaps. 26 and 30).[8,18] Seddon reported that only 8.6% of his patients with median nerve injuries achieved a satisfactory level of sensory function, and only 4.9% of his patients with ulnar nerve injuries achieved a satisfactory level of motor function.[17] Similar findings were noted by Woodhall.[19]

Several explanations have been provided to explain these results.[18] These include the shorter distance from site of injury to end-organ, the relatively easy identification of sensory and motor components of the radial nerve, minimizing the risk of fascicular mismatching even at arm level, and the relatively gross motor function of the radial innervated muscles as compared to the more precise and intricate ulnar-innervated intrinsic muscle function and the complex function of the median-innervated cutaneous mechanoreceptors.

REFERENCES

1. Allbritten FF. The surgical repair of the deep branch of the radial nerve. Surg Gynecol Obstet 1946; 82: 305–310.
2. Boswick JA, Schneewind J, Stomberg W. Evaluation of peripheral nerve repairs below the elbow. Arch Surg 1965; 90:50–51.
3. Brown PW. The time factor in surgery of upper extremity peripheral nerve injury. Clin Orthop Rel Res 1970; 68:14–21.
4. Brown PW. Factors influencing the success of surgical repair of peripheral nerves. Surg Clin North Am 1972; 52:1137.
5. Dellon AL, Mackinnon SE. Surgery of the peripheral nerve. New York: Thieme, 1988:121–122.
6. Granthan EG, Pollard C, Brabson JA. Peripheral nerve surgery: Repair of nerve defects. Ann Surg 1948; 127:696.
7. Labosky DA, Waggy CA. Apparent weakness of the median and ulnar nerves in radial nerve palsy. J Hand Surg [Am] 1986; 11:528–533.
8. Larsen RD, Posch JL. Nerve injuries in the upper extremity. Arch Surg 1958; 77:469–482.
9. Lundborg G. Nerve injury and repair. New York: Churchill-Livingstone, 1988:196–197.
10. Marble HC, Hamlin E, Watkins AL. Regeneration in the ulnar, median and radial nerves. Am J Surg 1942; 55:274–294.
11. Mayer JH, Mayfield FH. Surgery of the posterior interosseous branch of the radial nerve. Surg Gynecol Obstet 1947; 84:979–982.
12. Omer GE. Injury to nerves of the upper extremity. J Bone Joint Surg [Am] 1974; 56:1615–1624.
13. Omer GE. The evaluation of clinical results following peripheral nerve suture. In: Omer GE, Spinner M, eds. Management of peripheral nerve problems. Philadelphia: WB Saunders, 1980:431–442.
14. Pollock LJ, Davis L. Peripheral nerve injuries. Am J Surg 1932; 18:579–595.
15. Sakellarides H. A follow-up study of 172 peripheral nerve injuries in the upper extremity in civilians. J Bone Joint Surg [Am] 1962; 44:140–148.
16. Seddon H. Surgical disorders of the peripheral nerves, ed 2. New York: Churchill-Livingstone, 1975:303–307.
17. Seddon HJ. Peripheral nerve injuries. Medical Research Council Special Report Series No. 282. London: Her Majesty's Stationery Office, 1954. Cited in Omer GE, Spinner M, eds. Management of peripheral nerve problems. Philadelphia: WB Saunders, 1980:435.
18. Sunderland S. Nerves and nerve injuries, ed 2. New York: Churchill-Livingstone, 1978:838.
19. Woodhall B, Beebe GW. Peripheral nerve regeneration, a follow-up study of 3656 World War II injuries. Veterans Administration Medical Monograph. Washington DC: U S Government Printing Office, 1956:117–118.

29

Ulnar Nerve: Applied Anatomy and Operative Exposure

David B. Siegel
Richard H. Gelberman

AUTHORS' KEY POINTS

- The posterior branch of the medial cutaneous nerve of the forearm crosses the ulnar nerve from 6 cm proximal to 4 cm distal to the medial epicondyle and should be isolated proximally and protected throughout the operative field when exploring the ulnar nerve in the cubital tunnel.[14]
- A straight line drawn from the medial epicondyle to the radial margin of the pisiform outlines the course of the ulnar nerve in the forearm.
- The Martin-Gruber neural connection, from the median to ulnar nerve in the forearm, occurs in 15% of upper limbs and should be considered a possibility when there is preservation of distal ulnar nerve function following high ulnar nerve injury.
- The Riche-Cannieu connection occurs in the palm or thenar eminence of 50% of upper limbs and may account for the variable number of fingers involved in clawing, following low ulnar nerve injury.
- When using McConnell's medial approach to explore the ulnar nerve in the forearm, the interval between the flexor carpi ulnaris and flexor digitorum superficialis muscles should be developed first, rather than attempting initially to develop the interval between the flexor carpi ulnaris and flexor digitorum profundus.

ANATOMY

Ulnar Nerve in the Arm

The ulnar nerve arises directly from the medial cord of the brachial plexus. It contains fibers from the eighth cervical and first thoracic nerve roots and lies between the axillary artery laterally and the axillary vein medially (Fig. 29-1). At the inferior border of the subscapularis muscle, the nerve may receive fibers of the seventh cervical nerve root via the so-called lateral root of the ulnar nerve. This supplemental nerve arises from either the lateral cord or middle trunk.[22] The ulnar nerve de-

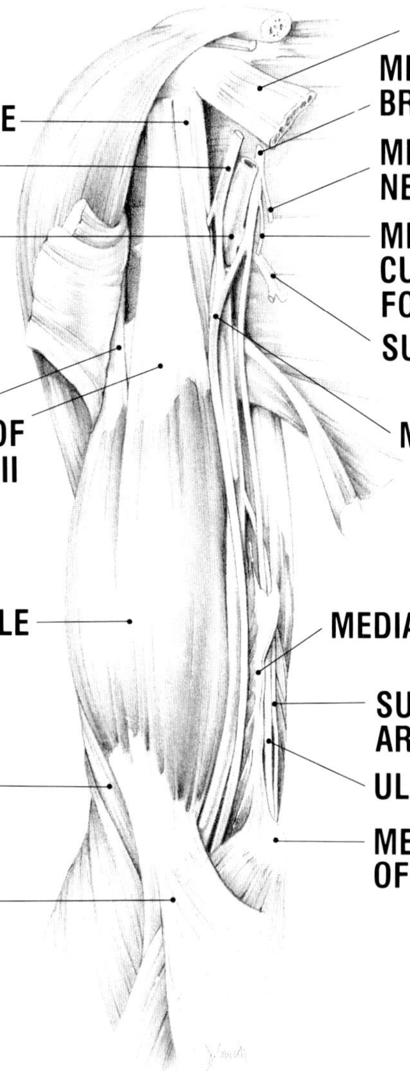

Figure 29–1. *The ulnar nerve arises from the medial cord of the brachial plexus and lies medial to the brachial artery and median nerve throughout the arm. It pierces the medial intermuscular septum with the superior ulnar collateral artery.*

scends in the arm posterior to the pectoralis major muscle and medial or posteromedial to the brachial artery. At the inferior border of the pectoralis major, the nerve diverges medially from the brachial artery and pierces the medial intermuscular septum, about 8 cm above the medial epicondyle.[7] The superior ulnar collateral artery, a branch of the brachial artery, pierces the medial intermuscular septum in conjunction with the nerve. Both descend distally and medially on the anterior surface of the medial head of the triceps muscle. The artery, joined by a branch of the inferior ulnar collateral artery at the medial supracondylar ridge, accompanies the ulnar nerve as it enters the interval between the medial epicondyle of the humerus and the olecranon. The nerve passes into the ulnar groove on the dorsal aspect of the medial epicondyle. While it does not innervate any muscles of the arm, it may innervate the flexor carpi ulnaris 0.5 to 1 cm above the medial epicondyle.

Potential Points of Compression in the Arm

Three potential points of compression of the ulnar nerve in the arm have been recognized:

1. Ulnar nerve fibers of the medial cord may be compressed at the level of the first rib as the nerve passes between the rib and the clavicle (see Chap. 84).[15]
2. About 8 cm proximal to the medial epicondyle, the nerve pierces the medial intermuscular septum. A thick fascial band, the arcade of Struthers, is present in 20% to 70% of upper limbs and extends from the medial head of the triceps muscle to the intermuscular septum.[18]
3. Hypertrophy of the medial head of the triceps may force the nerve anteriorly. With triceps muscle contraction, the nerve may be compressed around the medial epicondyle.

SUMMARY OF ANATOMICAL COMPRESSION POINTS OF THE ULNAR NERVE

ARM

1. First rib
2. Arcade of Struthers
3. Medial head of triceps muscle

ELBOW/FOREARM

1. Anconeus epitrochlearis muscle
2. Fibrous arcade between two heads of flexor carpi ulnaris
3. Osteophytes from the ulnohumeral joint
4. Elbow joint ganglia
5. Lipomata

HAND/WRIST

1. Palmaris brevis muscle
2. Fibrous origin of flexor digiti minimi
3. Anomalous muscles
4. Ulnar artery aneurysm or thrombosis
5. Distal ulnar tunnel ganglia

Variations

Although the ulnar nerve originates from the medial cord of the brachial plexus, it frequently receives fibers from the lateral cord, the middle trunk, or the anterior division of the middle trunk. These neural elements, collectively labeled the lateral root of the ulnar nerve, join the nerve at or just distal to the inferior border of the subscapularis muscle and provide innervation to the flexor carpi ulnaris muscle.[22] While ultimately the first branch of the ulnar nerve generally takes off within the cubital tunnel, variations in the articular and first muscular branches are common. The articular branch, normally the first branch of the nerve, exits from the main trunk in the ulnar groove and passes horizontally into the joint. One or several articular branches may exit the nerve in the arm, as far proximally as 1 cm above the medial epicondyle. The first muscular branch to the flexor carpi ulnaris muscle commonly exits immediately distal to the articular branch. However, division as high as 4 cm above the medial epicondyle has been reported.[10]

Ulnar Nerve at the Elbow and Forearm

Within the cubital tunnel, the ulnar nerve passes from the extensor surface of the arm to the flexor surface of the forearm (Fig. 29-2). This fibro-osseous tunnel, bordered medially by the elbow joint, is divided geographically into three parts.[2] The first part, the ulnar groove in the medial epicondyle, provides the entrance to the tunnel. A fascial arcade, which attaches to the medial epicondyle and the olecranon and connects the ulnar and humeral heads of origin of the flexor carpi ulnaris muscle, covers the nerve in the second part of the tunnel. The muscle bellies of the flexor carpi ulnaris form the third portion of the tunnel.

As the ulnar nerve crosses the medial surface of the elbow, it lies on the posterior and oblique portions of the ulnar collateral ligament. The distance between the medial humeral epicondyle and the olecranon is shortest with elbow extension and increases with elbow flexion.[21] The roof of the cubital tunnel, formed by the fascial arcade and the flexor carpi ulnaris, becomes taut with elbow flexion. The volume of the tunnel decreases as the elbow flexes, and pressure within it increases, even when the aponeurotic arch is not thickened (see Chap. 75).

In the first part of the cubital tunnel, the nerve provides one branch or several small articular branches to the elbow joint. In the second portion of the tunnel, two branches supply the flexor carpi ulnaris muscle. The first branch leaves the main trunk horizontally, and the second courses distally

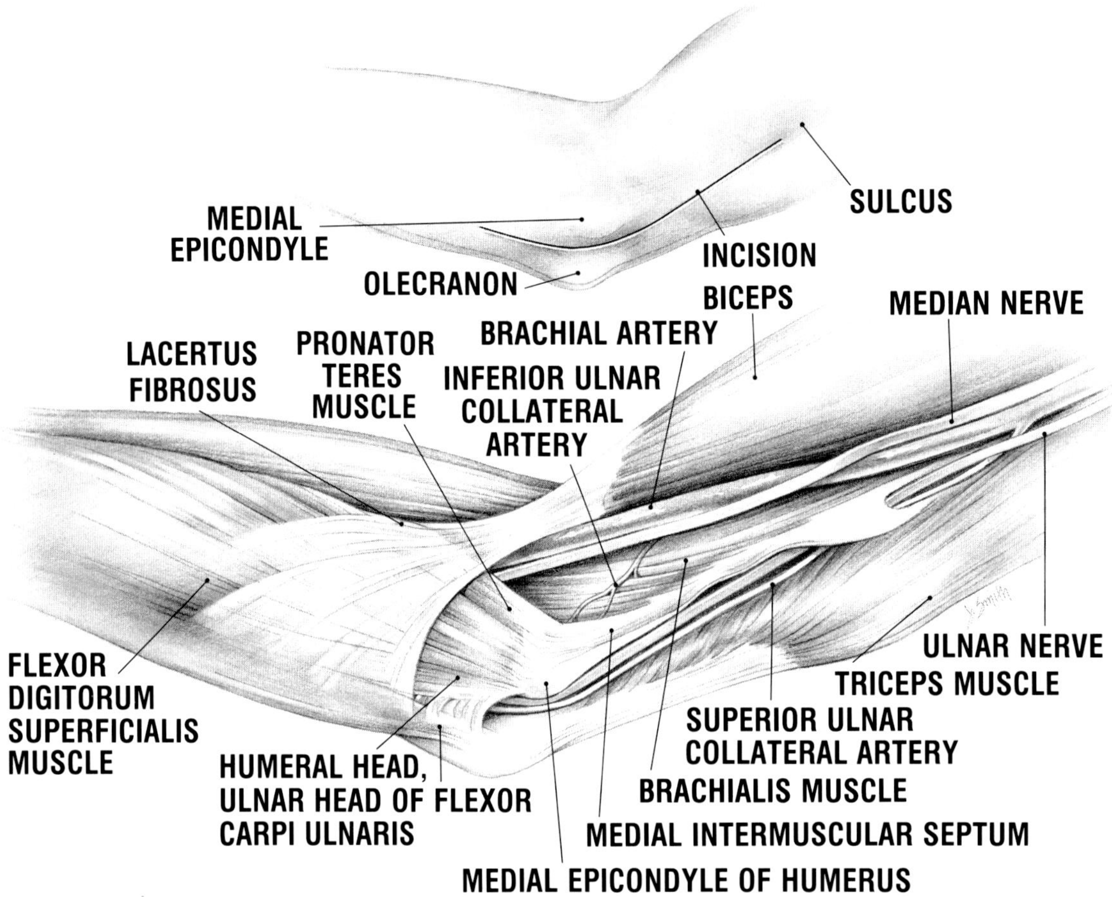

Figure 29–2. *Operative exposure of the ulnar nerve in the cubital tunnel is achieved with a straight incision that begins superiorly in the sulcus between the biceps and triceps muscles and extends distally to the groove between the medial epicondyle and the olecranon process. A branch of the medial antebrachial cutaneous nerve may be found crossing the incision within the subcutaneous tissue (See Text).*

for several centimeters before entering the muscle. As many as four flexor carpi ulnaris muscle branches have been reported, leaving the main nerve between 4 cm proximal and 10 cm distal to the medial epicondyle.[7] The first muscular branch to the flexor carpi ulnaris divides in 5% of limbs to supply the flexor digitorum profundus.[19]

As the ulnar nerve leaves the cubital tunnel, it lies between the flexor carpi ulnaris and flexor digitorum profundus muscles on the palmar surface of the latter (Fig. 29-3). The nerve maintains this relationship through the proximal to middle forearm. In the distal third of the forearm the nerve becomes superficial, lying just radial to the flexor carpi ulnaris muscle. **A straight line drawn from the medial epicondyle to the radial margin of the pisiform outlines the course of the nerve in the forearm.** The ulnar artery passes deep to the two bellies of the pronator teres, coursing medially to join the nerve in the middle third of the forearm. The nerve remains medial to the artery as the two course distally. After emerging from under the cover of the flexor carpi ulnaris, both nerve and artery pass radial to the pisiform, palmar to the transverse carpal ligament, and dorsal to the superficial palmar carpal ligament. The ulnar nerve divides into deep terminal and superficial palmar branches at the base of the hypothenar eminence.[3]

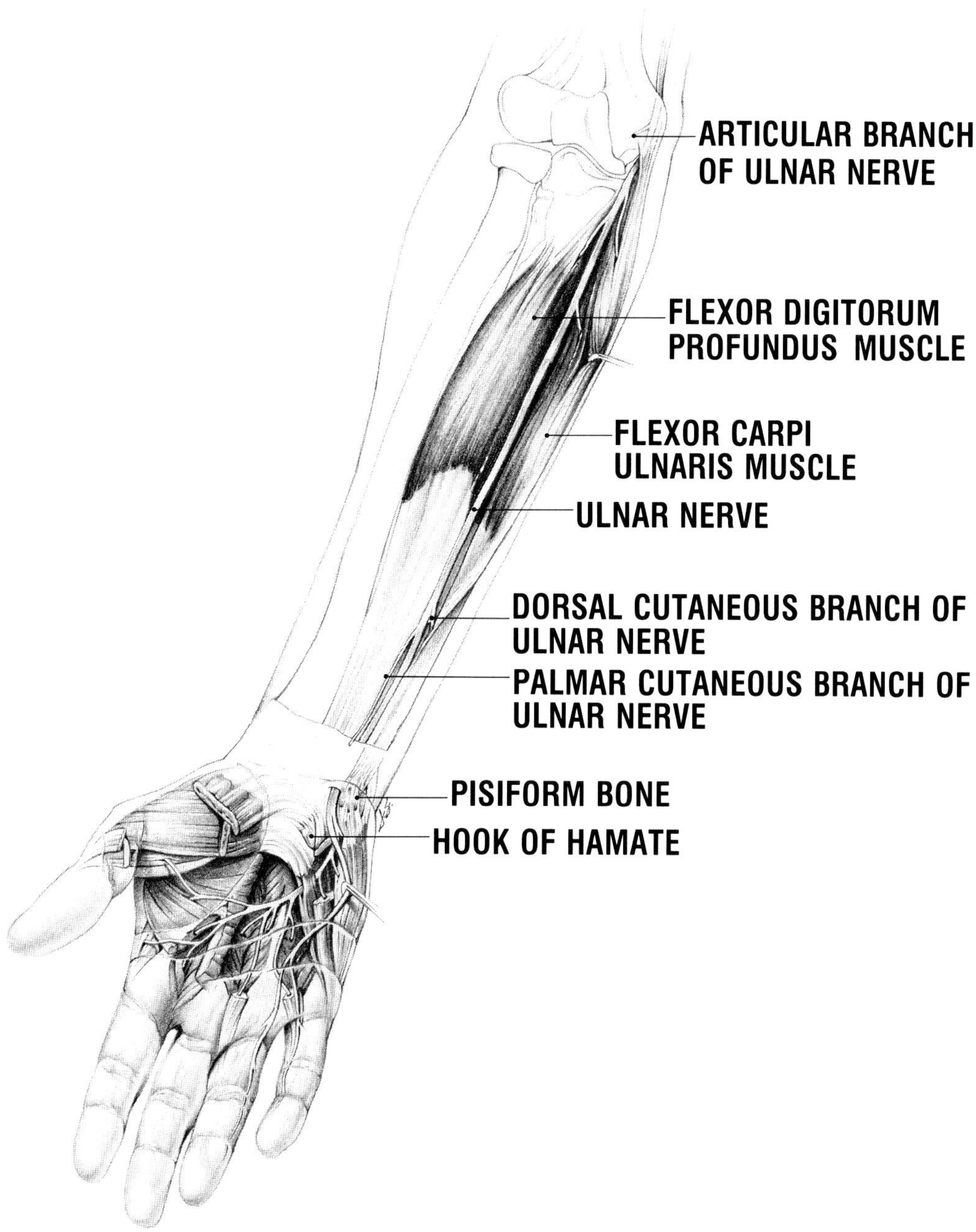

Figure 29–3. *The course of the ulnar nerve in the forearm and hand. Note specifically the relationship of the ulnar nerve to the flexor digitorum profundus and flexor carpi ulnaris muscles.*

The three branches of the ulnar nerve in the forearm are the muscular branch to the flexor digitorum profundus and the palmar and dorsal cutaneous branches. The motor branch to the ulnar half of the flexor digitorum profundus muscle arises 3 cm distal to the medial epicondyle and passes distally for about 2.5 cm before entering the muscle.[7] In 80% of upper limbs, a single branch supplies this muscle, and in about 20% two or more supply it. When there is no direct branch from the main nerve trunk, the flexor digitorum profundus may be supplied entirely by the median nerve or by the branch of the ulnar nerve to the flexor carpi ulnaris. Characteristically, the ulnar nerve supplies the flexor digitorum profundus to the ring and little fingers, and the median nerve supplies the index and long fingers. However, Sunderland documented this pattern in only 50% of upper limbs.[20] He found it more likely for the median nerve to innervate the ring and little fingers than for the ulnar nerve to innervate the long finger.

The flexor digitorum profundus muscle to the index finger is supplied by the median nerve only. The palmar cutaneous branch of the ulnar nerve arises at the junction of the middle and distal thirds of the forearm. It courses distally on or within the epineurium of the ulnar nerve or on the palmar surface of the ulnar artery. After perforating the antebrachial fascia immediately above the distal wrist flexion crease, it supplies the skin of the hypothenar eminence, the ulnar artery, and occasionally the palmaris brevis muscle. The dorsal cutaneous branch of the ulnar nerve arises 5 to 7 cm above the distal wrist flexion crease on the deep dorsal surface of the flexor carpi ulnaris. It pierces the fascia about 3 cm above the distal wrist crease, courses distally in the subcutaneous tissue, and divides into two dorsal digital nerves, supplying the skin on the dorsoulnar side of the hand, the little finger, and the ulnar half of the ring finger. Occasionally, a third digital nerve supplies the third dorsal web space, communicating with the dorsal sensory branch of the radial nerve.[12]

The medial cutaneous nerve of the forearm, containing fibers from the eighth cervical and first thoracic nerve roots, arises directly from the lower trunk or medial cord of the brachial plexus.[13] In the axilla it courses with the ulnar nerve between the axillary artery and vein. A small branch leaves the nerve to supply the skin over the biceps muscle and the elbow flexion crease. It descends along the medial surface of the brachial artery, piercing the antebrachial fascia in the middle third of the arm with the basilic vein. It divides into anterior and posterior branches about 15 cm proximal to the medial epicondyle. The anterior branch passes in front of the median cubital vein between the medial epicondyle and biceps tendon, supplying the palmar skin of the forearm. Its terminal branches join the palmar cutaneous branches of the ulnar and median nerves in the hand. The posterior branch of the medial cutaneous nerve of the forearm often crosses the ulnar nerve from 6 cm proximal to 4 cm distal to the medial epicondyle. It descends along the medial side of the basilic vein, supplying the dorsomedial skin of the forearm. Distally, it joins the dorsal cutaneous branch of the ulnar nerve.

Potential Points of Neural Compression at the Elbow and Forearm

The anconeus epitrochlearis, present in 1% to 30% of limbs, is a small anomalous muscle that may compress the ulnar nerve at the elbow immediately above the cubital tunnel.[6] It arises from the medial epicondyle, crosses over the ulnar nerve, and inserts into the medial border of the olecranon. It occasionally appears as an abnormal extension of the medial portion of the triceps muscle. The fibrous arcade, connecting the two heads of origin of the flexor carpi ulnaris muscle, may become thickened and fibrotic. Known as Osborne's band, it may compress the ulnar nerve, particularly with elbow flexion.[16] Osteophytes, ganglia emanating from the medial aspect of the joint, and lipomas also may compress the ulnar nerve within the cubital tunnel.[2]

Another potential point of compression in the proximal forearm, distal to the cubital tunnel, has been reported recently. Within the intermuscular fascia of the flexor–pronator origin is a common aponeurosis between the flexor digitorum superficialis to the ring finger and the humeral head of the flexor carpi ulnaris muscle.[9] The septum attaches to the medial surface of the coronoid process and medial epicondyle. It extends distally, attaching to the proximal ulna for 2 cm. The ulnar nerve passes posterior to the septum and may be compressed sharply during operative decompression and submuscular transposition of the ulnar nerve.

Variations

Anomalous connections between the median and ulnar nerves in the forearm are discussed in detail in Chapter 12. There is little deviation from normal in the course of the ulnar nerve from elbow to wrist, or in the division of its five branches. However, there is variation in the innervation of the flexor digitorum profundus muscle.[12] It is more common for the median nerve to innervate muscles in ulnar nerve territory than for the ulnar nerve to invade median nerve territory.[19] The medial cutaneous nerve of the forearm may arise from a common branch with the medial cutaneous nerve of the arm, the smallest branch of the brachial plexus.[10] It may arise from the lower trunk, the first thoracic nerve root, or the ulnar nerve itself. It communicates commonly with the intercostobrachial nerve in the axilla and the medial cutaneous nerve of the arm proximally.[11]

Ulnar Nerve in the Hand and Wrist

The ulnar nerve enters the hand through the distal ulnar tunnel. Four centimeters long, the tunnel begins at the proximal edge of the palmar carpal ligament.[3] The nerve lies medial to the ulnar artery, maintaining the relationship held in the forearm. It enters the tunnel dorsal to the palmar carpal ligament and palmar to the transverse carpal ligament and flexor digitorum profundus tendons. It courses radially to the pisiform, where it is covered by the palmaris brevis muscle. In the distal portion of the tunnel, the nerve lies between the pisohamate and pisometacarpal ligaments and opponens digiti minimi muscle dorsally, and hypothenar fat and fibrous arch palmarly. The nerve divides in the midportion of the tunnel into the superficial palmar cutaneous and deep motor branches (see Fig. 29-3).[3]

The superficial palmar branch exits the distal ulnar tunnel with the superficial terminal branch of the ulnar artery. It provides two small motor branches to the palmaris brevis muscle, after which it is purely sensory. After sending several small twigs to supply the skin on the medial side of the hand, the nerve divides into the proper digital nerve to the ulnar side of the little finger and the common palmar digital nerve to the fourth web space. At the level of the metacarpal shafts, the common digital nerve divides into two proper digital nerves. In the palm the nerves lie dorsal to the superficial palmar arch and palmar to the flexor tendons. Immediately after division, the proper digital nerves come to lie palmar (superficial) to the digital arteries. The neurovascular bundles are stabilized within the digits by the retaining skin ligaments, Cleland's dorsally and Grayson's palmarly. The proper palmar digital nerves supply the palmar skin of the fingers, as well as the skin distal to the distal interphalangeal joints dorsally.

The deep terminal branch of the ulnar nerve exits the distal ulnar tunnel dorsoulnar to the deep terminal branch of the ulnar artery. It passes around the hook of the hamate, under the fibrous arch of the hypothenar muscle origin. It passes between and innervates the abductor digiti minimi and flexor digiti minimi muscles, then pierces the opponens digiti minimi.[17] The nerve crosses the palm with the ulnar artery (the deep palmar arch). It innervates all of the interossei, the third and fourth lumbricals, the adductor pollicis, and the flexor pollicis brevis (Table 29-1). In addition, the

Table 29-1. *Level and Order of Innervation of Muscles Supplied by Ulnar Nerve*

Muscle	*cm From Medial Epicondyle (Shortest to Longest)*
Flexor carpi ulnaris	13.4–17.3
Flexor digitorum profundus	16.0–16.8
	cm From Radial Styloid
Abductor digiti minimi	3.3–3.6
Flexor digiti minimi	4.2–4.6
Opponens digiti minimi	4.4–4.6
Fourth web space interossei	5.6–6.1
Third web space interossei	6.1–6.5
Second web space interossei	7.1–7.5
Fourth lumbrical	7.5
Third lumbrical	7.5
Adductor pollicis (oblique head)	7.5–7.7
Adductor pollicis (transverse head)	7.7–7.8
First dorsal interosseous	8.2–8.3

(From Sunderland S, Hughes ESR. Metrical and non-metrical features of the muscular branches of the ulnar nerve. J Comp Neurol 1946;85:113–120, with permission.)

deep terminal branch provides sensory afferents to the ulnocarpal, intercarpal, and carpometacarpal joints.

Potential Points of Compression in the Hand and Wrist

The ulnar nerve may be compressed at several points within the distal ulnar tunnel.[3] The palmaris brevis muscle may be hypertrophied or may have a fibrous edge that compresses the nerve in the midportion of the distal ulnar tunnel. The origin of the flexor digiti minimi may compress the motor branch as it passes around the hook of the hamate. Anomalous muscles, such as a duplicated palmaris longus, may cross and constrict the nerve. Ulnar artery thrombosis or aneurysm is a well-documented cause of nerve compression.[23] Ganglia arising from the triquetral-hamate are reportedly the most common cause of compression.[14]

Variations

There are three major patterns of variability involving the ulnar nerve in the hand and wrist. Occurring in 50% to 77% of hands, the Riche-Cannieu communication (see Chap. 12) involves the deep terminal branch of the ulnar nerve and the motor branch of the median nerve.[10] It occurs commonly within the substance of the flexor pollicis brevis.[1,17] Recent reports demonstrated that the flexor pollicis brevis is innervated by the median nerve in about 35% of hands, the ulnar nerve in 50%, and both in 15%. The median nerve innervates the abductor pollicis brevis in 95%, the ulnar nerve in 2.5%, and both nerves in 2.5% of hands. The opponens pollicis muscle is supplied by the median nerve alone in 83%, by the ulnar nerve in 10%, and both in 7%.[4] Through the Riche-Cannieu communication, the median nerve may innervate the third lumbrical, or, rarely, all the lumbrical muscles.[19] In addition, the second lumbrical may be innervated by the ulnar nerve; in that circumstance, a low ulnar nerve lesion will lead to clawing of the ulnar three digits.

The most common connection is between the superficial sensory branch of the ulnar nerve in the palm and the common digital nerve to the third web space from the median nerve. This leads to dual innervation of the adjacent sides of the long and ring fingers. A similar connection may occur between the dorsal sensory branches of the radial and ulnar nerves. When present, a third dorsal digital branch from the ulnar nerve supplies the third web space in conjunction with the radial digital nerve, providing dual innervation.

The second pattern of variability concerns anomalous divisions of the nerve. The deep motor branch may divide proximal to the hook of the hamate. The radial division enters the carpal tunnel and rejoins the ulnar division distal to the hamate. Less commonly, the nerve may divide proximal to the pisiform, communicate with the dorsal sensory branch, or rejoin the nerve distal to the pisiform. In the event of nerve injury distal to an anomalous division, function will be partially preserved. The ulnar digital nerve to the ring finger may arise in the forearm, passing superficial to the distal ulnar tunnel. Similarly, the dorsal cutaneous branch may arise near the elbow, passing distally in the subcutaneous tissue to reach the hand.

The dorsoulnar aspect of the hand may be supplied, partially or entirely, by the radial nerve or the posterior cutaneous nerve of the forearm. The dorsal cutaneous nerve may deviate palmarly at the pisiform, join the superficial sensory branch, and supply the palmar surface of the little finger. Rarely, the posterior cutaneous nerve of the forearm, normally a branch of the radial nerve, arises from the ulnar nerve.

OPERATIVE EXPOSURE

Ulnar Nerve in the Arm (Extensile to Cubital Tunnel)

The medial approach provides the most extensile exposure of the ulnar nerve in the arm.[8] Cutaneous landmarks are the coracoid process, the medial intermuscular septum, and the medial humeral epicondyle. In the arm, the nerve lies medial to the brachial artery and coracobrachialis muscle. At the insertion of the coracobrachialis muscle into the humerus, the nerve curves medially toward the intermuscular septum. About 8 cm above the medial epicondyle, the nerve pierces the septum in conjunction with the superior ulnar collateral artery, coming to lie on the medial head of the triceps muscle. It descends to the cubital tunnel within the epimysium of the triceps.

Authors' Preferred Method

Operative exposure of the ulnar nerve throughout the upper extremity is accomplished with the patient positioned supine, with the arm on a hand table. The shoulder is abducted 90° and externally rotated, and the forearm is supinated and slightly flexed. The medial epicondyle and olecranon are marked, and the sulcus between the two is palpated. The coracoid process is palpated beneath the anterior fibers of the deltoid muscle, and its position is marked. The sulcus between the biceps and triceps is palpated and traced proximally to the inferior border of the pectoralis major tendon. A straight incision is made from this point distally, directed toward the interval between the medial epicondyle and olecranon (Fig. 29-4). The medial cutaneous nerve of the forearm, piercing the antebrachial fascia with the basilic vein, should be isolated and protected. The fascia is incised in line with the skin incision. The nerve is identified proximally, medial to the brachial artery, and is traced distally to the intermuscular septum (see Fig. 29-1). The septum is incised, exposing the nerve within the epimysium of the triceps. As there are no branches of the nerve in the arm, it is easily mobilized distally to the cubital tunnel. Retraction of the pectoralis major muscle along with the anterior fibers of the deltoid provides adequate exposure of the nerve proximally. The incision may be extended proximally over the pectoralis major tendon and into the deltopectoral interval toward the coracoid process. Release of the pectoralis major tendon from the humerus facilitates proximal exposure.

Ulnar Nerve in the Cubital Tunnel (Extensile to Arm and Forearm)

Exposure of the nerve within the cubital tunnel is achieved with a straight incision centered 1.5 cm posterior to the medial epicondyle. Cutaneous landmarks are the sulcus between the brachialis and triceps muscles proximally, the interval between the medial epicondyle and olecranon, and the medial border of the forearm between the flexor carpi ulnaris and flexor digitorum profundus muscles distally. The incision begins 8 cm proximal to the medial epicondyle and continues distally over the cubital tunnel into the forearm for 4 to 5 cm (see Fig. 29-2). The posterior branch of the medial cutaneous nerve of the forearm has a vari-

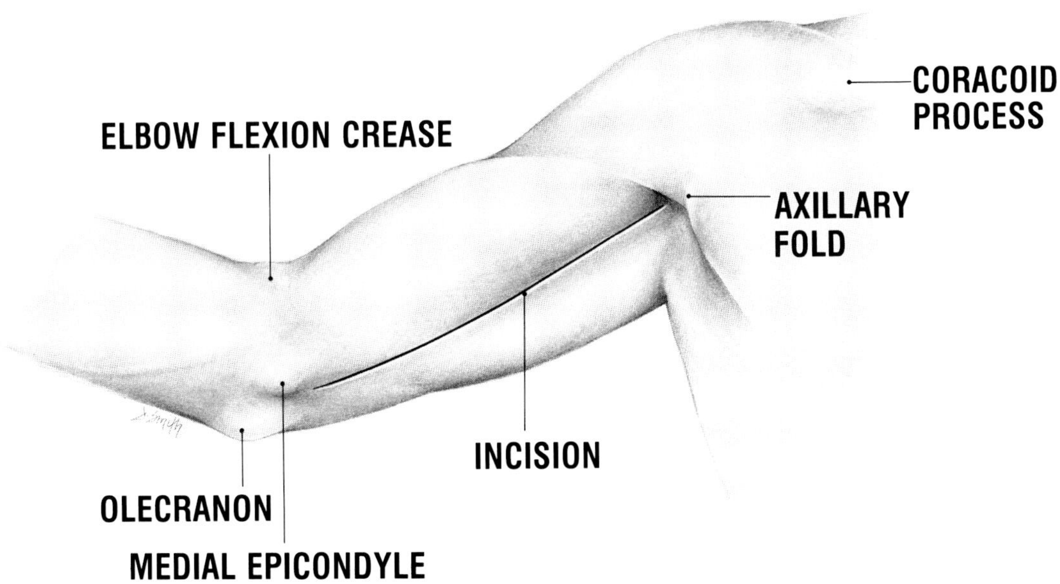

Figure 29–4. *A straight incision in the sulcus between the biceps and triceps muscles is used to expose the ulnar nerve in the arm.*

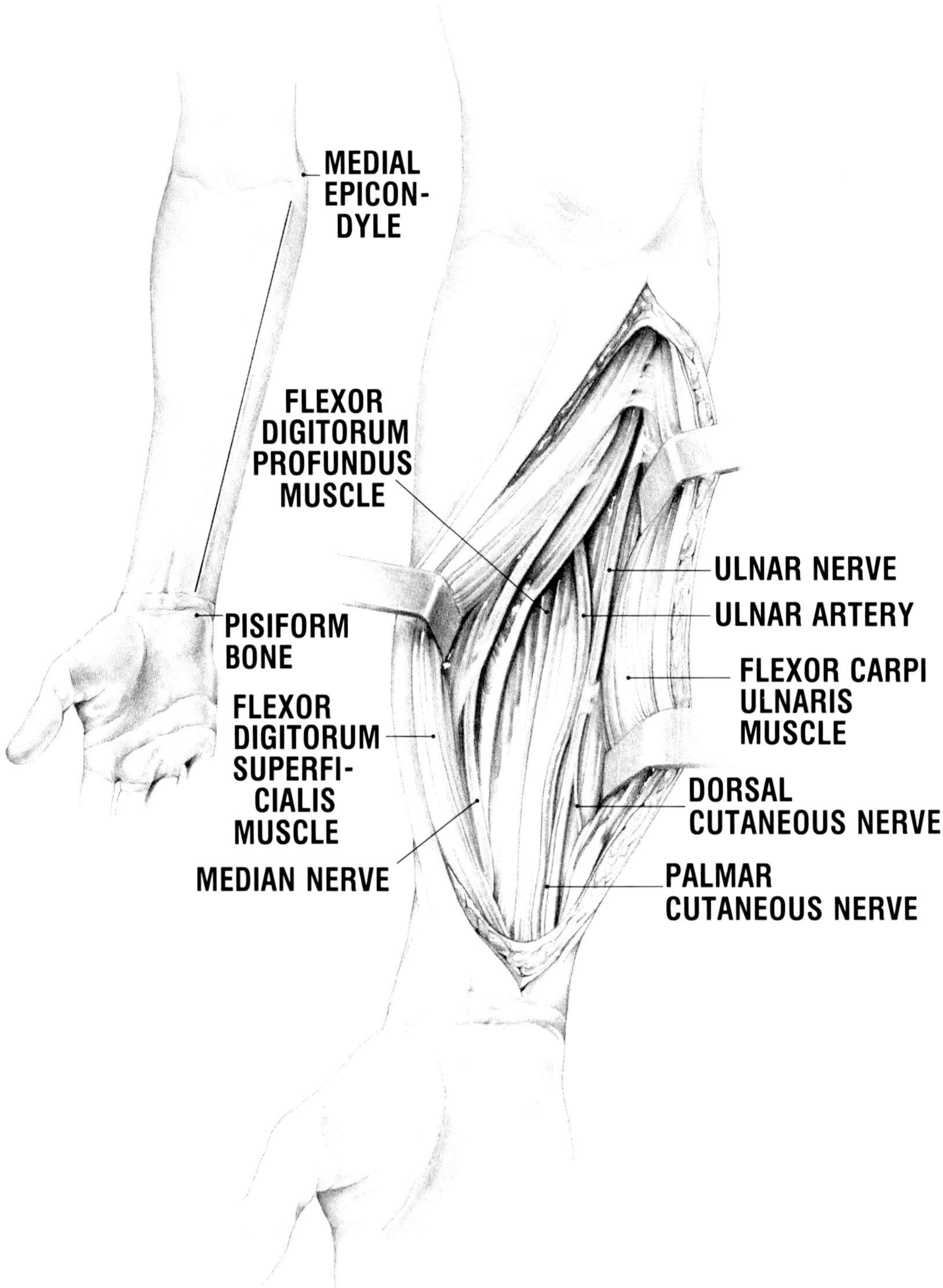

Figure 29–5. *A straight incision drawn from the medial epicondyle to the pisiform outlines the course of the ulnar in the forearm. Retraction of the flexor digitorum superficialis muscle and median nerve radially exposes the ulnar nerve and artery in the interval between the flexor carpi ulnaris and flexor digitorum profundus muscles.*

able course across the elbow and proximal forearm; it should be identified and protected. The ulnar nerve may be identified proximally as it pierces the medial intermuscular septum. In transposing the nerve, the surgeon excises the septum and observes that the nerve is not compressed by the arcade of Struthers.[11] The epimysium is incised to mobilize the nerve distally to the fascial arcade attached to the medial epicondyle and olecranon. The superior and inferior ulnar collateral arteries provide an anastomotic network around the elbow. The fascia between the two heads of origin of the flexor carpi ulnaris is incised, and the muscle bellies are separated 5 cm below their origin. Complete release of the nerve in the proximal forearm requires division of the common aponeurosis between the flexor digitorum superficialis to the ring finger and the humeral head of the flexor carpi ulnaris muscle.[9]

Ulnar Nerve in the Forearm (Extensile to Hand and Cubital Tunnel)

A straight line from the medial epicondyle to the radial margin of the pisiform marks the course of the ulnar nerve in the forearm. After exiting the cubital tunnel, the nerve comes to lie between the flexor carpi ulnaris and flexor digitorum profundus muscles. The nerve lies within the epimysium of the flexor digitorum profundus, joined by the ulnar artery in the middle third of the forearm. The nerve is exposed through a straight medial incision about 5 cm palmar to the subcutaneous border of the ulna.[8] The antebrachial fascia is incised in line with the skin incision, and the medial cutaneous nerve of the forearm is identified and protected. Initially, the interval between the flexor carpi ulnaris and flexor digitorum superficialis muscles is developed. The flexor carpi ulnaris is retracted from the flexor digitorum profundus, and the interval between these muscles is developed. The nerve is located between the flexor carpi ulnaris and flexor digitorum profundus (Fig. 29-5). If necessary, the flexor carpi ulnaris may be released from its proximal origin. The dorsal and palmar cutaneous branches may be found 5 to 7 cm above the distal wrist crease.

This approach is the same as that described by McConnell for combined exposure of the median and ulnar nerves in the forearm (see Chap. 25).

Anterior Approach, Combined with Exposure of the Radius and Median Nerve

The anterior approach for exposure of the median nerve, combined with exposure of the radius, may be extended to include the ulnar nerve (see Chap. 25 for details on the initial anterior approach in the proximal forearm). The interval between the mobile wad and the pronator teres muscle is developed. The fascial incision is continued distally along the radial border of the flexor carpi radialis. The superficial muscle group is retracted ulnarly, exposing the flexor digitorum superficialis muscle. Flexion of the fingers and wrist relaxes the muscle belies and facilitates exposure. At the ulnar margin of the flexor digitorum superficialis, the interval between this muscle and the flexor carpi ulnaris is developed. Elevation and radial retraction of the flexor digitorum superficialis exposes the flexor digitorum profundus and the ulnar neurovascular bundle.[5]

REFERENCES

1. Day MH, Napier JR. The two heads of the flexor pollicis brevis. J Anat 1961; 95:123–130.
2. Eversmann WW Jr. Entrapment and compression neuropathies. In: Green DP, ed. Operative hand surgery, ed 2, 1988:1441–1454.
3. Gross MS, Gelberman RH. The anatomy of the distal ulnar tunnel. Clin Orthop 1985; 196:238–247.
4. Harness D, Sekeles E. The double anastomotic innervation of the thenar muscles. J Anat 1971; 109: 461–466.
5. Henry AK. Extensile exposure, ed 2. New York: Churchill-Livingstone, 1973:94–111.
6. Hirasawa Y, Sawamura H, Sakakida K. Entrapment neuropathy due to bilateral epitrochleoanconeus muscles: A case report. J Hand Surg [Am] 1979; 4: 181–185.
7. Hollingshead WH. Anatomy for surgeons: Vol. 3, The back and limbs, ed 3. Philadelphia: Harper & Row, 1982:341–529.
8. Inglis AE. Surgical exposure of peripheral nerves.

In: Omer GE, Spinner M, eds. Management of peripheral nerve problems. Philadelphia: WB Saunders 1980:317–331.

9. Inserra S, Spinner M. An anatomic factor significant in transposition of the ulnar nerve. J Hand Surg [Am] 1986; 11:80–83.
10. Kaplan EB, Spinner M. Normal and anomalous innervation patterns in the upper extremity. In: Omer GE, Spinner M, eds. Management of peripheral nerve problems. Philadelphia: WB Saunders, 1980: 75–99.
11. Leffert RD. Anterior submuscular transposition of the ulnar nerves by the Learmonth technique. J Hand Surg [Am] 1982; 7:147–155.
12. Linell EA. The distribution of nerves in the upper limb, with reference to variabilities and their clinical significance. J Anat 1920–21; 55:79.
13. Masear VR, Meyer RD, Pichora DR. Surgical anatomy of the medial antebrachial cutaneous nerve. J Hand Surg [Am] 1989; 14:267–271.
14. McDowell CL, Henceroth WD. Compression of the ulnar nerve in the hand by a ganglion. J Bone Joint Surg [Am] 1970; 59:980.
15. Nichols HM. Anatomic structures of the thoracic outlet. Clin Orthop 1986; 207:13–20.
16. Osborne G. The surgical treatment of tardy ulnar neuritis. J Bone Joint Surg [Br] 1957; 39:782.
17. Rowntree T. Anomalous innervation of the hand muscles. J Bone Joint Surg [Br] 1949; 31:505–510.
18. Spinner M. Management of nerve compression lesions of the upper extremity. In: Omer GE, Spinner M, eds. Management of peripheral nerve problems. Philadelphia: WB Saunders, 1980:569–587.
19. Sunderland S. The innervation of the flexor digitorum profundus and lumbrical muscles. Anat Rec 1945; 93:317.
20. Sunderland S, Hughes ESR. Metrical and non-metrical features of the muscular branches of the ulnar nerve. J Comp Neurol 1946; 85:113–120.
21. Vanderpool DW, Chalmers J, Lanb DW, Whiston TB. Peripheral compression lesions of the ulnar nerve. J Bone Joint Surg [Br] 1968; 50:792–802.
22. Warwick R, Williams PL, eds. Gray's anatomy, ed 35 [Br]. Philadelphia: WB Saunders, 1973:1042–1445.
23. Weeks PM, Young VL. Ulnar artery thrombosis and ulnar nerve compression associated with anomalous hypothenar muscle. Plast Reconstr Surg 1982; 69: 130–131.

30

Ulnar Nerve Repair

James W. Strickland
Richard S. Idler
Jeanne L. DelSignore

AUTHORS' KEY POINTS

- The time interval from ulnar nerve repair to functional assessment is of prime importance. Maximal sensory recovery is expected in children by 2 years and in adults by 5 years. Maximal motor recovery may take as long as 5 to 7 years from the time of repair.
- In studies evaluating peripheral nerve injuries incurred in warfare, considering all levels of injury, functional motor recovery has been noted in 35% of cases (M4) and functional sensory recovery in 30% to 68% (S3).
- The estimated rate of ulnar nerve regeneration is 1.09 mm/day; motor recovery lags behind sensory return.
- Direct primary repair of the ulnar nerve with gaps of up to 2.5 cm is indicated. A significant deterioration in results is noted following direct repair when there are gaps of greater than 3 cm.
- The results of ulnar nerve repair distal to the elbow are superior to those carried proximally. The prognosis for intrinsic muscle return following above-elbow injuries in adults is poor.
- There is no significant difference between immediate and delayed ulnar nerve repair (within 6 months of injury).
- The rapidity and completeness of ulnar nerve recovery is considerably better in children than in adults, regardless of level of injury.
- Based on numerous clinical and experimental studies, there is no significant difference between group fascicular and epineural repair. Meticulous microsurgical technique that anatomically realigns the severed nerve is more important than suture technique.
- The nature or mechanism of injury correlates well with ultimate recovery. High-velocity or crushing injuries with extensive associated local damage can be expected to yield poorer results than sharp, clean lacerations. Fortunately, most civilian injuries are due to sharp lacerations, which predictably yield better results than wartime injuries.

HISTORICAL REVIEW

Many factors influence the results of peripheral nerve repair, including the age of the patient, site of injury, nature and severity of the injury, associated injuries, type of nerve (pure or mixed function), and delay prior to repair. In analyzing the results of peripheral nerve repair, the criteria for evaluation must be standardized, emphasizing reproducible objective findings. It is important for final assessment of results to occur only after a sufficient time interval to ensure a maximum level of recovery.

The most common system of evaluating results following peripheral nerve repair is that introduced by the British Medical Research Council (BMRC) in 1954 (see Chap. 27).[24] Since those criteria were established, various authors have modified the original recommendations; unfortunately, these modifications have not been consistent through the various retrospective studies, making it difficult to compare results.[6,15] Refinements of the motor classification system for evaluating results following ulnar nerve repair include:

- M2+: forearm and hand muscles all active, but the first dorsal interosseous cannot contract against resistance
- M3: forearm muscles, hypothenars, and first dorsal interosseous can contract against resistance
- M4: all muscles can contract against resistance, with some independent lateral movement of the fingers

Jongen suggested a refinement in the evaluation of sensory recovery, defining S3+ sensory recovery as less than 20 mm two-point discrimination and S4 recovery as less than 12 mm two-point discrimination with normal tactile gnosis.[6] Moberg, who felt that the BMRC sensory grading system was inadequate, proposed a more precise method of sensibility rating following median and ulnar nerve repair, suggesting additional rating levels between S3+ and S4.[14] Moberg described the following two-point discrimination distances: good, less than 12 mm; fair, 12 to 15 mm; poor, 15 to 20 mm; and bad, more than 20 mm. According to Moberg's system, a good result must demonstrate two-point discrimination of less than 12 mm, since greater distances require visual input to improve functional sensibility. Any return of 20 mm or greater (S3, according to the BMRC system) would be considered a bad result. Moberg's system does not address the issue of persistent pain or hyperesthesia and thus may not be as helpful in determining a successful result.

Most investigators agree that the primary determinant of function following ulnar nerve injury is motor recovery. The BMRC system attempted to eliminate, as much as possible, subjective elements of grading muscle function. In using the system, however, it is important that the examiner identify the presence of any cross-innervation, substitution, or trick movement in assessing muscle function. For some investigators, the BMRC system is too subjective. Gaul has proposed more objective evaluation of ulnar nerve recovery using the results of pinch and grip strength values, with comparison between the affected and unaffected extremity.[2]

Even when using a standardized system of evaluation, there is disagreement as to what constitutes a functional level of recovery. Useful or functional motor recovery has been defined anywhere from an M2+ level of recovery to an M4–5 level. Useful sensory recovery varies from S2 to S3–4. According to Omer, a good clinical recovery following ulnar nerve repair rates an S3 and M4 level of recovery.[16]

In evaluating series of ulnar nerve repairs, it is important to identify the level of injury. The BMRC has recognized this, and its system defines proximal and distal muscles for each peripheral nerve. Proximal muscles innervated by the ulnar nerve are the flexor carpi ulnaris and flexor digitorum profundus of the ring and little fingers. Distal muscles are the intrinsic muscles of the hand normally innervated by the ulnar nerve. Ulnar nerve lesions can, therefore, be subdivided into proximal and distal levels of injuries based on the muscle groups involved. Unfortunately, some series fail to make this distinction when summarizing functional results following ulnar nerve repair.

Allowing adequate time between repair and final follow-up is a critical factor in accurately assessing functional results following peripheral nerve repair. This time interval is influenced by the level of injury and the rate of regeneration. Stromberg evaluated sensory return in injuries of the median and ulnar nerves.[21] His findings revealed that maximum sensory recovery could be expected in children by 2 years after repair and in adults no less than 5 years after repair. Nicholson and Seddon felt that a maximum motor recovery was not present until at least 3 years after injury.[15] Others have argued the time interval for maximum muscle recovery following ulnar nerve injuries may be as long as 5 to 7 years.[5] Few studies investigating recovery following ulnar nerve repair have achieved this length of follow-up with significant numbers of patients.

Given the multitude of factors influencing results of peripheral nerve repair, the variability in length of follow-up, and the method of evaluation, it is difficult to compare studies evaluating results following ulnar nerve repair. Despite this difficulty, it is worthwhile to review these reports from the standpoint of their conclusions and the variables they identified as affecting their results.

Much of the early information concerning functional results following peripheral nerve repair was obtained by evaluating military casualties in World War II. These nerve repairs were performed prior to the era of microsurgical technique.

The two most important series were the British *Peripheral Nerve Injuries*, edited by Seddon,[24] and the American *Peripheral Nerve Regeneration*, edited by Woodhall and Beebe.[23] Most of the injuries covered in these series were produced by high-velocity projectiles or blast injuries. In addition, there was a high incidence of associated tissue injury. The American series noted that ulnar nerve injuries were associated with arterial injury in 23.4% of cases and with other nerve injury in 40.2% of cases. Seddon's report used the BMRC system for grading recovery of motor function; the American report used a modification of this system that consisted of seven levels.

Omer reviewed the overall results of these two studies.[16] Using the British system, a good result was defined as a motor recovery of M4–5 and sensory recovery to S3–4. According to Omer, the American report found a good level of motor recovery in 12.9% of cases and good sensory recovery in 31.4% following ulnar nerve repair. The British series documented a good motor recovery in 4.9% and a good sensory recovery in 30.8% following ulnar nerve repair. These results include all levels of injury and were not analyzed by the various factors known to influence results.

In contrast to studies evaluating combat peripheral nerve injuries, investigators evaluating civilian peripheral nerve injuries have dealt primarily with injuries produced by sharp laceration. These injuries not uncommonly involve adjacent tissues, specifically the ulnar artery and adjacent flexor tendons. Little attention has been paid to the potential impact of injury to these structures on evaluating final results. The presence of an intact arterial system has been shown by several investigators to be significant in achieving a good functional result.[6,20] Most studies reviewing results of ulnar nerve repair fail to mention information regarding the patency of the ulnar artery.

Studies in the past 35 years have had the benefit of microsurgical technique in performing nerve repair. Topographic mapping of severed nerves has been done by visual inspection,[12] electrodiagnostic testing,[8] and histochemical technique.[17] These techniques assist alignment of neural tissue with surgical fascicular or group fascicular repair, as well as the standard technique of epineural repair. To date, no clinical studies have proved the superiority of any one technique of nerve repair over another in similar clinical settings.

In 1942, Marble and colleagues reported a 10-year experience of upper extremity nerve injuries from the Massachusetts General Hospital.[11] About a third of the injuries involved the ulnar nerve. Twenty-one cases involving ulnar nerve repair were available for follow-up after a "sufficient" period of time. Most of these injuries were at wrist level. The criterion for a good result was the recovery of the useful hand for ordinary occupation and daily activities. Based on these guidelines, 90.4% of the evaluated patients obtained a good result. These authors noted surprisingly little functional impairment of the hand immediately following injury. They estimated that the rate of ulnar nerve regeneration was 1.09 mm/day. Motor recovery was found always to lag behind sensory return. In no case did they identify return of function to the third volar interosseous muscle. Their series included both primary and secondary nerve repair with no obvious difference in results.

In 1957, Nicholson and Seddon reported a minimum 3-year follow-up of 103 cases of ulnar nerve repair from the years 1941 to 1948.[15] Of the 163 cases of ulnar nerve injury, 98.6% were caused by sharp laceration. Associated injuries included the median nerve in 20.2% of cases and adjacent flexor tendons in 40.5% of cases. Results were evaluated using the BMRC system and divided among proximal, intermediate, and distal repairs. Distal repairs were those beyond the branches to the flexor digitorum profundus. Intermediate repairs occurred between the branches to the flexor carpi ulnaris and flexor digitorum profundus. Proximal repairs were above the branches to the flexor carpi ulnaris. Useful sensory recovery was felt to be S2+ and useful motor M2+. Review of the distal repairs demonstrated an M2 level of recovery in 81.7% and an M4 level of recovery in 35%. S2+ sensory recovery was present in 82.5% and S3 recovery in 68.5%.

The authors compared their results to the British *Peripheral Nerve Injury* study, in which an M2+ level of recovery was found in 87.5%, M4 in 16%, S2+ in 64.6% and S3 in 49.5% of cases. Only small numbers of repairs at the intermediate and proximal levels were available for evaluation. At 3-year follow-up in the intermediate group, an M2+ level or better was seen in seven of eight patients and S2+ level or better in five of nine patients. Results in proximal repairs evaluated at 3 years revealed an M2+ level or better in seven of nine patients and an S2 level or better in six of nine patients. Recovery was found to be better in children than in adults, particularly in children ages 10 years or less. No influence on the extent of nerve gap or mobilization of the nerve in preparation for repair could be identified as an influence on the results of ulnar nerve repair. No significant difference was found between the results of primary vs secondary repair. Most repairs in this study were performed within 6 months of injury, but repair after 6 months was not felt to be strongly adverse to recovery: M2+ or better motor recovery was found in 64.7% and S2+ or better recovery in 68.8% of ulnar nerve repairs performed 6 months or longer after injury.

In 1961, Stromberg and associates reported on sensory recovery after injury to the median and ulnar nerves.[21] Thirty-two of these cases involved the ulnar nerve and were available for follow-up more than 1 year after repair. Return of pinprick was found in 28 patients, light touch in 28 patients, two-point discrimination in 1, and tactile gnosis in none. As part of the evaluation of sensory recovery, ninhydrin and pick-up tests were performed. The appearance of sweating, as documented by the ninhydrin test, was found to correlate most closely with the return of pinprick and demonstrated a poor correlation with normal tactile gnosis. The Moberg pick-up test was found to be of little value in evaluating functional sensory recovery for injuries of the ulnar nerve but was of great value in evaluating recovery of median nerve sensory function. In long-term follow-up of sensory recovery in median and ulnar nerve injuries, Stromberg concluded that sensibility reaches a maximum in children by 2 years and in adults in no less than 5 years after repair.

In 1962, Sakellarides reported on a study of 172 upper extremity civilian nerve injuries.[18] In this study, 46.5% of the patients had an associated tendon injury, 14.7% an associated arterial injury, and 10% an associated fracture. In this series, there were 68 injuries of the ulnar nerve and 20 cases of combined median and ulnar nerve injury. Primary repair of the ulnar nerve was performed in 49 patients and secondary repair in 39 patients. Patient age ranged from 3 to 81 years; 26% of the cases involved school-aged children. Assessment of the results was based on level of injury and recovery using the BMRC system. Only patients with follow-up of 2 years or longer were included in the results. A good level of motor function was defined as M2+ or better, and sensory function was defined as good when it was S2+ or better.

In evaluating distal repairs following primary suture, 36% achieved a good or better motor recovery; after secondary repair 55% of the patients did so. M3 or better motor recovery was present in 5% of primary repairs and 10% of secondary repairs. Sensory recovery following distal repair was good or better in 42% of primary repairs and 53% of secondary repairs. Evaluation of high and intermediate repairs revealed a good level of motor recovery in 22% of primary repairs and 44% of secondary repairs. Sensory recovery in these groups revealed identical findings. In analyzing their results, the authors felt that secondary repair gave better results than primary repair, although they concluded that primary repair could be performed in appropriate situations.

In evaluating the delay of repair, motor recovery

no better than M2 was found in ulnar nerve repairs performed after a delay of 7 months or more. In evaluating the length of nerve defect, ulnar nerve injuries with a gap of 2.5 cm or less achieved good to excellent results in 76%; only 23% achieved good or excellent results in nerve gaps of 3 cm or more. Ulnar nerve repairs had good to excellent results in 80% of patients under 16 years of age but in only 30% of patients over 16 years of age.

In 1975, Seddon reported his experience with recovery of peripheral nerve injuries spanning a 25-year period.[19] He noted that the ulnar nerve was the most commonly repaired nerve. Evaluation was by the BMRC system; good motor recovery was defined as M3 or better and sensory recovery as S3 or better. His series documented results of 21 cases of primary ulnar nerve repair at wrist level and 267 cases of secondary repair of the ulnar nerve at all levels, including 179 cases involving the forearm and wrist. A good level of motor and sensory recovery following primary repair of the ulnar nerve at the wrist was found in 47.6%. A good level of recovery following secondary repair of the ulnar nerve at the forearm and wrist was found in 37.9%.

In 1976, Millesi reported on his results of interfascicular grafting of median, ulnar, and radial nerve injuries.[13] Using the BMRC criteria to evaluate ulnar nerve lesions, he rated a useful motor recovery as M2+ or greater. He reported on the results of 39 cases of ulnar nerve grafting at various levels of injury with various lengths of defects, including 12 cases of combined median and ulnar nerve grafting. An M2+ or better level of recovery was found in 87% of cases. An M3 level of recovery was found in 30.8% of cases with an average age of 43 years (± 16.6 years) and an average graft length of 6.4 cm (± 4.5 cm). A level of M4 or M5 was achieved in 47.9% of patients with an average age of 29.2 years (± 21 years) and a defect averaging 4.6 cm (± 2.2 cm).

In 1982, Gaul reported his evaluation of intrinsic motor recovery in 41 patients following ulnar nerve laceration.[2] Ages ranged from 2 years to 60 years; young patients were defined as those 18 years of age or less. Injuries were divided between high and low level. In evaluating results, Gaul departed from the BMRC system, which he felt was too subjective. Instead, he compared his results based on examination of specific intrinsic muscle recovery reported as an estimate of normal; presence or absence of clinical signs such as clawing, little finger abduction, and Froment's sign; and objective strength measurements obtained with a Jamar dynamometer and pinch gauge. Grip and pinch strengths were given as a percentage of values measured in the unaffected hand.

Follow-up of his patients ranged from 1 to 6 years. Unfortunately, it is difficult to compare his results with other studies because of his departure from the BMRC grading system.

Gaul did not note any influence of nerve gaps up to 5 cm or any adverse affect in delay of repair up to 6 months. He reported that following an ulnar nerve palsy, a decrease of 20% to 50% of normal lateral key pinch and 10% to 50% of normal grip strength could be expected. Variations in pinch and grip strength between the dominant and nondominant hand could be expected to be 10% to 15%.

It is interesting to note that in evaluating high ulnar nerve lesions in adults, no significant recovery of intrinsic motor function was documented. Among young patients with low-level injuries, nine of ten available for evaluation at 23 months following injury had favorable intrinsic motor recovery, with a mean key pinch of 86% of normal. In adults with low-level injuries, six patients were available for evaluation 26 to 51 months after injury; all six showed some level of intrinsic motor recovery, with a key pinch averaging 82% of normal, three-inch grip 78% of normal, and one-inch grip 65% of normal. Gaul concluded that results were superior in children.

The association of a median nerve laceration did not necessarily lead to a bad result. He could identify no adverse affect of associated flexor tendon injury and he recommended that a 2.5- to 5-year recovery period was necessary to adequately evaluate motor recovery following ulnar nerve repair.

In 1985, Leclercq reported on the association between results following ulnar nerve repair and the patency of the ulnar artery.[9] Her study documents a minimum 2-year follow-up in 40 patients undergoing primary nerve repair and 24 patients undergoing nerve grafting of the ulnar nerve. The age of the patients with direct repair averaged 30 years (range, 1 to 60 years). Among patients undergoing grafting of the ulnar nerve, ages ranged from 4 to 52 years, with an average of 26. Results were evaluated using the BMRC criteria, with a useful result defined as M3/S3 or better.

In the primary repair group, an M3 level of recovery was achieved in 81.5% of cases and an S3 level of recovery achieved in 74% of cases when the ulnar artery was intact or patent following repair. Results of primary repair in which the ulnar artery was ligated or thrombosed demonstrated an M3 level of recovery in 53% of cases and an S3 level of sensory recovery in 53.8% of cases. Results were even more impressive in evaluating the influence of patency of the ulnar artery on the results of ulnar nerve grafting. When the artery was intact or patent following repair, an M3 or S3 level of recovery was present in 73.3% of cases; a similar level of recovery was present in only 22.2% of cases of ulnar nerve grafting with a ligated or thrombosed ulnar artery. (Other investigators have noted a similar association between the results of nerve repair and vascular status.[20])

In 1987, Lijftogt and coworkers presented the results of microsurgical treatment of nerve injuries at wrist level. Their patients ranged in age from 3 to 63 years. The predominant mechanism of injury was glass laceration. There were 15 ulnar nerve lesions, 14 of which were associated with lacerations of the ulnar artery; 11 involved one or more flexor tendons. Ten of the patients underwent primary repair and five underwent nerve grafting for defects of 3 to 6 cm. All nerve grafts were carried out as secondary procedures, with all but one performed between 2 and 7 months following injury. Nerve repair was by group fascicular and supplemental epineural repair using 10-0 monofilament suture. Arterial repair was performed simultaneously when possible. Follow-up was available 2 or more years following surgery. The BMRC criteria were used for evaluation, and a good result was defined as an M4 and S3+ level of recovery.[10]

Among the primary repair group, an M4/S3 level of recovery was found in 50% of patients and an M3/S3 level of recovery in 40%. Among the patients undergoing nerve graft, an M3/S3 level of recovery was found in 80%; no patients achieved a good result. As other investigators have, Lijftogt and associates felt their best results were achieved in young patients, with almost complete recovery seen in patients younger than 10 years. Results were better in primary repair than in nerve grafting. The authors felt that no clear conclusion could be made regarding the results of their technique of nerve repair in comparison to previous studies.[10]

In 1988, Jongen and van Twisk reported on their results following primary repair of ulnar and median nerves at the wrist.[6] Their study included 10 patients with ulnar nerve injuries, all of whom were treated within 17 hours of injury. All the injuries were produced by sharp laceration. Follow-up evaluation was by the BMRC criteria, with a minimum follow-up of 2 years. A good result was defined as an M3/S3 level of ulnar nerve recovery. The technique of repair was epineural or combined group fascicular epineural. An M4/S3 level of recovery was reported in 30% and a fair level (M3/S3) in 60% of patients. The authors noted that a minimum 2-year level of recovery was probably insufficient to document a final status. As with other authors, they noted better results in children than in adults. No comparison of their technique of microscopic repair was made with other series.

RESULTS

In reviewing patients treated at our facility from 1979 to 1987, we identified 46 cases of ulnar nerve repair. Patients who had sustained simultaneous laceration of the median or radial nerve were excluded from the study. Fifteen cases were lost to follow-up. Using a minimal follow-up interval of 2 years for patients under 20 years of age and 3 years for patients over 20 years of age, 17 patients were available to return and be examined by one of the three authors (Table 30-1). The length of follow-up ranged from 2 to 9.2 years (average, 4.8 years). The patients ranged in age from 4 to 67 years (average, 28.4 years). Eight patients were younger than 20 years (range, 4 to 16 years); nine were older than 20 (range, 21 to 67 years).

In 11 patients, the mechanism of injury was a sharp laceration; broken glass was the most common cause. Six patients sustained crushing lacerations usually associated with high-velocity injuries, compound fractures, or the use of power equipment. The level of laceration was noted in each case and was divided into five levels: axilla, elbow, forearm, wrist, and hand. Three patients sustained ulnar nerve lacerations near the axilla or proximal arm, one patient had an injury about the elbow, six patients had forearm injuries, six patients had injuries at the wrist, and one had lacerated the ulnar nerve in the hand. Eleven patients had concomitant wrist and finger flexor tendon lacerations, six had ulnar artery lacerations, one had a brachial artery laceration, and two had forearm fractures.

Operative repair was carried out under the supervision of a hand surgeon. Ten nerves were treated using epineural repair and seven were repaired at the group fascicular level. The timing of repair was categorized into three groups. Repairs carried out within 24 hours of injury were classified as primary. Nerve repairs performed after 24 hours but before 21 days were categorized as delayed primary, and those performed after 21 days were considered secondary or reconstructive. Twelve patients underwent primary repair, four underwent delayed primary repair, and one underwent reconstructive repair. (The one patient who required reconstructive repair had initially been treated elsewhere with failed recognition of nerve involvement with the original injury. The patient required a sural nerve graft to restore continuity to the ulnar nerve.) In each case, an operating microscope was used for surgical repair.

Motor and sensory recovery were assessed according to the modified BMRC classification. In addition, objective measurements of pinch and grip strength expressed as a percentage of the opposite side were tabulated. Subjective evaluation was further obtained by asking patients their opinions about hand function and satisfaction. Using this grading system, a good result was defined as motor function of M4 or greater and sensory return of S3+ or greater; a fair result M3/S3; a poor result M2/S2; and a bad result M1 or less and S1 or less.

Good results of M4/S3+ were found in nine (52%) of the patients. A fair result occurred in five patients (29%). Two patients (12%) had poor results and one patient (7%) had a bad result. All of the patients who were less than 20 years old had good to excellent results, regardless of the level of injury or timing of repair. Among the adult population, there was one good result, five fair results, two poor results, and one bad result. The good result occurred in a 29-year-old male who had sustained a sharp laceration of the ulnar nerve at the level of the palm. Minimum follow-up among the three patients with a poor or bad result was 4.6 years. All had undergone primary repair of their ulnar nerve lacerations. The bad result occurred in a 26-year-old male who sustained a crushing-type laceration in the proximal arm with an associated brachial artery injury. The two poor results were a midforearm laceration with associated flexor tendon and ulnar artery injuries in a 21-year-old, and a crushing laceration at elbow level with no other associated injuries in a 66-year-old.

Excellent return of two-point discrimination was documented in the group of patients under 20 years of age: six of eight patients achieved two-point discrimination of 5 mm. None of the patients in the over-20 age group achieved this level of two-point discrimination. Return of pinch and grip strength expressed as a percentage of the uninvolved side was as follows in the various motor groups: M5 pinch 96%, grip 100%; M4 pinch 92%, grip 93%; M3 pinch 74%, grip 92%; M2 pinch 84%, grip 73%; and M1 pinch 68%, grip 41%. The patients' subjective assessment of function and satisfaction correlated well with the BMRC objective criteria for performance.

DISCUSSION

There has yet to be an ideal study of the results following ulnar nerve repair. Retrospective studies cannot control the multitude of variables known to influence the results of nerve repair. This limits the ability to compare studies as well as the ability to isolate and determine the influence of individual variables on nerve recovery following injury. Inability to control these same variables in the emergent trauma setting also makes prospective evaluation of nerve injuries difficult.

The primary importance of the ulnar nerve to the upper extremity is its contribution to the innervation of the intrinsic muscles of the hand. These muscles are crucial in balancing the extrinsic digital flexor and extensor muscles, controlling fine motor movement, and contributing to the force of grip and pinch. While assessing ulnar sensory function is easy, objective and quantitative analysis

Table 30–1. Ulnar Nerve Repair

	Injury Date	Age at Injury	Level	Mechanism	Associated Injuries	Surgery Date
1	12/08/81	4	wrist	laceration	FCU; FDS r, s; uln art; FDP I, r, s	same day
2	07/10/85	10	dist forearm	laceration	FCU; FDS r, s; FDP r, s	same day
3	06/03/87	4	prox arm	laceration		06/29/87
4	07/19/86	16	wrist	laceration		07/21/86
5	1982	12	wrist	laceration		01/16/84
6	07/21/87	16	mid forearm	crush, lac	compd fx forearm; FCU; FDS s, FDP i-s	07/31/87
7	06/08/81	12	prox arm	laceration	brachial art, med antebrach cut n	06/09/81
8	1984	12	mid forearm	laceration	FDP, FDS r, s	same day
9	04/07/80	40	wrist	laceration	FCU; FDS r, s; FDP I, r, s; uln art	same day
10	12/06/82	53	mid forearm	crush, lac	FCU; FDS s; uln art	same day
11	04/30/81	47	dist forearm	crush, lac	FCU; FDS I-s; ECU	same day
12	12/06/85	26	prox arm	crush, lac	brachial art	same day
13	08/07/85	48	wrist	laceration	FCU, FDP I, r, s; uln art	same day
14	05/14/82	21	mid forearm	laceration	FDS, FDP i-s; uln art	same day
15	03/10/84	29	palm	laceration	FDS r, s; FDP s	same day
16	01/30/82	67	wrist	crush, lac	FCU, FDP s; uln art	same day
17	11/21/83	66	elbow	crush, lac		11/27/83

	Timing of Repair	Type of Repair	Magnification	Follow-up (yrs)	Fine Touch	Pin Prick	2 Point (mm)	Sens BMRC	Grip (lbs) %
1	primary	epineural	microscope	6.600	+	+	5	S4	100
2	primary	epineural	microscope	4.000	+	+	5	S4	100
3	delayed primary	group fascicular	microscope	2.200	+	+	5	S4	100
4	delayed primary	epineural	microscope	3.000	+	+	5	S4	100
5	reconstr sural n graft	group fascicular	microscope	4.300	+	+	5–8	S3+	73
6	delayed primary	group fascicular	microscope	2.000	+	+	5–10	S3+	98
7	primary	epineural	microscope	6.830	+	+	5	S4	92
8	primary	epineural	microscope	5.600	+	+	5	S4	100
9	primary	epineural	microscope	9.200	+	+	10–20	S3+	89
10	primary	epineural	microscope	7.600	+	+	15–20	S3	95
11	primary	epineural	microscope	4.200	+	+	>20	S3	97
12	primary	group fascicular	microscope	4.600	–	–	–	S1	41
13	primary	epineural	microscope	3.800	+	+	15–20	S3	80
14	primary	group fascicular	microscope	7.200	+	–	>20	S2	95
15	primary	group fascicular	microscope	4.600	+	+	5–10	S3+	94
16	primary	epineural	microscope	6.300	+	+	>20	S3	74
17	delayed primary	group fascicular	microscope	4.500	+	+	8–15	S3+	100

(continued)

Table 30–1. *(continued)*

	Pinch (lbs) %	Motor BMRC	Function	Satisfaction	Froments	Clawing
1	100	M5	excellent	excellent	−	−
2	88	M5	excellent	excellent	−	−
3	100	M5	excellent	excellent	−	−
4	82	M4	excellent	excellent	−	−
5	100	M4	good	good	+	−
6	82	M4	excellent	excellent	+	−
7	100	M4	excellent	excellent	+	−
8	100	M4	excellent	excellent	+	−
9	82	M3	good	good	+	−
10	75	M3	good	good	+	−
11	67	M3	good	good	+	−
12	68	M1−	poor−	poor	+	+
13	78	M3	good	good	+	−
14	80	M2−	poor	poor	+	−
15	88	M4	good	good	+	−
16	66	M2−	poor	poor	+	−
17	69	M3	good	good	+	−

of individual muscles innervated by the ulnar nerve is quite difficult. Techniques for evaluation of ulnar motor function include observation of muscle bulk (most easily visualized in the hypothenar and first dorsal interosseous area); strength of individual muscle testing (ie, first dorsal interosseous, abductor digiti minimi, flexor digiti minimi, flexor digitorum profundus of the small and ring fingers); presence or absence of known deformities associated with ulnar nerve palsy (ie, Wartenberg's sign, clawing of the ring and small fingers, Froment's sign); and diminished grip and pinch strength. Assessment of individual muscle function and the detection of possible cross-innervation would most accurately be determined by selective electromyographic studies.

In the trauma setting of ulnar nerve injury, pre-injury assessment is unavailable. If the pre-injury status of ulnar nerve function is unavailable, then it is necessary to identify the deficit created by ulnar nerve injury to accurately assess final recovery. In the emergent situation, however, a careful, detailed examination of ulnar nerve function is rarely carried out. In addition, the function of the hand may be influenced by injuries other than the nerve injury, making interpretation of the physical examination difficult. Despite these limitations, an accurate examination prior to repair is helpful in identifying anomalous patterns of innervation to the intrinsic muscles, particularly in a setting where compensatory muscle strengthening and substitution cannot influence the examination. Further documentation of ulnar nerve injury may be possible following repair in the interval between recovery from injury to associated soft-tissue structures and the onset of reinnervation of the intrinsic muscles.

In following the patient over time, it might be possible to document a plateau in recovery of pinch and grip strength as well as noting a progression of intrinsic muscle atrophy prior to any documented recovery. Previous retrospective studies have not taken such an approach to longitudinal observation, and their conclusions regarding recovery may not accurately take into account anomalous patterns of innervation and compensatory substitution. While it may be impossible to perform a controlled prospective study of the results following ulnar nerve repair, a study that accurately examines and follows over time those tests available for assessment of ulnar nerve function may provide more accurate information regarding the variables influencing results.

By far the most significant factor determining outcome following nerve repair is the age of the patient at the time of injury. In the very young, this variable seems to outweigh the influence of other factors such as site and mechanism of injury. Recovery in adults remains compromised, and it is in this population that closer scrutiny of the variables influencing recovery following nerve injury is important. Variables beyond the surgeon's control are mechanism of injury, associated tissue injury, and site of injury. Most civilian ulnar nerve injuries permit immediate primary repair. Even in situations of segmental nerve loss and surrounding soft-tissue deficit, microsurgical techniques of reconstruction allow the creation of a well-vascularized bed acceptable for end-to-end repair or nerve grafting during the early post-injury period. Excessive delay in awaiting soft-tissue equilibrium now rarely occurs. While it is generally accepted that primary repair gives a better clinical result and delays greater than 6 months a poor clinical result, the effects of intermediate time delay during this period are uncertain.

The ulnar nerve is a mixed nerve containing both motor and sensory components. Most injuries to the nerve occur distal to the level of the elbow. At this level, the motor and sensory components are distributed in separate group fascicles. The internal topography of the ulnar nerve has been well studied, and topographical maps may be helpful in intraoperative alignment of the nerve.[5] In acute nerve repairs within 48 hours of injury, electrical stimulation of the distal motor unit may still be possible.[1,3,4] Efficient techniques of intraoperative histochemical staining have not been perfected.[1] Use of evoked sensory potentials or stimulation of the sensory component of the proximal nerve under local anesthesia with the patient awake are not yet commonly used.[3] Despite the theoretical advantages of operative techniques that accomplish repair at a fascicular or group fascicular level, experimental and clinical studies have been unable to prove their superiority over a well-performed epineural repair.

The patency of the adjacent ulnar artery has also been implicated as influencing recovery following ulnar nerve repair. In most situations, repair of the ulnar artery does not present a technical problem; however, it has been clearly shown that in the presence of an intact radial artery, maintaining patency of an ulnar artery repair at the level of the distal forearm or wrist may be difficult. The impact on final recovery of maintaining arterial patency in such a setting may be worth further investigation.

The most important element of recovery following ulnar nerve repair is the motor component. The minimal acceptable level of recovery should correct deformities of imbalance such as Wartenberg's sign, digital clawing, and Froment's sign. Most tendon transfers are performed to correct these deformities. Sensory recovery should at least provide protective sensation to the ulnar border of the hand. Improvement in fine motor activities is difficult to quantify. Tests used to evaluate hand function such as the Jebsen test are affected more significantly by sensory function than by motor function and have proven helpful in evaluating recovery following median nerve repair but of little value in assessing ulnar nerve function. Grip and pinch strength may be used as an indirect measurement of ulnar nerve recovery; however, improvement in these values without concomitant correction of deformities, reversal of intrinsic muscle atrophy, or electromyographic confirmation of recovery may be only a reflection of compensatory strengthening of non–ulnar-innervated musculature.

SUMMARY

Because of the large number of variables affecting the analysis of the results of peripheral nerve repair and the wide discrepancy in the methodology of assessing those results, scientifically credible information regarding functional recovery following ulnar nerve division and repair is difficult to gather and interpret. This chapter has reviewed the most meaningful published reports and, although comparisons between these studies are almost impossible, some general deductions may be made.

It is safe to say that meticulous microsurgical nerve repair techniques will improve the ultimate functional recovery following ulnar nerve interruption. While there is no demonstrable superiority of any single method of nerve suture, every effort should be made to accurately realign the nerve ends and to match fascicular elements in an effort to precisely restore the normal internal topography of the nerve at the particular level of division. Concomitant preservation or repair of the adjacent ulnar artery has also been shown to improve ulnar nerve recovery.

Evidence shows that direct repair of the ulnar nerve with gaps of up to 2.5 cm does not prejudice the final result, but there is a significant deterioration in recovery for repairs of gaps greater than 3 cm. Well-performed nerve grafts can lead to recovery that is reasonably comparable to direct suture; grafting is particularly suitable for situations in which there are wide gaps or long segments of nerve damage.

Ulnar nerve suture at distal levels outperforms more proximal repairs, and there is little likelihood of intrinsic muscle return following high interruption. Although the evidence is not entirely clear, it would appear that recovery following immediate or delayed ulnar nerve suture does not differ greatly, providing definitive repair is accomplished within 6 months of nerve division. Higher lesions may be better managed by delayed repair.

In all studies, the speed and quality of ulnar nerve recovery is substantially better in children than in adults. The time-honored concept that repaired nerves regenerate at about 1 mm/day appears to be a fairly reliable guide for assessing the progression of return following these injuries. It would also appear that both sensory and motor improvement can often be expected to occur over at least a 5-year period following ulnar nerve repair, and long-term evaluations may yield surprisingly good results.

In general, the recovery of ulnar nerve function following a sharp distal laceration in a young adult, managed by meticulous, tension-free microsurgical repair with concomitant arterial repair (if necessary), should lead to a reasonable recovery of sensation and intrinsic muscle function. A decrease of pinch and grip strength between 20% and 50% can be anticipated in almost all cases. Individual intrinsic muscles may have differing degrees of return, leading to alterations in the ability to use the involved hand for intricate activities that require equal and coordinated participation of these muscles.

REFERENCES

1. Engel J, Ganel A, Melamed R, Simon R, Farine I. Choline acetyltransferase for differentiation between human motor and sensory nerve fibers. Ann Plast Surg 1979; 4:376–380.
2. Gaul JS. Intrinsic motor recovery: A long-term study of ulnar nerve repair. J Hand Surg 1982; 7:502–508.
3. Gaul JS. Electrical fascicle identification as an adjunct to nerve repair. Hand Clinics 1986; 2:709–722.
4. Hakstian RW. Funicular orientation by direct stimulation: an aid to peripheral nerve repair. J Bone Joint Surg [Am] 1968; 50:1178–1186.
5. Jabaley ME, Wallace WH, Heckler FR. Internal topography of major nerves of the forearm and hand: A current review. J Hand Surg 1980; 5:1.
6. Jongen SJM, Van Twisk R. Results of primary repair of ulnar and median nerve injuries at the wrist: An evaluation of sensibility and motor recovery. Neth J Surg 1988; 40:86–89.
7. Kline DG, Hudson AR, Bratton BR. Experimental study of fascicular nerve repair with and without epineurial closure. J Neurosurg 1981; 54:513–520.
8. Kutz JE, Shealy G, Lubbers L. Interfascicular nerve repair. Orthop Clin North Am 1981; 12:277–286.
9. Leclercq DC, Carlier AJ, Khue T, Luc Depierreux, Lejeune GN. Improvement in the results in 64 ulnar nerve sections associated with arterial repair. J Hand Surg [Am] 1985; 10:997–999.
10. Lijftogt HJA, Dijkstra R, Storm van Leeuwen JB. Results of microsurgical treatment of nerve injuries of the wrist. Neth J Surg 1987; 39(6):170–174.
11. Marble HC, Hamlin E Jr., Watkins AL. Regeneration in the ulnar, median and radial nerves. Amer J Surg 1942; 55:274–294.
12. Millesi H. Different techniques of nerve grafting. In: Gorio A, Millesi H, Mingrino S, eds. Post-traumatic peripheral nerve regeneration: Experimental basic and clinical implications. New York: Raven, 1981:325–328.
13. Millesi H, Meissl G, Berger A. Further experience

with interfascicular grafting of the median, ulnar and radial nerves. J Bone Joint Surg [Am] 1976; 58: 209–218.

14. Moberg E. Surgical treatment for absent single-hand grip and elbow extension in quadriplegia: principles and preliminary experience. J Bone Joint Surg [Am] 1975; 57:196.
15. Nicholson OR, Seddon HJ. Nerve repair in civil practice: Results of treatment of median and ulnar nerve lesions. Brit Med J 1957; 2:1065–1071.
16. Omer GE Jr. Evaluation of clinical results following peripheral nerve suture. In: Omer GE Jr., Spinner M (eds). Management of peripheral nerve problems. Philadelphia: WB Saunders, 1980; 431–442.
17. Orgel MG. Epineurial vs perineurial repair of peripheral nerves. In: Terzis JK, ed. Clinics in plastic surgery: Symposium on peripheral nerve microsurgery. Philadelphia: WB Saunders, 1984:101–104.
18. Sakellarides H. A follow-up study of 172 peripheral nerve injuries in the upper extremity in civilians. J Bone Joint Surg [Am] 1962; 44:140–148.
19. Seddon HG. Surgical disorders of the peripheral nerves, ed 2. New York: Churchill-Livingstone, 1975:209–213.
20. Starkweather RJ, Neviaser RJ, Adams JP, Parsons DB. The effect of devascularization on the regeneration of lacerated peripheral nerves: An experimental study. J Hand Surg 1978; 3:163–167.
21. Stromberg WB, McFarlane RM, Bell JL, Koch SL, Mason ML. Injury of the median and ulnar nerves: 150 cases with an evaluation of Moberg's ninhydrin test. J Bone Joint Surg [Am] 1961; 43:717–730.
22. Sunderland S. Nerve and nerve injuries, ed 2. Edinburgh: Churchill-Livingstone, 1978:505–532.
23. Woodhall B, Beebe GW, eds. Peripheral nerve regeneration: A follow-up study of 3656 World War II injuries VA Medical Monograph. Washington DC: U.S. Government Printing Office, 1957:116.
24. Zachary RB. Results of nerve suture. In: Seddon HJ, ed. Peripheral nerve injuries. Medical Research Council Special Report Series No. 282. London: Her Majesty's Stationery Office, 1954:354–388.

31

Axillary Nerve

James A. Nunley
Gerard Gabel

AUTHORS' KEY POINTS

- The most common mechanism of injury of the axillary nerve is traction from trauma in the shoulder region.
- Spontaneous resolution is common, but exploration is indicated if recovery is not evident by 6 months.
- The level of injury is usually diffuse, frequently extending through the quadrilateral space, requiring anterior and posterior exposures.
- When neuronal continuity has been lost, direct repair is usually impossible due to the limited mobility of the axillary nerve. Nerve grafting is almost always required for tension-free repair.
- Postoperative prognosis is good for lesions repaired less than 6 months after injury.

Isolated axillary nerve palsy is a relatively uncommon injury, occurring only 0.3% to 6% as often as more diffuse injuries of the brachial plexus.[13,16] The most common mechanism of injury is traction or crushing from forces applied in an indirect, closed method (ie, shoulder dislocations or fractures, forceful depression–internal rotation of the shoulder).[3,8,11,13] Axillary nerve injury can also occur by open means such as operative procedures about the shoulder or penetrating injuries.[14] Other less common causes include the quadrilateral space syndrome,[15] nerve compression due to tumor, and toxic or autoimmune processes[5] (ie, toxic neuritis, poliomyelitis, brachial neuritis).

The primary deficit seen with an axillary nerve palsy is a dysfunction of the shoulder abductor mechanism due to paralysis of the deltoid muscle. The resultant weakness in shoulder abduction approaches 57%; shoulder flexion and extension are involved as well (49% and 15% respectively).[6] In five patients who had had complete deltoid excision for tumor procedures, Markhede found that active abduction was slightly limited (5°–15°).[9] He determined that abduction strength was decreased an average of 27% in different positions of abduction and flexion and that extension strength was reduced an average of 35% and 25%, respectively, at 45° and 90° of flexion. Overall functional impairment was thought to be minimal.

Other authors have also observed the restoration of complete or nearly complete abduction despite deltoid paralysis.[1,17] This was attributed to compensation on the part of the long heads of the biceps and triceps as well as the supraspinatus muscles.

In contrast to this assessment, Petrucci, reporting on 21 axillary nerve palsies, noted that deltoid paralysis "gravely affects the function of the upper limb."[13] Although objective strength or range of motion data were not provided, he observed that "the resulting loss has always been notable and has never been adequately replaced by substitution of other muscles."

The initial evaluation of an axillary nerve deficit includes assessment of the mechanism of injury (if post-traumatic) as well as the clinical course following the injury to help localize the level and assess the spontaneous course of the lesion. An atraumatic onset of axillary nerve paralysis may indicate a compressive, toxic, or autoimmune neuropathy.[4,5] Physical examination of a patient with an axillary nerve palsy will reveal absent deltoid contraction against resistance, followed by gradual atrophy of the deltoid muscle (Fig. 31-1) over 2 to 3 months. A region of decreased sensation may be present over the lateral aspect of the shoulder or upper arm, depending on the autonomous sensory distribution of the axillary nerve. Teres minor dysfunction may be present, depending on the level of the lesion. Initially, range of motion, especially abduction and flexion, is severely restricted (less than 90° each), but as compensatory mechanisms evolve over time, range of motion may be significantly restored, with excellent strength in all positions.

Examination of other muscle groups may reveal more diffuse involvement, indicating a more diffuse brachial plexus lesion. A Tinel's sign in the supraclavicular or infraclavicular region helps localize the level of injury. Sensory examination may be affected in the axillary nerve cutaneous distribution, but a complete sensory examination of the extremity is needed as well as a complete motor test. Radiographic examination of the cervical spine and shoulder girdle is indicated to rule out occult cervical spine injuries as well as shoulder fractures or dislocations.

Electromyographic evaluation may help localize an axillary nerve injury proximal or distal to the teres minor branch; more importantly, it may reveal other areas of involvement that are not apparent on examination. It may also indicate a lesion at a level of the brachial plexus other than the axillary nerve branch and may alter the prognosis and treatment.

Conservative management of an axillary nerve palsy includes physical therapy to maintain shoulder range of motion. The use of an arm sling or abduction splint and galvanic stimulation have been recommended to minimize traction on the nerve and to minimize denervation atrophy, but these are not of proven benefit.[2]

The anticipated course of axillary nerve injuries depends to a significant degree on the mechanism of injury. In a review of brachial plexus injuries associated with Putti-Platt or Bristow procedures, two axillary nerve injuries were identified that failed to resolve spontaneously.[14] At surgical exploration one nerve was entrapped in suture and the other in a focal area of dense scar tissue. Spontaneous recovery in the former and possibly the latter was unlikely. According to Bateman, a mechanism with a similarly poor prognosis is that of an "upward driving force directly into the armpit," crushing the nerve against the glenoid.[2]

In contrast to the unfavorable prognosis in these mechanisms, it has been shown that axillary nerve injuries associated with shoulder fractures and dislocations are quite common and have a generally favorable prognosis. Blom and Dahlback evaluated 73 patients who had suffered shoulder fractures or dislocations.[3] Twenty-four (33%) axillary nerve injuries were identified by electromyography; nine of these were complete and fifteen partial. Clinical recovery in all cases was uniformly good with no apparent residual loss, even in cases with initial complete denervation.

Leffert and Seddon, in a review of infraclavicular brachial plexus injuries associated with proximal humerus fractures or dislocations, also found a generally favorable prognosis for spontaneous recovery of axillary nerve function.[8] If the initial lesion involved diffuse injury to the brachial plexus, 93% of their patients demonstrated grade IV or V deltoid strength at review, but as the injury became more localized to the region of the axillary nerve, the prognosis was poorer. Of seven patients with posterior cord involvement, return of deltoid strength of grade IV or V was seen in only 71%. Of six patients with isolated axillary nerve injury, only one (17%) regained a similar degree of deltoid

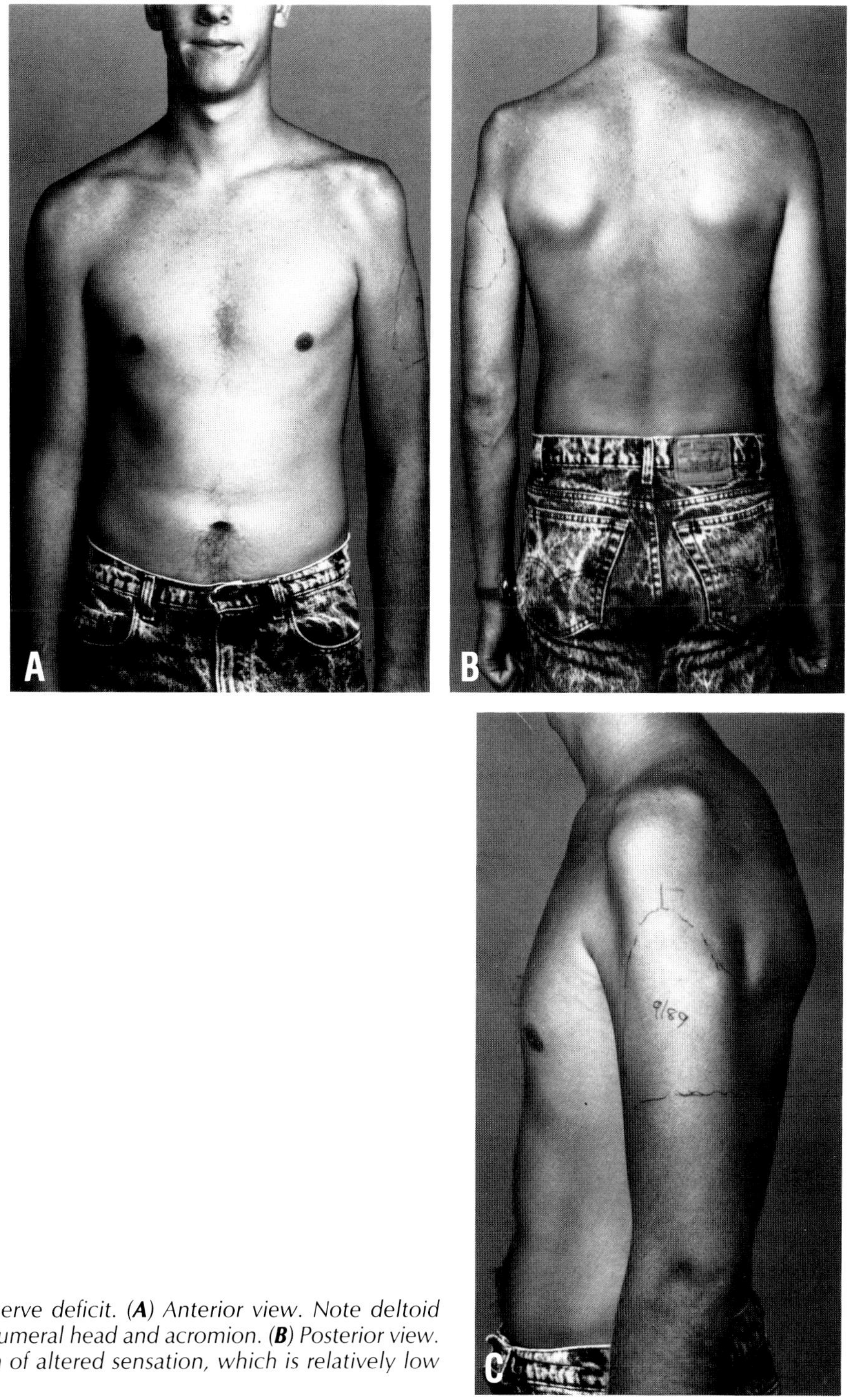

Figure 31–1. *Left axillary nerve deficit. (**A**) Anterior view. Note deltoid atrophy and prominence of humeral head and acromion. (**B**) Posterior view. (**C**) Lateral view. Note region of altered sensation, which is relatively low in this patient.*

function. This may represent patient referral bias rather than a true natural history of isolated axillary nerve paralysis.

The prognosis in isolated axillary nerve injuries associated with shoulder trauma probably lies somewhere between the incidence in Leffert's and Blom's reports, as in the experience of Watson-Jones, in which two of fifteen (13%) patients with axillary nerve injuries associated with shoulder dislocations had permanent paralysis.[17] Of the remaining thirteen patients, all but one recovered fully by 7 months.

The quadrilateral space syndrome, described by Cahill, represents an entrapment neuropathy of the axillary nerve in the quadrilateral space.[4] Symptoms consist of poorly localized anterior shoulder pain and paresthesias in a nondermatomal distribution in the upper extremity. Point tenderness is present at the posterior quadrilateral space, and the symptoms are reproduced by placing the shoulder in abduction and external rotation for one minute. Deltoid atrophy is rare (1%), and the neurological examination is otherwise normal. Electromyography is invariably normal. Subclavian arteriography may demonstrate posterior humeral circumflex arterial occlusion with the shoulder abducted and externally rotated. Reassurance and symptomatic measures (anti-inflammatory medication, physical therapy) are sufficient treatment in over 75% of cases, but some patients will continue to be symptomatic enough to warrant operative treatment. Since motor and sensory findings in this syndrome are uncommon, the diagnosis of quadrilateral space syndrome is relatively difficult to verify.

Finally, deltoid weakness in brachial neuritis has a good prognosis: over 90% of patients recover complete function, although the course may be protracted.[5]

INDICATIONS AND CONTRAINDICATIONS FOR SURGERY

The primary indication for surgical treatment of an isolated axillary nerve injury is that of persistent shoulder dysfunction due to axillary nerve paralysis. In patients who demonstrate minimal deficiency in range of motion and strength despite deltoid paralysis, the role of surgical treatment is less clear. Although excellent substitutive mechanisms for absent deltoid function have been demonstrated, restoration of normal strength, range of motion, and shoulder abduction mechanics have not been shown in any patient with this injury. The impact of this on the long-term function of the shoulder may be minimal in a sedentary or older patient, but in a young athletic patient or one who places significant demands on the shoulder, surgical treatment may be indicated despite adequate substitution because the long-term prognosis is uncertain.

The timing of surgical treatment varies; if no evidence of clinical or electromyographic recovery is seen at 2 to 3 months after injury, exploration should be performed. The maximum delay following injury for consideration of surgical treatment is not well defined; good return of deltoid function following neurolysis or nerve grafting has been realized with procedures as late as 6 to 8 months post-injury.[7,12,13] Recovery is unlikely after 12 months of denervation, and surgical treatment is of negligible benefit in this setting.

ANATOMY

The axillary nerve (Fig. 31-2) originates from the posterior cord of the brachial plexus in 80% of cases and from the posterior division of the upper trunk in the rest. The axillary nerve contains fibers from the fifth and sixth cervical roots and, in 10% to 15% of cases, the seventh cervical root as well. After branching from the plexus, the axillary nerve runs obliquely across the subscapularis muscle, turning sharply posteriorly in the region of the subscapularis musculotendinous junction. At this point the axillary nerve enters the quadrilateral space, accompanied by the posterior humeral circumflex artery. The borders of the quadrilateral space consist of the subscapularis and teres minor muscles superiorly, the long head of the triceps medially, the humerus laterally, and the teres major muscle inferiorly. The nerve branch to the teres minor muscle usually arises from the axillary nerve, either within the quadrilateral space or as the axillary nerve exits the quadrilateral space, and this

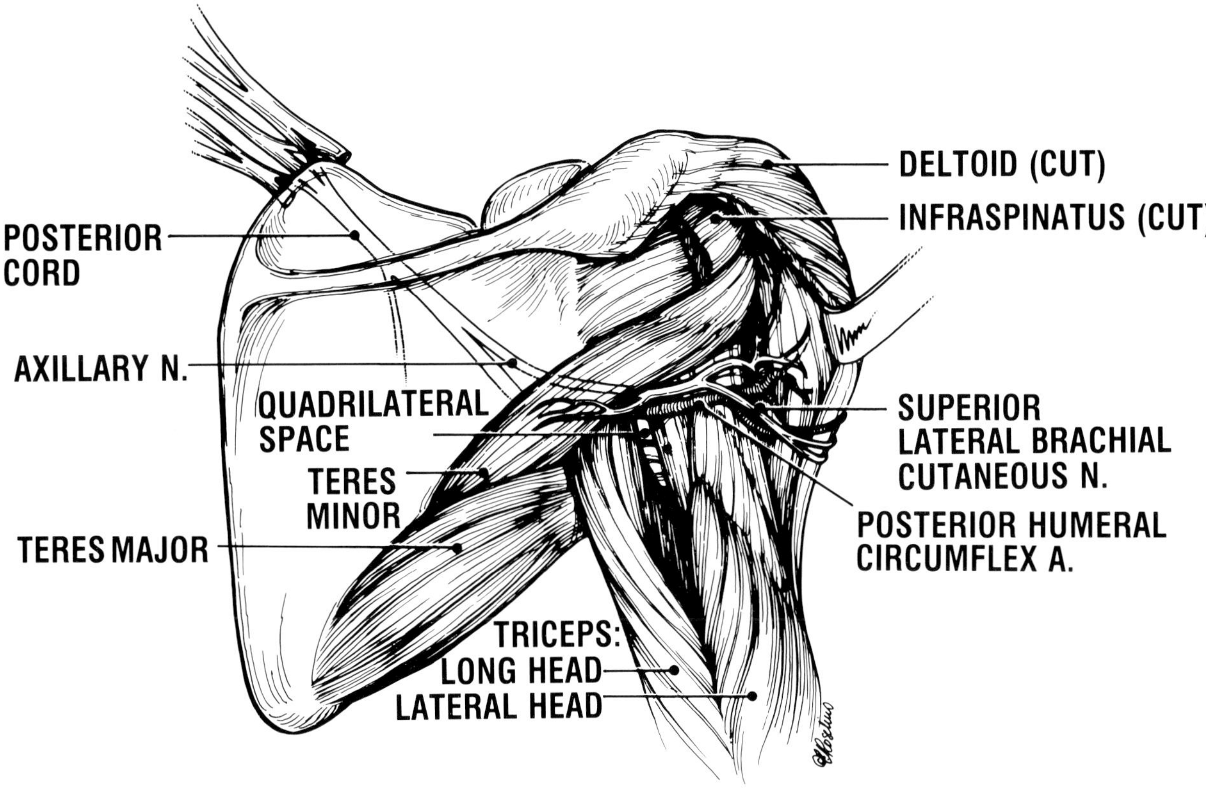

Figure 31–2. *Axillary nerve entering quadrilateral space after branching from posterior cord.*

branch then enters the inferior or posterior aspect of the teres minor muscle. The superior lateral brachial cutaneous nerve then branches from the axillary nerve, passing through or around the posterior head of the deltoid to innervate the skin on the lateral aspect of the shoulder. The axillary nerve and posterior humeral circumflex artery continue, intimately applied to the undersurface of the deltoid muscle in a neurovascular sheath, and it is from this area that the nerve fibers to the deltoid originate.

There are three notable variations: the branch to the teres minor may originate prior to the quadrilateral space; the lower subscapular nerve may originate from the axillary nerve rather than the posterior cord; and the branch to the teres minor may be as large or larger than the branch to the deltoid.

The fascicular anatomy of the axillary nerve in the axilla usually consists of one large fascicle.[15] As the nerve enters the quadrilateral space, three group fascicular bundles are seen: that to the deltoid, that to the teres minor, and the superior lateral brachial cutaneous nerve. Branching occurs as described above. Proximally, the fascicles (or fascicle) of the axillary nerve remain discrete (that is, they do not form plexi with any other fascicles) for at least 2 cm after joining the posterior cord.

The anatomical fixation of the axillary nerve within the quadrilateral space and on the undersurface of the deltoid muscle predisposes it to traction injury. Milton, in a cadaveric study of nerve injuries associated with shoulder dislocations, found that the axillary nerve was under significant tension "when it was stretched across the head of the humerus during the hyperabduction stage of dislocation."[11] In one of 15 cadavers, this maneuver resulted in nerve rupture 1 inch distal to the posterior cord. With the shoulder dislocated, Milton reproduced extreme tension in the nerve with adduction, internal rotation, and longitudinal traction. He concluded that reduction maneuvers should avoid this combination of positions to avoid iatrogenic axillary nerve injuries.

TYPES OF OPERATIONS

The choice of surgical method depends on the etiology of the axillary nerve deficit. This section will address the management of isolated axillary nerve injuries. Combined nerve injuries from more proximal brachial plexus trauma and those deficits secondary to viral autoimmune or toxic neuritis will not be discussed, nor will various tendon transfers that substitute for the paralyzed deltoid muscle.

The surgical options include:

1. Decompression
2. Neurolysis
3. Resection and neurorrhaphy
4. Resection and nerve grafting

Decompression

When the diagnosis of quadrilateral space syndrome can be established (which may be difficult), failure of conservative treatment can be managed by surgical decompression of the quadrilateral space. Cahill's technique involves a posterior approach with elevation of the deltoid off the spine of the scapula.[4] The teres minor tendon is then incised and reflected medially to gain exposure to the quadrilateral space, which is decompressed using blunt and sharp dissection. Fibrous bands traversing the quadrilateral space may be encountered and must be incised. Dissection is continued through the space to the origin of the posterior humeral circumflex artery. At this time, if the artery has a pulse with the arm abducted and externally rotated at least 110° and 45° respectively, then decompression is complete. In Cahill's series of eighteen operative cases, eight patients had "dramatic relief," eight "were improved but continued to have symptoms at night," and two were unimproved.[4]

Neurolysis

If at exploration the axillary nerve is found to be encased in scar tissue, internal neurolysis using the operating microscope may be sufficient if the fascicles are in continuity. Bateman recommended mobilization of the nerve from surrounding scar tissue and external neurolysis but gave no report of the results of this method.[2] Petrucci performed neurolysis alone in six patients with lesions in continuity with gratifying results (grade IV or V) in all patients with follow-up examination.[13] Richards reported one patient with an axillary nerve deficit following anterior shoulder surgery who underwent exploration and external neurolysis with resultant motor recovery of grade IV, V.[14] Our experience with internal neurolysis has also been uniformly good.

Resection and Neurorrhaphy

If focal injury to the axillary nerve is found at exploration, resection of the injured segment and nerve repair may be attempted. Because of the anatomical features of the axillary nerve, with a relatively brief free course on the subscapularis muscle and fixation of the nerve as it exits from the quadrilateral space, potential for mobilization of the nerve is very limited and neurorrhaphy is likely to be under tension without grafting. In none of Friedman's[7] or Petrucci's[13] cases was nerve repair without grafting possible. The only instance where neurorrhaphy is likely to be possible is if the nerve is accidentally lacerated during surgery, and this is recognized at the time. Similarly, a sharp penetrating injury to the axillary nerve may be repaired by primary neurorrhaphy, but any lesion that requires resection of more than 6 to 10 mm of axillary nerve should not be repaired without nerve grafting.

Resection and Nerve Grafting

Nerve repair under tension has been demonstrated to give uniformly poor results. As mentioned in the previous paragraph, the anatomy of the axillary nerve predisposes the nerve to require nerve grafting for a tension-free repair. This is especially true in light of the fact that the most common mechanism of injury is traction and the resultant zone of injury is usually diffuse.

Millesi described five cases of axillary nerve injuries that he explored.[10] All five required nerve grafting, as end-to-end repair was deemed untenable. One or two cable nerve grafts were used, and useful function was restored in four of the five patients.

Richards reported on one patient with a complete axillary nerve palsy following a Putti-Platt repair of the shoulder.[14] Exploration at 4 months revealed a suture around the nerve at the inferior margin of the shoulder joint. Resection of the involved nerve and sural nerve grafting resulted in full recovery of deltoid muscle bulk and strength.

Petrucci reported on 15 patients with isolated axillary nerve injuries treated by resection and nerve grafting.[13] One to three sural nerve grafts of 3 to 8 cm in length were used to effect a tension-free repair. Of the eight cases with adequate follow-up, all but one patient recovered grade IV or V abduction strength.

Friedman reviewed three cases of residual axillary nerve paralysis following brachial plexus injuries.[7] Each patient was found to have axillary neuromas (one in continuity). In none were fascicles in continuity present after microscopic internal neurolysis; therefore, resection and two sural nerve grafts of 4 to 6 cm were placed. Each patient regained grade IV or V deltoid function.

SURGICAL METHOD

After general anesthesia is obtained, the patient is placed in the lateral decubitus position. An anterior skin incision is made from the midclavicle, extending distally along the medial arm to the lower border of the pectoralis major muscle. The deltopectoral groove is opened, mobilizing the cephalic vein and the deltoid muscle. The superior aspect of the tendon of the pectoralis major muscle is divided as needed for exposure. In most patients it is unnecessary to divide the entire attachment of the pectoralis major, as retraction within the deltopectoral groove affords adequate exposure. The pectoralis minor muscle is then detached from the coracoid process, exposing the distal cords of the brachial plexus. The origin of the musculocutaneous nerve from the lateral cord is observed, since the axillary nerve originates from the posterior cord below the brachial artery at approximately the level of the musculocutaneous nerve's origin from the lateral cord. Each of these nerves branches from its respective cord at approximately the level of the coracoid process.

This approach allows exposure of the axillary nerve from its origin off the posterior cord to its entry into the quadrilateral space. Most injuries of the axillary nerve will be evident, at least in part, with the anterior exposure. Each of Friedman's three cases[7] and fourteen out of twenty-one of Petrucci's cases[13] demonstrated an injury proximal to entry into the quadrilateral space.

Should the lesion be confined to a region proximal to the quadrilateral space, repair using an anterior approach alone is sufficient. At this level the fascicular anatomy of the axillary nerve is that of a single bundle with no distinct orientation of those fibers destined for each of the three primary terminal branches.

Should the level of nerve injury extend into the quadrilateral space, which is usually the case, the patient's shoulder is then rolled anteriorly, and a second incision is made along the posterior border of the deltoid. Because the deltoid muscle is often atrophic, its posterior borders can be rolled forward without detaching its origin. The interval between the long and lateral heads of the triceps is developed to expose the quadrilateral and triangular spaces. The quadrilateral space and axillary nerve are identified through the posterior exposure.

If a neuroma-in-continuity is encountered, neurolysis using the operating microscope is performed. Intraoperative electroneurography may be a useful adjunct. If the neuroma extends through the quadrilateral space, resection and grafting is indicated, as neurolysis of the nerve within the quadrilateral space is very difficult and results are likely to be suboptimal. If neurolysis fails to reveal intact fascicles or if the injury to the axillary nerve is not in continuity, resection and nerve grafting are indicated. The axillary nerve is serially cut back proximally and distally from neuroma and glioma until normal-appearing fascicles are encountered. Proximally, the nerve may be dissected free from the posterior cord of the brachial plexus for at least 2 cm, if necessary, as plexus formation does not occur until higher in the posterior cord. Distally, the motor fascicles (usually a grouped fascicle) to the deltoid muscle may be isolated from the sensory and teres minor branches.

Two sural nerve grafts are threaded through the quadrilateral space bridging the anterior and posterior exposures. The grafts are anastomosed to the distal deltoid motor fascicles, and the posterior wound is closed in layers. The patient's shoulder is rolled posteriorly and the grafts identified through the anterior wound. The grafts are trimmed so as to be just long enough to permit shoulder movement without tension, and then are anastomosed to the proximal stump of the axillary nerve. The pectoralis muscles are repaired using previously placed Mersilene sutures, and the anterior wound is closed in layers. If grafting is performed, the shoulder is immobilized for 2 to 4 weeks in a shoulder immobilizer, and then progressive shoulder range-of-motion exercises are begun. If neurolysis is performed, the shoulder is immobilized for comfort only. In a report of his results of 25 grafts to isolated axillary nerve lesions, Narakas rated 60% excellent (M4+), 20% good (M4), 12% fair (M3), and 8% poor.[12]

COMPLICATIONS

No specific complications following axillary neurorrhaphy or grafting have been reported, but the period of immobilization required after operative treatment tends to produce shoulder stiffness and limited passive range of motion. It is of paramount importance that physical therapy overcome this as much and as soon as possible, as limited passive range of motion cannot be overcome by even a perfect recovery of deltoid strength.

REFERENCES

1. Babcock JL, Wray JB. Analysis of abduction in a shoulder with deltoid paralysis due to axillary nerve injury. Clin Orthop 1970; 68:116–120.
2. Bateman JE. Nerve injuries about the shoulder in sports. J Bone Joint Surg [Am] 1967; 49:785–792.
3. Blom S, Dahlback LO. Nerve injuries in dislocations of the shoulder joint and fractures of the neck of the humerus. Acta Chir Scand 1970; 136:461–466.
4. Cahill BR, Palmer RE. Quadrilateral space syndrome. J Hand Surg 1983; 8:65–69.
5. Dillon L, Hoaglund FT, Scheck M. Brachial neuritis. J Bone Joint Surg [Am] 1985; 67:878–880.
6. Fick R. Anatomie und mechanik der gelenke. Teil III. Spezielle Gelenk und Muskelmechanik. Gustav Fischer, Jena.
7. Friedman AH, Nunley JA, Goldner RD, Urbaniak JR. Repair of isolated axillary nerve lesions following infraclavicular brachial plexus injuries Neurosurgery 1990; 27(3):403–407.
8. Leffert RD, Seddon H. Infraclavicular brachial plexus injuries. J Bone Joint Surg [Br] 1965; 47:9–22.
9. Markhede G, Monastyrski J, Stener B. Shoulder function after deltoid muscle removal. Acta Orthop Scand 1985; 56:242–244.
10. Millesi H. Nerve grafts: Indications, techniques, and prognosis. In: Management of peripheral nerve problems. Philadelphia: WB Saunders, 1980:425–426.
11. Milton GW. The mechanism of circumflex and other nerve injuries in dislocation of the shoulder and the possible mechanism of nerve injuries during reduction or dislocation. Aust N Z J Surg 1953; 25–30.
12. Narakas AO. Lesions du nerf axillaire et lesions associées du nerf suprascapulaire. Revue Medicale de la Suisse Romande 1989; 109:545–556.
13. Petrucci FS, Morelli A, Raimondi PL. Axillary nerve injuries: 21 cases treated by nerve graft and neurolysis. J Hand Surg 1982; 7:271–278.
14. Richards RR, Hudson AR, Bertoia JT, Urbaniak JR, Waddell JP. Injury to the brachial plexus during Putti-Platt and Bristow procedures. Am J Sports Med 1987; 15:374–380.
15. Sunderland S, Marshall RD, Swaney WE. The intraneural topography of the circumflex musculocutaneous and obturator nerves. Brain 1959; 82: 116–118.
16. Sunderland S. The axillary nerve. In: Nerves and nerve injuries. New York: Churchill-Livingstone, 1978:845.
17. Watson-Jones R. Fractures in the region of the shoulder joint. In: Proceedings of the Royal Society of Medicine, 1936:1058–1072.

32

Spinal Accessory Nerve

Gerard Gabel
James A. Nunley

AUTHORS' KEY POINTS

- Excisional biopsy in the posterior triangle of the neck is the most common cause of unexpected spinal accessory nerve injury.
- Prognosis for spontaneous recovery in these iatrogenic injuries is poor.
- Early exploration (less than 3 months post-injury) is indicated.
- Direct repair or nerve grafting has a good prognosis when performed early (less than 3 months post-injury).

Spinal accessory nerve injury can occur following direct or indirect trauma, but the most common injury resulting in spinal accessory nerve deficit is iatrogenic.[12,14,23] The frequency of iatrogenic cases in earlier reports range from 0% in Kramer's series of World War I gunshot-wound victims[9] to 100% in Valtonen's series.[23] Unrecognized iatrogenic causation can be implicated in most series about 90% of the time, as in Norden's account of 16 injuries, 15 of which occurred during operative procedures.[12]

Procedures most frequently associated with accidental spinal accessory nerve injury include biopsy of lesions of the posterior triangle of the neck and excision of tuberculous cervical lymph nodes.[7,8,12,14,23–25] The incidence of spinal accessory nerve injury in biopsy and excision of cervical lymph nodes was 3% to 10% in series from the first half of this century. Fortunately, recognition of this problem and more attentive surgery has decreased the occurrence of accidental injury to the nerve. However, spinal accessory nerve injuries associated with biopsies of lipomas, lymph nodes, and other lesions in the posterior triangle are still reported.[13,14,23]

The most common operative procedure causing spinal accessory nerve paralysis today is dissection performed for carcinomas of the head and neck. In the classical operation of radical neck dissection, the nerve is intentionally sacrificed for oncologic principles, accepting the morbidity of loss of trapezial function in exchange for presumed better tumor control. Modified radical neck dissection, in which the spinal accessory nerve is preserved, has evolved in an attempt to decrease morbidity associated with the classical procedure. Analysis of recurrence rates and disease-free survival rates have not, for the most part, shown worse results when the modified procedure was used instead of the classical procedure.[16,18,19]

DIAGNOSIS

The diagnosis of spinal accessory nerve injury and attendant trapezius paralysis is sometimes difficult to ascertain soon after injury, especially when extensive dissection in the region of the shoulder and neck has been performed. When injury of the spinal accessory nerve occurs during a minor operative procedure, the resultant dysfunction is attributed to the nerve injury and not to the procedure itself. In such instances, pain in the shoulder and periscapular region is experienced, usually within several days.[23] The pain is exacerbated with use of the extremity, especially with tasks that place inferior traction on the shoulder girdle, or activities that require suspension of the arm by the shoulder. The pain may be experienced with minimal activity, such as hanging the arm freely at the side. Relief is obtained with maneuvers that passively elevate the extremity, such as using a sling or placing the arm on a rest or a table. About half of patients experience numbness or paresthesias radiating into the arm, forearm, or hand.

Physical examination reveals inferior translation of the shoulder (Fig. 32-1) and inferior and lateral rotation of the scapula on the chest wall as well as occasional winging of the scapula. Abduction is severely limited, especially soon after injury, with active abduction less than 90° in 80% to 90% of cases.[14,23] Atrophy is not evident for 2 to 3 months, but palpable contraction of the superior component of the trapezius is absent from the time of injury. (The middle and inferior components of the trapezius may still function due to anatomical considerations, which will be covered later.) Active elevation of the shoulder, the so-called "shrug" test, may be normal due to compensatory mechanisms provided, in particular, by the levator scapulae. Function of the sternocleidomastoid muscle is assessed by resisted rotation of the head toward the unaffected side. Examination of the operative incision (if present) and percussion for a Tinel's sign are performed. Further evaluation of the extremity includes a complete neurovascular examination.

Valtonen reported on 14 patients who sustained spinal accessory nerve injuries during superficial biopsies of benign lesions in the posterior triangle of the neck.[23] Twelve patients noted pain in the shoulder region within a few days of biopsy. At initial evaluation (usually within 1 to 2 weeks of the procedure) all patients had lowering of the shoulder, nine had inferolateral translation of the scapula, and thirteen had limited active abduction (less than 90°). Operative repair was not undertaken in any of these patients. Physical therapy, for symptomatic relief as well as for training of substitute mechanisms, was performed in each case. Only seven of the fourteen patients noted any relief with these measures, and in each of these the relief was transient.

Norden, in a review of sixteen patients, reported similar findings, except that ten patients described the pain as severe, three moderate, and one mild; two had no pain.[12] The pain was located in the shoulder or scapular region and radiated into the arm in two patients and into the hand and forearm in nine patients. Seven patients also complained of numbness or paresthesias in the shoulder or hand. Both pain and paresthesias were exacerbated with exertion, especially lifting or other activities that placed downward traction on the arm. Even the weight of the arm, if left hanging freely, was enough to cause severe symptoms. In most cases, pain was decreased or resolved when the arm was supported.

Further evaluation of spinal accessory nerve injury includes electromyographic study of the sternocleidomastoid, trapezius, and, if indicated, components of the brachial plexus.

Evaluation of the neck and shoulder following radical neck dissection is difficult due to the morbidity secondary to the procedure itself. Most authors cite paralysis of the trapezius muscle as the primary source of morbidity following classical radial neck dissection.[1,2,18,20] Studies that compare preservation and sacrifice of the spinal accessory nerve are conflicting in the incidence of pain and dysfunction, but most confirm superior results when the nerve is preserved. Short found shoulder pain in all patients after radial neck dissection and in 60% after modified radical dissection.[20] He also found a significant superiority in function with modified vs radical dissection. Saunders reported that 69% of modified and 50% of classical radical neck dissections were asymptomatic.[18] However, the incidence of severe pain was nearly five times as high following the classical procedure (33% vs 7%).

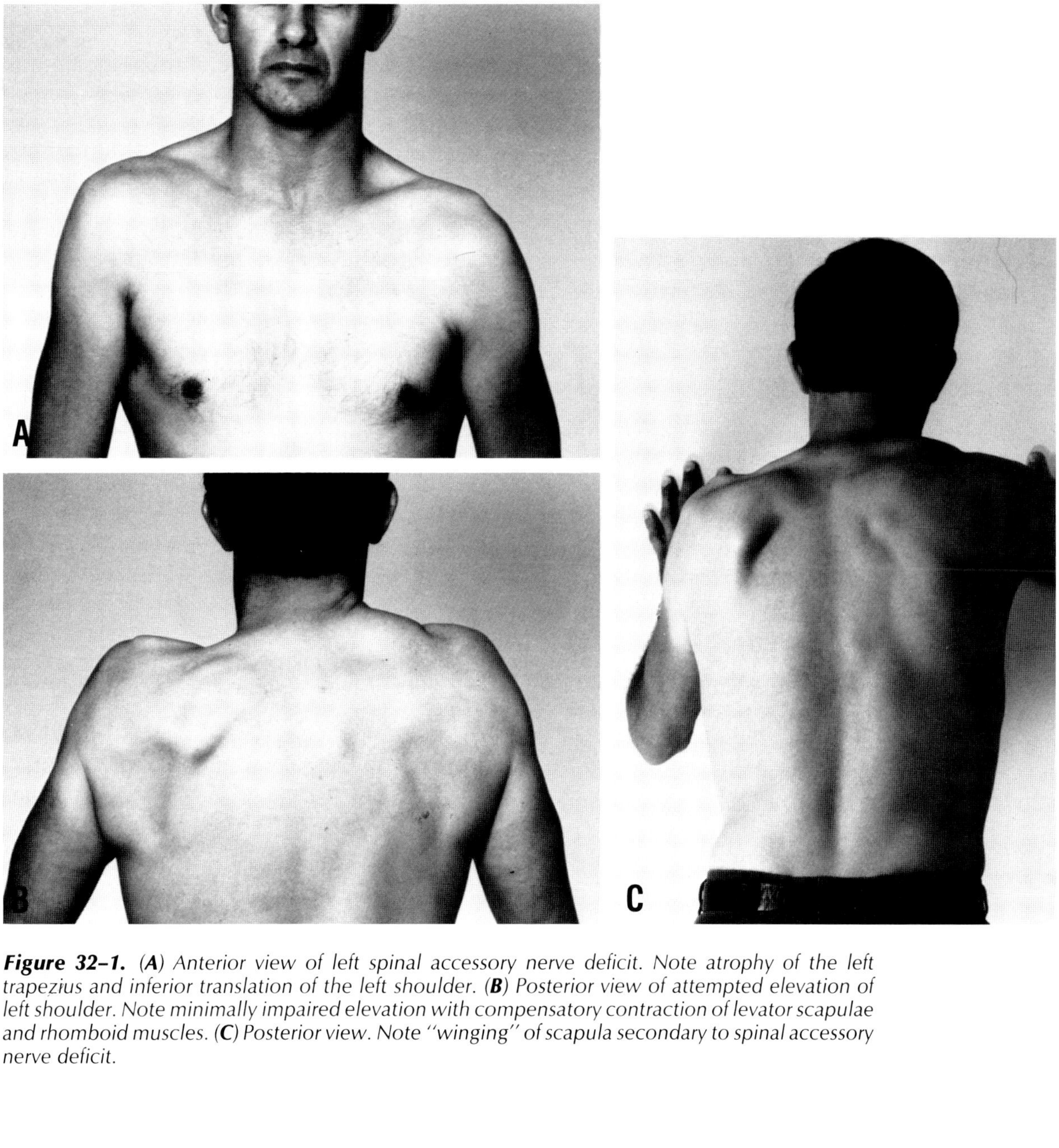

Figure 32–1. *(**A**) Anterior view of left spinal accessory nerve deficit. Note atrophy of the left trapezius and inferior translation of the left shoulder. (**B**) Posterior view of attempted elevation of left shoulder. Note minimally impaired elevation with compensatory contraction of levator scapulae and rhomboid muscles. (**C**) Posterior view. Note "winging" of scapula secondary to spinal accessory nerve deficit.*

Unfortunately, functional integrity of the spinal accessory nerve after modified radical neck dissection is unpredictable. Carenfelt and Eliasson[5] and Saunders[18] found paresis of the trapezius in 30% and frank paralysis in 20% after procedures in which preservation of the spinal accessory nerve was attempted. The variability in the incidence of spinal accessory nerve dysfunction after modified radical neck dissection may relate to the need for dissection in the region of the nerve. Leipzig found that dissection that involved only a portion of the spinal accessory nerve was less likely to result in objective loss of trapezius innervation than with more extensive perineural dissection.[11] In patients with neural dissection in the region of the posterior triangle alone, 12% had findings of trapezius denervation, compared to 50% of patients with a radical neck dissection whose nerve was maintained in continuity but dissected free throughout its course.

Overall, the results of modified vs classic radical neck dissection justify the use of the former when possible. Morbidity is significantly decreased when the spinal accessory nerve is preserved. However, spinal accessory nerve dysfunction can be expected in up to 50% of cases even when the nerve is in continuity.

ETIOLOGY AND PROGNOSIS

The natural history of spinal accessory nerve injury depends upon the cause of dysfunction. Woodruff reported trapezius denervation secondary to the use of an arm sling; recovery was complete at 1 year.[26] Eisen and Bertrand reported four cases of idiopathic spinal accessory nerve palsy, only one of which was followed for more than 3 months; that patient had complete recovery by 22 months.[6] Spillane reported on three patients with trapezius and sternocleidomastoid wasting of spontaneous onset, and none had any evidence of useful recovery at follow-up.[21] Norden reported on one patient who had blunt trauma (a ladder fell on the patient's shoulder) leading to trapezius palsy; that patient had no recovery at 6 years.[12]

Patterson reported an incident of spinal accessory nerve injury with trapezius muscle denervation and atrophy following inferior dislocation of the clavicle on the acromion.[15] The acromioclavicular joint injury was openly reduced, but the spinal accessory nerve injury was treated closed. At 1 year post-injury, the trapezius had completely recovered.

Spinal accessory nerve palsy following carotid endarterectomy has been attributed to traction injury due to lateral retraction on the superior aspect of the anterior border of the sternocleidomastoid muscle. Two patients described by Swann and Heros had sternocleidomastoid and trapezius palsies, which resolved over 6 months following carotid endarterectomy.[22]

The natural history of spinal accessory nerve injury following minor operative procedures in the posterior triangle of the neck is dismal. Combining the series of Woodhall,[25] Gordon,[7] and Valtonen,[23] only 2 of 35 patients demonstrated spontaneous recovery. In an attempt to assess prognosis in spinal accessory nerve palsy cases, Krogness suggested using serial nerve conduction latencies.[10] Normal latency from the mastoid process to the sternocleidomastoid and trapezius muscles were 2.3 and 3.5 msec, respectively. He reported on a patient followed for 11 months after biopsy of a lymph node whose latency to the trapezius decreased from 8 to 4.0 msec and whose trapezius showed some recovery. The deficiency of this method is that by the time serial latencies verify a poor prognosis for spontaneous recovery, the results of operative intervention are likely to be poor.

The reason for the poor prognosis in iatrogenic spinal accessory nerve injuries following minor operative procedures in the posterior triangle relates to the usual degree of injury to the nerve. Rarely is the deficit due to a traction injury, either neurapraxic or axonotmetic. Osgaard reviewed a series of patients with spinal accessory nerve injury following minor posterior triangle procedures.[14] Of nine patients who had operative exploration, all had complete transection of the nerve, several with apparent segmental defects.

The prognosis for maintenance or recovery of trapezius muscle function following neck dissections depends on the status of the nerve at the time of the procedure. If the nerve was resected during the procedure, severe dysfunction or no function is seen in the trapezius muscle. Function does not improve spontaneously. However, as illustrated by Carenfelt, patients whose nerves were not resected had a better prognosis.[5] Of 35 patients examined, 23 demonstrated minor or major paresis of trapezius muscles on early follow-up. Eight of these patients (35%) had complete resolution at long-term follow-up, six patients (26%) still exhibited complete paralysis, and nine patients had mild paresis of the trapezius.

The long-term consequences of trapezius palsy following minor posterior triangle procedures were evaluated in Valtonen's series of 14 patients.[23] Late evaluation of these patients (mean follow-up, 3.6 years) revealed persistent morbidity in 12 patients. Eleven patients either were disabled from work or seriously compromised in their vocational use of the affected extremity. Twelve continued to have shoulder girdle pain. Examination revealed persistent lowering of the shoulder in 12, trapezius atrophy in 11, and active abduction less than 90° in 11. Only one patient had spontaneous recovery of trapezius muscle function.

APPLIED ANATOMY

The spinal accessory nerve originates from rootlets from the medulla (the bulbar or cranial rootlets) and the upper cervical spine (usually from the first through sixth cervical segments). As the nerve exits the jugular foramen, it divides into internal and external rami. The internal ramus, composed of the cranial or bulbar portion of the nerve, joins the vagus nerve. The external ramus, composed of the spinal fibers, continues as the spinal accessory nerve proper. Descending between the internal carotid artery and internal jugular vein, the spinal accessory nerve passes anterior or posterior to the vein. Four to six centimeters below the mastoid process, the spinal accessory nerve gives branches to the sternocleidomastoid muscle while passing through the muscle (80%) or posterior to it (20%). The nerve then enters the posterior triangle of the neck (Fig. 32-2), the borders of which are the sternocleidomastoid muscle anteriorly, the trapezius posteriorly, and the clavicle inferiorly. The nerve leaves the posterior border of the sternocleidomastoid muscle just above the midpoint of the sternocleidomastoid muscle. In the posterior triangle, sensory branches from the third and fourth cervical segments may join the spinal accessory nerve before innervating the trapezius muscle.

The spinal accessory nerve traverses the posterior triangle between the superficial and deep (prevertebral) layers of the cervical fascia surrounded by dense fascia, fat, and lymphatic tissue. At a level approximately 3 to 5 cm medial to the clavicular insertion, the nerve passes beneath the trapezius, coursing inferiorly to give branches to

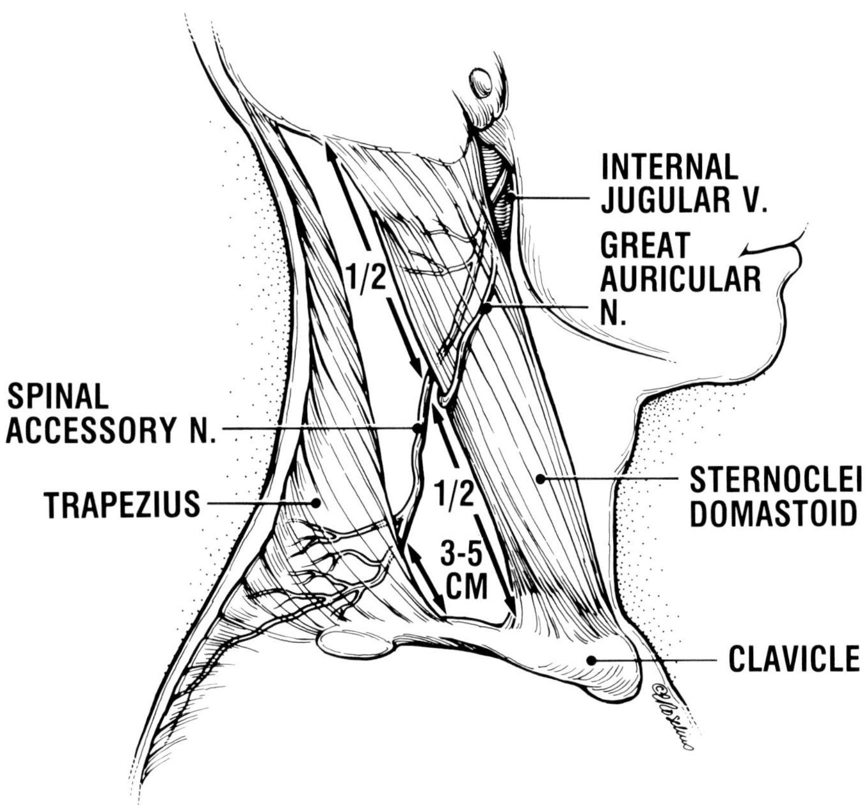

Figure 32–2. Posterior triangle of the neck. The anterior border is the sternocleidomastoid (SCM): the inferior border is the clavicle; and the posterior border is the trapezius. Note course and possible branching of the spinal accessory nerve (SAN). It exits the posterior margin of the SCM at midpoint between origin and insertion. The main trunk of the SAN enters the undersurface of the trapezius at 3 to 5 cm medial to clavicular insertion.

the three components of the trapezius.[4] The spinal accessory nerve may branch prior to passing beneath the anterior margin of the trapezius. In about half of patients, one, two, or three high branches occur, destined for the superior component of the trapezius.[4]

Variations of note deal primarily with the cervical plexus contributions in the posterior triangle. These roots (usually the second through fourth) consist probably of sensory fibers only. There is controversy over this, but most data including intraoperative cervical root stimulation supports a primarily sensory function. The cervical root contribution to the spinal accessory nerve may occur in the posterior triangle or as the spinal accessory nerve passes under the anterior margin of the trapezius.

TYPES OF OPERATIONS

Neurolysis

The nature of the injury to the spinal accessory nerve may leave the nerve in continuity. The dysfunction of the nerve may occur acutely due to closed trauma, traction during an operative procedure, or a shock effect (as in gunshot wounds). Dysfunction of the nerve may manifest itself later due to edema and cicatrix formation in the region of the nerve.

Bateman reported spinal accessory nerve injuries that occurred in sports, such as a blow from a hockey or lacrosse stick.[3] He said that exploration at 6 weeks with neurolysis usually gave extremely good results, but no data were provided.

Woodhall reviewed three patients with iatrogenic injuries who, at exploration, were found to have lesions in continuity with a positive response to electrical stimulation.[24] External neurolysis was performed in each case, with return of full muscle mass and strength.

Gordon described one patient who underwent exploration for a spinal accessory nerve deficit 4 months after cervical node biopsy.[7] The nerve was found to be tethered to the transverse process of C2. An internal and external neurolysis was performed. Range of motion and strength were improved on follow-up, but the degree of recovery was not stated.

Exploration and Direct Repair

The most frequent finding at operative exploration of the spinal accessory nerve for deficits following operative procedures in the posterior triangle is complete transection of the nerve. In these cases, the length of defect present after preparing the nerve ends may be small enough to allow direct repair. Woodhall said that the gap is "always small, 1 cm or less,"[25] but he reported resection of pathological segments of up to 3.5 cm[24] in preparation of the nerve. He recommended using a sling to elevate the shoulder, allowing repair with minimal tension. Of the four patients treated with this regimen, two had had a suture constricting the nerve, requiring resection of the affected segment. Three of the patients were followed, with good functional recovery noted and only minimal residual muscle atrophy. The interval between injury and repair and the length of follow-up were not specified.

Norden reported on three patients who had exploration and repair of the spinal accessory nerve.[12] Two of the nerves, one explored at 4 weeks and the other at 9 months post-injury, had complete resolution of trapezius paresis. One patient, explored at 4 months, had minimal functional improvement. Norden also reported on one patient in whom the distal portion of the spinal accessory nerve could not be found 18 months after injury. The proximal spinal accessory nerve stump was sutured to "a branch of the cervical nerves," and no recovery occurred.

Osgaard reviewed five patients who underwent exploration and repair.[14] In each case, the nerve ends could be mobilized and the repair accomplished in a tension-free fashion. Of the four with adequate follow-up, two had normal, pain-free function, one had improved function, and one had no return of function.

Exploration and Nerve Grafting

Because most of the minor operative procedures that cause spinal accessory nerve injury involve excisional biopsy (lipomas, lymph nodes, cysts), a segmental defect of the nerve is frequently encountered. The use of nerve grafts to bridge spinal accessory nerve defects following minor operative procedures has been reported by Osgaard.[14] Four patients were found to have defects prohibiting tension-free direct repair, but the defect length and nerve graft length were not specified. Sural nerve grafting was carried out; the number of grafts used was also not given. Three of the four patients had full recovery, while the other exhibited no recovery.

Authors' Preferred Method

Injury of the spinal accessory nerve and the resultant trapezius paralysis usually result in disruption of scapulothoracic motion and loss of the suspensory function of the upper trapezius muscle. Consequent dysfunction and pain may be severe. Although substitute mechanisms may develop, they are rarely complete. As the prognosis for spontaneous recovery of spinal accessory nerve function following minor operative procedures in the posterior triangle is poor, operative exploration is indicated in most cases. The period of observation that may be allowed is not well defined. Operative treatment at 3 months or less post-injury has resulted in excellent recovery in all six patients cited in the literature.[12,14,25] Operative treatment after 4 months has been less encouraging, with excellent results in 13% (one patient), good in 38% (three patients), and poor in 50% (four patients).[7,12,14] Although these numbers are small, they suggest that the period of observation should not exceed 3 months.

The patient is placed in a semi-sitting (lawnchair) position with the arm prepped free. An incision is planned based on the previous surgical scar (if present) or the location of maximal Tinel's sign (as determined preoperatively). An oblique incision is made, starting at the midpoint of the posterior margin of sternocleidomastoid muscle and extending inferiorly and laterally to a point approximately 4 cm from the clavicular insertion of the trapezius. The nerve stumps are usually located in the fibro-fatty subcutaneous tissue. It is important to clearly identify the accessory nerve proper both proximally and distally to avoid an erroneous repair. The accessory nerve is identified as it exits from beneath or through the midpoint of the posterior margin of the sternocleidomastoid muscle (Fig. 32-2). The great auricular nerve exits at the same point but courses anteriorly over the sternocleidomastoid muscle and must not be confused with the accessory nerve.

The accessory nerve distally is localized at the anterior margin of the trapezius 3 to 5 cm medial to the clavicular insertion (see Fig. 32-2). Branches to the trapezius, present in half the cases, are preserved.

If segmental nerve loss or retraction has not occurred, the stumps are resected to good tissue and repair performed with 9-0 nylon sutures. The nerve is approximately 3 mm in diameter at this level.[17] In cases where repair cannot be performed without undue tension, nerve grafting using one or two grafts is required. If the level of injury occurs distal to branching of the accessory nerve, one graft is used to restore continuity to the branches. In cases where these branches are relatively small compared to the main nerve, grafting is performed only to the main trunk. The length of graft required varies, however; the position of the head greatly influences the length. With the head in neutral position, the nerve measures 4 to 5 cm from the sternocleidomastoid to trapezius margins. However, with the head turned to the opposite shoulder it measures 9 to 10 cm. The length of graft is assessed with the head in a neutral position with sufficient length that tension is avoided. Redundancy of the nerve is avoided.

After completing the repair, subcutaneous tissue and skin are closed over a drain. The drain is removed on the 1st or 2nd postoperative day. Range of motion of the neck is limited by use of orthoses, such as a Philadelphia collar. A sling is worn to limit depression of the shoulder. The sling and collar are removed at 4 to 6 weeks and unlimited activity can be resumed. Clinical and electrical evidence of recovery take variable periods of time, depending on the level of the lesion.

REFERENCES

1. Anderson R, Flowers RS. Free grafts of the spinal accessory nerve during radical neck dissection. Am J Surg 1969; 118:796–799.
2. Ballantyne AJ, Guinn GA. Reduction of shoulder disability after neck dissection. Am J Surg 1966; 112:662–665.
3. Bateman J. Nerve injuries about the shoulder in sports. J Bone Joint Surg [Am] 1967; 49:785–792.
4. Caliot PH, Bousquet V, Midy D, Cabanie P. A con-

tribution to the study of the accessory nerve: Surgical implications. Surg Radiol Anat 1989; 11:11–15.

5. Carenfelt C, Eliasson K. Occurrence, duration and prognosis of unexpected accessory nerve paresis in radical neck dissection. Acta Otolaryngol 1980; 90: 470–473.
6. Eisen A, Bertrand G. Isolated accessory nerve palsy of spontaneous origin. Arch Neurol 1972; 27:496—502.
7. Gordon SL, Graham WP, Black JT, Miller SH. Accessory nerve function after surgical procedures in the posterior triangle. Arch Surg 1977; 112:264–268.
8. King RJ, Motta G. Iatrogenic spinal accessory nerve palsy. Ann R Coll Surg Engl 1983; 65:35–37.
9. Kramer F. Schussverletzungen der peripheren nerven. VII. Hirnnerven, Nerven des Kopfes und Rumpfes. Muschr Psychiat Neurol 1922; 53:344.
10. Krogness K. Serial conduction studies of the spinal accessory nerve used as a prognostic tool in a lesion caused by lymph node biopsy. Acta Chir Scand 1974; 140:7–11.
11. Leipzig B, Suen JY, English JL, Barnes J, Hooper M. Functional evaluation of the spinal accessory nerve after neck dissection. Am J Surg 1983; 146: 526–530.
12. Norden A. Peripheral injuries to the spinal accessory nerve. Acta Chir Scand 1946; 94:515–532.
13. Olarte M, Adams D. Accessory nerve palsy. J Neurol Neurosurg Psychiatry 1977; 40:1113–1116.
14. Osgaard O, Eskesen V, Rosenorn J. Microsurgical repair of iatrogenic accessory nerve lesions in the posterior triangle of the neck. Acta Chir Scand 1987; 153:171–173.
15. Patterson WR. Inferior dislocation of the distal end of the clavicle: A case report. J Bone Joint Surg [Am] 1967; 49:1184.
16. Roy PH, Beahrs OH. Spinal accessory nerve in radical neck dissections. Am J Surg 1969; 118:800–804.
17. Samardzic M. Reinnervation of avulsed brachial plexus using the spinal accessory nerve. Surg Neurol 1990; 33:7–11.
18. Saunders JR, Hirata RM, Jaques DA. Considering the spinal accessory nerve in head and neck surgery. Am J Surg 1985; 150:491–494.
19. Schuller DE, Reiches NA, Hamaker RC, et al. Analysis of disability resulting from treatment including radical neck dissection or modified neck dissection. Head Neck Surg 1983; 6:551–558.
20. Short SO, Kaplan JN, Laramore GE, Cummings CW. Shoulder pain and function after neck dissection with or without preservation of the spinal accessory nerve. Am J Surg 1984; 148:478–482.
21. Spillane J. Isolated unilateral spinal accessory nerve palsy of obscure origin. A report of three cases. Br Med J 1949; 2:365.
22. Swann KW, Heros RC. Accessory nerve palsy following carotid endarterectomy. J Neurosurg 1985; 63:630–632.
23. Valtonen EJ, Lilius HG. Late sequelae of iatrogenic spinal accessory nerve injury. Acta Chir Scand 1974; 140:453–455.
24. Woodhall B. Trapezius paralysis following minor surgical procedures in the posterior cervical triangle. Ann Surg 1952; 136:375–380.
25. Woodhall B. Operative injury to the accessory nerve in the posterior cervical triangle. Arch Surg 1957; 74:123–127.
26. Woodruff A. Unilateral spinal accessory nerve palsy caused by an arm sling. Br Med J 1950; 1:821–822.

33

Digital Nerves

John S. Gould

AUTHOR'S KEY POINTS

- Early primary suture of transected digital nerves without tension is common practice today. The results with delayed suture, however, may be equally satisfactory.
- Epineural and fascicular suture techniques provide equivalent results in digital nerves repaired with magnification.
- Results of digital nerve repair in children and in patients of all ages with distal levels of injury are superior.

Surgeons performing digital nerve repairs encounter the same problems as they do in repairing larger mixed nerves, including type of injury, alternatives of basic suture techniques, management of gaps, and variability of results. Digital nerve repairs are unique, however, in their small size (three to six fasciculi) and their pure sensory (and sympathetic) function.

APPLIED ANATOMY

Anatomically, the palmar digital nerves are the distal terminal branches of the median and ulnar nerves. While they lie deep to the vessels in the palm, they are palmar to them in the digits. The neurovascular bundles are found on either side of the digit just dorsal to Grayson's cutaneous ligaments and palmar to Cleland's. In the thumb, the digital nerves lie more palmar and closer to the midpalmar line. At the distal interphalangeal joint level and just distal to it, the palmar digital nerves divide into at least three and sometimes more branches, to the pulp and dorsally to the nail bed area. These pulp branches supply sensibility to areas beyond the midline of the pulp from either side. When one digital nerve is lost, the intact single nerve can provide a more extensive sensory territory, covering most of the pulp, presumably by peripheral sprouting. Just proximal to the proximal interphalangeal joint, the palmar digital nerve provides a dorsal branch that extends obliquely across the side of the joint to supply the skin on the dorsal distal digit. On the thumb, dorsal coverage is provided in variable patterns by superficial radial nerve branches, the lateral antebrachial cutaneous nerve, and branches of the median nerve from the digital nerves. Sympathetic fibers are supplied to adjacent arteries segmentally, and reciprocally minute vessels (vasa nervorum) are supplied to the nerves. The nerves also have an axial blood supply.

MODES OF INJURY

Digital nerves can be damaged by all the types of injuries that can happen to fingers and thumbs. They are exposed to transection by knives, other cutting tools, and glass; crush injuries in car doors, machinery, and heavy objects; avulsion; crush-avulsion; heat and cold injury; and bites and envenomizations. Nerve injuries are commonly associated with damage to tendons, bone, joints, adjacent vessels, and with all of the above in cases of complete amputation.

INDICATIONS FOR REPAIR

Indications for immediate or at least early repair (within 6 days) include all sharp cut or local crush (dull cut) injuries.[22] Avulsion or diffuse crush injuries are probably better managed by at least a 2-week delay, so that the surgeon may better determine the proper level of injury (see Chap. 24). Grossly untidy wounds warrant delay until they are at least secondarily clean. Replantation surgeons have taken some liberties with these concepts: they rely on the principle that a reasonable estimate of the level of damage can be made at the time of surgery, and that the subsequent risk to the adjacent repaired vessels when dissecting through scar during reoperation is greater than potential problems with primary nerve repair. Consequently, the replantation surgeon makes ample use of acute grafting and carries out later reconstruction in the event that nerve repair fails. Many authors, including Honner,[6] Buncke,[2] Seddon,[20] Boswick,[1] Larsen,[7] and Önne[17] support primary repair, noting specific indications for delay.

While Wallace[24] and Wallace and Copeland[25] state that spontaneous regeneration occurs in the distal digit, particularly at the distal interphalangeal joint level, obviating repair, most authors today repair digital nerves to at least the distal interphalangeal joint level. Tupper[23] and Mackinnon and Dellon[9] repair the distal branches, while Wilgis and Maxwell[28] have carried out grafting at the distal level to provide a superior sensory return.

TYPES OF OPERATIONS

Repair techniques include epineural and fascicular suture. In addition, nerve grafting (acute and delayed) using a variety of donors, vein graft conduits and polyglycolic acid conduits, vascularized nerve grafts, and reversed venous arterialized nerve grafts are indicated in specific circumstances. Most surgeons now use epineural suture technique, arguing that it is at least as effective as a grouped fascicular repair in larger mixed nerves. As digital fascicles are sensory, there is little risk of significant misorientation of fibers. In studies of fascicular repair, Tupper found that static two-point discrimination averaged 9.82 (14 cases) in one series and 7.63 (27 cases) in another (see Chap. 19).[23] Young, Wray, and Weeks[30] carried out a prospective review of 34 nerves in 27 patients with magnification and 9-0 or 10-0 suture technique. They performed 17 fascicular and 17 epineural repairs, and obtained identical results in both series.

Most hand surgeons use 3.5× to 4.5× loupe magnification or a microscope, with zoom capabilities up to 20×, to assist with operative repair. Grafting, conduits, and vascularized methods are almost always performed with a microscope, allowing the surgeon to trim nerve ends accurately, place sutures appropriately through outer or inner epineurium, coapt surfaces without gaps or buckling, and work comfortably with fine suture.

Most surgeons use 8-0 to 10-0 (22 μm) monofilament nylon or polypropylene suture with a 75- or 130-μm needle (see Chap. 17). The 3/8-circle arc is often preferred to the half circle, and longer cord lengths are commonly preferred. The BV taper-point needle is preferred to a cutting edge. Buncke still prefers to use straight needles for nerve repairs.[2]

While multiple suture techniques are used, the common denominators are that the repair is carried out without tension with joints either extended or flexed no more than 45°.[22] Nunley determines the length of graft to be used by placing the wrist in neutral and the digit in full extension at all three joints.[15] Any tension is taken off the repair with temporary stay sutures away from the repair line or with the VanBeek nerve holder (Fig. 33-1). In many cases, neither stay sutures nor special holders are used. In the epineural repair, near-and-far interrupted sutures are placed 180° apart (Fig. 33-2). The nerve is turned, using these long corner sutures, to repair the back wall interval followed by returning the nerve and closing the front wall (Fig. 33-3). While some authors use six to ten sutures for each nerve, most use fewer (typically four).

With the fascicular technique (Fig. 33-4), one or two sutures are used for each funiculus, placing the suture through the inner epineurium (previously called a perineural suture). The microscope and 10-0 sutures are needed for this method.

OVERCOMING DEFECTS IN DIGITAL NERVES

Nerve grafting has been strongly advocated by Millesi[10–12] for any gap and by most surgeons when the gap exceeds 1 cm. Donor nerves include the sural,[16,27] the lateral antebrachial cutaneous anterior branch of the medial antebrachial cutaneous,[15] the terminal articular branch of the posterior interosseous,[28] the dorsal cutaneous branch of the ulnar nerve,[5] digital nerves from the noncritical side of another digit,[27] digital nerves from nonreplantable digits, and the lateral femoral cutaneous nerve (see Chap. 38). As many procedures are now done under regional anesthesia, upper-extremity sources are often favored.

For short grafts, the posterior interosseous is a useful donor, but obtaining it means dissecting through the fourth extensor compartment. The antebrachial cutaneous nerves are subcutaneous and easily accessible, but incisions leave unsightly scars on the proximal volar forearm. While the lateral antebrachial cutaneous nerve is most popular, its branches can extend to innervate skin on the thumb. The dorsal cutaneous branch of the ulnar, lateral femoral cutaneous, and superficial radial nerves, if used, can leave painful neuromas, although authors advocating the first two choices do not report significant problems.[5] Even a sural nerve donor can lead to a painful neuroma.

Walton and coworkers[26] reported on the clinical use of vein conduits for defects of 1 to 3 cm. The vein diameter chosen is slightly larger than the diameter of the nerve. The vein lumen edge and epineurium are either sutured end-to-end or the nerve

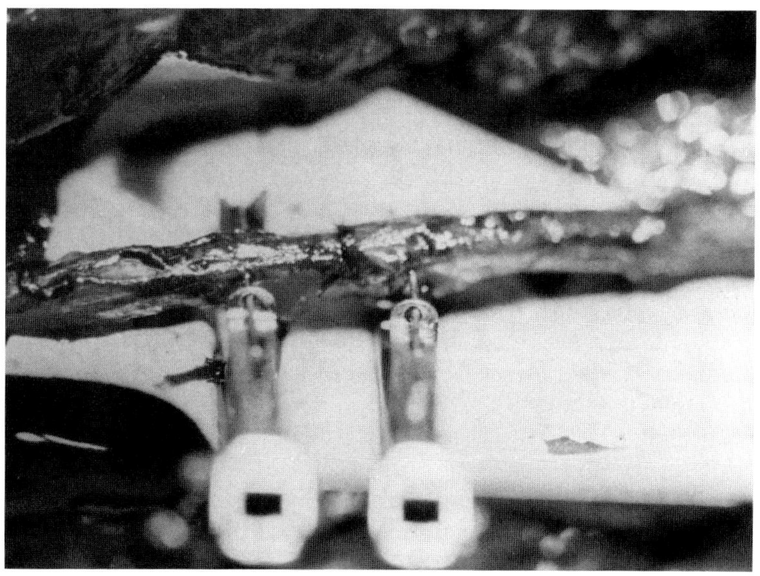

Figure 33–1. *The Van Beek holder–approximator.*

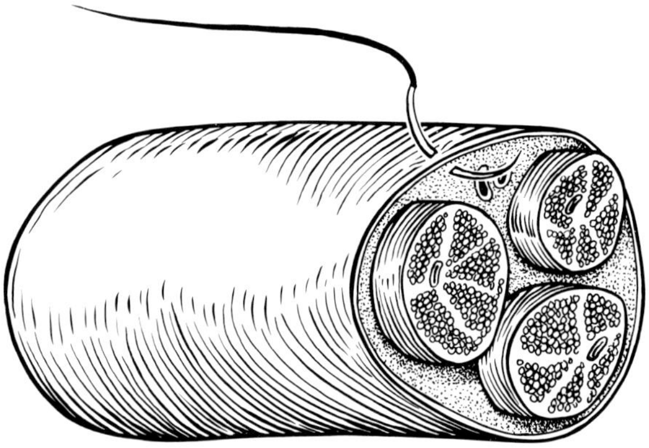

Figure 33–2. *The epineural (outer epineural) suture.*

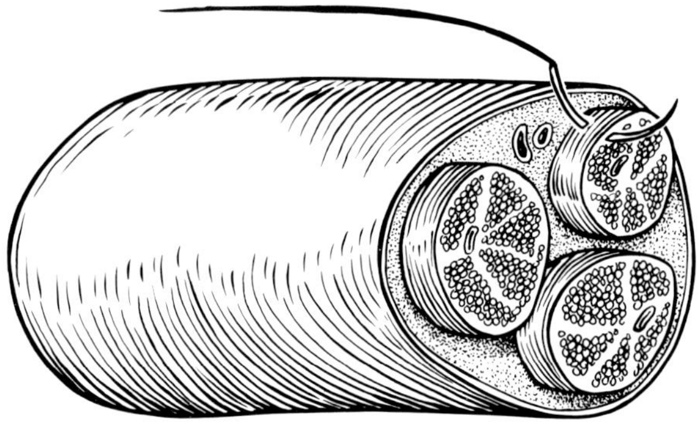

Figure 33–4. *The inner epineural (fascicular) suture.*

ends are placed within the vein lumen, and secured with mattress sutures taken through the vein wall, grasping the underlying epineurium of the nerve. Dellon and Mackinnon[3] reported recent work with polyglycolic acid biodegradable conduits for short nerve gaps. Mackinnon[8] reports superior results to those obtained with veins, apparently due to resistance to collapse of this material.

Rose and Kowalski[18] have reported promising results with vascularized nerve grafts (using the deep peroneal nerve accompanied by the dorsalis pedis artery) for scarred beds in fingers. The nerve and the artery segmental complex is interposed in the digital segmental gap and sutured end-to-end to the artery and nerve. More recently, these authors have reported success using the reversed venae comitantes of the dorsalis pedis, with the deep peroneal nerve, thus preserving the dorsalis pedis artery.[19]

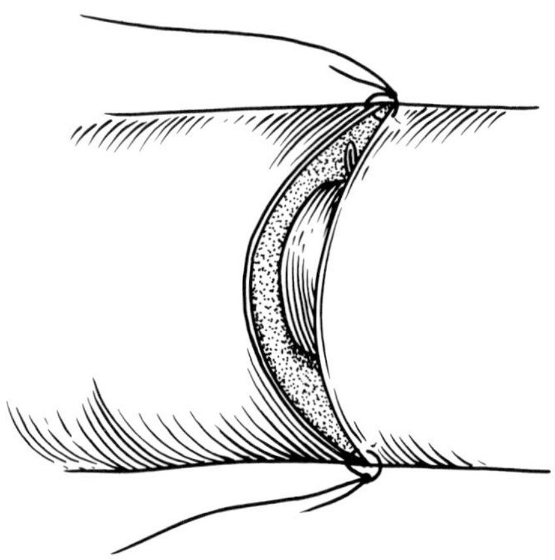

Figure 33–3. *The near-and-far 180° epineural suture, used for turning the nerve.*

Author's Preferred Method

When the gap is less than 1 cm, I carry out primary repairs of digital nerves, if the wound is tidy and the injury mode sharp or local crush. Unless a replantation is involved, this surgery is typically done electively the next day or so. The operative approach is dictated to some extent by the skin wound. A Bruner zigzag incision typically is used. With very distal wounds, a midaxillary incision helps expose branches.

The initial dissection is done with 4.5× loupes. In the palm and proximal digit, loupes are acceptable,[5] but for more distal lesions, the microscope is preferable. I prefer to use the microscope for all digital nerves because I feel more confident with the adequate trim and placement of sutures.

The repair is carried out over a colored plastic background with microsuction apparatus attached. This allows frequent irrigation and clearance of fluid. The exposure is performed with a tourniquet inflated. It is released prior to nerve suture to control intraneural bleeding. Nerve holders are not used. Epineural suturing is done with 9-0 or 10-0 monofilament nylon with a 75-μm, 3-mm cord length BV needle.

Nerve trim is done in a guillotine fashion with a single-edge razor blade over a moistened wooden tongue blade (Fig. 33-5). A silicone cutting board

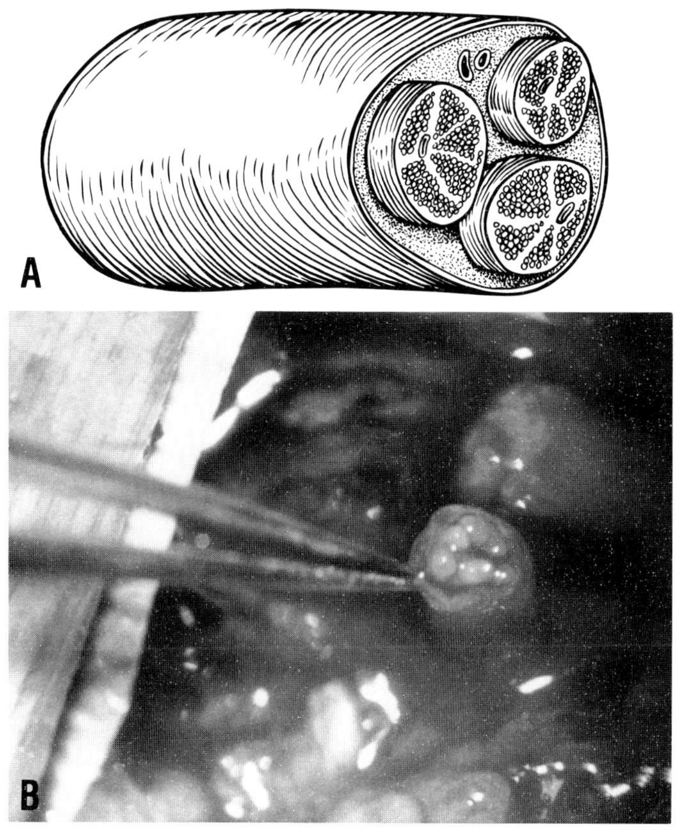

Figure 33–5. *The well-trimmed digital nerve. The fascicles are clearly visible. (**A**) Artist's rendition. (**B**) Clinical photograph.*

may also be used. A nerve of this size does not need a special holder, although the surgeon may hold the nerve with a moist sponge if desired. Epineural sutures are placed 180° apart with single sutures placed at 90° intervals on either side. Occasionally, an additional suture is used.

Isolating barrier materials are not placed around the nerve, although methylcellulose (Surgicel) has been used in the past (Fig. 33-6). The digit is immobilized for a month unless a tendon repair is done simultaneously. In this case, the controlled-motion method is used.

When I encounter a gap of 1 cm or greater (and on occasion a lesser gap when early mobilization is a concern), I use a nerve graft from the lateral antebrachial cutaneous donor site. If the gap is significant, I reverse the graft to avoid loss of axons. Other than that, the procedure is done in the same manner as direct repair.

Delayed repairs are done within 2 weeks if possible. Conduits and vascularized nerve grafts are investigational.

RESULTS

Nerve regeneration is followed by an advancing Tinel's sign, anticipating a progression of 1 to 3 mm per day. The result is tested for vibration with a tuning fork (rapidly adapting fibers), and when 256 cycles/second is reached, sensory re-education is begun (see Chap. 58). Additional evaluations include sharp/dull, moving two-point discrimination (rapidly adapting fibers), static two-point discrimination (Weber-Moberg),[10] and pressure threshold testing (Semmes-Weinstein monofilaments). Dellon argued that moving two-point discrimination is the best predictor of object recognition.[9,26] Although many authors test the autonomous zone of a digital nerve on the distal radial or ulnar pulp, the most reliable results can be achieved by blocking the uninvolved nerve with lidocaine and testing the involved side rapidly prior to spillover. The British Medical Research Council category S3+ to S4 is

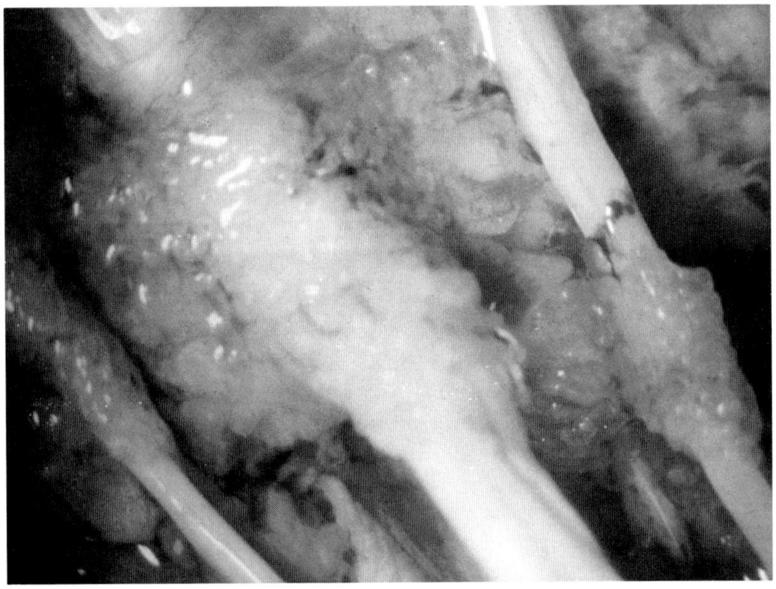

Figure 33–6. Nerve and tendon repairs completed, wrapped with methylcellulose (Surgicel). The barrier material is no longer used.

considered good by Moberg;[10] all lower categories represent fair and poor results. However, S4 represents static two-point discrimination of 6 mm or lower, and S3+ has a two-point discrimination of approximately 15 mm (or some testable two-point discrimination). Methods of reporting make some results difficult to evaluate.

Larsen[7] noted an S3+ rating in 65% of his patients; Seddon[20] had 43% of patients in this category, Buncke 60%,[2] Stromberg 8%,[21] Önne 36%,[17] and Boswick 13%.[1] Young, Wray, and Weeks had 88% in the S3+ category, with 34% in the S4 category.[30] Generally, one can conclude from existing reports that in patients under 20 years of age, 80% regain useful two-point discrimination with modern methods.[30] Over age 40, there is a reduced possibility of gaining useful two-point discrimination.

Wilgis and Maxwell reported on 12 interfascicular grafts in adults with nerves at the distal interphalangeal joint level or more distally.[28] In 67%, they had two-point discrimination of 6 mm. Typical grafts were 1.6 cm long (Fig. 33-7). Yamano and coauthors, using lateral antebrachial grafts in replanted digits, reported an average two-point discrimination of 10.5 mm.[29] Murakami, Ikuta, and Tsuge claimed better results in replanted digits when two nerves were repaired at the proximal phalanx level.[14] At the middle phalanx and distally, the number of nerves repaired (one or two) appeared unimportant. The results improved with more distal levels of repair.

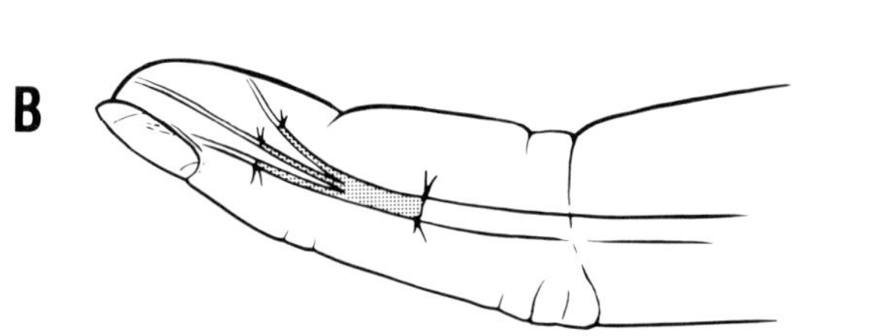

Figure 33–7. (**A**) Three major fascicles of digital nerve just distal to DIP joint, as described by Wilgis and Maxwell. One fascicle goes to the nail fold, the second to the tip of the digit, and the third to the pulp. (**B**) Nerve graft splayed distally and interposed between the digital nerve and its three distal fascicles. (Modified from Wilgis EFS, Maxwell GP. Distal digital nerve grafts: Clinical and anatomical studies. J Hand Surg 1979;4:439–443, with permission.)

Walton's vein graft conduits had 4 to 6 mm of moving two-point discrimination in 11 nerves; all late grafts failed (delays of 2, 6, and 9 months before repair).[26] Static two-point discrimination results were not provided. In Nunley's series, interpositional nerve grafts with the anterior branch of the medial antebrachial cutaneous nerve, 20 of 21 nerves had sharp and dull discrimination and 18 of 21 had two-point discrimination between 5 and 15 mm (average, 9 mm).[15] Rose and Kowalski, using vascularized nerve grafts, obtained two-point discrimination of 9.5 mm with grafts averaging 6.6 cm long.[18]

In my series, in a 3-year period, 169 nerves were repaired in 93 patients: 58 nerve repairs in replantation patients, 10 in digits with severe vascular compromise, and 101 in fingers with normal vascularity.[4] In the group with normal vascularity, the microscope (8–40× magnification) was used for 55 nerves, 4.5× loupes for 30, and 2.5× to 3.5× loupes for 16.

Most of the nerves were repaired within 1 month of injury: 16 were repaired within hours of injury, 37 between day 1 and day 7, 12 between day 8 and 14, and 15 between day 15 and 1 month. Nine were repaired between 1 and 3 months from the injury, and 12 were repaired between 3 months and 1 year. Despite delays, there was little difference in final results. Patients under age 10 achieved 5 mm of two-point discrimination, and patients between ages 11 and 60 achieved 7 mm two-point discrimination. In this series using the microscope, patients having 8-0 suture achieved average two-point discrimination of 8 mm (4–15 mm). When the 10-0 suture was used, the average was 6 mm (4–10 mm). With the 4.5× loupes using 8-0 suture, 8 mm (3–17 mm) was achieved; when the 2.5× to 3.5× loupes and 8-0 suture were used, the results were 7 mm (4–15 mm).

The results were biased by the routine use of the microscope for distal injuries, for branches, and in children. The measurements were made by an experienced hand therapist using Moberg's recommended technique, carrying out the testing in the autonomous zone of the nerve. Uninvolved nerves were not blocked with local anesthetic, however.

CONCLUSIONS

The information, to date, suggests that while meticulous technique is important, epineural repairs without tension or grafts can both have excellent results if patients are young (particularly children) and injuries are located in the distal digit. While microsurgical technique is a clearly positive factor, normal two-point discrimination is not commonly achieved in adults. It must be recognized that even patients with normal Semmes-Weinstein monofilament testing of 2.83, including those achieving relatively normal moving and static two-point discrimination, often still have significantly decreased sensibility. While even the best technology does not necessarily achieve normal sensibility, useful and superior functional results have become routine with today's methodologies for digital nerve repair.

REFERENCES

1. Boswick JA Jr, Schneewind J, Stromberg W Jr. Evaluation of peripheral nerve repairs below the elbow. Arch Surg 1965; 90:50–51.
2. Buncke HJ. Digital nerve repairs. Surg Clin North Am 1972; 52:1267–1285.
3. Dellon AL, Mackinnon SE. An alternative to the classical nerve graft for the management of the short nerve gap. Plast Reconstr Surg 1988; 82:849–856.
4. Gould JS. Digital nerve repairs with magnification techniques. Presented to Orthopaedic Section, Southern Medical Association Meeting, New Orleans, LA, Nov. 9, 1977.
5. Greene TL, Steichen JB. Digital nerve grafting using the dorsal sensory branch of the ulnar nerve. J Hand Surg [Br] 1985; 10:37–40.
6. Honner R, Fragiadakis EG, Lamb DW. An investigation of the factors affecting the results of digital nerve division. Hand 1960; 2:21–30.
7. Larsen RD, Posch JL. Nerve injuries in the upper extremity. Arch Surg 1958; 77:469.
8. Mackinnon SE. Surgical management of the peripheral nerve gap. Clin Plast Surg 1989; 16:587–603.
9. Mackinnon SE, Dellon AL. Surgery of the peripheral nerve. New York: Thieme, 1988:89–130.
10. Millesi H. Microsurgery of peripheral nerves. Hand 1973; 5:157–160.

11. Millesi H. Indication, technique, and results of nerve grafting. Handchirurgie (Suppl) 1977; 2:1–24.
12. Millesi H, Meissel G, Berger A. The interfascicular nerve-grafting of the median and ulnar nerves. J Bone Joint Surg [Am] 1972; 54:727–750.
13. Moberg E. Sensibility in reconstructive limb surgery. In: Fredricks S, Brady GS, eds. Symposium on the neurologic aspects of plastic surgery. St. Louis: CV Mosby, 1978:30.
14. Murakami T, Ikuta Y, Tsuge K. Relationship between the number of digital nerves sutured and sensory recovery in replanted fingers. J Reconstr Micro 1985; 1:283–286.
15. Nunley JA, Ugino MR, Goldner RD, Regan N, Urbaniak JR. Use of the anterior branch of the medial antebrachial cutaneous nerve as a graft for the repair of defects of the digital nerve. J Bone Joint Surg [Am] 1989; 71:563–567.
16. Omer GE, Spinner M. Management of peripheral nerve problems. Philadelphia: WB Saunders, 1980: 353–474.
17. Önne L. Recovery of sensibility and sudomotor activity in the hand after nerve suture. Acta Chir Scand [Suppl] 1962; 300:1–69.
18. Rose EH, Kowalski TA. Restoration of sensibility to anesthetic scarred digits with free vascularized nerve grafts from the dorsum of the foot. J Hand Surg [Am] 1985; 10:514–521.
19. Rose EH, Kowalski TA, Norris MS. The reversed venous arterialized nerve graft in digital nerve reconstruction across scarred bed. Plast Reconstr Surg 1989; 83:593–602.
20. Seddon H. Surgical disorders of the peripheral nerve. Edinburgh: Churchill Livingstone, 1975: 172–213.
21. Stromberg WB Jr, McFarlane RM, Bell JL, et al. Injury of the median and ulnar nerves. J Bone Joint Surg [Am] 1961; 43:717–730.
22. Sullivan DJ. Results of digital neurorrhaphy in adults. J Hand Surg [Br] 1985; 10:41–44.
23. Tupper J. Fascicular nerve repair. In: Jewett DL, McCarroll HR, eds. Nerve repair and regeneration. St. Louis: CV Mosby, 1980:320–328.
24. Wallace WA. The damaged digital nerve. Hand 1975; 7:139–144.
25. Wallace WA, Copeland RE. Variations in the nerves of the thumb and index finger. J Bone Joint Surg [Br] 1975; 57:491–494.
26. Walton RL, Brown RE, Matory WE Jr, Borah GL, Dolph JL. Autogenous vein graft repair of digital nerve defects in the finger: A retrospective clinical study. Plast Reconstr Surg 1989; 84:944–949.
27. Weckesser EC. The repair of nerves in the palm and the fingers. Clin Orthop 1961; 19:200–207.
28. Wilgis EFS, Maxwell GP. Distal digital nerve grafts: Clinical and anatomical studies. J Hand Surg 1979; 4:439–443.
29. Yamano Y, Namba Y, Hino Y, Hasegawa T, Ugawa A, Ise M. Digital nerve grafts in replanted digits. Hand 1982; 14:255–262.
30. Young L, Wray RC, Weeks PM. A randomized prospective comparison of fascicular and epineural digital nerve repairs. Plast Reconstr Surg 1981; 68: 89–92.

34

Facial Nerve Paralysis

Richard L. Fabian

AUTHOR'S KEY POINTS

- Motor function of the facial nerve elicits facial animation. Neurosensory control is mediated by the nervus intermedius.
- Loss of facial function is severely debilitating, both aesthetically and functionally. Accurate diagnosis precedes surgical intervention and rehabilitation.
- Restoration of facial nerve function is difficult and multifactorial. Facial form and functional rehabilitation surgery is characterized by variable results.
- Surgical techniques are divided into three classes of repair: neurophysiological, myophysiological, and static suspension. The selection of technique and the timing of surgery is determined by preoperative analysis. Technical success requires meticulous, properly selected surgical technique.

ANATOMY

The facial nerve has a motor and motor-sensory division (nervus intermedius) with important intracranial, intratemporal, and extracranial relationships. The extracranial facial nerve divides into the cervicotemporal and cervicofacial division, the motor innervation of the muscles of facial expression. The motor-sensory division of the facial nerve provides efferent and afferent neuropathways responsible for general and special sensory transmission of taste, proprioception, lacrimation, and intercommunication with the Vth, IXth, and Xth cranial nerves.

Intratemporal Course (Fig. 34-1)

The motor division and nervus intermedius emerge between the inferior peduncle and olive in the lower portion of the pons. The combined trunk passes through and enters the internal acoustic meatus accompanied by the vestibular and cochlear nerves, internal auditory artery, and internal auditory vein. Within the internal auditory canal, the facial nerve occupies the anterior–superior position. As it exits the internal acoustic fundus, the facial nerve curves anteriorly around the basal turn of the cochlea and enlarges into a bulbous expansion called the geniculate ganglion.

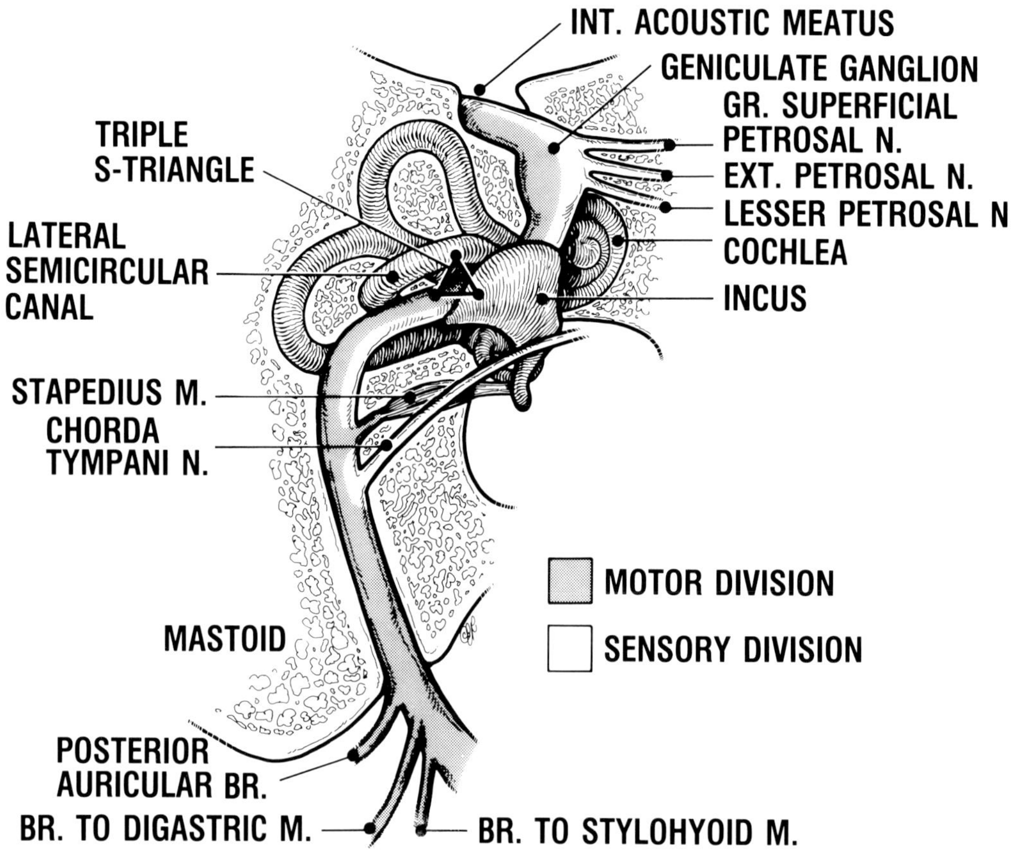

Figure 34-1. *Intratemporal course of the motor and sensory divisions of the facial nerve.*

From the anterior edge of the geniculate ganglion, the greater superficial petrosal nerve exits anteriorly and proceeds through the hiatus canal facialis.[15]

The first genu and subsequent horizontal portion of the facial nerve is characterized by an abrupt posterior direction change. In its horizontal portion, the facial nerve at first is positioned posterior–superiorly to the cochleariform process and proceeds to form the superior portion of the stapes niche. The nerve then curves laterally and inferiorly (the second genu) and descends through the mastoid portion of the temporal bone (vertical portion). During its descent, the vertical portion of the facial nerve gives off a small motor branch to the stapedius muscle and gives origin to the chorda tympani nerve.

Important relationships of the vertical portion of the facial nerve are its anterior caudate position to the lateral semicircular canals, its lateral position to the stapedius muscle, and its posterior medial location to the short process of the incus. The triangle consisting of the short process of the incus, the facial nerve, and the lateral semicircular canal is known as the "triple-S triangle."[9] This relationship is particularly important to the otologic temporal bone surgeon.

Extratemporal Course (Fig. 34-2)

After the facial nerve emerges from the stylomastoid foramen, one or two small motor branches are given off to the posterior belly of the digastric,

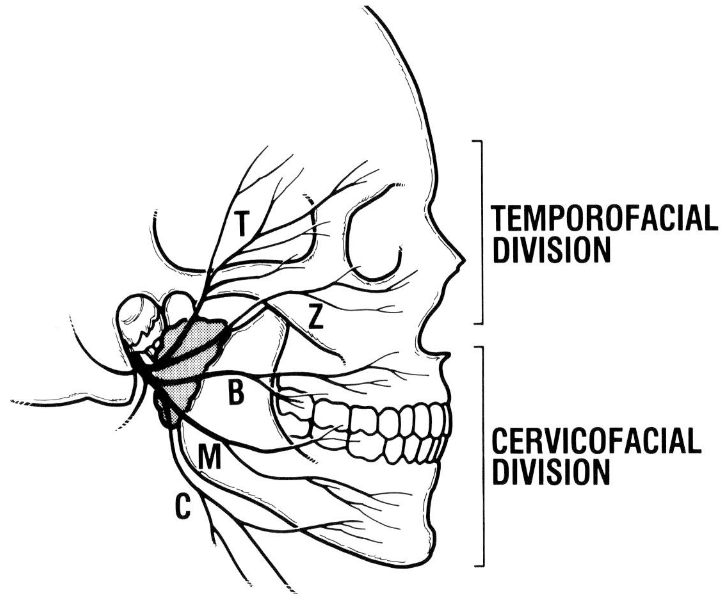

Figure 34-2. *Extratemporal (facial) divisions and motor branches of the facial nerve.*

stylohyoid, and auricular muscles. Before entering the superficial and deep portions of the parotid gland, the main trunk of the facial nerve is positioned between the mastoid tip and the base of the styloid process. Before dividing into an upper and lower division, the main trunk lies about 4 to 8 mm medial to the tympanomastoid fissure, lateral to the external carotid artery, and inferior to the triangular process of the cartilaginous external auditory meatus (cartilage pointer). The posterior facial vein is crossed by the facial nerve, which then divides into an upper trunk called the temporofacial division, and a lower trunk, the cervicofacial division. In the gland, terminal branching occurs. Although terminal branching is quite variable, a common pattern consists of two terminal branches from the upper division and three terminal branches from the lower.[8]

Temporofacial Division (Fig. 34-3)

The temporal branch appears at the upper border of the gland and runs superiorly and forward to innervate the frontalis muscle and superior fibers of the orbicularis oculi muscle. The second branch of the upper division is the zygomatic branch, which rises over the zygomatic bone at the junction of the anterior one third and posterior two thirds of the zygomatic process, innervating the orbicularis oculi muscle and muscles of the upper nose.

Cervicofacial Division

The buccal branch emerges anterior to the parotid gland, accompanied by an artery and parotid duct to innervate the buccinator, orbicularis oris, lower nasal muscles, and zygomatic and levator groups to the lips.

The mandibular branch emerges from the anterior border of the parotid gland to innervate the muscles of the upper and lower lip, as well as the risorius and platysma. The cervical branch appears at the most inferior border of the parotid gland, below the angle of the jaw. It proceeds to innervate the platysma, with terminal fibers contributing to the innervation of the chin and depressors of the lower lip.

Variations of the patterns of facial nerve peripheral branching have been well documented by Davis and colleagues.[8] It is important for the sur-

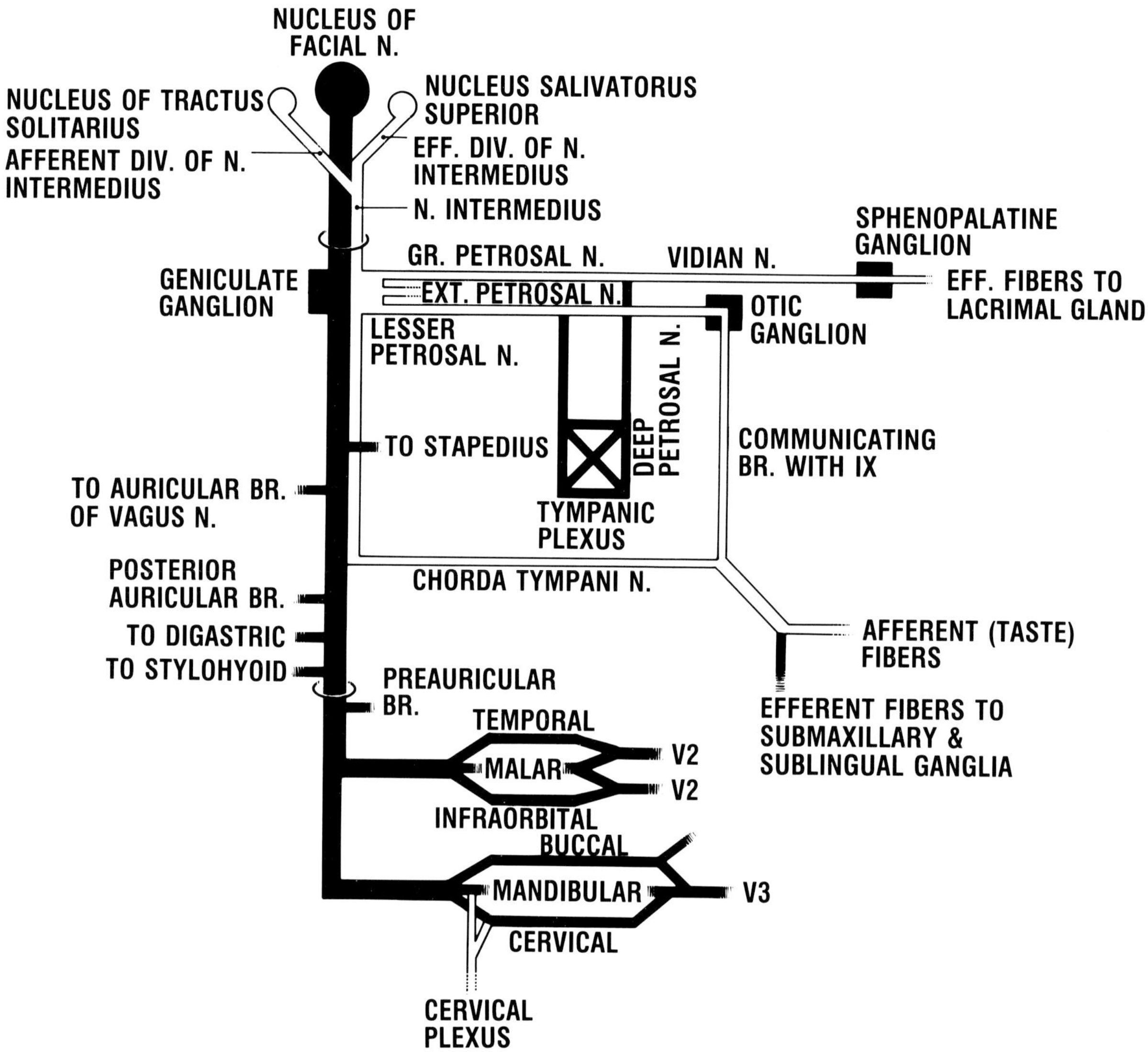

Figure 34-3. *Functional relationships of the sensory and motor divisions of the VIIth nerve.*

geon to be aware of the wide variation in peripheral branching and intercommunication between the temporal, zygomatic, and buccal branches. It is equally important to be aware of the virtually nonexistent peripheral intercommunication between the ramus mandibularis and other nearby branches of the facial nerve. This accounts for the low incidence of spontaneous reinnervation of the ramus mandibularis after total transection.

The neurophysiological composition of the facial nerve at the level of the pons and medulla and its subsequent entry in the internal acoustic meatus consists of a motor division and sensory division (nervus intermedius). The motor division consists of special visceral efferent fibers whose cells of origin lie in the motor nucleus of the facial nerve. These fibers run by way of the motor division of the facial nerve to subsequently innervate the muscles of facial expression, the accessory masticatory muscles (posterior belly of digastric and stylohyoid muscles), and the accessory auditory muscles (stapedius and auricular).

Nervus Intermedius (see Fig. 34-3)

The nervus intermedius forms a conduit for efferent and afferent fibers. The cells of origin of the general visceral efferent fibers originate in the superior salivatory nucleus. Preganglionic parasympathetic fibers destined for the submandibular and sublingual glands travel by way of the nervus intermedius through the chorda tympani nerve to the submandibular ganglion. Postganglionic fibers innervate the submandibular and sublingual glands. Preganglionic parasympathetic cells destined to innervate the lacrimal gland and glands of the nose and palate travel by way of the nervus intermedius through the greater superficial petrosal nerve to the sphenopalatine ganglion. Postganglionic fibers from the ganglion complete the neural connections.

General somatic afferents whose cells of origin are in the genicular ganglion are distributed to the proprioceptors of the face. Central fibers of the ganglion run by way of the nervus intermedius to the tractus solitarius and spinal tract of the trigeminal to terminate in the nucleus of the trigeminal and nucleus solitarii. General visceral afferents originate from cells in the geniculate ganglion and are distributed to provide sensation from the nose and soft palate via the greater superficial petrosal nerve. Central termination is in the nucleus solitarius. Special visceral afferent fibers providing taste from the anterior two thirds of the tongue originate in the geniculate ganglion and travel by way of the chorda tympani nerve. This nerve penetrates the petrotympanic fissure and joins the lingual nerve in innervating the anterior two thirds of the tongue. Central processes travel by way of the nervus intermedius to the medulla and pons and ultimately terminate in the nucleus solitarius.

The tympanic plexus, which lies on the promontory of the middle ear, is a network of intercommunication between the facial nerve, the glossopharyngeal nerve, and the vagus nerve.[17] Facial nerve contributions to the plexus arise in the geniculate ganglion. Preganglionic parasympathetic fibers from the inferior salivatory nucleus located in the medulla travel to the otic ganglion by the way of the IXth cranial nerve. Postganglionic fibers are distributed to the parotid gland by way of the auricular temporal nerve.

The lesser superficial petrosal nerve consists of fibers from the tympanic plexus as well as direct fibers from the nervus intermedius. Arnold's nerve, the auricular branch of the vagus nerve, innervates part of the external auditory canal and communicates with the tympanic plexus. A wide variety of intercommunication of the facial nerve between the Vth, IXth, and Xth cranial nerves accounts for the variety of sensory and autonomic aberrations associated with facial nerve paralytic states of varying etiologies.[3,25] This relationship may also explain the occasional reports of spontaneous return of facial recovery following division of the facial nerve.[18]

DIAGNOSIS AND CLINICAL CONSIDERATIONS

The clinical evaluation of a facial nerve paralysis requires the following information:

1. Cause, location, and degree of facial nerve paralysis
2. Association with other neurological and pathophysiological deficits
3. Chronology of the facial nerve paresis
4. Diagnostic testing
5. Age, medical evaluation, prognosis for medical recovery, and psychosocial status of the patient.

Etiology and Neuroanatomical Classification

The general categories of facial nerve paralysis are congenital, traumatic, infectious, metabolic, neoplastic, iatrogenic, and idiopathic. The differential diagnosis in each category has been well documented, and the reader is referred to the appropriate texts and articles dealing with this subject.[18,28] *The three most frequent cases of facial nerve paralysis, in order of occurrence, are Bell's palsy, trauma, and neoplasia.*

The neuroanatomical classification of facial nerve paralysis is divided into central, intratemporal, and extracranial.

Central Paralysis

SUPRANUCLEAR PARALYSIS

Central paralysis of the supranuclear type is characterized by a paralysis of the lower face. Sparing of the forehead occurs because of bilateral innervation of the upper portion of the face and forehead by crossed and uncrossed cortical bulbar tracts. Muscle tone and spontaneous involuntary facial motion are preserved as well as taste and lacrimation. The diagnosis is substantiated by the absence of Bell's phenomenon, the presence of other neural abnormalities such as hemiplegia, retention of the R1 of the blink test, and normal facial nerve peripheral electrophysiological testing.[20]

NUCLEAR PARALYSIS

Nuclear paralysis is characterized by total facial paralysis and interruption of essential connections to the facial nuclei that are responsible for initiating involuntary expressions of anger or surprise. Taste and salivation are preserved.

INFRANUCLEAR PARALYSIS

Central paralysis of the infranuclear type relates to lesions of the posterior fossa such as meningioma or acoustic neuroma. This type of paralysis is characterized by incomplete to complete facial paralysis with absence of taste, lacrimation, and salivation; various degrees of neurological deficiencies of the Vth, IXth, Xth, and XIth cranial nerves; and aberration of unilateral vestibular and cochlear function.

INTRATEMPORAL PARALYSIS

Intratemporal facial paralysis within the internal auditory canal and proximal to the horizontal portion (inclusive of the geniculate ganglion) results in a facial paralysis with hyperacusis and loss of taste, lacrimation, and salivation. Disruption of the vestibular and cochlear portions of the VIIIth cranial nerve may be involved, depending on the level of the internal auditory canal involved. Intratemporal horizontal segment facial paralysis is associated with hyperacusis, diminished salivation and taste, and preservation of lacrimation. Persistent stapedius muscle function and taste with no evidence of external extracranial disease typifies a lower vertical segment interruption.

EXTRATEMPORAL PARALYSIS

Extratemporal paralysis is a pure motor deficit of one or more branches of the facial nerve and their innervation of the muscles of facial expression. Lacrimation, salivation, taste, and stapedius muscle function is preserved.

Characteristics of Facial Motor Paralysis

The clinical presentation of the degree of facial paralysis may vary. Complete paralysis is characterized by the loss of all motor activity to the muscles of facial expression, either unilateral or bilateral. Partial facial paralysis implies the loss of one or more of the peripheral branches of the facial nerve. Another variation of partial paralysis is seen in supranuclear lesions, in which there is a dense lower facial paralysis with preservation of the frontalis muscle.

The clinical assessment of facial paralysis documents the following findings:

1. Volitional and involuntary movement
2. Symmetry at rest
3. Symmetry with volitional and involuntary movement
4. The degree, strength, and quality of muscle movements related to each peripheral nerve branch.

The movement initiated by each branch is as follows:

- Frontalis: frontalis forehead contraction and brow elevation
- Zygomatic: orbicularis oculi lid contraction and upper nasal grimacing
- Buccal: lower nasal grimacing, elevation and lateral displacement of the lower lips

- Mandibular: lateral displacement of the lower lips, puckering-depression of the lower lip
- Cervicalis: grimacing and depressing of the lower lip.

Other associated findings are the degree of drooling, sagging of the lower lip, ectropic depression of the lower lid, the presence or absence of inflammatory changes of the eye, the presence of Bell's phenomenon, the absence of tears, corneal ulceration, and ocular pain.

Chronology

The time course in the evolution of the facial paralysis is important in establishing an accurate diagnosis and treatment parameters. Only after a complete diagnostic assessment has been done can the efficacy of surgical intervention be considered.

The basic evaluation of all patients with a facial nerve paresis consists of the following steps:

1. Complete history and general physical evaluation
2. Complete head and neck and neurological evaluation
3. Hematologic, chemical, and hormonal testing
4. Other medical tests (eg, urinalysis, cerebrospinal fluid tap, chest x-ray, electrocardiogram) as appropriate
5. Specific radiographic tests (head, temporal bone, neck computed tomography scans or magnetic resonance imaging)
6. Site of lesion testings
7. Multidiscipline consultation
8. Psychological assessment.

Subsequent special testing (eg, arteriography and ultrasound) may be indicated.

DIAGNOSTIC ASSESSMENT

The first assessment by the clinician includes observation and careful recording of the volitional and spontaneous activity of the motor division of the facial nerve. These records, along with nervous intermedius testing, allow the clinician to classify the type and degree of paralysis. To supplement the recordings of subjective movement observations, still photographs and video documentation provide greater objectivity and clarity.

Salivary Flow Test

The evaluation of general visceral efferent fibers passing through the chorda tympani nerve to the submandibular gland is the intent of this test. A small polyethylene tube is used to cannulate both submandibular ducts on the undersurface of the tongue. After oral stimulation with lemon juice, the volume flow of both sides is recorded. A reading of less than 25% of the normal-side secretion rate, recorded for 2 minutes at three separate intervals, shows a degenerative facial paralysis and suggests a lesion proximal to the vertical portion of the facial nerve.

Taste Test

Special visceral afferent fibers from the anterior tongue that mediate taste are tested using natural stimulants to elicit salt, sour, and sweet sensations. Normal and abnormal side responses are recorded and compared. More objective testing is elicited with an electrogustometer; over 250 microamperes suggests a severe degenerative state.

Stapedius Muscle Reflex

The basis for this test is the fact that sound louder than 85 decibels results in the reflex contraction of the stapedius muscle in both ears. Stapedius muscle contraction results in an increase in acoustic impedance due to the stiffening of the middle ear conduction mechanism. If the impedance bridge recording from the side in question fails to record an increase after auditory stimulation of the opposite (normal) ear, a lesion of the facial nerve exists proximal to the stapedius nerve. Variable results will be found in brain stem disease, incomplete paralysis, demyelinating multifocal diseases, or disease directly affecting the muscle and tendon itself.

Lacrimation (Schirmer) Test

Special visceral efferents by way of the greater superficial petrosal nerve provide parasympathetic innervation to the lacrimal glands and glands of the nose. After emptying both lacrimal sacs by direct pressure, two standardized strips of filter paper are bent and placed in the lower lid fornix of both eyes. The patient is given ammonia to breathe, and the degree of tearing from each eye is recorded after 3 minutes. A major difference (>60%) between sides and less than 15 mm of tear absorption indicate a facial nerve lesion at or proximal to the geniculate ganglion.

Nerve Excitability Testing

Direct peripheral facial nerve testing compares both sides using the minimal amperage necessary to produce a visible movement of a specific muscle group of the whole face. Points of stimulation should be consistent. Main trunk stimulation is elicited anterior to the mastoid tip, inferior to the ear lobe, and posterior to the angle of the mandible. The frontalis branch is located two fingerbreadths posterior to the lateral edge of the eyebrow. The zygomatic branch is stimulated at the junction of the anterior one third and the posterior two thirds of the zygomatic arch. The buccal branch lies half the distance between a line drawn from the external ear canal and commissure of the mouth. The mandibular branch stimulates at the mandibular notch. A rapidly rising stimulus to the limits and beyond the subjective comfort level after 72 hours from the onset of paralysis usually predicts a severe axonotmesis.

The maximal stimulation test uses the maximal tolerable square wave pulse that can be tolerated by the patient. A finding of less than 25% motor response on the abnormal side indicates a greater than 90% loss of fibers and severe long-standing facial paralysis.

Neither of these tests is sensitive until the 3rd day after severe insult to the facial nerve.

Electroneurography

Electroneurography measures evoked summation potentials of the facial muscles after applying a nerve stimulus. A response of less than 10% to 25% of the normal side shows a severe degenerative state. A blink response test requires stimulation of both supraorbital nerves. The R1 response (initial motor response) recorded on the side of stimulation reflects a short reflex loop through the medulla and pons. The longer response, R2, is multisynaptic through the pons, and its nucleus, the Vth nerve, medulla, and pons are assessed.

Electromyography

After 10 days, the appearance of fibrillation potentials and the absence of voluntary motor activity substantiate complete degeneration. Reappearance of this activity is the earliest evidence of regeneration and recovery.

Other Tests

The evolution of the diagnostic process will guide the surgeon's choice of tests, but in most cases computed tomography (CT) and magnetic resonance imaging of the entire course of the facial nerve with whole brain sections are essential. Bone destruction and fracture are best delineated by CT scanning. The main difficulty with electrical testing is that only the distal portion of the facial nerve can be assessed; therefore, detection and identification of axonal loss are delayed by at least 72 hours.[20,29] The complexity and variations with the other site of lesion tests add to the difficulty sometimes encountered in assessing the location, degree, and nature of the neuronal pathology. With long-standing paralysis, muscle biopsy permits objective analysis of the end organ and the degree of atrophy present.

OPERATIVE REPAIR

Principles

The general factors that guide the clinician in deciding on operative repair are as follows:

1. The nature and etiology of paralysis
2. Location
3. Type of paralysis
4. Duration of paralysis
5. The patient's overall medical condition.

The *nature and cause* of a facial nerve paralysis relate to the neuroanatomical location of the facial nerve lesion. Central paralysis may be the result of the congenital abnormalities, intracranial trauma, neoplasms of the intracranial cavity, progressive systemic degenerative nervous system disease, or vascular abnormalities. Facial nerve paralysis originating within the temporal bone is most commonly a result of Bell's palsy. Other considerations include bacterial and viral infections; middle ear and mastoid disease such as cholesteatoma; neoplasms of the middle ear and mastoid and temporal bones; trauma; and iatrogenic causes. Extracranial facial paralysis is often generated by trauma, tumors of the parotid and surrounding tissue, and iatrogenic causes. The nature of the paralysis often dictates the appropriate surgical response.

The *location* of the paralysis also has a direct bearing on the choice of surgical treatment. In general, central division of the facial nerve is not amenable to direct intervention. Intratemporal facial paralysis is a surgically correctable process. Two major procedures considered in the repair of intratemporal facial nerve paralysis are decompression of the facial nerve and reapproximation of a severed nerve.[20] Extracranial facial nerve paralysis is the most amenable to surgical correction; several techniques are available to rehabilitate the paralyzed face.

The *chronology* of the paralysis is important because immediate paralysis is usually related to a clear causation (often iatrogenic or traumatic in nature). In cases where objective and subjective information indicates that progressive acute neuronal degeneration may be potentially reversible, immediate surgical exploration of the facial nerve is indicated. The general indications for acute surgical exploration are as follows:

1. A substantiated diagnosis of immediate paralysis consistent with VIIth nerve compression or nerve interruption (eg, iatrogenic, traumatic, or neoplastic)
2. Radiographic, neurophysiological, and myophysiological testing confirming absolute or evolving neurotmesis.

Once the patient's medical condition has been stabilized and all appropriate testing and evaluation has been tabulated, immediate surgical intervention for the divided nerve is the treatment of choice.

Delayed facial paralysis requires more cognitive skill and evaluation to avoid unnecessary surgery and further injury to the facial nerve. In general, the factors that influence surgical intervention in delayed paralysis are as follows:

1. Substantiation by testing that facial paralysis is progressing from neurapraxia to complete axonotmesis
2. Recognition that a previously diagnosed delayed paralysis was, in fact, immediate paralysis
3. Proper identification of the nature and etiology of the facial paralysis, which is potentially correctable by surgical intervention.

The duration of an existing facial paralysis and subsequent attempts at surgical rehabilitation relate directly to the following factors:

1. Atrophy and loss of end organs (muscles of facial expression) will not respond to neurophysiological surgical reconstruction techniques.
2. Progressive myoneurodegenerative disease contraindicates the use of nerve transposition, such as VIIth, XIIth, or XI-to-VII repairs.
3. Clinical and diagnostic testing of long-standing paralysis must document persistent, complete

degeneration in cases where natural regeneration may occur.

The overall medical condition, age, sex, and psychosocial characterization of the patient, as well as the etiology of the facial paralysis, directly affect the decision as to whether the patient is a candidate for surgical rehabilitation, as well as the type of procedure. Patients of markedly advanced age, those with rapidly progressing disease with poor prognosis for survival, and those who are medically unstable or poor anesthetic risks can often be eliminated from serious consideration for direct or indirect facial nerve rehabilitation surgery.

Table 34-1 classifies the operative repairs available for correcting acute and chronic facial paralysis. The complexity of facial nerve rehabilitation requires the communication, cooperation, and skill of a multidisciplined team. Team members include a neurosurgeon, neurologist, otolaryngologist/head and neck surgeon, plastic surgeon, and ophthalmologist. Although the variety of surgical procedures offers the patient with a paralyzed face a reasonable expectation of some meaningful form of rehabilitation, the fact remains that the totally paralyzed face will never be completely normal.[14] Ideal dynamic restoration implies the return of facial symmetry and volitional and spontaneous coordinated facial motion.

Regeneration of the facial nerve, spontaneously or by direct surgical repair, often results in the loss of controlled synchronized facial movement. Periods of involuntary spasm and inappropriate muscle group contraction (synkinesis) is not unusual. Clinical observations, as well as indirect animal research on the cat by Tomander and Gacek, indicate a random mixing of facial nerve fibers at various portions of the facial nerve and a lack of spatial orientation.[11]

Although the clinician cannot predict the degree and quality of facial motion and restoration, the dynamic procedure that holds the best promise for near-normal rehabilitation is dynamic reneurotization of the facial muscles using direct ipsilateral VIIth nerve repair techniques.

Table 34–1. *Classification of Operative Repair*

- **I.** Neurophysiologic (dynamic)
  - **A.** VIIth-to-VIIth repair, ipsilateral
    1. Primary end-to-end anastomosis
    2. Graft interposition
    3. Transposition
  - **B.** VIIth-to-VIIth repair, contralateral (nerve crossover)
  - **C.** XIIth to VIIth transfer
- **II.** Myophysiologic (dynamic)
  - **A.** Masseter transfer
  - **B.** Temporalis transfer
  - **C.** Digastric transfer
  - **D.** Free microvascular transfer (gracilis muscle)
- **III.** Static (adynamic)
  - **A.** Fascia lata suspension
  - **B.** Rhytidectomy
  - **C.** Browlift
  - **D.** Blepharoplasty
- **IV.** Adjuvant procedures
  - **A.** Tarsorrhaphy
  - **B.** Gold lid implant
  - **C.** Nasolabial fold plasty
  - **D.** Lip mucosal fold resection
  - **E.** Contralateral myectomy and neurectomy

Facial Incisions

- Facial incisions are placed in cosmetically accepted zones.
- Low tension and fine sutures ensure minimal facial scar exposure.

Cosmetically sensitive procedures require incisions to be placed in a cosmetically acceptable area without compromising the surgical procedure. Low-tension closure is best accomplished by using subcutaneous and dermal, long-life but absorbable sutures such as Vicryl or Maxon. Rapidly absorbing 6-0 mild chromic is used for epithelial closure. High-tension areas may be strengthened by the addition of a buried subcuticular running monofilament suture. Depending on the technique used, this may be removable or permanent; if permanent, a clear monofilament suture is recommended. Because of the vascularity of the face and the degree of undermining that is often used, a Silastic suction catheter is recommended.

NEUROPHYSIOLOGICAL DYNAMIC REPAIR

With few exceptions, most peripheral facial nerve paralytic states secondary to neurotmesis and degeneration of the facial nerve will recover to some degree if anatomical continuity is present or has been reestablished. Unfortunately, the degree and quality of facial motion after reinnervation is never absolutely normal. Full scrutiny of the reanimated face will always indicate some degree of asymmetry, uncoordination in voluntary and involuntary motion, and often some degree of synkinesis. Lack of spatial orientation of facial nerve fibers, fiber intermixing, and diminished axonal load means that the reanimated state will be imperfect to some degree after reinnervation.

The best result that can be expected after complete deinnervation is the maintenance or reestablishment of recontinuity of the facial nerve from its central motor nucleus to its end plate receptor. The ipsilateral VIIth-to-VIIth repair is best achieved, if technically possible, by primary end-to-end anastomosis. In pathologic states where end-to-end anastomosis is not technically possible, graft interposition is recommended. Isolated injuries to various divisions or their subdivisions can often be rehabilitated by transposing the adjacent division and subdivision. Recent reports indicate that excellent functional results may be achieved with contralateral VIIth-to-VIIth repair (nerve crossover) where ipsilateral VIIth-to-VIIth repair is no longer possible.[1,10,26] Long interposition grafts between the paralyzed and nonparalyzed segment across the midface have met with variable success.[24,27]

Although this technique clearly has excellent potential, a high degree of patient selectivity and individual analysis limits its use to a relatively small group of patients. Likewise, the possibility of weakening of the normal side (even temporarily) often dissuades the patient from serious consideration on a subjective basis. The final theoretical disadvantage of this technique is the considerably diminished axon load that can be delivered from a peripheral facial nerve branch across a long graft to a paralytic area.

Ipsilateral VIIth-to-VIIth Repair

- The site of facial nerve transection or crush injury is identified. Under magnification, the injured distal and proximal nerve ends are trimmed back to a cleanly divided epineural fascicular segment using a sharp scalpel or microvascular scissors.
- Primary end-to-end repair cannot be successfully achieved under tension. Injuries within the temporal bone require complete decompression of the facial nerve distal and proximal to the zone of injury. Rerouting in order to achieve a primary tension-free anastomosis is often necessary. Peripheral facial nerve injuries may require identification of the pes, upper and lower divisions, as well as subdivisions, depending on the nature of the injury and the location of the repair.
- In cases where a primary end-to-end anastomosis cannot be done, graft interposition is indicated. The most commonly used graft for interposition repairs is the greater auricular nerve and its branches. In cases where a graft longer than 7 cm is needed, where the greater auricular nerve is unavailable, or where there is a significant size discrepancy between the diameters of the facial nerve and graft, the sural nerve is an easily harvested second choice.

Indications

This technique is indicated when the surgeon has identified a distal and proximal facial nerve that can be bridged by a direct, transposition, or cable nerve graft.

Technique

Primary end-to-end anastomosis or graft interposition is achieved using an operating microscope or, as a second choice, magnifying loupes. The field should be free of blood. The anastomosis should be carried out against a colored background, often a 3-inch square of sterilized blue plastic drape. Blunted edges of epineurium are carefully trimmed from the underlying fasciculi posterior to the edge of transection for about 0.5 to 1 mm. Fine jeweler's forceps, middle-ear scissors, or curved microvascular scissors minimize the trauma to the distal ends of the graft or primary nerve transection site.

Various suture materials have been recommended, but I think that 8-0 monofilament or silk using a double-armed spatula allows the surgeon the most practical and technically maneuverable suture for this repair.

Injuries involving the pes or pes–division junction require at least four sutures at 45° intervals. The suture is carefully placed through the epineurium of the nerve ends or nerve-to-graft interface. Other areas of epineural dehiscence may be filled in with additional 8-0 suture material or 10-0 monofilament. All areas of anastomosis must be carefully protected from suction drains or suture injury during the closure of the incisions.

In cases of ablative surgery for neoplasm, the use of postoperative radiation therapy has not been demonstrated to interfere with the repair and reinnervation process.[19] Except for ramus mandibularis injuries, injuries to peripheral branches of the facial nerve beyond the midcheek area of the face are not permanent. The wealth of distal arborization will usually result in a spontaneous reanimation of the weakened segments. Despite this fact, small peripheral branches, when visualized and available for repair, are repaired with 10-0 suture material.

Patients are warned not to expect reinnervation for at least 6 to 8 months after graft or primary ipsilateral repair. Passive facial movement is recommended during the waiting period. A realistic expectation of the degree of recovery should be discussed early, as well as the possibility of synkinesis.

The principles of end-to-end anastomosis and graft interposition relate to transposition procedures in isolated peripheral VIIth-to-VIIth repairs. The most common site of transfer is from the peripheral arborization of the midface and buccal division to the zygomatic periorbital division of the facial nerve. Before the surgeon commits to dividing the buccal branch segment and subsequently transposing it to the zygomatic segment, peripheral arborization of the midface regions is identified and demonstrated with selective facial nerve stimulation. In repairs using a transposition technique, the patient is warned to expect transient weakness in a previously normal area of the face; full recovery will occur.

Intratemporal Bone Facial Nerve Identification

- The transmastoid facial nerve recess approach allows the surgeon access to the intratemporal facial nerve from the geniculate ganglion to the stylomastoid foramen.
- The middle cranial fossa identification of the facial nerve allows the surgeon access to the intratemporal facial nerve from the geniculate ganglion to the brain stem.

The two surgical techniques most commonly used in the exploration of the intratemporal course of the facial nerve are the transmastoid and middle cranial fossa approaches. After a standard postauricular incision, a simple mastoidectomy, preservation of the posterior canal wall, and exposure of the middle ear and its contents through the facial nerve recess allow the surgeon access to the horizontal and vertical portions of the facial nerve. Subsequent decompression of the facial nerve is carried out with a high-speed diamond drill. Full exploration of the horizontal portion of the facial nerve to the region of the geniculate ganglion usually requires the temporary dislocation of the incus. In cases of trauma, assessment of the tympanic membrane and middle ear ossicles, as well as the integrity of the oval and round windows, eliminates the potential concomitant existence of an ossicular discontinuity or inner ear fistula.

The middle cranial fossa approach enables the surgeon to assess the facial nerve from the geniculate ganglion and first genu to the internal auditory meatus. Nerve continuity and the potential for facial nerve edema usually require the splitting of the facial nerve sheath with a sickle knife or middle ear scissor to compensate for actual or potential edema following decompression. The ideal repair for complete interruption is a direct end-to-end anastomosis. Long segment neuronal loss may necessitate a VIIth nerve rerouting procedure to gain length for a direct repair.[16] When end-to-end repair is impossible, cable grafting is the treatment of choice.

The potential complications of intratemporal facial nerve decompression and repair are:

1. Instrument or drill injury to the facial nerve, middle ear, or inner ear structures

2. Cerebrospinal fluid leak
3. Infection, the most serious of which is meningitis
4. Injury to the labyrinth or cochlea, resulting in temporary or complete loss of hearing and persistent vertigo.

Extracranial Facial Nerve Identification

The trunk of the extracranial portion of the facial nerve is located in the anatomical pocket bounded by the posterior belly of the digastric, the tragal pointer, the tympanomastoid suture line, and the mastoid tip.

Identification of the facial nerve as it emerges from the stylomastoid foramen is well known to the surgeon trained in head and neck surgery. Because of the loss of nerve excitability, however, the use of a facial nerve stimulator intraoperatively may not be feasible. Strict adherence to anatomical markers allows for timely and accurate exposure of the facial nerve, its trunk, and its branches.

A standard parotidectomy incision is recommended (Fig. 34-4). This consists of a preauricular limb carried to the mastoid tip. A secondary vertical limb extends forward from the mastoid tip inferiorly, across the midportion of the sternocleidomastoid to lie 3 cm anterior and inferior to the angle and lower border of the mandible. If identification of the hypoglossal is contemplated, this incision is lengthened to the midhyoid region, three fingerbreadths below the lower border of the mandible. Deep dissection to the pretragal plane results in the identification of the perichondrium of the tragus. The parotid–masseteric fascia is separated from the mastoid tip. The posterior aspect of the tail of the parotid is mobilized and dissected away from the anterior border of the sternocleidomastoid muscle. Blunt dissection is used to separate the parotid tail deep to the mastoid tip until the posterior belly of the digastric muscle is identified. The tragal and conchal perichondrium is followed deeply while dividing and cauterizing all small veins and arteries between the parotid–masseteric fascia and perichondrium. The triangular process of the conchal cartilage, posterior belly of the digastric muscle, and the indentation between the tympanic bone and mastoid tip serve as important landmarks to the facial nerve. The pes or main trunk of the facial nerve occupies the immediate posterior compartment of the tympanomastoid fissure, inferior to the tragal pointer, deep to the mastoid tip, and lateral to the digastric muscle. Just prior to its division into the upper and lower divisions, the pes is invested by an extension of parotid tissue and a fibrofascial layer. Separation of this tissue in the direction of the expected course of the facial nerve will avoid inadvertent injury.

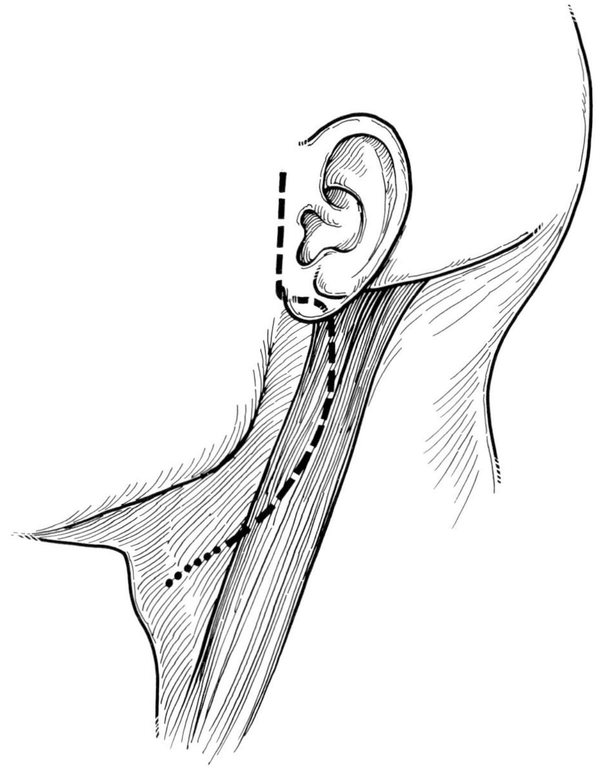

Figure 34-4. *Standard parotidectomy incision with anterior extension. The VIIth and XIIth nerves can be identified.*

In cases where grafting is contemplated, the identification and harvesting of sensory branches of the second and third cervical nerves is recommended. The most common branch selected is the great auricular nerve, which exits from behind the sternocleidomastoid muscle about 5 cm inferior to the mastoid tip. As it courses in an anterior–superior direction, the nerve lies deep to the subcutaneous fat and is partially invested by the parotid–masseteric fascia. As the nerve approaches the lobule of the ear, it lies posterior–lateral to the external jugular vein and divides into two branches posterior and anterior to the external auditory canal. Further dissection uncovers secondary and tertiary divisions. Harvesting of the sensory branch and its divisions should match the complexity of repair elicited or contemplated.

Hypoglossal Nerve Identification (Fig. 34-5)

- Anteriorly, the hypoglossal nerve is in the floor of the submaxillary triangle.
- Posteriorly, the hypoglossal nerve is anterior to the transverse process of the first cervical vertebra.

To identify the hypoglossal nerve, the incision is carried forward to the midhyoid level. Dissection is deepened through the platysma muscle fibers until the anterior border of the digastric muscle and inferior capsule of the submaxillary gland are identified. The fascia immediately overlying the capsule of the gland is incised. By blunt dissection, the inferior aspect of the submaxillary gland is separated from the floor of the submaxillary triangle. Retraction of the gland superiorly and the mylohyoid fibers anteriorly will reveal the upper and forward course of the hypoglossal nerve on the floor of the submaxillary triangle. Dissection of the nerve in its forward course toward the tongue is often accompanied by bleeding due to the presence of two vena communicantes. Traced posteriorly, the hypoglossal nerve courses across the external and internal carotid arteries and relates directly to the occipital branch of the parotid gland. The transverse process of the first cervical vertebra can be felt. Immediately anterior to the transverse process of the first cervical vertebra are the internal jugular vein, internal carotid artery, vagus, hypoglossal nerve, and XIth cranial nerve. Care should be used in this region to avoid injuring these structures.

Sural Nerve Grafts

The sural nerve is selected from cable grafting in cases where length and diameter cannot be matched by alternative donor nerves. Nerve graft requirements longer than 8 cm, such as those used with cross-facial nerve grafting, require the harvesting of sural nerves. The ipsilateral leg is prepped and draped from thigh to toes. A tourniquet is applied to dilate the saphenous vein and its tributaries. A 3-cm incision is made posterior and superior to the lateral malleolus. The saphenous vein and accompanying sural nerve are identified. The sural nerve usually lies deep and anterior to the vein. Once identified, the nerve and its branches are transected and dissected away from the surrounding structures. More than 30 cm is usually available.

For speed, efficiency, and safety, the initial incision is enlarged superiorly as a continuous incision until the desired length of nerve has been achieved. Closure consists of subcutaneous and intradermal 4-0 chromic catgut sutures, followed by subcuticular 5-0 nylon. A continuous gauze wrap dressing to the extremity is followed by an elastic bandage.

Facial–Hypoglossal Transfer (see Fig. 34-5)

Hypoglossal facial nerve transfer provides a powerful high-load reinnervation of the facial muscles.[2] Innervation of just the lower division results in a more cosmetically and functionally efficient facial rehabilitation.[6,7]

Indications

Indications for facial–hypoglossal transfer are are follows:

1. Any facial paralytic state where the proximal segment is unavailable for primary or cable-grafting repair. Examples of this loss include acoustic neuroma surgery, temporal bone injuries, oncologic surgical ablation of the temporal bone, central motor paralysis, and periparotid and adjacent regional surgery in which sufficient peripheral divisions of the facial nerve are available for transfer.
2. Failure of VIIth-to-VIIth repair clinically and by electrical testing at 12 months after injury and repair.
3. End-stage Bell's palsy with failure to achieve meaningful voluntary motion.

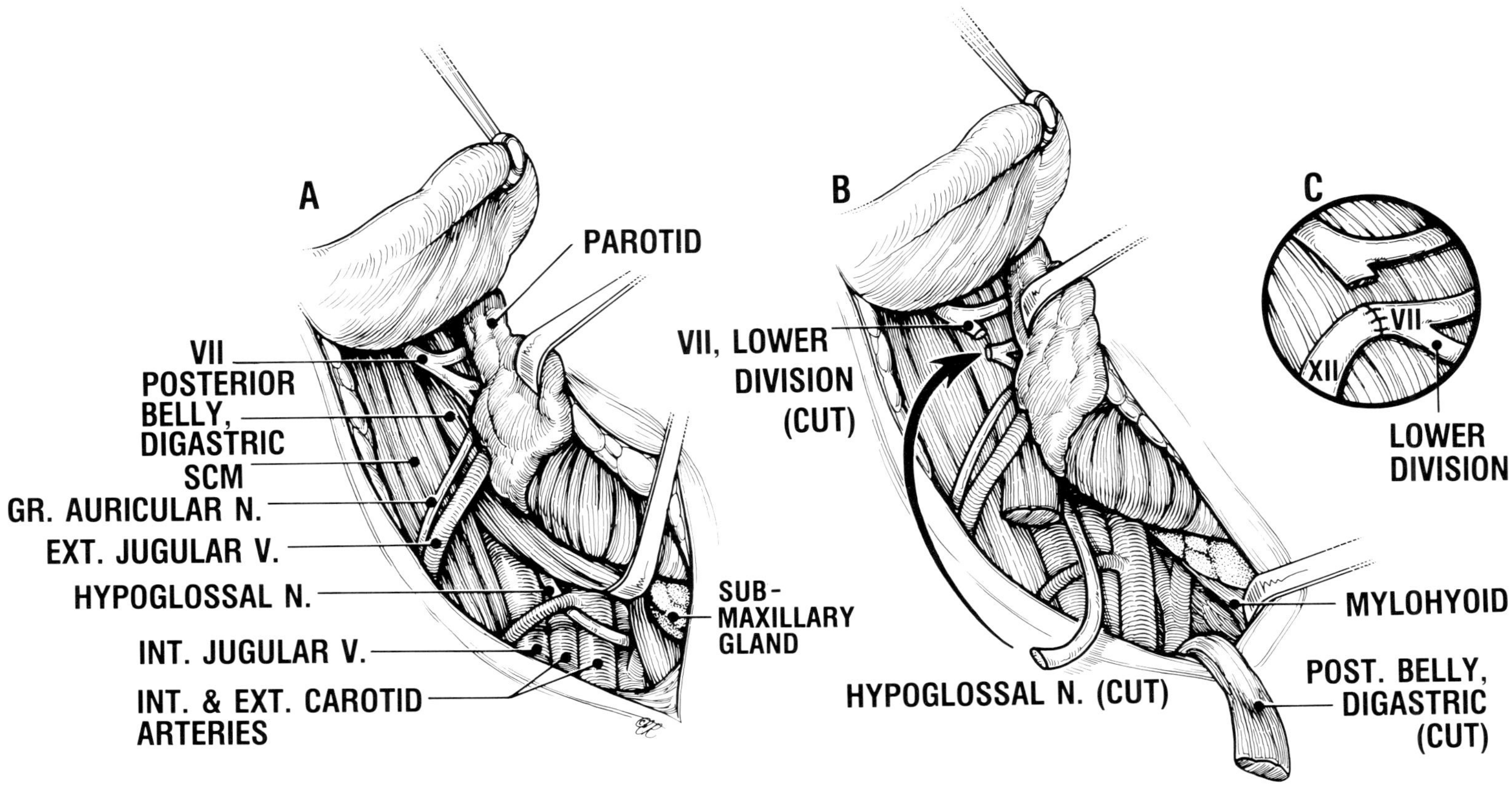

Figure 34-5. *Anatomical relationships of the XIIth cranial nerve. Axis of rotation to VIIth nerve pes indicated by arrow. XII to VII nerve transfer complete.*

Technique

Before the transfer, the pes of the facial nerve and the hypoglossal nerve as previously described must be identified. The essential pivot point upon which the axis of rotation of the hypoglossal nerve will occur lies immediately anterior to the transverse process of the first cervical vertebra. Care should be taken in this region to avoid injuring the jugular vein, the XIth cranial nerve, the vagus nerve, and internal carotid artery. A malleable stainless steel ruler is used to measure the distance from the transverse process to the point of anastomosis. This area usually is in the vicinity of the stylomastoid foramen and pes of the facial nerve. This measurement is recorded, and an additional 1 to 2 cm of hypoglossal nerve is added to avoid tension at the suture line. In cases where transfer to the separate upper and lower divisions is needed, peripheral arborization of the hypoglossal nerve or a division of its main trunk into two separate branches can be done using a disposable cornea knife. The hypoglossal nerve is transected, usually within the floor of the submaxillary triangle. The nerve is carefully dissected away from the underlying structures in a posterior direction. Care is taken to avoid bleeding from the vena communicantes that accompany the nerve. Dissection is sometimes easier if the digastric muscle, under which the hypoglossal nerve passes, is divided.

Following mobilization of this nerve, the nerve is transferred to the area of anastomosis. As with direct VIIth-to-VIIth transfer, a colored background and careful sharp preparation of the nerve ends for grafting are done. I recommend using 8-0 monofilament or 8-0 silk with a spatula diamondpoint needle for epineural repair.

Because of the high axonal load and inappropriate contraction of the upper division muscles of the face, a superior cosmetic result is achieved with reinnervation of the lower division of the facial nerve only. Realistic expectations should be addressed early. The first evidence of clinical reinnervation is noted by subtle but objective improvement in symmetry and tone at rest. Volitional movements, once identified, are refined by careful patient education. Volitional activity is usually initiated by the conscious pressure of the tongue against the inner aspect of the teeth. Subsequent coordination of this activity with the volitional movement of the normal face is refined by practice and long sessions in front of a mirror.

Facial–hypoglossal transfer often is combined with ancillary adjuvant procedures such as temporalis muscle transfer, rhytidectomy, and browlifts.

Complications

Complications may include the following:

1. Failure to achieve the necessary cosmetic and functional result
2. Hemorrhage
3. Infection
4. Injury to adjacent structures and transfer, such as the vagus and accessory nerve, internal jugular vein, and carotid artery
5. Synkinesis.

MYOPHYSIOLOGICAL DYNAMIC MUSCLE TRANSFER

Temporalis Muscle Fascial Transfer and Suspension[21,22]

- The temporalis muscle flap provides a static and potentially functional muscle sling for suspension of the lower eyelid and rehabilitation of the lower face.
- The temporalis muscle transfer may be used as the sole modality of rehabilitation, either early for "babysitting" the face during reneurotization or late as a primary modality of rehabilitation.
- Function depends on preserving reinnervation to the muscle, a function of the IVth cranial nerve.
- Early overcorrection is important to longevity.

Indications

The indications for temporalis muscle transposition are:

1. Failure of spontaneous or iatrogenic ipsilateral facial nerve regeneration after 18 to 24 months of observation
2. Facial paralysis and loss of facial mimetic muscles following ablation cancer surgery
3. Contraindication of XIIth-to-VIIth or cross-facial nerve reinnervation due to patient choice,

neurological status (central nervous system or demyelinating disease), or elderly age group
4. Facial muscle atrophy.

Temporalis dynamic muscle suspension offers the patient symmetry at rest, learned but limited voluntary motion of the paralytic side, and replacement of facial atrophy due to loss of the facial mimetic muscles. Limitations relate to the patient's inability to develop spontaneous symmetrical facial movements and loss of consistent full range of facial mimetic motion of a predictable nature.

Anatomy

The temporalis muscle inserts into the anterior border of the coronoid process and passes under the zygomatic arch in a fan shape to occupy the temporal fossa overlying the frontoparietal squamous suture line and greater wing of the sphenoid bone. The nerve supply is derived from the deep temporal branches of the mandibular nerve. This nerve enters the muscle about 1 cm inferior and posterior to the zygomatic arch and divides into three branches. The temporalis fascia is a strong layer of aponeurotic tissue that covers the upper three fourths of the temporalis muscle. Superiorly, a single sheet attachment occurs at the superior temporal line of the skull. Inferiorly, the fascia splits into lateral and medial sheets, which invest the lateral and medial margins of the upper border of the zygoma. The action of the temporal muscle is to elevate and retract the mandible.

Technique (Fig. 34-6)

A general anesthetic is given, preferably through the nasotracheal route because this avoids distortion of the oral commissure. The smallest endotracheal tube compatible with good anesthetic tech-

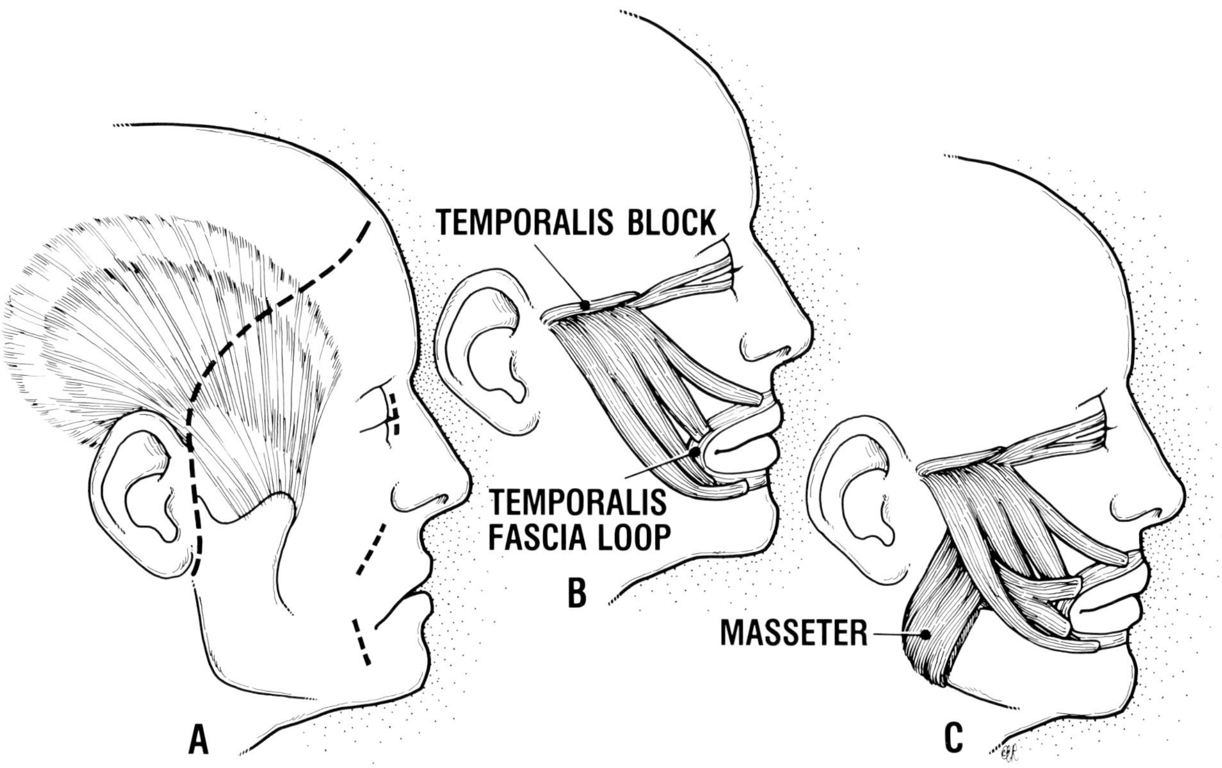

Figure 34-6. *(**A**) Facial and scalp incisions. (**B**) Temporalis muscle transfer completed. (**C**) Combined temporalis/masseter muscle completed.*

nique is recommended. In cases where this is not technically possible, a standard orotracheal intubation with the endotracheal tube placed in the neutral midline position is acceptable.

After protecting both eyes with scleral shells, the face and scalp are prepped with a Betadine soap and solution and draped in the usual fashion. Exposure of the contralateral face is recommended in order to judge the effectiveness of the temporalis pull and its effects on the contralateral face. In patients with markedly ptotic facial skin, a standard rhytidectomy incision is extended superiorly in the hair-bearing temporal portion of the scalp to the mid-vertex position. In patients where a coronal incision and browlift is contemplated, this incision may be extended across the vertex to the contralateral side, down to the level of the root of the contralateral helix. In younger patients who would not benefit from a concomitant rhytidectomy, the incision is modified to span from the mid-pretragal region to the vertex behind the hairline.

Accessory incisions include the following anatomical areas of the facial skin:

1. The ipsilateral nasolabial crease line
2. A vermilion skin junctional incision of the upper and lower lip in the midline plan
3. An incision medial to the inner canthus of the eye.

The dissection, which is superficial to the parotid–masseteric fascia, is extended anteriorly to a line drawn from the midbody of the zygoma to the midbody of the mandible. Superior dissection extends over the temporalis fascia posterior to the level of the posterior auricular sulcus and anterior to the anteriormost projection of the temporalis line. The nasolabial incision is deepened to expose the attachments of the zygomaticus major, minor, and levator muscles as they insert on the orbicularis oris muscle. Vermilion lip incisions are deepened until fibers of the orbicularis oris muscle can be identified.

A horizontal incision is made through the temporalis fascia immediately above the zygomatic arch. Vertical anterior and posterosuperior incisions of the fascia are then directed to the temporal line. The temporalis fascia is carefully dissected from the underlying temporalis muscle to a point about 1 cm inferior to the attachment of the temporalis fascia at the temporal line. Quilting mattress sutures of 4-0 white Dacron are used to plicate the base of the temporalis fascia to the underlying temporalis muscle superiorly.

An incision is made posterior to the temporalis muscle to the underlying bony calvarium. By blunt and sharp dissection, the temporalis muscle is reflected off the calvarium to about 1 cm superior to the zygomatic arch. Care is taken not to damage the innervation entering the muscle from the infratemporal fossa.

Muscle fascial strips are designed to suspend the upper and lower eyelids with the remaining muscle fascial bulk destined to suspend and attach to the region of the orbicularis oris muscle. A single strip of temporal fascia, 1 cm at its widest, is removed from the posterior portion of the reflected temporalis muscle. The underlying posterior segment of temporalis muscle is dissected away from the main body of the muscle in order to be directed along the base sulcus of the reflected muscle. The purpose of this technique is to diminish the step-off created immediately above the zygomatic arch when the temporalis muscle is dissected inferiorly. An alternate technique is to place a silicone sponge at the point of temporalis muscle reflection.

The segment of temporalis fascia removed from the muscle is fixed in a continuous loop to the orbicularis oris at the philtrum of the upper lip and midportion of the lower lip, as well as the muscle immediately lateral to the commissure of the lip. This is facilitated by creating a superior tunnel subcutaneously above the vermilion border of the upper lip and a concomitant tunnel in the lower lip region.

Superior temporalis muscle strips are tunneled to the previously fixated perioral orbicularis oris fascial loop at the following locations:

- 0.5 cm lateral to the philtrum
- 0.5 cm superior and 0.5 cm inferior to the commissure
- 1 cm lateral to the midportion of the lower lip.

Care is taken to tunnel each of these fascial muscle strips through the previously undermined segment of skin between the midportion of the cheek and nasolabial incision. Fixation of the fascial muscle slings to these points is established with buried inverted 4-0 Dacron sutures.

Eyelid tunnels are created 4 mm above the upper and lower lash line from the lateral to medial canthus. Muscle fascial strips are directed lateral to medial and fixed to the medial canthal tendon with 4-0 Dacron. All fascial muscle strips to the upper and lower lip, as well as the eyelid region, are sutured under tension to cause overcorrection of the upper and lower lips and appropriate suspension of the eyelids. This is accomplished by folding and plicating the fascial strips with 4-0 Dacron.

The anterior border of the masseter muscle is then defined as it attaches to the inferior rim of the mandible. A 2.5 cm segment of masseter muscle is cleaved from its attachment anteriorly and inferiorly to the body of the mandible. A concomitant 4-cm vertical incision is made to allow an anterior strip of masseter muscle to be passed forward. A tunnel is created to the lower lip, and the masseter muscle is carried around the previously placed temporalis lower lip fascial strip. This pulley arrangement is tightened by suturing the masseter muscle strip to its main body posteriorly. The effect of this maneuver is to create a posterior–inferior pull on the commissure, widening the lateral commissure of the lip. The previously undermined facial skin is retracted in a superior–posterior direction, and a complementary rhytidectomy (facial skin excision) is executed.

Plication of the submuscular aponeurotic system (SMAS) or available deep fascia overlying the residual facial musculature is directed in a superior direction using 3-0 Mersilene. A medium-large Silastic suction drain is placed below the skin of the scalp and facial cheek area and brought out through a separate stab wound in the postauricular area. Fixation sutures of 3-0 nylon are placed in the anterior helical root area and inferior mastoid tip area to support the skin of the face. Subcutaneous closure with 3-0 chromic catgut is followed by skin closure with skin clips in the temporoparietal incision and scalp neck incision. Skin closure is completed with 6-0 mild chromic sutures in the preauricular and postauricular incisions. A tight pressure dressing of layered cotton under a flexible stocking over the cheek, preauricular, postauricular, and temporoparietal areas is recommended.

Younger patients with dominant overpull of the quadratus levator superiorus and zygomaticus major muscles on the contralateral side, as determined by preoperative evaluation, may be weakened by complementary incisions made intraorally catching the attachment of zygomatic major and levators from the orbicularis oris. As previously mentioned, a complementary forehead lift may be constructed by dissecting the scalp behind the hairline to the suprabrow area.

Voluntary muscle movement rehabilitation is not recommended for 2 weeks, to minimize the chance of detaching the fascial connections. Once facial edema has subsided and adequate healing has taken place, the patient is encouraged to develop volitional muscle rehabilitation. With the patient looking into a mirror, a forced smile and concomitant clenching of the teeth will initiate a major temporalis contraction. Further refinements in volitional movement relate to the technical effectiveness of the repair and individual abilities.

Masseter Transfer (Fig. 34-7)

- Masseter muscle innervation enters the mid-muscle mass from its posterior surface.
- Superior movement of the angle of the mouth may be available if deinnervation of the muscle is avoided.
- A visible lateral upper neck incision is usually necessary to harvest the masseter muscle.[5,13,23]

Indications

Indications for masseter transfer are complementary dynamic suspension of oral commissure and correction of isolated deanimation to midface and oral commissure.

Anatomy

The masseter muscle is the major muscular elevator of the mandible, which in conjunction with the medial and lateral pterygoid muscles plays its major role in chewing. It arises from the superficial and

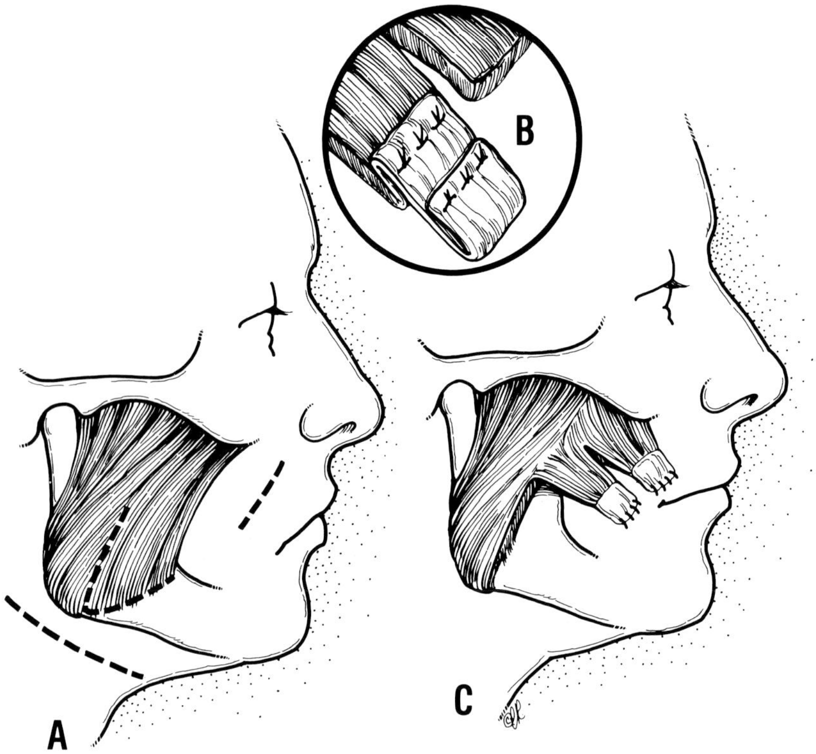

Figure 34-7. *Masseter muscle transfer with fascial extensions.*

deep cortex of the zygomatic arch. The muscle then descends along the lateral surface of the ramus to the angle of the mandible and the posterior third of the mandible body. The nerve supply is derived from the masseteric branch of the mandibular nerve. This branch reaches the deep surface of the muscle by passing through the mandibular notch and enters the muscle at a point equidistant between the mandibular notch and the angle of the mandible.

Technique

The primary importance of a masseter transfer is for suspension and potential reanimation of the oral commissure. This procedure may be used alone or in conjunction with a temporalis muscle transfer, static facial sling, or rhytidectomy. The exposure of the masseter muscle may therefore take place through a standard rhytidectomy incision or by way of a direct incision placed below the angle of the mandible and extending forward to the midportion of the body of the mandible in a natural crease line.

In the direct approach, the incision is carried deep to the platysma muscle with subsequent superior dissection to the posterior body of the mandible and angle region. The skin and subcutaneous tissue overlying the masseter muscle is elevated.

Attachments to the body of the mandible of the anterior half of the masseter muscle are sharply divided through periosteum to the underlying cortical surface of the mandible. A vertical incision is made through the body of the muscle, separating the anterior from the posterior half of the muscle. The height of this separation should be no greater than half the distance between the mandibular notch and the angle of the mandible. Further dissection carries a risk of loss of blood supply and trigeminal innervation. The separated anterior half of this muscle belly is then stripped away from its attachments to the ramus and body of the mandible.

A second vertical incision is then made to allow for a two-slip insertion into the oral commissure region. Because of the friability of the muscle bellies and the possibility that more length may be required to reach the point of attachment at the oral commissure, fascia lata or temporalis muscle strips are plicated over the anterior and posterior half of each masseteric slip using 4-0 Tevdek or Dacron. Further strengthening can be ensured by plicating the fascial loop to itself beyond the muscle belly. A nasolabial incision is made on the ipsilateral side, and dissection is deepened to identify the attachment of the zygomaticus major and minor muscles and quadratus levator superioris.

The two muscle fascial slips are then sutured to the point of attachment of the elevators and retractors of the oral commissure as they insert into the orbicularis oris muscle. This attachment is constructed using 4-0 Dacron suture material. A continual oversewing technique is recommended to minimize the chances of postoperative repair dehiscence. As with other static or dynamic repairs, overcorrection of the superior and inferior commissure region is desirable.

As with all facial undermining procedures, I prefer the use of medium-sized Silastic catheter drains under continual suction during the first 24 to 48 hours. Skin closure is with subcutaneous and subdermal 4-0 chromic catgut sutures, followed by a subcuticular 4-0 nylon and 6-0 mild chromic epidermal closure.

Complications

Complications include bleeding, infection, and injury to the parotid duct.

Digastric Transfer

- The digastric muscle pull in a lateral inferior direction makes it an excellent adjuvant repair for lower lip rehabilitation.
- The anterior belly is innervated by the Vth cranial nerve.

Indications

Indications for digastric transfer include an isolated injury to the ramus mandibularis branch of the facial nerve, and as an adjuvant procedure to correct the loss of lip depressor function.

Anatomy

The digastric muscle consists of two bellies connected by a common tendon. The posterior belly arises from the mastoid notch, coursing forward and medially crossing the vagus, accessory, and hypoglossal nerves and the occipital, internal carotid, external carotid, and facial arteries. The common tendon by which it is joined to the anterior belly is attached to the corner of the hyoid bone by a slip of fascia. The anterior belly runs forward and upward anteriorly from the cornu of the hyoid bone, and attaches to the lower border of the mandible near the midline. The posterior belly of the muscle is innervated by a branch of the facial nerve, while the anterior belly is innervated by the mylohyoid nerve branch of the trigeminal nerve. The primary function of the digastric is to elevate the hyoid or to depress the mandible.

Technique

A curvilinear incision about 4 cm long is made two fingerbreadths below the anterior body of the mandible. This incision is carried deeply through the platysma muscle to expose the inferior border of the submaxillary gland and the entire anterior belly of the digastric muscle, its tendon, and part of the posterior belly. Care should be taken to avoid injuring the facial vessels and the hypoglossal nerve, which lies immediately below the anterior belly.

Division of the anterior belly at its attachment to the mandible has two major limitations. One is that transferring this muscle to the depressors of the lip often results in a foreshortened muscle that cannot adequately reach the area of appropriate attachment. A second limitation is that dissection of the anterior belly results inevitably in deinnervation of the muscle and a possible loss of blood supply. I prefer a transection of the posterior belly of the digastric muscle at its midpoint, attachment of a temporalis or fascia lata fascial loop to the blunt edge of the muscle, and plication to the lower lip depressor muscle group, as previously mentioned in other procedures.

The common tendon is detached carefully from the cornu of the hyoid bone, and an anterior dissection of the anterior belly is extended to the midportion of the anterior belly. Further dissection is not recommended because of possible interference with innervation and blood supply. A long muscle strip with common tendon is then transferred to the lower lateral corner of the orbicularis oris at the point of attachment of the depressors of the lip. The muscle fascial end is then plicated to the depressor group using 4-0 Dacron. Appropriate overcorrection of the lower lip depressor action is created by reattaching the common tendon to the hyoid bone with Silastic tubing. An excellent choice for this tubing is a retinal band commonly used in retinal surgery.

Using a large curvilinear atraumatic needle, which is passed under the common tendon of the digastric and under the hyoid bone at the point of the desired attachment, the retinal band is threaded through this area and tied over the digastric tendon. Three loops are recommended to ensure attachment to the hyoid bone. Suture materials such as Tevdek and Dacron are not recommended because they may devascularize the distal portion of the muscle. A standard Silastic suction drain is placed and wound closure is completed.

Complications

Complications include injury to facial vessels and the hypoglossal nerve.

Free Microvascular Transfer—Gracilis Muscle

Several reports have appeared on the use of free muscle transfers such as the gracilis muscle in cases where reinnervation and atrophic loss of the muscles of facial expression have occurred. Advances in microvascular surgery have allowed the skillful team to transfer muscle successfully, but no report to date has shown persistent success or a major advantage of a combination of nerve crossover and free muscle transfer over other standard procedures. The major disadvantage of this technique is that it requires numerous operations, and variable results have been reported. Although the future of more refined facial reanimation may emerge from techniques of this kind, their use as a standard approach has not been demonstrated.[12,30]

STATIC OR ADYNAMIC FACIAL REHABILITATIVE SURGERY

Fascia Lata Sling

- The main effect of a fascia lata sling is to provide facial symmetry at rest.
- Combining a static sling with a browlift and facelift maximizes static rehabilitation of the face.
- Overcorrection and generous mattress suturing prevent detachment and weakening of the repair.

Indications

Indications include the following:

1. Muscle-wasting disease with facial paralysis
2. "Babysitting": a temporary facial sling to produce symmetry with spontaneous return of facial function expected
3. Central nervous system instability (eg, post-stroke).

Fascia lata suspension, rhytidectomy, browlift, and blepharoplasty may be used alone or in combination to establish the static suspension of the face and brow. The goal is to achieve symmetry at rest and less deformity during animation of the normal side. Fascia lata suspension, rhytidectomy, browlift, and blepharoplasty are often used as a one-stage procedure when other methods, such as myophysiological or neurophysiological dynamic suspension, are impossible. The operative description will include all four methods of reconstruction.

The patient is given a general anesthetic through a nasotracheal tube. The entire neck and face, bilaterally, extending to the vertex of the scalp, is prepped with Betadine soap and Betadine solution. In a similar manner, the ipsilateral thigh, from the patella to the groin, is prepped and draped.

Standard Incisions

The rhytidectomy incision proceeds from a point at the anterior base of the helix in a natural skin crease and descends in the pretragal region around the undersurface of the ear lobule to the posterior articular area. The posterior incision continues on the posterior articular skin, one fingerbreadth from the postauricular sulcus to the midconchal region. The incision is directed posteriorly to 1 cm within the hairline over the mastoid tip to the occipital prominence. Dissection is deepened to the subcutaneous plane inferiorly to the midportion of the sternocleidomastoid muscle, anteroinferiorly to the midportion of the mandible and posterior edge of the submaxillary gland, and anteromedial over the cheek and zygomatic process to the junction of the zygomatic arch with the lateral orbital rim. To allow for the temporalis muscle for facial suspension, the rhytidectomy incision is then extended superiorly in the hairline to the point equidistant between the vertex of the cranium and the forehead hairline junction. This incision is developed to the underlying temporalis fascia, then anteriorly to the lateral supraorbital ridge.

Secondary incisions are made in the nasolabial crease and in the upper and lower vermilion borders of the lip and medial canthal area, as previously described in the temporalis muscle transfer technique. Meticulous control of bleeding is recommended, using bipolar electrocauterization for small bleeders and direct ligation for all large bleeding points.

Fascia Lata

The thigh is internally rotated. The strongest point of fascia lata is anatomically located over the lateral side of the thigh. In this area, tendinous longitudinal fibers attach superiorly to the iliac crest and inferiorly to the lateral condyle of the tibia. Its function is to provide for insertion of the right part of the gluteus maximus muscle, as well as for the tensor muscle of the fascia lata.

A vertical incision about 5 cm long is made superior to the lateral condyle of the tibia and popliteal fossa. Dissection is carried down through the subcutaneous tissue through the fibrofatty layer to identify the tractus iliotibialis. The skin overlying the fascia is dissected superiorly for about 10 cm. A vertical incision is made in the fascial tract, and long strips of fascia are removed with a fascial stripper. Fascial strips at least 3 cm wide will avoid fragmentation and provide plentiful tissue for reconstruction. These strips are placed on a cork board and covered with moist saline or a physiological solution that prevents desiccation.

Skin closure over a Silastic suction drain consists of subcutaneous and subdermal 4-0 chromic catgut sutures followed by interrupted horizontal mattress sutures of 4-0 nylon. Fine line epithelial closure can then be accomplished with continuous 6-0 mild chromic. A wrap-around gauze pressure dressing from the knee to the upper thigh is recommended in addition to suction drainage to avoid hematoma formation and to minimize superficial venous thrombosis.

Two fascial strips with two distal limbs are fashioned. One strip suspends the upper and lower eyelid; the other suspends and retracts the upper and lower commissure of the lips. A continual subcutaneous fascial strip is tunneled from the philtrum of the upper lip to the oral commissure and subsequently through the subcutaneous tract of the lower lip to the midplane. As described with the temporalis muscle transfer, this continual fascial strip is fixed to the underlying fibers of the orbicularis oris muscle with 4-0 Dacron or 4-0 clear monofilament nylon sutures. Also as described in the temporalis muscle transfer, fascial strips are threaded through subcutaneous tunnels in the upper and lower lid near the palpebral margin, crossed, and sutured to the medial canthal tendon through a separate vertical incision with 4-0 Dacron or buried 4-0 clear monofilament nylon sutures. The upper lid fascial strip is then sutured to the temporalis fascia posterosuperior to the superior root of the helix. These are then plicated and tied over the temporalis fascia through two horizontal incisions. The purpose of the loop-and-plication method is to provide adequate pull to overcorrect and mimic the actions of the zygomaticus major muscle group and its actions on the commissure, and to prevent weakening this pull in the postoperative period.

The third fascial suspender is attached to the lower lip fascial strip and fixed to the depressor muscles of the lower lip. The fascia strip is interdigitated and woven through the lateral aspect of the depressor angular oris muscle, brought superiorly, and attached to the temporalis fascia and zygomaticus suspension fascial strip superiorly. Overcorrection of the lower and upper lip, as well as the oral commissure, is strongly recommended because of the tendency of antagonistic contralateral facial muscle pull to reverse the surgery's desired effect.

The skin of the face, scalp, and neck is then retracted in a superior posterior direction, and redundant skin overlying the pinna is carefully excised. Major points of attachment, including the rhytidectomy, occur at the root of the helix anteriorly and a point immediately superior and posterior to the postauricular crease and mastoid tip. These fixation sutures are usually 3-0 Tevdek or 3-0 monofilament nylon. A single medium Silastic drain is placed under the facial neck flap and brought out through the posterior occipital scalp limb of the rhytidectomy incision. Closure of the rhytidectomy incision is as follows:

1. Subcutaneous and subdermal layers with interrupted 3-0 and 4-0 chromic catgut sutures
2. Hairline anterior and posterior scalp incisions with stainless steel clips
3. Preauricular and postauricular incision skin closure with 6-0 mild chromic.

Browlift (Fig. 34-8)

- A browlift can be achieved through a coronal or suprabrow incision.
- Natural deep horizontal crease lines can be used in selected cases.
- Plication of the dermis to the frontalis fascia prevents early disrepair and unwanted asymmetry. Bilateral repair will ensure improved symmetry.

A browlift on the weakened side consists of a predetermined excision of crescentic skin above the affected eyebrow to bring the weakened side in compliance symmetrically with the nonparalyzed brow. This predetermined excision relates preoperative measurements taken at rest and during animation.

An incision is made at the junction of the brow with the skin from medial to lateral. This incision is deepened and the periosteum overlying the suprabrow area is identified. Care is taken not to injure the supratrochlea or supraorbital area. The lower brow is then elevated to its appropriate position. The browlift is maintained by placing at least

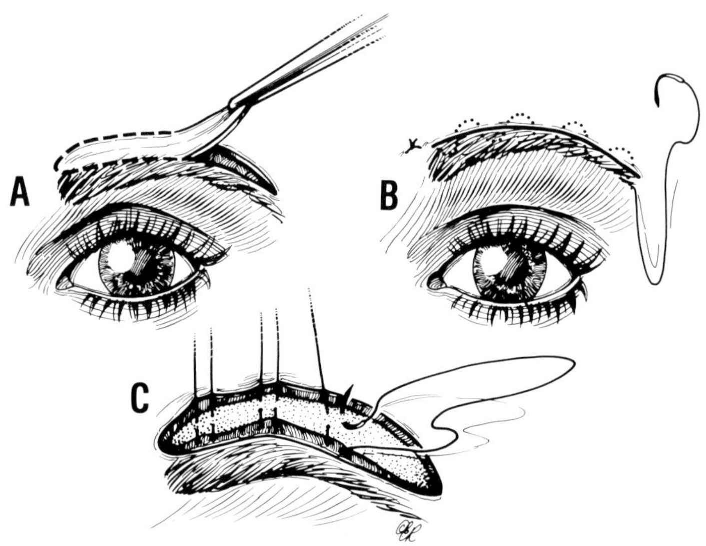

Figure 34-8. *Supraorbital browlift incision and repair.*

four clear 4-0 monofilament nylon sutures between the periosteum of the suprabrow area and the subcutaneous, subdermal layer of the brow area. Full closure of the brow incision consists of subcuticular 4-0 monofilament nylon suture, followed by the skin closure using running 6-0 mild chromic sutures. Nasolabial and periorbital incisions are closed similarly to those described under the temporalis muscle suspensory technique.

Although standard blepharoplasty of the upper and lower eyelids can be completed during the facial suspension procedure, I prefer to delay this technique until the results of the browlift and suspension have been observed for 3 months. I also defer the procedure because I believe that a blepharoplasty of the contralateral lid is often necessary and that local anesthesia ensures more refined cosmetic, functional, and symmetrical results.

Complications

Complications include the following:

1. Hematoma
2. Infection
3. Herniation of thigh muscles
4. Loss of suspension due to dehiscence of repair
5. Injury to parotid duct
6. Hypertrophic scarring
7. Failure to achieve facial symmetry or desired effect
8. Anesthesia (sensation loss) in face and brow
9. Corneal injury
10. Hair loss.

Adjuvant Procedures

Gold Weight Lid Tarsorrhaphy (Fig. 34-9)

- Creating a supratarsal pocket with preservation of the levator will avoid a ptosis.
- A skin incision is made 8 mm above the supratarsal fold.

The consistently essential procedures in facial paralysis are those directed to the short- and long-term protection and cosmesis of the eye. Patients with a poor Bell's phenomenon, frequent conjunctivitis, iritis, corneal pain or ulceration, lower lid ectropion, or exposure keratosis are best treated by procedures that offer protection to the eye. To this end, a popular procedure is a gold implant in the eyelid, a procedure easily carried out in the office.[4]

Gradated gold weights are taped to the eyelid until the appropriate closure of the eyelid produces the desired endpoint of protection and cosmesis with a ptosis of less than 3 mm. Under sterile conditions, a small incision is made 2 mm above the lash line at the midportion of the lower lid. An alternate incision is made in the tarsal–supratarsal fold. The inferior incision is dissected to the tarsal plate and a supratarsal pocket is created. The gold implant is placed 3 to 4 mm above the lid margin in a supratarsal pocket and sutured deeply to the underlying tarsal plate. The suture material most commonly used is 8-0 Ethilon or 7-0 Vicryl on a P1 needle. The supratarsal or lid margin incision is then closed in layers, using 7-0 Vicryl for the

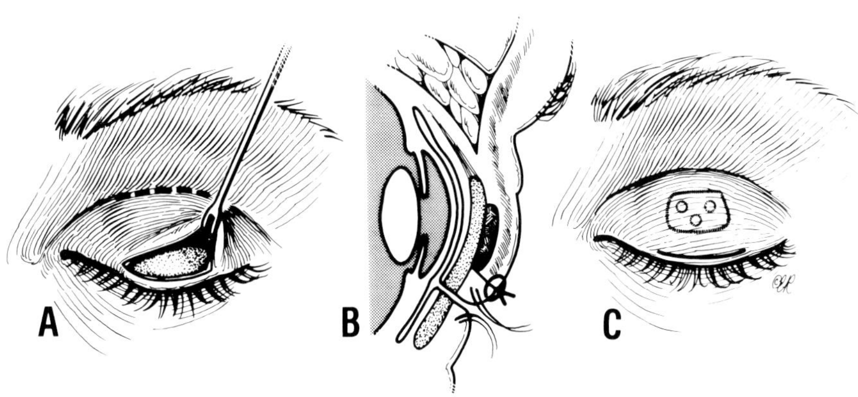

Figure 34-9. *Gold lid implant procedure.*

muscle and subcutaneous layer and a continuous 6-0 mild chromic for the skin closure. The patient is warned that mild edema may occur for about 24 hours.

Tarsorrhaphy

- A lateral tarsorrhaphy is the best assurance of eye protection in a dense facial nerve paralysis.
- At least 5 mm of lid mucosa at parallel, opposite locations in the upper and lower lids ensures lid adhesion.
- At least 21 days should be allowed for proper lid adhesion before the continuous bolstered suture is removed.

Although the cosmetic effect of standard tarsorrhaphy is inferior to that of a gold implant, many patients with dry eyes, corneal ulceration, iritis, or conjunctivitis are not good candidates for gold weight implantation. In such cases, a standard tarsorrhaphy is highly recommended. Tarsorrhaphy is a simple procedure that can be performed in the office with a minimum of instrumentation. The patient is placed in a supine position. Under good illumination, the eye is anesthetized with proparacaine. The lateral third of the eyelid is infiltrated with 1% xylocaine and 1:100,000 epinephrine, taking care to anesthetize the supratarsal and subconjunctival tarsal area and the upper and lower lids laterally. A 5- to 7-mm strip of palpebral mucosa is removed with a No. 11 scalpel blade from the upper and lower eyelids. The segment of demucosalization of the upper lid corresponds in location and length to that of the lower lid. A small gap is left between the lateral canthus and the tarsorrhaphy to allow for a easy division when reinnervation has occurred. Sutures of 4-0 silk (Davis and Geck) using a DO-1 double-arm spatula needle are passed in a looping fashion through a previously cut Silastic retinal band. The suture is passed through the lower lid incision through a second retinal band, looped, and then passed through the lower lid to the upper lid incision and retinal band. The suture is tied over the retinal band. Buckling of the retinal band is avoided; a slight eversion of the lash line is the desired effect. At least six knots are tied because of this repair tends to dehisce. Antibiotic ophthalmic ointment is applied to the tarsorrhaphy area for about 3 weeks. Suture removal is not recommended before the end of the 3 weeks, to avoid premature dehiscence of the repair.

Nasolabial Fold Plasty, Lip Mucosal Fold Resection, and Contralateral Myectomy

Nasolabial fold plasty, lip mucosal fold resection, and contralateral myectomy and neurectomy are adjuvant procedures that can sometimes be used at the end-stage correction of the paralyzed face. Indications for these procedures relate to the results of previous procedures. Long-standing paralysis involving the lower face may often result in a redundancy of inner lip mucosa, a common source of irritation and injury during chewing. Correcting this redundant mucosa will often improve this constant source of irritation to the patient. A common occurrence following a fascial or temporalis muscle sling procedure is the redundancy of skin in the region of the newly created nasolabial fold. In order to achieve cosmetic balancing with the normal side, this area may be corrected by a selective resection of skin. After a sling or suspension procedure, a partial loss of suspension may result in a loss of the nasolabial fold. Suspension tension may be strengthened by crescentic resection of the previous scar and adjacent skin along the lines of the natural nasolabial fold crease. Dissection to the underlying muscle and subsequent elevation of a superior and inferior skin flap often exposes dehisced fascial strips. Plication of the underlying muscle and fascial strips superiorly with 5-0 or 4-0 clear Ethilon, followed by a reconstruction of the nasolabial fold, reestablishes appropriate symmetry of the upper lip commissure region.

Contralateral myectomy is sometimes necessary because of the overpull by the normal side, particularly in the region of the oral commissure. Because the degree of weakening cannot be accurately controlled, most patients are reluctant to accept this procedure.

A recent development is the use of botulinum toxin in spastic dysphonia, blepharospasm, hemifacial spasm, and torticollis. Undoubtedly the use of this material will be extended to correcting the overpull of the normal side in facial paralysis. It has the advantage of being a simple and controllable technique and for the most part is reversible in a 6- to 8-month period. This technique is currently investigational and is not recommended for clinical use.

REFERENCES

1. Anderal H. Reconstruction of the face through cross-facial nerve transplantation in facial paralysis. In: Converse JM, ed. Reconstructive plastic surgery, ed 2. Philadelphia: WB Saunders, 1977:1848–1867.
2. Baker DC, Conley JJ. Facial nerve grafting, a 30-year retrospective review. Clin Plast Surg 1979; 6: 343–369.
3. Bischoff EPE. Microscopic analysis of anastomosis between the cranial nerves. In: Sachs E, Valtin EW (trans). The facial nerve. Hanover, NH: University Press of New England, 1977:43–76.
4. Bojrab DI. Upper-eyelid gold weight implantation. Insights in Otolaryngology. St. Louis: CV Mosby, 1989:4.
5. Castro DE, Correi P, Zani R. Masseter muscle rotation in the treatment of inferior facial paralysis. Plast Reconstr Surg 1973; 52:370–373.
6. Conley J. Hypoglossal crossover: 122 cases. Trans Am Acad Otolaryngol 1977; 84:763–768.
7. Conley JJ, Baker DC. Surgical treatment of extra-temporal facial paralysis: An overview. Head Neck Surg 1978; 1:12–23.
8. Davis RA, Ansen BJ, Puddinger JM, Kirth RE. Surgical anatomy of the facial nerve and parotid gland based upon a study of 350 cervical facial halves. Surg Gynecol Obstet 1956; 102:385–412.
9. Donaldson JA, Ansen BJ. Symposium on disease and injury of the facial nerve. Otolaryngologic Clinics of North America. Philadelphia: WB Saunders, 1974; 7:289–308.
10. Freilinger G. A new technique to correct facial paralysis. Plast Reconstr Surg 1975; 56:44–48.
11. Gacek RR, Radpour S. Fiber orientation of facial nerve: An experimental study in the cat. Laryngoscope 1982; 93:547–556.
12. Harii K. Microneurovascular free muscle transplantation for reanimation of facial paralysis. Clin Plast Surg 1979; 6:361–375.
13. Hastings S. Transplantation of anterior half of masseter muscle for facial paralysis. Proceedings of the Royal Society of Medicine 1920; 13:64–65.
14. House JW, Brachmann DE. Facial nerve grading system. Otolaryngol Head Neck Surg 1985; 93: 146–147.
15. Kullman GL, Dyck PJ, Cody DTR. Anatomy of the mastoid portion of the facial nerve. Arch Otolaryngol Head Neck Surg 1971; 93:29–33.
16. May M. Total facial nerve exploration: Transmastoid extra-labyrinthine and subtemporal results. Laryngoscope 1979; 89:906–916.
17. May M. The facial nerve. Anatomy of the facial nerve for the clinician. New York: Thieme, 1986: 21–62.
18. May M. Anatomy of the facial nerve for the clinician. The facial nerve. New York: Thieme, 1986:57–59.
19. Miehlke A. Surgery of the facial nerve. Philadelphia: WB Saunders, 1973:240–262.
20. Neal J. Progressive supranuclear palsy. Brain 1972; 95:693–704.
21. Rubin L. Reanimation of the paralyzed face. St. Louis: CV Mosby, 1977:340–352.
22. Rubin L. Temporalis and masseter muscle transposition. New York: Thieme, 1986:665–669.
23. Sachs ME, Conley JJ. Intraoral masseter muscle transposition. Arch Otolaryngol Head Neck Surg 1982; 108:397–410.
24. Samii M. Rehabilitation of the face by VIIth nerve substitution. In: Fisch U, ed. Facial nerve surgery. Birmingham: Aesculapius Publishing Company, 1977:206–208.
25. Sato H. Aberrant neurons in the facial nerve trunk. Arch Otorhinolaryngol 1973; 206:69–76.
26. Scarmella FLF. Preliminary report on facial nerve anastomosis. Read before the Second International Symposium on Facial Nerve Surgery, Osaka, Japan, 1970.
27. Smith JW. A new technique in facial animation. Transactions of the Fifth International Congress of Plastic and Reconstructive Surgery, Australia. Washington DC: Butterworths, 1971.
28. Spector GS. Mimetic surgery for the paralyzed face. Laryngoscope 1984; 95:1494–1522.
29. Sunderland S, Bradley KC. Deinnervation atrophy of the distal stump of the severed nerve. J Comp Neurol 1950; 93:401.
30. Tucker MH. Restoration of selective facial nerve function by nerve muscle pedicle technique. Clinical Plastic Surgery 1979; 6:293–300.

35

Peripheral Nerve Injuries to the Lower Extremity

Michael B. Wood

AUTHOR'S KEY POINTS

- *Traction injuries* involve a spectrum from neurapraxia to axonotmesis to neurotmesis. Since early repairs of disrupted nerves following traction injuries do not have a favorable prognosis because of the diffuse region of nerve injury, it is best initially to observe these neuropathies. Operative exploration is reserved for cases that fail to demonstrate spontaneous recovery by 6 months post-injury.
- *Laceration injuries*, in contrast, are associated with neurotmesis lesions with a localized site of nerve damage. Injuries of this sort have a favorable prognosis for recovery following repair or graft reconstruction. Early operative exploration (within 6 weeks post-injury) is advised.
- Peroneal nerve palsy is the most common lower extremity complete nerve injury. The extent of nerve trauma may include traction, compression, focal ischemia, and laceration. Anticipated neuropathology is correlated with the history and mechanism of injury. Indications for observation versus operative exploration are based on the likelihood of an in-continuity vs a neurotmesis lesion. Most traction, compression, and focal ischemia lesions of the peroneal nerve demonstrate spontaneous partial or complete recovery.
- The sciatic nerve is topographically differentiated proximally into posterior tibial and common peroneal divisions. An incomplete sciatic nerve palsy may present clinically as either an isolated peroneal neuropathy (most commonly) or posterior tibial neuropathy. In the former instance, electromyographic evidence of a posterior tibial neuropathy or involvement of the hamstrings helps establish the level of injury.
- Femoral neuropathy often results from iatrogenic operative injury. Patients present with vague complaints of knee or gait weakness or instability. There are only minor sensory symptoms.
- To clinically localize neuropathies of the lower extremity, it is essential to know the sensory distribution of the lateral femoral cutaneous (L1, L2, L3), saphenous (femoral nerve), sural (posterior tibial and common peroneal nerves), lateral sural cutaneous (common peroneal nerve), superficial peroneal, deep peroneal, and posterior tibial sensory distributions, as well as the motor distribution of the femoral, superior and inferior gluteal, posterior tibial, deep and superficial peroneal nerves. See Figures 35-1 and 35-2.

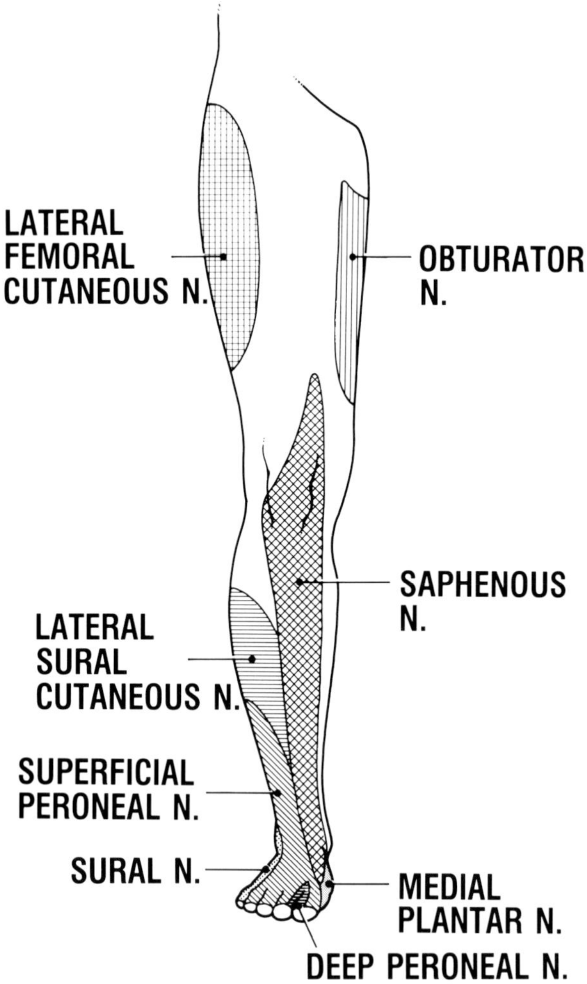

Figure 35-1. *Anterior aspect of the lower extremity, showing cutaneous territories of some of the important peripheral nerves or their branches.*

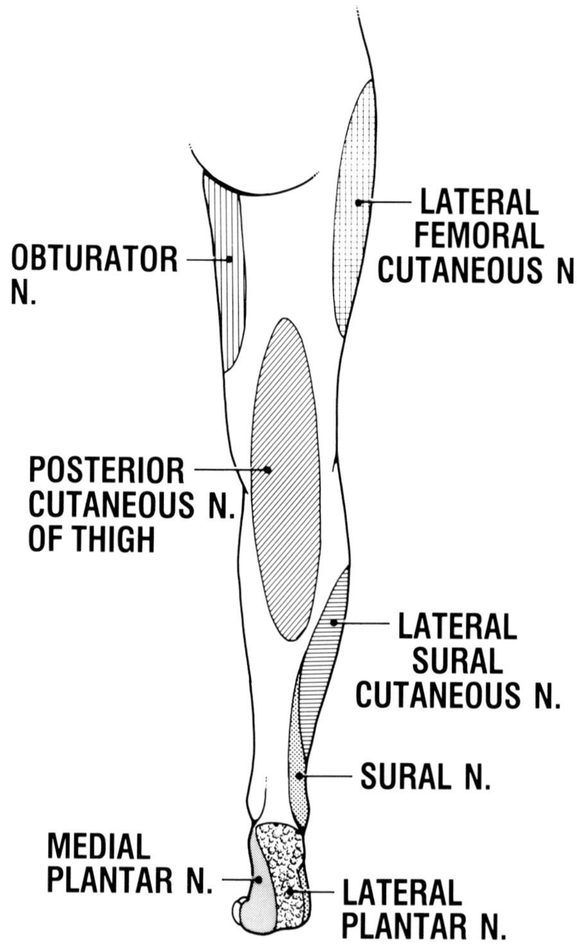

Figure 35-2. *Posterior aspect of the lower extremity, showing cutaneous territories of some of the important peripheral nerves or their branches.*

Peripheral nerve injuries involving the lower extremity have received little attention in the literature, compared with upper extremity nerve deficits. Although lower extremity injuries are relatively common (particularly in association with penetrating trauma, open fractures, hip or knee dislocations, and iatrogenic operative accidents), firm principles of management have not been developed. Recent advances in diagnostic evaluation, microsurgical technique, and rehabilitation modalities, as well as a trend toward limb salvage for traumatic and neoplastic conditions, has prompted contemporary interest in lower extremity peripheral nerve operative management. It has become clear that with appropriate patient selection, repair or reconstruction of peripheral nerve injuries in the lower limb may be rewarding in terms of functional recovery. Therefore, no longer is a generalized nihilistic treatment approach to these injuries justified. The functional impact, prognosis, and therapeutic implications of lower limb peripheral nerve lesions vary with the specific nerve affected and the mechanism of injury, and often these two factors may be related.

LUMBOSACRAL PLEXUS (Fig. 35-3)

While partial injuries to the lumbosacral plexus are common, they often escape detection. Lesions of this sort are encountered in patients with pelvic fractures, particularly when the sacrum or sacroiliac joint is involved.[15] When associated with pelvic fractures, the mechanism of lumbosacral injury is usually traction. The prognosis for spontaneous recovery following fracture reduction and stabilization is favorable. However, a poor prognosis is associated with traction injuries to the brachial plexus. The difference is probably due to the fact that the lumbosacral nerve roots are protected, in part, by the bony structure of the pelvis, which is very resistant to marked displacement relative to the spine.[8] The brachial plexus, on the other hand, is made up of poorly protected nerve roots subjected to wide displacement by the cervical spine or upper limb, or both. Lumbosacral nerve deficits may also result from penetrating trauma, although this more often causes neurotmesis lesions. In such cases, the extent of neurologic functional loss may be difficult to ascertain initially because of the coexistence of more dramatic injuries involving the intra-abdominal viscera and great vessels.

There have been only sporadic case reports of the functional outcome of lumbosacral plexus reconstruction.[11] Definitive statements regarding prognosis following operative repair of such lesions are therefore impossible to make. However, from an empirical standpoint, the results of lumbosacral reconstruction approximate those of brachial plexus reconstruction, if one allows for the greater distance required for regenerating axons to reach their motor or sensory end organs in the lower limb.

Author's Preferred Method

Neurotmesis lesions may warrant secondary exploration with consideration of nerve graft

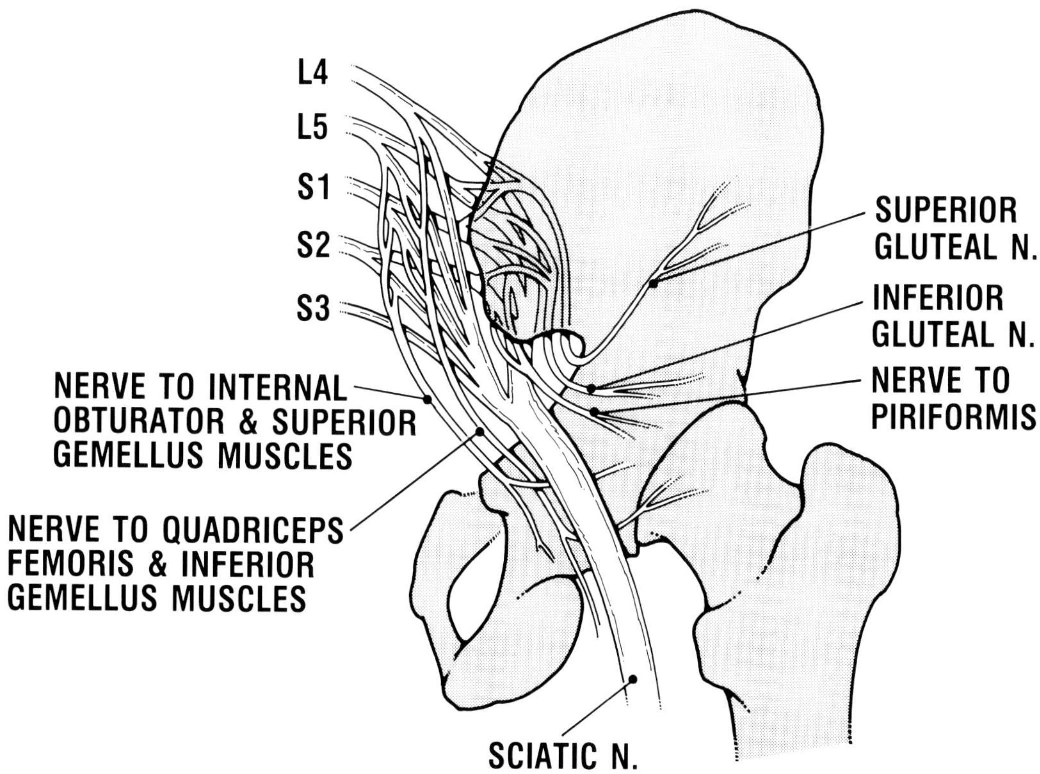

Figure 35-3. *Lumbosacral plexus distribution.*

reconstruction 1 to 3 months post-injury (Fig. 35-4). The specific indications for operative intervention in such cases include a high index of suspicion of anatomical disruption of a portion of the lumbosacral plexus and a fixed and functionally significant neurologic deficit confirmed both by clinical examination and electrodiagnostic studies, in a patient who is otherwise stable in regard to associated injuries. The surgeon must anticipate the need for a nerve graft donor site and possibly a limited sacral laminectomy, ideally using intraoperative electrodiagnostic studies.

SCIATIC NERVE (Fig. 35-5)

The sciatic nerve may be injured at any level from the pelvic outlet at the sciatic notch to its division into the common peroneal and posterior tibial nerves. Because of its course and its somewhat vulnerable location, mechanisms of injury vary and include traction, direct contusion, injection, and laceration. Traction lesions result from displaced pelvic fractures and traumatic hip hyperflexion injuries.[15] Traction neuropathies also result from acutely lengthening the lower extremity, particularly after correcting longstanding hip contractures in the course of hip arthroplasty.[18] A relatively common cause of sciatic nerve injury is a posterior hip dislocation or fracture dislocation, which produce both traction injury and direct contusion to the nerve (see Chap. 43). Often the amount of traction and contusion that occurs with hip dislocations is asymmetrically distributed to the nerve, resulting in what appears to be a common peroneal nerve palsy clinically. This is probably because the common peroneal division of the sciatic nerve is

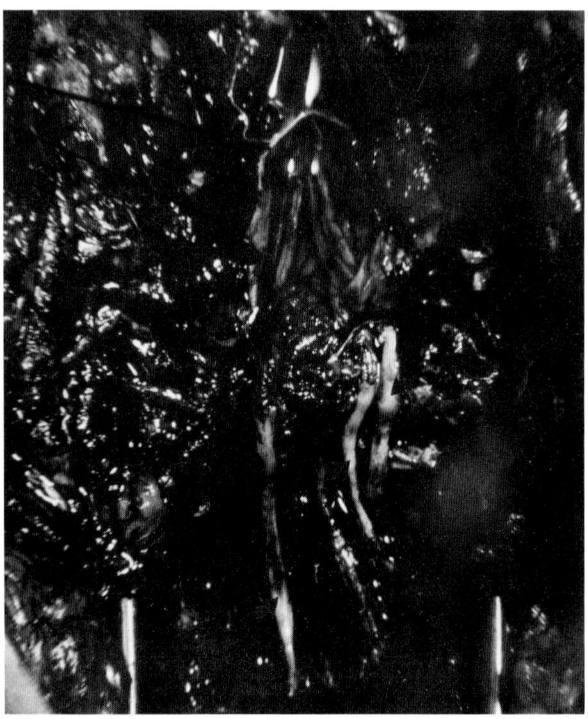

Figure 35-4. *Avulsion neurotmesis injury to lower lumbosacral plexus. Sacral laminectomy. Reconstruction of multiple sacral nerve roots with autologous sural nerve grafts (arrows).*

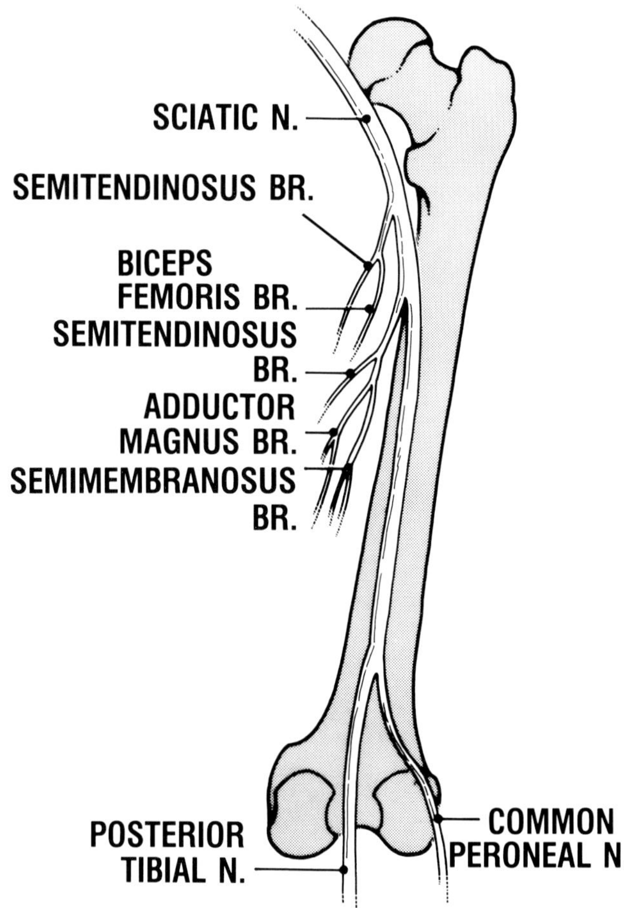

Figure 35-5. *Sciatic nerve distribution.*

relatively fixed at the neck of the fibula and hence more prone to stretch injury.

Injection injuries to the sciatic nerve resulting from hypodermic injections have become much less common in recent years due to increased awareness of the problem by health-care providers. The extent of nerve damage is related to both the volume and content of the injected material.[4] Direct laceration occurs from penetrating injuries, sharp fractured bone edges, and operative iatrogenic injuries.

The deficit resulting from complete sciatic neuropathy is profound for both motor and sensory function.[5] Partial motor loss is managed by orthotic support for the foot and ankle. However, sensory loss, involving all but a small region of the foot, leads to trophic ulceration, deep infection, and in some instances eventual limb amputation. Therefore, the major goal of treatment of sciatic nerve lesions is to restore protective sensibility to the foot without concomitant disabling dysesthesias.

Author's Preferred Method

Of all the lower extremity nerve injuries, the management of sciatic nerve lesions is the least controversial. Nerves injured by traction mechanisms, where the likelihood of direct laceration by a fractured bone fragment is low, are observed for signs of recovery for 3 months post-injury. The absence of clinical or electromyographic signs of reinnervation after this interval is an indication for exploration. If an in-continuity lesion is encountered, the decision to limit intervention to neurolysis as opposed to resection and graft reconstruction is based on the extent to which fascicular detail of the nerve is preserved at the injury site, as well as the presence of electrical conduction across the injured segment (see Chap. 42). If the sciatic nerve is asymmetrically injured, consideration of resection and graft reconstruction is limited to the severely involved portion of the nerve only.

Lacerations of the sciatic nerve are repaired or reconstructed in virtually all cases. The repair is performed as early as possible, depending on the care needed for associated injuries. Sharp lacerations without a concomitant fracture or other significant soft-tissue loss are repaired directly within a few days. Slight delays in repair minimize the technical problems related to nerve end retraction and fibrosis as well as distortion of fascicular cross-sectional detail at the time of neurorrhaphy. In lacerations resulting from blunt trauma or those associated with an element of crush or traction injury, operative intervention is delayed for 3 to 4 weeks. This delay allows more accurate demarcation of injured nerve ends at the time of surgery and thus permits more precise resection of the injury site to healthy nerve substance both proximally and distally.

The surgeon undertakes direct neurorrhaphy or nerve graft reconstruction based on the ease of coaptation of resected nerve ends. In general, if the two prepared nerve ends can be coapted by a single 8-0 nylon suture while maintaining the knee in a position of mid-flexion, direct neurorrhaphy is undertaken.[20]

If this is not the case, reconstruction using the technique of interfascicular nerve grafting is indicated (see Chap. 37).[12] The ipsilateral sural nerve is taken as a donor, since it most likely will be nonfunctional. If more nerve graft substance is required, contralateral sural nerve or ipsilateral superficial peroneal nerve is used. The length of interposed nerve graft segments should slightly exceed that of the deficit when all involved joints are placed in neutral position. After securing the grafts at both ends, graft cables are initially splayed out for maximal contact with the soft-tissue bed for effective graft revascularization (Fig. 35-6).

Sciatic nerves injured by hypodermic-needle injections are observed for 6 weeks to 3 months. Many of these injuries spontaneously improve, particularly if they involve only a portion of the nerve cross-sectional area and a small volume of injectate, and do not involve sclerosing substances. There are no data to support immediate nerve exploration and intraneural neurolysis with debridement of injected material. If spontaneous recovery is not evident by 3 months post-injection, exploration and neurolysis is indicated. Excision of the damaged nerve segment with nerve graft reconstruction is warranted if complete nerve destruction is encountered.

FEMORAL NERVE (Fig. 35-7)

The femoral nerve has a relatively abbreviated course in the lower extremity, dividing into its various terminal branches at about the level of the inguinal ligament. It is injured most frequently by penetrating trauma to the groin region and iatro-

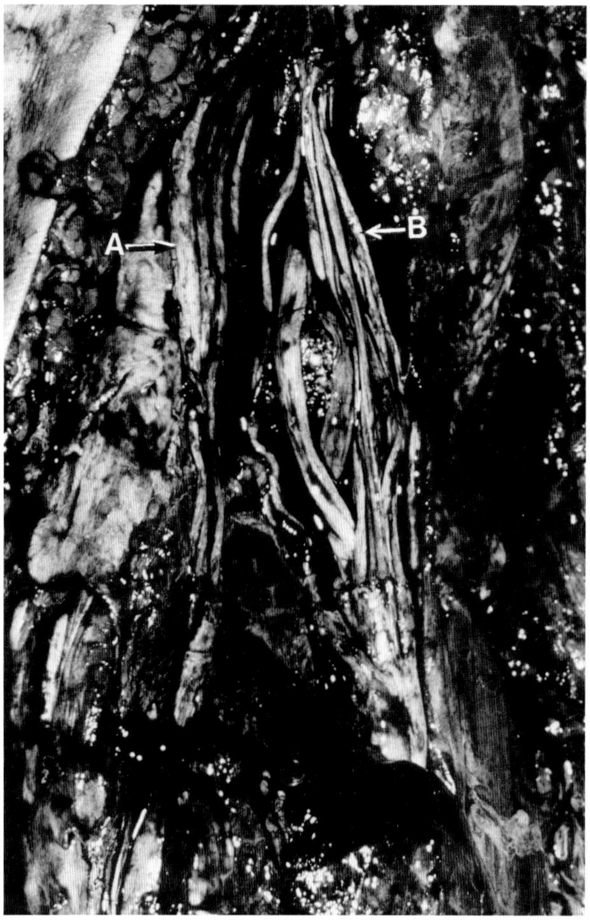

Figure 35-6. *Sciatic nerve reconstruction using interfascicular grafting technique with multiple autologous sural nerve segments. At left, common peroneal division (**A**); at right, posterior tibial nerve division (**B**).*

genically during herniorrhaphy, saphenous vein ligation, anterior hip exposure, and other proximal thigh procedures.[17] In the upper leg the femoral nerve consists of multiple terminal branches; therefore, partial neuropathy is not unusual. Presenting complaints are frequently ill-defined and vague. If complete neuropathy is present, obvious quadriceps weakness is present, with inability to extend or stabilize the knee during gait, plus a sensory deficit in the anterior thigh and in the saphenous nerve distribution of the leg and ankle. In the patient with only partial motor palsy, however, only part of the quadriceps is paralyzed and some ability to extend and stabilize the knee is maintained.

Treatment is individualized depending on the neurologic deficit and likely cause. The prognosis for recovery of motor function following femoral nerve repair is favorable. This is most likely related to the fact that terminal nerve branches are primarily motor in function and, when injured in the groin region, are in close approximation to muscle end organs. Further, most femoral nerve injuries result from sharp lacerations or other very localized trauma mechanisms.

Author's Preferred Method

If there is little or no motor weakness and a painless sensory deficit, treatment is not indicated. In some cases, with only very mild motor weakness, a compensatory progressive-resistance strengthening program for the remaining functional quadriceps muscle is all that is required. Extremities with significant quadriceps muscle weakness, or complete paralysis, particularly those sustaining iatrogenic or sharp penetrating lacerations, are explored. Direct neurorrhaphy, practical in sharp well-defined lesions, is facilitated by gentle hip flexion. More extensive defects require graft reconstruction. The saphenous nerve branch of the femoral nerve is an ideal donor choice for the graft, if it is nonfunctional.

OBTURATOR NERVE

The obturator nerve is primarily motor in function and has only a short course in the lower extremity. It divides above the inguinal ligament into anterior and posterior divisions. Injuries to the obturator nerve are rare. When present, they cause weakness of thigh adduction.[13] Depending on the extent of injury, the resultant disability may be moderate to negligible.[16] Although no data are available concerning prognosis, the results of repair are expected to be good because the obturator nerve is predominantly motor very close to its muscles of innervation.

Author's Preferred Method

Indications for repair depend on the mechanism of injury and the perceived disability. Localized sharp lacerations to the obturator nerve, or either of its

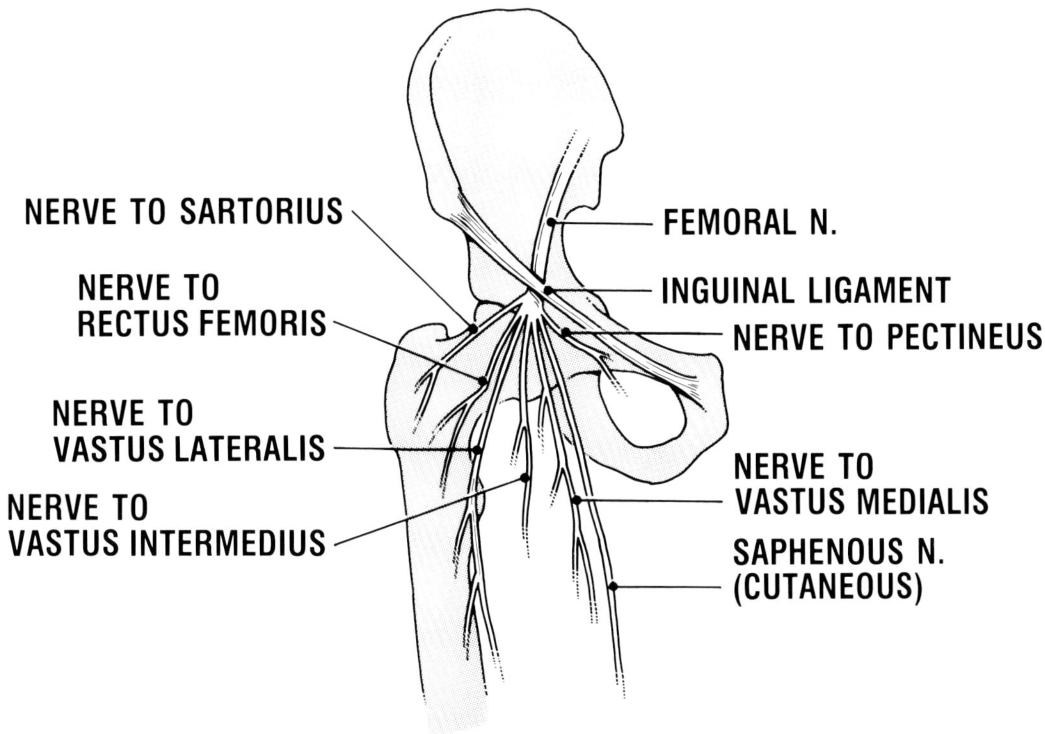

Figure 35-7. *Femoral nerve distribution.*

divisions, that cause moderate functional loss are indications for repair or reconstruction.

POSTERIOR TIBIAL NERVE (Fig. 35-8)

The posterior tibial nerve may be injured at any point from the distal thigh, where it originates from the sciatic nerve, to its divisions into medial and lateral plantar nerves in the foot. This nerve is particularly vulnerable to injury at the popliteal fossa and the ankle. Partial posterior tibial neuropathies are common and are often associated with post-traumatic or post-ischemic deep posterior compartment syndromes of the leg. Complete lesions of the posterior tibial nerve, however, are more often a result of direct injury. This may be a neurotmesis lesion from penetrating trauma, traction/avulsion injury in cases of knee or ankle dislocation, or complete lesion in continuity resulting from lesser degrees of traction, as may be associated with displaced tibial fractures.

Goals of treatment for posterior tibial nerve injuries vary with the level of injury. A complete nerve lesion at any level from distal thigh to ankle results in dense sensory deficits over the plantar aspect of the foot.[10] Expected problems with this sensory deficit, however, are substantially less than those seen with a sciatic palsy. The preserved sensibility from the superficial and deep peroneal nerve divisions and any preserved sensibility in the sural nerve distribution (depending on the level of posterior tibial nerve injury and presence or absence of innervation provided by the peroneal communicating nerve branch of the sural nerve) decrease the risks of trophic ulceration, despite the fact that most of the plantar aspect of the foot is anesthetic.

Motor deficits resulting from posterior tibial nerve injury are markedly different if the lesion is in the distal thigh above the gastrocnemius muscle

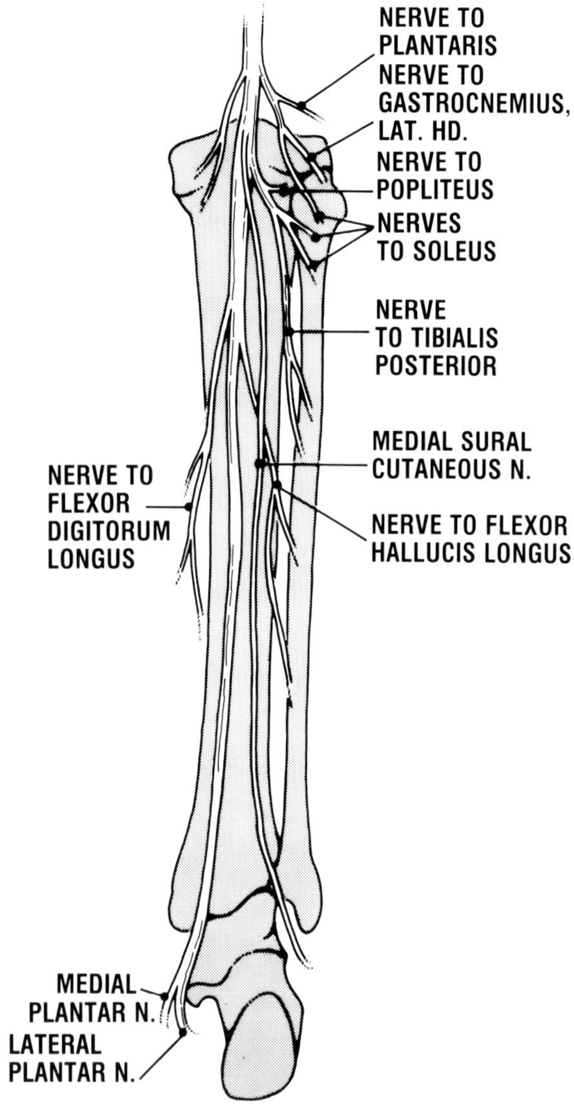

Figure 35-8. *Posterior tibial nerve distribution.*

motor branch compared to injuries in the popliteal fossa. With injuries in the thigh, ankle plantar flexion is extremely weak, being present only as a result of peroneus longus and brevis function. With injuries in the popliteal fossa, strong ankle plantar flexion is preserved. With injuries at levels below the mid-tibia, toe flexion and strong ankle inversion are maintained. When the posterior tibial nerve is injured at this distal level, orthotic support of the foot and ankle is not required. A troublesome problem often seen with posterior tibial nerve injuries, and particularly with incomplete lesions, whether treated or untreated, is that of painful dysesthesias in the foot.[6] These symptoms may preoccupy the patient and supersede complaints or disabilities related to paralysis or plantar sensibility deficits.

Author's Preferred Method

The principles of management are similar to those discussed for the sciatic nerve. If a posterior tibial nerve injury is thought to be the result of traction, observation is recommended for 3 to 6 months. There is perhaps less urgency to proceed with posterior tibial nerve exploration than with the sciatic nerve, because the nerve injury site is significantly more distal in the limb, closer to terminal end organs. Those posterior tibial nerve injuries thought likely to be neurotmesis injuries are repaired by direct neurorrhaphy early (1–3 days) for sharp injuries or undergo delayed (1 month) repair or nerve graft reconstruction if crushed or avulsion mechanisms were involved (Fig. 35-9). The technical principles of repair or nerve grafting discussed for sciatic nerve injuries apply to this nerve as well.

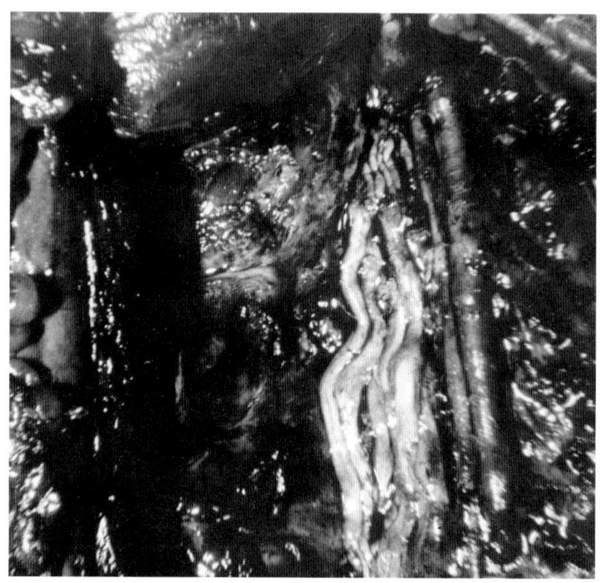

Figure 35-9. *Posterior tibial nerve reconstruction using interfascicular grafting technique with multiple autologous sural nerve segments.*

MEDIAL/LATERAL PLANTAR NERVES

The largest terminal branches of the posterior tibial nerve, arising within or distal to the tarsal tunnel, are the medial and lateral plantar nerves. These nerves are injured, either together or separately in the foot, as a result of penetrating trauma. Injury to either nerve may also occur from a surgical mishap in the course of subtalar joint exposure, plantar fasciotomy or fasciectomy, or intrinsic muscle flap transposition.[1] The indications for operative repair of lesions to either nerve depend on the patient's specific complaints, which may include sensory deficit, intrinsic muscle palsy, or troublesome neuroma. In general, the deficit seen with injury to both medial and lateral plantar nerves is less than that seen with posterior tibial nerve injury because of preserved heel sensibility and unimpaired sensibility in the sural nerve distribution. Therefore, the indications to proceed with nerve repair for the purposes of sensory recovery are not especially compelling, particularly when only a single nerve (medial or lateral plantar) is affected. Neuroma symptoms, perhaps the most significant complaint, may be of sufficient magnitude to preclude weight bearing altogether (Fig. 35-10). In such cases, nerve repair or reconstruction by grafting may not relieve neuroma symptoms, even when successful motor and sensory recovery is noted.

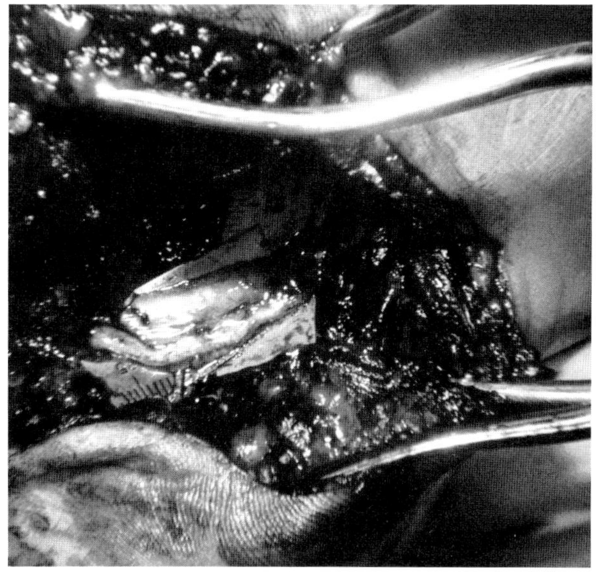

Figure 35-10. *Medial plantar nerve reconstructed with two sural nerve graft segments. Patient had prior laceration with neuromatous pain complaints sufficient to prevent weight bearing.*

Author's Preferred Method

When the patient's complaints focus primarily on painful neuroma symptoms, sensory hypesthesia or intrinsic motor paralysis are lesser problems in comparison. In such cases, proximal neurectomy of the affected branch or neuroma transposition may be a more prudent treatment option than that of repair. Nerve repair or reconstruction for the intended goal of motor or sensory recovery is a valid consideration for either medial or lateral plantar branch. The technical principles are identical to those discussed previously.

PERONEAL NERVE (Fig. 35-11)

Peroneal neuropathy is the most common lower extremity nerve palsy, accounting for 15% of all peripheral nerve injuries in one series.[3] The common peroneal nerve, or its superficial and deep divisions at the neck of the fibula, are particularly vulnerable to either indirect or direct injury by penetrating trauma, compression, or traction. This is related to a number of factors, including the facts that the nerve is superficially located (overlying the bony prominence of the fibular head), that it is tethered distally by motor branches and the fibrous arcade at the fibula neck, and that the peroneal nerve has a low ratio of epineural to fascicular cross-sectional area.[21]

While the common peroneal nerve, or its deep and superficial divisions, may be injured at any level, in the vast majority of cases the lesion is at the distal thigh or knee level. A variety of mechanisms account for injury at the knee, including penetrating trauma; lacerations from displaced femoral, fibular, or tibial fracture fragments; and traction with or without avulsion from varus or hyperextension knee ligament injuries. Displaced distal femur and proximal tibia fracture fragments may also injure the peroneal nerve. The peroneal nerve seems particularly prone to injury from iatrogenic accidents during the course of lateral knee

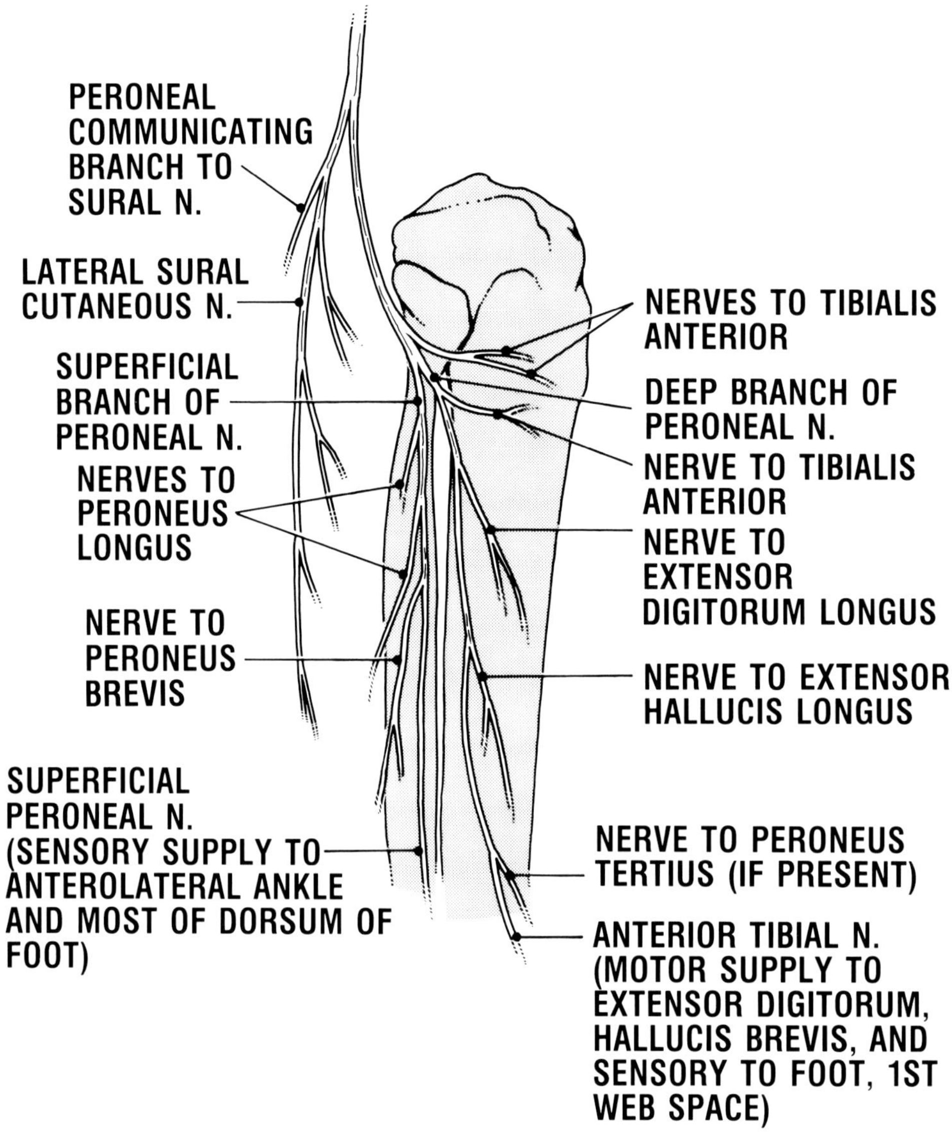

Figure 35-11. *Common peroneal nerve distribution.*

ligament repair, lateral meniscectomy, upper tibial osteotomy, knee arthroplasty, and even arthroscopic procedures.[21]

The functional deficit resulting from peroneal nerve injury depends greatly on whether a single division of the nerve or both are affected. A lesion involving the common peroneal nerve or both superficial and deep divisions results in paralysis of the peroneal muscles (ankle eversion) as well as paralysis of the anterior compartment muscles (ankle and toe extension). This results in both a slapfoot gait and an unbalanced ankle favoring inversion, due to the unopposed activity of the tibialis posterior muscle. Thus, in the absence of orthotic support, the patient experiences frequent ankle sprains and awkwardness in clearing the foot from the floor. The sensory disturbance is confined to only a portion of the dorsum of the foot and the anterolateral ankle region and is of little functional significance.

If only part of the peroneal nerve is injured, the deep division is most commonly affected. The deficit is paralysis of toe and ankle extension. Peroneal muscle control is preserved. Thus, although a drop-foot gait occurs, the ankle remains well balanced with much less of a tendency toward recurrent sprains and injury. Sensory deficit, which is confined to the first web space in the foot, may be barely noticed by the patient. Involvement of only the superficial division leads to an unbalanced ankle but with less of a tendency to recurrent injury because foot drop is not present. Often this deficit is well tolerated by the patient; in fact, the chief complaint relates to hypesthesias along the dorsum of the foot, or painful neuromas at the site of injury.

The deep and superficial nerve divisions over most of the length of the leg are covered and protected generously by muscles. Thus, injury between knee and ankle results chiefly from penetrating trauma. Functional deficit depends on the level of the lesion and the extent of direct muscle or tendon transection. In the distal leg and ankle region, the terminal portions of the deep and superficial peroneal nerves are superficial, becoming more vulnerable to injury. At this distal level, however, the functional consequence of nerve injury is much less significant than that noted with injury at more proximal levels. In fact, painful neuromas at the transection site are frequently the most troublesome complaints.

Author's Preferred Method

The management of peroneal nerve palsy depends on several factors, including the level and mechanism of injury, the extent of paralysis, and the availability of palliative treatment alternatives, including orthotics or tendon transfer. Exploration within a few days after injury is warranted in cases of sharp penetrating trauma (knife or glass) or in cases of known or suspected direct iatrogenic nerve injury in the course of operative intervention about the knee. Sharp, well-localized injuries to the peroneal nerve, if explored early, are treated by direct neurorrhaphy (Fig. 35-12). The criteria for using direct neurorrhaphy are the same as those outlined for the sciatic nerve. It is extremely difficult to compensate for loss of length of the

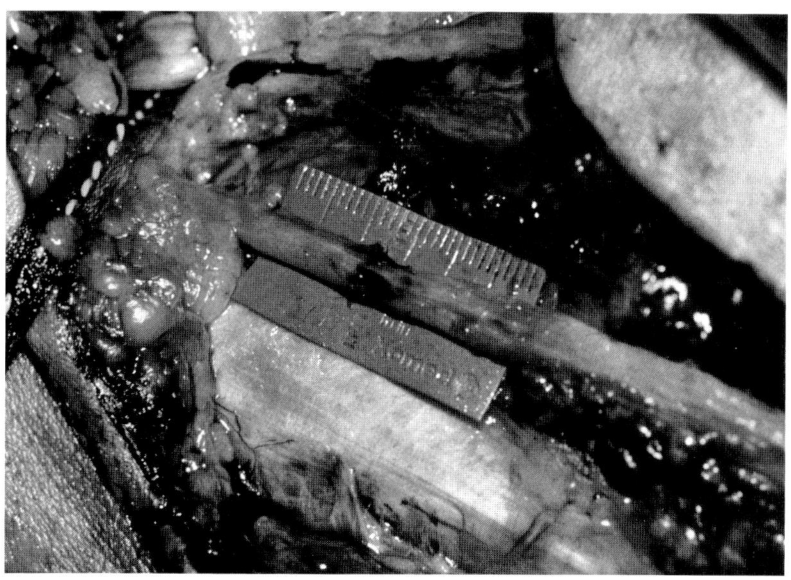

Figure 35-12. *Direct epineural neurorrhaphy of common peroneal nerve 8 days after accidental laceration during arthroscopic meniscectomy.*

peroneal nerve because of its anatomical location. Therefore, in limbs where some resection of nerve ends is required, or in limbs where treatment delay has allowed retraction and fibrosis of nerve ends, primary repair is usually impossible; in such patients, nerve graft reconstruction is carried out.

At the level of the knee, traction and compression injuries are common. Because each has a reasonable potential for spontaneous recovery, a closed injury at this level warrants observation for 3 to 6 months.[2,7,19] If surgery is indicated for management of associated fractures or ligament injuries, the nerve is, at the same time, explored to document the extent of injury. If nerve disruption is confirmed, reconstruction is carried out 1 month post-injury. This delay allows time for demarcation of the injured zone of nerve ends.

If, on the other hand, an in-continuity lesion is confirmed, observation for up to 6 months is warranted. If at 6 months neurologic recovery has not occurred, exploration is indicated.

In patients where the status of nerve integrity is unknown, exploration is considered at 3 to 6 months post-injury if there has been no evidence of recovery. When an in-continuity lesion is encountered at exploration, the potential for progressive neurologic recovery is assessed. This is best done by inspecting the nerve at the injury site and by using intraoperative electrodiagnostic studies. A nerve that is intact on inspection (preserved fascicular detail without a localized site of fascicular disruption) and has preserved conduction across the injury zone is observed for signs of neurologic recovery.

On the other hand, when there is a focal area of damage and no evidence of fascicular continuity or preserved electrical conduction, the injured segment is resected to healthy fascicles both proximally and distally. In these cases, reconstruction by interfascicular nerve grafting is warranted (Fig. 35-13). The choice of donor nerve for this purpose depends on the sensibility defect in the affected limb. If, in the affected limb, the sural nerve has also been transected, it may be used as a donor nerve distal to the injury site. However, if there is a sensibility defect in the distribution of the superficial peroneal nerve but the ipsilateral sural nerve is functional, it should be maintained to provide sensibility to the dorsolateral aspect of the foot. In such cases, the contralateral sural nerve is a better donor choice.

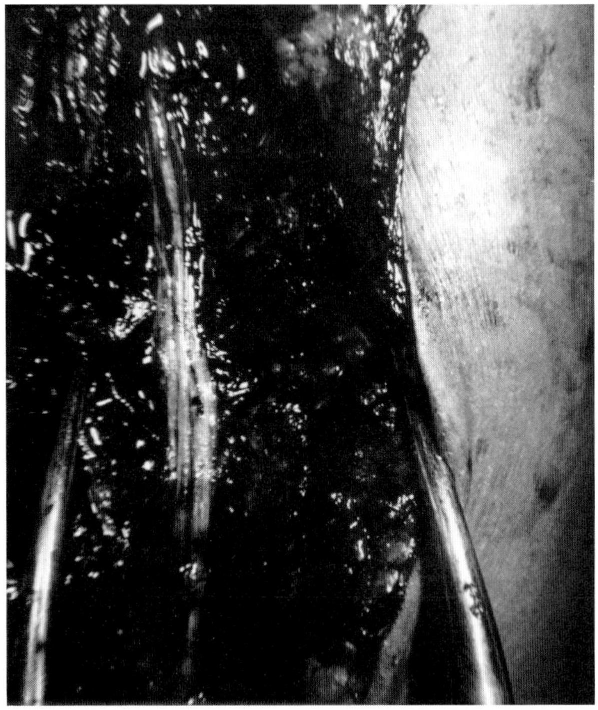

Figure 35-13. *Common peroneal nerve reconstruction using interfascicular grafting technique with multiple autologous sural nerve segments. (Arrows indicate proximal and distal nerve graft coaptation sites.)*

In my experience the results of nerve grafting are related in part to the length of defect to be reconstructed. Graft lengths of 8 cm or less have a reasonable expectation for recovery if they are done within 6 months post-injury.[21] The degree of motor recovery decreases when graft lengths exceed 8 cm and when there is a delay in treatment (see Chaps. 24 and 39). For defects exceeding 15 cm, nerve grafting is indicated only in unusual circumstances; in such cases, palliative procedures involving a tendon transfer or an orthotic device are preferable.

Simultaneous tendon transfer is considered in patients undergoing nerve graft reconstruction of defects exceeding 8 cm less than 6 months post-injury (or shorter defects if treatment is delayed beyond 9 months). The preferred tendon transfer procedure for common peroneal nerve palsy is posterior tibial transfer to either anterior tibial tendon or the middle cuneiform bone (Fig. 35-14) (see Chap. 53). This procedure removes a

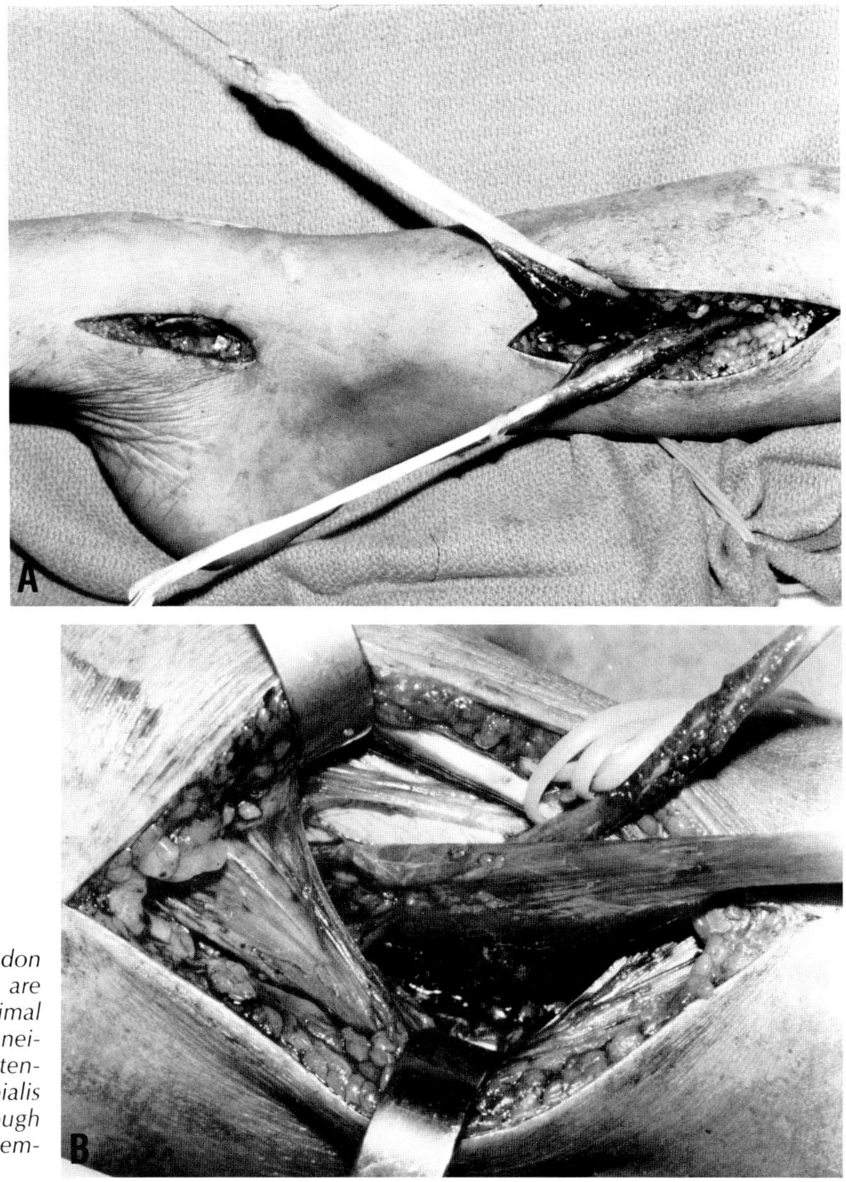

Figure 35-14. *(**A**) Posterior tibial tendon and flexor digitorum longus tendon are isolated and withdrawn through proximal wound prior to transfer to middle cuneiform and extensor digitorum longus tendons, respectively. (**B**) Passage of tibialis posterior tendon and muscle through window in tibiofibular intraosseous membrane.*

deforming force (ankle inversion) and restores ankle extension. In many patients, however, tendon transfer alone does not obviate the need for a supportive orthosis, since it does little to improve ankle stability. In patients with paralysis of the deep peroneal nerve division only, ankle balance is not a problem. Inversion provided by the posterior tibial tendon is balanced by intact ankle everters (peroneal muscles). Thus, ankle balance is best left undisturbed. In such patients, an appropriate choice for tendon transfer is the medial gastrocnemius with an attached strip of tendo Achillis to the anterior tibial tendon (Fig. 35-15) with or without flexor digitorum longus to extensor hallucis and digitorum longus tendons.

The alternative to tendon transfer is the use of

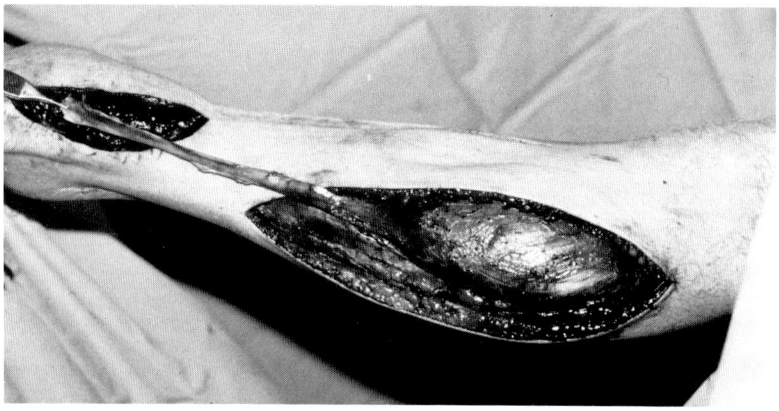

Figure 35-15. *Medial gastrocnemius transfer to tibialis anterior tendon for isolated deep peroneal palsy.*

an orthosis to assist ankle extension and control ankle imbalance or instability. The most useful and least cumbersome orthosis is the posterior polypropylene splint (Fig. 35-16). This device accommodates to most footwear and alleviates the slap-foot gait while simultaneously controlling ankle instability. For heavier activity it may not be sufficiently strong; in such cases, a shoe-mounted double-upright dorsiflexion-assist hinged ankle splint is recommended.

For nerve defects exceeding 15 cm, or in those cases without recovery more than 1 year post-injury, tendon transfer alone or an orthosis is considered. Injuries distal to the knee require individual consideration for treatment. The degree of functional loss related to nerve injury vs that of direct muscle or tendon injury is taken into account. Nerve repair or reconstruction distal to the mid-tibia is not advised, except when symptoms related to a painful neuroma are debilitating.

SAPHENOUS NERVE

The saphenous nerve, a cutaneous branch of the femoral nerve, has a superficial position in the distal medial thigh. It has no motor component. It supplies sensibility from the anterior medial knee to the anterior medial ankle (see Fig. 35-1). While injury to this nerve does not result in a profound functional sensory deficit, it may lead to a troublesome neuroma (Fig. 35-17). In such a case, initial management is directed to desensitization measures or friction massage. If ineffective, proximal neurectomy, allowing the sectioned nerve end to retract into deep tissues, is recommended. This nerve is expendable and may be used as a source of nerve graft material.

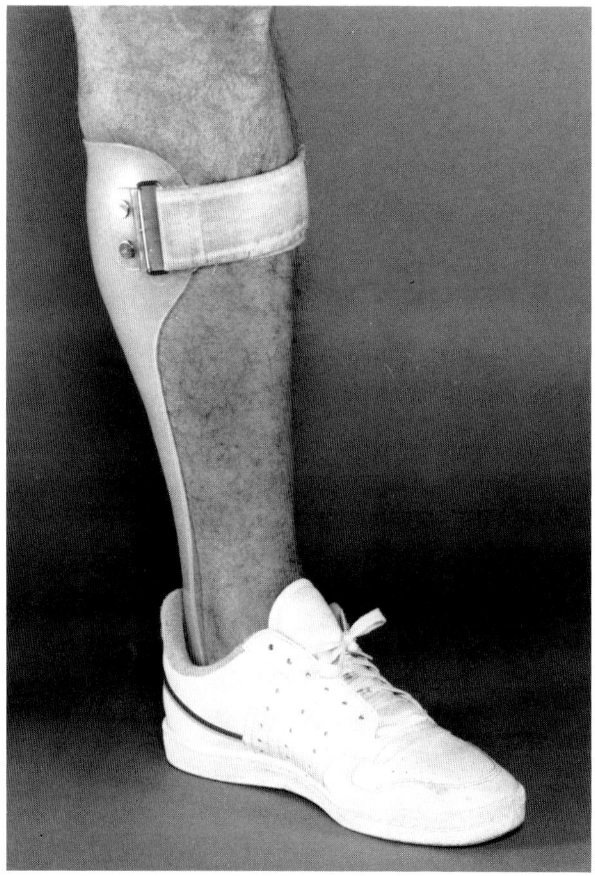

Figure 35-16. *A polypropylene orthosis is useful for palliative management of peroneal nerve palsy.*

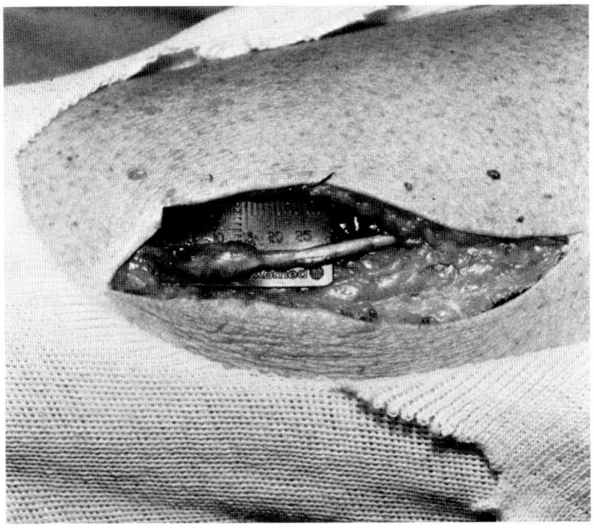

Figure 35-17. *This saphenous neuroma was isolated and excised because of troublesome neuroma symptoms unresponsive to desensitization therapy.*

SURAL NERVE

The sural nerve supplies sensibility to the distal lateral leg, lateral ankle, and lateral foot, usually as far distally as the fifth toe. It has no motor component. It originates from the medial sural cutaneous nerve (a branch of the posterior tibial nerve) alone in 20% of patients; in the remaining 80%, the sural nerve is formed by union of the medial sural cutaneous nerve with the peroneal communicating branch of the common peroneal nerve or the lateral sural cutaneous nerve in the distal third of the leg.[14] The chief importance of the sural nerve and its tributaries (medial sural cutaneous, peroneal communicating branch) is as a source of nerve graft material (see Chap. 38) and its accessibility for diagnostic peripheral nerve biopsy. Rarely, following injury, a painful neuroma results. Management principles are as outlined for the saphenous nerve.

LATERAL FEMORAL CUTANEOUS NERVE

Neuropathy of the lateral femoral cutaneous nerve is relatively common and is better known as *meralgia paresthetica.* In most instances, pathology occurs near the anterior superior iliac spine, and symptoms resolve with time. While the nerve may be injured at any point throughout its course, most commonly it is transected during harvest of anterior iliac bone grafts, during elevation of groin flaps, or while making an incision in the anterolateral thigh. Occasionally, troublesome, painful neuroma symptoms result following laceration.[9]

REFERENCES

1. Aldea PA, Shaw WW. Lower extremity nerve injuries. Clin Plast Surg 1986; 13:691–699.
2. Berry H, Richardson PM. Common peroneal nerve palsy: A clinical and electrophysiological review. J Neurol Neurosurg Psychiatry 1976; 39:1162–1171.
3. Clark DF. External popliteal nerve injuries. Illinois Med J 1930; 58:117–121.
4. Clark K, Williams PE, Willis W, McGavron W. Injection injury of the sciatic nerve. In: Ojemann RG, ed. Clinical neurosurgery, vol. 17. Baltimore: Williams & Wilkins, 1970:111–124.
5. Clawson DK, Seddon HJ. The late consequences of sciatic nerve injury. J Bone Joint Surg [Br] 1960; 42:213–225.
6. Hattrup SJ, Wood MB. Delayed neural reconstruction in the lower extremity: Results of interfascicular nerve grafting. Foot Ankle 1986; 7:105–109.
7. Highet WB, Holmes W. Traction injuries to the lateral popliteal nerve and traction injuries to peripheral nerves after suture. Br J Surg 1943; 30:212–233.
8. Huittinen VM. Lumbosacral nerve injury in fracture of the pelvis. A postmortem radiographic and pathoanatomical study. Acta Chir Scand 1972 (suppl); 429.
9. Kapell HP. Lower extremity lesions. In: Omer GE Jr, Spinner M, eds. Management of peripheral nerve problems. Philadelphia: WB Saunders, 1980:626–638.
10. Kline DG. Operative management of major nerve lesions of the lower extremity. Surg Clin North Am 1972; 52:1247–1265.
11. Meyer VE. Specific problems of skeletal management in upper limb replantation. In: Urbaniak J, ed. Microsurgery for major limb reconstruction. St. Louis: CV Mosby, 1987:56–61.
12. Millesi H. Nerve grafts: Indications, techniques, and prognosis. In: Omer GE Jr, Spinner M, eds. Management of peripheral nerve problems. Philadelphia: WB Saunders, 1980:410–430.

13. Millesi H. Lower extremity nerve lesions. In Terzis J, ed. Microreconstruction of nerve injuries. Philadelphia: WB Saunders, 1987:239–251.
14. Ortiguela ME, Wood MB, Cahill DR. Anatomy of the sural nerve complex. J Hand Surg [Am] 1987; 12:1119–1123.
15. Patterson FP. Neurological complications of fractures and dislocations of the pelvis. J Trauma 1972; 12:1013–1024.
16. Siliski JM, Scott RD. Obturator nerve palsy resulting from intrapelvic extrusion of cement during total hip replacement. J Bone Joint Surg [Am] 1985; 67: 1225–1228.
17. Simon KJ, Goodrich A. Femoral neuropathy: A case report and topic review. Orthopedics 1984; 7: 1841–1844.
18. Weber ER, Daube JR, Coventry MB. Peripheral neuropathies associated with total hip arthroplasty. J Bone Joint Surg [Am] 1976; 58:66–69.
19. White J. The results of traction injuries to the common peroneal nerve. J Bone Joint Surg [Br] 1968; 50:346–350.
20. Wood MB. Atlas of reconstructive microsurgery. Rockville, MD: Aspen, 1990:13–35.
21. Wood MB. Peroneal nerve palsy: Results of surgery. Clin Orthop (accepted for publication).

VII

NERVE GRAFTING

36 Overcoming Defects in Peripheral Nerves

37 Indications and Techniques of Nerve Grafting

38 Donor Nerves for Grafting

39 Results of Nerve Grafting

40 Vascularized Nerve Grafts

41 Nerve Grafting Through Resorbable Tubes

36

Overcoming Defects in Peripheral Nerves

Thomas Trumble

AUTHOR'S KEY POINTS

- The four major methods for overcoming nerve defects to achieve end-to-end coaptation are in situ mobilization, rerouting and transposition, joint positioning, and bone shortening.
- Elongation of nerve to overcome gap formation should be limited to 8% to 10% to avoid neural ischemia. Although nerves have increased stiffness when the repairs are delayed, the vascularity of the nerves is increased so that the same degree of elongation can be tolerated without causing neural ischemia.
- Mobilization by stripping mesoneurial attachments is safely carried 8 to 12 cm along each end of the nerve. Larger nerves tolerate greater lengths of mobilization than smaller ones. The ratio that represents the maximal amount of mobilization possible before neural ischemia occurs is 1:45 (diameter of the nerve:length mobilized).
- Maintaining tension on unrepaired nerves initially minimizes the amount of nerve mobilization needed secondarily for repair.
- Recommendations for overcoming a segmental defect in peripheral nerve have been determined for immediate repair of acute injuries. With a prolonged interval to repair, the increased shortening of the nerve causes a sixfold increase in the deficit that must be overcome (1.1 diameters in acute repairs vs 6.3 diameters of the original nerve in delayed repairs).

Defects in peripheral nerves result from injuries that cause acute segmental loss of nerve, from delayed repairs that allow retraction of nerve ends, and from lesions-in-continuity and tumors that require segmental nerve resection. Surgeons face several important choices as they attempt to obtain functional return in the treatment of nerve lesions with significant gaps. I have found an algorithm for repair of peripheral nerve injuries helpful (Fig. 36-1).

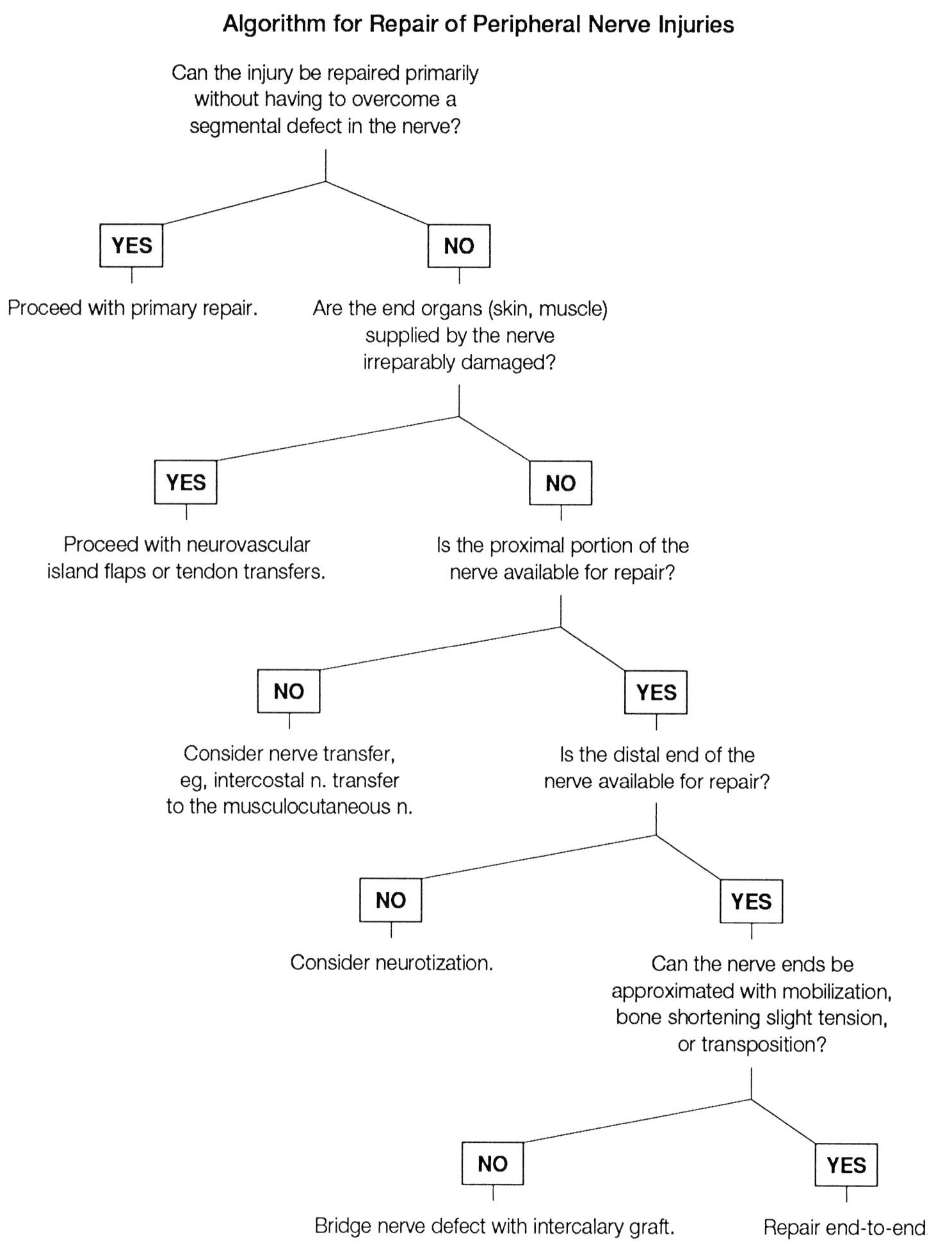

Figure 36–1. *The different methods for reconstructing peripheral nerve injuries are outlined in this algorithm.*

NERVE INJURIES CAUSING SIGNIFICANT GAPS

The Distal End of the Nerve and the Sensory or Motor End-Organs are Irreparably Damaged

Motor or sensory reinnervation may be impossible due to concomitant injury (eg, crush, burn,) to muscle or skin in the distribution of an injured nerve. The delay between initial injury and repair or the proximal nature of an injury also may make nerve reconstruction impossible.[20] In these cases tendon transfers or cutaneous transfers in the form of neurovascular island pedicle flaps are the most useful methods of salvage (see Chap. 56).[11]

Reinnervation of Distal Tissues by Nerve Reconstruction

When the proximal and distal ends of transected nerve cannot be reapproximated, autogenous nerve grafts from a distant donor site are most commonly used to bridge the defect. Some complex injuries allow reconstruction of one nerve using an adjacent irreparably injured nerve.[14,24] The donor nerve can be transferred as a pedicle graft (Fig. 36-2),[24] a vascularized graft (see Chap. 40),[21] or a nonvascularized fascicular graft. When injury to the proximal end of the nerve precludes the use of nerve grafts, nerve transfers may permit reinnervation, particularly of motor end-organs. When injury to the distal nerve end (with or without additional trauma to the proximal nerve end) precludes the use of a graft or transfer, neurotization (embedding the distal end of the nerve directly into recipient muscle) can restore some motor function.[5,25] Either the originally injured nerve or a previously uninjured transferred nerve is used for this procedure (see Chap. 55).

OVERCOMING NERVE GAPS FOR END-TO-END COAPTATION

There are four techniques for overcoming gaps for the purpose of achieving direct coaptation of nerve ends: nerve stump mobilization, nerve rerouting and transposition, joint positioning, and bone shortening.

Nerve Mobilization In Situ

Mobilization involves the release of constricting fascia, division of mesoneural attachments, dissection or division of nerve branches that tether nerve, and occasionally epineurolysis. The fundamental objective of mobilizing nerve stumps is to provide additional length in order to decrease tension on the repair site.

Nerve Repair Under Tension

The major problem associated with repairing peripheral nerve under tension is the difficulty in determining the critical tension limits insofar as both repair site integrity and nerve stump blood supply are concerned. Experimental and clinical studies have reported varying safe limits, depending on the criteria used. A range of acceptable nerve elongation of 4% to 25% has been proposed in clinical studies.[9,12,15] In experimental studies, some authors noted that 15% elongation caused a consistent loss of motor function, and others noted a decrease in blood flow by microscopic evaluation and laser Doppler technique when nerve was elongated by that amount.[4,6,15] Other investigators noted that dissection of as little as 3 cm of nerve resulted in significantly decreased blood flow,[19] and others found increased scar formation with 2 cm of nerve dissection.[22]

McLaren confirmed a correlation between ischemia, tension, and nerve function.[16] As little as 5N tension decreased nerve blood flow and nerve conduction velocity (NCV), both of which recovered when tension was released. Studies by Lundborg and Rydevik demonstrated the anatomy of the vascular pathways and showed that the blood flow decreased with as little as 5% elongation, and complete loss of blood flow occurred with 15% elongation (Figs. 36-3, 36-4).[15] In acutely repaired injuries, the elongation failure caused by suture pull-out occurs at a 17% increase in length.[6] Therefore, neural ischemia, not suture pull-out strength, is the limiting factor in nerve elongation

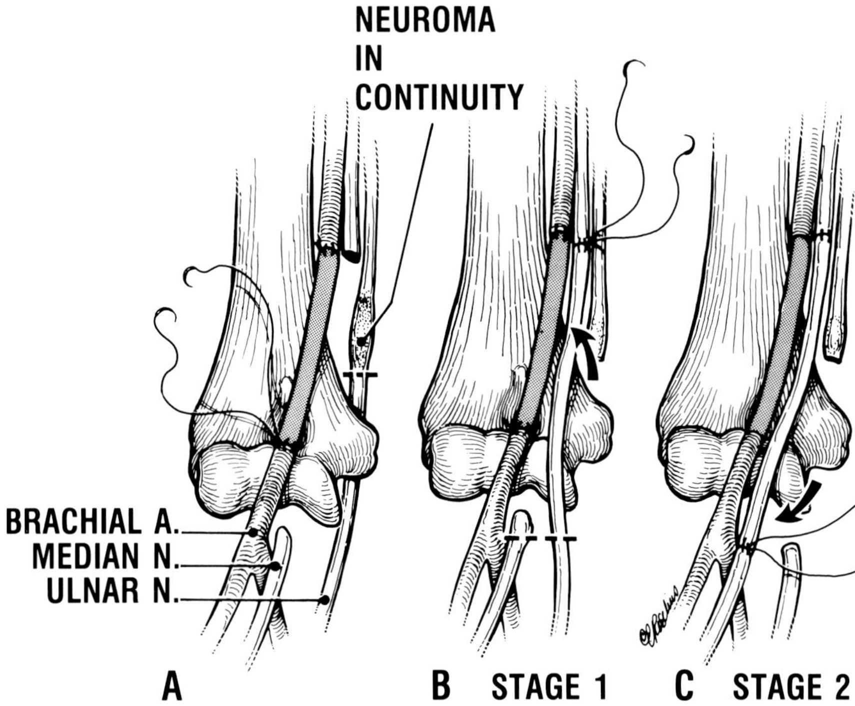

Figure 36–2. *The median nerve can be reconstructed using salvage portions of the ulnar nerve. (**A**) Missile injury of the right arm which destroyed the brachial vessels and the median nerve and injured the ulnar nerve in continuity. Complete median and ulnar paralysis. Immediate repair of the brachial artery with a vein graft from the leg. (**B**) Three months later first stage of an ulnar-to-median nerve–pedicle graft, with anterior transposition of the ulnar nerve. (**C**) After a further 2 months, bridging operation completed. Fourteen months after the injury: all median-innervated muscles are at level 4 except pronator teres and abductor pollicis brevis, both 0. Sensibility 3+. (Reproduced with permission from Seddon HJ. Surgical disorders of peripheral nerves, ed 2. Edinburgh: Churchill Livingstone, 1975:250–315.)*

during acute repairs. The limit for elongation of unscarred peripheral nerves has now been established as 8% to 10%, a point at which Lundborg and Rydevik have shown blood flow decreased by 50%.

With delayed repair of nerves with segmental defects in which fibrosis and wallerian degeneration have taken place, elasticity decreases by as much as 50% (Fig. 36-5). Studies of the modulus of elasticity of repaired nerves under tension have shown that the nerve adapts to tension with increasing cross-sectional area and increasing tissue compliance.[1]

Recent in vivo biomechanical studies have confirmed that both acutely and chronically divided nerves demonstrate viscoelastic properties (Fig. 36-6).[6] The stress relaxation of peripheral nerves directly correlates with the increase in neural blood flow over time (Fig. 36-7). It should be noted that the baseline blood flow in previously divided nerves is significantly higher than in acutely divided nerves (Fig. 36-8), probably as the result of ingrowth of small vessels. Laser Doppler flowmetry measurements show that the blood flow in both recently and previously divided nerves can recover within 30 minutes due to stress relaxation of the nerve following 8% elongation, but not 15% elongation (Fig. 36-8). Using an animal model, acute division resulted in a nerve gap equivalent to 1.0 diameters (4.4% of the length) of the intact nerve, whereas previous division caused a deficit equivalent to 6.3 diameters (27.8% of the intact length of the nerve). Acute and delayed repairs failed at approximately 16% to 17% elongation. For either

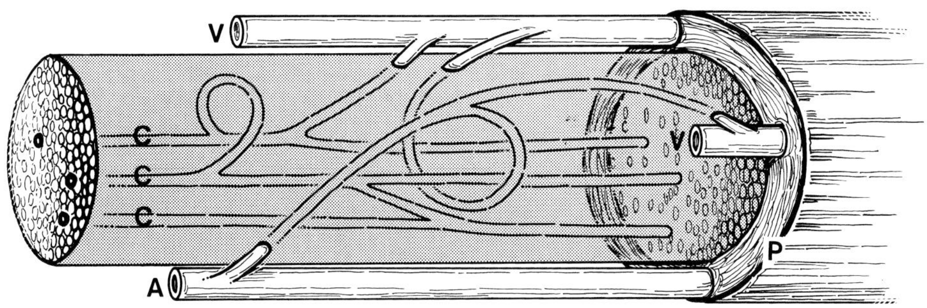

Figure 36–3. The pattern of vessels is highlighted in this schematic drawing of the intrafascicular microvascular architecture. Note the capillary loops, sometimes arranged in planes perpendicular to the long axis of the nerve. Arrows indicate the direction of flow. P, perineurium; A, arteriole; V, venule; C, capillary. (Reproduced with permission from Lundborg G, Bränemark PI. Microvascular structure and function of peripheral nerves. Vital microscopic studies of the tibial nerve of the rabbit. Adv Microcirc 1968;1:66–88.)

type of repair, ischemia, not the strength of the repair, is the limiting factor in nerve elongation.

Clinical Assessment of Nerve Elongation

Author's Preferred Method

The tolerable limit for nerve mobilization can be determined clinically by placing methylene blue dye markers on the nerve prior to mobilization. Because the proximal and distal ends of the nerve move at different rates after tension is applied, the percentage of elongation is calculated by the following formula:[15]

$$[(A' - B') - (A - B)/(A - B)] \times 100$$

(A − B) represents the original length, and (A′ − B′) represents the length after elongation.

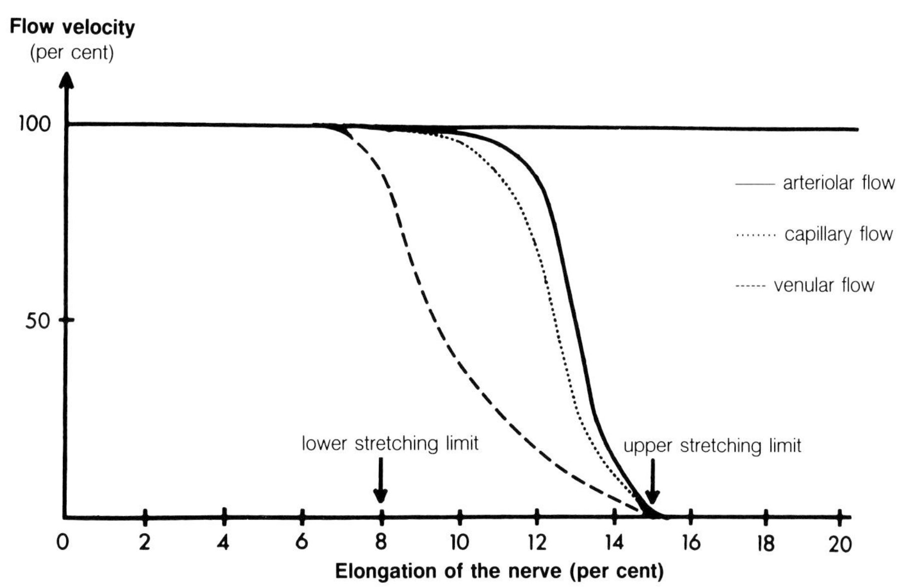

Figure 36–4. The effects of tension on the microvascular flow in rabbit tibial nerve are demonstrated in this graph. The flow velocity in the different components of the vascular bed was estimated by sight. (Reproduced with permission from Lundborg G, Rydevik B. Effects of stretching the tibial nerve of the rabbit: A preliminary study of the intraneural circulation and barrier function of the perineurium. J Bone Joint Surg [Br] 1973;55:395.)

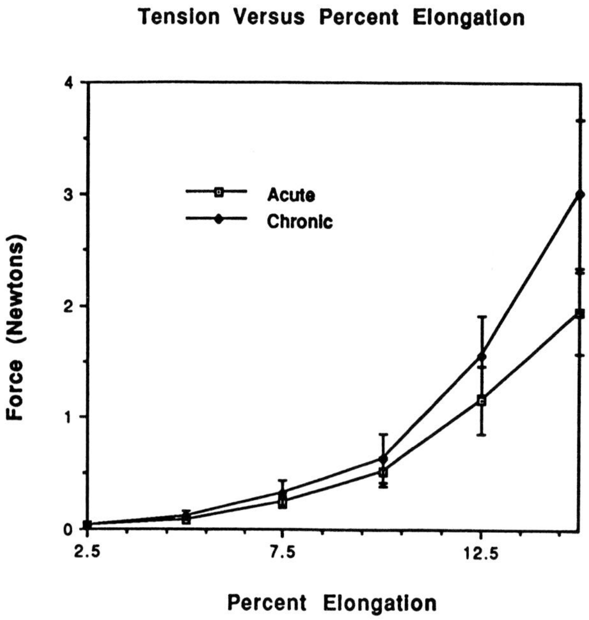

Figure 36–5. The previously divided nerves (chronic injuries) demonstrate increased stiffness, particularly from 12.5% to 15% elongation of the nerve.

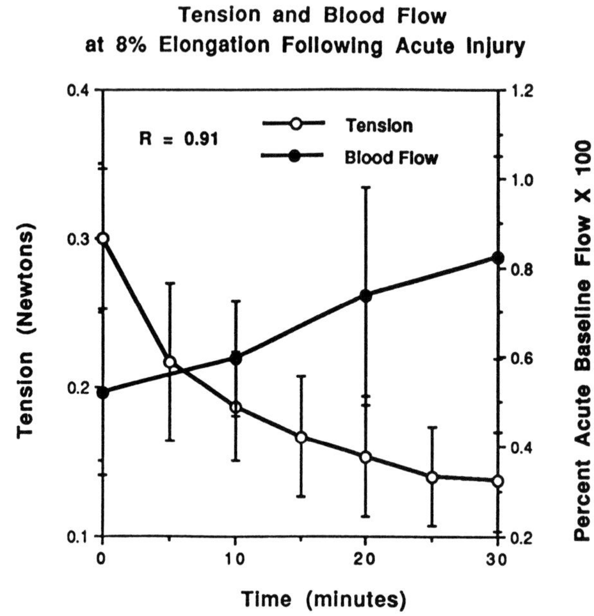

Figure 36–7. There is a direct correlation between tension and blood flow. As the tension decreases, there is an increase in blood flow over time.

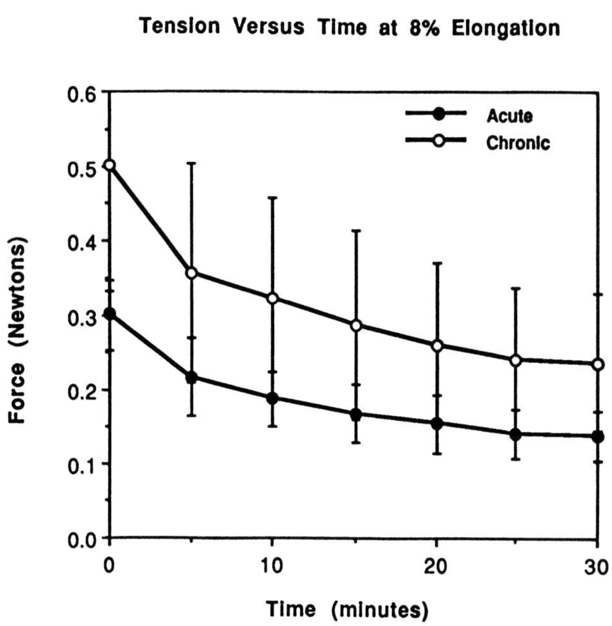

Figure 36–6. Both acutely and chronically injured nerves demonstrate viscoelasticity with significant decrease in stress over time following 8% elongation.

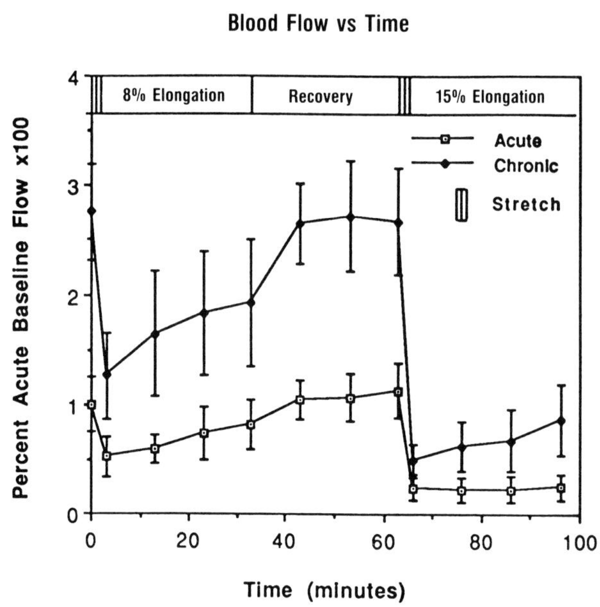

Figure 36–8. Previously divided (chronic injuries) nerves have a higher baseline blood flow than acutely divided nerves. Following 8% elongation, both groups have a substantial recovery of blood flow. However, 15% elongation results in a profound ischemia with much less recovery in blood flow.

From a practical standpoint, this technique is most helpful in determining whether to graft a defect that appears borderline for end-to-end coaptation. A convenient length (eg, 5 cm) along the proximal and distal ends of the nerve is marked with methylene blue. If a change in length greater than 10% of the original length occurs (eg, 0.5 cm), nerve grafting should be used to bridge the defect.

Nerve Rerouting and Transposition

The technique of transposition moves a nerve from its original bed to a site that allows a more direct course. The procedure can provide several additional centimeters of length and allows transfer to a well-vascularized bed free of mechanical impingement when the original nerve bed is no longer suitable (eg, elbow fracture with transaction of the ulnar nerve that requires transposition for the combined effects of preventing nerve impingement by internal fixation devices and overcoming defects in order to accomplish tension-free repair).

The following sites are most appropriate for nerve transposition:

- Ulnar nerve at the elbow
- Recurrent motor branch of ulnar nerve at wrist (into carpal tunnel)[2]
- Median nerve at the elbow (with release of the lacertus fibrosus, pronator teres muscle, and flexor digitorum sublimus muscle)
- Common peroneal nerve at the proximal fibula (with partial or complete resection of the fibular head)

Joint Positioning

The use of joint positioning to decrease tension on the repair site is common. The acceptable levels of joint flexion were determined empirically by early investigators who, during World Wars I and II, accrued a large volume of clinical experience with massive injuries to peripheral nerves.[3,7,8,24,26] Table 36-1 lists the general limits established for positioning joints to overcome small- to moderate-sized gaps.

The greatest reductions in tension at the repair site occur with positioning the joints closest to the site of injury. When used in conjunction with nerve rerouting, tension is further reduced, especially in situations where the nerve lies in an eccentric position relative to the center of rotation of a joint that has one plane of motion. For example, anterior transposition of the ulnar nerve not only increases length by mobilization but also multiplies the effect by moving the nerve inside the center of motion of the elbow so that a smaller radius of flexion is required.

Table 36-1.

Joint Position	Length Gained (cm)
Wrist 40° dorsiflexion or palmar flexion	2
Elbow 90° flexion	4
Shoulder abduction (to 90°)	2
Knee 90° flexion	5
Ankle 10° flexion (planar or distal)	2

One conservative method for correcting joint position postoperatively starts 2 to 3 weeks after repair and allows a 10° per week increase in joint motion. An alternate technique requires dividing the total amount of flexion necessary for overcoming the gap into thirds. At 2-week intervals, the joint is extended one third of the total amount of flexion at each interval, beginning at the second week post-repair. By 6 weeks the joint is fully extended.

OVERCOMING SPECIFIC NERVE DEFECTS

Defects in the Brachial Plexus

The brachial plexus is formed from five spinal roots (C5–T1) and comprises three trunks, anterior and posterior divisions, three cords, and multiple terminal nerves. The nerves that enter muscle shortly after they branch—the suprascapular, dorsal scapular, medial and lateral pectoral, axillary, and subscapular—tether the plexus to the muscles of the shoulder girdle, making mobilization of the brachial plexus difficult.

Only lateral bending of the neck and shoulder positioning (abduction for upper and adduction for lower plexus injuries) decreases tension on the brachial plexus significantly. These techniques are not practical, however, in most circumstances. Shoulder positioning can provide 2 cm of nerve length, although adduction (lower trunk repair) is the most practical. For these reasons, nerve grafting is usually the preferred treatment when significant defects in the brachial plexus exist.

Defects in the Median Nerve

The median nerve, the terminal nerve of the medial and lateral cords containing axons from the spinal roots of C6–T1, accompanies the brachial artery into the forearm by passing beneath the lacertus fibrosus, traveling between the two heads of the pronator teres muscle. The nerve dives deep to the flexor digitorum superficialis muscle at the edge of the muscle fascia. It then travels between the flexor digitorum superficialis and flexor digitorum profundus muscles, becoming more superficial in the distal portion of the forearm. It enters the hand through the carpal tunnel.

Injury at Arm Level

The lack of muscular branches in the arm facilitates mobilization of the median nerve at this level. Release of the pectoralis major muscle insertion at the humerus provides exposure but does not substantially increase the length available for repair. Elbow flexion and release of the lacertus fibrosus, humeral head of the pronator teres muscle, and flexor digitorum superficialis muscles ("pronator syndrome release") provides anterior translation of the nerve, which combined with elbow flexion decreases tension of the repair site significantly (Fig. 36-9). Shortening of the humerus is an option, particularly in patients who have sustained fractures. A maximum of 5 cm of humeral shortening is acceptable.[26]

Gradual elongation of nerve repaired under tension occurs to a greater extent in segments proximal and distal to the repair site.[1] Patients in whom extreme joint positioning has been required post-repair may develop a Tinel's sign, at or slightly distal to the repair, that stops advancing as efforts to extend the joint are carried out. If this occurs, excessive tension may be inhibiting or preventing nerve regeneration.

With the advancement of internal fixation techniques to stabilize fracture fragments and allow early motion, nerve grafts have allowed the earlier and more vigorous therapy necessary to regain joint motion, particularly when concomitant intra-articular fractures are present.

Bone Shortening

This technique is applicable to the upper extremity only. Humeral shortening, used most commonly, facilitates both radial and median nerve end-to-end repair and is indicated most often when multiple nerves have been injured and a comminuted fracture is present. Because of the greater distance between an injury at arm level and the muscles supplied by the ulnar nerve, shortening the humerus to overcome a segmental defect in the ulnar nerve is indicated in children and adolescents or when concomitant repair of the median or radial nerve can be accomplished.

Author's Preferred Method

While the literature is inconclusive regarding the optimal method for overcoming defects, a series of guidelines can be established.

Peripheral nerve stumps are mobilized by stripping mesoneural attachments up to a distance of 8 to 12 cm, depending on the diameter of the nerve. As the maximal limit for acceptable mobilization is achieved, the surgeon should remember Lundborg's guideline about keeping the ratio of nerve diameter to length of mobilized segment less than 1:45.[15] In most instances elongation of nerve by 8% to 10% is the safe limit in acute or delayed repairs. The surgeon should expect a gap equivalent to 1.0 nerve diameters in acute repairs and 6.3 diameters in delayed repairs. This limit can be determined by marking the nerve prior to repair with methylene blue as described previously.

The limits for joint positioning for gaining additional length are 90° for the knee and elbow and 40° for the wrist. Safe limits for joint positioning are lower when there is considerable

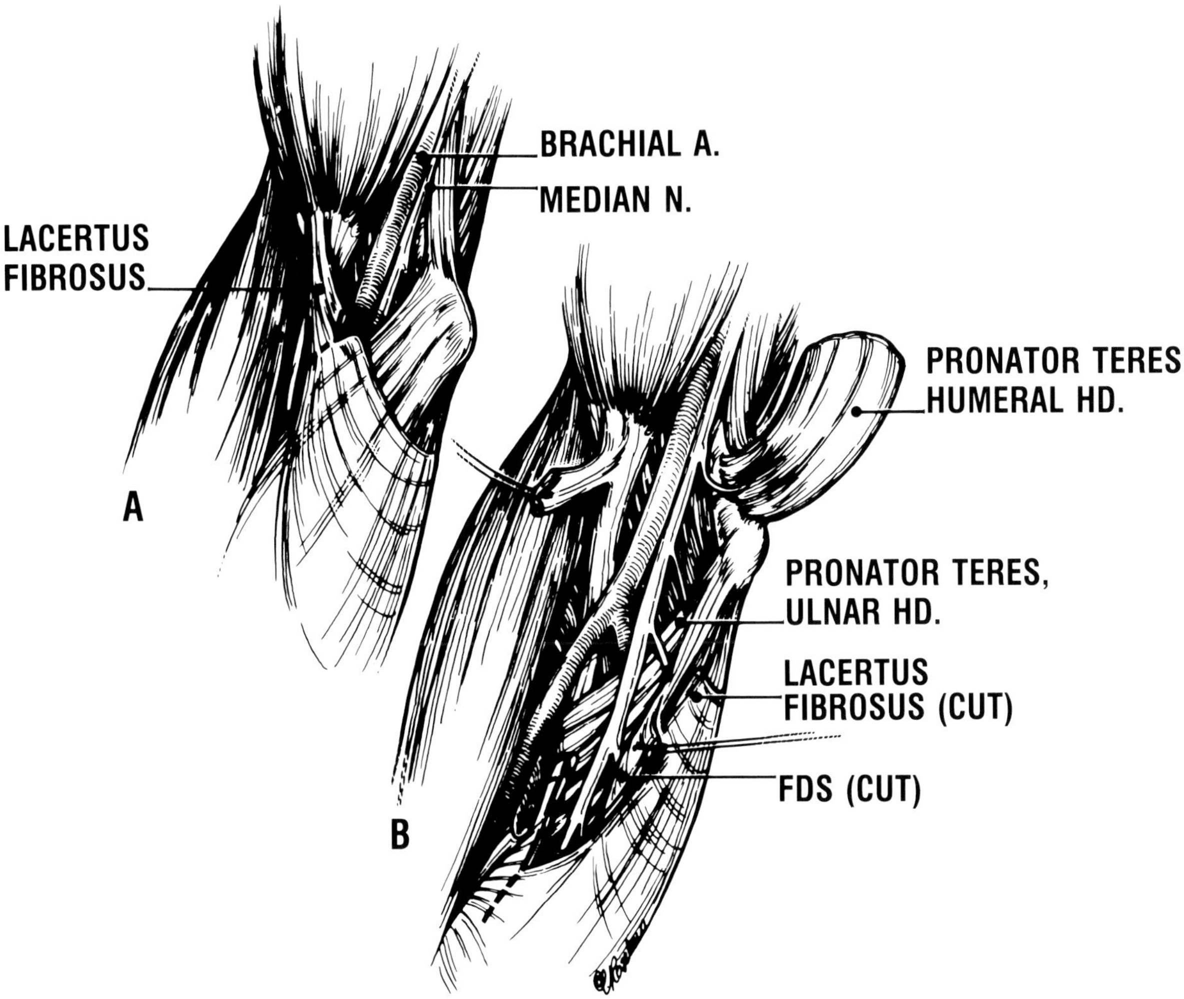

Figure 36–9. *(**A**) The lacertus fibrosus is divided as the first step of a pronator-level release of the median nerve. (**B**) With the additional release of the humeral head of the pronator teres muscle and the fascia and muscular origin of the flexor digitorum sublimus (FDS), further length of the median nerve can be gained.*

scarring, preventing satisfactory nerve repair site excursion. Safe limits in these cases are reduced to 45° elbow flexion, 30° knee flexion, 30° wrist flexion or extension, and 10° plantar flexion of the ankle. If tension persists and bone shortening is not indicated, nerve grafting is required.

Injury at Elbow Level

For mobilization of the nerve at the elbow, the pronator syndrome release described above is used. While the elbow may be flexed to a maximum of 90°, it is difficult to operate on a nerve in this position, and trauma occurs later as efforts to straighten the elbow are carried out. Thus, a safer limit of 45° is preferred. Intraneural dissection of motor branches from the main trunk of the nerve, especially those to the pronator teres muscle and flexor digitorum superficialis, carried out over several centimeters, provides additional length. Total increase in length with a combination of these techniques is 4 to 6 cm (Table 36-2).

Table 36–2.

Median Nerve

I. Maximum length gained with upper extremity position (cm)

Shoulder adduction	2.5
Elbow flexion	3–4
Wrist flexion	2–3

II. Maximum length gained with anterior transposition of the nerve or humeral oestotomy (cm)

Site of Injury	Length Gained
Arm	5.0 with osteotomy
Elbow	2.0 with transposition
Forearm (proximal)	2.0 with transposition

III. Maximum length gained from mobilization of nerve (cm)

Site of Injury	Length Gained
Arm	5
Elbow	4
Forearm: proximal	3
middle	4
distal	3
Wrist	2.5

IV. Total length gained with combination of techniques (cm)

Site of Injury	Gap Closed Without Grafting
Arm	5 (10 with humeral osteotomy)
Elbow	6
Forearm: proximal	6
middle	5
distal	4
Wrist	2.5

Injury at Forearm Level

Proximally, the nerve is deep to the flexor digitorum superficialis, but distally the nerve becomes more superficial as it passes the musculotendinous junction. There are motor branches from the proximal half of the nerve, making mobilization in this region more difficult. The pronator syndrome release, along with dissection of the nerve's motor branches, is often necessary. For mid-forearm injuries, elbow flexion, wrist palmar-flexion, or both, gain 4 to 6 cm.

Injury at Wrist Level

The wrist is the most common site of median nerve injury. A particular concern in this region is the need for satisfactory soft-tissue coverage of the nerve. Occasionally cutaneous pedicle flaps (eg, groin or abdominal flaps) are necessary to provide the quality of skin coverage necessary to allow nerve regeneration. Carpal tunnel release and mobilization of the nerve are the initial methods for gaining length. Wrist flexion provides an additional 1 to 2 cm of length. Table 36-2 shows, from a composite of clinical data, the maximal lengths that can be overcome in the acute setting with nerve mobilization and joint positioning.[8,18,19,23,26]

Defects in the Ulnar Nerve

The ulnar nerve, the terminal branch of the medial cord of the brachial plexus, contains nerves from three spinal roots (C7–T1). In the middle third of the arm, the nerve departs from the axillary sheath, piercing the medial intramuscular septum. At the level of the elbow, the nerve passes just posterior to the medial epicondyle of the humerus. The nerve enters the forearm by diving deep between the two heads of the flexor carpi ulnaris. The nerve courses beneath a fascial band as it passes between the two heads of the flexor carpi ulnaris muscle. There are several motor branches to the flexor carpi ulnaris muscle at this level. The nerve then travels between the flexor digitorum sublimus and the flexor digitorum profundus through the remaining length of the forearm. Five to seven centimeters proximal to the ulnar styloid, the dorsal sensory nerve branches to supply sensation to the dorsum of the hand. The ulnar nerve crosses the wrist in Guyon's canal, where it gives off motor branches to the hypothenar eminence as well as the recurrent motor branch.

Injury at Arm Level

Since there are no significant motor branches in the arm, extensive mobilization at this level is indicated. As with the median nerve, humeral shortening can help overcome gaps in the ulnar nerve when there has been a fracture, segmental loss, or malunion of the humerus requiring osteotomy. The amount of return of motor function is weighed against the morbidity associated with humeral osteotomy. Resection of the anterior portion of the intramuscular septum and transposition of the ulnar nerve provides 4 to 5 cm of length beyond that gained by mobilization. Elbow flexion and shoulder adduction add more length, especially once the nerve has been transposed (Table 36-3).

Injury at Elbow Level

Often, for injuries at this level, transposition of the ulnar nerve serves a dual purpose: it removes the nerve from the site of mechanical impingement and provides additional length. Transposition of the ulnar nerve may be carried out as described in Chapters 77, 78, and 80. Release of the fascia of the flexor carpi ulnaris, dissection of the motor branches, and flexion of the elbow to 45° provide added length.

Table 36–3.

Ulnar Nerve

I. Maximal length gained with upper extremity position (cm)

Shoulder adduction	1–2
Elbow flexion	2–4
Wrist flexion	2

II. Length gained with transposition of nerve (cm)

Site of Injury	Length Gained
Arm	3–4
Elbow	4
Forearm: proximal	2
middle	2
Distal and wrist (Boyes' technique)	1–2

III. Length gained with mobilization of nerve (cm)

Site of Injury	Length Gained
Arm	2
Elbow	1
Forearm: proximal	1
middle	2
distal	2
Wrist	1

IV. Total length gained with combination of techniques (cm)

Site of Injury	Gap Closed Without Grafting
Arm	6
Elbow	6–8
Forearm: proximal	4–5
middle	3–4
distal	4
Wrist	3–4

Injury at Forearm or Palm Level

The more proximal defects in the forearm are difficult to manage because of motor branches to the flexor carpi ulnaris and flexor digitorum profundus. However, proximal defects can be overcome more easily by anterior transposition than can mid-forearm or distal nerve defects. Distally, with flexion of the wrist and dissection of the dorsal sensory branch, several centimeters of mobilization can be achieved. Mobilization of the nerve within the palm is extremely difficult due to the many critical sensory and motor branches.

Additional length is gained by transposition of the deep motor branch of the ulnar nerve into the carpal canal. Guyon's canal is released by dividing the pisohamate ligament (Fig. 36-10*A*). The attachment of the hypothenar muscles to the hamate is also released. The ulnar artery is identified and mobilized, and the deep motor branch is separated from the superficial branch by dissection of its epineural sheath. The motor and sensory branches are separated to a point 1 or 2 cm proximal to the pisiform (Fig. 36-10*B*). The transverse carpal ligament is released, and the deep motor branch is transposed into the carpal canal by placing it palmar to the ulnar artery (Fig. 36-10*C*).

Guidelines for maximal lengths that can be overcome in the acute setting are listed in Table 36-3.[7–9,18,24,26]

Defects in the Radial Nerve

The radial nerve, the terminal nerve of the posterior cord of the brachial plexus, receives contributions from C5 to C8 and sometimes T1. The nerve exits the brachial plexus and continues posteriorly to enter the spiral groove of the humerus. In this location it is most susceptible to injury when the humerus is fractured. It is the most commonly injured nerve in the arm. The nerve then courses laterally, where it pierces the intramuscular septum to lie between the brachialis and brachioradialis. Just distal to the elbow, the nerve divides into a sensory branch and the posterior interosseous nerve, which dives into the supinator muscle. At this juncture there is usually a thick band of fascia (arcade of Froshe) that the posterior interosseous nerve passes beneath. The posterior interosseous

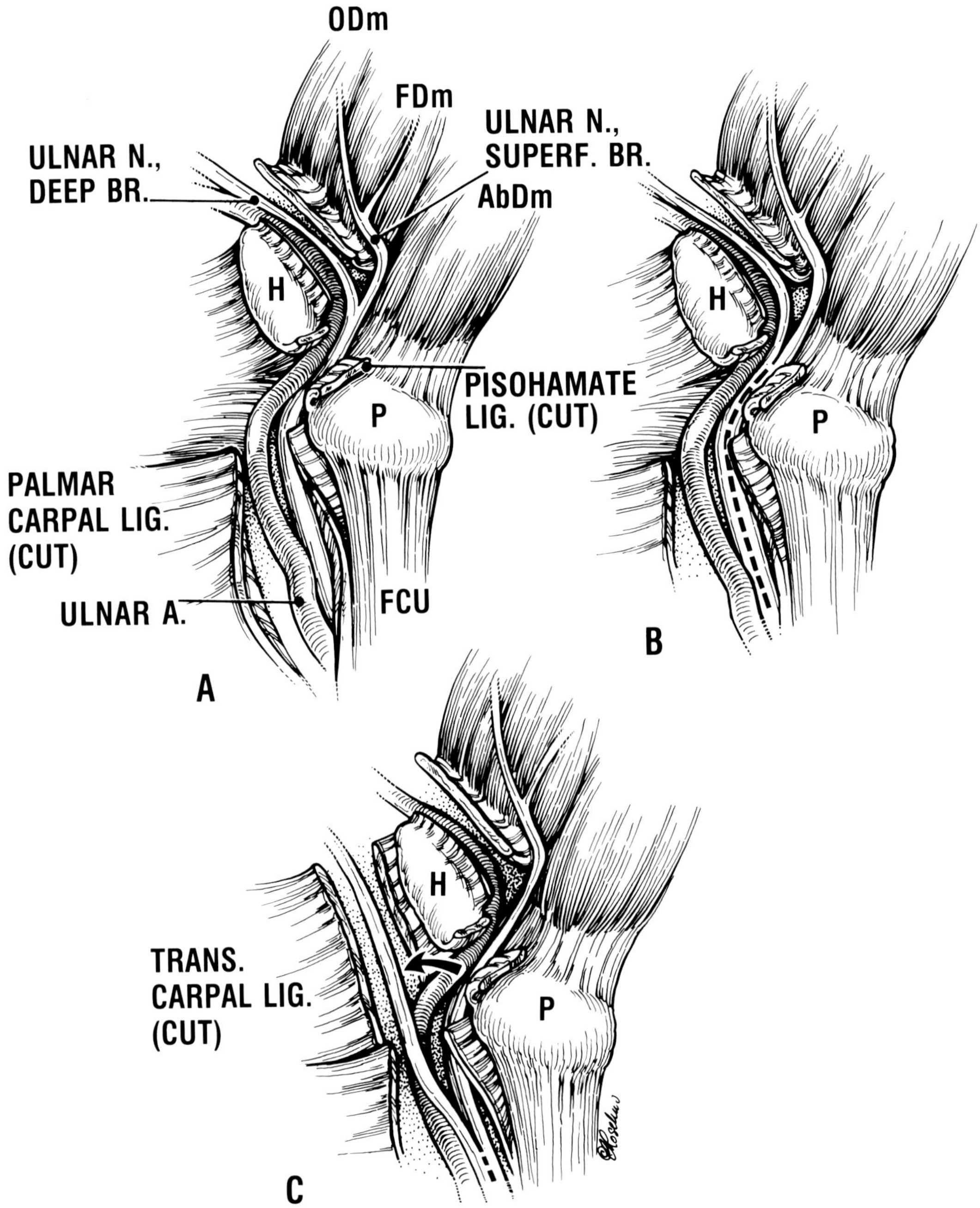

Figure 36–10. *(**A**) In order to transpose the deep motor branch of the ulnar nerve into the carpal tunnel, the pisohamate and the volar carpal ligament are first divided. (**B**) Dissection of epineural sheath allows the two branches of ulnar nerve to be separated to a site proximal to the pisiform. (**C**) The deep branch is then transposed palmar to the branch of the ulnar artery to the superficial palmar arch. AbDm, abductor digiti minimi; FCU, flexor carpi ulnaris; FDm, flexor digiti minimi; H, hamate; ODm, opponens digiti minimi; P, pisiform.*

nerve then branches to supply all the muscles in the dorsal compartment of the forearm. Repair is particularly difficult when posterior interosseous nerve has been injured in the area where it branches. The sensory branch of the radial nerve travels along the underside of the brachioradialis muscle and tendon. Approximately 4 cm from the radial styloid, the sensory branch travels dorsal to the brachioradialis tendon and branches to innervate the skin on the dorsal and radial aspect of the hand.

Injury at Arm Level

Because of the motor branches to the triceps proximally and the bifurcation into sensory and posterior interosseous nerve branches distally, it is difficult to obtain significant length by mobilization of the radial nerve. By dissecting the motor branches both proximally and distally, 1- to 2-cm gaps can be overcome. Flexion of the elbow and release of the intramuscular septum provides another 2 cm. If the radial nerve has been injured in the arm at the time of fracture of the humerus, shortening the bone or transfer anteriorly through the fracture site allows increased mobilization (Table 36-4).[7–9,18,24,26]

Humeral osteotomy effectively provides an additional 5 cm of radial nerve length. The anterolateral approach is indicated (Fig. 36-11). The interval between the brachioradialis and brachialis muscles is developed to expose the distal humerus, identifying the radial nerve. Dissection is extended proximally in the interval between triceps and brachialis. The anterior surface of the humerus is scored with an osteotome to serve as a guide for maintaining correct rotational alignment. Parallel transverse osteotomies are made with an oscillating saw (see Fig. 36-7). A segment of bone is removed and the humerus stabilized with a 4.5-mm dynamic compression plate. The osteotomies can be made in an oblique fashion, if the amount of exposure permits, to maximize the surface area of bone contact. With either technique, bone graft should be added. When a proximal osteotomy is indicated, a blade plate can be fashioned using a semitubular plate. (Repairs of the radial nerve are performed once the humerus has been stabilized.) A posterior

Table 36-4. *Maximal Gaps That Can Be Overcome for Radial Nerve*

I. Length gained with upper extremity position (cm)

Shoulder adduction	1.5
Elbow flexion	3–4

II. Length gained with transposition or humeral osteotomy (cm)

Site of Injury	Length Gained
Arm: Humeral osteotomy	5
Transposition with release of intermuscular septum	1

III. Length gained with mobilization of nerve (cm)

Site of Injury	Length Gained
Arm	2
Forearm: posterior interosseous branch	0.5
sensory branch	2

IV. Total length gained with combination of techniques (cm)

Site of Injury	Gap Closed Without Grafting
Arm	4–6 (9–10 with humeral osteotomy)
Forearm: posterior interosseous branch	0.5
sensory branch	2

plaster splint is used to protect the osteosynthesis site. Elbow motion is initiated at an early interval.

Injury at Forearm Level

The posterior interosseous nerve branches shortly after it dives into the supinator muscle in the proximal portion of the forearm. At this level it is difficult to repair the nerve, even in the acute setting. With chronic injuries, retraction of nerve ends into the muscle belly compounds difficulties in obtaining direct nerve repair. Either nerve grafts or tendon transfers are indicated, depending on the patient's age and the interval to injury. The superficial branch of the radial nerve runs along the underbelly of the brachioradialis muscle. Release of the

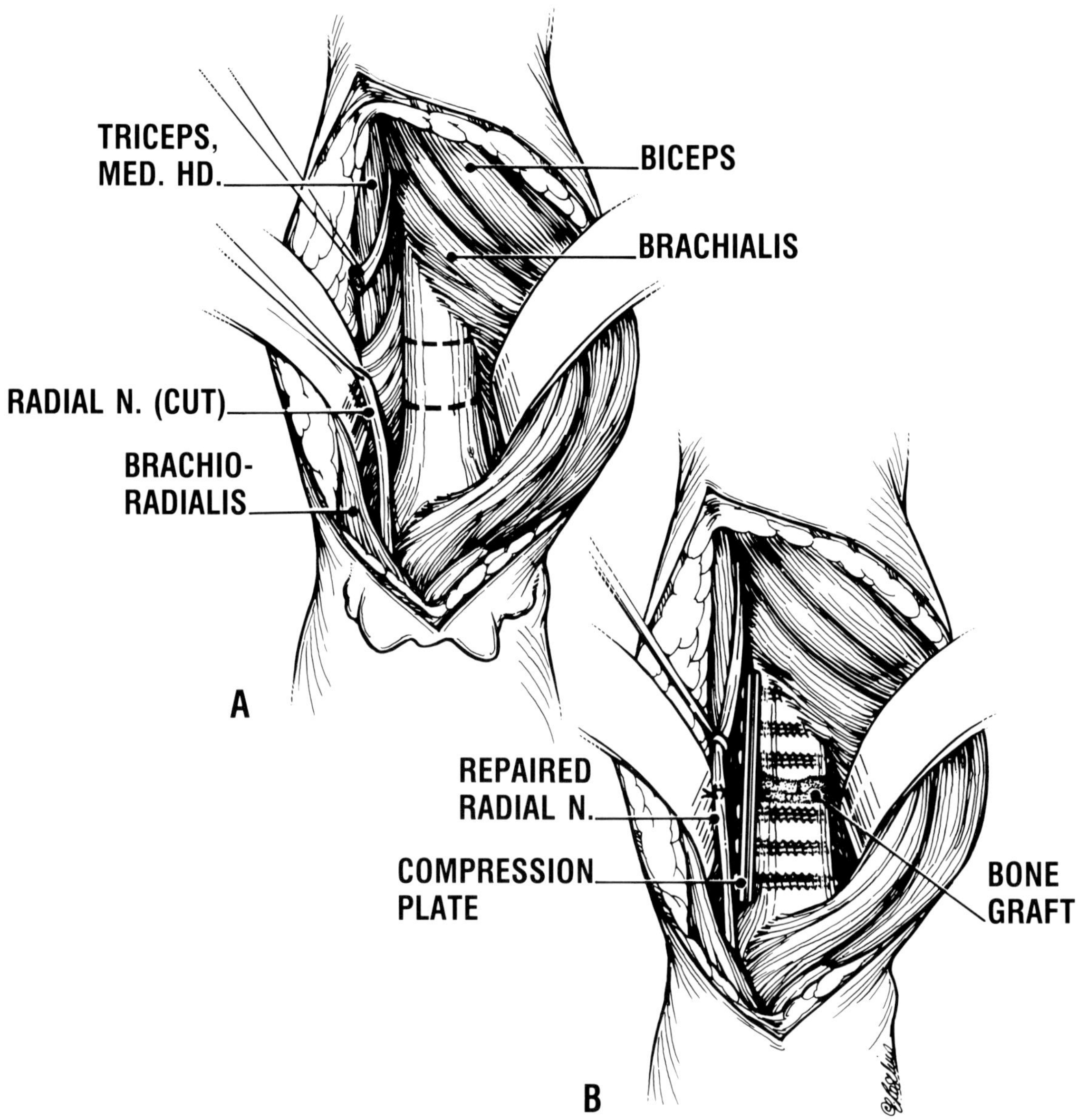

Figure 36–11. *(**A**) In the anterolateral approach to the humerus, the interval between the biceps and brachialis muscles distally and the biceps and triceps muscles proximally is used. (**B**) The humerus is shortened using parallel or oblique osteotomies, stabilized with cortical screws, and augmented with iliac crest bone graft.*

fascial attachments to the distal portion of the brachioradialis, in conjunction with mobilization of the nerve along its long course in the forearm, provides 1 cm of additional length. Guidelines for maximal gaps that can be overcome in the acute setting for the radial nerve are shown in Table 36-4.[7–9,18,24,26]

Defects in the Musculocutaneous Nerve

The musculocutaneous nerve, the terminal branch of the lateral cord of the brachial plexus, contains nerve fibers from C5 and C6. After leaving the brachial plexus, the nerve passes beneath the coracoid and enters the coracobrachialis muscle, 6 to 8 cm below the tip of the coracoid process. The nerve branches at this point to supply the coracobrachialis, biceps brachii, and brachialis muscles.

Injury at Arm Level

Because the nerve travels only a short distance before supplying three muscles, only limited mobilization is possible. Detaching the coracobrachialis from the tip of the coracoid decreases some tension on the repair site in this region. Dissection of the motor branches provides additional length. Guidelines for acute nerve defects that can be repaired are given in Table 36-5.[7–9,18,24,26]

Defects in the Sciatic Nerve

The sciatic nerve is composed of two lumbar and three sciatic roots (L4, L5, S1–S3). The nerve exits the pelvis via the sciatic notch and travels deep to the piriformis muscle. As it courses by the piriformis it becomes more superficial and posterior in orientation. At this site it lies deep to the gluteus medius and superficial to the obturator internus and superior gemellus muscles. Farther distally in the thigh it passes deep (anterior) to the long head of the biceps femoris. Except for the branch to the short head of the biceps femoris, all of the branches from the sciatic nerve exit from the medial side of the nerve to innervate the rest of the hamstring muscles (semitendinosus, semimembranosus, and long head of the biceps) (Fig. 36-12). More distally a medial branch arises to innervate the adductor magnus muscle.

Injury at Thigh Level

Dissection along the lateral aspect of the sciatic nerve provides a 1- to 2-cm increase in length. Intraneural dissection of motor branches from the main portion of the nerve further decreases repair site tension. Guidelines for overcoming nerve gaps in the acute setting are given in Table 36-6.[7–9,18,24,26]

Defects in the Tibial and Peroneal Nerves

The anatomy of the bifurcation of the sciatic nerve into the tibial and peroneal nerves varies greatly. Often the bifurcation occurs in the distal third of the thigh. The peroneal nerve gives off a branch to the short head of the biceps in this case. The tibial (or medial side of the sciatic) nerve provides a medial branch to supply the adductor magnus. The tibial nerve continues distally between the two heads of the gastrocnemius muscle. It disappears

Table 36–5. *Guidelines for Acute Nerve Defects That Can Be Repaired*

I. Length gained with upper extremity position (cm)
Shoulder adduction 0.5–1.5

II. Length gained with mobilization of nerve (cm)

Site of Injury	Length Gained
Shoulder/arm	1–2

III. Total length gained with combination of techniques (cm)

Site of Injury	Gap Closed Without Grafting
Shoulder/arm	2

Table 36–6. *Guidelines for Overcoming Sciatic Nerve Gaps*

I. Length gained with upper extremity position (cm)
Hip extension 1
Knee flexion 3–4

II. Length gained with mobilization of nerve (cm)

Site of Injury	Length Gained
Buttock to upper third of thigh	6
Middle third of thigh	2–3
Distal third of thigh	2–3

III. Total length gained with combination of techniques (cm)

Site of Injury	Gap Closed Without Grafting
Buttock to upper third of thigh	7
Middle third of thigh	5
Distal third of thigh	5

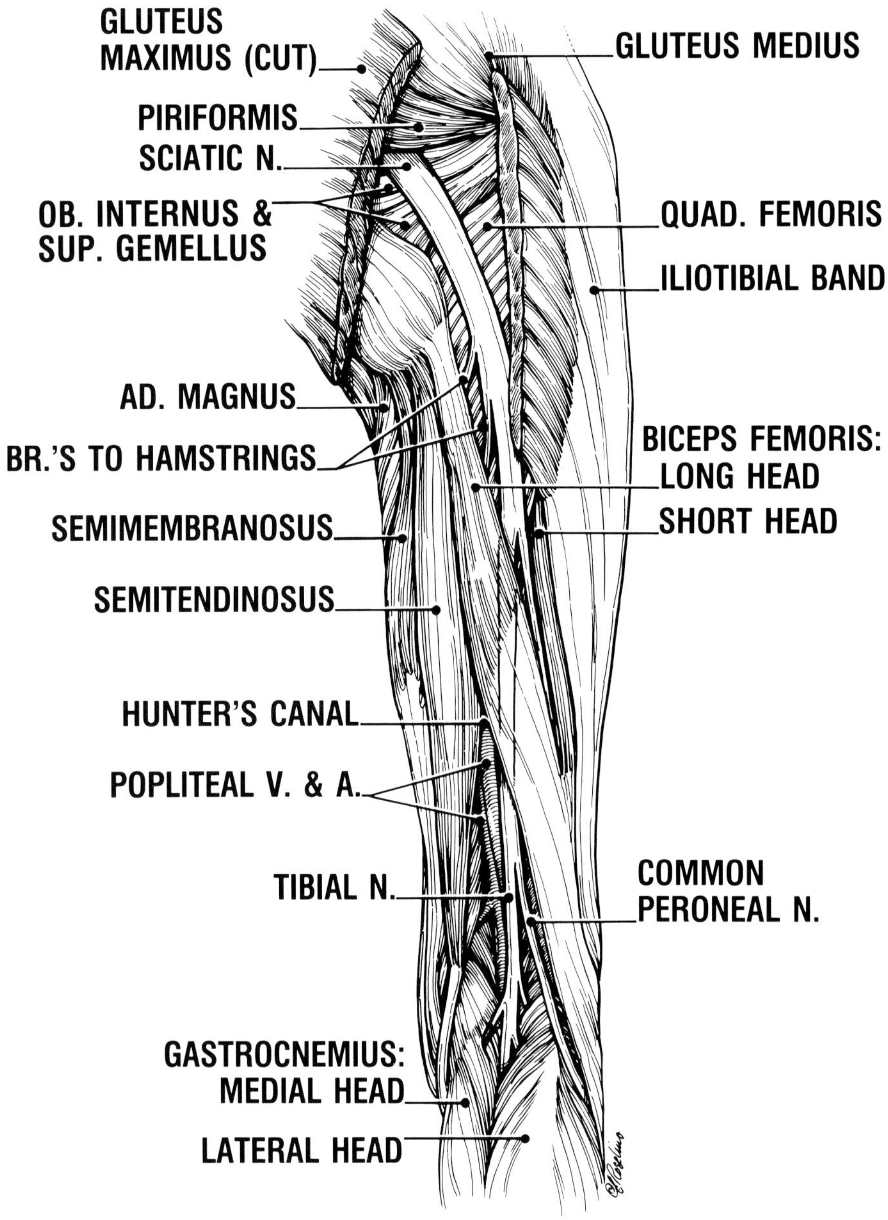

Figure 36–12. *Only the nerve branches to the short head of the biceps femoris exit from the lateral side of the sciatic nerve. Nerve injuries in the area adjacent to Hunter's canal frequently involve the femoral artery as well.*

beneath the soleus muscle and lies superficial to the posterior tibial muscle, where it is accompanied by the posterior tibial artery. The common peroneal nerve is more prone to injury than the posterior tibial nerve because it travels to the lateral side of the leg, staying superficial to the lateral head of the gastrocnemius muscle and the neck of the fibula. It is anchored between its site of bifurcation from the sciatic nerve and its course around the proximal fibula. Distal to the fibular neck it bifurcates into the deep and superficial peroneal nerves.

Injury at Thigh Level

In most people the tibial and peroneal branches of the sciatic nerve can be separated to nearly the middle third of the thigh. This provides substantial increases in length when only one branch has been injured. If necessary, the branch to the short head of the biceps femoris can be sacrificed. The peroneal and tibial nerves are supplied extensively by both the popliteal artery and perforating branches from adjacent muscles, allowing mobilization over considerable lengths.

Injury at Knee and Leg Level

Branching veins and arteries in the popliteal space overlying the tibial nerve make mobilization difficult. Nerve branches to the gastrocnemius muscle, soleus muscle, and the remaining muscles in the posterior compartment of the leg limit the extent of mobilization. Intraneural dissection of motor branches provides 1 or 2 cm of additional length. Flexion of the knee greatly increases the length, but caution is necessary to avoid problems of restricted motion and later tension on the repair site with knee extension.

Additional length of the peroneal nerve is obtained by partial resection of the fibular head to allow the nerve to be transposed anteriorly. Release of the fascia of the tibialis anterior muscle and dissection of the motor branches of the deep peroneal nerve also increase the length available for repair. Guidelines for maximal defects that can be repaired in the acute setting are given in Table 36-7.[7–9,18,24,26]

Defects in the Femoral Nerve

The femoral nerve emerges from the lumbar plexus (L2–L4). It courses anterior to the psoas muscle and accompanies the iliac artery. It enters the anterior aspect of the thigh deep to the inguinal ligament, accompanied by the femoral artery. Just distal to the inguinal ligament it divides into cutaneous sensory branches and muscular branches supplying the quadriceps femoris muscle and sartorius muscle.

Injury at Thigh Level

The femoral nerve is damaged most often by hematomas and tumors that distend the psoas muscles, compressing the nerve. Occasionally, penetrating lesions injure the nerve at this level. In the

Table 36–7.

Tibial and Peroneal Nerves

I. Length gained with lower extremity position (cm)

Knee flexion	3–4
Ankle: Plantar flexion (tibial)	1–2
Dorsiflexion (peroneal)	1

II. Length gained with transposition (cm)

Site of Injury	Length Gained
Common peroneal: Knee level	2
Leg level	1

III. Length gained with mobilization (cm)

Site of Injury	Length Gained
Distal thigh: Tibial	2
Peroneal	2
Knee level: Tibial	0–1
Peroneal	0–1
Leg level: Tibial	1
Peroneal	1

IV. Total length gained with combination of techniques (cm)

Site of Injury	Gap Closed Without Grafting
Distal thigh:	
Tibial	5
Peroneal	5
Knee level:	
Tibial	4–6
Peroneal	4–5
Leg level:	
Tibial	2
Peroneal	2–3

Table 36–8.

I. Length gained with lower extremity position (cm)

Hip flexion	3–4
Knee extension	1

II. Length gained with mobilization of nerve (cm)

Site of Injury	Length Gained
Groin	2–3
Proximal thigh	2

III. Total length gained with combination of techniques (cm)

Site of Injury	Gap Closed Without Grafting
Groin	6
Proximal thigh	4

thigh, mobilization is difficult because of multiple muscular branches. Hip flexion and knee extension decrease tension on the nerve somewhat. Maximal acute nerve defects that can be overcome by mobilization and joint positioning are listed in Table 36-8.[7-9,18,24,26]

REFERENCES

1. Bora FW, Richardson S, Black J. The biomechanical responses to tension in a peripheral nerve. J Hand Surg 1980; 5:21–25.
2. Boyes JH. Repair of the motor branch of the ulnar nerve in the palm. J Bone Joint Surg [Am] 1955; 37: 920.
3. Brooks D. The place of nerve grafting in orthopaedic surgery. J Bone Joint Surg [Am] 1955; 37:299–305.
4. Brown RA, Pedowitz RA, Kwan MK, et al. The effects of stretching upon conduction properties in the rabbit tibial nerve. Trans of the 35th Annual Meeting of the Orthopaedic Research Society, 1989.
5. Brunelli G, Monini L. Direct muscular neurotization. J Hand Surg [Am] 1985; 10:993–997.
6. Clark WL, Trumble TE, Hollis J, Swiontkowski MF. A comparison of peripheral nerve elongation following acute and chronic injury. J Hand Surg (submitted for publication)
7. Forrester-Brown M. The possibilities of suture after extensive nerve injury. J Orthop Surg 1921; 19: 277.
8. Grantham EG, Pollard C, Brabson JA. Peripheral nerve surgery: Repair of nerve defects. Ann Surg 1948; 127:696.
9. Highet WB, Sanders FK. The effects of stretching nerves after suture. Br J Surg 1943; 30:355–369.
10. Learmonth JR. Technique for transplanting the ulnar nerve. Surg Gynecol Obstet 1942; 75:729.
11. Littler JW. Neurovascular island transfer in reconstructive hand surgery. Transactions of the International Society for Plastic Surgery, 2nd Annual Congress, London, 1959:175.
12. Liu CT, Benda CE, Lewey FH. Tensile strength of human nerves: An experimental physical and histologic study. Arch Neurol Psychiatry 1948; 59: 322–336.
13. Longo F, Hayman EG, Davis GE, et al. Neurite-promoting factors and extracellular matrix components accumulating in vivo within nerve regeneration chambers. Brain Res 1984; 309:105–117.
14. Louis DS, Eckenrode JF. Autogenous nerve pedicle graft in the forearm. J Hand Surg [Am] 1986; 11: 703–706.
15. Lundborg G, Rydevik B. Effects of stretching the tibial nerve of the rabbit: A preliminary study of the intraneural circulation and the barrier function of the perineurium. J Bone Joint Surg [Br] 1973; 55:390–401.
16. McLaren AC. Peripheral nerve response to tension. Transactions of the 35th annual meeting of the Orthopaedic Research Society, Las Vegas, Nevada, 1989;14:24.
17. Mitchell SW, Morehouse GR, Keen WW. Gunshot wounds and other injuries of nerves. Clin Orthop Related Res 1982; 163:2–7.
18. Nicholson OR, Seddon HJ. Nerve repair in civil practice: Results of median and ulnar nerve lesions. Br Med J 1980; 2:1065–1071.
19. Ogata K, Manske PR, Lesker PA. The effect of surgical dissection on regional blood flow to the ulnar nerve in the cubital tunnel. Clin Orthop Related Res 1985; 193:195–198.
20. Omer GE. Reconstructive procedures for extremities with peripheral nerve defects. Clin Orthop Related Res 1982; 163:80–91.
21. Restrepo Y, Merle M, Michon J, Follegut B, Petry D. Vascular nerve grafts using an empty perineural tube. Microsurgery 1983; 4:105–112.
22. Rodkey WG, Cabaud E, McCarroll HR. Neurorrhaphy after loss of a nerve segment: Comparison of epineurial suture under tension versus multiple nerve grafts. J Hand Surg 1980; 5:366–371.
23. Seddon HJ. The practical value of peripheral nerve repair. Proc R Soc Med 1949; 42:427.
24. Seddon HJ. Surgical disorders of peripheral nerves, ed 2. Edinburgh: Churchill-Livingstone, 1975:250–315.
25. Sorbie C, Proter TL. Reinnervation of paralyzed muscles by direct motor nerve implantation. J Bone Joint Surg [Br] 1969; 51:156–164.
26. Souttar HS. Some points arising in nerve injuries. Br Med J 1917; 2:817.

37

Indications and Techniques of Nerve Grafting

Hanno Millesi

AUTHOR'S KEY POINTS

- Two factors have recently improved the results of nerve grafts. First, the two sites of coaptation are sutured without tension. Second, when cutaneous nerve segments are used to bridge defects in major nerve trunks, individual fascicles are separated by interfascicular microsurgical dissection so that coaptation is performed individually for each fascicle or fascicle group.
- Mechanical considerations are key to the success of free nerve grafts. The length of a nerve graft is determined by the maximal distance between the two stumps, with coaptation performed in an extended position of the limb without tension.
- The results of nerve grafting using short grafts are inferior to end-to-end repair under similar degrees of tension.
- Vascularized nerve grafts are less sensitive to tension, as they maintain a gliding tissue surface and do not need adhesions for revascularization.
- Free nerve grafts are revascularized by spontaneous vascularization from vessels of the recipient site; those vessels establish connections with vessels within the grafts. As the relationship between tissue mass and surface must be favorable, the graft must be thin.
- If a complex primary repair is carried out after a severe injury, a nerve defect may be bridged with a primary nerve graft, but this is the exception rather than the rule. Nerve grafting is generally performed secondarily.
- If the straight line connecting proximal and distal nerve stumps extends directly across scar tissue, or is crossed by a contracting scar, this area is bypassed. A longer graft is used to avoid placing the graft in a scarred bed.
- In defining the two nerve stumps clinically, all efforts are made to coapt corresponding areas, recognizing the original orientation of the stumps and applying existing knowledge of intraneural topography. Orientation in space is determined by dissecting the proximal stump until the next major branch exits the nerve. Similarly, the distal stump is followed until major branching is noted.
- For a nerve the diameter of which is smaller than that of the nerve graft, only part of the graft is used. This is accomplished by longitudinal dissection of the donor nerve. Fibrin clotting provides a sufficient coapting force to maintain union without suture for these small grafts.

HISTORY

The first nerve graft in humans was performed by Albert in 1876.[4] Foerster[35] used cutaneous nerve segments to secure survival after free grafting, and Bielschowsky and Unger[9] demonstrated better survival with cutaneous nerve grafting compared to free grafting of nerve trunks. While successful nerve grafting was reported by Bunnel[23] and Ballance and Duel,[8] Seddon[81] developed the technique of cable grafting. Several cutaneous nerve segments were packed together by sutures or adhesives, creating a graft of the same size as the nerve under repair. Other techniques include vascularized nerve grafts, first recommended by Strange in 1947: if two parallel nerves, such as the median and ulnar nerves, are injured, one may be repaired at the expense of the other, transferring a segment as a pedicle flap with preservation of its circulation.[84]

Because the results of earlier procedures were less than satisfactory, nerve grafting was used as a salvage procedure, only after all other possibilities for managing nerve defects (eg, transposition, mobilization, and maximal approximation by flexion of adjacent joints) had been exhausted. However, it became apparent that end-to-end repair under tension carried a high percentage of failure, especially if the defect was large.[68,76]

The results of nerve grafting became more reliable after two reasons for earlier failures were recognized. First, if a free nerve graft is used to overcome a nerve defect, the two sites of coaptation are coapted without any tension, not only during surgery but also in the period of mobilization.[60–62] Second, if cutaneous nerve segments are used as grafts for bridging defects in major nerve trunks, it is better to separate individual major fascicles and fascicle groups by interfascicular microsurgical dissection and to perform the coaptation individually for each of these fascicles and fascicle groups, instead of packing cutaneous nerve segments together to form a cable graft. The grafts are individually located and have much more surface for contact with recipient sites. A great deal of the surface of the individual nerve graft is lost for revascularization if it is in contact with another nerve graft.[63–65]

Taylor considered using nerve trunks to bridge nerve defects, revascularizing the graft immediately by microvascular anastomosis.[90] Lundborg opened a new dimension in his experiments, showing that nerve tissue proceeds from one stump to another if an empty interval is provided (see Chap. 7).[50]

BIOLOGY

To better understand the problems associated with nerve grafting, some basic considerations regarding nerve regeneration are reviewed.

End-to-End Nerve Repair

After clean transection and ideal nerve repair, the endoneurium and nerve fibers of the proximal stump are normal. Axon sprouts grow out laterally or terminally. In the distal stump, wallerian degeneration takes place and axon and myelin sheaths disappear. The only remnant of nerve fiber remaining is the basal membrane, which is filled with Schwann cells. The endoneural framework is normal.

Axon sprouts must cross the space between the two stumps (Fig. 37-1). When they reach the distal stump, waiting Schwann cells provide them with an ideal environment as they proceed along the distal stump. This process can be termed nerve–nerve neurotization (in contrast to nerve–muscle or muscle–muscle neurotization).

Fresh Autologous Nerve Grafts

An autologous nerve graft behaves like a distal stump after it is removed from the donor nerve. Wallerian degeneration occurs and axons and myelin sheaths disappear. The connective tissue framework is normal. If the nerve graft survives the grafting procedure, Schwann cells remain viable.[3]

In this case, axon sprouts entering the proximal end of the nerve graft are exposed to the same conditions as they would be in a distal stump and can proceed along the graft. The only difference from end-to-end nerve repair is the fact that axon sprouts must extend across another barrier between the distal end of the graft and the distal stump. This is

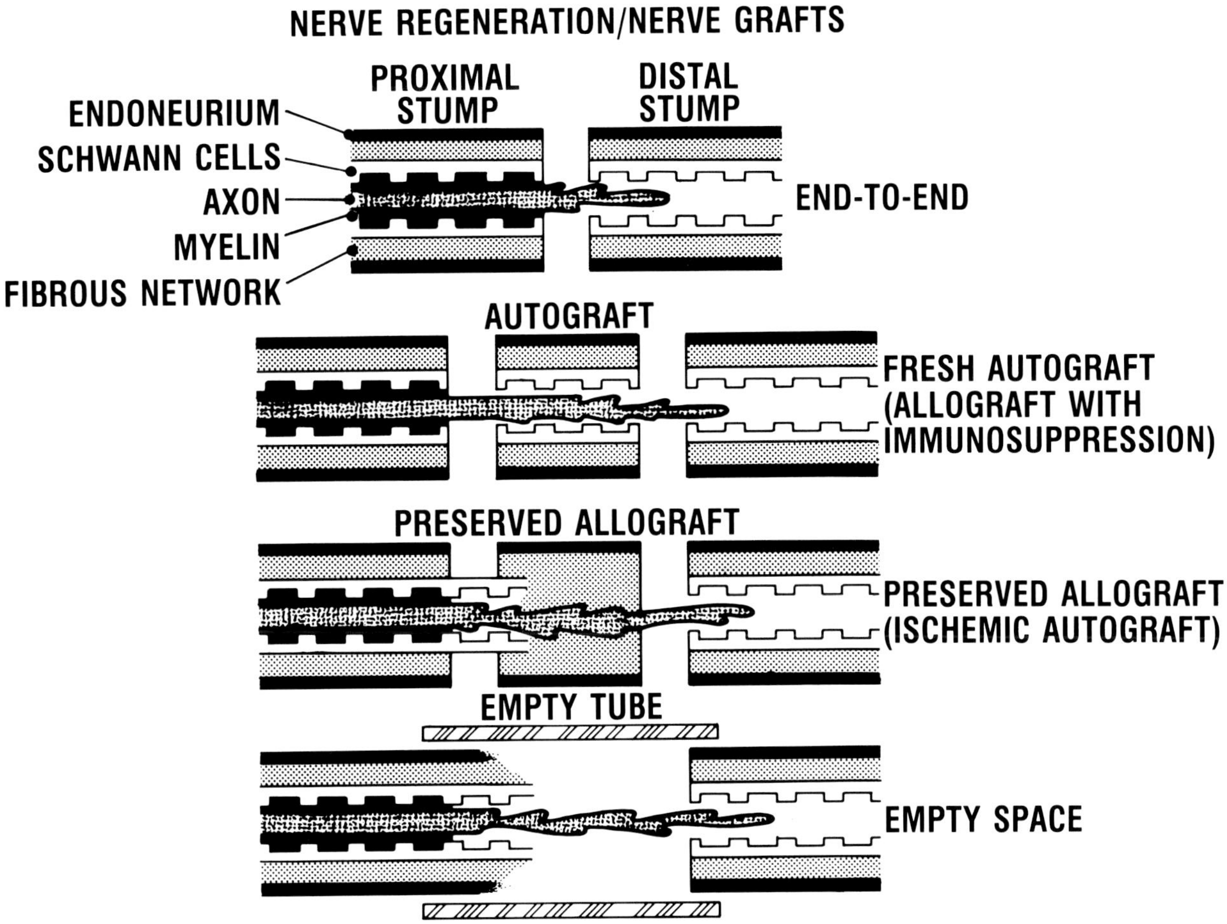

Figure 37–1. *Nerve regeneration following nerve grafts.*

nerve-to-nerve neurotization; the nerve graft behaves like a railbed for axons, providing them with all they need by the activity of the Schwann cells.

Preserved Allografts

Researchers in the early 1970s tried to bridge nerve defects with allografts, preserved either in cialite solution,[2] by lyophilization, by deep freezing,[44,96,97] or by treatment with ionizing irradiation.[53,54] These grafts are the opposite extreme from successful autologous nerve grafts. While they do not contain living cells, they maintain a collagen framework. They are neurotized from the proximal stump by axon sprouts growing into the grafts in the company of Schwann cells, endothelial cells, and capillary and perineural fibroblasts that produce a perineural sheath around a group of axon sprouts. Schröder and Seiffert called this *neuromatous neurotization*.[78] After neurotization, the framework is completely changed and consists basically of connective tissue and minifascicles. These preserved allografts behave like a rail for a neuroma to grow along (see Fig. 37-1).

Autograft With Damage Due to Ischemia

If an autograft fails due to ischemia, Schwann cells do not survive. Fibrous tissue prevails and the original tissue framework is lost. Such a graft is also neurotized by neuromatous neurotization because of delayed spontaneous revascularization. This might be due to the following:

A relatively avascular recipient site
Contact of a graft with another free graft
The poor relationship between diameter of the graft and surface area available for spontaneous revascularization.

Fresh Allograft Under Immunosuppression

A fresh allograft under immunosuppression should behave like an autograft. It may become functional if fibroblasts and Schwann cells are gradually replaced by host cells. If there is an immunologic reaction, fibrosis develops.

Neurotization Along an Empty Space

Lundborg and Hansson demonstrated the growth of axons along an empty space within a mesothelial chamber.[50] Previously, veins and other types of tubes had been used with the same objectives. It is well documented that axons reach the distal stump through such empty spaces, but a question remains as to whether this is the consequence of a proceeding neuroma (neuromatous neurotization[78]) or creation of new normal nerve tissue. In this case, normal endoneural framework must be regenerated. Tissue consisting mainly of minifascicles can be regarded as neuromatous neurotization.

CLASSIFICATION OF NERVE GRAFTS

So many different techniques of nerve grafting are available that a classification system is required.

Origin of Grafts

In the vast majority of cases, grafts from the same individual are used (*autografts*). An *isograft* is a graft from an identical twin. *Allografts* are harvested from individuals from the same species, *xenografts* from individuals of different species. Allo- and xenografts cause an immunologic reaction that must be suppressed by immunosuppressive treatment. Mackinnon and associates[51] and Schaller and coworkers[77] had considerable success in experiments using allografts coupled with cyclosporin A treatment.

Donor Nerves

A cutaneous nerve or a nerve trunk can be used as a nerve graft. Harvesting a *cutaneous nerve* does not cause significant functional loss (see Chap. 38). It is essential to transect cutaneous nerves as far proximally as possible beneath fascia to avoid irritation of the stump; otherwise, painful neuromas may form. Cutaneous nerves show a favorable relationship between tissue mass and surface area, and they survive the process of free grafting well.

Because harvesting a *major nerve trunk* causes an important loss of function, trunks should be used only if the nerve is situated in an amputation stump and the muscles the nerve usually innervates have been lost, or if the chances of reneurotization of the nerve trunk are negligible. For example, this is the case with the ulnar nerve following brachial plexus lesions where the C8 and T1 roots have been avulsed. Trunk grafts are too thick to survive free grafting, even in a well-vascularized recipient site. Circulation must therefore be maintained or immediately restored (*vascularized nerve grafts*). If free grafting of a nerve trunk is planned, the epifascicular epineurium is removed and the nerve trunk divided into fascicle groups, which are then grafted individually (*split trunk graft*).

Mechanical Aspects

This aspect of nerve repair and reconstruction is often neglected. If a certain amount of nerve tissue has been destroyed, a well-defined nerve defect is present. This defect is increased by resection of damaged or fibrotic nerve tissue in the proximal and distal stumps. The distance between the two stumps varies according to the position of adjacent joints. It is *minimized* by flexing adjacent joints to approximate the two nerve stumps as much as possible. It is *maximized* by extending adjacent joints, separating the two stumps as far as possible. The length of the nerve graft is selected according to the maximal, minimal, or any transient distance between the two stumps according to joint position.

If the minimal distance is selected, the graft will be rather short and, on limb mobilization, the two sites of coaptation will be exposed to tension. In this case, the advantages of using a short graft are countered by the serious disadvantage of creating two unfavorable sites of coaptation. Free nerve grafts are particularly sensitive to tension. The results of nerve grafting using short grafts are inferior to end-to-end repair under similar degrees of tension.

If nerve grafts are selected according to the maximal distance between the two stumps, coaptation can be performed in the extended position without tension. Optimal healing conditions are provided for both sites of coaptation. On mobilization, there is no tension at the sites of coaptation. The graft, having formed adhesions in an extended position, must only crimp to adapt to the flexed position of adjacent joints.

A common error is selecting a length of graft that is correct according to the maximal distance between two stumps, but then immobilizing the limb by flexing adjacent joints. In this case the nerve graft forms the adhesions required for survival in flexion, and will not be able to elongate to its original length when mobilization starts. Thus, the sites of coaptation will be exposed to considerable tension.

Vascularized nerve grafts are less sensitive to tension because they maintain their gliding tissue surface and do not need adhesions for revascularization. The graft length is selected according to the maximal distance between the two stumps, and the limb is immobilized in that position for about 10 days.

Circulation

Spontaneous Revascularization

Free nerve grafts are revascularized by spontaneous revascularization from vessels of the recipient site, which establish connections with vessels within the grafts. The recipient site must have sufficient vascularity, and, as the relationship between tissue mass and surface must be favorable, the graft must not be too thick. Because spontaneous revascularization occurs through the formation of adhesions at the recipient site, the graft is fixed to the recipient site and cannot adapt to different positions of the limb by passive movement. If the graft survives, Schwann cells survive and the graft behaves like a distal stump. Otherwise, Schwann cells do not survive, and the graft becomes fibrotic (see Autograft with Damage Due to Ischemia).

Preserved Circulation

If the circulation is preserved, all cellular elements survive. Strange performed nerve transplantation with preserved vascularity, using neighboring nerve as a pedicle flap.[84] A nerve segment supplied by a well-defined vascular pedicle can be transferred on its pedicle, preserving the circulation as an *island flap*. An example is the transposition of the ulnar nerve on the superior collateral ulnar artery in managing a defect following a brachial plexus lesion.

Revascularization by Microvascular Anastomosis

Nerve segments with well-defined vascular pedicles can be transferred as free tissue transfers with arterial and venous anastomoses. Circulation is immediately restored and there is no danger of cell damage, provided the anastomoses remain patent. If vascular occlusion occurs, however, the transplanted nerve tissue is not as effective as a free graft. The major advantage of vascularized nerve grafts is the fact that they are independent of the vascularity of the recipient site and that the gliding tissue remains intact (see Chap. 40). Not only are these grafts much less sensitive to tension, the selection of appropriate length is not as important.

Since the number of available nerve trunks is limited (an amputation stump or irreparable nerve damage must be present), techniques have been developed to transplant cutaneous nerves as vascularized nerve grafts.[32,34,43,94]

TECHNIQUE OF FREE NERVE GRAFTING

Overview

If a complex primary repair of tissues following a severe injury is planned, a nerve defect may be bridged by a nerve graft. However, this is the exception; as a rule, nerve grafting is a secondary procedure. The two fundamentally different situations can be distinguished.

If primary care of the wound is performed at the same institution by a member of the same team, the anatomical situation is known. At the primary procedure, the tendons are repaired, the skin defect covered, and the osseous injury treated. The two stumps and the defect in nerve are defined and their locations are well known. The patient is scheduled for early secondary repair. In this situation, the two nerve stumps are explored by minimal exposure. *A connection between the site of the two stumps is established by tunnelling in good soft-tissue environment.* A complete exploration of all structures is unnecessary. Special care is taken to avoid placing nerve grafts in contact with repaired tendons. The nerve grafts are introduced into these tunnels and suturing is performed at two distant operative sites.

If the patient has been cared for in another institution and the anatomical situation is unclear, a more extensive exposure is indicated to clarify the anatomical situation, to define the extent of damage, and to evaluate the recipient site.

The incisions follow the general rules of plastic surgery. In the upper extremity, the shoulder joint is abducted, the elbow joint extended, and the wrist joint extended slightly. In the lower extremity, the hip joint is maintained in neutral, the knee joint is extended, and the ankle joint is held in neutral position. Prepping and draping is done in a way that allows extension of exposure, if necessary. Also, the patient is positioned to facilitate access to presumptive donor nerves.

If possible, incisions crossing the future course of the nerve graft are avoided, because constriction by subsequent scar is one of the major reasons for failure of the procedure. For example, I prefer a midlateral incision along the ulnar side of the forearm and wrist for median and ulnar nerve repair, instead of a palmar incision. In this approach, a tension-free skin closure can be achieved by applying a split-thickness skin graft on the ulnar aspect of the wrist joint.

If the straight line that connects the two stumps directly extends across scar tissue or is crossed by a contracting scar, I prefer to bypass this area, using a longer graft, rather than to put the graft in a scarred bed. If bypassing the area is impossible, the situation is improved by plastic procedures prior to nerve repair. In extreme cases, a vascularized nerve graft is selected, as it functions independently of the recipient site.

The disadvantage of nerve grafting is the fact that the regenerating axon sprouts must cross two sites of coaptation. Scar tissue at the distal site of coaptation may block the crossing of axons from the graft to the distal stump. In the early days of grafting, this was the rule; therefore, resection of the distal suture site was performed in a second stage in grafts longer than 3 or 4 cm.[22] Bosse then suggested that the proximal coaptation be performed solely in the first stage, with the distal coaptation secured after an interval had elapsed after the graft had been neurotized.[12,13] With microsurgical techniques, blockage at the distal site occurs rarely. In the first 50 nerve grafts I performed, blocks occurred and had to be treated in seven cases (14%), but since then the percentage has become much lower. For this reason I do not think that two-stage nerve grafting is justified, but the surgeon should keep this possibility in mind before declaring a grafting procedure a failure. Blockage at the distal coaptation site is recognized by the presence of a constant Tinel's sign at the level of the distal end of the graft. Resection and coaptation between graft and newly prepared distal stump salvages the result.

Donor Nerves

The most commonly used donor nerve is the *sural nerve* (see Chap. 38). It originates from the tibial nerve, forming a separate fascicle group within the trunk of this nerve as far proximally as the popliteal fossa. It is located subfascially, between the medial and lateral heads of the gastrocnemius muscle. It perforates the fascia in the middle of the calf and is then located in subcutaneous tissue, following the small saphenous vein. It usually receives a branch from the lateral sural cutaneous nerve. Strictly speaking, the sural nerve starts after the two sources have met. Very often the peroneal branch is very small and is not encountered during harvesting. In 20% of cases, the contribution from the peroneal nerve is quite important and then, of course, both nerves are harvested. In rare cases, the whole nerve originates from the peroneal nerve.

The sural nerve is 30 to 40 cm long and is easily located behind the lateral ankle. The preferred method of excision is to define the nerve behind the lateral ankle through a small incision. A second incision is made 3 cm proximally, and the nerve is located in that area. The nerve is then transected at the distal incision. By gentle traction on the nerve in the proximal incision, the surgeon determines whether there are distal branches present; if so, they are transected. The nerve is then withdrawn easily from the proximal incision. Local traction at the second incision allows palpation of the course of the nerve. The surgeon determines whether there is an important peroneal contribution. The nerve is transected at the most proximal level, just distal to the popliteal fossa, where the proximal stump disappears under the fascia between the two heads of the gastrocnemius muscle. I always excise the whole nerve, even if only a small segment is needed.

With some experience, it is easy to excise the nerve with the patient lying on his or her back, the lower extremity flexed at the hip and knee, and the ankle dorsiflexed. It is unnecessary to excise the nerve with the patient in the prone position before the nerve to be repaired is explored. Some surgeons prefer longitudinal excisions from the popliteal fossa to the area behind the lateral ankle. Several instruments (nerve strippers) have been designed for excising the sural nerve through one or two incisions. If the nerve is formed only from the tibial nerve, this works well, but if there is a major contribution from the peroneal nerve, this portion is destroyed by stripping.

The sural is an ideal nerve, as it usually starts as a monofascicular nerve. Along its course, the number of fascicles increases, and at the very end it contains many small fascicles. If a short nerve defect is to be bridged, and the whole length of the sural nerve is excised, segments of the sural nerve are selected that offer the most favorable match with the fascicular groups being connected.

The second choice for nerve graft tissue is the *medial antebrachial cutaneous nerve* (see Chap. 38). It is formed from the medial cord of the brachial plexus and follows the brachial vein, entering the subcutaneous space in the middle of the upper arm. It divides into anterior and posterior branches. The nerve is exposed by making three transverse incisions along the medial aspect of the upper arm, or by a mediolateral longitudinal incision. A nerve graft of about 20 cm can be harvested. I do not use this nerve when there is an ulnar nerve lesion because the sensory territory of this nerve may overlap the ulnar nerve's territory.

The third choice is the *lateral femoral cutaneous nerve* (see Chap. 38), which is located just medially and caudally to the spina iliaca ventralis where it exits the abdominal wall. It proceeds in a lateral, distal direction on the ventral lateral aspect of the thigh. It is harvested through several transverse incisions. A 30-cm-long graft can be obtained.

The *dorsal antebrachial cutaneous nerve*, a branch of the radial nerve, is located on the lateral aspect of the distal half of the upper arm. It extends to the dorsal side of the forearm. A 15- to 20-cm-long graft can be harvested. I do not use this nerve if the medial antebrachial cutaneous nerve has been excised.

The *lateral antebrachial cutaneous nerve* is defined lateral to the biceps tendon. It is excised through several transverse incisions. I have no experience with using this nerve. I would not use it if the medial antebrachial cutaneous nerve had been excised.

The *superficial radial nerve* can be excised as a long nerve graft from its formation to its branching in the distal forearm. It follows the brachioradialis tendon. I have used this nerve in cases of brachial plexus lesions when I was very short of grafts; otherwise, I would not touch it due to its known tendency to form painful neuromas in peripheral nerve lesions.

The *saphenous nerve* can be excised to a length of about 40 cm on the medial aspect of the thigh and the leg. It can also be used as a vascularized nerve graft. I do not use this nerve if the sural nerve has been excised.

Exploration and Definition of the Two Nerve Stumps

One of the major challenges in nerve repair in general is to connect the corresponding areas of the proximal and distal stumps.

Recently researchers have demonstrated both fascicle specificity of the outgrowing axons and end-organ specificity (see Chap. 13).[17–21,71,72,80] Clinically, all efforts are undertaken to coapt corresponding areas. Therefore, it is extremely important to recognize the original orientation of the two nerve stumps in space: only then can the knowledge of intraneural topography be applied. Orientation in space is recognized by dissecting the proximal stump until the next major branch leaves the nerve. In a similar way, the distal stump is followed until major branching is noted. If the defect is located in a peripheral portion of the nerve (eg, in the distal forearm) the median and ulnar nerves are followed until they divide. By retrograde tracing on the surface of the nerve trunk, a clear image of the intraneural topography of the distal stump is obtained. From Sunderland's studies we know that the fascicular pattern of a nerve changes rapidly along its course (see Chap. 14).[86–88] In contrast to the fascicular pattern, the group pattern remains constant over much longer distances.[45,98] If the fascicular pattern of the distal stump, and the orientation in space of the proximal stump have been defined, a good estimation can be made of areas in the proximal stump that must be united with corresponding areas in the distal stump.

Techniques used to differentiate between motor and sensory fibers are helpful (see Chap. 16).[36,42,74,92] However, with proximal-level injuries, where more help is needed, fascicles usually contain a mixture of motor and sensory fibers. For example, the motor fibers forming the posterior interosseus nerve are diffusely distributed in the radial nerve in the midarm. Studies on intraneural topography have demonstrated that nerve fibers for this nerve are more highly concentrated along the dorsal aspect of the radial nerve trunk.[86] With a long defect of the radial nerve, I would, therefore, coapt the nerve grafts connected distally with the posterior interosseus nerve, with the dorsal aspect of the radial nerve trunk proximally.

Restoration of Continuity

After exploration, the two nerve stumps are prepared. All neuromatous tissue is resected until normal nerve tissue is encountered. The dissection increases the distance between the two stumps. The number of segments of the cutaneous donor nerve necessary to cover the cross-section of the nerve to be repaired is defined. The length of each graft segment harvested is 10% longer than the distance between the two stumps in the respective extended neutral positions of adjacent joints. The nerve graft is harvested and transected into segments of the estimated length. I transect the donor graft under the microscope with serrated scissors, which transect the nerve layer by layer and fascicle by fascicle. Epineural tissue is shifted away from exposed fascicles to avoid the capping of fascicles by epineural tissue. Meyer's forceps are particularly useful for this task.[59]

The next step is to approximate one end of the nerve graft to a well-defined point in the proximal stump. This end is then coapted carefully to the fascicular tissue at this spot. The same maneuver is performed at the distal end. According to the size and the fascicular pattern of the nerve to be repaired, these basic steps are performed in different ways.

In a *small nerve* of the approximate diameter of the cutaneous nerve graft, the two stumps are prepared by repeated transection until normal tissue is encountered. One nerve graft is sufficient. The nerve graft is approximated to the nerve stumps by one suture, which is anchored into the epineurium of the graft and the epineurium of the stump. This suture allows the surgeon to handle the nerve graft without touching it, allowing approximation of the graft to the stump and achieving coaptation of the fascicular tissue. According to the anatomical situation, usually second and third sutures are necessary to secure and maintain coaptation.

For a *very small nerve*, the diameter of which is smaller than the nerve graft, only part of the graft is used, prepared by longitudinal dissection of the donor nerve. The two ends of the tiny nerve graft are placed in contact with the proximal and distal stumps. After 20 minutes, normal fibrin clotting provides sufficient coapting force to maintain the coaptation without a suture. In such cases the tensile strength is increased by application of homologous fibrinogen as an adhesive. If tension is zero, as it should be, the clot alone is sufficient.

In a *nerve trunk larger than the nerve graft*, the preparation is done according to the fascicular pattern. Five basic types of fascicular patterns can be distinguished (Fig. 37-2):

1. The monofascicular pattern, in which the nerve consists of one large fascicle
2. The oligofascicular pattern, with up to four large fascicles
3. The oligofascicular pattern, with five or more fascicles of a manageable size (about the size of the nerve graft)
4. The polyfascicular pattern, with more than 10 or 12 smaller fascicles arranged in groups
5. The polyfascicular pattern, with many small fascicles that are diffusely arranged.

At proximal levels, peripheral nerves very often have monofascicular or oligofascicular patterns with a few large fascicles. Toward the periphery, short distances of polyfascicular patterns without group arrangement and with considerable fiber exchange are followed by longer segments with polyfascicular patterns with group arrangement and not much fiber exchange.

Segments with monofascicular or oligofascicular patterns with a few large fascicles contain a high percentage of fascicular tissue and very little nonfascicular tissue in cross-section. These stumps are prepared by resection until normal tissue is noted. Resection of epifascicular epineurium is unnecessary. Cutaneous nerve graft segments are approximated and coapted to the large fascicles until the exposed cross-sectional surface is completely covered. The objective is to provide more than one graft segment to cover the cross-sectional surface of one fascicle (fascicular coaptation 1:2, 1:3, etc.) (Fig. 37-3*A*).

In a segment with an oligofascicular pattern with 5 to 12 fascicles, about the size of the nerve graft, optimal coaptation is achieved if one graft is coapted to one fascicle (fascicular coaptation). In these segments, the relationship between fascicular and nonfascicular tissue is less favorable for the fascicular tissue. To avoid coapting a graft to nonfascicular tissue, epifascicular tissue is resected and fascicles are isolated. One end of one graft is approximated by one suture to the selected fascicle. The suture secures the epineurium of the graft to the interfascicular epineurium remaining on the surface of the isolated fascicle. To minimize operative manipulation, the fascicles are transected at different levels. After the first graft has been coapted, the subsequent grafts are supported lat-

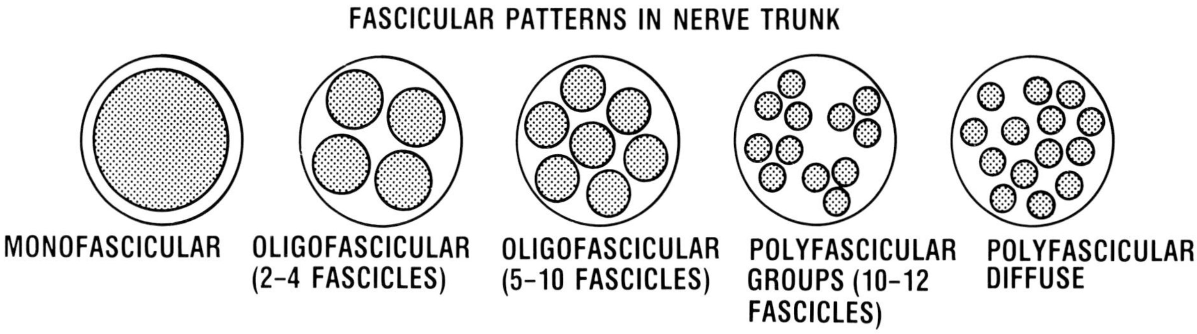

Figure 37–2. *Fascicular patterns in the nerve trunk.*

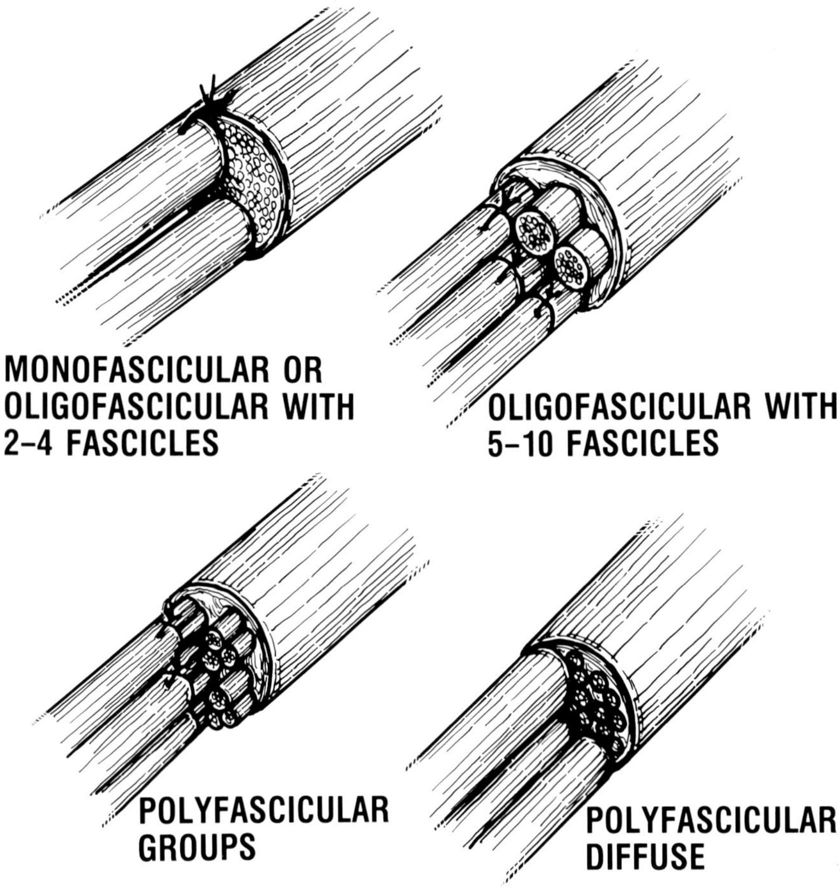

Figure 37–3. *Methods of coaptation.*

erally by the graft already in situ and the neighboring protruding fascicles. The approximation suture is generally sufficient for approximation, coaptation, and maintenance of coaptation. Only if the graft does not coapt well, due to rotation, is a second suture necessary (Fig. 37-3*B*).

In a segment with a polyfascicular pattern with group arrangement, the exposed cross-sectional surface of the nerve consists of fascicle groups or individual large fascicles that are separated from each other by interfascicular epineurium. These groups are preformed and not artificially created by the surgeon. The percentage of nonfascicular tissue is very high and, therefore, resection of the epineural tissue helps avoid incorrect coaptation. As with the oligofascicular pattern with 5 to 12 manageable fascicles, interfascicular dissection is performed to isolate the fascicle groups. Dissection extends from proximal to distal, from neuroma to normal tissue. The epineurium is resected. Following the intraneural vessels the fascicle groups are isolated. Fascicles are followed toward the neuroma and are transected precisely where they lose their normal appearance. Again, the transection is performed at different levels. In the same way as with the fascicular coaptation, one end of the nerve graft is approximated to each fascicle group by one suture, anchored in the epineurium of the graft and the interfascicular epineurium of the group. Usually one suture provides satisfactory coaptation. Grafts and fascicle groups protruding at different lengths from the stumps support the neighboring graft by side-by-side contact (Fig. 37-3*C*).

In the case of a fascicular pattern without group arrangement, the relationship between fascicular tissue and nonfascicular tissue is very unfavorable. The danger of incorrect coaptation is high. However, since there are no preformed spaces to isolate groups, interfascicular dissection is not performed. The stump is prepared by resection. Each graft is coapted with a certain area of the cross-section according to our knowledge of intraneural topography (Fig. 37-3*D*).

If the grafts are long enough and there is no longitudinal tension present, additional measures to maintain coaptation are unnecessary. Over the past years, the additional use of fibrin glue has been recommended by several researchers who tried to use tissue glue as the only method of maintaining coaptation; ultimately they concluded that better results were achieved if the glue was combined with sutures (see Chaps. 20 and 22).[30,33,47,66] Alnot and Benfrech[6] and Narakas[67] united the ends of individual nerve grafts by tissue collagen, creating one stump of the same size as the nerve to be repaired. This stump is then coapted by epineural sutures to the proximal, then distal, stumps. The step of approximation is simplified at the expense of exactness of coaptation. While at the extremities these nerve grafts resemble cable grafts, the disadvantage of cable grafts is avoided because the grafts remain isolated except at their ends.

Wound Closure

In locations where a tourniquet can be applied, the dissection is performed under tourniquet. I deflate the tourniquet and obtain hemostasis before doing the grafting procedure itself. Wound closure is performed carefully to avoid shearing forces. This phase is critical: the repair may be disrupted if skin closure is performed without necessary care, or if the position of the limb during the operation is not maintained immediately after wound closure by application of a cast before the patient awakens. Immobilization must be done in the extended position, similar to that maintained during the operation. Immobilization in a flexed position changes the location of the graft and creates tension at the sites of coaptation as the patient starts moving the limb again. Postoperatively the limb is immobilized for 10 days; thereafter, the patient moves freely.

VASCULARIZED NERVE GRAFTS

Transfer as a Pedicle Flap

Strange suggested in 1947 that the ulnar nerve be transferred as a pedicle flap to restore the continuity of the median nerve if both nerves had long defects.[84] The ulnar nerve was cut distally and its distal end sutured to the median nerve. After the blood supply had been reestablished at this end, the proximal end of the nerve was transected and transferred to the distal end of the median nerve, where coaptation was performed. Shelden modified this technique by transferring the ulnar nerve into the defect of the median nerve in an orthodromic manner.[82] One study followed three of these cases for 15 years after surgery.[49] All cases showed some improvement in sensibility, but the result was not objectively convincing. Chase used cutaneous nerves (medial antebrachial and medial brachial) in a similar way.[24]

Nerve trunks usually cannot be used as donors because of the loss of function that occurs as a result of excising the nerves. This problem is not important in cases of brachial plexus lesions if the roots C8 and T1 are avulsed and regeneration along the ulnar nerve cannot be expected. In those cases, the ulnar nerve can be used as a donor nerve in several ways.

Bonney and associates transferred the ulnar nerve along with the ulnar artery and observed the return of biceps muscle function to a level better than M3 in 9 of 12 cases (75%).[11] Terzis and colleagues[93] reported excellent recovery after transfer of the ulnar nerve, based on the superior ulnar collateral artery, as described by Breidenbach and Terzis[14,15] and Kuenzel and coworkers.[48] This transfer can be performed as a free vascularized graft with microvascular anastomosis or as an island flap. The superior ulnar collateral artery is usually located 1 to 4 cm distal to the lower border of the pectoralis major muscle, arising from the humeral artery. Terzis and colleagues reported excellent recovery in several cases.[93]

Anderl and Hussl also applied this technique successfully.[7] Alnot and Benfrech[6] achieved elbow flexion of M3 or better in 15 of 18 cases, a remarkably good result.[7,69] In 15 cases the ulnar

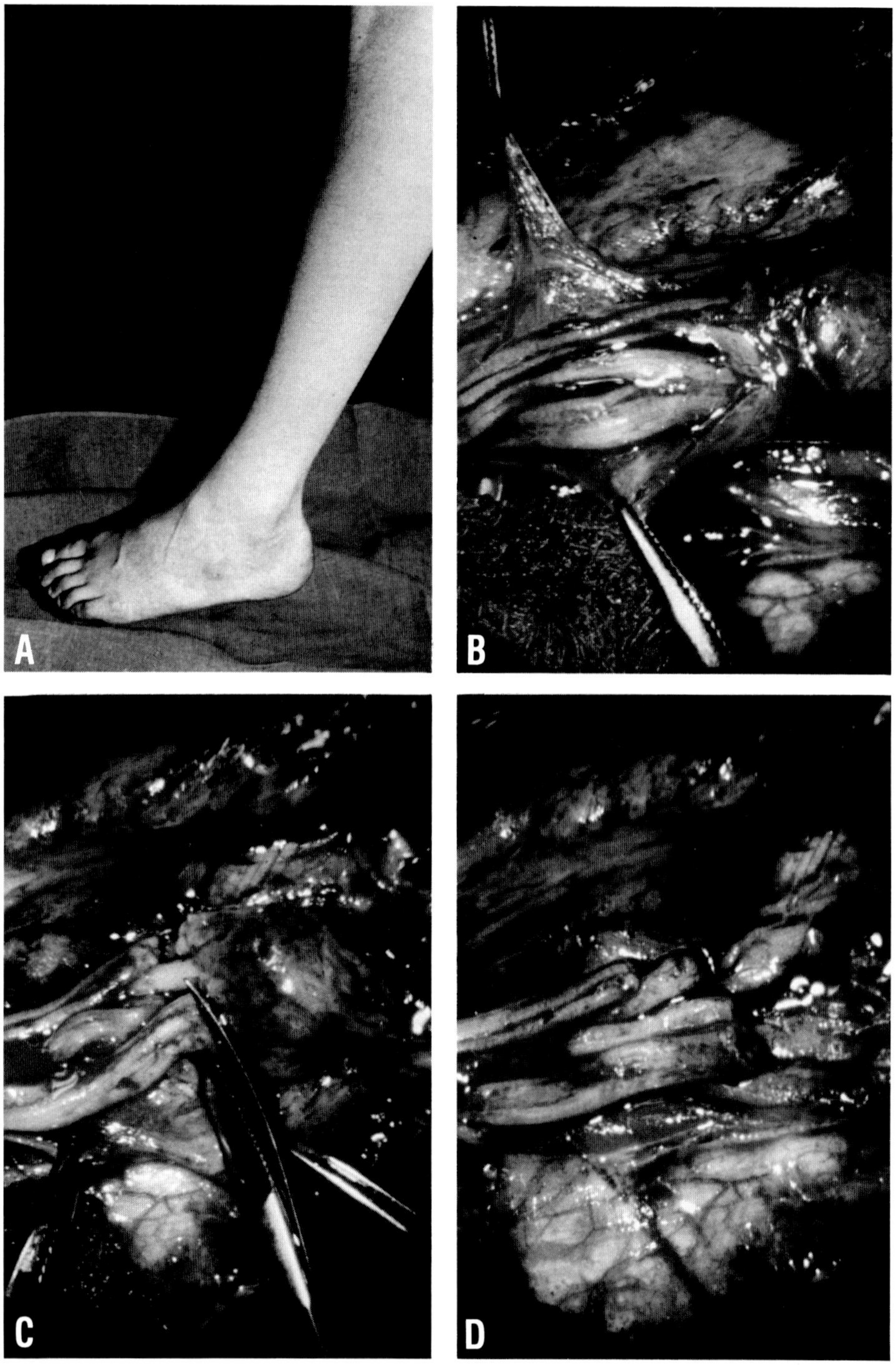

Figure 37–4. *(**A**) Complete palsy of peroneal nerve–innervated muscles after transection of the peroneal nerve. (**B**) Proximal stump of the peroneal nerve. The neuroma is on the right. Proximal to the neuroma, epifascicular epineurium is transected and the fascicle groups are separated by interfascicular dissection. (**C**) Transection of each fascicle group in the transient zone between normal tissue and neuroma. (**D**) After interfascicular dissection, the proximal stump is divided into four fascicular groups.*

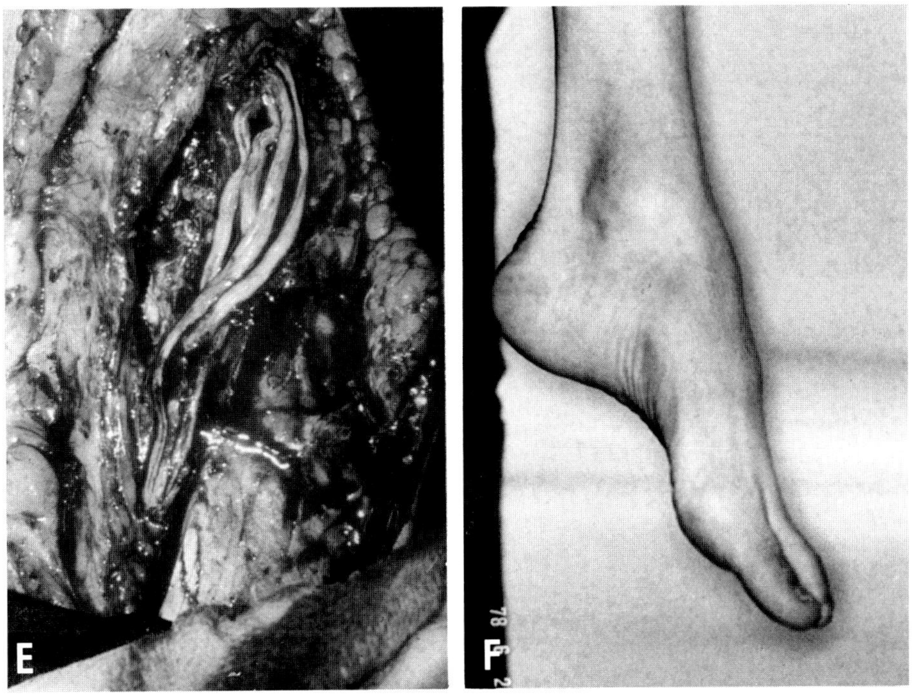

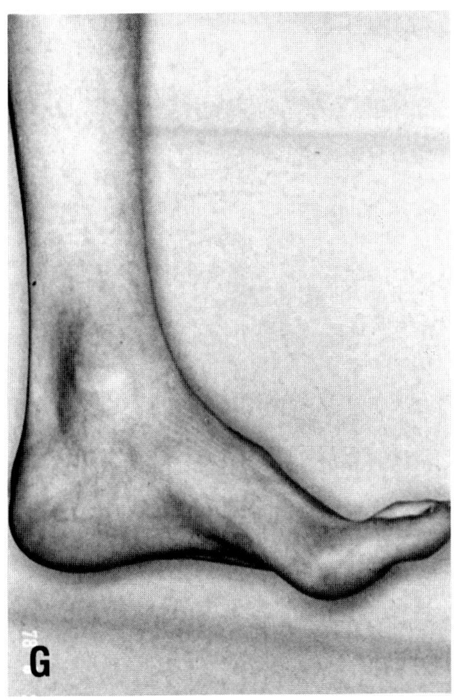

Figure 37–4. (Continued) (***E***) The four fascicular groups are connected by four segments of the sural nerve to corresponding fascicular groups of the distal stump. Note the individual positioning of each graft segment. (***F, G***) Postoperative results.

nerve was transferred as one segment with vascular anastomosis to the transverse cervical artery and its concomitant veins. The dorsal branch of the ulnar nerve was coapted with the suprascapular nerve. In three cases the nerve itself was transected with careful preservation of the paraneurium and vessels. In this way the nerve can be transferred in two segments, one being united with one spinal nerve (eg, C5), the other being coapted to another spinal nerve (eg, C6). In some of these cases, function of M3 with the flexor digitorum superficialis was achieved.

I have used vascularized nerve grafts in eight cases to neurotize the biceps muscle at the same time that free nerve grafts were used to neurotize the triceps muscle. In four of these cases the biceps had better function than the triceps, in two cases the functional result was equal, and in two cases the triceps was innervated in a better way by free grafts than the biceps by the vascularized nerve grafts.

Oberlin and associates reported on two cases of median nerve repair by free vascularized nerve grafts.[69] In one, the flexor digitorum superficialis achieved function of M4; in the other, function to M1 was achieved only in the flexor carpi radialis. In three other cases they restored continuity between the medial portion of the sciatic nerve and the tibial nerve by transferring the peroneal nerve as a vascularized nerve graft (vascularized by the third perforator of the profunda femoris artery). In all three cases there was return of function in the triceps surae of M4, but no other tibialis-innervated muscle achieved sufficient function for a tendon transfer to be performed. The coaptation in all these cases had been performed by epineural sutures.

Cutaneous Nerves

Since nerve trunks can be used only in rare cases to overcome peripheral nerve defects, many studies have been performed to explore the possibility of transferring cutaneous nerves. The first vascularized nerve graft, performed by Taylor, used the superficial radial nerve.[90]

To overcome the differences in caliber, techniques have been developed to use cutaneous nerves in several segments. If the paraneurium, including all the vessels, is carefully preserved, the nerve can be transected without damaging the circulation. The following nerves have been used:

1. Superficial branch of the radial nerve.[89,90] Usually a 23-cm-long graft can be obtained; the pedicle is 6.4 cm long. The nerve is supplied by the radial artery, which must be sacrificed. Taylor performed this operation in three cases to restore the continuity of the median nerve.[89] Protective sensibility returned but there was no return of motor function.
2. Sural nerve. Fachinelli and associates developed a technique to transfer the sural nerve based on the superficial sural artery, which originates either from the popliteal artery or from the medial or lateral sural artery.[34,39] A 35-cm-long graft can be obtained; the pedicle of the sural artery is 4.8 cm long. Gilbert reported on one case in which a defect of the median nerve was bridged by four segments of the sural nerve.[39] There was return of protective sensibility but not of motor function.

Doi and colleagues bridged defects in the median and ulnar nerves by transferred the sural nerve based on a cutaneous or a muscular branch of the peroneal artery and vein.[32] A skin island permitted observation of survival. Their results were no better than could have been achieved by free nerve grafts.

Townsend and Taylor developed a new concept in which the saphenous vein was excised in connection with the sural nerve.[94] An adequate segment of the vein was sutured into an arterial defect, and simultaneously the nerve repair was performed. They reported encouraging results in seven cases.

A similar concept was developed by Gu and coworkers.[43] With a simultaneous vascular and nerve defect, a combined graft consisting of the small saphenous vein and the sural nerve was transferred. The vein was sutured in a reversed manner into the arterial defect and the sural nerve was used to overcome the nerve defect. This technique was applied in 14 cases. In one radial nerve repair, a motor result of M4 to M5 was achieved. Motor recovery of M3 or better was observed in only two of eight ulnar repairs and in one of five median nerve repairs.

Rose and Kowalski repaired digital nerves in severely scarred fingers by transferring the deep peroneal nerve as a vascularized graft based on the dorsalis pedis artery.[75] In these cases, not only was the nerve restored in its continuity, but the blood supply to the finger in general improved as well.

Overview

The use of vascularized nerve grafts raises a basic question: Is the vascularized nerve graft just one form of nerve grafting that has its specific indications, or is the vascularized nerve graft so much better than a free nerve graft that it should become the treatment of choice in all circumstances?[91] Despite many attempts, significant benefits from vascularized nerve grafts have not been demonstrated experimentally.[55,70] While reports have shown rapid neurotization of vascularized grafts, with earlier signs of recovery, the results have not differed significantly from free nerve grafts.[5,10,37,38,56–58] The results published by Doi and associates[32] and Gu and colleagues[43] are no better than could have been achieved with free nerve grafts. The same is true for the reports of Oberlin and coworkers for the median and sciatic nerves.[69] Using the ulnar nerve as a vascularized nerve graft has special merit in brachial plexus lesions with avulsion of C8 and T1 roots.[11,69,93]

The advantages of vascularized nerve grafts are:

- Since the circulation is preserved or reestablished immediately, formation of adhesions to the recipient site is not a condition for survival.
- Because the paraneurium is preserved, vascularized nerve grafts are not as sensitive to longitudinal traction and tension at the sites of coaptation as are free nerve grafts.
- Vascularized nerve grafts are independent of the vascularity of the recipient site.
- More nerve fibers can be placed into the defect.
- The overall circulation of the recipient site (such as a scarred finger) is improved simultaneously.

ALTERNATIVES TO NERVE GRAFTING

Elongation of Nerve Tissue

Like other tissues, a peripheral nerve can be elongated by the gradual inflation of a tissue expander. Animal experiments have demonstrated that this is possible.[1,29] However, if the elongation is performed too quickly, nerve function is impaired. The results of Van Beek's three cases were not convincing.[95]

Providing Free Space For Neuromatous Neurotization

Based on Lundborg and Hansson's observations with the mesothelial chamber, different techniques have been used to allow axons to advance from proximal to distal stumps.[50] Several researchers have demonstrated the successful bridging of nerve gaps by autologous vein grafts.[16,25,26,73,85] Sparmann achieved encouraging experimental results, but the final outcome remained below the level of control autologous nerve grafts.[83] Chiu and Strauch compared end-to-end nerve repairs, autologous nerve grafts, and autologous vein conduits for digital nerve defects and concluded that autologous venous nerve conduits were valid for the treatment of defects of nonessential cutaneous nerves with short gaps.[27] My personal experience with autologous venous nerve conduits is favorable.

Biodegradable nerve conduits have been tested by various researchers; Dellon and Mackinnon found them a valid alternative to the management of short nerve gaps (see Chaps. 20 and 22).[28,31,52,79]

Providing an Autologous Tissue Framework for Neuromatous Neurotization

Keynes and associates[46] and Glasby and colleagues[40,41] used longitudinal freeze-degenerated muscle to provide a framework for outgrowing nerve fibers. They observed a higher number of axons in the distal stump with muscle interposition than with autologous nerve grafts. Unfortunately, they did not report on functional recovery. This does not necessarily mean that the interposed muscle has a better prospect for improved results, especially as the microphotographs show abundant collagenization of the autologous nerve grafts, indicating that they did not survive well.

I have used freeze-thawed muscle grafts on a few occasions. While I can confirm that this tissue becomes neurotized, the results appear inferior compared to free nerve grafts. Sparmann has reported favorable experimental results.[83]

SUMMARY

The autologous free cutaneous nerve graft remains the workhorse for the management of peripheral nerve defects, but vascularized nerve grafts are a valid alternative in selected cases. The application of allogenic nerve grafts might become a reality in the future. Alternatives to nerve grafting may develop into acceptable alternatives in less important nerves.

No matter what method is used, the technique must be meticulously performed, a point that is often overlooked. The most frequent errors include the use of cutaneous nerve grafts as free nerve grafts that are packed together; these have a poorer chance of survival without fibrosis. Also, grafts are not always harvested in sufficient lengths to avoid tension. Often limbs with nerve grafts are immobilized in flexed positions, creating unfavorable conditions for the graft once the limb is remobilized.

REFERENCES

1. Adson HM, Van Beek AL, Smith DO. Generation of nerve length with tissue expander. Presented at the 42nd annual meeting of the American Society for Surgery of the Hand, San Antonio, 1987.
2. Afanasieff A. Premieres résultates de 20 homogreffes de nerfs conservés par le cialit (main et avant-bras). Presse Méd 1967; 27:1409–1410.
3. Aguayo AJ, Attiwell M, Trecarten J. Abnormal myelination in transplanted trembler mouse Schwann cells. Nature 1977; 265:73.
4. Albert E. Einige Operationen am Nerven. Wien Med Presse 1885; 26:1285.
5. Alnot JY, Oberlin C, Bellaicke H. Vascularized ulnar nerve transfer in total palsy of the brachial plexus. Paper presented at the 10th international meeting of the Groupe d'Avancement de la Microchirurgie and the 7th annual meeting of the Deutschsprachige Arbeitsgemeinschaft für Mikrochirurgie der peripheren Nerven und Gefässe (DAM), Strasbourg, 1984.
6. Alnot YY, Benfrech E. Les autogreffes nerveuses. Problèmes techniques actuels. Ann Chir Main 1989; 8:291–295.
7. Anderl H, Hussl H. Erfahrungen mit vaskularisierten Nerventransplantaten. Paper presented at the annual meeting of the Deutsche Arbeitsgemeinschaft für Mikrochirurgie der peripheren Nerven und Gefäße, Berne, 1986.
8. Ballance C, Duel AB. Operative treatment of facial palsy by the introduction of nerve grafts into the fallopian canal and by other intratemporal methods. Arch Otolaryngol 1932; 15:1.
9. Bielschowsky M, Unger E. Überbrückung großer Nervenlücken. Beiträge zur Kenntnis der Degeneration und Regeneration peripherer Nerven. J Psychol Neurol (Leipz) 1918; 22:267.
10. Birch R. Personal communication at the Symposium sur le plexus brachial, Lausanne, 1984.
11. Bonney G, Birch R, Jamieson AM, Eames RA. Experience with vascularized nerve grafts. In: Terzis JK. Microreconstruction of nerve injuries. Philadelphia: WB Saunders, 1987:403.
12. Bosse JP. Personal communication at the International Symposium on Microsurgery, Guaruja, 1979.
13. Bosse JP. Discussional remark. In: Gorio A, Millesi H, Mingrino S, eds. Post-traumatic peripheral nerve regeneration (experimental basis and clinical implications). New York: Raven, 1981:347.
14. Breidenbach WP, Terzis JK. Vascularized nerve grafts. Essay Contest. American Soc Plast Reconstr Surg, 1983.
15. Breidenbach WP, Terzis JK. The anatomy of free vascularized nerve grafts. Clin Plast Surg 1984; 11:65.
16. Brunelli G, Fontana C, Jäger G, Bartolaminelli P, Baudet F. Chemotactic arrangement for regrowing motor and sensory axons of vein grafts. Paper presented at the 3rd Congress of the International Federation of Societies for Surgery of the Hand, Tokyo, 1986. Abstract 18-2, p. 161.
17. Brushart TM. Specific sensory motor tropism in peripheral nerve regeneration. Paper presented at the annual meeting of the Sunderland Society, Vienna, 1986.
18. Brushart TM, Henri EW, Mesulam MM. Reorganization of muscle afferent projections accompanies peripheral nerve regeneration. Neuroscience 1981; 6:2053.
19. Brushart TM, Mesulam MM. Alteration in connections between muscle and anterior horn motor neurons after peripheral nerve repair. Science 1980; 208:603.
20. Brushart TM, Seiler WA. Selective reinnervation of distal motor stumps by peripheral motor axons. Exp Neurol 1987; 97:289.
21. Brushart TM, Tarlow EC, Mesulam MM. Specificity

of muscle reinnervation after epineurial and individual fascicular suture of the rat sciatic nerve. J Hand Surg 1983; 8:248–253.
22. Bsteh FX, Millesi H. Zur Kenntnis der zweizeitigen Nerveninterplantation bei ausgedehntem peripheren Nervendefekt. Klin Med 1960; 15:571–578.
23. Bunnel S. Surgery of nerves of the hand. Surg Gynecol Obstet 1927; 44:145.
24. Chase RA. Reconstructive procedures after irreversible nerve damage in the upper extremity. Clin Neurosurg 1970; 17:142.
25. Chiu DTW. Autogenous vein graft as a conduit for nerve regeneration. Surg Forum 1980; 31:550.
26. Chiu DTW, Janecka I, Krizek TJ, Wolff M, Lovelace RE. Autogenous vein graft as a conduit for nerve regeneration. Surgery 1982; 91:226.
27. Chiu DTW, Strauch B. A prospective clinical evaluation of autogenous vein grafts used as nerve conduits for distal sensory nerve defects of 3 cm or less. Plast Reconstr Surg 1990, in press.
28. Collin W, Donoff RB. Nerve regeneration through collagen tubes. J Dental Res 1984; 63:987.
29. D'Anjou B, Allieu Y, Cenac P, Sanz J. Expansion nerveuse. Ann Chir Main 1989; 8:336–337.
30. Daverio PJ, Krupp S. Sutureless nerve anastomosis. Transactions of the 8th Congress of Plastic and Reconstructive Surgery, 1983.
31. Dellon AL, Mackinnon SE. An alternative to the classical nerve graft for the management of the short nerve gap. Plast Reconstr Surg 1988; 82:849.
32. Doi K, Kuwata N, Kawakami F, Tamaru K, Kawai S. Free vascularized sural nerve graft. Microsurgery 1984; 5:175.
33. Egloff DB, Narakas AO. Anastomose nerveuse par fibrinocollage. Rapport clinique préliminaire. Ann Chir Main 1983; 2:101–115.
34. Fachinelli A, Masquelet A, Restrepo J, Gilbert A. The vascularized sural nerve: Anatomy and surgical approach. Int J Microsurg 1981; 3:57.
35. Foerster O. Die Schußverletzung der peripheren Nerven und ihre Behandlung. Z Orthop Chir 1917; 36:310.
36. Freilinger G, Gruber H, Holle J, Mandl H. Zur Methodik der sensomotorisch differenzierten Faszikelnaht peripherer Nerven. Handchirurgie 1975; 7:133.
37. Gilbert A. Personal communication at the Symposium on Clinical Frontiers in Microsurgery, Anaheim, 1981.
38. Gilbert A. Vascularized nerve grafts. Paper presented at Reconstructive Microsurgery, Oklahoma City, 1982.
39. Gilbert A. Vascularized sural nerve graft. Clin Plast Surg 1984; 11:73–77.
40. Glasby MA, Gilmore JA, Gschmeissner SE, Hems TEJ, Miles LM. The repair of large peripheral nerves using skeletal muscle autografts: A comparison with cable grafts in the sheep femoral nerve. Brit J Plast Surg 1990; 43:169–178.
41. Glasby MA, Gschmeissner SE, Hitchcock RJI, Huang CLH, DeSouza BA. A comparison of nerve regeneration through nerve and muscle grafts in rat. Neuro-Orthopedics 1986; 2:21.
42. Gruber H, Zenker W. Acetylcholinesterase: Histochemical differentiation between motor and sensory nerve fibers. Brain Res 1973; 51:207.
43. Gu Y-D, Wu M-M, Zheng Y-H, Li H-R, Xu Y-N. Arterialised venous free sural nerve grafting. Ann Plast Surg 1985; 15:332.
44. Hiles RW. Freeze-dried irradiated nerve homografts: A preliminary report. Hand 1972; 4:79.
45. Jabaley ME, Wallace WH, Heckler FR. Internal topography of major nerves of the forearm and hand: A current review. J Hand Surg 1980; 5:1–18.
46. Keynes RJ, Hopkins WG, Huang LH. Regeneration of mouse peripheral nerves in degenerating skeletal muscle, guidance by residual muscle fiber membrane. Brain Res 1984; 295:275.
47. Kuderna H. Die Fibrinklebung peripherer Nerven. In: Nigst H, ed. Nervenwiederherstellung nach traumatischen Läsionen. Stuttgart: Hippokrates, 1985:78–94.
48. Künzel KH, Fischer C, Anderl H. The ulnar nerve as vascularized nerve transplant. I. Anatomy: Arterial vascular supply. J Reconstr Microsurg 1986; 2:174.
49. Louis DS, Eckenrode JF. Autogenous nerve pedicle graft in the forearm. J Hand Surg [Am] 1986; 11: 703–706.
50. Lundborg G, Hansson HA. Regeneration of the peripheral nerve through a preformed tissue space. Brain Res 1979; 178:573.
51. Mackinnon SE, Hudson AR, Falk RE, Hunter DA. The allograft response, an experimental model in the rat. Ann Plast Surg 1985; 14:334.
52. Madison R, DaSilva CF, Dikes P, Sidman RL, Chiu TH. Increased rate of peripheral nerve regeneration using bioabsorbable nerve guides and laminin-containing gel. Exp Neurol 1985; 88:767.
53. Marmor L. Regeneration of peripheral nerve defects by irradiated homografts. Lancet 1963; 1:1911.
54. Marmor L. Regeneration of peripheral nerves by irradiated homografts. J Bone Joint Surg [Am] 1964; 46:383.
55. McCullough CJ, Gagay O, Higginson DW, Sandin BM, Crow JC, Sebille A. Axon regeneration and vascularization of nerve grafts, an experimental study. J Hand Surg [Br] 1984; 9:323–327.

56. Merle M. Greffes vascularisées. Paper presented at the Symposium sur le plexus brachial, Lausanne, 1984.
57. Merle M, LeBreton E, Bour C, Maneaud M, Marin-Braun F. Free vascularized nerve transfer in brachial plexus injuries. Paper presented at the 10th international meeting of the Groupe d'Avancement de Microchirurgie and 7th annual meeting of the Deutschsprachigen Arbeitsgemeinschaft für Mikrochirurgie der peripheren Nerven und Gefäße (DAM), Strasbourg, 1984.
58. Merle M, LeBreton E, Foucher G, Bour C, Marin-Braun F. Vascularized nerve grafts: First results. Paper presented at the Inaugural Meeting of the American Society for Reconstructive Microsurgery, Las Vegas, 1985.
59. Meyer VE, Smahel J. The surgical cut surface of peripheral nerves. Int J Microsurg 1980; 2:187.
60. Millesi H. Zum Problem der Überbrückung von Defekten peripherer Nerven. Wien Med. Wschr 1968; 118:182.
61. Millesi H. Die Eingriffe and den Hand- und Fingernerven. In: Wachsmuth W, Wilhelm A, eds. Allgemeine und spezielle chirurgische Operationslehre: Die Operationen an der Hand, Vol. 10/3. Berlin-Heidelberg-New York: Springer-Verlag, 1972:226–250.
62. Millesi H. Healing of nerves. Clin Plast Surg 1977; 4:459–473.
63. Millesi H, Ganglberger J, Berger A. Interfaszikuläre Nerventransplantation mit Hilfe der mikrochirurgischen Technik. In: Transactions of the 4th International Congress of Plastic and Reconstructive Surgery, Rome, 1967. Amsterdam: Excerpta Medica, International Congress Series 174, pp 56–59.
64. Millesi H, Meissl G, Berger A. The interfascicular nerve grafting of the median and ulnar nerves. J Bone Joint Surg [Am] 1972; 54:727–750.
65. Millesi H, Meissl G, Berger A. Further experiences with interfascicular grafting of the median, ulnar and radial nerves. J Bone Joint Surg [Am] 1976; 58: 209–218.
66. Narakas A. The use of fibrin glue in repair of peripheral nerves. Orthop Clin North Am 1988; 19: 187–199.
67. Narakas A. Les greffes nerveuses: Expérience clinique. Ann Chir Main 1989; 8:302–311.
68. Nicholson R, Seddon HJ. Nerve repair in civil practice. Results of treatment of median and ulnar nerve lesions. Brit Med J 1957; 2:1065.
69. Oberlin C, Alnot JY, Comtet JJ. Les greffes nerveuses tronculaires vascularisées. Technique et résultat de 27 cas. Ann Chir Main 1989; 8:316–323.
70. Pho RWH, Lee YS, Rujiwetpongstore V, Pang M. Histological studies on the vascularized nerve graft and conventional nerve graft. J Hand Surg [Br] 1985; 10:45–48.
71. Politis MJ. Specificity in mammalian peripheral nerve regeneration at the level of the nerve trunk. Brain Res 1985; 328:271–276.
72. Politis MJ, Ederle K, Spencer PS. Tropism in nerve regeneration in vivo, attraction of regenerated axons by diffusable factors derived from cells in distal nerve stumps of transected peripheral nerves. Brain Res 1982; 253:1–12.
73. Rigoni G, Smahel J, Chiu DTW, Meyer VE. Veneninterponat als Leitbahn für die Regeneration peripherer Nerven. Handchirurgie 1983; 15:227.
74. Riley DA, Lang DH. Carbonic anhydrase activity of human peripheral nerves: Possible histochemical aid to nerve repair. J Hand Surg [Am] 1984; 9:112–120.
75. Rose E, Kowalski TA. Restoration of sensibility of unesthetic scarred digits with free vascularized nerve grafts from the dorsum of the foot. J Hand Surg [Am] 1985: 10:514.
76. Sakellarides H. A follow-up study of 173 peripheral nerve injuries in the upper extremity in civilians. J Bone Joint Surg [Am] 1962; 44:240.
77. Schaller E, Mailänder P, Becker M, Walter GF, Berger A. Nervenregeneration im autologen und allogenen Transplantat des N. ischiadicus der Ratte mit und ohne Immunosuppression durch Cyclosporin A. Handchirurgie 1988; 20:7.
78. Schröder JM, Seiffert KE. Die Feinstruktur der neuromatösen Neurotisation von Nerventransplantaten. Virch Arch [B] 1970; 5:219.
79. Seckel BR, Chiu TH, Nyilas E, Sidman RI. Nerve regeneration through synthetic biodegradable nerve guides: Regulation by a target organ. Plast Reconstr Surg 1984; 74:173.
80. Seckel BR, Ryan SE, Gagne JR, Tin Ho Chiu CST, Watkins E. Target-specific nerve regeneration through a nerve guide in the rat. Plast Reconstr Surg 1986; 78:793.
81. Seddon HJ. The use of autogenous grafts for the repair of large gaps in peripheral nerves. Brit J Surg 1947; 35:151.
82. Shelden C, Pudenz H, McCarty S. Two-stage autograft repair of extensive median and ulnar nerve defects. J Neurosurg 1947; 4:492–496.
83. Sparmann M. Die Bedeutung des sogenannten Leitschieneneffektes für die Regeneration peripherer Nerven über Defektstrecken. Eine tierexperimentelle Untersuchung am N. peronaeus des Kaninchens. Habilitationsschrift aus dem Fachbereich 3, Klinikum Charlottenburg, der Freien Universität Berlin, 1987.

84. Strange FG St. C. An operation for nerve pedicle grafting: Preliminary communication. Brit J Surg 1947; 34:423.
85. Strauch B, Rosenberg B, Brunelli F, Ferder M, DeMoura W. Autogenous vein graft substitute in long segment nerve defects. Paper presented at the Inaugural Meeting of the American Society for Reconstructive Microsurgery, Las Vegas, 1985.
86. Sunderland S. The intraneural topography of the radial, median and ulnar nerve. Brain 1945; 68:243.
87. Sunderland S, Ray JL. The intraneural topography of the sciatic nerve and its popliteal divisions in man. Brain 1948; 71:242.
88. Sunderland S, Marshall RD, Swaney WE. The intraneural topography of the circumflex, musculocutaneous and obturator nerve. Brain 1959; 82:116.
89. Taylor GI. Nerve grafting with simultaneous microvascular reconstruction. Clin Orthop 1978; 133:56–70.
90. Taylor GI, Ham F. The free vascularized nerve graft. Plast Reconstr Surg 1976; 57:413–426.
91. Terzis JK. Sensibility and motor re-education. Paper presented at Reconstructive Microsurgery, Oklahoma City, 1982.
92. Terzis JK. The use of carbonic anhydrase in the sensory motor differentiation of peripheral nerve trunks. Paper presented at the Symposium sur la plexus brachial, Lausanne, 1984.
93. Terzis JK, Liberson WT, Maragh HA. Motorcycle brachial plexopathy. In: Terzis JK, ed. Microreconstruction of nerve injuries. Philadelphia: WB Saunders, 1987:361–384.
94. Townsend PLG, Taylor GI. Vascularized nerve graft using composite arterialised neurovenous system. Brit J Plast Surg 1984; 37:1–17.
95. Van Beek A. Presentation at the annual meeting of the American Society of Microsurgery, Seattle, 1989.
96. Weiss P. Functional nerve regeneration through frozen dried nerve grafts in cats and monkeys. Proc Soc Exp Biol 1943; 54:277.
97. Weiss P, Taylor AC. Repair of peripheral nerves by grafts of frozen dried nerves. Proc Soc Exp Biol 1943; 52:326.
98. Williams HB. Peripheral nerve injuries in children. In: Kernahan DA, Thomson HG, Bauer BS, eds. Symposium on Pediatric Surgery. St. Louis: CV Mosby, 1982:266–282.

38

Donor Nerves for Grafting

James A. Nunley

AUTHOR'S KEY POINTS

- Selection of a donor nerve graft takes into consideration three factors: the cross-sectional area of the recipient nerve, the total length of nerve defect, and donor site morbidity.
- The four prime sources of donor nerve in the upper extremity are the dorsal cutaneous branch of the ulnar nerve, the medial antebrachial cutaneous nerve, the lateral antebrachial cutaneous nerve, and the terminal posterior interosseous nerve.
- When total defects exceed 10 to 12 cm, lower-extremity grafts are obtained.
- The medial antebrachial cutaneous nerve is located by marking a point 2 cm distal and 2 cm lateral to the medial epicondyle. The lateral antebrachial cutaneous nerve lies just lateral to the biceps tendon in the antecubital fossa. Dissection of the posterior interosseous nerve is deep, below the extensor tendons and muscles in the midline of the distal forearm. The dorsal cutaneous branch of the ulnar nerve is isolated 4 cm proximal to the wrist crease. The nerve courses from palmar to dorsal, lying mid-axially, at the level of the ulnar styloid.
- From each sural nerve, 40 cm of nerve graft can be obtained. The nerve is located 1 cm posterior and 1 cm superior to the tip of the lateral malleolus.

Nerve grafting has become widely used for making up gaps in many upper- and lower-extremity nerves.[5] Thanks to the pioneering efforts of Millesi[12–14] and others, the results of nerve grafting have justified their continued use in clinical practice.[15,27] Most surgeons now agree that a nerve should not be repaired under tension and that if tension exists between two nerve ends it is best to insert a graft.[12,19,26] The polarity of the nerve graft does not seem to make a significant difference.[23]

The question still remains of where to obtain a donor nerve graft. Currently there are only two types of nerve grafts in clinical use, nonvascularized and vascularized autografts,[3] although other materials have been tried experimentally.[1,2,4] This chapter will deal exclusively with nonvascularized conventional nerve grafts.

REQUIREMENTS FOR NERVE GRAFT

An ideal donor nerve graft would exactly match the recipient neural defect with respect to axon count, branching patterns, and internal topogra-

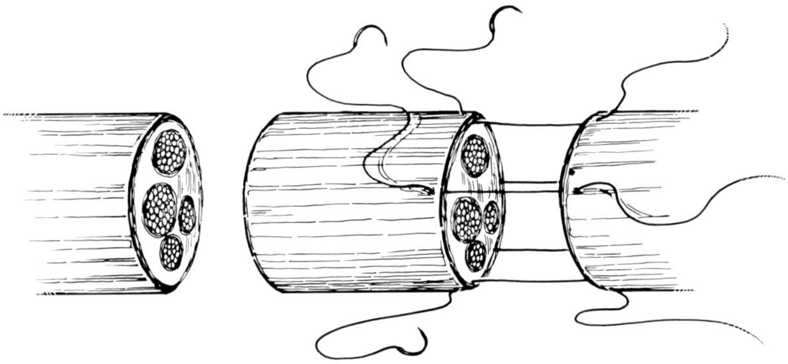

Figure 38–1. *Trunk graft.*

phy, but this is rarely possible. When choosing a donor graft, the surgeon must assess the cross-sectional area of the recipient nerve, the total length of the neural defect, and donor site morbidity.

Cross-Sectional Area

It is possible, but not desirable, to replace a segment of a large nerve such as the upper trunk of the brachial plexus with a single donor nerve that has a cross-sectional area and fascicle count approximately equal to the neural defect (Fig. 38-1). Seddon used the median antebrachial cutaneous nerve where it exits the brachial plexus as a donor nerve graft for defects in the brachial plexus; however, the results were poor and he attributed the failures to central necrosis of the donor nerve graft.[20,21] When using a large nerve as a graft, the central area of the graft rarely becomes vascularized, and neural regeneration is poor.[7,10]

A more popular technique for replacement of major nerves with large cross-sectional areas involves the use of multiple cable grafts (Fig. 38-2).

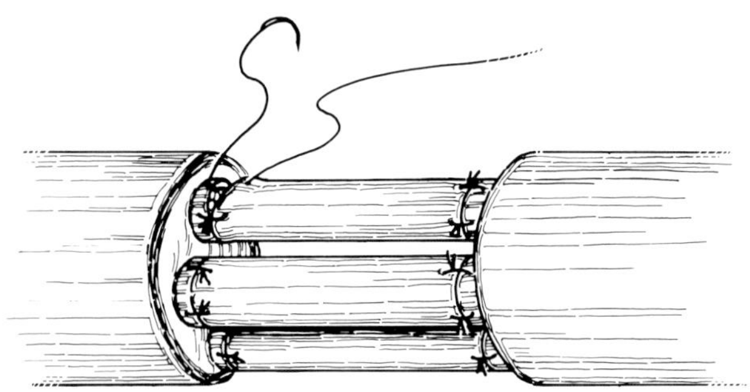

Figure 38–2. *Cable nerve graft.*

Each cable contains a single strand of donor nerve (eg, sural) that has a finite number of axons and neural tissue. By using multiple small cables, the surgeon can dissect a large nerve internally into multiple groups or bundles of fascicles and can repair individual groups or bundles of nerve fibers to single cable grafts, thus performing a precise anatomic repair.[27] Since each cable is in close proximity to a blood supply by diffusion, revascularization is rapid.[13]

Length of Donor Grafts

In small nerves such as the digital nerve, the overall length of graft needed is a reflection of the actual neural defect. Many times, only one cable or, in some cases, only one fascicle is needed for grafting the defect. However, in larger nerves such as the median nerve in the forearm, the length of donor graft will be the product of the actual length of the gap and the number of cables needed to fill the cross-sectional area. Often the sural nerve will be selected as the donor graft over other more conveniently located nerves because of the vast length of graft material that it has available (Table 38-1).

Donor Site Morbidity

Under ideal circumstances, the donor site for a nerve graft would be conveniently located in the same extremity as the defect so that regional anesthesia could be used. However, it is often impossible, because of length requirements, for the donor and recipient sites to be in the same extremity.

Ideally, the area of hypesthesia and anesthesia from the donor nerve is minimal and is not in a

Table 38–1. *Donor Nerve Graft*

Nerve	*Length*	*Donor Morbidity*	*Difficulty of Dissection*
Dorsal cutaneous branch of ulnar	4–6 cm	++	+
Medial antebrachial cutaneous (below elbow)	8–10 cm	+	+
Lateral antebrachial cutaneous (below elbow)	10–12 cm	++	+
Posterior interosseous (terminal portion)	4–6 cm	0	+++
Sural	20–40 cm	+	++
Lateral femoral cutaneous	10–20 cm	+++	+++

+, least; ++, intermediate; +++, most.

critical area for sensibility. For example, a defect in the digital nerve has been replaced by the medial antebrachial cutaneous nerve, the lateral antebrachial cutaneous nerve, and the dorsal cutaneous branch of the ulnar nerve. If the digital nerve to receive the graft is in the thumb, then the lateral antebrachial cutaneous nerve would not be satisfactory since it often contributes to the volar and dorsal radial sensation of the thumb. If the digital nerve graft is in the small finger, the dorsal cutaneous branch of the ulnar nerve is a poor choice since it contributes to sensibility of the small finger.

Ideally, the donor nerve is subcutaneous, not close to any significant structure, and the nerve graft dissection does not interfere with function. Although the terminal portion of the posterior interosseous nerve has been used as a graft for a digital nerve, dissecting this nerve requires a deep plane: the extensor tendons are retracted and the extensor retinaculum usually must be divided. This nerve, when used as a graft, has the potential to interfere with finger and wrist function because of tendon dissection.

UPPER-EXTREMITY DONOR NERVES

Grafting of neural defects is much more commonly performed in the upper than the lower extremity. There are four main sources of donor nerve located in the upper extremity: the medial antebrachial cutaneous nerve,[16] the lateral antebrachial cutaneous nerve,[11,24,25] the terminal posterior interosseous nerve,[29] and the dorsal cutaneous branch of the ulnar nerve.[9] All four of these donor nerves may be used as graft tissue for replacement of digital nerves, but only the medial and lateral antebrachial cutaneous nerves have enough length to be useful in replacing *small* defects in the median, ulnar, and superficial radial nerves. When the total defect in the median, ulnar, or radial nerve exceeds the critical length of 10 to 12 cm, then another donor nerve (usually the sural) is selected.

Medial Antebrachial Cutaneous Nerve

The medial antebrachial cutaneous nerve (MACN) exits the brachial plexus and courses along the medial aspect of the arm. Above the elbow it is too large to be suitable for grafting, but just above the elbow it divides into an anterior and posterior division.[16] The MACN is harvested below the elbow, where the nerve lies in the subcutaneous tissues. It is found by extending the elbow and measuring two fingerbreadths below the medial epicondyle in line with the flexor carpi ulnaris and then moving up two fingerbreadths toward the middle of the forearm (Fig. 38-3). Either the anterior or posterior division may be taken. The area of hypesthesia and anesthesia is shown in Figure 38-4.

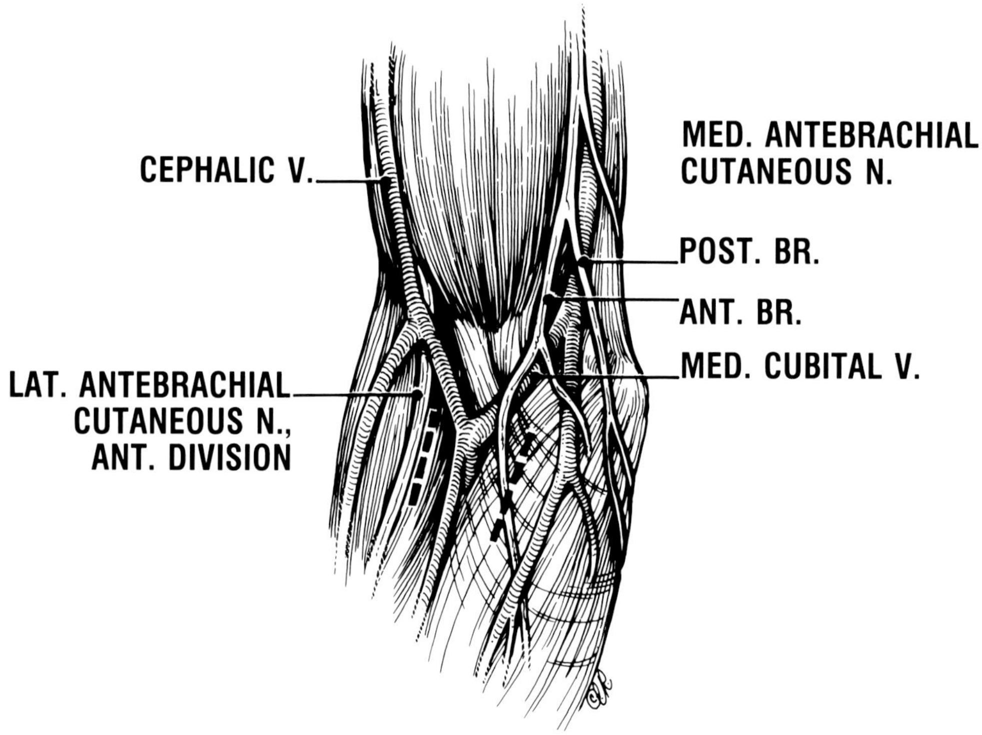

Figure 38–3. *Anterior view of the elbow demonstrating skin incisions for isolation of medial antebrachial cutaneous nerve and lateral antebrachial cutaneous nerve.*

Lateral Antebrachial Cutaneous Nerve

The lateral antebrachial cutaneous nerve (LACN) is the terminal sensory portion of the musculocutaneous nerve. This nerve exits the arm just lateral to the biceps tendon where it lies on top of the brachialis muscle. The LACN divides into anterior and posterior divisions at the elbow crease. This nerve is subcutaneous, and either division may be taken for grafting (see Fig. 38-3).[11,24,25] The dis-

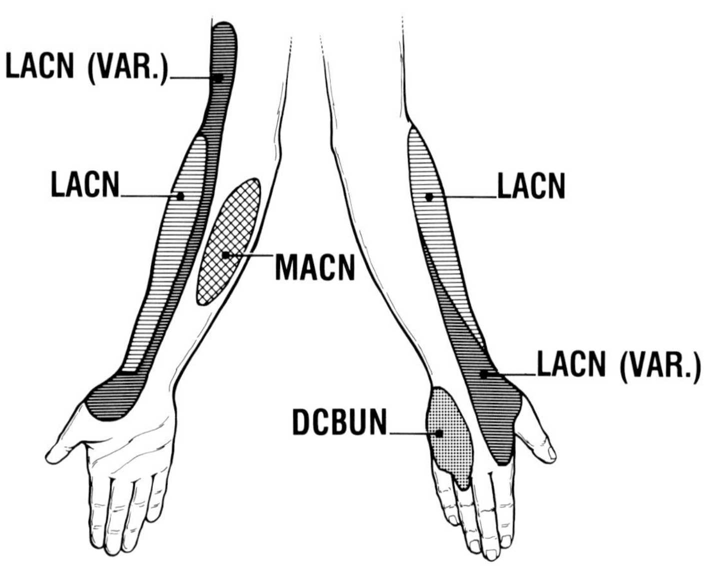

Figure 38–4. *Anterior and posterior view of the forearm indicating areas of hypesthesia from use of donor nerves in the upper extremity. MACN, medial antebrachial cutaneous nerve; LACN, lateral antebrachial cutaneous nerve; DCBUN, dorsal cutaneous branch of the ulnar nerve.*

advantage to this nerve graft is the occasional loss of sensibility in the thenar area. For this reason, it is not a good donor nerve for the median nerve, the digital nerve in the thumb, or the superficial radial nerve.

Posterior Interosseous Nerve

The posterior interosseous nerve (PIN) is primarily a motor nerve, but after giving off its final motor branches to the "outcropper" muscles, it courses with the posterior interosseous artery to the wrist, where it partially innervates the wrist joint (Fig. 38-5). This nerve may be taken as a nerve graft from the last motor branch all the way to the wrist crease. This is a useful nerve for grafting in the digit,[29] but its dissection is deep below the extensor tendons and muscles, which could in some cases result in scarring and loss of function.

Dorsal Cutaneous Branch of Ulnar Nerve

The ulnar nerve gives off its dorsal cutaneous branch approximately 4 cm proximal to the wrist crease. This nerve then courses from palmar to dorsal, becoming quite superficial at the level of the ulnar styloid. The dorsal cutaneous branch of the ulnar nerve (DCBUN) is usually harvested 1 to 2 cm distal to the ulnar styloid so that the resected end will be dorsal, and not near the distal ulna, which is a frequently traumatized area (see Fig. 38-5). The DCBUN is useful in grafting small defects in the digital nerves,[9] but it should not be used for grafts to the small finger because this nerve provides sensibility to the small finger.

LOWER-EXTREMITY DONOR NERVES

Although it would be possible to use any cutaneous nerve from the lower extremity as a nerve graft, the sural nerve is the generally preferred donor nerve in the leg. The sural nerve is the most commonly used donor nerve for peripheral nerve grafting, primarily because it provides such generous lengths of expendable nerve and because of its ease of harvesting.[17] There is some morbidity to harvesting a sural nerve; Staniforth and Fisher reported that 44% of their patients complained of loss of sensibility over the lateral aspect of the foot and ankle.[22] While 42% of Staniforth's patients complained of calf tenderness, only 16% had significant pain. Wood reported that 6.1% of his patients had neuromas producing symptoms in the donor legs, and 9.1% of patients were dissatisfied with the altered sensibility in the foot.[17]

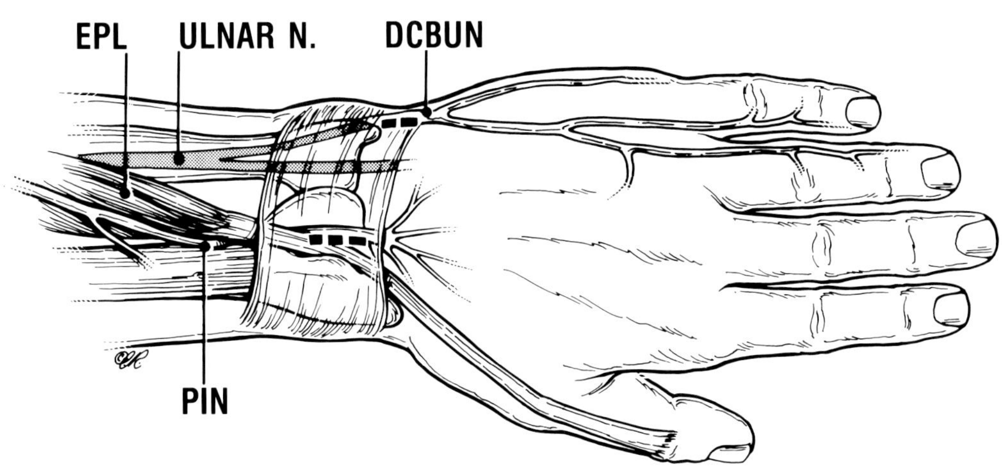

Figure 38–5. *Dorsal view of the wrist showing skin incisions for dorsal cutaneous branch of the ulnar nerve (DCBUN) and posterior interosseous nerve (PIN).*

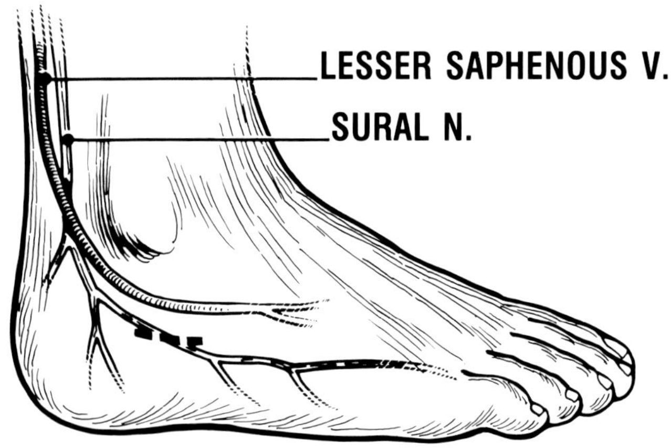

Figure 38–6. *Lateral view of the leg demonstrating incision used to harvest the sural nerve.*

Sural Nerve

The sural nerve is harvested either above or below the ankle. When harvested below the ankle, the sural nerve is removed from along the lateral border of the foot, in line with the peroneal tendons (Fig. 38-6). This portion of the sural nerve has been used for grafting digital nerves.[6] However, it is a poor choice for replacing a digital nerve, for several reasons: there are several better choices in the up-

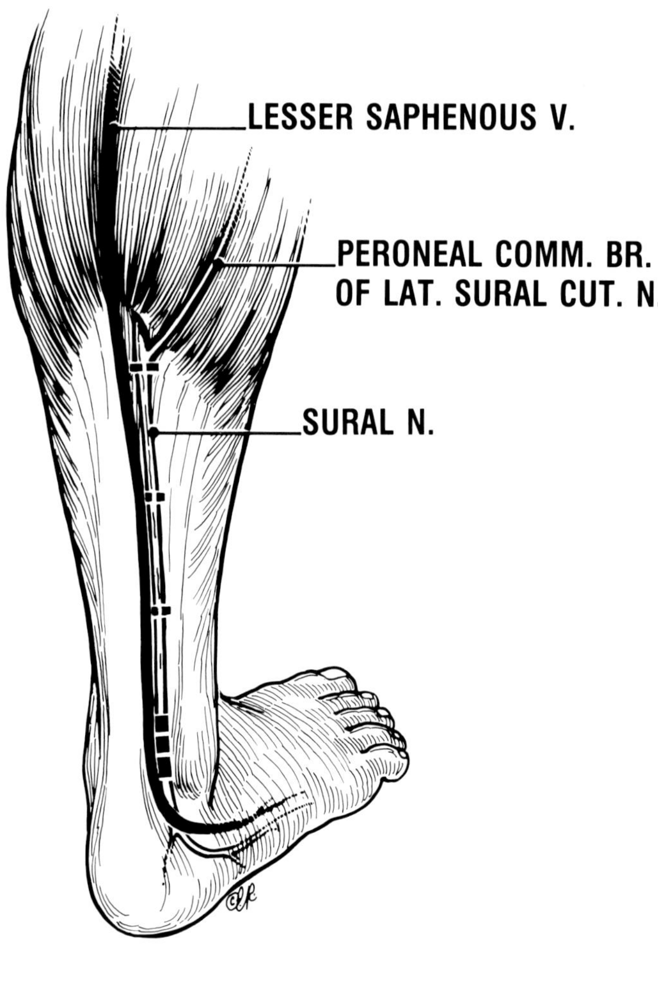

Figure 38–7. *The sural nerve is harvested beginning with a longitudinal incision above and posterior to the lateral malleolus. The remainder of the nerve is taken through multiple small horizontal incisions.*

per extremity, regional or local anesthesia cannot be used, and the donor scar along the lateral border of the foot can be irritating when wearing certain types of shoes.

The sural nerve is typically harvested above the ankle and is used in major nerve grafting procedures where 30 to 40 cm of donor nerve are needed.[8] The first step is to place a pad beneath the donor-side buttock to internally rotate the leg, since this nerve is located posteriorly in the calf (Fig. 38-7). A thigh tourniquet is used to provide a bloodless field. A longitudinal incision is made one fingerbreadth posterior to the lateral malleolus and 1 cm superior to the tip of the lateral malleolus. This skin incision is designed to avoid contact with conventional footwear.

The sural nerve is found in the subcutaneous tissues adjacent to the lesser saphenous vein. It is transected distally and held in a moist sponge. Gentle traction is applied, and the remaining portion is harvested by making multiple small transverse incisions in the skin proximally. It is possible to harvest the sural nerve by making one long incision, but this is unnecessary. The sural nerve may also be harvested with a stripper, but this is a delicate procedure and injury to the nerve graft can occur.[18,28] The dissection of this nerve graft must be atraumatic. By applying traction to the free end of the nerve, each new skin incision can be planned up the leg. As the nerve is located *beneath* the fascia in the middle of the leg, the fascia is divided to gain adequate length. The sural communicating branch of the peroneal nerve joins the main sural nerve in the midcalf area, and this branch is divided to mobilize the nerve higher in the leg.

Lateral Femoral Cutaneous Nerve

The lateral femoral cutaneous nerve (LFCN) is an independent branch of the lumbosacral plexus; after coursing through the pelvis, this nerve enters the thigh and becomes subcutaneous. The LFCN usually pierces the fascia lata 2 cm below and slightly medial to the anterior superior iliac spine (ASIS), becoming subcutaneous just distal to the sartorius muscle. The LFCN then runs down the anterior lateral aspect of the thigh to the knee. This nerve is harvested for use as a graft by finding the nerve at the level at which it becomes subcutaneous and then tracing it distally.[30] The initial skin incision is begun just inferior and medial to the ASIS, and the LFCN can then be harvested over many centimeters, either through one long incision or, as with the sural nerve, through multiple small transverse incisions.

REFERENCES

1. Ashley FL, Murphy JE, Morgan SC, et al. Axon growth through irradiated median and ulnar nerve homografts in primates. Plast Reconstr Surg 1968; 42:313.
2. Barnes R, Bacsich P, Wyburn GM, et al. A study of the fate of nerve homografts in man. Br J Surg 1946; 34:34.
3. Birch R, Dunkerton M, Bonney G, Jamieson AM. Experience with the free vascularized ulnar nerve graft in repair of supraclavicular lesions of the brachial plexus. Clin Orthop Rel Res 1988; 237:97–104.
4. Bora FW, Bednar JM, Osterman AL, Brown MJ, Sumner AJ. Prosthetic nerve grafts: A resorbable tube as an alternative to autogenous nerve grafting. J Hand Surg [Am] 1987; 12:685–692.
5. Brooks D. The place of nerve grafting in orthopaedic surgery. J Bone Jt Surg [Am] 1955; 37:299.
6. Buncke HJ Jr. Digital nerve repairs. Surg Clin North Am 1972; 52:1267–1285.
7. Bunnell S, Boyes JH. Nerve grafts. Am J Surg 1939; 44:64.
8. Doi K, Kuwata N, Kawakami F, Tamaru K, Kawai S. The free vascularized sural nerve graft. Microsurgery 1984; 5:175–184.
9. Greene TL, Steichen JB. Digital nerve grafting using the dorsal sensory branch of the ulnar nerve. J Hand Surg [Br] 1985; 10:37–40.
10. Holmes W. Histological observation on the repair of nerves by autografts. Br J Surg 1947; 35:167.
11. McFarlane RM, Mayer JR. Digital nerve grafts with the lateral antebrachial cutaneous nerve. J Hand Surg 1976; 1:169–173.
12. Millesi H. Microsurgical nerve grafting. Int Surg 1980; 65:503–508.
13. Millesi H. Nerve grafting. Clin Plast Surg 1984; 11: 105–113.
14. Millesi H, Meissl G, Berger A. The inter-fascicular nerve-grafting of the median and ulnar nerves. J Bone Joint Surg [Am] 1972; 54:727–750.
15. Moneim MS. Interfascicular nerve grafting. Clin Orthop Rel Res 1982; 163:65–74.
16. Nunley JA, Ugino MR, Goldner RD, Regan N, Ur-

baniak JR. Use of the anterior branch of the medial antebrachial cutaneous nerve as a graft for the repair of defects of the digital nerve. J Bone Joint Surg [Am] 1989; 71:563–567.
17. Ortiguela ME, Wood MB, Cahill DR. Anatomy of the sural nerve complex. J Hand Surg [Am] 1987; 12:1119–1123.
18. Rindell K, Telaranta T. A new atraumatic and simple method of taking sural nerve grafts. Ann Chir Gynaecol 1984; 73:40–41.
19. Rodkey WG, Cabaud HE, McCarroll HR Jr. Neurorrhaphy after loss of a nerve segment: Comparison of epineurial suture under tension versus multiple nerve grafts. J Hand Surg 1980; 5:366–371.
20. Seddon HJ. The use of autogenous grafts for the repair of large gaps in peripheral nerves. Br J Surg 1947; 35:151.
21. Seddon HJ. Nerve grafting. J Bone Joint Surg [Br] 1963; 45:447–461.
22. Staniforth P, Fisher TR. The effects of sural nerve excision in autogenous nerve grafting. Hand 1978; 10:187.
23. Stromberg BV, Vlastou C, Earle AS. Effect of nerve graft polarity on nerve regeneration and function. J Hand Surg 1979; 4:444–445.
24. Tank MS, Lewis RC Jr, Coates PW. The lateral antebrachial cutaneous nerve as a highly suitable autograft donor for the digital nerve. J Hand Surg 1983; 8:942–945.
25. Tenny JR, Lewis RC. Digital nerve-grafting for traumatic defects: Use of the lateral antebrachial cutaneous nerve. J Bone Joint Surg [Am] 1984; 66: 1375–1378.
26. Terzis J, Faibisoff B, Williams HB. The nerve gap: Suture under tension versus graft. Plast Reconstr Surg 1975; 56:166–170.
27. Urbaniak JR. Fascicular nerve suture. Clin Orthop Rel Res 1982; 163:57–64.
28. Wessberg GA. Atraumatic harvesting of the sural nerve. J Oral Maxillofac Surg 1985; 43:237.
29. Wiglis EGS, Maxwell GP. Distal digital nerve grafts: Clinical and anatomical studies. J Hand Surg 1979; 4:439–443.
30. Yamano Y, Namba Y, Hino Y, Hasegawa T, Ugawa A, Ise M. Digital nerve grafts in replanted digits. Hand 1982; 14:255–262.

39

Results of Nerve Grafting

Gary K. Frykman
Kevin Gramyk

AUTHORS' KEY POINTS

- The compiled results of nerve grafting in the upper extremity display an inverse relationship with age, graft length, and delay between injury and grafting.
- Patient age is the best predictor of the results of nerve grafting.
- Level of injury has a significant effect on the results of grafting of all three upper extremity nerves.
- Graft length has a marked effect on the recovery of median nerve function following grafting. Of grafts less than 5 cm, 95% obtained useful recovery; only 66% of those over 10 cm did so.
- The recovery of ulnar nerve function overall is more favorable than is sometimes depicted.
- Lower-extremity nerve grafts achieved less favorable recovery than reported in the upper extremity, but some cases obtained useful motor control and protective sensation.

In this chapter, information from published studies on nerve autografts using nonbiological suture materials and performed under magnification is presented to provide a basis for assessing the usefulness of this technique and to allow comparison with other nerve reconstruction methods. The results are summarized in tables and figures to facilitate understanding and discussion.

The use of autografts for nerve repair has increased steadily since the late 1920s. Several techniques have been developed because of the inadequacies of end-to-end repair. In 1928, Bunnell found that regeneration through autogenous nerve grafts occurred as rapidly as with direct end-to-end suture repair.[6] The results of Millesi's experimental work showed no significant differences in nerve recovery between direct repair and nerve grafting, provided there was no tension along the suture lines and conditions were favorable (ie, adequate vascular supply, healthy soft-tissue bed, etc).[22,23] In recent years, nerve grafting has become the most frequently used alternative procedure for bridging nerve defects.[26]

While nerve grafting was described in experimental form in 1810,[29] Albert[1] first described the clinical use of nerve grafting in 1885 (he used a xenograft to overcome a 3-cm median nerve gap). The long-term results of this procedure were not reported.

Attempts by surgeons to salvage nerves interrupted by penetrating trauma in World War I using nerve grafts were largely unsuccessful. Although some early results indicated success with nerve-grafting techniques[5,7] subsequent reports were not as promising.[4,7,9,20,40,44] Surgeons tended to avoid the procedure and instead used end-to-end repair. Among the methods used, singly or in combination, were bone shortening, nerve mobilization, and flexion of adjacent joints.

Interest in nerve grafting was renewed when Bunnell reported experience with digital nerve grafts in the late 1920s.[6] In 1927 Bunnell reported on a successful nerve graft for reconstructing the facial nerve.[5]

The largest studies reporting on nerve repair and grafting were gathered from World War II experience. The technique used for reconstruction of most injuries during this time was trunk grafting without microscopic magnification. Seddon reported on the experience in Great Britain with 699 nerve injuries, 8.6% of which were treated by nerve grafts.[27,35,36] In the United States, Woodhall and Beebe reported that grafts had been used in only 30 of 3415 nerve injuries.[49]

The poor results achieved initially in the World War II cases have been attributed to the fact that nerve grafting was reserved for those cases where methods for direct end-to-end repair could not be used.[27,35,36,49] Also, it was performed only in the most severe injuries with the longest gaps. The use of large-diameter donor nerves may have been another significant factor contributing to initially poor results. Grafts with a diameter greater than 3 mm, such as the peroneal or ulnar nerves, while technically easy to suture, are subject to central necrosis from inadequate early revascularization.[37]

Interfascicular nerve grafting, introduced by Millesi, involves the coaptation of the donor cutaneous nerve graft to a single small recipient nerve, such as a digital nerve, or to a group of fascicles of a larger nerve.[24] Others have referred to this method as a group fascicular nerve graft[45] or

Table 39–1. *Studies Included in Chapter 39 Results*

Author	***Digital***	***Median***	***Ulnar***	***Radial***
Frykman/Cally, 1988[10]	X	X	X	X
Haase, 1981[11]	—	X	X	—
Hirasawa/Katsumi/Tokioka, 1986[15]	X			
Ito/Hirotani/Yamamoto, 1976[16]		X	X	
McFarlane/Mayer, 1976[21]	X			
Millesi/Meissl/Berger, 1972[24]		X	X	
Millesi/Meissl/Berger, 1976[25]		X	X	X
Moneim, 1982[26]	X	X	X	X
Nunley et al, 1989[28]	X			
Rose/Kowalski, 1985[31]	X			
Rose/Kowalski/Norris, 1989[32]	X			
Samii/Waagner, 1975[34]		X	X	X
Stellini, 1982[39]	X	X	X	X
Tenny/Lewis, 1984[43]	X			
Walton/Finseth, 1977[44]		X	X	X
Wilgis/Maxwell, 1979[46]	X			
Yamano, 1982[50]			X	X
Yamano/Namba/Hino, 1982[51]	X			

Table 39–2. *Studies Without Individual Patient Data*

Digital Nerve Grafts

	N	*Gap (mm)*	*Age (yr)*	*≥S3 (%)*	*<S3 (%)*
Seddon, 1947[35]	15	30–80	adult	42	58
Brooks, 1955[4]	17	>20		47	18
Young, 1980[52]	27	>20	15–57	100	0
Beazley et al, 1984[2]	12	10–15	0.5–71	58	42
Mackinnon/Dellon, 1988[19]	31	10–15	18–64	94	6
Berger et al, 1988[3]	Unknown	10–16	Unknown	80	20

Median Nerve Grafts

	N	*Gap (mm)*	*Age (yr)*	*Motor Recovery*	*Sensory Recovery*
Seddon, 1974[35]	11	50–150	adult	M4 = 18%, M3 = 36%	S3+ = 18%, S3 = 45%
Brooks, 1950[4]	33	>70		M3 = 69%	S3 = 69%, S2 = 21%
Tallas et al, 1978[42]	6	40–150		82% ≥ M3	S3+ = 33%
Haase et al, 1980[12]	30	10–230	6–73	Low: 90% ≥ M3	97% ≥ S2+
	7	10–230	6–73	High: 57% ≥ M3	71% ≥ S2+
Young, 1980[52]	11	>20	15–57	73% ≥ M3	100% ≥ S3
Sedel/Bricout, 1982[38]	19		11–71	37% very good, 32% good, 26% fair, 5% nul	
Beazley et al, 1984[2]	5	40–60	0.5–71	M2+ average	S2 average
Wiswe et al, 1987[48]	45		av = 28	60% very good, 20% good	42% very good, 16% good

Ulnar Nerve Grafts

	N	*Gap (mm)*	*Age (yr)*	*Motor Recovery*	*Sensory Recovery*
Tallas et al, 1978[42]	10	30–70		M4 = 30%, M3 = 50%, M2 = 20%	S3+ = 20%, S3 = 40%, S2+ = 20%
Haase et al, 1980[12]	14	15–70	9–73	Low: 93% ≥ M3	71% ≥ S2+
	12	15–70	9–73	High: 50% ≥ M3	75% ≥ S2+
Young, 1980[52]		>20	15–57	25% ≥ M3 (n = 4)	78% ≥ S3 (n = 9)
Sedel/Bricout, 1982[38]	16		11–71	25% very good, 56% good, 12% fair, 6% nul	
Beazley et al, 1984[2]	6	20–70	0.5–71	M2 average	S1 average
Wiswe et al, 1987[48]	46		av = 28	22% very good, 46% good	26% very good, 39% good

Radial Nerve Grafts

	N	*Gap (mm)*	*Age (yr)*	*Motor Recovery*	*Sensory Recovery*
Sedel/Bricout, 1982[38]	10		11–71	20% very good, 40% good, 30% fair, 10% nul	
Beazley et al, 1984[2]	4	40–100	0.5–71	M3 average	S2 average
Wiswe et al, 1987[48]	46		av = 28	100% very good	

N, *number of grafts.*

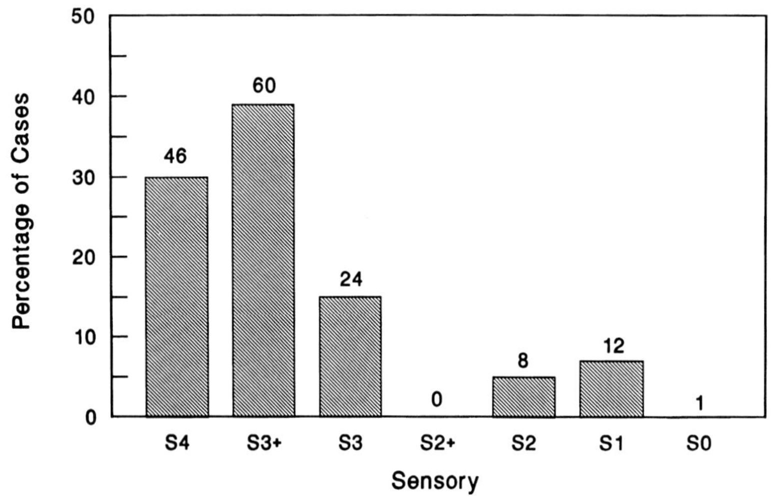

Figure 39–1. *Digital nerve grafting. Results of 151 nerve grafts. (Reprinted with permission from Department of Veterans Affairs.)*

funicular graft.[41] Magnification and attention to the internal anatomy of the nerve are important to success with this technique.[8,47]

The factors affecting results following nerve repair described in Chapter 24 may also be applied to results from nerve grafting. These factors will not be discussed fully here, but the four most important factors are the patient's age, the length of the gap, the time delay from injury to nerve grafting, and the level of the injury (proximal or distal).

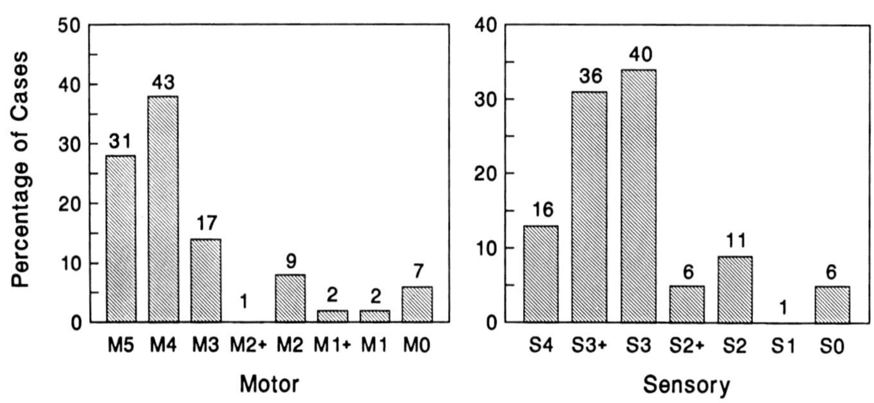

Figure 39–2. *Median nerve grafting. Results of 112 grafts for motor loss and 116 grafts for sensory loss. (Reprinted with permission from Department of Veterans Affairs.)*

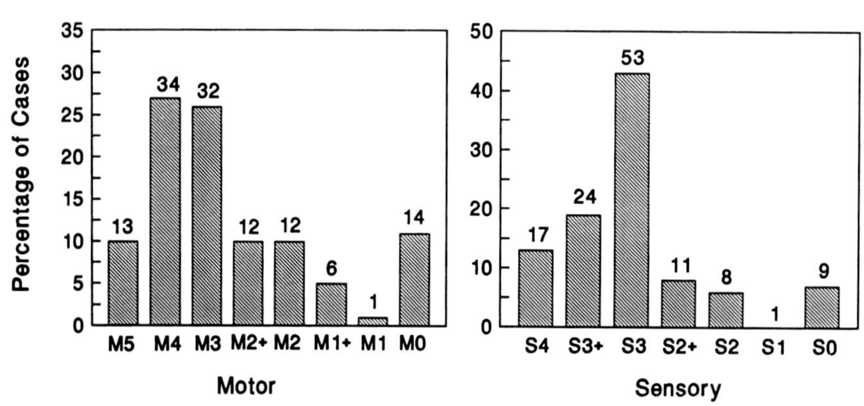

Figure 39–3. *Ulnar nerve grafting. Results of 124 grafts for motor loss and 123 grafts for sensory loss. (Reprinted with permission from Department of Veterans Affairs.)*

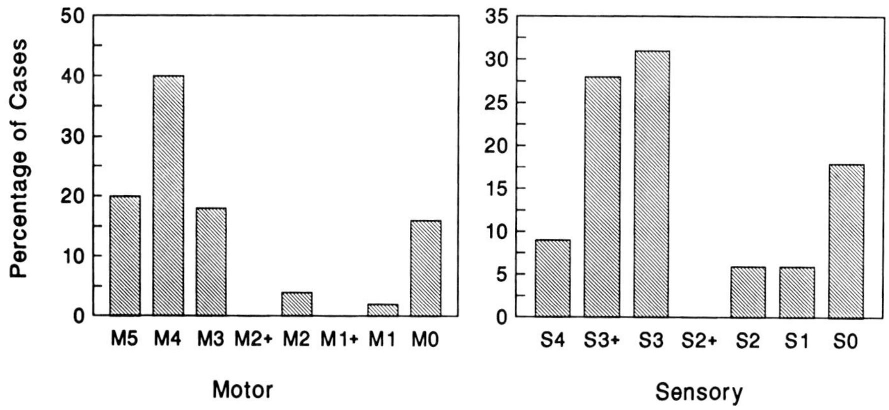

Figure 39-4. *Radial nerve grafting. Results of 50 grafts for motor loss and 32 grafts for sensory loss. (Reprinted with permission from Department of Veterans Affairs.)*

METHODOLOGY

A review of the published literature on nerve grafting was performed (Table 39-1). To ensure the most reliable and meaningful results, only those cases that met the following criteria were used:

1. The results of each patient were described, allowing classification of motor and sensory recovery separately for mixed nerves.
2. Subgroups of age, time delay before grafting, and graft length were noted.
3. A minimum follow-up of 1 year after the nerve grafting procedure was reported.

The results described here were obtained by evaluating those studies that met all criteria. The results from studies prior to 1972 using the older methods of trunk grafting are not included, as they do not meet the criteria outlined above. Several other nerve grafting studies that published secondary data were excluded from analysis because the methods of presentation used by the authors did not meet the criteria noted above. The results of these studies are summarized in Table 39-2.

In our study the overall results for each nerve in the upper extremity are presented in graphic form (Figs. 39-1 to 39-4). We further divided the results for each individual nerve to look at the effect of age, gap length, and delay for digital nerves. In addition, we added level of injury and separated motor and sensory recovery for median, ulnar, and radial nerves. The subgroups for age, gap length, and delay have been chosen somewhat arbitrarily, by looking for trends or divisions in the data. Brachial plexus grafts were not analyzed, as they are covered separately in Chapters 90 through 94.

Sensory results are reported in Tables 39-3 and 39-4,using Highet and Sanders' scheme[14] with Mackinnon and Dellon's modification[18] (S3 is defined as static two-point discrimination of 15 to 20 mm, S3+ as sensory return of 7 to 15 mm, and S4 for sensory return of 2 to 6 mm). We use the term "useful" return of sensation to describe those cases with S3 or greater. We use the term "useful" motor recovery for M3 or better.

Table 39-3. *Classification of Motor Recovery*

Grade	***Motor Recovery***
M0	No contraction
M1	Return of perceptible contraction in the proximal muscles
M1+	Proximal muscles contract against gravity but intrinsics paralyzed
M2	Same as in M1+ with perceptible intrinsic contraction
M2+	Proximal and distal muscles are all active against gravity
M3	Return of function in both proximal and distal muscles to such a degree that all important muscles are sufficiently powerful to act against gravity
M4	All muscles act against strong resistance and some independent movements are possible; some intrinsic weakness
M5	Full recovery in all muscles

Table 39-4. *Classification of Sensory Recovery*

Grade	Sensory Recovery
S0	No sensory recovery
S1	Recovery of deep cutaneous pain sensibility
S2	Recovery of superficial pain sensibility
S2+	As in S2, but with overresponse
S3	Recovery of pain and touch sensibility with disappearance of overresponse Two-point discrimination >15 mm
S3+	As in S3, but localization of the stimulus is good Two-point discrimination 7–15 mm
S4	Complete recovery Two-point discrimination 2–6 mm

RESULTS OF NERVE GRAFTING

Digital Nerve

Of the 151 cases presented, 88% achieved useful (S3 or better) sensory recovery and 69% achieved some two-point discrimination (Fig. 39-1). Table 39-5 shows that the results deteriorate with age. All patients under age 20 achieved some two-point discrimination, and up to age 40 all patients achieved useful sensory recovery. Over age 40, 63% achieved useful recovery. Graft lengths of less than 50 mm were found to have nearly an 80% chance of returning some two-point discrimination.

A delay before grafting of greater than 6 months did not appear to affect the results significantly, as 90% of these had useful recovery. Therefore, grafting digital nerves after 6 months' delay should

Table 39-5. *Digital Nerve Grafting: Sensory Recovery*

	S4	S3+	S3	S2+	S2	S1	S0	N
AGE (yrs)								
<20	11	9	0	0	0	0	0	20
(%)	55	45	0	0	0	0	0	
20–39	24	35	12	0	0	0	0	71
(%)	33	49	17	0	0	0	0	
≥40	8	16	12	0	8	12	1	57
(%)	14	28	21	0	14	21	1	
GAP (mm)								
<30	27	31	11	0	4	0	0	73
(%)	37	42	15	0	5	0	0	
30–49	11	16	4	0	0	2	1	34
(%)	32	47	12	0	0	6	2	
≥50	8	10	6	0	3	10	0	37
(%)	21	27	16	0	8	27	0	
DELAY (months)								
0–6	32	41	15	0	4	12	1	105
	30	39	14	0	4	11	0	
>6	11	19	7	0	4	0	0	41
	27	46	17	0	9	0	0	

N, *number of nerve grafts.*

not be discouraged. *Patient age at the time of grafting was the best predictor of final recovery.*

Median Nerve Motor Recovery

Median nerve grafting achieved 81% useful (M3 or better) motor return (see Fig. 39-2). However, this result may not be due entirely to median nerve regeneration because at least 30% to 40% of low median nerve injuries have sufficient ulnar innervation of the thenar muscles to have functional opposition of the thumb.[33] Thus, about half of this group would have satisfactory thumb opposition with no median reinnervation of the thenar muscles. Of the patients under age 20, 88% had useful motor return (Table 39-6). Although motor return deteriorates after age 40, 64% of this subgroup achieved useful results.

Gap length had a marked effect on motor recov-

Table 39–6. *Median Nerve Grafting: Motor Recovery*

	M5	M4	M3	M2+	M2	M1+	M1	M0	N
AGE (yrs)									
<20	14	14	2	0	2	0	0	2	34
(%)	41	41	6	0	6	0	0	6	
20–39	12	15	4	0	2	1	0	3	37
(%)	32	41	11	0	5	2	0	8	
≥40	4	9	6	1	5	1	1	2	29
(%)	14	31	21	3	17	3	3	7	
GAP (mm)									
<50	15	19	3	0	0	1	0	1	39
(%)	38	49	8	0	0	2	0	2	
50–99	14	16	14	1	5	1	2	3	56
(%)	25	29	25	2	9	2	3	5	
≥100	2	8	0	0	3	0	0	2	15
(%)	13	53	0	0	20	0	0	13	
DELAY (months)									
0–6	14	20	7	0	4	1	1	0	47
(%)	30	43	15	0	8	2	2	0	
>6	9	12	4	1	5	1	0	7	39
(%)	23	31	10	2	13	2	0	18	
LEVEL									
High	2	4	4	1	4	1	2	1	19
(%)	11	21	21	5	21	5	11	5	
Inter	10	16	6	0	2	1	0	0	35
(%)	29	46	17	0	5	2	0	0	
Low	9	13	5	0	1	0	0	5	33
(%)	27	39	15	0	3	0	0	15	

Level: high (above elbow), intermediate (forearm), low (wrist).
N, number of nerve grafts.

ery: 95% of grafts of less than 5 cm obtained useful recovery, but only 66% of gaps greater than 10 cm did so. When the time delay before grafting was greater than 6 months, 24% fewer patients had useful recovery. About 50% of high median nerve grafts, 92% of intermediate-level (forearm), and 81% of low (wrist) median nerve grafts obtained useful results. The unexpectedly better results from intermediate- over low-level injuries may be due to the relatively small number of intermediate grafts in the studies and also the fact that 15% of low median nerve grafts had no return of motor function.

Median Nerve Sensory Recovery

For median nerve sensory grafts, 79% overall achieved useful sensory recovery (see Fig. 39-2). The marked effect of patient age is again noted (Table 39-7), as 27% of patients under age 20 achieved S4 sensory recovery but no patients over

Table 39–7. *Median Nerve Grafting: Sensory Recovery*

	S4	S3+	S3	S2+	S2	S1	S0	N
AGE (yrs)								
<20	10	17	9	0	1	0	0	37
(%)	27	46	24	0	2	0	0	
20–39	3	11	14	2	6	0	2	38
(%)	7	29	37	5	16	0	5	
≥40	0	3	14	4	3	1	4	29
(%)	0	10	48	14	10	3	14	
GAP (mm)								
<50	9	11	13	2	4	0	2	41
(%)	21	26	31	4	9	0	4	
50–99	6	20	19	3	6	1	3	58
(%)	10	34	32	5	10	1	5	
≥100	1	4	8	1	1	0	0	15
(%)	6	26	53	6	6	0	0	
DELAY (months)								
0–6	5	18	16	1	5	0	2	47
(%)	10	38	34	2	10	0	4	
>6	2	8	15	5	5	1	4	40
(%)	5	20	37	12	12	2	10	
LEVEL								
High	0	5	10	0	3	0	1	19
(%)	0	26	52	0	15	0	5	
Intermediate	2	10	16	2	3	0	2	35
(%)	6	28	46	6	8	0	6	
Low	11	11	9	0	3	0	3	37
(%)	29	29	24	0	8	0	8	

Level: high (above elbow), intermediate (forearm), low (wrist).
N, number of nerve grafts.

age 40 did so. While 98% of patients under age 20 had useful sensory recovery, only 58% of patients over age 40 achieved the same results.

Increased gap length correlated inversely with S4 sensory return; however, 85% of grafts with a length of greater than 100 mm achieved useful results. A delay of greater than 6 months before grafting lowered the number of cases achieving useful recovery by 20%.

No patients with a high median nerve graft achieved normal two-point discrimination, but nearly a third of those with low injuries did so.

Ulnar Nerve Motor Recovery

Recovery of ulnar nerve function was more favorable than is sometimes depicted. Overall, 63% of ulnar nerve repairs had return to M3 or better function, and 75% achieved useful sensory recovery (Fig. 39-3). Useful motor recovery was found in 75% of patients under age 20, 66% of those age 20 to 39, and nearly half of those over age 40 (Table 39-8). A gap greater than 100 mm significantly reduced the M4 (good) and M5 (excellent) results from 46% to 9%. Neither a delay of greater than

Table 39–8. *Ulnar Nerve Grafting: Motor Recovery*

	M5	*M4*	*M3*	*M2+*	*M2*	*M1+*	*M1*	*M0*	*N*
AGE (yrs)									
<20	8	15	7	5	4	0	0	2	41
(%)	19	36	17	12	9	0	0	4	
20–39	3	8	9	2	2	1	0	5	30
(%)	10	26	30	6	6	3	0	16	
≥40	1	3	7	1	2	1	1	6	22
(%)	4	13	31	4	9	4	4	27	
GAP (mm)									
<50	9	15	9	6	4	1	1	6	51
(%)	17	29	17	11	7	1	1	11	
50–99	4	10	9	2	4	0	0	6	35
(%)	11	28	25	5	11	0	0	17	
≥100	0	1	6	1	1	1	0	1	11
(%)	0	9	54	9	9	9	0	9	
DELAY (months)									
0–6	7	6	9	5	6	0	0	2	35
(%)	20	17	25	14	17	0	0	5	
>6	4	13	13	2	3	2	1	8	46
(%)	8	28	28	4	6	4	2	17	
LEVEL									
High	2	11	8	2	7	2	0	5	37
(%)	5	29	21	5	18	5	0	13	
Intermediate	2	4	11	7	1	3	0	2	30
(%)	6	13	36	23	3	10	0	6	
Low	0	10	9	3	3	1	1	4	31
(%)	0	32	29	9	9	3	3	12	

Level: high (above elbow), intermediate (forearm), low (wrist).
N, number of nerve grafts.

6 months before nerve grafting nor the level of injury significantly affected the result.

Ulnar Nerve Sensory Recovery

Useful ulnar nerve sensory recovery was achieved in 87% of patients under age 20 and about 70% of those over age 20 (Table 39-9). A gap of less than 50 mm resulted in useful sensory recovery in 83% of the cases, but useful recovery was achieved in 20% fewer cases when a gap of greater than 100 mm existed. Little difference in sensory return was found for high vs low levels of injury. Cases with a delay of less than 6 months resulted in 87% useful results compared with 71% in those with delay of greater than 6 months.

Radial Nerve Motor Recovery

Seventy-eight percent of radial nerve reconstructions resulted in useful motor function, but in 16% of cases no motor recovery occurred (Fig. 39-4).

Table 39–9. *Ulnar Nerve Grafting: Sensory Recovery*

	S4	S3+	S3	S2+	S2	S1	S0	N
AGE (yrs)								
<20	9	10	16	2	1	0	2	40
(%)	22	25	40	5	2	0	5	
20–39	2	7	12	2	4	0	3	30
(%)	6	23	40	6	13	0	10	
≥40	2	3	15	2	2	0	4	28
(%)	7	10	53	7	7	0	14	
GAP (mm)								
<50	11	12	22	2	3	0	3	53
(%)	20	22	41	3	5	0	5	
50–99	2	4	16	2	3	0	5	32
(%)	6	12	50	6	9	0	15	
≥100	0	4	3	2	1	0	1	11
(%)	0	36	27	18	9	0	9	
DELAY (months)								
0–6	6	7	17	0	0	0	4	34
(%)	17	20	50	0	0	0	11	
>6	3	10	19	5	5	0	2	44
(%)	6	22	43	11	11	0	4	
LEVEL								
High	4	8	12	1	4	0	6	35
(%)	11	22	34	2	11	0	17	
Intermediate	2	2	23	2	0	1	0	30
(%)	6	6	76	6	0	3	0	
Low	5	7	14	3	2	0	1	32
(%)	15	21	43	9	6	0	3	

Level: high (above elbow), intermediate (forearm), low (wrist).
N, number of nerve grafts.

These patients were either over age 40, had gaps greater than 100 mm, or sustained high levels of injury (Table 39-10).

All of the patients under age 20 or with grafts less than 50 mm had M3 or better return of function. Eighty-one percent of patients with a delay before grafting of less than 6 months had useful motor recovery. Sixty percent of grafts in the arm, 75% of those below the extensor carpi radialis longus, and all grafts of the posterior interosseous nerve obtained useful function.

Radial Nerve Sensory Recovery

While radial sensory recovery was achieved to the S3 level in all those under age 20, the number of cases was small (Table 39-11). All patients with gap lengths of less than 50 mm had S3+ return, but only 56% of those with gaps greater than 100 mm had useful sensory recovery. A delay of more than 6 months did not significantly affect the sensory recovery. Sensory recovery for the mixed radial nerve above the elbow was poor, with only 30% obtaining useful sensory recovery.

Table 39–10. *Radial Nerve Grafting: Motor Recovery*

	M5	*M4*	*M3*	*M2+*	*M2*	*M1+*	*M1*	*M0*	*N*
AGE (yrs)									
<20	3	5	1	0	0	0	0	0	9
(%)	33	55	11	0	0	0	0	0	
20–39	5	10	3	0	2	0	0	2	22
(%)	22	45	13	0	9	0	0	9	
≥40	2	4	5	0	0	0	1	1	13
(%)	15	30	38	0	0	0	7	7	
GAP (mm)									
<50	5	3	1	0	0	0	0	0	9
(%)	55	33	11	0	0	0	0	0	
50–99	6	14	4	0	0	0	1	1	26
(%)	23	53	15	0	0	0	3	3	
≥100	1	2	4	0	2	0	0	2	11
(%)	9	18	36	0	18	0	0	18	
DELAY (months)									
0–6	6	9	5	0	0	0	1	1	22
(%)	27	40	22	0	0	0	4	4	
>6	4	10	4	0	2	0	0	2	22
(%)	18	45	18	0	9	0	0	9	
LEVEL									
Above ECRL	5	7	4	0	1	0	1	5	23
(%)	21	30	17	0	4	0	4	21	
Below ECRL	1	1	1	0	0	0	0	1	4
(%)	25	25	25	0	0	0	0	25	
PIN	2	1	0	0	0	0	0	0	3
(%)	66	33	0	0	0	0	0	0	

Level: ECRL (extensor carpi radialis longus), PIN (posterior interosseous nerve).
N, number of nerve grafts.

Table 39–11. *Radial Nerve Grafting: Sensory Recovery*

	S4	S3+	S3	S2+	S2	S1	S0	N
AGE (yrs)								
<20	0	0	5	0	0	0	0	5
(%)	0	0	100	0	0	0	0	
20–39	1	6	3	0	2	0	1	13
(%)	7	46	23	0	15	0	7	
≥40	2	2	2	0	0	1	1	8
(%)	25	25	25	0	0	12	12	
GAP (mm)								
<50	0	2	0	0	0	0	0	2
(%)	0	100	0	0	0	0	0	
50–99	1	5	9	0	1	1	0	17
(%)	5	29	52	0	5	5	0	
≥100	2	1	1	0	1	0	2	7
(%)	28	14	14	0	14	0	28	
DELAY (months)								
0–6	1	4	4	0	1	1	0	11
(%)	9	36	36	0	9	9	0	
>6	2	4	6	0	1	0	2	15
(%)	13	26	40	0	6	0	13	
LEVEL								
Above ECRL	0	2	1	0	0	1	4	8
(%)	0	25	12	0	0	12	50	
Below ECRL	0	0	0	0	1	1	0	2
(%)	0	0	0	0	50	50	0	

Level: ECRL (extensor carpi radialis longus).
N, number of nerve grafts.

Lower-Extremity Nerve Grafts

Table 39-12 summarizes 28 cases of lower-extremity nerve grafts. In no case was there better than S2 sensory recovery. As expected, the recovery is much poorer than that reported in the upper extremity. Hattrup and Wood reported M3 recovery in three patients in their series of four deep peroneal nerve grafts.[13] Some cases did obtain useful motor recovery and protective sensation.

DISCUSSION

The results showed digital nerve grafting to be very rewarding, with 90% useful results and 70% with some return of two-point discrimination. Even delays up to 6 months or a gap up to 50 mm were associated with 80% good (S3+) or excellent (S4) results. Digital nerve grafting is highly successful when done by competent peripheral nerve surgeons.

Overall, useful motor return in median and radial nerve grafting was about 80% and about 60% for ulnar grafts. This difference should not discourage attempts at reconstructing ulnar nerve injuries. Increased age had a significant affect on decreasing motor recovery in all three nerves. A gap of greater than 100 mm or a delay of greater than 6 months did not affect ulnar motor recovery but did have a negative effect on median or radial results. Level of injury had a significant effect on motor recovery in all three nerves.

Table 39–12. *Lower Extremity Nerve Grafts*

	N	*Nerve*	*Motor Recovery*	*Sensory Recovery*
Platt, 1919[30]	1	Sciatic	No regeneration	No recovery
MacCarthy, 1951[17]	1	Tibial	Moderate	
Sedel/Bricout, 1982[38]	8	Sciatic	38% very good, 25% good,	13% fair, 25% nul
Beazley et al. 1984[2]	1	Sciatic	M0	S0
	1	Peroneal	M3	—
Hattrup/Wood, 1986[13]	3	Sup. Peroneal	M4 = 1, M2+ = 1, M2 = 1	—
	1	Deep Peroneal	75% ≥ M3	—
	1	Com. Peroneal	Poor	—
	2	Plantar	—	1 good, 1 poor
Frykman/Cally, 1988[10]	1	Tibial	M0	S1
	1	Plantar	—	S2
	1	Peroneal	M1	S2

N, *number of grafts.*

From these results, surgeons can expect that virtually 100% of the posterior interosseous nerve grafts, 80% of low median nerve grafts, and 60% of low ulnar nerve grafts will obtain useful recovery. Just over one half of high median and ulnar grafts and two thirds of high radial nerve grafts will achieve useful motor return.

Unexpectedly, no significant difference was found in motor recovery from high to low ulnar nerve injuries. Also, a delay of greater than 6 months had little effect on motor return, but most of the grafts were done in the first 12 months after injury.

Median and ulnar nerve grafts had about the same (79% vs 75%) sensory recovery. Age had the greatest effect on sensory recovery, with about 25% of median and ulnar nerve grafts obtaining S4 return in the under-20 age group; less than 7% over age 20 achieved normal two-point discrimination. However, about 90% of patients under age 20 in all three nerves had some two-point discrimination return, and 58% to 75% of those over age 40 had useful sensory return. A gap greater than 10 cm had a significant effect on radial sensory recovery but not so on median and ulnar sensory recovery. A delay of greater than 6 months before grafting had no effect on motor recovery and only a slight effect on sensory results.

The effect of age, gap, delay, and level of injury on nerve graft recovery varied somewhat with the nerve. As with direct nerve repairs, the results of nerve grafting deteriorate with increasing age, gap, delay, and higher levels of injury. The most important effect on nerve recovery after grafting is age, closely followed in importance by gap length, level of injury, and delay. However, the effect of gap and delay were much greater in sensory than motor recovery, and level of injury had a greater effect on motor than sensory recovery.

The above conclusions, while not absolute, are based on the data compiled from published reports. More studies with larger series and longer follow-up are needed, with more uniform methods of classifying injury and level of recovery.

Also of note is that the reported nerve grafting series generally have been performed by microsurgeons experienced in peripheral nerve surgery. Thus, they represent the best realistic results obtained to date with current techniques of interfascicular nerve grafting. The results are not ideal, but they represent a marked advance over techniques of nerve grafting in use 20 to 25 years ago. The present results support the use of the techniques and methodology developed by Millesi nearly 20 years ago (see Chapter 37). Interfascicular nerve grafting remains the contemporary method of choice for bridging significant nerve defects.

REFERENCES

1. Albert E. Einige Operationen an Nerven. Wien Med 1885; 26:1285.
2. Beazley WC, Milek MA, Reiss BH. Results of nerve grafting in severe soft tissue injuries. Clinical Orthopaedics and Related Research 1984; 188:208–212.
3. Berger A, Mailander P, Schneider W, Becker M. Sensory recovery by different techniques, presented at the 3d International Hand Surgery Symposium, Tokyo, April 1988.
4. Brooks D. The place of nerve grafting in orthopedic surgery. J Bone Joint Surg [Am] 1955; 37:299–326.
5. Bunnell S. Suture of facial nerve within temporal bone with report of first successful case. Surg Gynecol Obstet 1927; 45:7.
6. Bunnell S. Repair of nerves and tendons of the hand. J Bone Joint Surg 1928; 10:1–16.
7. Bunnell S, Boyes JH. Nerve grafts. Am J Surg 1939; 44:64–75.
8. Chow JA, Van Beek AL, Bilos ZJ, Meyer DL, Johnson MC. Anatomical basis for repair of ulnar and median nerves in the distal part of the forearm by group fascicular suture. J Bone Joint Surg [Am] 1986; 68:273–280.
9. Davis L, Cleveland DA. Experimental studies in nerve transplants. Ann Surg 1934; 99:271–283.
10. Frykman GK, Cally D. Interfascicular nerve grafting. Orthop Clin North Am 1988; 19:71–80.
11. Haase J. Interfascicular nerve grafting of peripheral nerve lesions. Childs Brain 1981; 8:9–17.
12. Haase J, Bjerre P, Simesen K. Median and ulnar nerve transection treated with microsurgical interfascicular cable grafting with autogenous sural nerve. J Neurosurg 1980; 53:73–84.
13. Hattrup SJ, Wood MB. Delayed neural reconstruction in the lower extremity: Results of interfascicular nerve grafting. Foot Ankle 1986; 7:105–109.
14. Highet WB, Sanders FK. The effects of stretching nerves after suture. Br J Surg 1943; 30:355.
15. Hirasawa Y, Katsumi Y, Tokioka T. Evaluation of sensibility after sensory reconstruction of the thumb. J Bone and Joint Surg [Br] 1986; 67:814–819.
16. Ito T, Hirotani H, Yamamoto K. Peripheral nerve repairs by the funicular suture techniques. Acta Orthop Scand 1976; 47:283–289.
17. MacCarthy CS. Two-stage autograft for repair of extensive damage to the sciatic nerve. J Neurosurg 1951; 8:319.
18. Mackinnon SE, Dellon AL. Nerve repair and nerve grafting; surgery of the peripheral nerve. New York: Thieme, 1988:89–129.
19. Mackinnon SE, Dellon AL. Nerve grafting in the lower extremity, in preparation.
20. Mayo-Robson AW. Nerve grafting as a means of restoring function in limbs paralysed by gunshot or other injuries. Br Med J 1917; 1:117.
21. McFarlane RM, Mayer JR. Digital nerve grafts with the lateral antebrachial cutaneous nerve. J Hand Surg 1976; 1:169–173.
22. Millesi H. Interfascicular grafts for repair of peripheral nerves of the upper extremity. Orthop Clin North Am 1977; 8:387–404.
23. Millesi H. Interfascicular nerve grafting. Orthop Clin North Am 1981; 12:287–301.
24. Millesi H, Meissl G, Berger A. The interfascicular nerve-grafting of the median and ulnar nerves. J Bone Joint Surg [Am] 1972; 54:727–750.
25. Millesi H, Meissl G, Berger A. Further experience with interfascicular grafting of the median, ulnar and radial nerves. J Bone Joint Surg [Am] 1976; 58:209–218.
26. Moneim MS. Interfascicular nerve grafting. Clin Orthop 1982; 163:65–74.
27. Nicholson OR, Seddon HJ. Nerve repair in civil practice: Results of treatment of median and ulnar nerve lesions. Br Med J 1957; 2:1065–1071.
28. Nunley JA, Ugino MR, Goldner RD, Regan N, Urbaniak JR. Use of the anterior brandh of the medial antebrachial cutaneous nerve as a graft for the repair of defects of the digital nerve. J Bone Joint Surg [Am] 1989; 71:563–567.
29. Phillipeaux JM, Vulpian A. Note sur les essais de greffe d'un troncon de nerf lingual entre les deux bouts de l'hypoglosse. Arch Physiol Norm Pathol 1817; 3:618.
30. Platt H. On the results of bridging gaps in injured nerve trunks by autogenous fascial tubulization and autogenous nerve grafts. Br J Surg 1919; 7:384–389.
31. Rose EH, Kowalski TA. Restoration of sensibility to anesthetic scarred digits with free vascularized nerve grafts from the dorsum of the foot. J Hand Surg [Am] 1985; 10:514–521.
32. Rose EH, Kowalski TA, Norris MS. The reversed venous arterialized nerve graft in digital nerve reconstruction across scarred beds. Plast Reconstr Surg 1989; 83:593–604.
33. Rowntree T. Anomalous innervation of the hand muscles. J Bone Joint Surg [Br] 1949; 31:505–510.
34. Samii M, Waagner D. Ergebnisse der autologen nerven transplatationen bei lasionen kranialer and peripherer nerven. Therapeutische Umschau 1975; 32:453–460.
35. Seddon HJ. The use of autogenous grafts for repair of large gaps in peripheral nerves. Br J Surg 1947; 35:151–167.

36. Seddon HJ. Nerve grafting. J Bone Joint Surg [Br] 1963; 45:447.
37. Seddon H. Surgical disorders of the peripheral nerves. Baltimore: Williams & Wilkins, 1972:299–314.
38. Sedel L, Bricout N. Resultats des greffes de gros troncs nerveux. Sem Hop Paris 1982; 58:1569–1574.
39. Stellini L. Interfascicular autologous grafts in the repair of nerves; eight years experience. Br J Plast Surg 1982; 35:478–482.
40. Stopford JSB. The treatment of large defects in peripheral nerve injuries. Lancet 1920; 2:1296–1327.
41. Sunderland S. Nerves and nerve injuries, ed 2. Edinburgh: Churchill-Livingstone, 1978:603–636.
42. Tallas R, Staniforth P, Fisher TR. Neurophysiological studies of autogenous nerve grafts. J Neurol Neurosurg Psychiatry 1978; 41:677–683.
43. Tenny JR, Lewis RC. Digital nerve grafting for traumatic defects. Use of the later antebrachial cutaneous nerve. J Bone Joint Surg [Am] 1984; 66:1375–1379.
44. Walton R, Finseth F. Nerve grafting in the repair of complicated peripheral nerve trauma. J Trauma 1977; 17:793–796.
45. Wilgis EFS. Nerve repair and grafting. In: Green DP. Operative hand surgery, ed 2. New York: Churchill-Livingstone, 1988:1385–1393.
46. Wilgis EF, Maxwell GP. Distal digital nerve grafts: Clinical and anatomical studies. J Hand Surg 1979; 4:439–443.
47. Williams HB, Jabaley ME. The importance of internal anatomy of the peripheral nerves to nerve repair in the forearm and hand. Hand Clin 1986; 2:689–707.
48. Wiswe VI, Müller D, Vitzthum HE, Minda R, Lampe J. Spätergebnisse nach Behandlung peripherer Nervenverletzungen der oberen Extrimität. Zent bl Neurochir 1987; 48:335–342.
49. Woodhall B, Beebe WG. A follow-up study of 3656 World War II injuries. In: Peripheral nerve regeneration. Veterans Administration medical monograph. Washington DC: US Government Printing Office, 1956.
50. Yamano Y. Electrophysiological study of nerve grafting. J Hand Surg 1982; 7:588–592.
51. Yamano Y, Namba Y, Hino Y, et al. Digital nerve grafts in replanted digits. Hand 1982; 4:255–262.
52. Young VL, Wray CR, Weeks PM. The results of nerve grafting in the wrist and hand. Ann Plast Surg 1980; 5:212–215.

40

Vascularized Nerve Grafts

Warren C. Breidenbach
Brent Graham

AUTHORS' KEY POINTS

- Experimental models show that nonvascularized nerve grafts undergo a 72-hour period of ischemia; vascularized nerve grafts do not.
- A definite indication for a vascularized nerve graft is a poorly vascularized recipient bed. More controversial indications are proximal lesions, large gaps, and compromised recipient beds.
- Before microsurgical transfer, the following must be determined: the anatomy of the donor nerve, the method by which blood supply will be maintained to each cable, and how the vascularized nerve graft will be monitored.
- There are no conclusive studies that indicate the superiority of vascularized nerve grafts, except in scarred recipient beds.
- The sural nerve is used for peripheral nerve reconstruction, the ulnar nerve for brachial plexus reconstruction (but only if there is a preganglionic lesion at C8–T1).

In 1976 Taylor and Ham introduced the concept of the vascularized nerve graft (VNG) as a free tissue transfer.[31] This innovative technique was presented to improve the results of nerve grafting. Since then, there has been considerable debate regarding the value of this procedure. Indications for the technique are not well defined, operative techniques for transferring a nerve with its blood supply are poorly understood, and the anatomy of potential donor nerves continues to be redefined yearly. Thus, no clear superiority of final results has been shown.

The purpose of this chapter is to present current information on vascularized nerve grafting. Experimental and clinical evidence for and against VNGs is presented, and based on these studies indications for the use of VNGs are determined. The anatomy of donor VNGs is explained, and operative techniques, which must be followed carefully to ensure nerve blood supply, are described. The reader should realize that the indications, appropriate donor nerves, and techniques are likely to change.

There is little doubt that VNGs will continue as a viable method of peripheral nerve reconstruction in certain situations. What remains unclear is whether they will find wider application or will remain a technique with only limited application.

EXPERIMENTAL RESULTS

Reconstructing a nerve gap using a nonvascularized nerve graft (NNG) involves the transfer of living tissue. The NNG is transferred without its blood supply and therefore requires revascularization from its recipient bed. An ingrowth of blood supply is necessary to ensure the survival of Schwann cells and to avoid intraneural fibrosis. If the NNG is treated in some manner (radiation, freezing, or prolonged ischemia), Schwann cells die and long-term grafting results are poor.[29] Therefore, nerve grafting is seen as a transfer of not only the structural components of nerve (endoneural tubes and fascicles) but also the transfer of Schwann cells. For this reason, NNGs are indicated only in recipient beds that allow rapid revascularization.[29,21,22]

Theoretically, VNGs improve results by increasing the number of Schwann cells surviving the procedure, by decreasing intraneural fibrosis, and by increasing the rate of axonal regeneration.[5,6] Most animal experiments have examined either these underlying assumptions or functional results of VNGs vs NNGs.

There appears to be a consensus that even in a well-vascularized bed, the NNG undergoes a period of ischemia, which is avoided by maintaining vascularization. Studies compared blood flow in VNGs and NNGs using the same experimental model, the canine saphenous nerve.[7,17,18,27] Using radioactive isotopes, blood flow in both types of grafts was examined quantitatively. The results indicated that the NNG suffered a 3-day period of ischemia postoperatively, during which the VNG maintained blood flow. By day 3, the NNG started to revascularize, and this proceeded rapidly. Interestingly, both nerve grafts showed a marked increase in blood flow, to values higher than normal. The NNG blood flow actually surpassed that of the VNG by day 7. A high rate of blood flow was maintained for 6 weeks, at which time it returned to normal levels. The cause and significance of this phenomenon remains unexplained.

The advantages of VNGs are assumed to result from maintained blood flow. Experimental studies show that blood flow in the VNG is superior to that of the NNG only during the first 3 days following surgery. Therefore, the adverse effects of Schwann cell death and increased intraneural fibrosis, if they exist, must be initiated during this period.

Interestingly, few experiments have directly examined the underlying changes present in VNGs. There have been no published studies demonstrating a superior number of Schwann cells in a VNG compared to a NNG. In part, this may be due to the difficulty in counting Schwann cells. Likewise, no studies directly address the extent of intraneural fibrosis present in NNGs compared to VNGs.

A few studies have addressed the question of axonal regeneration: Koshima and Harii examined axonal regeneration in NNGs and VNGs of the rat sciatic nerve.[15,16] These studies were carried out in poor recipient beds. Long-term studies did not show any significant difference between NNGs and VNGs with respect to fiber density or diameter. Evidence of a significantly improved rate of axonal maturation was found, however, in the VNGs.

Similar results were reported by Restrepo and colleagues, who used a rabbit model to examine myelin sheath thickness in VNGs and NNGs placed in normal recipient beds.[23] Although the authors did not statistically analyze the results, their data showed a greater axonal density and average diameter both at the midpoint and distal regions of the VNGs than in comparable areas of the NNGs. They determined that the rate of axonal regeneration of the VNG was approximately double that of the NNG between the 9th and 14th week following surgery.

Data that conflicts with the findings of these studies have been reported by other authors. McCullough and coworkers compared VNGs to NNGs in compromised and normal recipient beds using rat sciatic nerves.[19] These experiments demonstrated that revascularization of NNGs was significantly delayed when the graft was isolated from the surrounding bed. Eventually, however, NNGs in a poor bed completely revascularized by ingrowth of vessels from both ends. Further, there was no difference in the rate of axonal regeneration, or the size or duration of action potentials between VNGs and NNGs.

In a somewhat different rat sciatic nerve model, Seckel and coworkers found no difference between VNGs and NNGs in a normal recipient bed with respect to the size of regenerating fibers.[26] In fact, the myelin sheath was found to be thicker in the NNGs.

Comparing these studies demonstrates some of the problems in reaching conclusions from experimental results. These studies used different animals, different measuring techniques, and different experimental conditions, making direct comparison of experimental data difficult.

Another point worth noting is that these experiments used different recipient beds: in some cases the bed was scarred, in others normal. The issue of what constitutes an appropriate recipient bed for the design of an informative experiment remains controversial. Some surgeons feel that the only indication for a VNG is a badly scarred recipient bed, one that will not support an NNG. Others want to investigate the possibility that a VNG is superior to an NNG even in a normal recipient bed. If the latter is true, it would greatly expand the indications for VNGs.

Few studies have compared the functional results of VNGs to those of NNGs, but two experiments have addressed this issue. In the first study, VNGs and NNGs of the median nerve of the rabbit were carried out in a normal recipient bed.[28] Functional results were evaluated by testing muscle strength. These results showed a 20% greater strength in muscles re-innervated by a VNG. In the other study, VNGs and NNGs in a normal recipient bed were compared using the rat sciatic nerve.[12] Gait analysis was carried out as a measure of function. Again the VNG demonstrated results superior to the NNG.

In conclusion, there is little doubt that an NNG undergoes a period of ischemia lasting about 3 days, but whether this significantly alters the number of Schwann cells is unknown. It seems unlikely that this should produce any marked intraneural fibrosis as long as the NNG is placed in a good recipient bed. In a poor recipient bed, severe intraneural fibrosis can be anticipated that might be avoided with a VNG.

Experimental findings regarding axonal regeneration are contradictory. In some experiments VNGs were superior to NNGs, while in others the opposite was found. However, in those experiments that examined function, results seem to indicate a superiority for VNGs, even when they were used in normal recipient beds. These results are still preliminary, however, and further work is obviously needed. Table 40-1 summarizes most of the studies examining these issues.

INDICATIONS FOR VASCULARIZED NERVE GRAFTING

The indications for a VNG are determined by evaluating the recipient bed, the anatomical position of the lesion (proximal or distal), and the size of the nerve gap.

Recipient beds may be classified into three types: scarred, compromised, and normal. A badly scarred bed is found in deep dermal burns, electrical injuries, and Volkmann's ischemic contracture. A compromised bed consists of an incompletely scarred bed, as found following gunshot wounds, multiple reconstructive surgeries, and crush injuries. A normal bed is that found following a simple laceration.

Since an NNG must revascularize to survive, a definite indication for a VNG is a scarred recipient bed. NNGs are used in compromised and normal recipient beds because these beds, although scarred to some extent, can revascularize the graft. Experiments from our laboratory examined the use of NNGs vs VNGs in a compromised recipient bed. In two experiments, VNGs produced superior results to NNGs in minimally scarred recipient beds.[12,28] This finding implies that a VNG might be indicated regardless of the state of the recipient bed. We are now clinically investigating this possibility by using VNGs in compromised recipient beds.

Theoretically, large gaps and proximal lesions would benefit more from reconstruction with

Table 40–1. *Summary of Experiments of Vascularized Nerve Grafts*

Author	***Animal***	***Nerve***	***Recipient Bed***	***Evaluation***	***Conclusion***
Koshima and Harii[15]	rat	sciatic	scarred	24 weeks	axonal growth VNG > CNG
Townsend and Taylor[32]	canine	sural (arterialized venous)	normal	9 weeks	VNG > CNG
Settergren and Wood[27]	canine	saphenous	normal	6 weeks	blood flow CNG > VNG
Lux et al.[18]	canine	saphenous	normal	3 days	blood flow VNG > CNG
McCullough et al.[19]	rat	sciatic	normal and scarred	24 days	CNG = VNG
Seckel et al.[26]	rat	sciatic	normal	6 weeks	CNG = VNG
Shibata et al.[28]	rabbit	median	normal	6 months	VNG > CNG
Kanaya et al.[12]	rat	sciatic	normal	6 months	VNG > CNG
Restrepo et al.[23]	rabbit	sciatic	normal	15 weeks	VNG > CNG

VNG, vascularized nerve graft; CNG, conventional nerve graft.

VNGs, but this remains experimentally unproved.

In conclusion, the one clearly established indication for a VNG is a badly scarred recipient bed. As the vascularity of the bed improves, the indications for a VNG become more controversial. Still to be investigated is the possibility of achieving better results by using VNGs in compromised beds and in situations where there are large nerve gaps and more proximal lesions.

TECHNIQUES OF VASCULARIZED NERVE TRANSFER

Several technical points must be considered before carrying out a VNG transfer, including the following:

- The anatomy of the nerve's blood supply
- The method of vascularizing the nerve graft
- Methods of forming cable grafts while maintaining vascular supply
- Monitoring the VNG.

There are only six potential VNGs. Tables 40-2 and 40-3 review the pertinent anatomy for each of the donor nerves. Of the six potential VNGs, the nerves most commonly used are the sural, saphenous, and superficial radial.

The sural nerve has an unreliable pedicle coming from the popliteal fossa.[5] Because the pedicle is not reliable, Doi and colleagues developed an alternate procedure in which the sural nerve is harvested with the fascia that is supplied by the vessels coming through the lateral posterior crural septum.[8,9] These vessels are more reliable than the blood supply coming from the popliteal fossa.

Table 40–2. *Nerves and Vessels That May Be Used as Vascularized Nerve Grafts*

Nerve	***Blood Supply***
Superficial radial	Radial
Ulnar	Superior ulnar collateral
Sural	Superficial sural
Anterior tibial	Anterior tibial
Superficial peroneal	Superficial peroneal
Saphenous	Saphenous

(From *Breidenbach WC, Terzis JK. The blood supply of vascularized nerve grafts. J Reconstr Microsurg 1986; 3:43, with permission.)*

Table 40–3. *Cadaver Dissection Results of Donor Vascularized Nerve Grafts*

Nerve	No. of Dissections	% Suitable as VNG	Artery (mm)		Artery Pedicle Length (cm)		Vein (mm)		Vein Pedicle (cm)	
			Average	Range	Average	Range	Average	Range	Average	Range
Superficial radial	20	100	3.6	2.5–5.5	6.4	3.5–13	2.5	1.0–5.0	6.4	3.5–13
Ulner	25	96	1.8	0.8–2.5	4.9	3–9	1.9	1–3	4.0	1–8
Sural	20	30	1.2	1.1–1.4	5.0	3–7	1.3	0.8–1.9	4.8	3–7
Anterior tibial	20	95	4.4	3.1–5.5	4.2	3–7	3.4	1–5	4.2	3–7
Superficial peroneal	20	90	1.7	0.9–2.5	4.1	3–5	1.9	0.6–3.2	4.0	2–6
Saphenous	20	80	2.0	1.0–2.7	3.1	2.5–6	2.1	1.1–2.8	4.6	2.5–9
Lateral antebrachial cutaneous nerve of the forearm	20	30	1.81	0.8–2.9	3.17	1.5–5	1.8	1.1–3.0	3.2	1.5–5

(From *Breidenbach WC, Terzis JK. The blood supply of vascularized nerve grafts. J Reconstr Microsurg 1986; 3:43, with permission.)*

The superficial radial nerve requires sacrifice of the radial artery; this has recently been shown to be the dominant artery of the hand in many patients and therefore should not be sacrificed if avoidable.[14]

The saphenous nerve requires a large dissection, and its pedicle is absent in as many as 20% of patients.[5]

The ulnar nerve may only be used as a VNG in brachial plexus reconstruction where roots C8 and T1 have suffered preganglionic avulsion.

Both the tibial and superficial peroneal nerves provide relatively short nerve grafts, and the former requires sacrifice of a major lower-extremity vessel.[5]

Because of these problems, surgeons have sought alternate ways to vascularize nerve grafts.[11,24,25,32] Two new methods have been developed for supplying blood to nerves. The first uses only the artery associated with the nerve (arterialized VNG) and does not use the associated vein. Reconstruction is completed in a manner that allows arterialized blood to enter the artery, and the nerve is used to reconstruct the recipient nerve defect.

The second method uses only the vein associated with the nerve (arterialized venous nerve graft) and does not use the artery. Here arterialized blood enters the vein. The vein–nerve complex is reversed from its normal anatomical orientation so that the vein may bridge the arterial gap, while the associated nerve is used to bridge the nerve gap.

How the circulatory system functions in either of these nerve grafts is not understood. Obviously, the arterialized VNG will allow blood to enter the nerve, but it is unclear by what mechanism venous drainage occurs. With the arterialized venous nerve graft, how the blood enters the nerve is not well understood.

A few experimental and clinical reports have investigated these methods of vascularizing nerve grafts, all reporting good results.[11,24,25,32] One recent experimental study demonstrated adverse effects on the circulatory function of the nerve with the arterialized venous nerve graft.[1] Using the rabbit median nerve model, blood flow was found to cease by 72 hours, and severe damage to the blood nerve barrier was demonstrated. At present, the use of arterialized vascularized or arterialized venous nerve grafts should be approached with caution.

Another technical problem in transferring VNGs is the formation of *cable grafts*. Initial clinical studies using VNGs placed the nerve as a single strand in the defect, but this resulted in a large discrepancy in the size of donor and recipient nerves. Accordingly, methods were developed to allow the surgeon to form cables out of a single VNG. This cannot be accomplished, however, until the surgeon fully understands the relationship between the nerve and its blood supply.

Nerve blood supply is categorized as either *extrinsic* or *intrinsic*. Extrinsic vessels lie outside and intrinsic vessels lie within the epineurium. Unfortunately, not all extrinsic vessels are suitable for microsurgical transfer (Fig. 40-1). Many vessels that directly enter the nerve are small myocutaneous, periosteal, or fascial branches. Other extrinsic vessels are large and course longitudinally with the nerve, supplying it through the vasa nervorum. These large, longitudinal vessels are more advantageous for surgical transfer and are called the *dominant system*. Each nerve in the body may be categorized as having no, one, or multiple dominant systems (Fig. 40-2). The medial brachial cutaneous and medial antebrachial cutaneous nerves of the forearm, for example, do not have a dominant system; their blood supply comes from small musculocutaneous and fascial vessels. The superficial radial nerve has one dominant system, the radial artery. The ulnar nerve has multiple dominant systems (the ulnar and superior ulnar collateral arteries).

When the dominant system runs the whole length of the nerve, the nerve can easily be formed into cables (Fig. 40-3). Fachinelli and coworkers introduced the concept of folding the vascularized nerve graft and transecting only the nerve, so that each segment of nerve receives its blood supply from the vasa nervorum.[10] The resulting segments of nerve are then grafted into place side by side forming cables, with blood flowing to each cable from the intact dominant system.

When the dominant system runs less than the whole length of the nerve, forming cables is more difficult because a long segment of nerve is not di-

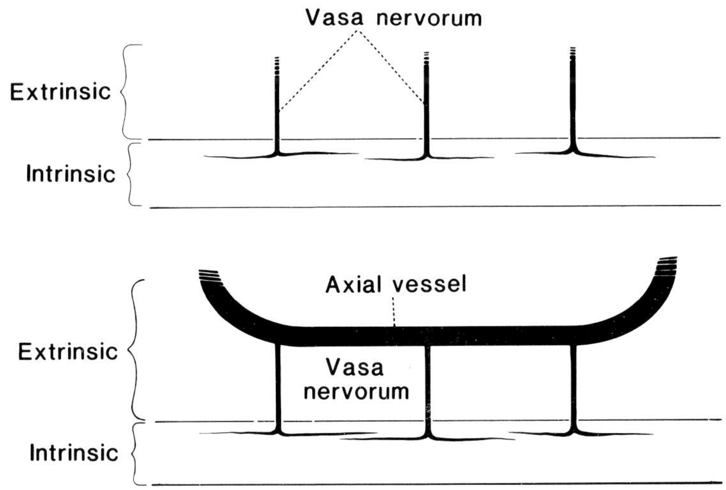

Figure 40–1. *Blood supply to nerves. Extrinsic vessels lie outside and intrinsic lie inside the epineurium. Note two types of extrinsic vessels. Those shown in the upper diagram arise from fascial, musculocutaneous, and periosteal vessels. The second type, shown in the lower diagram, arises from axial vessels. This axial vessel is referred to as the* dominant system. *Vasa nervorum refers to any nutrient vessel of a nerve. (From Breidenbach WC, Terzis JK. The blood supply of vascularized nerve grafts. J Reconstr Microsurg 1986;3:43, with permission.)*

rectly supplied with blood. When such a nerve is elevated as a vascularized nerve graft, this long segment (called the *free segment*) is supplied with blood only by the nerve's intrinsic system (Fig. 40-4). The portion of the nerve supplied by the dominant system can still be separated into cables, but the free segment of nerve cannot be divided in the same manner into cables without interrupting its intrinsic blood supply (Table 40-4).

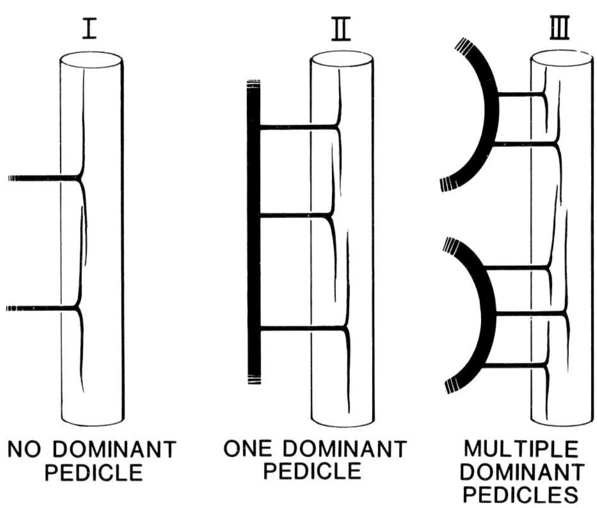

Figure 40–2. *Classification of blood supply to nerves. (From Breidenbach WC, Terzis JK. The blood supply of vascularized nerve grafts. J Reconstr Microsurg 1986;3:43, with permission.)*

A method of folding and transecting the free segment while maintaining blood supply has been reported.[5] The nerve epineurium is transected longitudinally under the microscope, keeping the epineural vessels intact. The fascicles of the nerve are transected transversely while visualizing the epineurial vessels to ensure they are not severed (Figs. 40-5, 40-6). The senior author has performed this procedure clinically a number of times and has seen bleeding from the transected ends of nerve. The extent of blood flow maintained through a folded epineurial system has been studied experimentally and found to be sufficient.[13]

The final technical problem in transferring the vascularized nerve graft is monitoring the vessel anastomosis. Most, if not all, of the VNG donors have an associated skin flap. The superficial radial, saphenous, ulnar, and sural nerves are associated with the forearm, saphenous, medial arm, and fasciocutaneous lateral leg flaps respectively; in other words, the vessels that supply the nerve seem to be the same vessels that supply the flaps.

If the VNG is transferred with an associated skin flap, the best method of monitoring the vessel anastomosis is by determining the flow in the skin flap. With the sural nerve, for example, the vessels in the posterior crural septum supply both the skin and the nerve. Therefore, if this nerve were selected for a VNG, some of the skin of the lateral leg would also be elevated and used as a monitor. The senior author has used skin islands as monitors

Table 40–4. *Results of Measurements From Cadaver Dissections of Donor Vascularized Nerve Grafts*

Nerve	Origin to Entry of Blood Supply (cm)		Length Pedicle Runs With the Nerve (cm)		Graft Length (cm)		Nerve Length Before First Branching		Nerve Length Before Last Motor Branch		Special Measurements (cm)
	Average	Range	Average	Range	Average	Range	Average	Range	Average	Range	
Superficial radial	9.0	4.5–14	11.8	9–17.5	23.8	20–28	21.3	18–24	NA	NA	Average 26.3* Range 22–29
Ulnar	16.6	14–20	10.5	4–15	55.7	46–62	29.7	16–38	NA	NA	Average 57.8* Range 48–64 Average 17.8† Range 14–22
Sural	—	—	—	—	—	—	—	—	—	—	—
Anterior tibial	6.4	4–8	NA	NA	24.6	19–30	—	—	10.7	6–22	NA
Superficial peroneal	8.4	6–12	9.1	3–18	23.6	14–30	—	—	7.7	1–12	Average 10.7‡ Range 7–15
Saphenous	27.4	17–42	13.2	17–23	40.4	31–49	23.2	6–39	NA	NA	NA
Lateral antebrachial cutaneous nerve of the forearm	—	—	4.1	1–9	34	19–41	—	—	NA	NA	NA

* *Length of extremity (cm).*
† *Medial epicondyle to origin of blood supply in cm.*
‡ *Cm below head of fibula at which pedicle joins the nerve.*
— *No measurement obtained.*
NA, measurement not applicable.
(From *Breidenbach WC, Terzis JK. The blood supply of vascularized nerve grafts. J Reconstr Microsurg 1986; 3:43, with permission.)*

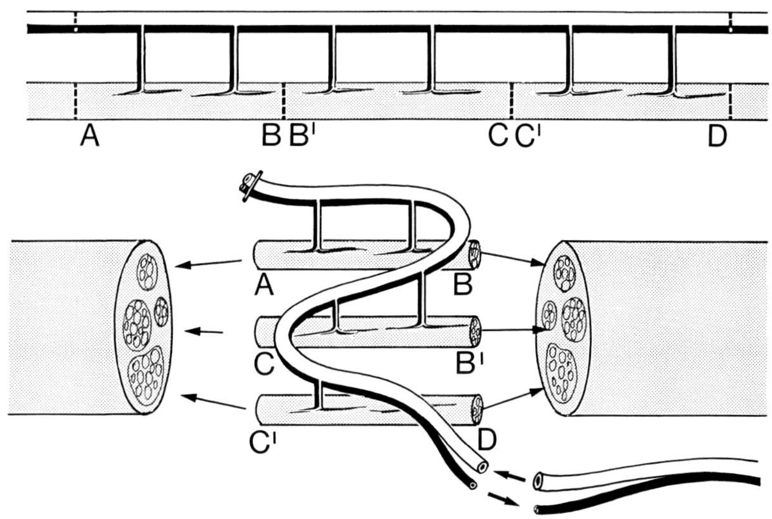

Figure 40–3. *The method presented in Fachinelli et al[10] by which a nerve with a dominant blood supply may be cut and folded into cables and transferred as a vascularized nerve graft. (From Breidenbach WC, Terzis JK. The blood supply of vascularized nerve grafts. J Reconstr Microsurg 1986;3:43, with permission.)*

with the saphenous (saphenous flap) and sural (skin island based on the intermuscular septum) VNG.

CLINICAL STUDIES

Table 40-5 lists the most important clinical studies to date investigating VNGs. Most of these studies found VNGs to be superior to NNGs, but unfortunately the conclusions cannot be accepted as irrefutable. None of these studies was conducted in a randomized, blind, prospective manner, nor is this likely to happen considering the difficulties of classifying nerve injuries (crush, laceration, avulsion), controlling patient population (age), controlling operative technique (epineural vs group fascicular repair), and most importantly quantifying functional results.

Therefore, the best method available for evaluating VNGs vs NNGs is a critical review of the

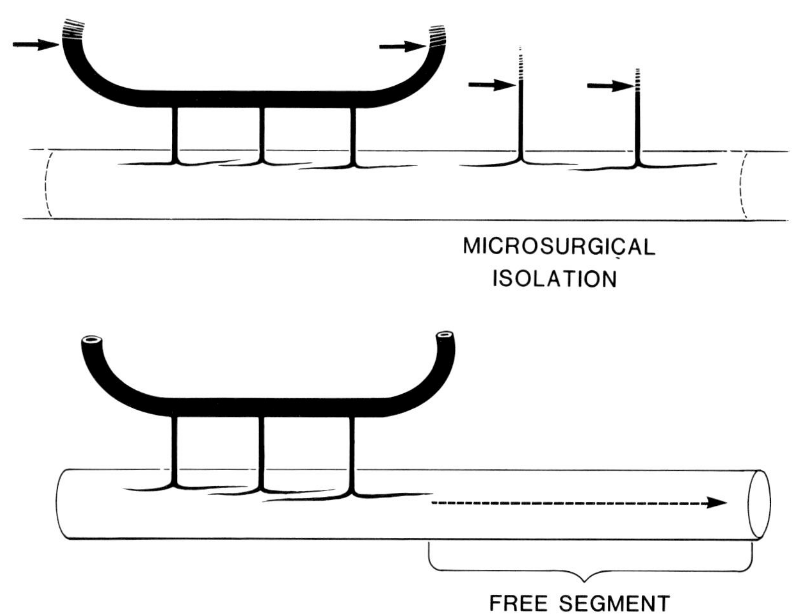

Figure 40–4. *All extrinsic vessels must be transected, as indicated by arrows in the upper diagram, in order to transfer a nerve microsurgically. Microsurgical anastomosis is carried out only on the dominant vessel. The free segment of the nerve, which was supplied by fascial, musculocutaneous, or periosteal vessels, must now be supplied by intrinsic vessels fed from the dominant pedicle. (From Breidenbach WC, Terzis JK. The blood supply of vascularized nerve grafts. J Reconstr Microsurg 1986;3:43, with permission.)*

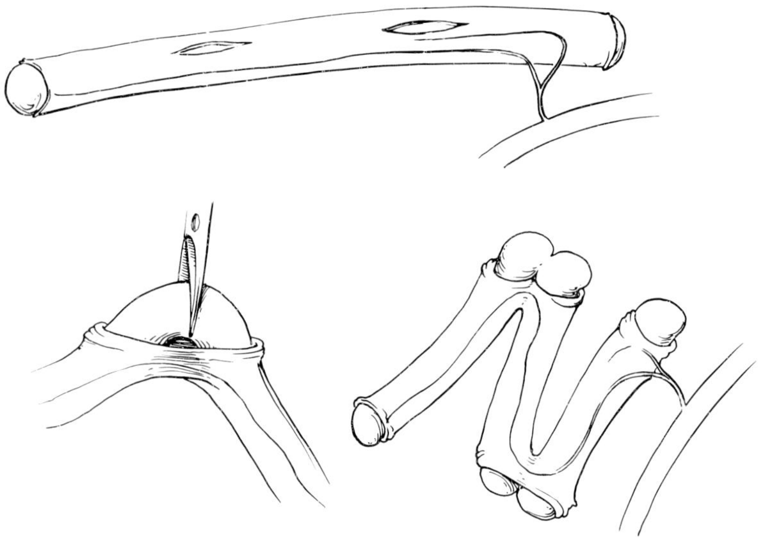

Figure 40-5. *In order to form vascularized cables epineurium is transected longitudinally; then the nerve is transected transversely.*

literature, being fully aware of the limitations within each study. The first three studies reported in Table 40-5 used VNGs to reconstruct peripheral nerve defects below the brachial plexus.[30,10,31] One of these studies did not provide follow-up data; the other two concluded that VNGs were superior to NNGs. Careful review, however, reveals that the number of cases was small, that follow-up was adequate (about 2 years) but not complete (5 years is preferable), and that there were no controls.

Bonney and colleagues and Merle and associates both used the ulnar nerve for brachial plexus reconstruction but reached different conclusions.[2,20] Bonney believed that reconstruction using VNGs produced results superior to NNGs; the number of cases studied was sufficient, but there were no reported controls. Merle concluded that although function returns more rapidly with VNGs, the final results were the same as those obtained with NNGs. Again, the number of patients studied was adequate, but there were no controls. These encouraging reports indicate that VNGs may have benefits in brachial plexus reconstruction, but the results are inconclusive.

Doi and associates used the vascularized sural nerve graft in 16 patients.[9] Follow-up was short and there were no controls. As the main purpose of the paper was to introduce a new method of harvesting a vascularized sural nerve graft, the authors did not draw definite conclusions regarding the superiority of VNGs.

The remaining studies used arterialized venous

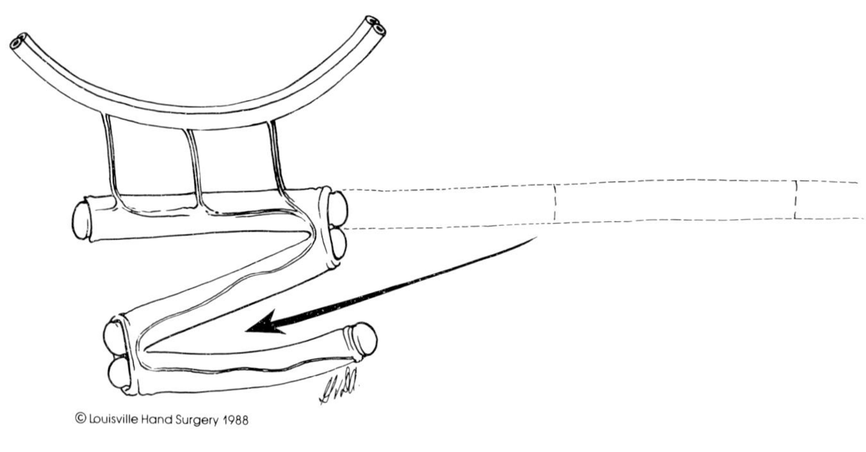

Figure 40–6. *How to form vascularized cables when the dominant pedicle does not run the whole length of the nerve. Dotted line represents the original position of the free segment. The epineurium is transected longitudinally and then the nerve transversely. Blood supply is maintained through the folded epineurium.*

Table 40–5. *Clinical Studies of Vascularized Nerve Grafts*

Author	Indications for VNG	Donor Nerve	No. of Cases	Control	Follow-up	Results
Taylor[30]	Volkmann's contracture	Superficial radial	3	no	9 mo–2 yr	VNG superior
	Electrical burns	Median and ulnar				
Fachinelli et al.[10]	Volkmann's contracture	Sural	6	no	none	not stated
Bonney et al.[2]	Brachial plexus	Ulnar nerve	12	no	6–28 mo	VNG superior
Merle et al.[20]	Brachial plexus	Ulnar nerve	8	no	?–2 yr	VNG = CNG
Townsend and Taylor[32]	Trauma Electrical burns Facial paralysis	Arterialized venous sural	7	no	6 mo–3.5 yr	VNG superior
Rose and Kowalski[24]	Previous failed digital nerve grafts	Deep peroneal arterialized	6	yes	28 mo	VNG superior
Rose et al.[25]	Complex digital injuries	Deep peroneal arterialized venous	12	yes	6 mo–2 yr	VNG superior
Doi et al.[9]	Scarred bed Brachial plexus	Sural	16	no	2–31 mo	not stated
Gu et al.[11]	Scarred bed Large defect	Sural arterialized venous	14	no	1.6–4.6 yr	VNG > CNG

or arterialized VNGs.[11,24,25,32] Each reports superior results for the vascularized grafts. The basic physiology, however, of the microcirculation in these nerve grafts remains unclear. Until this is better understood, these results should be interpreted cautiously.

Therefore, while there is some evidence that VNGs may be superior to NNGs in peripheral nerve reconstruction, this conclusion is based on studies that lack controls and often have inadequate numbers of patients and inadequate follow-up.

OPERATIVE TECHNIQUE

Authors' Preferred Method

Selecting a donor VNG depends on the clinical situation. The senior author has advocated the use of the saphenous nerve as the best VNG for peripheral nerve reconstruction.[4] Only during the last year has the sural nerve graft been used based on the intermuscular septal vessels as described by Doi and associates.[9] At present, this is our choice for peripheral nerve reconstruction.

The sural nerve is used on the leg contralateral to the injured upper extremity. The patient is positioned supine with the hips rotated to a lateral decubitus position. The sural nerve donor leg is positioned upward. The leg is flexed to 90° and then supported. In this fashion two teams can work, one harvesting the sural nerve while the other prepares the recipient site.

A Doppler is used to identify the vessels in the posterior crural septum. According to the anatomical work carried out by Doi and associates, the sural nerve has two dominant pedicles.[8,9] The inferior pedicle arises from the peroneal artery, the superior from the posterior tibial. The skin island that will serve as the monitor is positioned over these perforators. A curvilinear incision is then initiated at the distal leg posterior to the lateral malleolus over the sural nerve (Fig. 40-7). The incision is carried down through skin and subcutaneous tissue until the sural nerve and short saphenous vein are identified. The incision is then extended proximally toward the skin island. It encompasses the skin island and then proceeds immediately to the popliteal fossa. A large subcutaneous flap is developed above the level of

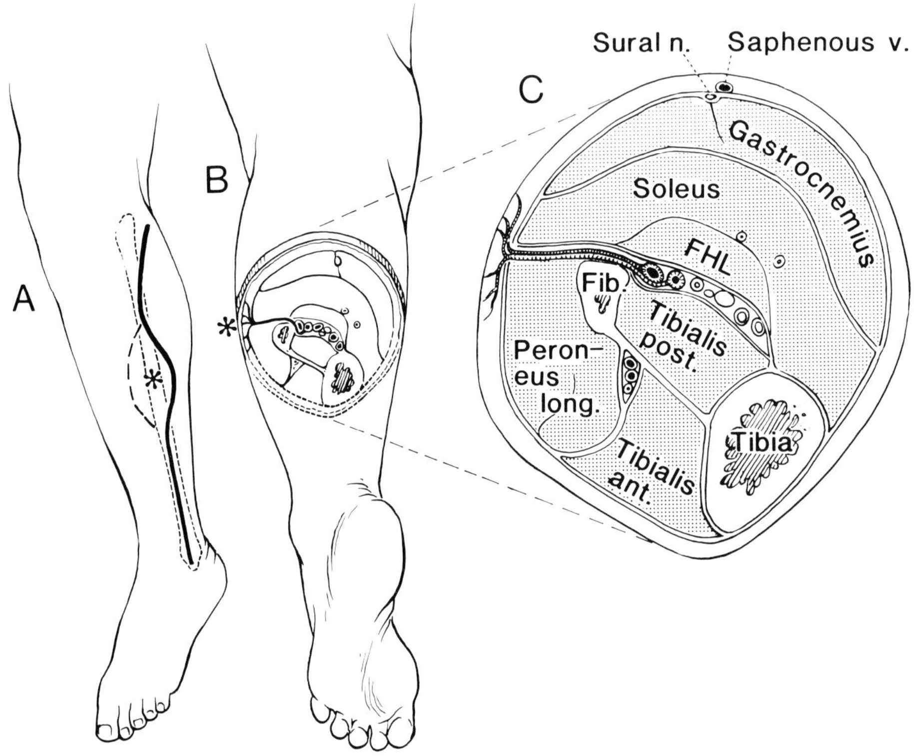

Figure 40–7. ***A, B,*** *and* ***C*** *all refer to the left leg.* ***A*** *shows the lateral view. Solid line indicates the opening incision. Asterisk shows the skin island over the intermuscular septum.* ***B*** *and* ***C*** *show a cross-section of the leg.*

the fascia from lateral to medial (Fig. 40-8). An incision is made on the medial side of the short saphenous vein and carried deep to the fascia. The short saphenous vein and sural nerve are identified proximally and distally and transected. (Often the sural nerve dives deep to the gastrocnemius and will need to be dissected from the muscle substance.)

As the proximal nerve is identified, care is taken to visualize any pedicle. In 30% to 60% of cases, a pedicle arises from the popliteal or sural vessels, which may be used as an alternative pedicle if the intermuscular septum's vessels are damaged.[5,10]

The next step is to approach the posterior crural septum. Dissection is carried deep to the fascia back toward the intermuscular septum (see dotted lines in Figs. 40-8 and 40-9) until the vessels are identified. Sometimes it is helpful to identify the vessels first by making an incision anterior to the skin island and then piercing the fascia and dissecting posterior toward the intermuscular septum until the vessels are identified. The most important issue is to identify the vessels within the intermuscular septum. These vessels vary in origin, course, and size. In some cases they can come directly through the muscle, not through the intermuscular septum.[33] In some cases the superior vessel, arising from the posterior tibial, and in others the inferior vessel, arising from the peroneal, is dominant.[8,9] If the recipient vessel is large, the inferior pedicle should be used. This pedicle is followed down to the peroneal vessel and a section of the peroneal vessel used. The peroneal vessel is a vessel of larger diameter than those in the intermuscular septum. The vascularity of the leg is checked before sacrificing the peroneal vessels because in a few cases the peroneal vessel provides the dominant blood supply to the foot.

The fascia to the nerve is handled appropriately. Only some of the nerve's fascia is preserved, since it can make the flap too bulky. The fascia is preserved between the skin island and the nerve (Fig. 40-10). A fascial edge of 2 to 3 mm is left on both sides of the sural nerve as it extends both proximally and distally from this central segment.

After the nerve has been elevated on the fascial

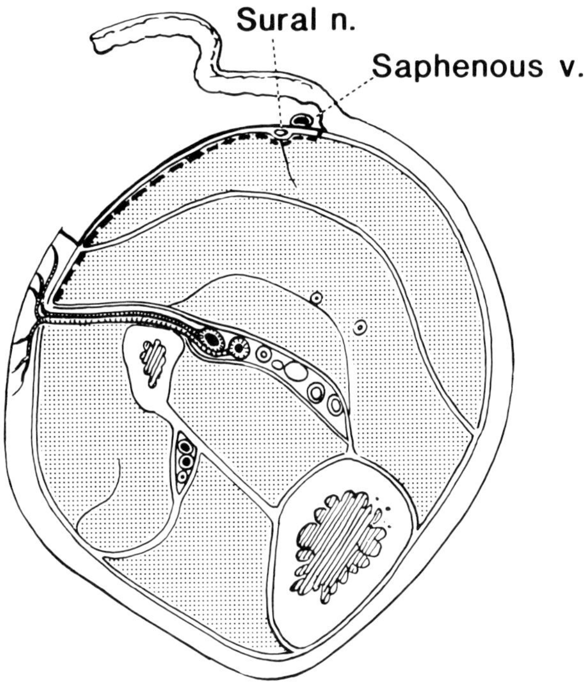

Figure 40–8. *Subcutaneous skin flap is elevated. Dotted line indicates where the next dissection should proceed, below the fascia starting medial to the short saphenous vein.*

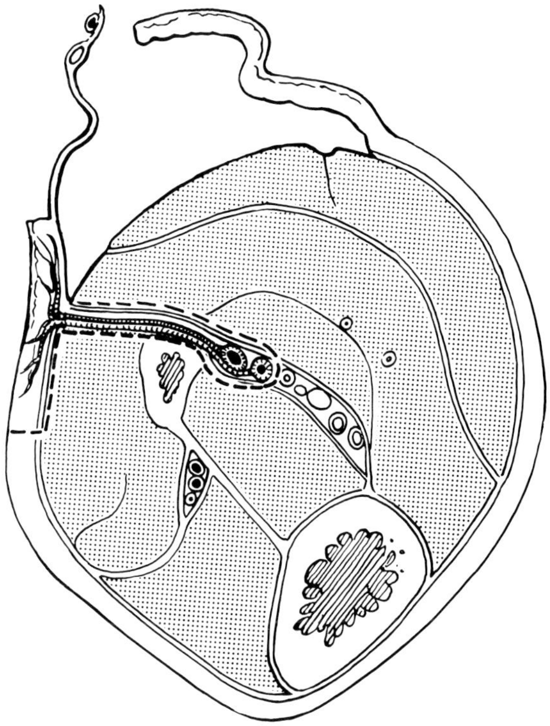

Figure 40–9. *Fascia, including the sural nerve, is elevated to the posterior crural intermuscular septum. Dissection should now proceed along the dotted line.*

segment and the appropriate pedicle isolated, it is transected. The vascularized nerve complex consisting of skin island, fascia, and nerve (see Fig. 40-10) is then transferred to the recipient site.

Attention first is turned to insetting the flap. Once the skin island has been inset and stabilized, the emphasis is on carrying out the microvascular anastomoses. After completion of the anastomoses, both the flap and the nerve are checked for the presence of bleeding. Once it is firmly established that circulation is present, nerve reconstruction is carried out. Great care must be taken in maintaining nerve blood flow to each of the cable segments of the sural nerve. The sural nerve is divided into cables attached either to the epineurium of the nerve or to the fascial segment (Fig. 40-11). This is accomplished by measuring the nerve defect and determining the number of cables required. Median and ulnar nerve reconstruction at the level of the mid-forearm normally requires three or four cables. The length of each cable is then measured, the microscope is brought into the field, and the nerve is teased out from the fascia. The fascia is left attached to the central cable. Proximally and distally the nerve extends beyond the fascia. These segments are made into cables as previously described. A longitudinal incision is made in the epineurium, and the nerve is transected transversely. In this fashion epineural blood supply is maintained (see Fig. 40-11). The segments supplied by epineural vessels only are then folded. The nerve segments are placed in the defect, and nerve repair is carried out under the microscope. Bleeding is visualized from each of the segments.

At completion of the nerve repairs, the wound is closed, and the flap is monitored constantly. We monitor all flaps with a photoplethysmograph at the time of closure and for 4 days thereafter. All nerve graft reconstructions are splinted postoperatively for 3 to 4 weeks.

Vascularized Ulnar Nerve Graft

The most commonly used vascularized donor nerve in brachial plexus reconstruction is the ulnar nerve. In those brachial plexus cases where preganglionic

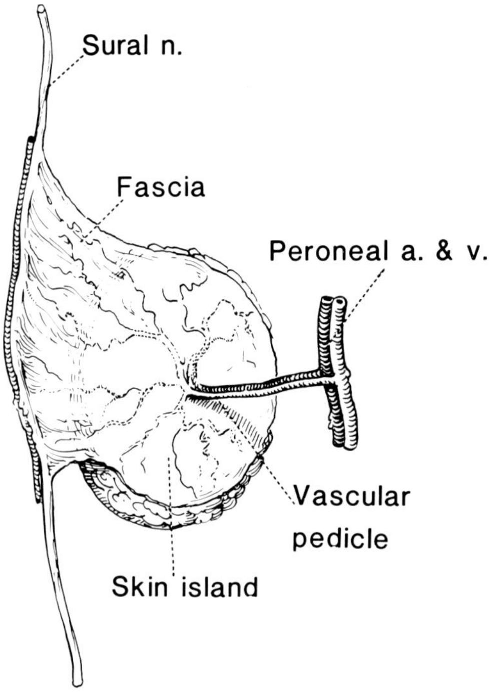

Figure 40–10. *View from the bottom of skin–fascia–nerve complex. Note that in this preparation a portion of the peroneal vessels was used.*

lesions of C8 and T1 have been firmly established, the ulnar nerve is used as a pedicle or free VNG.

Authors' Preferred Method

First, the supraclavicular brachial plexus is thoroughly explored. This requires visualization of the C8 and T1 avulsed root or empty foramina in order to establish that a preganglionic lesion is present. We do not believe that myelography or somatosensory tests indicating avulsion of C8 and T1 is sufficient evidence to sacrifice the ulnar nerve. Direct visualization of the brachial plexus is also recommended. Along with this, obviously, there must be some postganglionic lesions at C5, C6, or C7 in order to have sufficient proximal nerve for reconstruction.

Next, the infraclavicular exploration is carried out and the most proximal portion of the normal nerves are identified. In this manner the nerve gap that is present can be determined. After considering the size of the gap, the nature of the bed, the status of the proximal nerve roots at C5, C6, and C7, and the presence of a preganglionic lesion at C8 and T1, a decision is made regarding utilization of the ulnar nerve as a VNG. If one elects to proceed, the ulnar nerve is harvested.

An incision is made at the level of the cubital tunnel and carried proximally. The ulnar nerve is exposed in the same manner as in ulnar nerve subcutaneous transposition at the elbow. Once the ulnar nerve is identified at the level of the cubital tunnel, dissection is carried proximally. Several centimeters proximal to the cubital tunnel, the superior ulnar collateral artery and vein will normally be visualized. These run on the inner aspect of the nerve (as viewed by the surgeon) and terminate by connecting with the branches of the ulnar recurrent vessels (Fig. 40-12). The ulnar nerve is elevated out of its bed. In order to do this, the branches holding it to the ulnar recurrent vessels are transected. Dissection is then carried in

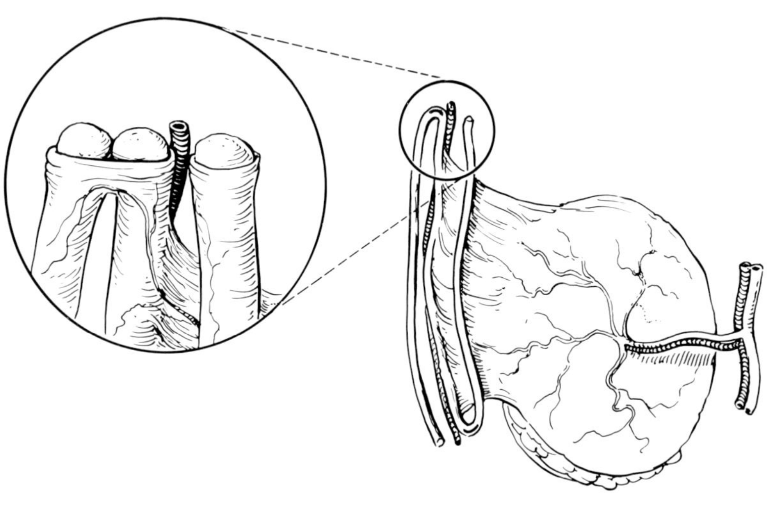

Figure 40–11. *How blood supply is maintained to each of the segments. The middle cable is supplied by the fascia, while the two remaining cables are supplied through the epineurium. The full-view diagram shows the longitudinal transection in the epineurium prior to nerve transection. The blow-up view shows the nerve after transection with epineurium intact.*

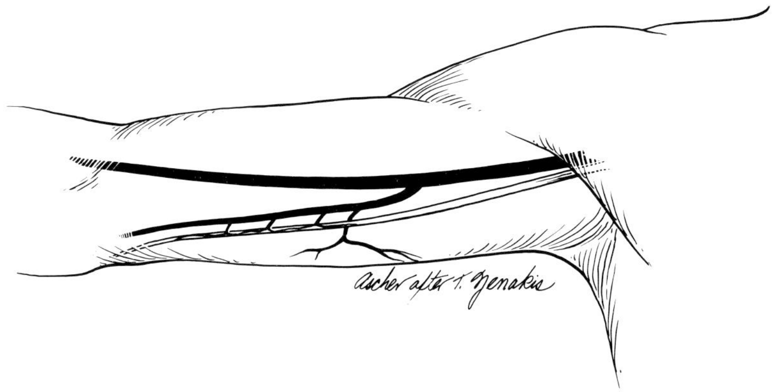

Figure 40–12. *Right arm viewed from the medial aspect. Brachial artery is shown with superior ulnar collateral artery supplying the ulnar nerve and skin.*

a proximal direction, maintaining the superior ulnar collateral vessels on the nerve with a cuff of tissue around the whole neurovascular complex. Dissection may be difficult because of the multiple branches to the surrounding muscle, which must be transected.

Two anatomical structures are carefully sought as the dissection proceeds from distal to proximal. First and most important, the superior ulnar collateral artery's origin from the brachial artery is identified. This normally arises 14 to 22 cm above the medial epicondyle.[5] Therefore, it may originate as high as the axilla. The vein starts in the same region or slightly lower, coming from the plexus formed by the basilic and brachial veins. These vessels then proceed in a medial direction to join the nerve. They run with the nerve on its inner deep side for 4 to 15 cm before turning away, always above the cubital tunnel.

The second important group of structures to visualize are the vessels running from the superior ulnar collateral vessel out to the medial skin. These vessels are used to make a skin island monitor. In only 80% of cases does a vessel run directly from the superior ulnar collateral vessels to the skin. In the remaining 20% of cases the vessel comes directly off the brachial vessels, making a skin island monitor impossible.[3]

Once the superior ulnar collateral artery origin from the brachial vessels has been identified, dissection proceeds rapidly in a more proximal direction until the ulnar nerve joins the brachial plexus. At this point the nerve is transected. Dissection then starts from the level of the cubital tunnel distally. The flexor carpi ulnaris fascia and muscle is split and the nerve is harvested from the level of the elbow to the wrist. Great care is taken not to damage the ulnar artery that is not harvested with the distal ulnar nerve. Once the distal ulnar nerve has been elevated, it is transected at the level of the wrist.

The whole length of the ulnar nerve may be used, obtaining a nerve graft length of 55.7 cm. The proximal and distal portions without extrinsic blood supply are dissected, leaving the epineurium intact to protect the epineural vessels. If these vessels are damaged, the portion of the nerve without extrinsic blood supply may not survive. A decision is then made as to whether the nerve is used as a pedicle nerve graft or free VNG. This decision depends on the amount of the nerve graft tissue necessary to reconstruct the defect. If only one proximal root is intact, a pedicle nerve graft is sufficient.

The superior ulnar collateral vessels are left attached to the junction with the brachial vessels. The nerve graft is rotated in such a fashion that the distal end, which is a free segment, is brought up into a position to reconstruct the defect. The epineurium is cut longitudinally and the nerve transversely to maintain epineural blood flow. In this fashion blood supply of the nerve graft is maintained and the nerve defect is reconstructed.

In cases where several proximal nerve roots are available for reconstruction and nerve gaps are large, 30 to 40 cm of large-caliber nerve graft may be necessary. In this case the nerve is transferred as a free VNG. As described in previous sections, the nerve is transferred based on its superior ulnar collateral vessels. Recipient vessels in the neck are identified; often the transverse cervical is used as the artery. The external or internal jugular may serve as the recipient vein by using an end-to-side anastomosis. Following establishment of blood flow, nerve graft reconstruction is carried out. The ulnar nerve is divided into cables corresponding to each of the defects to be reconstructed, using the techniques described above. Once the nerve cables are constructed, nerve repairs are carried out in standard fashion under the microscope.

In the event of a missed vascular thrombosis, the vascularized ulnar nerve is converted to a nonvascularized graft. Since the ulnar nerve has a large diameter it becomes a trunk graft, which undergoes central necrosis. The results of trunk grafting are inferior to cable NNGs.[2]9 Therefore, thrombosis in a vascularized ulnar nerve graft will produce results inferior to those obtained with conventional nerve grafting. To avoid this, the vascularized ulnar nerve graft is monitored when possible.

CONCLUSION

Reasonable experimental and some clinical evidence shows that a VNG performs superior to a conventional nerve graft under certain conditions. In a badly scarred recipient bed a VNG is clearly indicated; with proximal nerve lesions, large gaps, and a compromised recipient bed, a VNG may be useful.

Six potential donor vascularized nerves exist. At present, we feel that the sural nerve based on the intermuscular perforators, as described by Doi and associates,[9] represents the best choice for peripheral nerve reconstruction. In brachial plexus injuries with preganglionic lesions of C8–T1, a vascularized ulnar nerve graft is indicated.

Whichever donor nerve is used, the surgeon must become familiar with the anatomy of the nerve's blood supply, methods of maintaining vascular supply while forming cables, and techniques of monitoring the nerve.

REFERENCES

1. Arakaki A, Tsai TM, Firrell J, Breidenbach WC. Vascular perfusion of experimental arterialized venous nerve grafts. Presented to the American Society for Reconstructive Microsurgery, Seattle, 1989.
2. Bonney G, Birch R, Jamieson AM, Eames RA. Experience with vascularized nerve grafts. Clin Plast Surg 1984; 11:137–142.
3. Breidenbach WC, Adamson W, Terzis JK. Medial arm flap revisited. Ann Plast Surg 1987; 18:156–164.
4. Breidenbach W, Terzis JK. The anatomy of free vascularized nerve grafts. Clin Plast Surg 1984; 11: 65.
5. Breidenbach WC, Terzis JK. The blood supply of vascularized nerve grafts. J Reconstr Microsurg 1986; 3:43.
6. Breidenbach WC, Terzis JK. Vascularized nerve grafts: An experimental and clinical review. Ann Plast Surg 1987; 18:137.
7. Daly PJ, Wood MB. Endoneural and epineurial blood flow evaluation with free vascularized and conventional nerve grafts in the canine. J Reconstr Microsurg 1985; 2:45.
8. Doi K, Kuwata N, Kawakami F, Tamaru K, Kawai S. The free vascularized sural nerve graft. Microsurg 1984; 5:175.
9. Doi K, Kuwata N, Sakai K, Tamaru K, Kawai S. A reliable technique of free vascularized sural nerve grafting and preliminary results of clinical applications. J Hand Surg [Am] 1987; 12:677.
10. Fachinelli A, Masquelet A, Restrepo J, Gilbert A. The vascularized sural nerve. Int J Microsurg 1981; 3:57.
11. Gu YD, Wu MM, Zheng YL, Li HR, Xu YN. Arterialized venous free sural nerve grafting. Ann Plast Surg 1985; 15:332–339.
12. Kanaya F, Breidenbach WC, Tsai TM, Firrell J. Functional results of vascularized vs nonvascularized nerve grafting. Presented to the American Society for Reconstructive Microsurgery, Seattle, 1989.
13. Kanaya F, Firrell J, Breidenbach WC. Blood flow of segmentally cut and folded vascularized rabbit sciatic nerve. Presented to the American Society for Reconstructive Microsurgery, Baltimore, 1988.
14. Kleinert JM, Fleming S, Abel C, Firrell J. Radial and ulnar artery dominance in normal digits. J Hand Surg [Am] 1989; 14:504.
15. Koshima I, Harii K. Experimental study of vascularized nerve grafts: Morphometric study of axonal regeneration of nerves transplanted into silicone tubes. Ann Plast Surg 1985; 14:235–243.
16. Koshima I, Harii K. Experimental study of vascularized nerve grafts: Multifactorial analysis of axonal regeneration of nerves transplanted into an acute burn wound. J Hand Surg [Am] 1985; 10:64–72.
17. Lind R, Wood MB. Comparison of the pattern of early revascularization of conventional vs vascularized nerve grafts in the canine. J Reconstr Microsurg 1986; 2:229.

18. Lux P, Breidenbach WC, Firrell J. Determination of temporal changes in blood flow in vascularized and nonvascularized nerve grafts in the dog. Plast Reconstr Surg 1988; 82:133–142.
19. McCullough CJ, Grady O, Higginson DW, et al. Axon regeneration and vascularization of nerve grafts: An experimental study. J Hand Surg [Br] 1984; 9:323.
20. Merle M, Lebreton E, Froucher G, et al. Vascularized nerve grafts: Preliminary results. Presented to the American Society for Reconstructive Microsurgery, Las Vegas, 1985.
21. Millesi H, Meissl G, Berger A. The interfascicular nerve grafting of the median and ulnar nerves. J Bone Joint Surg [Am] 1972; 54:727–750.
22. Millesi H, Meissl G, Berger A. Further experience with interfascicular grafting of the median, ulnar and radial nerves. J Bone Joint Surg [Am] 1976; 58: 209–219.
23. Restrepo Y, Merle M, Michon J, Folliguet B, Barrat E. Free vascularized nerve grafts: An experimental study in the rabbit. Microsurgery 1985; 6:78–84.
24. Rose EH, Kowalski TA. Restoration of sensibility to anesthetic scarred digits with free vascularized nerve grafts from the dorsum of the foot. J Hand Surg [Am] 1985; 10:514–521.
25. Rose EH, Kowalski TA, Norris MS. The reversed venous arterialized nerve graft in digital nerve reconstruction across scarred beds. Plast Reconstr Surg 1989; 83:593.
26. Seckel BR, Ryan SE, Simons JE, Gagne RG, Watson E. Vascularized vs nonvascularized nerve grafts: An experimental structural comparison. Plast Reconstr Surg 1986; 78:211–220.
27. Settergren CR, Wood MB. A comparison of blood flow in free vascularized vs nonvascularized nerve grafts. J Reconstr Microsurg 1984; 1:95.
28. Shibata M, Tsai T-M, Firrell J, Breidenbach WC. Experimental comparison of vascularized and nonvascularized nerve grafting. J Hand Surg [Am] 1988; 13:358–365.
29. Sunderland S. Nerves and nerve injuries, ed 2. Edinburgh: Churchill-Livingstone, 1978: 626–629.
30. Taylor IG. Nerve grafting with simultaneous microvascular reconstruction. Clin Orthop 1978; 133:56.
31. Taylor IG, Ham FJ. The free vascularized nerve graft. Plast Reconstr Surg 1976; 57:143.
32. Townsend PLG, Taylor GI. Vascularized nerve grafts using composite arterialized neuro-venous systems. Br J Plast Surg 1984; 37:1.
33. Wei FC, Chen HC, Chuang CC, Noordhoff MS. Fibular osteoseptocutaneous flap: Anatomic and clinical application. Plast Reconstr Surg 1986; 78: 191.

41

Nerve Grafting Through Resorbable Tubes

Mark A. Urban
F. William Bora, Jr.

AUTHORS' KEY POINTS

- Nerve grafting with bioresorbable tube material is technically simpler and requires less operating time than conventional grafting with autogenous nerve tissue.
- This type of grafting does not sacrifice host nerve tissue, avoids the loss of other nerve function, and eliminates the need for a second operation for tube removal because it is bioresorbable.
- Ideally, bioresorbable tube material should allow incorporation of pharmacological agents that promote nerve regeneration (such as nerve growth factors) or inhibit scar formation (such as cis-hydroxyproline) during nerve regeneration.

BACKGROUND

The treatment of a segmental defect in an injured peripheral nerve poses a challenge to the surgeon. Conventional options for repair include nerve mobilization, suture under tension, joint positioning, and nerve grafting.[9] Suture under tension impairs axonal regeneration secondary to diminished intrafascicular circulation and creation of scar tissue.[9,63,91] Even suture with minimal tension yields a less-than-ideal result, as the inflammatory reaction created by the original injury and by the suture itself causes a fibroblastic reaction leading to neuroma formation.[5,8,38]

Weiss reviewed several early reports of materials wrapped around nerve repair sites to improve functional results from treatment.[96] These materials, used between 1880 and 1943, included bone, artery, vein, gelatin, fascia, fat, epineurium, agar, trachea, casein, feather quill, rubber, dura, muscle, parchment, tantalum, and others for sutureless repair of severed nerves. None of the methods appeared clearly superior. Later investigators found that wrapping the neurorrhaphy site with other types of sleeves, including Millipore,[4,13,14] Silastic ("Ducker cuff"),[22,23,61] Micropore adhesive tape (Steri-Strips),[26] collagen,[27,37] or a biodegradable polylactic/polyglycolic acid cuff[80] decreased the ingrowth of surrounding scar tissue, but electrophysiological and functional return were not improved.

Most surgeons have repaired a nerve gap with an intercalary segment of autogenous nerve tissue. Rather than closing a segmental defect under tension, autogenous nerve grafting has been the recommended treatment when a gap is encountered.[54,62,66,88,89,91] Unfortunately, this method creates a donor-site sensory defect, increases operating time, is technically inconvenient,[21] and yields unpredictable results.

NERVE REGENERATION THROUGH TUBULAR PROSTHESES

The past decade has seen the revival of attempts to span a nerve gap with an artificial tubular material. Successful regeneration of up to 20 mm in rats[34,57,67,68,100] and up to 3 cm in monkeys[20,54,55] has been observed. Application of this method for human use has not been reported, although research in this direction is underway. Campbell and coworkers wrapped Millipore tubes around peripheral nerve grafts in three patients in 1961, but their results were not described in detail.[14] All subsequent studies have used animal models.

The temporal and spatial events that allow regenerating neurons to cross a gap have been outlined histologically in silicone tubes[25,31,33,40–42,46,49,69,84,85,94,96,97,101] and vascularized pseudosynovial sheaths[48,50,51] implanted in mice and rats. By 7 to 8 days, these chambers are filled with an amorphic mass of fibrin/fibronectin and trapped erythrocytes (blood clot), loosely binding the severed nerve ends together. Capillary ingrowth begins by the 9th day, bringing neutrophils and macrophages into the sequestered environment. By 10 to 12 days, the mass begins to organize, with the central fibrin core shrinking from the tubular wall (syneresis) and forming its own "epineurium" of collagen layers, surrounded by a clear liquid. The composition of this liquid is unknown, although it may include neurite-promoting factors (NPFs) and other proteins immunochemically distinct from laminin and fibronectin, all important for nerve regeneration.[42,49,52] Laminin now appears on the fibrin strands as they reorganize in a longitudinal fashion. Unmyelinated axons begin to sprout and creep along this scaffolding by 2 weeks, followed shortly by Schwann cells that wrap around them.

Whether the axons create their own endoneurial tubes or follow previously established endoneurial tubes is controversial. Cabaud and associates[11] found that although some old endoneurial tubules persisted in monkey ulnar nerves up to 6 weeks after transection and epineurial suture, they were not always used as conduits for regenerating neurites; most new fibers passed down *new* tubules. Other investigators, however, found that up to 12 weeks after introducing an acellular allograft across sciatic nerve gaps in rodents, regenerating axons always grew out through the *inner* surface of basal lamina scaffolds; they were never seen outside the scaffolds.[28,32]

In rodents, fasciculation can be seen by the 3rd week, and by 5 weeks myelinated axon/Schwann cell units penetrate the distal stump. The number and diameter of axons increase over time, with regeneration occurring in all major fiber groups. Complete remyelination occurs between 4 and 6 weeks, in a proximal-to-distal gradient (Fig. 41-1). Unfortunately, these axons attain only 40% of their normal diameter and nerve-conduction velocity, even after 10 months.[25]

The mechanism whereby regeneration across a gap takes place is an active area of current research. Given the proper microenvironment,[47] neurites at the end of the proximal stump are drawn onto the fibrin scaffolding by neuronotrophic factors including nerve growth factor (NGF)[16,29,45] and a heterogenous population of other growth factors (eg, laminin, fibronectin, apolipoprotein E, basic fibroblast growth factor, delta-1 acid glycoprotein, and ganglioside-GM_1)[1,10,21,28,42,45,69,81,86,90] with some of these proteins specific for each neuron type.[43,44] The exact source of such growth factors, whether degenerating Schwann cells, fibroblasts, reticuloendothelial cells, or some other factor or cell type in the distal stump, is unknown.

Early in this century, Cajal suggested that humoral factors in the distal stumps of transected peripheral nerves exert a "neurotropic" effect on regenerating axons.[12] Later, however, the concept that "contact guidance" and not neurotropism was responsible for neuronal development became the accepted dogma for nearly 40 years, supported by

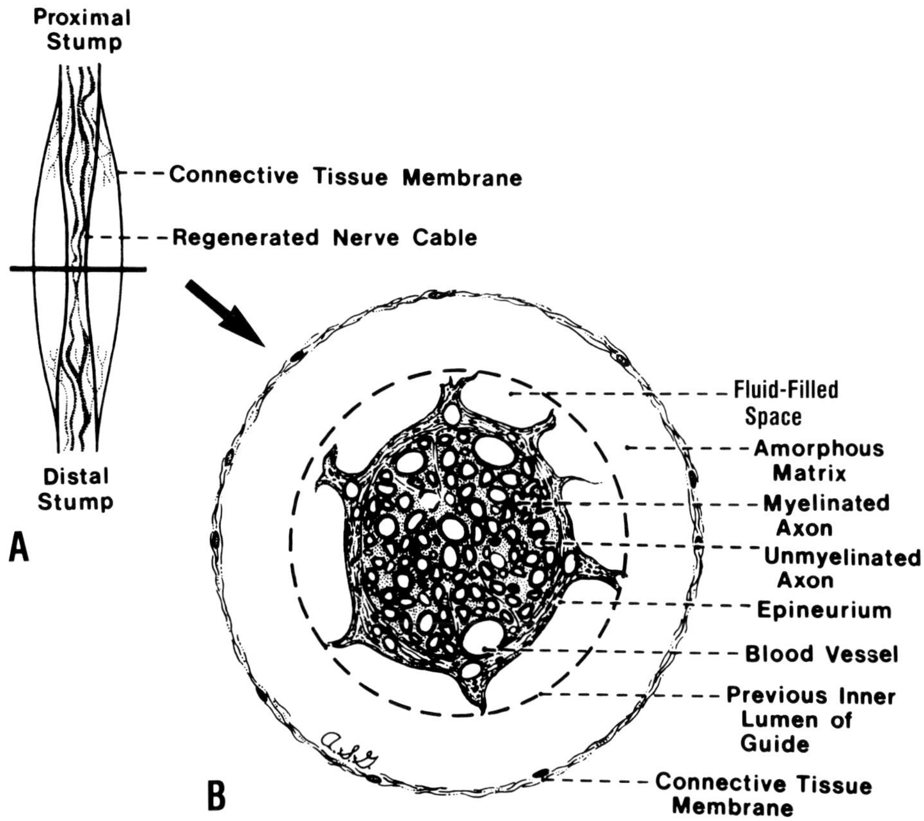

Figure 41–1. *(**A**) Schematic representation of a bioresorbable tube graft 3 months postoperatively with regenerated nerve segment. (**B**) Note regenerated nerve cable including blood vessels, myelinated and unmyelinated nerve fibers, regenerated epineurium, minimal scar tissue, and degradated guidance tube. (From Seckel BR, Chiu TH, Nyilas E, Sidman RL. Nerve regeneration through synthetic biodegradable nerve guides: Regulation by the target organ. Plast Reconstr Surg 1984;74:173–181, with permission.)*

experiments done by Weiss in 1944.[98] He demonstrated that regenerating nerve fibers growing down a Y-shaped arterial graft and encountering either degenerated nerve, tendon, or fat showed no specificity. Later investigators, however, felt that the results were influenced significantly by immunologic rejection of the graft or interference by arterial adventitia. Using Y-shaped silicone sleeves, this concept has now been refuted, as nerve "tissue specificity"[53] has been effectively demonstrated in rats and cats[78,102] and corroborated in primates as well.[56]

In more elaborate studies, nerves regenerated across gaps leading to either different peripheral nerve sensory branches (eg, peroneal vs tibial),[77,87] different motor branches (eg, tibial nerve/interosseous muscle vs peroneal nerve/tibialis anterior muscles),[79] or motor vs sensory branches only in a mixed nerve;[10] preferential axonal specificity was evident. Such "fascicular specificity"[53] may be mediated by target-derived neuronotrophic factors,[86,87] relating the ability of end-organ tissues to determine their own correct reinnervation ("end-organ specificity"[53]).

Recent studies with silicone[3,24,67] and mesothelial[47,54] tubes have analyzed the electrophysiological aspects of nerve regeneration across an artificial gap. The extent and rate of recovery have been shown to follow closely that of nerves regenerating after either primary neurorrhaphy or autografting. However, even under experimental conditions, muscle compound action potentials and nerve conduction velocities attain only 25% to 60% of their normal values.[24,54,67] After 10 months of regeneration, axons regain only a fraction of their normal size, which is felt to be the primary factor limiting return of normal physiologic activity.[25]

Unfortunately, silicone elastomer, acrylic copolymer (Silastic), polyethylene, and polytetrafluoroethylene (Gore-Tex) tubular prostheses, all excellent experimental materials for studying nerve regeneration, have one major problem when they are used clinically. Although they are biologically inert, nonresorbable tubes themselves eventually create chronic nerve compression by compromising the blood supply to the tissue within the tube.[3,54,59,68] They also damage the nerve and adjacent tissue by prolonged cuff movement and neuroma formation at the proximal end of the tube.[3,37,80] New materials are needed.

THE BIORESORBABLE NERVE GRAFT

Reid and colleagues were the first to use synthetic bioresorbable cuffs in an attempt to improve primary neurorrhaphy in dog ulnar and peroneal nerves.[80] Their polylactic/polyglycolic acid copolymer sleeves degraded after 8 to 12 weeks, inciting little inflammatory reaction and effectively limiting fibrosis from the external environment. However, the authors saw no difference in nerve conduction velocity or electromyography. They did show, however, that such material had a controlled rapid degradation, was nontoxic, provided a smooth lubricating surface for nerve regeneration, was easily fabricated, and could be altered at the time of surgery.

Molander and coworkers were the first to document nerve regeneration across an experimental gap in rabbit tibial nerves using synthetic, bioresorbable polyglactin 910 (Vicryl) meshed tubes.[64,65] This material, as well as polyglycolic acid (Dexon), both then in use as new suture materials, elicited a minimal tissue phagocytotic response and were resorbed by 90 to 120 days.[18] As previous tubular methods had shown, polyglactin 910 provided orientation for regenerating nerve fibers and allowed innervation of the distal stump. The resorbed tube was completely replaced by a new connective tissue sleeve after 8 weeks, reduced ingrowth of scar tissue from surrounding structures, and decreased neuroma formation. Use of such a material was also found to be technically simple, applied no tension to the epineurium of either proximal or distal stumps, and sacrificed no other nerves, as was required in autografting. Only minor clinical, histologic, and electrophysiological differences between using a resorbable tube and a nerve graft were seen.[64]

Other investigators have also studied nerve regeneration through bioresorbable tubes. The most common materials have been D,L-polylactic acid (PLA)[19,30,58–60,86,87] and polyglycolic acid (Dexon, PGA).[20,21,30,82] Several composites of 50% to 90% PLA or 75% PGA and copoly[1,4-butylene-(1:1)-D,L-lactate/D,L-hydroxysuccinate], copoly[1,6-hexylene-(1:1)-L-lactate/succinate], low-molecular-weight L-poly(lactic acid), or poly(2,3-butylene succinate)[30] have also been used, as well as alzamer* polyorthoester.[6]

Da Silva and colleagues noted that two thirds of motor nuclei and one third of sensory nuclei were retrogradely labeled by horseradish peroxidase stain after 6 weeks of regeneration across poly-D,L-lactate grafts in mice, indicating axonal transport in regenerated neurons across this material.[19] Seckel and coworkers found that after 3 months, approximately 40% of axons regenerated across a 10-mm gap in rat sciatic nerves, with complete resorption of the tubular graft material and without neuroma formation; active plantar flexion returned by this time, demonstrating at least partial return of motor function.[86,87]

Dellon and Mackinnon used polyglycolic acid grafts to span a gap of up to 3 cm in monkey ulnar nerves. Their results showed no significant difference in mean fiber diameter, action potential amplitude, or nerve conduction velocity between bioresorbable nerve grafts and autografts; these values were found, however, to be significantly less than normal (only 30%).[20] Rosen and coworkers also found similar myelinated axonal diameters with

* *Alza Corporation, Palo Alto, CA 94303-0802*

less disorganization at the repair site when polyglycolic acid grafts were compared to suture repair in rats.[82]

Bora and colleagues used a resorbable alzamer polyorthoester tube across severed cat sciatic nerves.[6] This material was unique because it could be impregnated with other substances, serving as a vehicle for trophic factors, anti-scar agents, or antibiotics. Their tubes were saturated with 10% cis-hydroxyproline (Fig. 41-2*A*). After 12 weeks, axons passed through a 15-mm gap and reinnervated end-organ muscle, as demonstrated by electrophysiological testing and fast axonal transport kinetics; no electrophysiological difference was seen between use of the resorbable grafts and autogenous nerve grafts. Addition of cis-hydroxyproline was also felt to improve slightly the efficiency of regeneration (Figs. 41-2*B*,*C*).

Using a variety of tubular diameters and compositions, Henry and coworkers saw "successful regeneration" through only about half of the tubes they tested, but an increased chance of regeneration as tubular diameter increased.[30] Because they undergo slow hydrolysis, bioresorbable grafts imbibe water and with time undergo swelling, wall deformation, and possible complete collapse.[30,87] The more biodegradable a graft, the more likely these investigators found it to undergo distortion and luminal narrowing, possibly leading to failure from nerve compression.

Bioresorbable tube grafts are technically simpler to implant than conventional autografts, the current "gold standard" in bridging a peripheral nerve gap. They do not require sacrifice of other host nerves and therefore do not cause sensory loss or formation of painful neuromas. They are biodegradable and do not require a second operation for graft removal to prevent long-term problems with nerve compression at the graft site. On the axon level, they may allow a more accurate anastomosis of individual transected peripheral nerve fibers than either primary neurorrhaphy or autografting, especially in mixed-component nerves.[21,53] Recent experiments have demonstrated that return of functional and electrophysiological parameters is at least as good after tube grafting as after autografting. The bioresorbable tube graft is indeed an attractive alternative.

CHARACTERISTICS OF THE IDEAL GUIDANCE SYSTEM

No currently available method has returned function of a transected nerve to its original state. Surgeons have encountered one common problem in all methods of nerve repair: the formation of excess scar tissue at the repair site. Substantial work has been done with chemical anti-inflammatory agents, the most promising of which is cis-hydroxyproline.[6,7,9,17,38,39,70,75,76] Alpha, alpha-dipyridyl,[7,17] beta-aminopropionitrile,[7,71–74] colchicine,[17] and D-penicillamine,[7,15,17,36] at least when administered systemically in doses required to reduce inflammation, have proven too toxic for this purpose. Beta-aminopropionitrile and D-penicillamine can induce hypersensitivity reactions.[17]

The proline analogue cis-hydroxyproline, an inhibitor of collagen synthesis, is preferentially incorporated into the protocollagen molecule,[83] preventing normal collagen triple-helical formation from this precursor[92,93] and thereby decreasing cellular collagen extrusion.[83] Early reports of this inhibitor focused on its ability to diminish scar tissue around sites of tendon repair,[7,39] but later it was also found to be effective in reducing neuroma formation at neurorrhaphy sites[6,38] and in increasing motor nerve conduction velocity[70] and regeneration.[74,76] No toxicity was noted.[38,39,75]

Ideally, tube material should be porous so as to allow the addition of an anti-scar agent such as alzamer incorporating 10% cis-hydroxyproline. This tube is made of polyorthoester, releasing its anti-scar agent by zero-order kinetics from direct hydrolysis. Degradation products of this tube are biodegradable and nonantigenic, forming cyclohexanedimethanol and 4-hydroxybutyrate. The former is excreted in the urine, and the latter is a natural intracellular metabolite. The rate of hydrolysis can be delayed from its baseline of 10 to 14 days to 5 to 6 weeks by adding 2% sodium bicarbonate.[6]

Another method of increasing axonal regeneration has been by prefilling tubular prostheses with matrix precursors or neuronotrophic factors prior to implantation.[16,57–59,69,90,99,100,103] Also, an increase in regeneration has been seen by making tubes more semipermeable, thereby allowing influx

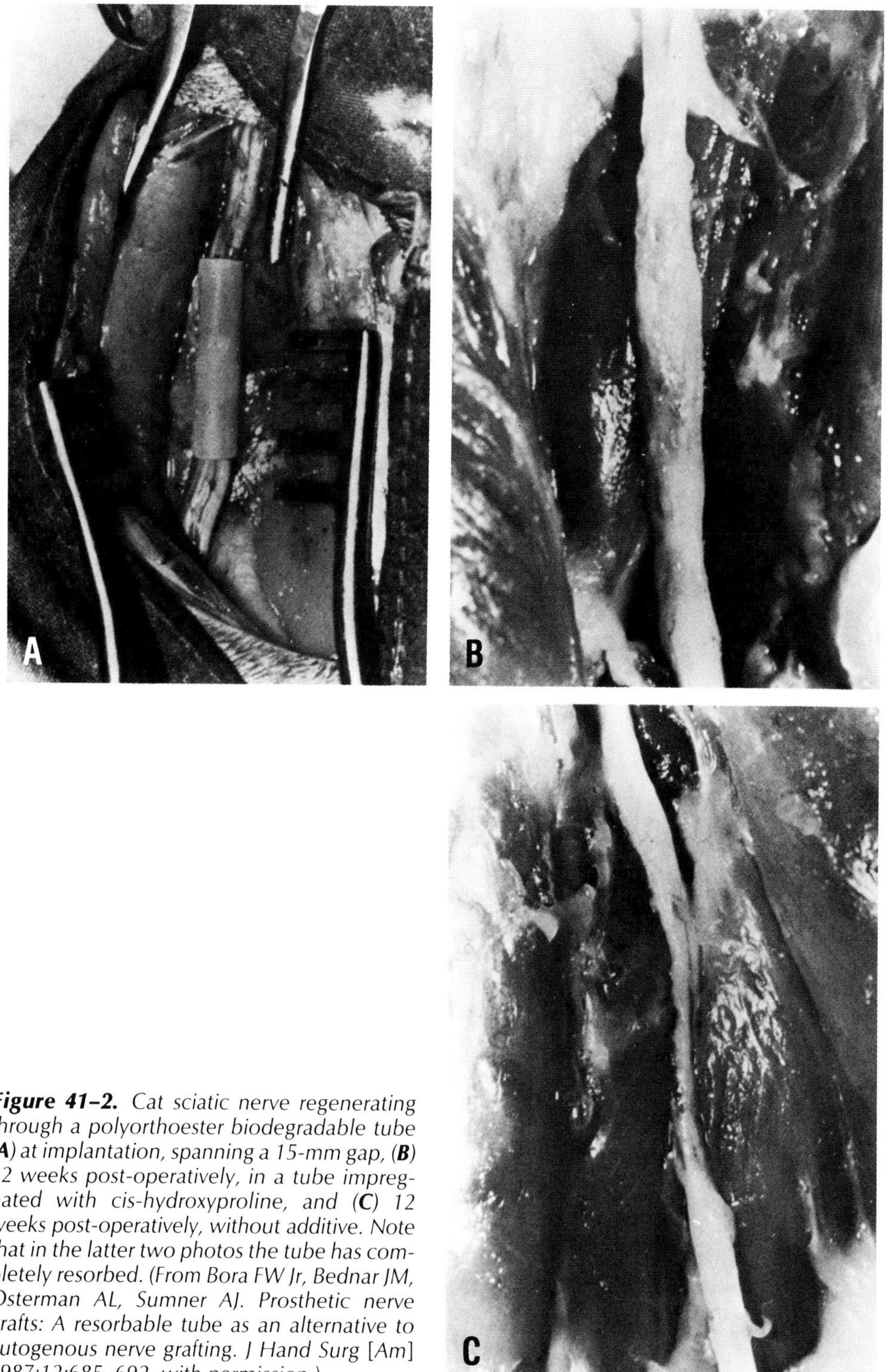

Figure 41–2. *Cat sciatic nerve regenerating through a polyorthoester biodegradable tube (**A**) at implantation, spanning a 15-mm gap, (**B**) 12 weeks post-operatively, in a tube impregnated with cis-hydroxyproline, and (**C**) 12 weeks post-operatively, without additive. Note that in the latter two photos the tube has completely resorbed. (From Bora FW Jr, Bednar JM, Osterman AL, Sumner AJ. Prosthetic nerve grafts: A resorbable tube as an alternative to autogenous nerve grafting. J Hand Surg [Am] 1987;12:685–692, with permission.)*

of extracellular nutrients while preventing escape of neuronotrophic factors.[1,4,33–35] Both of these methods rely on the observation that an orderly fibrin scaffold created between transected nerve ends guides sprouting axons across the gap; early and more orderly formation of this matrix may allow quicker and more complete regeneration of these neurons. It is important that this scaffold be orderly, because disorganized matrices have been reported to diminish regeneration.[2,95,99]

SURGICAL TECHNIQUE

Authors' Preferred Method

After the standard introduction of anesthesia, adequate exposure of the involved nerve should allow definition of normal nerve tissue proximal and distal to the injured nerve segment. The ends of each nerve stump should be cleanly trimmed back to nerve tissue with an acceptable fascicular pattern; a #11 blade supported by a sterile tongue-blade platform can be used for this surgical maneuver (Fig. 41-3*A*). The damaged nerve tissue is removed, defining the deficient area to be grafted. A tube whose inner diameter will accommodate postoperative swelling (approximately 0.5 to 1.0 mm larger than that of the involved nerve) should be chosen; it should be cut to a length that places 5 mm of nerve within each end of the tube. A gap of up to 3 cm may be tolerated in monkeys;[20] limits in humans are unknown.

Under either loupe or microscopic magnification, each end of the nerve is then sutured by two 9-0 nylon epineurial stitches passing from the tube out through the epineurium (Fig. 41-3*B*). No further manipulation of the nerve is necessary. Closure is made in the standard fashion and the limb immobilized for 3 weeks.

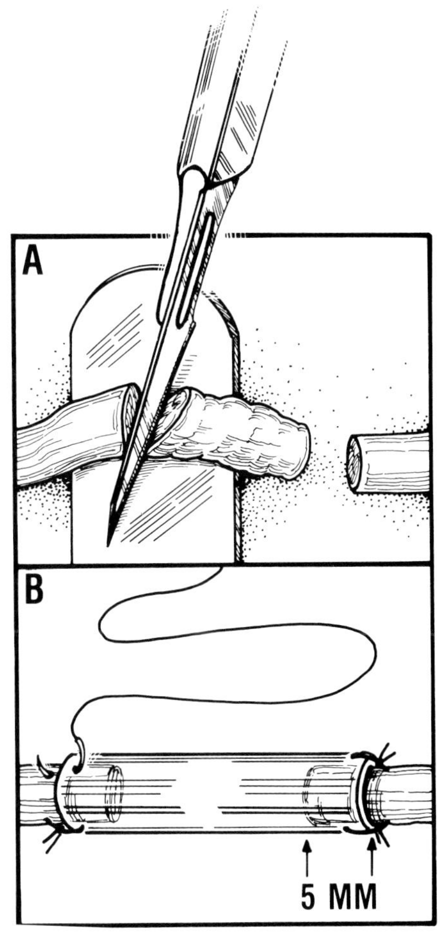

Figure 41–3. *Technique of nerve repair. (**A**) The involved nerve ends are isolated and trimmed cleanly with a No. 11 blade, and the distance between the tension-free ends is measured. (**B**) Two 9-0 sutures are used to attach each nerve end to the tube.*

FUTURE RESEARCH

Researchers are seeking the ideal nerve regeneration and guidance system for returning function after treatment of peripheral nerve injuries. Based on experiments reported to date, future efforts should concentrate on using topical neuronotrophic factors, anti-scar drugs, and agents that enhance early axon regeneration. Drugs that stimulate and accelerate the production of axoplasm by the anterior horn motor nuclei and dorsal root ganglion sensory nuclei may also prove to help functional return after treatment. New materials should leave transected nerve ends free from suture, reduce extraneural fibrous invasion at the graft site, be readily vascularized, and be permeable to both oxygen and other soluble nutrients. They should be nontoxic, have low antigenicity, be biodegradable, and maintain stable wall configurations. They should also be simple to use, flexible, inexpensive, and readily available. Synthetic bioresorbable tube grafts fulfill most of these criteria.

Future research must concentrate on the use of these materials in humans. Results from these efforts, if found to be as promising as those in animal models, including primates, will suggest an attractive alternative to an autologous nerve graft or primary suture under tension for a peripheral nerve gap.

REFERENCES

1. Aebischer P, Guenard V, Winn SR, Valentini RF, Galletti PM. Blind-ended semipermeable guidance channels support peripheral nerve regeneration in the absence of a distal nerve stump. Brain Res 1988; 454:179–187.
2. Aebischer P, Valentini RF, Winn SR, Kunz S, Sasken H, Galletti PM. Regeneration of transected sciatic nerves through semi-permeable nerve guidance channels: Effects of extracellular matrix protein additives. Trans Am Soc Artif Intern Organs 1986; 32:474–477.
3. Ashur H, Vilner Y, Finsterbush A, Rousso M, Weinberg H, Devor M. Extent of fiber regeneration after peripheral nerve repair: Silicone splint vs suture, gap repair vs graft. Exp Neurol 1987; 97:365–374.
4. Bassett CAL, Campbell JB, Husby J. Peripheral nerve and spinal cord regeneration: Factors leading to success of a tubulation technique employing Millipore. Exp Neurol 1959; 1:386–406.
5. Bora FW Jr. Peripheral nerve repair in cats: The fascicular stitch. J Bone Joint Surg [Am] 1967; 49:659–666.
6. Bora FW Jr, Bednar JM, Osterman AL, Brown MJ, Sumner AJ. Prosthetic nerve grafts: A resorbable tube as an alternative to autogenous nerve grafting. J Hand Surg [Am] 1987; 12:685–692.
7. Bora FW Jr, Lane JM, Prockop DJ. Inhibitors of collagen biosynthesis as a means of controlling scar formation in tendon injury. J Bone Joint Surg [Am] 1972; 54:1501–1508.
8. Bora FW Jr, Pleasure DE, Didizian NA. A study of nerve regeneration and neuroma formation after nerve suture by various techniques. J Hand Surg 1976; 1:138–143.
9. Bora FW Jr, Richardson S, Black J. The biomechanical responses to tension in a peripheral nerve. J Hand Surg 1980; 5:21–25.
10. Brushart TME, Seiler WA IV. Selective reinnervation of distal motor stumps by peripheral motor axons. Exp Neurol 1987; 97:289–300.
11. Cabaud HE, Rodkey WG, Nemeth TJ. Progressive ultrastructural changes after peripheral nerve transection and repair. J Hand Surg 1982; 7:353–365.
12. Cajal SR. Degeneration and regeneration of the nervous system. London: Oxford University Press, 1928.
13. Campbell JB, Bassett CAL, Girado JM, Seymour RJ, Rossi JP. Application of monomolecular filter tubes in bridging gaps in peripheral nerves and for prevention of neuroma formation: A preliminary report. J Neurosurg 1956; 13:635–637.
14. Campbell JB, Bassett CAL, Husby J, Thulin CA, Feringa ER. Microfilter sheaths in peripheral nerve surgery: A laboratory report and preliminary clinical study. J Trauma 1961; 1:139–158.
15. Chamson A, Frey J. Effects of D-penicillamine on collagen biosynthesis by fibroblast cell cultures. Clin Exp Pharmacol Physiol 1985; 12:549–555.
16. Chen YS, Wang-Bennett LT, Coker NJ. Facial nerve regeneration in the silicone chamber: The influence of nerve growth factor. Exp Neurol 1989; 103:52–60.
17. Cohen, IK. Can collagen metabolism be controlled: Theoretical considerations. J Trauma 1985; 25:410–412.
18. Craig PH, Williams JA, Davis KW, et al. A biologic comparison of polyglactin 910 and polyglycolic acid synthetic absorbable sutures. Surg Gynecol Obstet 1975; 141:1–10.
19. Da Silva CF, Madison R, Dikkes P, Chiu TH, Sidman RL. An in vivo model to quantify motor and sensory peripheral nerve regeneration using bioresorbable nerve guide tubes. Brain Res 1985; 342:307–315.
20. Dellon AL, Mackinnon SE. An alternative to the classical nerve graft for the management of the short nerve gap. Plast Reconstr Surg 1988; 82:849–856.
21. Dellon AL, Mackinnon SE. Basic scientific and clinical applications of peripheral nerve regeneration. Surg Annu 1988; 20:59–100.
22. Ducker TB, Hayes GJ. Experimental improvements in the use of Silastic cuff for peripheral nerve repair. J Neurosurg 1968; 28:582–587.
23. Ducker TB, Hayes GJ. Peripheral nerve injuries: A comparative study of the anatomical and functional results following primary nerve repair in chimpanzees. Milit Med 1968; 133:298–302.
24. Fields RD, Ellisman MH. Axons regenerated through silicone tube splices. I. Conduction properties. Exp Neurol 1986; 92:48–60.
25. Fields RD, Ellisman MH. Axons regenerated through silicone tube splices. II. Functional morphology. Exp Neurol 1986; 92:61–74.

26. Freeman BS, Perry J, Brown D. Experimental study of adhesive surgical tape for nerve anastomosis. Plast Reconstr Surg 1969; 43:174–179.
27. Gibby WA, Koerber HR, Horch KW. A quantitative evaluation of suture and tubulization nerve repair techniques. J Neurosurg 1983; 58:574–579.
28. Gulati A. Evaluation of acellular and cellular nerve grafts in repair of rat peripheral nerve. J Neurosurg 1988; 68:117–123.
29. Gundersen RW, Barrett JN. Neuronal chemotaxis: Chick dorsal-root axons turn toward high concentrations of nerve growth factor. Science 1979; 206: 1079–1080.
30. Henry EW, Chiu TH, Nyilas E, Brushart TM, Dikkes P, Sidman RL. Nerve regeneration through biodegradable polyester tubes. Exp Neurol 1985; 90:652–676.
31. Hurtado H, Knoops B, Van Den Bosch De Aguilar P. Rat sciatic nerve regeneration in semipermeable artificial tubes. Exp Neurol 1987; 97:751–757.
32. Ide C, Tohyama K, Yokota R, Nitatori T, Onodera S. Schwann cell basal lamina and nerve regeneration. Brain Res 1983; 288:61–75.
33. Jenq CB, Coggeshall RE. Nerve regeneration through holey silicone tubes. Brain Res 1985; 361: 233–241.
34. Jenq CB, Coggeshall RE. Permeable tubes increase the length of the gap that regenerating axons can span. Brain Res 1987; 408:239–242.
35. Jenq CB, Jenq LL, Coggeshall RE. Nerve regeneration changes with filters of different pore size. Exp Neurol 1987; 97:662–671.
36. Junker P. D-Penicillamine effects on inflammatory and normal connective tissues: Studies on collagen, glycosaminoglycans and nucleic acids with particular reference to antirheumatoid therapy. Dan Med Bull 1985; 32:87–103.
37. Kline DG, Hayes GJ. The use of resorbable wrapper for peripheral nerve repair: Experimental studies in chimpanzees. J Neurosurg 1964; 21: 737–750.
38. Lane JM, Bora FW Jr, Pleasure D. Neuroma scar formation in rats following peripheral nerve transection. J Bone Joint Surg [Am] 1978; 60:197–203.
39. Lane JM, Bora FW Jr, Prockop DJ, Heppenstall RB, Black J. Inhibition of scar formation by the proline analog cis-hydroxyproline. J Surg Res 1972; 3:135–137.
40. Le Beau JM, Ellisman MH, Powell HC. Ultrastructural and morphometric analysis of long-term peripheral nerve regeneration through silicone tubes. J Neurocytol 1988; 17:161–172.
41. Le Beau JM, Powell HC, Ellisman MH. Node of Ranvier formation along fibres regenerating through silicone tube implants: A freeze-fracture and thin-section electron microscopic study. J Neurocytol 1987; 16:347–358.
42. Longo FM, Hayman EG, Davis GE, et al. Neurite-promoting factors and extracellular matrix components accumulating in vivo within nerve regeneration chambers. Brain Res 1984; 309:105–117.
43. Longo FM, Manthorpe M, Skaper SD, Lundborg G, Varon S. Neuronotrophic activities accumulate in vivo within silicone nerve regeneration chambers. Brain Res 1983; 261:109–117.
44. Longo FM, Skaper SD, Manthorpe M, Williams LR, Lundborg G, Varon S. Temporal changes of neuronotrophic activities accumulating in vivo within nerve regeneration chambers. Exp Neurol 1983; 81:756–769.
45. Lumsden AGS, Davies AM. Earliest sensory nerve fibres are guided to peripheral targets by attractants other than nerve growth factor. Nature 1983; 306:786–788.
46. Lundborg G, Dahlin LB, Danielsen N, et al. Nerve regeneration in silicone chambers: Influence of gap length and of distal stump components. Exp Neurol 1982; 76:361–375.
47. Lundborg G, Dahlin LB, Danielsen N, et al. Nerve regeneration across an extended gap: A neurobiological view of nerve repair and the possible involvement of neuronotrophic factors. J Hand Surg 1982; 7:580–587.
48. Lundborg G, Dahlin LB, Danielsen NP, Hansson HA, Larsson K. Reorganization and orientation of regenerating nerve fibres, perineurium, and epineurium in preformed mesothelial tubes—An experimental study on the sciatic nerve of rats. J Neurosci Res 1981; 6:265–281.
49. Lundborg G, Gelberman RH, Longo FM, Powell HC, Varon S. In vivo regeneration of cut nerves encased in silicone tubes: Growth across a 6-mm gap. J Neuropath Exp Neurol 1982; 41:412–422.
50. Lundborg G, Hansson HA. Regeneration of peripheral nerve through a preformed tissue space. Preliminary observations on the reorganization of regenerating nerve fibres and perineurium. Brain Res 1979; 178:573–576.
51. Lundborg G, Hansson HA. Nerve regeneration through preformed pseudosynovial tubes: A preliminary report of a new experimental model for studying the regeneration and reorganization capacity of peripheral nerve tissue. J Hand Surg 1980; 5:35–38.
52. Lundborg G, Longo FM, Varon S. Nerve regeneration model and trophic factors in vivo. Brain Res 1982; 232:157–161.
53. Mackinnon SE. Discussion on target-specific nerve

regeneration through a nerve guide in the rat, by Seckel BR, Ryan SE, Gagne CST, Chiu TH, Watkins E Jr. Plast Reconstr Surg 1986; 78:799–800.

54. Mackinnon SE, Dellon AL. A comparison of nerve regeneration across a sural nerve graft and a vascularized pseudosheath. J Hand Surg [Am] 1988; 13:935–942.
55. Mackinnon SE, Dellon AL, Hudson AR, Hunter DA. Nerve regeneration through a pseudosynovial sheath in a primate model. Plast Reconstr Surg 1985; 75:833–839.
56. Mackinnon SE, Dellon AL, Lundborg G, Hudson AR, Hunter DA. A study of neurotrophism in a primate model. J Hand Surg [Am] 1986; 11:888–894.
57. Madison RD, Da Silva CF, Dikkes P. Entubulation repair with protein additives increases the maximum nerve gap distance successfully bridged with tubular prostheses. Brain Res 1988; 447:325–334.
58. Madison R, Da Silva CF, Dikkes P, Chiu TH, Sidman RL. Increased rate of peripheral nerve regeneration using bioresorbable nerve guides and a laminin-containing gel. Exp Neurol 1985; 88: 767–772.
59. Madison RD, Da Silva C, Dikkes P, Sidman RL, Chiu TH. Peripheral nerve regeneration with entubulation repair: Comparison of biodegradable nerve guides vs polyethylene tubes and the effects of a laminin-containing gel. Exp Neurol 1987; 95: 378–390.
60. Madison R, Sidman RL, Nyilas E, Chiu TH, Greatorex D. Nontoxic nerve guide tubes support neovascular growth in transected rat optic nerve. Exp Neurol 1984; 86:448–461.
61. Midgley RD, Woolhouse FM. Silastic sheathing technique for the anastomoses of nerves and tendons: A preliminary report. Canad Med Ass J 1968; 98:550–551.
62. Millesi H, Meissl G, Berger A. Further experience with interfascicular grafting of the median, ulnar, and radial nerves. J Bone Joint Surg [Am] 1976; 58:209–218.
63. Miyamoto Y. Experimental study of results of nerve suture under tension vs nerve grafting. Plast Reconstr Surg 1979; 64:540–549.
64. Molander H, Engkvist O, Hagglund J, Olsson Y, Torebjork E. Nerve repair using a polyglactin tube and nerve graft: An experimental study in the rabbit. Biomaterials 1983; 4:276–280.
65. Molander H, Olsson Y, Engkvist O, Bowald S, Eriksson I. Regeneration of peripheral nerve through a polyglactin tube. Muscle Nerve 1982; 5:54–57.
66. Moneim M. Interfascicular nerve grafting. Clin Orthop 1982; 163:65–74.
67. Muller H, Shibib K, Friedrich H, Modrack M. Evoked muscle action potentials from regenerated rat tibial and peroneal nerves: Synthetic vs autologous interfascicular grafts. Exp Neurol 1987; 95: 21–33.
68. Muller H, Shibib K, Modrack M, Friedrich H. Nerve regeneration in synthetic and autogenous interfascicular grafts. II. Morphometric analysis. Exp Neurol 1987; 98:161–169.
69. Muller H, Williams LR, Varon S. Nerve regeneration chamber: Evaluation of exogenous agents applied by multiple injections. Brain Res 1987; 413:320–326.
70. Nachemson AK, Lundborg G, Myrhage R, Rank F. Nerve regeneration and pharmacological suppression of the scar reaction at the suture site: An experimental study on the effect of estrogen-progesterone, methylprednisolone acetate and cis-hydroxyproline in rat sciatic nerve. Scand J Plast Reconstr Surg 1985; 19:255–260.
71. Nelson JM, Diegelmann RF, Cohen IK. Effect of beta-aminopropionitrile and ascorbate on fibroblast migration. Proc Soc Exp Biol Med 1988; 188: 346–352.
72. Ninomiya T, Kobayashi EO. Studies on deficiency of Schwann cell basal lamina and deformation of collagen fibres induced by beta-aminopropionitrile in cultures of developing rat peripheral neurons. J Anat 1985; 143:1–15.
73. Peacock EE Jr, Madden JW. Some studies on the effect of beta-aminopropionitrile on collagen in healing wounds. Surgery 1966; 60:7–12.
74. Peacock EE Jr, Madden JW. Some studies on the effects of beta-aminopropionitrile in patients with injured flexor tendons. Surgery 1969; 66:215–223.
75. Pleasure D, Bora FW Jr, Lane J, Prockop D. Regeneration after nerve transection: Effect of inhibition of collagen synthesis. Exp Neurol 1974; 45: 72–78.
76. Pleasure D, Bora W, Lane J, Prockop D. Acceleration of nerve regeneration by inhibition of collagen synthesis. Neurology 1974; 24:363.
77. Politis MJ. Specificity in mammalian peripheral nerve regeneration at the level of the nerve trunk. Brain Res 1985; 328:271–276.
78. Politis MJ, Ederle K, Spencer PS. Tropism in nerve regeneration in vivo. Attraction of regenerating axons by diffusible factors derived from cells in distal nerve stumps of transected peripheral nerves. Brain Res 1982; 253:1–12.
79. Politis MJ, Steiss JE. Electromyographic evaluation of a novel surgical preparation to enhance nerve-muscle specificity that follows mammalian periph-

eral nerve trunk transection. Exp Neurol 1985; 87:326–333.

80. Reid RL, Cutright DE, Garrison JS. Biodegradable cuff and adjunct to peripheral nerve repair: A study in dogs. Hand 1978; 10:259–266.
81. Riopelle RJ, Boegman RJ, Cameron DA. Peripheral nerve contains heterogenous growth factors that support sensory neurons in vitro. Neurosci Lett 1981; 25:311–316.
82. Rosen JM, Hentz VR, Kaplan EN. Fascicular tubulization: A cellular approach to peripheral nerve repair. Ann Plast Surg 1983; 11:397–411.
83. Rosenbloom J, Prockop DJ. Incorporation of cis-hydroxyproline into protocollagen and collagen. J Biol Chem 1971; 246:1549–1555.
84. Scaravilli F. Regeneration of the perineurium across a surgically induced gap in a nerve encased in a plastic tube. J Anat 1984; 139:411–424.
85. Scaravilli F. The influence of distal environment on peripheral nerve regeneration across a gap. J Neurocytol 1984; 13:1027–1041.
86. Seckel BR, Chiu TH, Nyilas E, Sidman RL. Nerve regeneration through synthetic biodegradable nerve guides: Regulation by the target organ. Plast Reconstr Surg 1984; 74:173–181.
87. Seckel BR, Ryan SE, Gagne RG, Chiu TH, Watkins E Jr. Target-specific nerve regeneration through a nerve guide in the rat. Plast Reconstr Surg 1986; 78:793–798.
88. Seddon HJ. The use of autogenous grafts for the repair of large gaps in peripheral nerves. Brit J Surg 1947; 35:151–167.
89. Seddon HJ. Nerve grafting. J Bone Joint Surg [Br] 1963; 45:447–461.
90. Shine HD, Harcourt PG, Sidman RL. Cultured peripheral nervous system cells support peripheral nerve regeneration through tubes in the absence of distal nerve stump. J Neurosci Res 1985; 14: 393–401.
91. Terzis J, Faibisoff B, Williams HB. The nerve gap: Suture under tension vs graft. Plast Reconstr Surg 1975; 56:166–170.
92. Uitto J, Dehm P, Prockop DJ. Incorporation of cis-hydroxyproline into collagen by tendon cells. Failure of the intracellular collagen to assume a triple-helical conformation. Biochim Biophys Acta 1972; 278:601–605.
93. Uitto J, Prockop DJ. Incorporation of proline analogues into collagen polypeptides: Effects on the production of extracellular protocollagen and on the stability of the triple-helical structure of the molecule. Biochim Biophys Acta 1974; 336:234–251.
94. Uzman BG, Villegas GM. Mouse sciatic nerve regeneration through semipermeable tubes: A quantitative model. J Neurosci Res 1983; 9:325–338.
95. Valentini RF, Aebischer P, Winn SR, Galletti PM. Collagen- and laminin-containing gels impede peripheral nerve regeneration through semipermeable nerve guidance channels. Exp Neurol 1987; 98:350–356.
96. Weiss P. The technology of nerve regeneration: A review. Sutureless tubulation and related methods of nerve repair. J Neurosurg 1944; 1:400–450.
97. Weiss P, Taylor AC. Histomechanical analysis of nerve reunion in the rat after tubular splicing. Arch Surg 1943; 47:419–447.
98. Weiss P, Taylor AC. Further experimental evidence against "neurotropism" in nerve regeneration. J Exp Zool 1944; 95:233–257.
99. Williams LR. Exogenous fibrin matrix precursors stimulate the temporal progress of nerve regeneration within a silicone chamber. Neurochem Res 1987;12: 851–860.
100. Williams LR, Danielsen N, Muller H, Varon S. Exogenous matrix precursors promote functional nerve regeneration across a 15-mm gap within a silicone chamber in the rat. J Comp Neurol 1987; 264:284–290.
101. Williams LR, Longo FM, Powell HC, Lundborg G, Varon S. Spatial-temporal progress of peripheral nerve regeneration within a silicone chamber: Parameters for a bioassay. J Comp Neurol 1983; 218: 460–470.
102. Williams LR, Powell HC, Lundborg G, Varon S. Competence of nerve tissue as distal insert promoting nerve regeneration in a silicone chamber. Brain Res 1984; 293:201–211.
103. Williams LR, Varon S. Modification of fibrin matrix formation in situ enhances nerve regeneration in silicone chambers. J Comp Neurol 1985; 231:209–220.

VIII

NERVE LESIONS IN CONTINUITY

42 Nerve Lesions in Continuity

42

Nerve Lesions in Continuity

Leo T. Happel
David G. Kline

AUTHORS' KEY POINTS

- The diagnosis of a nerve lesion in continuity indicates gross continuity of the peripheral nerve, including the damaged segment. Such a lesion may or may not regenerate well enough spontaneously to achieve significant functional recovery. As a result, more sophisticated methods for management must be considered (compared to those used for repair of completely transected nerves).
- Nerve lesions in continuity, induced most frequently by contusion or stretch mechanisms, are graded 1 through 4. The prognosis for spontaneous recovery depends upon maintenance of endoneural and connective tissue elements within nerve.
- Measuring the compound nerve action potential (CNAP) determines the functional status of a segment of nerve, facilitating clinical decision making. This technique can be applied reliably and safely with minimal effort.
- The presence or absence of the CNAP is the single most important determinant for clinical intraoperative testing in the early months after nerve injury.
- An absent CNAP indicates the necessity for resection and repair of a lesion in continuity; the presence of a response indicates that a better result can be achieved with neurolysis of the whole nerve or, in selected cases, split repair of only those fascicles that are damaged.

Peripheral nerve injuries that leave the nerve in continuity present complex challenges in both diagnosis and management. These injuries represent 60% to 70% of all peripheral nerve injuries.[9] This chapter discusses the grading and management of the various types of nerve lesions in continuity.

Total loss of anatomical continuity following injury is rarely associated with spontaneous recovery. Such cases require operative treatment rather than conservative management. In contrast, the lesion that leaves the nerve in some degree of anatomical continuity is associated with a wide range of internal derangement of nerve. It is not surprising that the clinical course of this kind of injury is associated with a broad range of outcomes. Some nerves recover completely in time without treatment, while others show some functional return but less than might be achieved with operative repair. Some nerves show no improvement and have decreasing levels of function when managed conservatively.[5,13] An accurate evaluation of the lesion in continuity is essential, not just at one time but at several points over the complete course of anticipated recovery.

Electrical testing of nerve and muscle provides detailed information on the extent of injury. Serial studies are used to follow progress, but even this information may not adequately portray the status of recovery at 2 to 3 months after injury, the precise time when information is most needed. Thus, nerve function must be evaluated more directly than conventional electromyographic (EMG) techniques allow in the early stages after injury. For many years, we have used direct measurement of nerve electrical activity from operatively exposed nerves to determine the extent of function remaining in various portions of nerve and also to obtain an indication of the effectiveness of any spontaneous regeneration that might be in progress. The description of these methods, below, emphasizes the effectiveness of this method in facilitating decision making during surgery, when the prospects for regeneration are optimal.

NEUROPATHOLOGY

A wide spectrum of distortion of internal anatomy of nerve is included under the term "lesion in continuity." The term indicates that some neural structures remain intact and implies that additional considerations are required for management compared to completely transected nerves. In considering the normal anatomy of a large peripheral nerve, the surgeon considers multiple membrane-bounded compartments, non-neural cellular components, a vascular component, and an axonal membrane component. A partial injury is one that alters—rather than totally obliterates—these components.

Sunderland's grading scale for lesions in continuity ranges from mild internal derangement of some of these structures (grade 1) to severe changes that profoundly affect all aspects of nerve (grade 4).[18] Between these extremes is a variety of conditions that constitute partial injuries.

The mechanism of injury may not always relate to the extent of anatomical change. For example, a sharp yet partial penetration of nerve may sever some fascicles and contuse the remaining fibers. Such a lesion may lead to progressive changes, with decreasing function in areas adjacent to severed fibers. This is especially the case if the perineural barrier has been interrupted.[13] Less commonly, vascular loss may lead to progressive neural loss due to alteration of the blood–nerve barrier and to edema.[16] Other unknown humoral factors may play a role as well. After several weeks, there may be a return of function in those portions of nerve left partially intact by the injury but affected secondarily. Recovery of transected fibers, without operative intervention, is less certain and quantitatively inconsistent.[5] The final outcome of recovery depends on the total degree of morphologic damage to the nerve at the time of injury.

Most lesions in continuity are induced by contusion or stretch, mechanisms that affect the entire cross section of the nerve. When the insult is slight, there is little or no discernible change in internal structure. Instead, there is a functional lesion due to a reversible block in conduction. Loss of function may last only hours or days. In some neurapraxic lesions, axons have localized thinning and evidence of localized segmental demyelination. These Sunderland grade 1 lesions generally have effective spontaneous recoveries.[18] In more severe injuries that are still primarily neurapraxic, there may be a few fibers sufficiently injured to undergo Wallerian degeneration with attendant denervational changes in distal musculature. While axon continuity may be lost in a few fibers (axonotmetic changes) there is good maintenance of endoneural and connective tissue framework. These axons usually regenerate well over a period of months. Denervational changes detected electromyographically are only transient.

From a clinical perspective, it is remarkable that, in mild injuries with mild axonotmetic changes, clinical manifestations are primarily a result of reduced motor function, with little detectable sensory loss.[3] While function is not lost entirely, weakness is apparent. Return of full or nearly full function almost always occurs. Unfortunately, only a small fraction of injuries are this benign. Most often, these result from prolonged compression or mild stretch injuries.

More commonly, the lesion in continuity disrupts axonal membranes but spares the multiple membranous compartments and cellular components of nerve.[17] In these Sunderland grade 2 lesions, while there is abundant wallerian degeneration of all disrupted axons, the fascicular framework remains, facilitating regrowth of axons. In the course of regeneration, the remaining Schwann cells proliferate. Regeneration may proceed effectively at a good pace. Under these conditions, sprouting of growing axonal tips is not as pronounced as in more severe lesions, and the regrowing fibers retain sufficient caliber to become effective. As with grade 1 lesions, grade 2 injured nerves usually recover effectively without operative intervention, although the process requires many months. The completeness of regeneration and the time required are subject to other variables, such as the location of injury and the specific nerve involved.

With more severe injuries, the histologic patterns show not only axonal loss but also breakdown of the connective tissue elements of nerve. Grade 3 injuries, a mixture of axonotmetic and neurotmetic lesions, also have a vascular component, with hemorrhage and edema. The latter may eventually lead to an even more severe problem: necrosis of nerve at the injury site.[16] Spontaneous recovery from an injury of this degree may or may not occur, depending on the amount of connective tissue disruption. With severe grade 3 lesions, regrowing fibers tend to branch more and wander farther from their original courses. The finer fibers do not achieve the level of function originally provided, and regeneration often is aberrant.

Grade 4 lesions represent injuries of greater severity in which complete loss of both extrafascicular and intrafascicular frameworks of nerve occur. There is a greater degree of scarring with haphazard deposition of connective tissue and, as a result, an even more formidable barrier to the regrowth of axons. Operative resection of a lesion such as that shown in Figure 42-1 is indicated to provide the best chance for successful axon regrowth.[7,10]

CLINICAL ELECTROPHYSIOLOGY

Electrical studies of a grade 1 lesion, where the problem is primarily neurapraxic, are very helpful. They may provide diagnostic information even in the early postinjury period. As might be expected, stimulation proximal to the lesion produces little or no distal motor activity, indicating complete conduction block. However, anatomical continuity of axons can be demonstrated by stimulation distal to the area of injury, which shows good motor activity. While the nerve has good compound nerve action potentials (CNAPs) proximal and distal to the lesion, CNAPs are absent across the area of

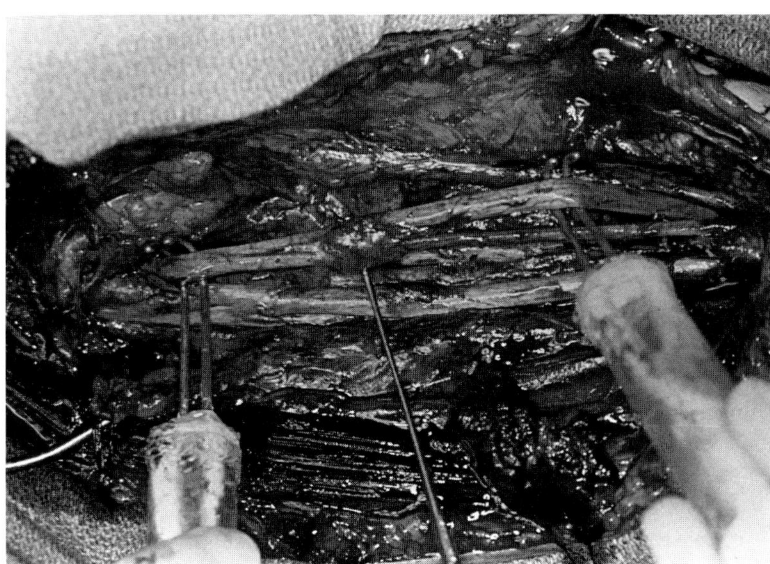

Figure 42–1. *Intraoperative stimulation and recording across a neuroma in continuity of a brachial plexus element secondary to gunshot wound. No CNAP was transmitted at 4 months post injury. The lesion (pointer) was resected and histologic study showed a Sunderland grade 4, or neurotmetic, lesion. (From Kline DG, Hachett ER, Happel L. Review of surgical lesions of the brachial plexus. Arch Neurol 1985;43:170, with permission.)*

conduction block. Electrical studies are not done within 72 hours of injury, as even completely transected fibers may retain some excitability before undergoing Wallerian degeneration.[14] In addition, needle EMG examination of the grade 1 lesion shows only rare denervational changes in muscles supplied by the injured nerve.[6]

More severe injuries (grades 2, 3, and 4) show similar effects on EMG, as all of these lesions affect the integrity of the axonal membrane. Within these groups, however, are both injuries that recover spontaneously and those that do not recover. A single electrophysiological assessment 2 to 3 weeks after injury cannot discriminate between these categories. The clinical distinction is important, as grade 3 and 4 injuries are unlikely to recover well without operative intervention.

All three of these grades of injury show evidence of profound loss of motor axons.[6] These features include markedly reduced or absent muscle activity as the EMG needle is inserted. In addition, fibrillation potentials are seen, representing the action potentials of single muscle cells that are no longer part of a motor unit. The muscle membranes fire because, after denervation, they are hypersensitive to even minute levels of acetylcholine. In addition, even a maximal voluntary effort by the patient fails to evoke significant muscle electrical activity. Electrical stimulation distal to the injury does not evoke a response.

Serial EMG studies allow grade 2 injuries to be distinguished from more severe insults. Conventional techniques applied 12 weeks or more after injury allow detection of early phase regeneration.[4] Timing may vary, based on the location of the injury and its proximity to target muscles. Some injuries require more time for adequate electrical studies to be carried out, since conventional EMG techniques depend on some muscle reinnervation.[14]

By 6 to 10 weeks after grade 2 injuries and some grade 3 injuries, large numbers of regenerating fibers may have regrown well past the injury site. Their presence can be demonstrated with a CNAP with stimulation proximal to the lesion.[10] This is achieved with some accuracy by transcutaneous stimulation and recording with the computer-averaging techniques available in many newer EMG machines. In this way, the progress of nerve regeneration can be tracked along the nerve's anatomical route until contact with muscle is finally achieved.

Even after the nerve has reached its target muscle, recovery of voluntary movements may lag behind electrically evoked responses by 2 to 6 weeks. Computer-averaging techniques are quite sensitive, allowing for recordings from nerves that are still a considerable distance away. Nonetheless, the uncertainties of transcutaneous nerve stimulation and recording raise the possibility of misleading observations.

For many years we have used direct recordings of evoked nerve activity during operative exploration of an injured nerve as a means of evaluating the lesion in continuity (Fig. 42-2).[8,12] This method, not subject to the problems inherent in transcutaneous techniques, provides an accurate evaluation of regenerating fibers through a lesion in continuity and permits an early evaluation and distinction of the grade 2 injury from grades 3 or 4. Grade 3 and 4 injured nerves do not show the CNAP distal to the injury site. The absence of the CNAP distal to the injury after 6 to 10 weeks is a strong indication of grade 3 or worse pathology. Although some fine fiber regeneration may occur spontaneously in severe grade 3 or even grade 4 injuries, the return of meaningful function is unusual. At 12 weeks such fibers produce minuscule CNAPs that are far smaller than successfully regenerating fibers and are easily distinguished from them.

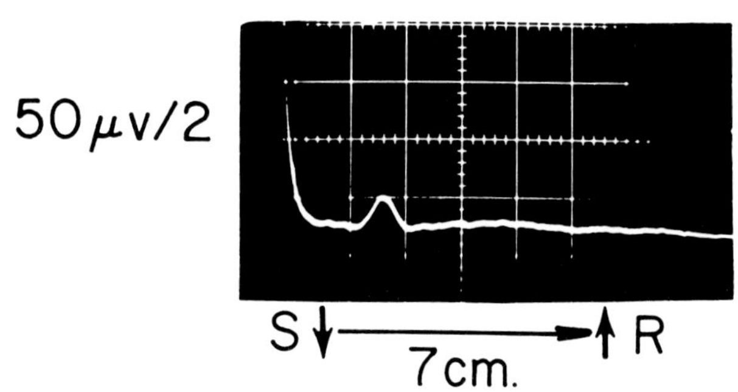

Figure 42–2. *Example of a CNAP recorded from an injured but satisfactorily regenerating nerve. Amplification was 50 V/div and time base was 2 msec/div. Stimulating electrodes were placed proximal to the lesion and recording electrodes distal. Interelectrode distance was 7 cm and conduction velocity approximated 25 m/sec.*

The use of operative recordings of the CNAP to evaluate lesions in continuity requires some understanding of the electrophysiology of the CNAP. Both theoretical and practical considerations are included here to provide a basis for operative recording.

ELECTROPHYSIOLOGY OF THE CNAP

The compound action potential of a peripheral nerve is the product of both the active events in many nerve membranes and the passive properties of the tissue that surrounds them. Thus, both active and passive processes are important determinants of stimulation characteristics. They also affect the characteristics of the action potentials that are recorded.

The following section considers both of these aspects of neural electrical characteristics. A theoretical perspective will be used initially, to explain the basis for the behavior of the CNAP for the purpose of testing the function of exposed nerve. This method is useful in evaluating segments of nerve during surgery and can give the surgeon a solid physiological basis for deciding whether to resect a lesion in continuity (Fig. 42-3).

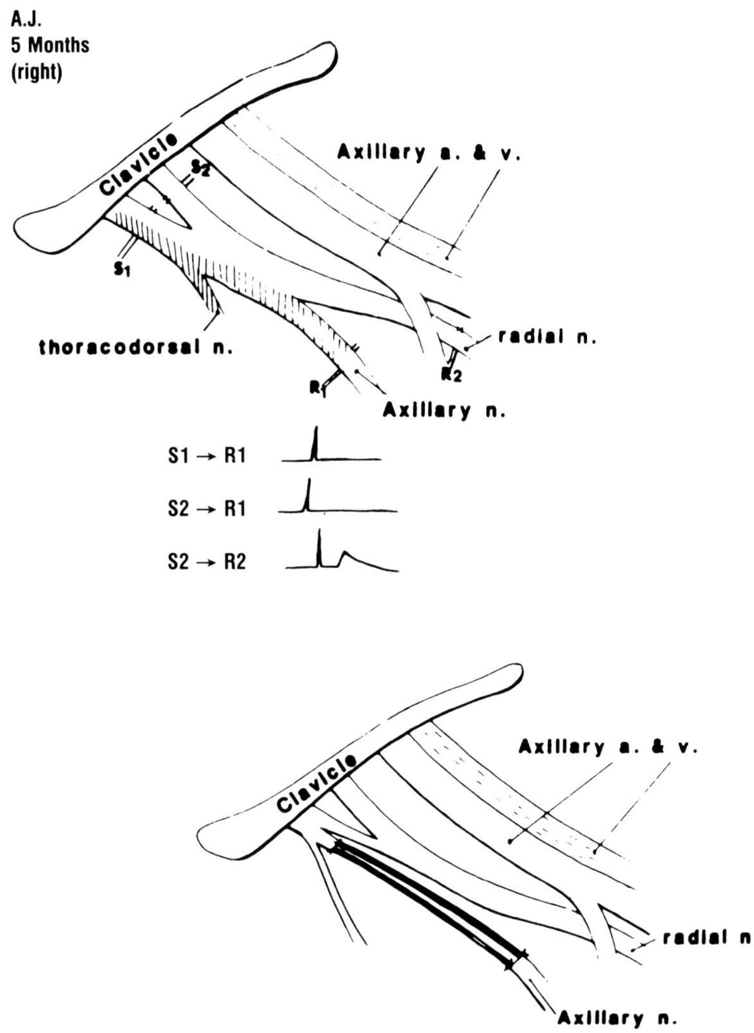

Figure 42–3. *Example of recordings made from brachial plexus injured by stretch. Deltoid remained completely paralyzed by clinical examination for 5 months. EMG showed severe denervational changes. No CNAP could be recorded from the posterior cord to axillary nerve, whereas posterior cord to radial nerve did show a CNAP. Posterior cord to axillary segment was resected and replaced by several interfascicular grafts harvested from sural nerve.*

Theoretical Considerations

Stimulation of excitable membranes with an electrical pulse occurs when certain parameters exceed a specific threshold value. Thus, a sufficient current flowing for an adequate length of time causes excitation in some of the axons within the whole nerve. Those axons that respond to the lowest stimulus do so because the resistance and capacitance associated with them is small. Medium-sized fibers appear to have the lowest threshold, large fibers are next, and small unmyelinated fibers have the highest threshold.[1] Since these axons do not behave uniformly, the CNAP shows graded amplitude over a range of stimulus intensities. The size of the CNAP recorded is related to the number of axons stimulated. Once an intensity of stimulation that activates all of the axons has been reached, the CNAP attains maximum amplitude.

The passive characteristics of axons, as well as the characteristics of the tissue that surrounds them, play a role in the stimulation of nerve. Axons with high capacitance, due either to large surface area (large diameter) or thin membrane (abnormal or regenerating membrane), are more difficult to excite.[19] The duration of the stimulus pulse is a parameter that determines whether the stimulus is adequate for excitation to occur because the duration affects the energy content of the stimulus pulse.

Figure 42-4 shows the relationship between the intensity of the stimulus required for a maximal CNAP and its duration. For normal, healthy nerve, shortening the duration of the stimulus to less than 0.3 msec requires that the intensity be increased, due to the fact that the stimulus must represent an adequate amount of energy. If some of the energy is removed (eg, decreased duration) it can be replaced with increased intensity. As stimulus duration decreases below 0.1 msec this phenomenon becomes quite pronounced, and markedly elevated intensities must be used in compensation. Finally, at extremely short durations (below 0.01 msec) even very high intensities fail to produce excitation in most axons. In this case, the passive properties of tissue capacitance and resistance prevent the stimulus from depolarizing the membrane.

Abnormal axons usually possess abnormal excitability characteristics. Figure 42-4, which shows that injured or regenerating axons are more sensitive to changes in the duration of short pulses, demonstrates that even higher intensities of stimulation may be required for excitation. Durations shorter than 0.1 msec may require very high intensities to produce excitation in many of these abnormal axons. The lower limit of stimulus duration in abnormal axons is significantly longer than that for normal nerve. This difference is due primarily to changes in the passive characteristics of the abnormal axonal membrane.

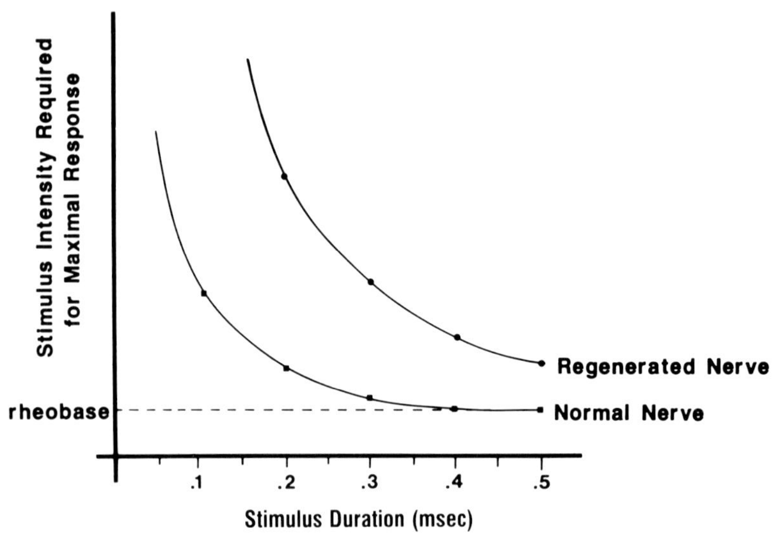

Figure 42–4. *Stimulus intensity–duration relationship for normal and regenerated nerves. As duration of the stimulus pulse decreases, greater intensities are required for a maximal CNAP. The effect is more pronounced in abnormal nerves.*

The tissue surrounding the axon is also considered in determining the efficacy of a given stimulus. The capacitance and resistance of soft tissue serves to shunt stimulating current away from the axonal membrane. Thus, the more abundant the volume of this tissue, the more intensity will be required for stimulation, as only a fraction of the stimulating current reaches the membrane. This is particularly important for nerve fibers embedded in scar tissue or within a tumor. Stimulation in these cases may require several times the normal amount to achieve excitation of axons, particularly when short-duration pulses are used.

Passive characteristics also are significant in recordings made of the CNAP. The surrounding soft tissue shunts electrical currents away from the recording electrodes, making the response small and difficult to record. The CNAP from unhealthy nerve may require very high amplification and low background noise levels for successful recordings to be made. Recently, techniques of recording using computer signal averaging have increased sensitivity to the point where the CNAP can be recorded at skin level from nerves that are several centimeters deep.

While averaging may be helpful in difficult situations, it can be misleading under some circumstances. Additional surrounding tissue can distort the recording in addition to reducing its amplitude. The less tissue involved, the more accurately the recorded response reflects the collective activity of fibers within a peripheral nerve. For this reason, recordings made directly from the nerve are a better basis for judging axonal function than recordings made at skin level.

Within a given myelinated axon, conduction of the impulse occurs as one region of active membrane, involving several nodes of Ranvier, excites adjacent nodes of Ranvier. The distance between nodes, and the number of nodes that respond as a unit, are factors that determine the velocity at which impulses are conducted. The time required to reproduce the action potential at each node also plays a major role in determining conduction velocity.[15] Anatomically, in a healthy nerve, the relationship between fiber diameter and internodal distance is fixed. This establishes a relationship between fiber diameter and conduction velocity. The diameter of the axon, which affects the flow of electrical current down the length of the axon, plays a role in establishing the number of nodes that behave as a unit. The combination of these effects is manifested in the distribution of conduction velocities among myelinated axons.

Variability in conduction velocity is more apparent as longer segments of nerve are surveyed, since the amount of time involved allows for dispersion of activity along the length of various axons (Fig. 42-5). Detailed studies of the distribution of conduction velocities have provided a basis for re-

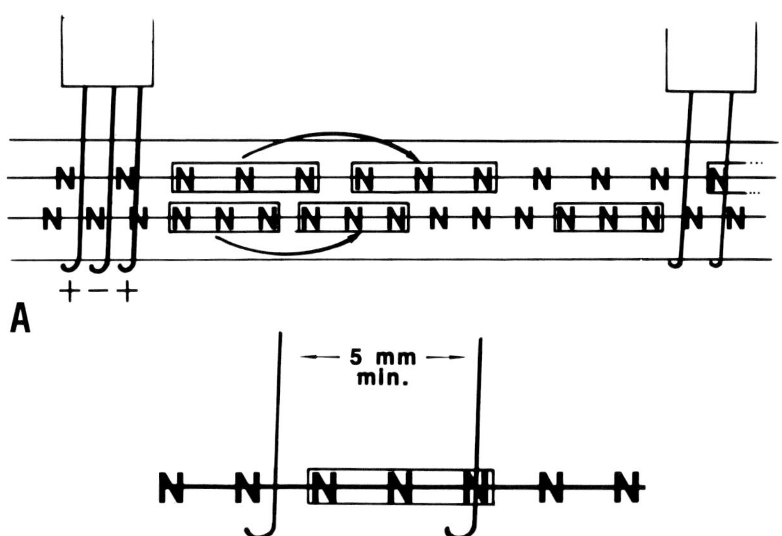

Figure 42–5. *(**A**) Conduction of the action potential from one group of several nodes of Ranvier to an adjacent group in different fibers. Differences in the internodal distances between fibers spread the length of active membrane as longer lengths of nerve are considered. (**B**) Proper spacing of recording electrodes ensures only one contact with active membrane and one reference.*

lating the shape of the CNAP to the histologic composition of the axons that make up the whole nerve.[2] Figure 42-3 shows this relationship between electrical characteristics and nerve structure. The shape of the CNAP changes with distance between stimulating and recording electrodes for the same reason; the difference is conduction velocities.

The length of active nerve is also a function of how far the evoked CNAP has traveled. As shown in Figure 42-5, the length of nerve containing active fibers is fairly small near the point of stimulation, since the action potentials are produced synchronously. As the distance is increased, however, more temporal dispersion occurs at greater distances. The differences in conduction velocity involve more length along the nerve.

When recordings are to be made, this factor is considered. Two electrodes placed along the length of nerve make contact with both active and inactive regions of nerve; that is, the distance between the two recording electrodes is sufficiently large so that the active region of the nerve does not encompass both electrodes at the same time. Should both electrodes contact active nerve, the potential difference between them is reduced and the amplitude of the recorded CNAP is less. If the distance between the electrodes is sufficiently small, they might be isopotential and fail to give any indication of underlying nerve activity. This subject is discussed further in the section on practical considerations.

The presence of a CNAP in a segment of peripheral nerve is direct evidence of viable axons. This information—the presence or absence of a CNAP—best facilitates decisions on how to treat the nerve. Other information concerning the character of an observed response supports this observation. The amplitude of the action potential is clearly indicative of the number of axons within the nerve, as long as the stimulus is sufficient to activate them all. Maximal stimulus intensity is determined by observing the threshold response and increasing the stimulus until the action potential reaches maximum amplitude. At this intensity, all the axons are stimulated. Thus, the amplitude of the response seen is an indirect reflection of the number of axons. To ensure activation of all axons, a slightly supramaximal stimulus is used.

In addition to the number of axons present, it is possible as well to measure the status of those axons. Conduction velocity measurements provide insights into the fiber sizes making up the nerve, as Kimura explained.[6]

Practical Considerations

Intraoperative stimulation and recording from peripheral nerve is easy and safe and leaves no residual effects, but the surgeon must exercise care to ensure the desired results.

Electrodes

Metal contact with intact nerve is generally innocuous until electrical currents are applied. At this point, the electrolysis that occurs during stimulation must be kept to a minimum; thus, the type of metal used for electrodes becomes significant. Active metals, such as silver, are avoided, as the deposition of silver salts over time is toxic to nerve. Noble metals, such as platinum, are desirable because of their relative chemical inactivity, but they are costly. Stainless steel alloys (in particular, medical-grade stainless steel) are a reasonable compromise. Stainless steel electrode wires can be embedded easily in a plastic handle and attached to wires connected to instrumentation. The electrodes are bent like a shepherd's crook so that the nerve can be suspended in the crook, away from other tissue (see Fig. 42-1). The plastics used should be stable at high temperatures so that autoclaving is possible; Teflon and Delrin brands work well. In addition, epoxy cements are carefully selected to withstand autoclaving and water absorption.

Stimulating electrode wires applied to the nerve are separated by a distance greater than 3 mm to allow sufficient current spread to excite the many axons in the whole nerve. With larger-diameter nerves, the electrode separation is increased to 5 to 7 mm to accommodate additional tissue volume. If stimulating electrodes are too close together, they do not allow current to flow through the volume of nerve, and stimulation of many fibers is not achieved.

The stimulation of an intact nerve in situ presents an unusual set of circumstances. Figure 42-6 illustrates how applying a potential difference with two electrodes along the length of a nerve creates two current paths. First, there is a current in the gap between the two electrodes; second, there is a current flowing away from the electrodes, through the nerve, through the tissues of the body, and back to the other electrode. The latter current path is problematic, as a current along the length of the nerve will be recorded together with the CNAP. This produces excessive stimulus artifact and, when the distance between stimulating and recording electrodes is short, may obscure the action potential.

A solution is shown in Figure 42-6. Three stimulating electrodes are used with the outermost connected together. In this arrangement, while the application of a potential difference between the inner and outer electrodes still produces two current paths, neither involves the whole nerve. The reduction in stimulus artifact achieved in this way permits even very small action potentials in injured or regenerating nerves to be seen.

The use of a tripolar electrodes also serves to limit the spread of stimulating current longitudinally along nerve. The latter is undesirable, as misleading observations are made when sufficient current spreads several centimeters away from the stimulating point. While there may be no viable axons at the point of stimulation, the spread of current may excite distant axons, leading to the production of a CNAP. This phenomenon could lead to the false inference of excitable axons at the point of stimulation. The surgeon must use caution, especially at higher stimulus intensities, to prevent this possibility from occurring.

The configuration of the recording electrodes also is important to the successful evaluation of the electrical characteristics of peripheral nerve. The selection of electrode material is not critical for the stimulating electrodes. While the noise characteristics may not be the best available, stainless steel electrodes are still a very cost-effective solution. Two wire electrodes along the nerve, with a separation of at least 3 to 5 mm, work well. If these electrodes are moved too close together, the amplitude of the recorded action potential will be reduced; thus a larger distance, 5 mm, is recommended. Note that if a long length of nerve is being studied (25–30 cm), this 5-mm electrode separation may be increased still further, since the length of active nerve also increases due to differences in conduction velocity in the axons comprising the nerve. Ideally, the separation of the recording electrodes permits one to contact inactive regions

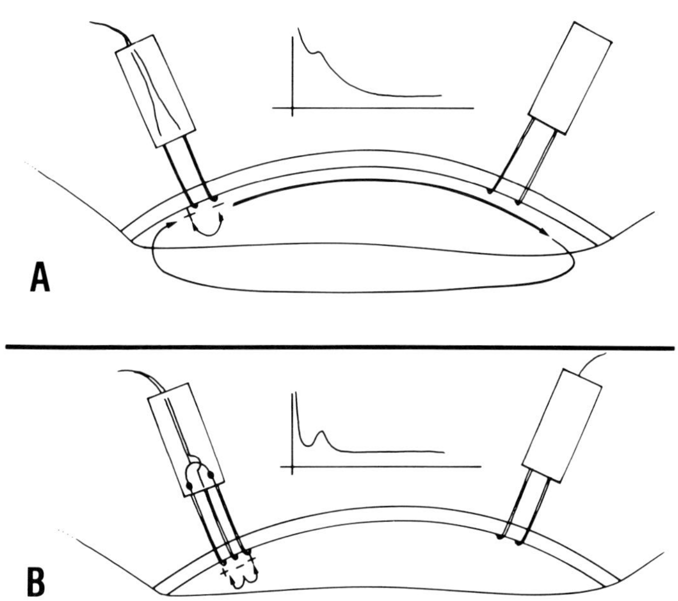

Figure 42-6. *(**A**) Bipolar stimulating electrodes produce two current paths—one between the electrodes and the other along the length of the nerve and through the body. This produces excessive stimulus artifact, as illustrated in the recording. It also produces spread of stimulation. (**B**) Tripolar stimulating electrodes with outermost terminals connected. Current paths can no longer involve the whole nerve, and thus stimulus artifact is reduced, making the CNAP more apparent.*

while the other records from the active region. If both electrodes are in contact with the parts of the nerve that are active, the response can still be recorded, but its amplitude may be significantly reduced. Proper separation facilitates recording.

Figure 42-7 shows that the distance between stimulating and recording electrodes affects recordings of the CNAP. When this distance is very short (less than 4 cm), the resistance and capacitance between the stimulating and recording electrodes permits an excessive amount of stimulus artifact to appear. This artifact obscures the CNAP. In addition, the CNAP requires little conduction time. It appears very shortly after stimulus, during a period when the artifact is still prevalent. The artifact obscures the CNAP, making measurements difficult. Simply increasing the distance will substantially reduce both problems.

Applying a ground to the subject is essential to obtaining a proper recording, especially in the operating room. The purpose of a ground is to eliminate, or markedly reduce, electrical noise induced in the subject's body. Grounding is accomplished by attaching a large surface-area electrode to the subject's body, preferably in a region not too far from the site of stimulation and recording. The ground is attached to the recording instrument in the appropriate place, thus preventing artifact from masking the CNAP.

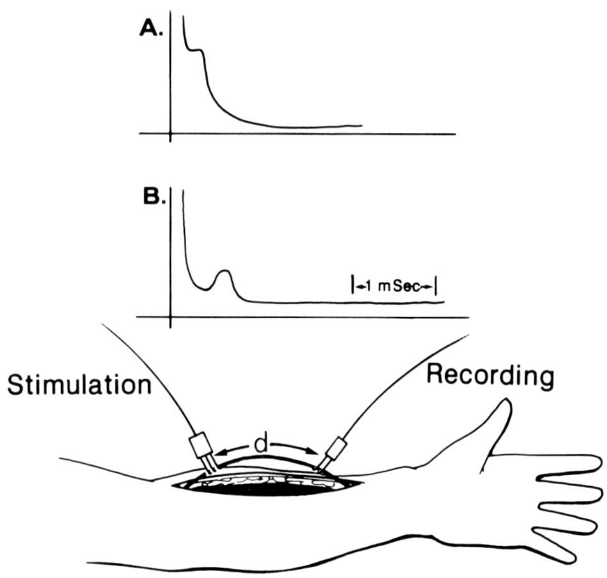

Figure 42–7. *Effect of distance (d) between stimulating and recording electrodes on the CNAP. (**A**) When d is very short, the CNAP is superimposed on the stimulus artifact. (**B**) As d is increased, the greater conduction time allows separation of CNAP from stimulus artifact.*

Only one ground is attached to the subject, and when it is attached, it is important to ensure that no other ground is also attached. If two grounds are attached at the same time, an electrical current may occur between them.

Electrosurgical units for cutting and coagulation are routinely used in operative procedures on peripheral nerves. The ground or return electrode used in conjunction with these instruments makes an excellent ground for recording. At the time stimulation and recording of the CNAP is begun, the electrosurgical unit is turned off and the return electrode connection is transferred to the recording instrument. In this way, safe grounding technique is observed and unwanted noise is suppressed. This provides a quick and easy solution to the problem of grounding.

Equipment

Many types of equipment can be used to stimulate and record the CNAP. EMG machines such as the TECA Model TD-20 are self-contained and are convenient for routine use. However, they lack some flexibility in terms of the selection of stimulation parameters and filter settings on the recorder. Other instruments, such as systems composed of stimulators and isolators (eg, the Grass Instruments Model S-44 and SIU-6 and oscilloscope recorders such as the Tektronix 7000 series), are flexible but more complicated to use: they require interconnection to synchronize the oscilloscope sweep with the stimulus pulse. If a system is assembled from individual components, the surgeon should pay particular attention to stimulus isolation for reasons of electrical safety and also for reducing stimulus artifact.

Stimulus artifact is reduced by separating the cables connecting the stimulating and recording electrodes with the instrumentation. Capacitance between these wires, as they are led off a sterile surgical field, can produce profound stimulus artifact in the recording. A distance of several inches between each cable and the stimulating and recording electrodes is adequate. While shielded cable may be used for the recording electrode, it should not be used for the stimulator as it causes a loss of isolation.

Most instruments used to stimulate and record the CNAP have filters on the recorder. While these may be used to minimize the amount of background noise, they can become a problem in themselves if not properly set. The objective is to eliminate as much background noise as possible without damaging the recorder's ability to recover from the stimulus pulse. Applying the stimulus to the nerve presents the recorder with a large transient. This transient affects the amplifying electronics, usually saturating the inputs. Some time is necessary for recovery, depending partly upon the high-frequency filter setting. The lower settings for the high-frequency filter increase the amount of stimulus artifact seen and even affect the CNAP itself (Fig. 42-8). High-frequency filter settings are set at 2500 Hz or higher to minimize the stimulus artifact. Low-frequency filter settings also may produce similar problems and are set in the range of 5 to 10 Hz or lower, if possible.

Many instruments also have 60-Hz notch filters for reducing or eliminating induced artifact. Interference usually originates in devices with electric motors or from fluorescent lighting. The 60-Hz notch filter is not used for CNAP recordings, as the filter itself can generate a wave resembling the CNAP. It is advisable to unplug motor-driven devices and to turn off fluorescent lights to eliminate the problem of background 60-Hz interference.

The selection of stimulation parameters also may minimize the problem of stimulus artifact. At shorter durations (less than 0.2 msec) the artifact for a specific intensity of stimulation decreases. This may allow a clear recording of the action potential in normal nerve. As duration is decreased below 0.05 msec, the intensity of stimulation is markedly increased, however, and the combination of effects may detract from this method of reducing artifact. A compromise setting for duration is reached that does not require such intensity that artifact levels increase profoundly. In general, durations of approximately 0.08 to 0.1 msec accomplish this.

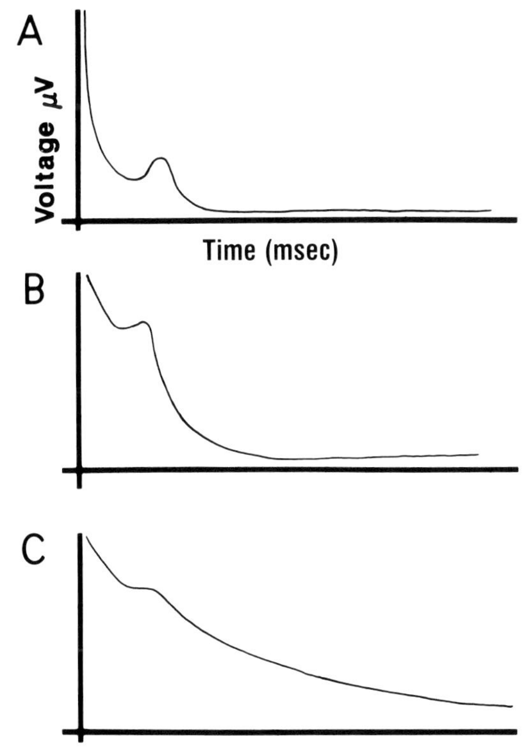

Figure 42-8. *Effect of filters on recordings of CNAP. (**A**) Recording with high-frequency filter setting above 2500 Hz. (**B**) Recording with high-frequency filter setting at 1000 Hz. (**C**) Recording with high-frequency filter setting at 500 Hz. Effects of overfiltering are to increase stimulus artifact and reduce amplitude of CNAP. Adjusting low-frequency filter settings improperly may produce similar phenomena or eliminate the CNAP altogether.*

The intensity–duration relationship is more pronounced with injured or regenerating nerve than with normal nerve. The technique of stimulating with short-duration pulses to reduce stimulus artifact also permits an elementary estimate of the status of any viable axons within a segment of nerve. Very small axons, which may represent an unproductive degree of regeneration, are not excited by short-duration pulses unless the intensity is very high. This observation leads to the conclusion that even though fine fibers are present, significant regeneration has not occurred at the level being tested. This facilitates discrimination between fibers with potential for significant regeneration and fibers with little or no potential.

As high-intensity stimulation is required under the specific circumstances described above, caution is exercised to prevent injury to the nerve being tested. Most commercially available EMG machines can furnish more stimulus than necessary. Stimulus pulses above approximately 40 V can cause electrical burns when the stimulus frequency is high and durations are long. At intensities above 40 V, the surgeon must be careful to keep the frequency below about 2/sec and the duration 0.1 msec or less. At these settings, high intensities can be used safely.

The intensity of stimulation required for normal, healthy nerve is between 3 and 15 V, a small fraction of the range setting for the typical EMG instrument. Abnormal nerve may require over 100 V when durations as short as 0.02 to 0.05 msec are used. When EMG instrumentation is used during an operative procedure, stimulation will generally require a relatively low setting, since electrodes are placed in direct contact with nerve.

Technique

The process of stimulating and recording begins with low levels of stimulation (3–5 V) and moderate sensitivity on the recorder (200–500 uV/cm). Stimulus intensity and recorder sensitivity are alternately increased until a response is seen or the nerve is judged inexcitable. With the intensity control on the stimulator at its lowest setting, the nerve is suspended in the crook of the stimulating and recording electrodes (thus supported, it is not in contact with other tissues or fluid pools). Usually the stimulating electrodes are placed proximally and the recording electrodes distally, because the size of the nerve increases proximally and fibers from distal regions become covered by fibers from more proximal distributions. Stimulating distally activates fibers that are more deeply buried in nerve and hence are more difficult to record with proximal electrodes. Adequate proximal stimulation, in contrast, activates all of the fibers distally.

Stimulating intensity is slowly increased to the range where a response is expected (usually above 3–5 V). If no response is seen, the intensity of the stimulus is increased to levels described previously. Amplification levels on the recorder are also increased to a maximum sensitivity of 20 uV/cm. At this sensitivity even small responses should be apparent. Figure 42-11 outlines this process.

Usually enough nerve is exposed proximal to a lesion in continuity so that both stimulation and recording can be done, initially, proximal to the lesion. If the electrodes and instrumentation are working properly, a CNAP is readily recorded. Then the electrodes are moved into the lesion site and below to see what happens to the CNAP. If a proximal segment is unavailable for study (such as with buttock-level sciatic nerve lesions or root-level brachial plexus lesions), the surgeon must be content with stimulating and recording across the lesion or, on occasion, even stimulating the lesion itself and recording below it.

The presence of muscle activity distal to the point of stimulation and in the distribution of the nerve being stimulated suggests that the nerve is being excited. If a response still is not seen, the stimulus intensity is decreased and the instrumentation checked again by placing both the stimulating and the recording electrodes on a segment of nerve known to be viable. This may be either a length of the same nerve proximal to a focal injury site or an adjacent nerve. The presence of activity in a proximal segment of nerve with no activity across distal parts is convincing evidence of a lack of functional axonal continuity in the nerve. Performed routinely, if clinical conditions permit, this method develops confidence in using the technique.

There is a natural inclination to use the averaging capabilities on many modern EMG machines, but the increased sensitivity obtained with averaging techniques can enhance the recording of activity from small numbers of very fine fibers. This may lead to the erroneous conclusion that an observed CNAP indicates significant activity in a nerve where the electrical activity is actually minimal. In general, averaging techniques are unnecessary during operative recordings of the CNAP. When we use averaging, we always ensure that a CNAP is present on a single evoked trace before averaging a number of traces to make a record.

In the case of nerve that appears partially damaged, individual fascicles can be dissected longitudinally and tested in the same manner as described above.[20] Each component of nerve can thus be treated individually. Under these circumstances some fascicles or groups of fascicles may conduct while other may not. Such findings indicate that a "split repair" of the nonconducting fascicles should be carried out (Fig. 42-9).

The amplitude of the CNAP recorded can vary from almost 2 mV to about 20 uV, depending on the status of the nerve and other factors. The sensitivity of the recorder used should cover this range. Initially, as stimulation commences, the recorder is set to display potentials in the range of 200 to 500 uV; changes in this setting are determined by the observations made. If no response is seen at the most sensitive settings (20 uV/cm), the stimulus intensity is raised until the upper limits of stimulation range are reached. No response under these conditions indicates an absence of adequate axonal membranes in the segment of nerve being tested.

The presence or absence of the CNAP is the single most important determinant for clinical intraoperative testing in the early months after injury. An absent CNAP usually indicates the necessity for resection and repair of a lesion in

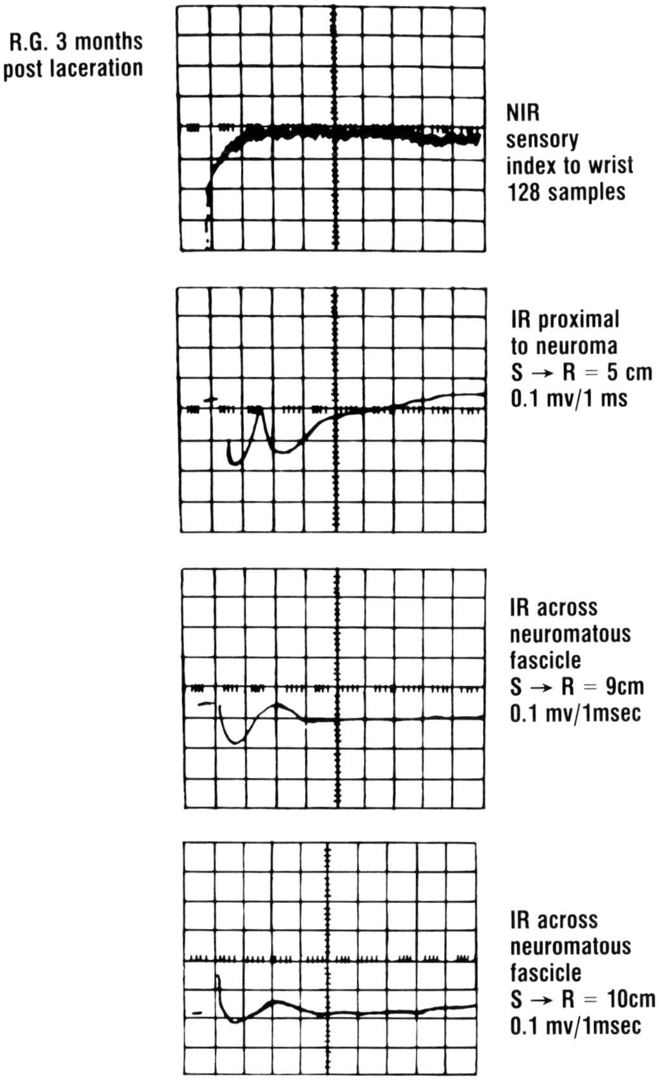

Figure 42–9. *Partial lacerating injury to median nerve at wrist, preserving continuity, studied intraoperatively at 3 months. Noninvasive skin-level recording across lesion showed no response (top inset) and EMG showed denervation of abductor pollicis brevis and opponens pollicis. CNAP was recorded proximal to the lesion (second inset). A good CNAP could be intraoperatively recorded across the lesion and, in fact, when the nerve was split into fascicles, most conducted a CNAP (see insets 3 and 4). These were neurolysed only, while those without a CNAP were resected and repaired.*

continuity, while the presence of a response indicates that a better result can be achieved with neurolysis or repair of only the damaged fascicles.

Particular care is taken to avoid confusing distant muscle action potentials with the CNAP. Muscle action potentials generally are larger in amplitude, have a longer latency than the CNAP, and also are longer in duration. They also may appear polyphasic. Potentials with a duration greater than 2 msec could represent muscle action potentials and should be carefully distinguished. Muscle activity is not seen in cases where anesthetic considerations require the use of neuromuscular blocking agents, but the CNAP persists. Muscle activity also may move the cables attaching the recording electrodes to the instrumentation, creating an artifact that might resemble the CNAP. These cables must be arranged so that they do not move.

Both normal and abnormal CNAPs are easily distinguished from evoked muscle activity. Large, normal CNAPs and small, regenerating CNAPs may occasionally be seen in the same setting (Fig. 42-10.).

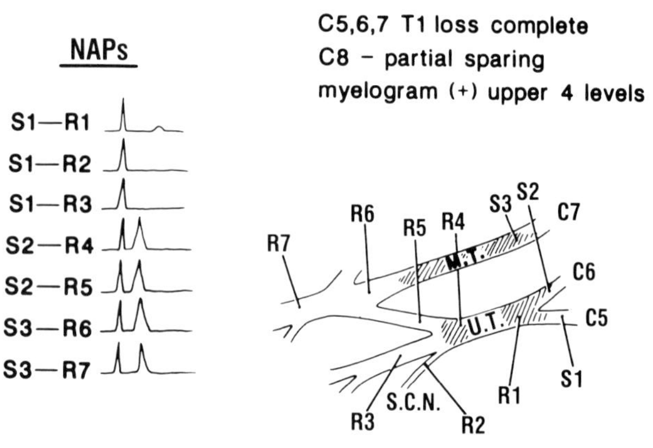

Figure 42-10. *A variety of intraoperative recording observations made from a severe brachial plexus stretch injury. C5 root to upper trunk (S1 to R1) shows a regenerative potential. Regeneration had not yet reached supraclavicular nerve (S1 to R2) and no response was seen. Absence of a response from C5 to anterior division of upper trunk (S1 to R3) also illustrates this point. Recordings made by stimulating either the C6 or C7 roots and recording distally (S2 or S3 to R4/R5 or R6/R7) show large, rapidly conducting (60–70 msec) CNAPs. These potentials from sensory fibers are an indication of very proximal injury, sparing the connection between dorsal root ganglia and sensory fiber but disconnecting the roots from spinal cord.*

Proficiency in recording the CNAP during an operative procedure comes with experience and acclimation to the technique. In a matter of minutes, this method can determine the functional status of a segment of nerve and thus can facilitate clinical decisions. Results can be achieved reliably and safely with minimal effort. Figure 42-11 illustrates the steps involved in recording the CNAP.

Authors' Preferred Method

The following case study illustrates the authors' preferred method of treatment for nerve lesions in continuity.

A 27-year-old right-handed male was thrown from his motorcycle and sustained contusions and abrasions at the tip of the shoulder. Initially he could not move his arm, but over the next few weeks he regained finger flexion and hand intrinsic motion. A myelogram done 1 month postinjury showed a meningocele on the C8 nerve root. At 5 months postinjury, there was no supraspinatus or infraspinatus, deltoid, biceps, brachioradialis, or triceps muscle function. There was weak pronation, absent supination and wrist extension with weak wrist flexion and fair finger flexion. Finger and thumb extension were weak but present. Grade V intrinsic function was present, including the hypothenar, thenar, interosseous, and lumbrical muscles. Latissimus dorsi muscle function was absent. The pectoralis major was graded 3/5. The scapula did not wing and the diaphragm was not elevated abnormally by chest X-ray. EMG showed extensive paraspinal deinnervation as well as complete deinnervation in the C5, C6, and C7 spinal nerve root distribution.

At operative exploration 5 months postinjury, spinal nerves, trunk, and truncal divisions were dissected free from scar but found to be in continuity. Stimulating spinal nerves and recording from more distal trunk divisions and proximal cords gave flat traces for outflow from C5 and C6. Small CNAPs were recorded from C7 to distal middle trunk and division and conducted at 30 msec, indicating early regeneration of C7 to the middle trunk. Excellent CNAPs were recorded by stimulating the lower trunk and recording from medial cord. Therefore, neurolysis was confined to C7 and its distal components. CNAPs were not recorded by stimulating C5 and C6 roots and recording from distal upper trunk or its anterior and posterior divisions.

Distal spinal roots, upper trunk, and proximal

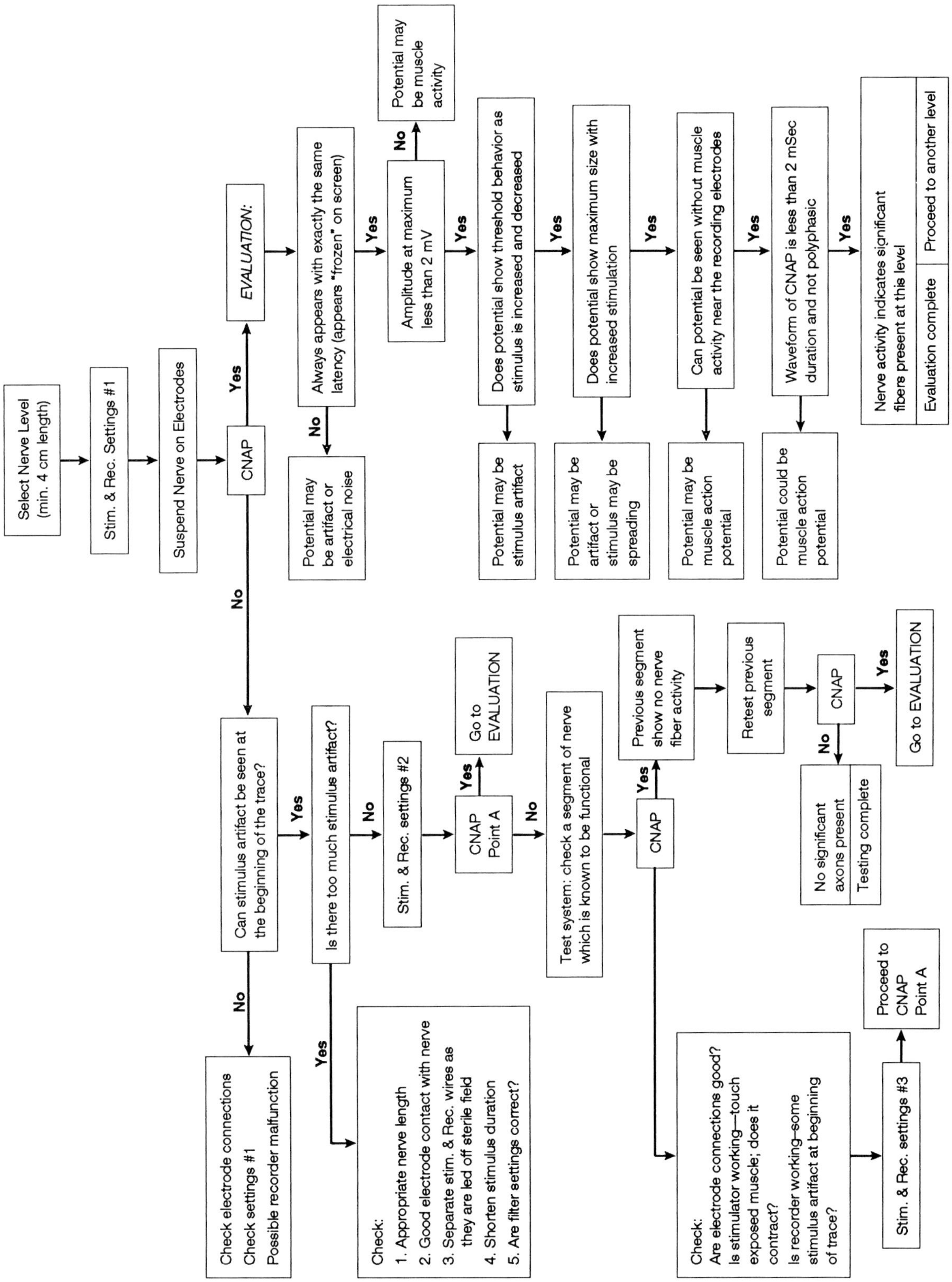

Figure 42–11. *Author's preferred method of performing operative recordings.*

upper trunk anterior and posterior divisions were sectioned back to healthier tissue. Stimulation of the existing C5 and C6 spinal roots in their foramina gave readily evoked cortical responses. A sural nerve graft was harvested and five 3-inch grafts were placed from proximal C5 and C6 spinal nerves to distal upper trunk, anterior and posterior divisions. Histologic study of resected segments showed neurotmesis with severe scar and internal disruption.

Over the first year postoperatively, the triceps returned and wrist extension and flexion improved. Some further finger and thumb extension occurred but remained weak. By 4.5 years postoperatively, the supraspinatus has achieved grade 3–4/5, infraspinatus is trace, and deltoid is 3/5, with abduction to 60° but not beyond. Biceps is 3–4/5, brachioradialis is 2–3/5, and supination is 3/5.

REFERENCES

1. Dawson GD. The relative excitability and conduction velocity of sensory and motor nerve fibers in man. J Physiol [Lond] 1956; 131:436–451.
2. Dorfman L et al. Conduction velocity distributions: A population approach to electrophysiology of nerve. New York: WR Liss, 1981:1–10.
3. Gilliatt RW, Sears TA. Sensory nerve action potentials in patients with peripheral nerve lesions. J Neurol Neurosurg Psychiatry 1958; 21:109–118.
4. Grundfest H, Oester YT, Beebe GW. Electrical evidence of regeneration. In: Woodhall B, Beebe GW, eds. Peripheral nerve regeneration. Washington DC: US Government Printing Office, 1956:203–240.
5. Hudson AR, Kline DG. Progression of partial injury to peripheral nerve. Part 2: Light and electron microscopic studies. J Neurosurg 1975; 42:15–22.
6. Kimura J. Electrodiagnosis in diseases of nerve and muscle: Principles and practice. Philadelphia: FA Davis, 1983:34–61.
7. Kline DG. Evaluation of the neuroma-in-continuity. In: Omer GE Jr, Spinner M, eds. Management of peripheral nerve problems. Philadelphia: WB Saunders, 1980:450–461.
8. Kline DG, DeJonge BR. Evoked potentials to evaluate peripheral nerve injuries. Surg Gynecol Obstet 1968; 127:1239–1250.
9. Kline DG, Hackett ER. Reappraisal of timing for exploration of civilian peripheral nerve injuries. Surgery 1975; 78:54–65.
10. Kline DG, Hackett ER. The neuroma-in-continuity: A management problem. In: Wilkins RH, Rengachary SS, eds. Neurosurgery. New York: McGraw-Hill, 1984:1864–1870.
11. Kline DG, Hackett ER, Happel L. Review of surgical lesions of the brachial plexus. Arch Neurology 1985; 43:170–181.
12. Kline DG, Hackett ER, May PR. Evaluation of nerve injuries by evoked potentials and electromyography. J Neurosurg 1969; 31:128–136.
13. Kline DG, Hudson AR, Hackett ER, Bratton BR. Progression of partial injury to peripheral nerve. Part 1: Periodic measures of muscle contraction strength. J Neurosurg 1975; 42:1–14.
14. Kline DG, Nulsen FE. The neuroma-in-continuity: Its preoperative and operative management. Surg Clin North Am 1972; 52:1189–1209.
15. Lafontaîne S, Rasminsky M, Summer AJ, Saida T. Conduction block in rat myelinated fibres following acute exposure to anti-galactocerebroside serum. J Physiol [London] 1982; 323:287–306.
16. Lundborg G. Structure and function of the intraneural microvessels as related to trauma, edema formation, and nerve function. J Bone Joint Surg [Am] 1975; 57:938–948.
17. Seddon HJ. Surgical disorders of the peripheral nerves. Baltimore: Williams & Wilkins, 1972:68–88.
18. Sunderland S. Nerves and nerve injuries, ed 2. Edinburgh: Churchill-Livingstone, 1978:127.
19. Waxman SG. Physiology and pathobiology of axons. New York: Raven, 1978:131–132.
20. Williams HB, Terzis JK. Single fascicular recordings: An intraoperative diagnostic tool for the management of peripheral nerve lesions. Plast Reconstr Surg 1976; 57:562–569.

IX

NERVE INJURY ASSOCIATED WITH FRACTURES AND OTHER TRAUMA

43 Peripheral Nerve Injuries Associated With Fractures and Dislocations

44 Nerve Injury Associated With Fractures in Children

45 Nerve Injuries Associated With Gunshot Wounds of the Extremities

46 Thermal Injury of Peripheral Nerve

47 Nerve Injury Associated With Devascularizing Trauma

43

Peripheral Nerve Injuries Associated with Fractures and Dislocations

David B. Siegel
Richard H. Gelberman

AUTHORS' KEY POINTS

- Nerve injuries occur at the time of fracture (primary nerve injury), after manipulation (secondary nerve injury), and after application of tight circular dressings. Neurapraxia is the most common primary nerve injury associated with fractures and dislocations. Axonotmesis is seen less commonly, and neurotmesis is least commonly observed.
- The spontaneous neural recovery rate following isolated nerve injuries associated with closed fractures is 85%. The spontaneous recovery rate following open injuries is lower (65%–70%). Ninety percent of those nerves that recover following closed injuries do so by 4 months. Between 4 and 6 months after the fracture, an additional 5% recover spontaneously.
- Immediate nerve exploration is indicated as follows: when the fracture requires internal fixation; if there is an associated vascular injury; after open fracture where operative debridement is performed; or if the fracture is irreducible. For primary nerve injury where operative management is not required to treat the fracture, early exploration of the nerve is not indicated. Following secondary nerve injury, early exploration of the nerve is recommended.
- Spiral oblique fractures at the junction of the middle and distal thirds of the humeral diaphysis with proximal, lateral displacement of the distal fragment (described initially by Holstein and Lewis[13]) are not currently considered an indication for early nerve exploration.
- The sciatic nerve is most commonly injured following posterior fracture-dislocation of the hip joint. Compared to other fractures and dislocations with primary nerve injury, the presence of this fracture pattern is an indication for early exploration of the nerve. The peroneal component of the sciatic nerve is more vulnerable to injury than is the tibial component.

The preferred management of patients with peripheral nerve injuries associated with fractures or dislocations has generated considerable controversy. Despite the great interest in this area, an acceptable protocol for treatment based on experimental or prospective clinical studies has not been provided. While retrospective clinical reviews constitute the majority of literature on this subject, a thoughtful approach to this problem has emerged based on a correlation of pertinent specific information regarding regional anatomy, fracture patterns, and associated injuries.

Seddon's classification is recommended for categorizing nerve injuries associated with fractures and dislocations (see Chap. 7).[31] Neurapraxia (focal demyelination without axonal degeneration) is the most common type of injury associated with fractures and dislocations. Axonotmesis (nerve fiber interruption with Schwann sheath preservation) is seen less commonly; neurotmesis (severe axonal disorganization or division) is least commonly observed.[24] There is general agreement that while spontaneous partial or complete nerve recovery occurs following neurapractic or axonotmetic lesions, operative repair is required to regain function following neurotmetic injuries.

The surgeon's responsibility is to differentiate those lesions that recover spontaneously from those that require operative repair. Early exploration of nerves that have undergone neurapraxia or axonotmesis is not indicated, however, as partial or complete recovery generally occurs spontaneously. On the other hand, failure to repair a transected nerve subjects a patient to unnecessary delays in reestablishment of axonal continuity and end-organ reinnervation.

Nerve injuries may occur at the time of fracture (primary nerve injury), after manipulation (secondary nerve injury), or after application of tight circular dressings. Tardy nerve palsy occurs secondary to angular deformity, skeletal instability, partial growth-plate arrest, and with exuberant callus or heterotopic bone.[39]

Incidence

The incidence of nerve injury associated with fractures and dislocations is unknown, as most series reported are from tertiary referral centers. The incidence is higher following dislocations than fractures, which is believed to be secondary to the traction force applied to the nerve following dislocations. About 80% to 90% of nerve injuries associated with fractures occur in the upper extremity.[24] The nerve most commonly injured is the radial nerve, with a reported incidence of up to 16% with humeral fractures.[28]

DENERVATION FOLLOWING FRACTURES AND DISLOCATIONS

Peripheral nerve and end-organ changes occurring after nerve injury are of fundamental importance when considering management. While muscle atrophy is determined experimentally by measuring the percentage loss of muscle weight, decrease in muscle fiber size, and cross-sectional area (see Chap. 5), clinically only extremity volume and circumference have been used to document changes following fractures with nerve injury. One month after denervation, there is about 30% muscle atrophy; by 2 months 50% to 60%; and by 3 months 60% to 80%. After 3 months, equilibrium is reached and further detectable atrophy is minimal. Cross-sectional area diminishes 80% to 90% by 90 days.[39,40]

The histologic changes following muscle denervation have been well described (see Chap. 5). While the morphological changes observed within the first year after denervation are believed to be reversible, irreversible degenerative changes are observed 3 years after denervation.[4] Clinically, the loss of function after varying periods of denervation can be estimated based on Woodhall and Beebe's determination that 1% function is lost for every 6 days of denervation.[48] However, other changes commonly observed with complete muscle paralysis, such as venous stasis and edema, have been noted to further increase interstitial fibrosis, reducing function.

Sensory end-organ alterations after denervation have not received the same degree of attention as have changes in muscle. The area of sensory loss diminishes with time, even without reinnervation. This may be due to local nerve sprouting from nerves in uninjured adjacent areas.[39] It is generally agreed that prompt nerve repair following a neurotmetic lesion yields the best functional outcome, as prolonged denervation leads to progressive end-organ deterioration. Experimental studies have demonstrated that the biochemical, histologic, physiological, and functional changes in muscle or sensory end organs are reversed completely if nerve repair is accomplished within 6 to 12 months of denervation.[39] Empirically, nerve repair is rarely successful after 18 months for motor nerves and after 3 to 5 years for sensory nerves.

Reinnervation and Recovery

Most nerves injured by fracture fragments recover spontaneously. The spontaneous recovery rate is 85% after closed fractures and 65% to 70% after open injuries. In a prospective study, Omer noted an 83% rate of spontaneous recovery in isolated upper extremity nerve injuries associated with fractures and dislocations.[24] Of those nerves that recovered, 90% did so by 4 months. This supports the concept that neurapractic lesions predominate. Nerves did not recover spontaneously beyond 7 months after injury (Fig. 43-1). Of all upper extremity neural injuries, about 72% recovered spontaneously by 4 months. An additional 5% recovered between 4 and 6 months. After 6 months, only an additional 6% recovered.[24]

The prognosis for spontaneous neural recovery following dislocation is poorer than that following fracture. It has been observed that traction associated with dislocations is more likely to cause neurotmesis or axonotmesis, whereas fractures more often cause neurapraxia. Nerves injured with dislocations or juxta-articular fractures are subject to traction because the nerve is frequently tethered to the joint capsule by fascial bands (eg, posterior interosseous nerve adjacent to the radiocapitellar joint). Proximal injuries have a poorer prognosis for motor and sensory recovery than do distal injuries; the cause is not well understood.[39]

Reinnervation profiles are performed regularly following neural injury. Tinel's sign is sought and its location precisely noted. One of the earliest signs of muscle recovery is tenderness of involved muscles. Manual muscle grading, as proposed by the British Medical Research Council (see Chap. 25), is performed. Contractures are prevented with therapy and splinting.[40]

Management

Radiographs include joints proximal and distal to the fracture. Correlating the fracture pattern, degree of comminution, and level of injury with regional peripheral nerve anatomy aids in determining the type of nerve damage. Provisional fracture

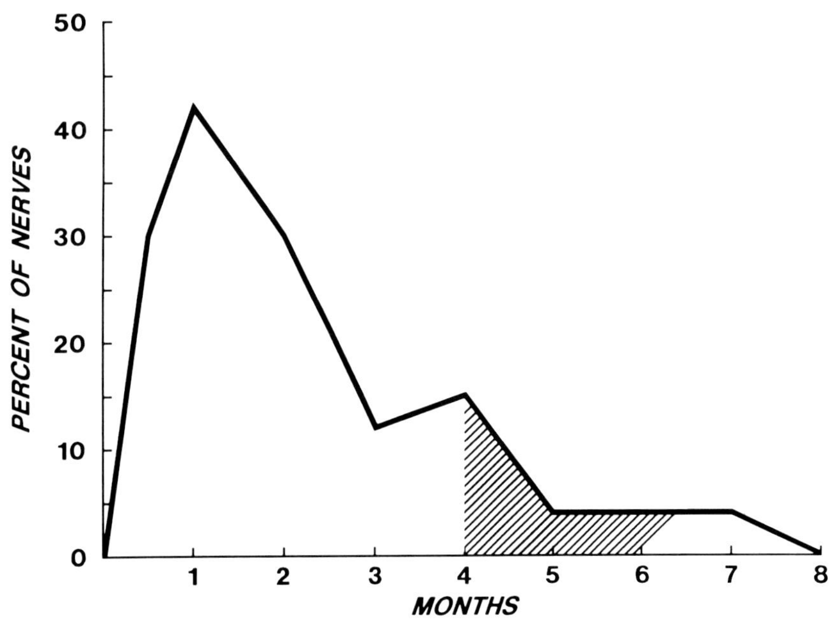

Figure 43-1. *Time course for spontaneous neural recovery following isolated closed fractures and dislocations. Ninety percent of the nerves that recovered spontaneously did so by 4 to 6 months. The shaded area indicates the time for operative exploration following isolated nerve injury associated with fractures and dislocations.*

stabilization with splints minimizes further nerve damage. Neurological function is examined after manipulative reduction and splinting. Paralyzed limbs are supported, avoiding circumferential constricting dressings. Because of their superficial location as they cross their respective joints, the ulnar and common peroneal nerves are most vulnerable to direct compressive injuries from limb swelling after fracture.

Immediate operative nerve exploration is indicated in several specific situations. First, if the fracture requires internal fixation, the nerve is explored at the time of skeletal stabilization. Irreducible fractures and those associated with vascular injuries are included in this group. Second, open fractures where operative debridement is performed should include nerve exploration. Early exploration is not recommended after isolated closed injuries.[24,28] The advantages of early surgery include ease of dissection, removal of structures that may cause nerve entrapment, fracture stabilization to minimize subsequent nerve damage, and ease of nerve repair. A spontaneous recovery rate of 80% to 90%, however, precludes early surgery except under the preceding circumstances.

Secondary Nerve Injury

The management of secondary nerve injury following fracture-fragment manipulation is controversial. The concept that neurotmesis may occur with fracture reduction is based on theoretical rather than well-supported clinical data. At operative exploration for secondary paralysis, Shah and Bhatti found no evidence of nerve severance in eight cases.[33] One nerve was trapped within the fracture, and three nerves were compressed by fracture fragments. While no definitive studies have conclusively demonstrated substantial benefits from early exploration, this approach has become commonly accepted practice. We continue to recommend it, although more definitive data supporting this approach are required.

Electrophysiological studies assess neural function at intervals during the post-injury period. With all three types of injury there are immediate conduction blocks at the sites of injury. Following neurapractic injuries, distal conduction velocity remains normal. Slowing of conduction velocity may be demonstrated across the lesion after 1 to 3 weeks. Subsequently, recruitment of motor units is seen on electromyography. After axonotmesis, conduction velocity may be preserved distally for 7 days. Denervation changes are seen on electromyography after 2 to 5 weeks. Reinnervation potentials frequently appear after 6 to 8 weeks.

During the first week after injury, electrophysiological studies cannot differentiate the three types of injury. After 2 to 3 weeks, preservation of distal conduction velocities helps differentiate neurapraxia from axonotmesis and neurotmesis. After 6 to 8 weeks, the appearance of reinnervation potentials distinguishes axonotmesis from neurotmesis. The presence of evoked potentials may be used to distinguish axonotmesis from neurotmesis.[32] However, studies that fail to demonstrate return of neural function do not preclude spontaneous recovery, as prolonged conduction block may occur after either neurapraxia or axonotmesis.

Author's Preferred Method

After isolated, closed fractures, we prefer nonoperative management of primary neural injuries. Early operative nerve exploration is carried out in the following circumstances:

- Open fractures where the dissection necessary for nerve exploration does not increase significantly the magnitude of the surgery
- Fractures associated with vascular injuries
- Situations where open reduction and internal fixation are warranted.

Six weeks after injury, electrophysiological studies are obtained and are repeated preoperatively to determine if neural recovery that is not evident clinically has occurred. If there is no evidence of recovery, nerve exploration is carried out 4 to 6 months after injury.

RADIAL NERVE PALSY WITH HUMERAL SHAFT FRACTURES

Applied Anatomy

The radial nerve, the largest branch of the posterior cord of the brachial plexus, enters the arm between the long and medial heads of the triceps muscle (see Chap. 27).[43] It courses across the posterior aspect of the arm, separated 1 to 5 cm from the humerus by fibers of the medial head of the triceps muscle.[47] The nerve pierces the lateral intermuscular septum 10 cm above the lateral epicondyle. As the nerve approaches the lateral supracondylar ridge, it comes into contact with the spiral groove of the humerus, where it courses for about 3 cm. It does not lie directly within the groove, however. The spiral groove provides the origin of the posterior fibers of the brachialis muscle. The radial nerve lies in the interval between the brachialis and brachioradialis muscles before crossing the radiocapitellar joint to enter the forearm.[43]

The consistent anatomical relationship of the radial nerve and the humerus in the mid-diaphysis indicates that factors other than direct injury by bone fragments cause radial nerve palsy. The nerve is bound tightly as it pierces the lateral intermuscular septum. Angular deformities and traction to unstable humerus fracture fragments cause acute compressive neural changes. Similarly, because the nerve is tethered by the lateral intermuscular septum, traction injuries may be caused by acute angular deformity.

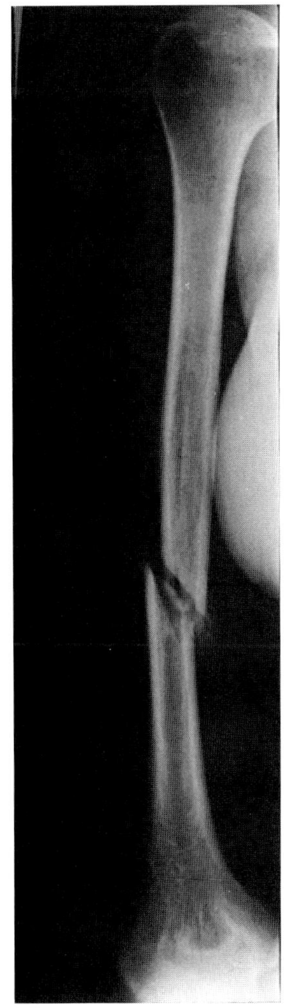

Figure 43–2. *Radiograph demonstrating the fracture pattern most commonly associated with radial nerve palsy.*

Incidence

The incidence of radial nerve palsy accompanying fracture of the humerus is about 11% (range, 2%–16%).[28,33] Three quarters of neural injuries are primary, and the rest occur after manipulation (these data include complete and partial lesions). About 10% of injuries occur with fractures in the proximal third of the humerus, 60% with those in the middle third, and 30% with those in the distal third (Fig. 43-2).[28] Although mid-diaphyseal fractures are associated most commonly with radial nerve palsy, oblique fractures of the distal third of the humerus have generated the greatest interest.[13]

Nerve Exploration

Reports of early exploration have noted occasional nerve impalement by bone fragments.[25] Less commonly, the nerve has actually been severed by bone fragments.[13] One particular fracture pattern has been associated with a high percentage of direct neural injuries: Holstein and Lewis noted that spiral oblique fractures at the junction of the middle and distal third of the humeral diaphysis with proximal, lateral displacement of the distal fragment often impale the radial nerve (Fig. 43-3).[13] They also noted that the nerve was often entrapped by fracture fragments and was likely to be further damaged during fracture healing, bound in either scar tissue or fracture callus. These findings were corroborated by Packer and associates.[25] However, larger and more recent studies have failed to substantiate earlier studies and have concluded that

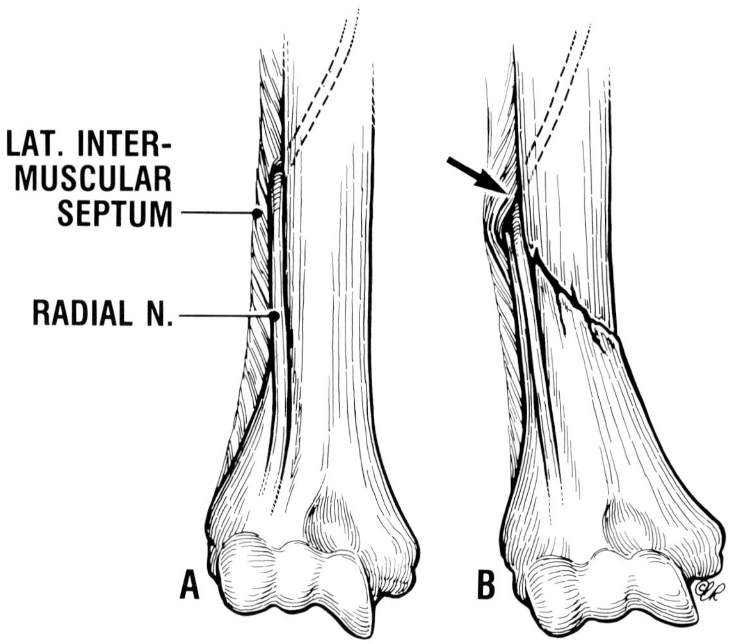

Figure 43–3. *(**A**) The normal anatomy of the radial nerve as it pierces the lateral intermuscular symptom. (**B**) The Holstein-Lewis fracture pattern causes entrapment of the radial nerve as it pierces the lateral intermuscular symptom. The arrow notes the area of entrapment, which is above the distal, lateral bone spike.*

early exploration is not warranted with Holstein-Lewis fracture patterns.[16,20,28]

Investigators examining the efficacy of early exploration have observed that nerves have been transected in 12% of cases; following open fractures, the rate of transection is 20%.[25,33] Recovery following early exploration leads to satisfactory functional return in 70% of patients. In contrast, the rate of spontaneous return of function without exploration is about 83% (range, 70%–100%).[24] The 17% failure rate of spontaneous recovery closely approximates the 12% rate of transected nerves found with exploration. Therefore, it can be inferred that more than 90% of radial nerves that are not transected demonstrate spontaneous functional recovery. Delayed exploration in those patients who have not had spontaneous return of function after 4 to 6 months has demonstrated a 20% rate of nerve division and a 5% rate of nerve entrapment in callus.[28]

The results of radial nerve suture repair following fracture-induced neurotmesis are variable. Omer reported that 25% of patients recovered after repair of sharp transections of the radial nerve above the elbow, but no recovery was seen following suture of nerves injured by fractures.[24] Pollock reported one successful neurorrhaphy[28] and Gurdjian and Smathers reported three patients with functional recovery following repair.[11] For detailed data on the results of radial nerve repair, see Chapter 28.

Authors' Preferred Method

Immediate exploration of nonfunctional radial nerves is recommended for the following conditions only:

- When operative debridement and fracture stabilization are required for open fractures or in the multiple trauma patient
- In fractures with associated vascular injuries
- In irreducible fractures.

Early nerve exploration is not indicated after closed isolated injuries. If a neurapractic lesion has occurred, recovery of all muscles is anticipated. Muscle return may occur simultaneously or nonsequentially. After axonotmesis, however, the order of muscle recovery is as follows: brachioradialis, extensor carpi radialis longus, extensor carpi radialis brevis, supinator, extensor digitorum communis, extensor carpi ulnaris, abductor pollicis longus, extensor pollicis brevis, and extensor pollicis longus.[39] As the nerve injury does not necessarily occur at the site of the fracture, using Seddon's clinical observation that neural recovery occurs at a rate of 1 mm/day may not predict accurately the timing of reinnervation of the most proximal muscles.[31] Although it has been suggested that the radial nerve should be explored 6 weeks post-injury, there does not appear to be any clinical or experimental support for this approach.[20,28,34] This is an inadequate period within which to expect spontaneous recovery and may be a most difficult period, technically, for exploration. Electrophysiological studies are obtained 6 weeks after injury and are repeated preoperatively. A more appropriate waiting period after closed injury is 4 to 6 months. There is no proven benefit of waiting for spontaneous recovery beyond 7 months. During this period, an advancing Tinel's sign may aid in monitoring recovery, but its absence does not imply absence of recovery. The operative approach to the radial nerve and humeral shaft is described in Chapter 27.

POSTERIOR INTEROSSEOUS NERVE PALSY WITH MONTEGGIA LESIONS

Applied Anatomy

The posterior interosseous nerve is the deep branch of the radial nerve, dividing from the main nerve trunk at the level of the lateral epicondyle. It crosses the radiocapitellar joint, to which it is attached by fibrous bands, and enters the substance of the supinator muscle. It courses from the flexor to the extensor surface of the forearm, dividing the two laminae of the supinator muscle. Although the nerve is normally separated from the radius by the deep head of the supinator muscle, occasionally it comes in contact with the radius itself at the level of insertion of the deep head.[36,43] After exiting the distal edge of the supinator muscle, the nerve divides to innervate the deep and superficial muscles of the extensor forearm.

Classification

The posterior interosseous nerve is the nerve most commonly injured following Monteggia fracture-dislocations.[5] This lesion, classified by Bado into four types, includes an ulnar shaft fracture with dislocation of the radial head.[2] Type I, with anterior angulation of the ulnar shaft and anterior radial head dislocation, occurs in 60% of cases. Type II, with posterior angulation of the ulna and posterior or posterolateral dislocation of the radial head, occurs in 15%, and Type III, with lateral or anterolateral dislocation, occurs in 20% of Monteggia lesions. Type IV is rare (5%) and consists of an anterior radial head dislocation with proximal radial and ulnar fractures.

Biomechanical studies have demonstrated that the most likely mechanism causing the injury is forced pronation with axial loading.[10] This becomes important when considering the cause of nerve injury associated with this fracture pattern.

Incidence

The incidence of posterior interosseous nerve injury with Monteggia fracture-dislocations varies from 3% to 43%.[2,5,7,15] The radial nerve itself is injured in as many as 10% of Monteggia lesions.[7,15] Unlike radial nerve injuries associated with humeral fractures, most posterior interosseous nerve palsies occur at the time of injury and not after manipulative reduction. Bruce and colleagues, however, reported a 14% incidence of secondary posterior interosseous nerve palsy.[7] One study noted an increased incidence of nerve palsy with Bado type II injuries.[15] Two cases of tardy posterior interosseous nerve palsy following Monteggia fracture-dislocations with unreduced radial heads have been reported.[1,18] In both cases nerves were found tented and attenuated over the dislocated, deformed radial heads. Two cases of nerve palsy associated with irreducible radial head dislocations have been reported in which the posterior interosseous nerve was found blocking reduction.[22,37] In both cases the nerve was found wrapped around the posterior aspect of the anteriorly dislocated radial head. Both patients recovered full neural function.

The posterior interosseous nerve is tethered in the region of the radial head by four structures: fibrous bands from the radiocapitellar joint, the radial recurrent leash of vessels, the arcade of Frohse, and the fibrous origin of the extensor carpi radialis brevis muscle.[36] These are thought to represent the anatomical sites of neural compression in radial tunnel syndrome (see Chap. 23). Because the posterior interosseous nerve wraps around the radial neck, radial head dislocation may cause a traction injury or an acute compressive injury at any of the four anatomical locations (Fig. 43-4). Further, forced pronation, thought to be the mechanism causing the Monteggia lesion, may lead to compression by the fibrous origin of the supinator (the arcade of Frohse), a structure present in 30% of cadaveric limbs.[36]

Reduction of the radial head restores the nerve to its normal location and relieves that component of neural compromise secondary to acute compression. If the radial head dislocates anteromedially, the posterior interosseous nerve may be displaced around the posterolateral aspect of the radial neck, in which case it may be a component blocking reduction.

Authors' Preferred Method

The recommendations for immediate and delayed neural exploration following other fractures and dislocations may be applied to Monteggia lesions. The operative approach is dictated by the direction of radial head displacement. For Bado type I injuries, the anterior approach is recommended; for types II through IV, the combined posterior approach to the radius and posterior interosseous nerve is used (see Chap. 27). Occasionally, anterior and posterior incisions are required. Open reduction with internal fixation of the ulna and closed reduction of the radial head are performed. If the radial head is not congruently aligned, then open reduction is carried out with posterior interosseous nerve exploration. Similarly, neural exploration is carried out after secondary injuries.

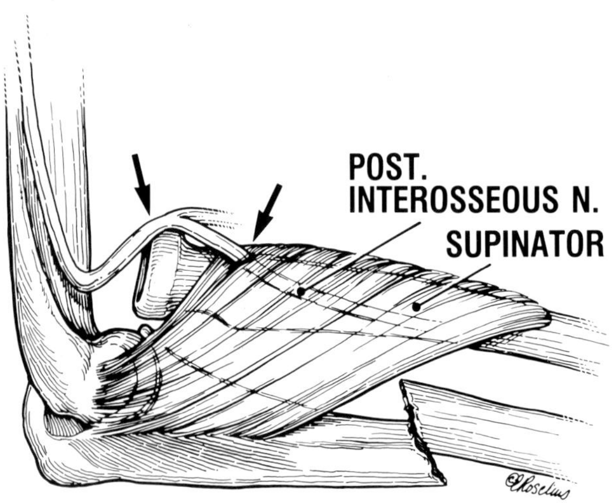

Figure 43-4. *Anterior Monteggia fracture dislocation causing acute traction injury of the posterior interosseous nerve.*

AXILLARY NERVE INJURY FOLLOWING SHOULDER DISLOCATION

Applied Anatomy

The axillary nerve arises from the posterior cord of the brachial plexus, lateral to the radial nerve and posterior to the axillary artery. It crosses the anterior surface of the subscapularis muscle, turns posterolaterally at the inferolateral border of that muscle, and enters the quadrangular space accompanied by the posterior humeral circumflex artery and veins. The boundaries of this space are the teres minor muscle superiorly, the neck of the humerus laterally, the teres major muscle inferiorly, and the long head of the triceps muscle medially. At the lateral border of the subscapularis muscle, the nerve lies in close proximity to the inferior glenohumeral joint capsule, which it supplies with sensory fibers. As the nerve exits the quadrangular space, it divides into anterior and posterior branches. The anterior branch supplies the anterior and middle portions of the deltoid muscle. The posterior branch supplies the teres minor muscle and the posterior portion of the deltoid muscle. The superior lateral cutaneous nerve of the arm is the terminal branch of the posterior division.[43]

Incidence

Because of its proximity to the joint capsule, the axillary nerve is the most commonly injured nerve associated with anterior glenohumeral dislocations. Radial, median, ulnar, and musculocutaneous nerve injuries, as well as brachial plexus palsies, have been described following anterior shoulder dislocation.[3,17] These specific nerve injuries are differentiated from the "dead arm syndrome" associated with recurrent anterior subluxation of the glenohumeral joint, the cause of which is unknown.[30] The anatomical relationship of the axillary nerve to the glenohumeral joint accounts for the high incidence of nerve injury with anterior dislocations (Fig. 43-5). The nerve is subject to traction as well as direct compressive forces when the humeral head displaces anteriorly. The humeral head pushes the subscapularis muscle anteriorly, causing pressure on the nerve. Further, because the nerve turns posteriorly around the inferolateral border of the subscapularis muscle, anterior displacement of this muscle causes a traction injury. Anterior dislocations account for 98% of shoulder dislocations, of which 85% are subcoracoid.[21,29] Neural injury following closed posterior dislocations is rare. However, displaced fractures of the surgical neck of the humerus may cause direct neural injury within the quadrangular space.

The incidence of neural injury following isolated acute anterior shoulder dislocation is 14% (range, 2%–35%).[17,37] The incidence is higher in patients older than 45 years. Isolated axillary nerve lesions, occurring in 10% to 20% of dislocations, account for about 80% of these neural injuries.[3,6] It appears that the incidence increases directly with the thoroughness of the examiner. In the most carefully documented study of patients with neural injury following anterior shoulder dislocations, Blom and Dahback found electromyographic evidence of axillary nerve dysfunction in 32% of all patients (approaching 50% in patients older than 50 years).[3] Axillary nerve injury combined with radial and musculocutaneous nerve injury occurred in two of their 24 patients. The lower incidence reported in other studies may be related to failure to recognize associated neural injury, or to the fact that electromyographically detected lesions are not all clinically apparent. About 40% are complete injuries, the rest partial.[6]

Evaluation of Deltoid Muscle Function

Axillary nerve function in patients with anterior shoulder dislocation is determined by direct palpation of the deltoid muscle with isometric voluntary contraction. Direct palpation is also used to

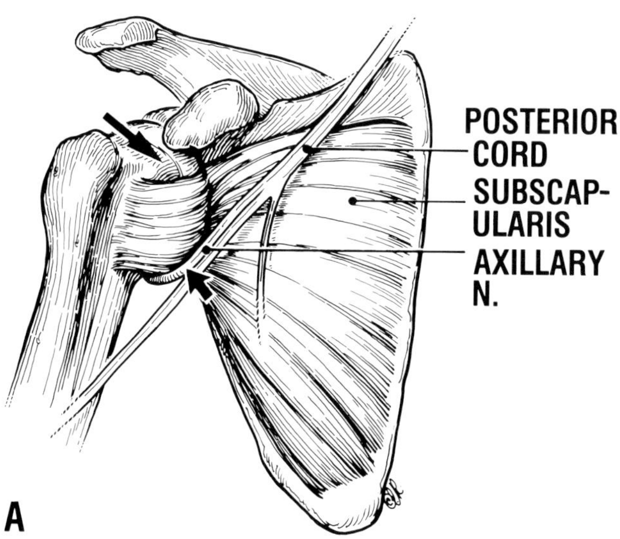

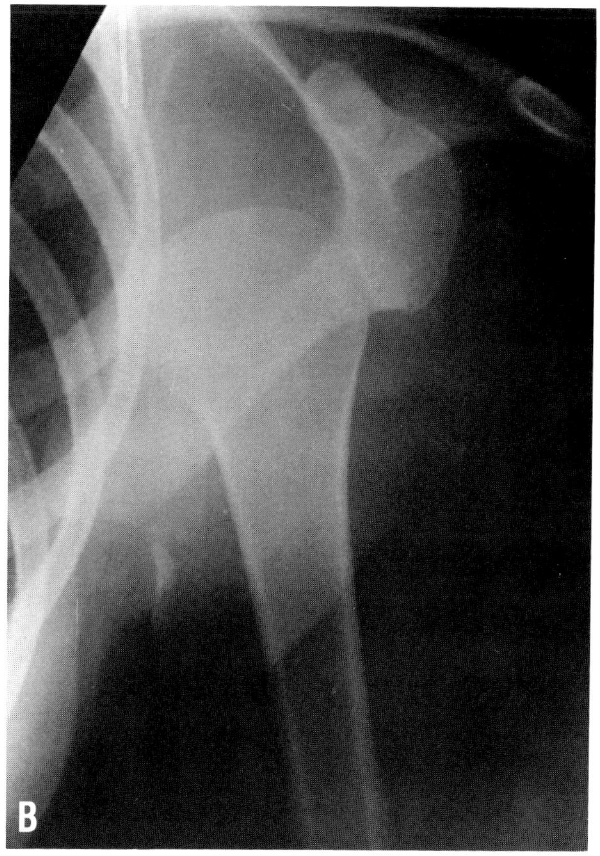

Figure 43–5. *(**A**) Pressure from the humeral head causes an acute compressive neuropathy of the axillary nerve. Note that the axillary nerve passes inferior to the caudal margin of the subscapularis muscle. The arrow points to the anteriorly dislocated humeral head. (**B**) Radiograph demonstrating an anterior shoulder dislocation.*

differentiate deltoid muscle paralysis from rotator cuff tear. The two lesions may occur concurrently.[27] Even when patients have severe pain, contraction of the deltoid muscle may be demonstrated if axillary nerve function is intact. Sensory testing for axillary nerve function is unreliable, as there is no true autonomous zone for lateral brachial cutaneous nerve.[3] After reduction, a repeat neurological examination is performed.

After reduction is accomplished, the arm is supported in a sling. In patients with axillary nerve paralysis the patient's age and associated injuries determine the length of time the shoulder is immobilized. The shoulder is brought through a full range of motion daily. During recovery the arm is not forcibly abducted, in an effort to avoid further traction on the nerve. A sling that supports the deltoid muscle at its normal resting length helps avoid overstretching muscle fibers.

Prolonged disability following shoulder dislocation has been attributed in part to axillary nerve palsy. Although full shoulder abduction may be accomplished with a paralyzed deltoid muscle, disability is significant, as the rotator cuff muscles cannot replace deltoid function completely. Patients with persistent deltoid paralysis can abduct their shoulders by rotating the scapula using the trapezius, rhomboid, and serratus anterior muscles. The glenohumeral joint is dynamically stabilized by the supraspinatus muscle and long head of the biceps muscle. At more than 90° elevation, the clavicular portion of the pectoralis major muscle assists in abduction. Paralysis of the teres minor muscle does not appear to be clinically significant.

Recovery

Spontaneous recovery of nerve function is the rule. Blom and Dahback noted that all of their patients recovered deltoid function, most within 6 weeks.[3] Watson-Jones noted an 85% spontaneous recovery rate: about 65% of patients recovered within 6 months and an additional 20% within 1 year after injury.[45] Brown noted uniform recovery in a series of 76 patients; most regained complete function.[6] With reinnervation, muscle contractions are first noted in the posterior deltoid, followed by the middle and anterior portions.

Nerve Exploration

If electrophysiological tests fail to demonstrate reinnervation of the deltoid muscle within 6 months of injury, operative exploration is recommended. Of patients who do not have deltoid contraction by 6 months, only 20% spontaneously recover function. While earlier exploration with nerve grafting has recently been advocated for patients with axillary palsy after dislocation, this approach is not firmly supported by other data in the literature.[6,27,30]

Authors' Preferred Method

We manage patients with primary axillary nerve injury after shoulder dislocation with immediate gentle closed reduction. Failure to obtain a congruent closed reduction, with associated nerve injury, is an indication for exploration. Axillary nerve function is examined with electrophysiological tests 6 weeks after injury. If reinnervation is not demonstrated by 6 months, the nerve is explored operatively.

SCIATIC NERVE INJURY WITH TRAUMATIC HIP DISLOCATION AND FRACTURE-DISLOCATION

Applied Anatomy

The sciatic nerve is the largest nerve emanating from the sacral plexus. It exits the pelvis with the piriformis muscle through the greater sciatic foramen, which is formed by the greater sciatic notch superiorly and the sacrospinous ligament inferiorly. After crossing the ischial spine, it passes behind the posterior capsule of the hip joint, separated from the capsule by the gemelli and obturator muscles. It wraps around the lateral aspect of the ischial tuberosity posterior to the quadratus femoris muscle and enters the posterior aspect of the thigh.[43]

The anatomical proximity of the sciatic nerve to the hip joint makes it susceptible to injury following posterior dislocation. Most sciatic nerve injuries occur primarily at the time of dislocation, but secondary injury and tardy sciatic nerve palsy secondary to heterotopic bone formation are not rare. For reasons that are not completely understood, the peroneal component is more likely to sustain injury than the tibial component. Sunderland theorized that this was due to the funicular pattern within the nerve.[39] The peroneal nerve is composed of fewer and larger bundles, with less connective and adipose tissue than the tibial nerve. He postulated that the dislocated femoral head presses directly on the nerve fibers of the peroneal nerve, but injury to the tibial nerve is dampened by the interstitial connective and adipose tissue.[39]

Classification

The Thompson-Epstein classification of posterior dislocations and fracture-dislocations is useful for prognosis and treatment.[41] Type I is dislocation without acetabular fracture. Types II through IV have an associated acetabular rim or floor fracture, and type V is associated with femoral head fracture. With type I posterior dislocations, there is direct compression of the sciatic nerve where it crosses the posterior hip joint capsule (Fig. 43-6). With fracture-dislocation (types II–IV) the posterior acetabular fragment may directly penetrate and impale the nerve.[38] Because the sciatic nerve is tethered as it exits the greater sciatic foramen, it has inadequate excursion to move away from the displaced femoral head, and an acute neural compressive lesion occurs.

The incidence of primary sciatic nerve injury with posterior dislocation or fracture-dislocations is 12% (range, 6%–20%).[9,12,14,23,38,41] It occurs three times more often with type II through IV injuries than with type I injuries.[12] The precise incidence of secondary or tardy sciatic nerve palsies has not been reported.

Authors' Preferred Method

As this is thought to represent an acute compressive neuropathy, prompt reduction is required to minimize that component of the insult due to ischemia. After reduction is accomplished, computed tomography is used to assess joint congruity and displacement of bone fragments. If reduction is congruent and bone fragments do not lie posterior to the joint, operative exploration of the nerve is not indicated. If the joint is not reduced congruently or if there are displaced bone fragments in the region of the greater sciatic notch or posterior acetabulum, operative exploration of the nerve is carried out. A specific fracture pattern that requires early exploration is one with displaced posterior acetabular bone fragments, where there is an associated primary sciatic nerve injury. At exploration, these fragments have been found commonly compressing or impaling the nerve. On the other hand, Nicoll found that the sciatic nerve was always in continuity.[23] Zachary and Roaf noted that recovery following exploration was better than that occurring spontaneously.[9]

Our recommendation for treatment of primary sciatic nerve injury associated with posterior fracture-dislocations of the hip is early nerve exploration and decompression. Secondary paralysis is also an indication for operative nerve exploration. Tardy sciatic nerve palsy secondary to heterotopic bone formation is treated by external neurolysis.

After reduction, an effort is made to reduce tension on the injured sciatic nerve. This is best accomplished by positioning the hip in extension and the knee in flexion. Slings and balanced suspension splints increase pressure on the nerve posteriorly and are therefore not recommended. A therapy program designed to minimize contractures optimizes the chances for functional recovery after reinnervation.

Functional recovery occurs in 65% of patients.[9,12] Recovery for peroneal nerve–innervated muscles is worse than for tibial nerve–innervated muscles. Many patients, however, require prolonged use of braces and ultimately undergo tendon transfers to restore motor function (see Chap. 53).

PERONEAL NERVE PALSY COMPLICATING FRACTURES AND DISLOCATIONS OF THE KNEE

Applied Anatomy

The sciatic nerve divides 10 cm above the knee into the tibial and common peroneal nerves. Lateral to the popliteal artery and vein, the common peroneal nerve descends obliquely across the plantaris muscle and then lies in the interval between the lateral head of the gastrocnemius muscle and the biceps femoris tendon. After crossing the inferior lateral genicular artery and soleus muscle, the nerve turns anteriorly behind the fibular head. It crosses the fibula neck under cover of the peroneus longus muscle. At the midlateral or anterior portion of the fibular neck, the nerve divides into

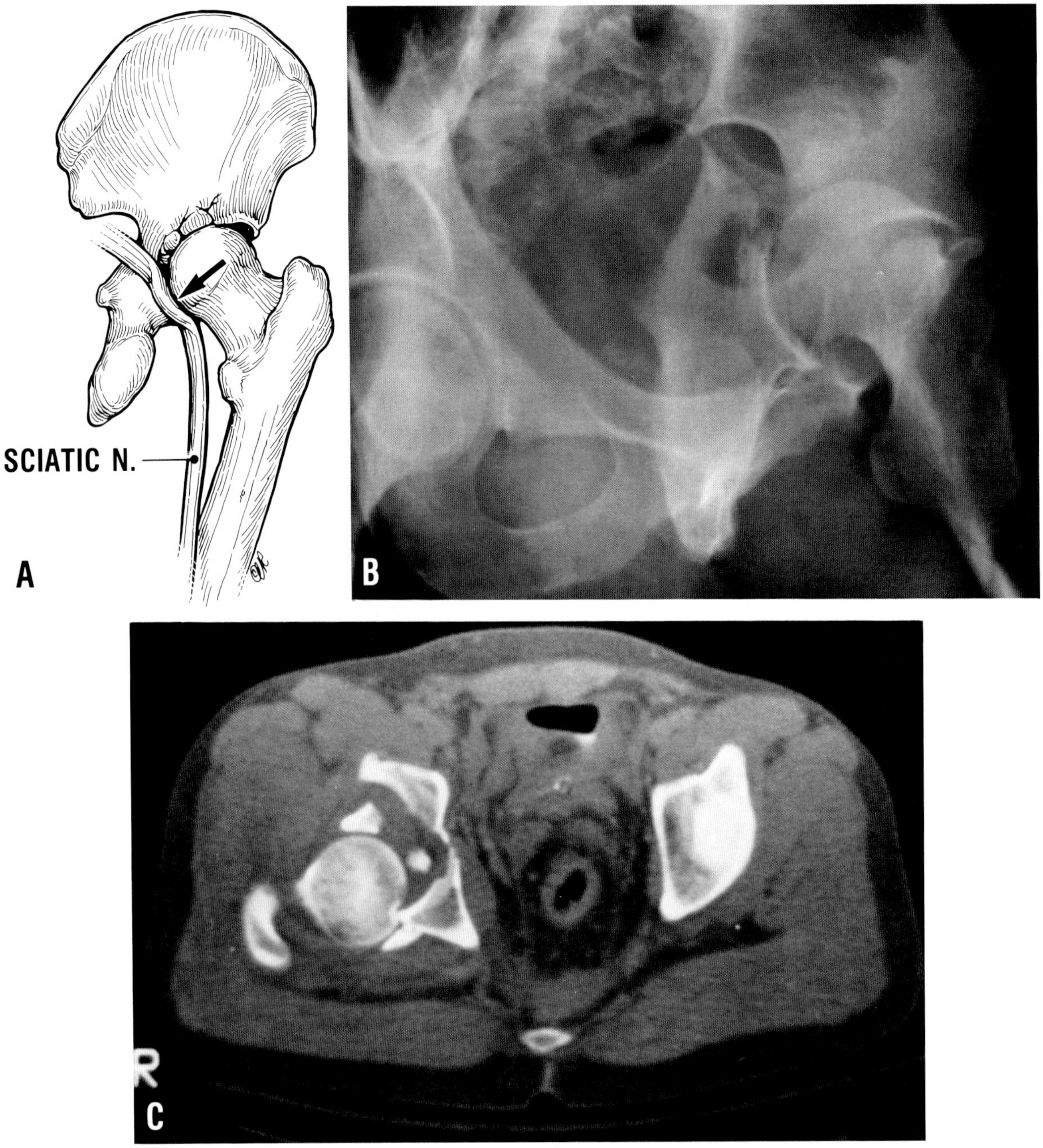

Figure 43–6. (***A***) *Posterior fracture dislocation of the hip causes direct compression of the sciatic nerve after it exits the greater sciatic notch. The arrow denotes the area of maximum compression of the sciatic nerve.* (***B***) *The oblique (Judet) view of the acetabulum demonstrates the posterior displaced acetabular fragments impinging on the greater sciatic notch posteriorly.* (***C***) *Computed tomographic scan demonstrating posterior fracture dislocation with displacement of the femoral head posteriorly and fracture fragments of the posterior lip of the acetabulum.*

deep and superficial branches. Branches of the deep peroneal nerve supply the anterior tibial compartment muscles and provide cutaneous sensation to the first web space of the foot. The superficial peroneal nerve supplies the peroneus longus and brevis muscles with cutaneous sensation to the lateral portion of the calf and dorsum of the foot.[43]

Sunderland found that the blood supply to the peroneal nerve was precarious in the region of the fibular neck.[39] In 88% of the nerves he dissected, the major intraneural vessels occupied a superficial exposed position. Most nerves had no arteriae nervorum or only a single vessel that reached the peroneal nerve in the popliteal fossa. In patients with vascular insufficiency, the blood supply was further compromised. Sunderland also found that the peroneal nerve contained less adipose and interstitial connective tissue than other nerves.[39]

Incidence

Because of its proximity to the fibular head and superficial location as it crosses the fibular neck, the peroneal nerve is particularly vulnerable to injury with proximal fibular fractures, tibiofibular dislocations, tibial plateau fractures, knee dislocations, and supracondylar femur fractures. The nerve may also be injured by a direct impact to the fibular head. Tight circular dressings commonly cause peroneal nerve palsy because of the nerve's superficial location at the knee. The incidence of peroneal nerve palsy following knee dislocation is 16% to 18%.[19,46]

Neural injury, associated with arterial injury in 20% to 35% of cases, occurs secondary to traction from acute angular deformity (Fig. 43-7). Because of the high associated incidence of vascular injuries and the high-energy trauma causing these injuries, compartment syndromes are also considered in the differential diagnosis of peroneal nerve loss.

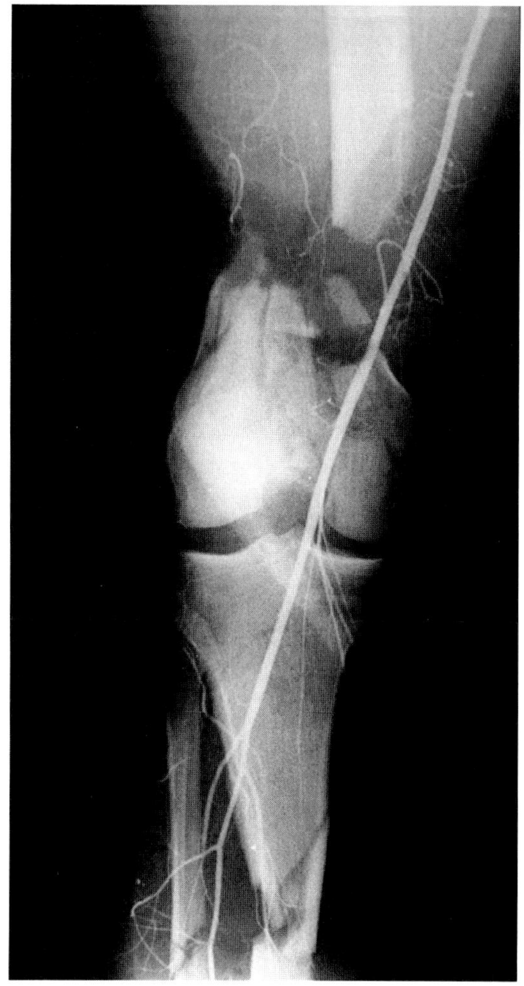

Figure 43–7. *Arteriogram of a 21-year-old man with open femoral and tibial fractures (floating knee). There was an associated complete common peroneal nerve palsy. At the time of operative treatment, his peroneal nerve was explored and found to be in continuity. Spontaneous recovery was first noted 7 months following injury.*

Treatment

Peroneal nerve palsy following *proximal tibiofibular joint dislocation* occurs in 5% of cases and is more common with posterior than superior or anterior dislocations.[8] The injury results either from direct trauma to the fibular head or through force transmitted through the ankle after a parachute-type landing.[19] Open reduction of the fibular head is indicated if closed treatment fails to achieve congruent reduction.[26] Operative exploration of the peroneal nerve is carried out if open reduction is performed, but is not required if closed manipulation is successful.

Fibular head fractures are caused by direct blows or by torsional stress to the ankle with or without angular stresses to the knee joint.[44] When the fracture is caused by a direct blow, the peroneal nerve is frequently contused or injured by subsequent swelling. Traction may result in neurapractic, axonotmetic, or neurotmetic injuries. Electrophysiological studies are obtained if return of function is not evident by 6 weeks. Nerve exploration is carried out between 4 and 6 months after injury if there is no return of function and no evidence of an advancing Tinel's sign.

Adduction and hyperextension knee-joint injuries are associated with acute traction injuries to the peroneal nerve.[42,46] While early exploration of the nerve has been advocated, this approach is not well supported in the literature. Delayed peroneal nerve palsy occurs following application of casts and tight circular dressings and by external pressure from positioning in bed. Unlike the median nerve in the carpal tunnel, the peroneal nerve does not travel through a compartment where increased interstitial pressure is a potential mechanism of injury. Therefore, treatment does not require operative decompression, but rather removal of dressings or repositioning. For a detailed discussion of operative treatment for peroneal nerve injuries, see Chapter 86.

Authors' Preferred Method

When peroneal nerve palsy complicates injuries about the knee, early operative exploration of the nerve is done only under specific conditions. When peroneal nerve injury is associated with injury to the popliteal artery, the nerve is explored at the time of arterial reconstruction. When open reduction and internal fixation of a fracture or dislocation is performed, and nerve exploration would not significantly increase the magnitude of the operative procedure, the nerve is isolated, inspected, and decompressed. At the time of debridement of open fractures, peroneal nerve exploration is done if this does not alter the operative approach.

After peroneal nerve injuries associated with isolated fractures and dislocations that are treated satisfactorily by nonsurgical means, electrophysiological studies are obtained 6 weeks after injury. If return of function is not seen by 4 to 6 months, repeat studies are obtained. Operative exploration is carried out at 4 to 6 months if clinical and electrical findings indicate that function is not returning.

REFERENCES

1. Austin R. Tardy palsy of the radial nerve from a Monteggia fracture. Injury 1975; 7:202–204.
2. Bado JL. The Monteggia lesion. Clin Orthop 1967; 50:71–80.
3. Blom S, Dahback LO. Nerve injuries and dislocations of the shoulder joint in fractures of the neck of the humerus. Acta Chir Scand 1970; 136:461–466.
4. Bowden REM, Gutman E. Denervation and reinnervation of human voluntary muscle. Brain 1944; 67:273–280.
5. Boyd DH, Boals JC. The Monteggia lesion. Clin Orthop 1969; 66:94–100.
6. Brown JT. Nerve injuries complicating dislocations of the shoulder. J Bone Joint Surg [Br] 1952; 34: 526–532.
7. Bruce HE, Harvey JP, Wilson JC. Monteggia fractures. J Bone Joint Surg [Am] 1974; 56:1563–1576.
8. Crothers DC, Johnson JTH. Isolated acute dislocation of the proximal tibiofibular joint. J Bone Joint Surg [Am] 1973; 55:181–183.
9. Epstein HC. Traumatic dislocations of the hip. Clin Orthop 1973; 92:116–142.
10. Evans EM. Pronator injuries of the forearm with special reference to the anterior Monteggia fracture. J Bone Joint Surg [Br] 1949; 31:578–588.
11. Gurdjian ES, Smathers HM. Peripheral nerve injury in fractures and dislocations of long bones. J Neurosurg 1945; 2:202–206.
12. Hirasawa Y, Oda R, Nakatani K. Sciatic nerve paralysis in posterior dislocation of the hip. Clin Orthop 1977; 126:172–175.
13. Holstein A, Lewis GB. Fractures of the humerus with radial nerve paralysis. J Bone Joint Surg [Am] 1963; 45:1382–1388.
14. Huckstep RL. Neglected traumatic dislocation of the hip. J Bone Joint Surg [Br] 1971; 53:355–362.
15. Jessing P. Monteggia lesions and their complicating nerve damage. Acta Orthop Scand 1975; 46:601–609.
16. Kettlekamp DB, Alexander H. Clinical review of radial nerve injury. J Trauma 1967; 7:424–432.
17. Leffert RD, Seddon H. Infraclavicular brachial plexus injuries. J Bone Joint Surg [Br] 1965; 47:9–22.
18. Lichter RL, Jacobsen T. Tardy palsy of the posterior interosseous nerve with a Monteggia fracture. J Bone Joint Surg [Am] 1975; 57:124–125.
19. Lord CD, Coults JW. A study of typical parachute injuries occurring in 250,000 jumps at the para-

chute school. J Bone Joint Surg [Am] 1944; 26:547–557.
20. Mast JW, Spiegel PG, Harvey JP Jr, Harrison C. Fractures of the humeral shaft: A retrospective study of 240 adult fractures. Clin Orthop 1975; 112: 254–262.
21. McLaughlin HL, MacLellan DI. Recurrent anterior dislocation of the shoulder. II. A comparative study. J Trauma 1967; 7:191–201.
22. Morris AH. Irreducible Monteggia lesions with radial nerve entrapment. J Bone Joint Surg [Am] 1974; 56:1744–1746.
23. Nicoll EA. Proceedings and reports of councils and associations: Traumatic dislocation of the hip joint. J Bone Joint Surg [Br] 1952; 34:503–505.
24. Omer GE. Injuries to nerves of the upper extremity. J Bone Joint Surg [Am] 1974; 56:1615–1624.
25. Packer JW, Foster RR, Garcia A, Grantham SA. The humeral fracture with radial nerve palsy: Is exploration warranted? Clin Orthop 1972; 88:34–38.
26. Parkes JC, Zelko RR. Isolated acute dislocation of the proximal tibiofibular joint. J Bone Joint Surg [Am] 1973; 55:177–180.
27. Pasila M, Kiviluoto O, Jaroma H, Sundholm A. Recovery from primary shoulder dislocation and its complication. Acta Orthop Scand 1980; 51:257–262.
28. Pollock FH, Drake D, Bovill EG, Day L, Trafton P. Treatment of radial neuropathy associated with fractures of the humerus. J Bone Joint Surg [Am] 1981; 63:239–243.
29. Rowe CR. Prognosis in dislocations of the shoulder. J Bone Joint Surg [Am] 1956; 38:957–977.
30. Rowe CR, Zarins B. Recurrent transient subluxation of the shoulder. J Bone Joint Surg [Am] 1981; 63: 863–872.
31. Seddon H. Surgical disorders of the peripheral nerves. Edinburgh: Churchill-Livingstone, 1975: 250–287.
32. Sethi RK, Thompson LL. The electromyographer's handbook. Boston: Little, Brown, 1989:159–179.
33. Shah JJ, Bhatti NA. Radial nerve paralysis associated with fractures of the humerus. Clin Orthop 1983; 172:171–176.
34. Shaw JH, Sakellarides HT. Radial nerve paralysis associated with fractures of humerus. J Bone Joint Surg [Am] 1967; 49:899–902.
35. Spar I. A neurologic complication following Monteggia fracture. Clin Orthop 1977; 122:207–209.
36. Spinner M. The arcade of Frohse and its relationship to posterior interosseous nerve paralysis. J Bone Joint Surg [Br] 1968; 50:809–812.
37. Stevens JH. Brachial plexus paralysis. In: Codman EA, ed. The shoulder. Brooklyn, NY: G. Miller, 1934:332–381.
38. Stewart MJ, McCarroll HR, Mulhollan JS. Fracture dislocation of the hip. Acta Orthop Scand 1975; 46: 507–525.
39. Sunderland S. Nerves and nerve injuries. Edinburgh: Churchill-Livingstone, 1978:188–235.
40. Sunderland S, Ray LJ. Denervation changes in mammalian striated muscle. J Neurol Neurosurg Psychiatry 1950; 13:159–162.
41. Thompson VP, Epstein HC. Traumatic dislocation of the hip. J Bone Joint Surg [Am] 1951; 33:746–778.
42. Towne LC, Blazina ME, Marmor L, Lawrence JF. Lateral compartment syndrome of the knee. Clin Orthop 1971; 76:160–168.
43. Warwick R, Williams PL, ed. Gray's anatomy, ed 35 [Br]. Philadelphia: WB Saunders, 1973:1037–1047.
44. Watson-Jones R. Styloid process of the fibula in the knee joint with peroneal palsy. J Bone Joint Surg 1931; 13:258–260.
45. Watson-Jones R. Fractures and joint injuries. London: Churchill-Livingstone, 1982:890–910.
46. White J. The results of traction injuries to the common peroneal nerve. J Bone Joint Surg [Br] 1968; 50:346–350.
47. Whitson RO. Relation of the radial nerve to the shaft of the humerus. J Bone Joint Surg [Am] 1954; 36: 85–88.
48. Woodhall B, Beebe GW. Peripheral nerve regeneration. Veterans Administration Medical Monograph. Washington DC: US Government Printing Office, 1956:340.

44

Nerve Injury Associated With Fractures in Children

Joseph P. Dutkowsky
James R. Kasser

AUTHORS' KEY POINTS

- Immediate neurological examination of the child with an extremity fracture is a fundamental part of initial assessment. In the distressed child who cannot be examined completely, specific observations on extremity function are recorded.
- For nerve injuries occurring with humeral shaft fractures, observation rather than operative exploration is recommended. If there is no recovery of nerve function by 4 months, exploration is carried out. If nerve palsy follows closed reduction, early operative exploration is indicated.
- Median and radial nerve palsies are most often associated with supracondylar fractures. Forward displacement of the proximal humeral fragment may partially or completely transect the radial or median nerves and brachial artery. The anterior interosseous nerve may be involved selectively. Prolonged delay in recovery, or delayed onset of nerve palsy following fracture healing, raises concern of nerve transection or entrapment in fracture callus.
- Percutaneous pin fixation of supracondylar humeral fractures is associated with a 2.8% incidence of iatrogenic nerve palsy. The insertion of two lateral pins is recommended for stabilization in order to avoid injury to the ulnar and radial nerves.
- Symptoms and signs of tardy ulnar nerve palsy may be noted following lateral condyle non-unions. In 40% of cases, symptoms developed 20 to 30 years following injury. The treatment of choice after establishing the diagnosis is ulnar nerve transposition.

Orthopedic surgeons in emergency care spend a large amount of time treating children with fractures. Nerve injuries are associated with about 2.5% of extremity fractures in children. They are over two times more likely to be found with upper-extremity fractures than lower-extremity fractures.[53] Injuries to nerves associated with fractures result from contusion, stretch, partial or complete laceration, or incorporation of the nerve into the fracture callus, and may be partial or complete. Nerve injury may occur during the initial trauma, during reduction, in traction, during fixation, or in the recovery period, or it may be delayed several years. Accordingly, the importance of a thorough neurological examination of a child with an extremity fracture upon presentation, immediately following treatment, and during the recovery period cannot be overemphasized. At times, a complete neurological examination cannot be performed on a distressed child following injury. In these cases that fact should be noted and specific observations should be recorded of the upper-extremity function that can be elicited.

Treatment of nerve injuries of extremity fractures in children vary from observation to immediate exploration and repair. The purpose of this chapter is to enhance the reader's clinical acumen in the anticipation and discovery of these nerve injuries and to provide a foundation for rational treatment plans based on the published experience of several generations of clinicians.

BIRTH INJURIES

Brachial plexus palsies may be diagnosed at birth in association with an upper-extremity fracture. It is likely that both lesions are evidence of a difficult delivery, not that the nerve injury is secondary to the fracture. One possible exception is a report of an isolated radial nerve injury in association with a humerus fracture at birth.[53] When there is a fracture at birth, the clinician should perform a thorough neurological evaluation of the newborn.

The treatment for brachial plexus injuries at birth is observation, for the most part (see Chap. 95). Reconstructive surgery is reserved for functional deficits noted with increasing age (see Chap. 96).

PROXIMAL HUMERUS FRACTURES

Nerve injuries associated with fractures and dislocations about the shoulder in adults are not uncommon, but nerve palsies following proximal humeral fractures in children are rare. Fractures that occur through the proximal humeral growth plate are at a level that is proximal to the region in which nerves lie directly adjacent to bone; thus nerve injury is unlikely. An exception is the axillary nerve, which lies posterior to the proximal humeral growth plate. However, since proximal humerus fractures in children generally angulate anteriorly and laterally, axillary nerve injury is rare. Only six cases of nerve injuries associated with proximal humerus fractures in children have been reported in the literature.

Two patients were treated with open reduction without osteosynthesis. In one case the patient experienced marked weakness in the arm and hand with ulnar paresthesias in the affected extremity. Follow-up examination revealed proximal muscular atrophy. In the second case the patient had slight muscular atrophy and weakness of the affected extremity.[96] Unfortunately, it cannot be discerned from the article whether nerve injury occurred at the time of initial trauma or following treatment. Of note, the same author reported 38 fractures treated by closed reduction, olecranon pin traction, or hanging cast or supporting bandage that were associated with nerve palsies. Of the six cases treated with open reduction and a supporting bandage, two were associated with nerve injuries.

Of the four cases of nerve injury following closed reductions, two involved the radial nerve.[18,71] Both extremities were treated by delayed operative exploration and neurolysis and subsequent improvement was noted. Another patient developed complete median and ulnar nerve palsies following closed reduction. After the fracture healed, the humerus was explored and the median nerve was found to be twisted and bound by scar. Neurolysis was performed. The ulnar nerve, trapped in fracture callus, was divided and repaired. The author reported a good outcome.[71] The final case was that of a patient with a severely comminuted surgical neck fracture of the humerus in which the brachial plexus was trapped between the fracture fragments. The patient underwent operative exploration but regained little function.[137]

The finding, in these four cases, of nerve entrapment in fracture sites related to a closed reduction supports a recommendation that nerve loss, occurring at the time of closed reduction, is best treated by operative exploration.

The treatment of displaced proximal humerus fractures in children may require a salute-type shoulder spica cast. In such a spica cast, in which the arm is brought anteriorly into a position of forward flexion, stretch is placed on the axillary nerve. This may result in a temporary axillary nerve palsy.

Nerve injuries associated with proximal humerus fractures in children are rare. If one is noted at the time of the patients' presentation it is appropriate to treat it conservatively. Nerve exploration is indicated if no improvement is noted after 4 months of observation. If nerve palsy is noted following closed reduction, early exploration is justified.

HUMERAL SHAFT FRACTURES

The course of the radial nerve in relation to the humerus gives it special vulnerability to injury when fractures of the humeral shaft occur (see Chap. 27).[142] The reported incidence of radial nerve injury in humeral shaft fractures in patients of all ages ranges from 1.8% to 16%.[99] The incidence of injury in skeletally immature individuals has not been determined. Traditionally, the injury is thought to occur most frequently in spiral fractures of the distal third of the humerus, as illustrated in Figure 44-1.[56] However, some have found the incidence of radial nerve palsy accompanying acute humeral shaft fractures to be evenly divided between midshaft and distal third fractures, as well as between spiral, oblique, and transverse fractures.[14,68,106,121]

Much discussion in the literature has been focused on the treatment of radial nerve injuries associated with humeral shaft fractures in adults. There are no reports that deal with the timing of treatment in children. However, since these fractures are not physeal injuries and the fracture patterns and anatomy are essentially the same,[55] it seems prudent to extend the clinical experience with adult humeral shaft fractures to children (see Chap. 43).

In a radial nerve palsy occurring with an open humeral shaft fracture or a fracture requiring open reduction and internal fixation, most authors recommend that the nerve be explored and repaired primarily during the initial operation.[120,121] Few authors favor delayed repair after fracture callus has had time to develop.[106] In the case of a closed humerus fracture associated with a radial nerve injury there is less consensus; strong statements have been made for and against early operative exploration. Some authors argue that early exploration helps in determining the prognosis and facilitates planning for neurorrhaphy, secondary repair, tendon transfers, and eventual rehabilitation. These authors also argue that nerve repair is technically easier in the acute stages before callus has formed. In addition, they feel that a reduced and internally fixed humerus helps prevent further radial nerve trauma during fracture healing.[11,21,38,43,56,99] A few authors have recommended observation for patients with incomplete nerve palsies.[99]

Authors who support observation and delayed exploration cite the desire to avoid potential surgical complications such as wound infection, osteomyelitis, delayed union, non-union, and iatrogenic injury to the radial nerve.[13,17,23,68,121,134] Most agree with initial observation, except for cases of nerve palsy following closed reduction.[14,121] They also point out that, in patients with complete radial nerve lesions associated with humeral shaft fractures that are explored immediately, only 12% of nerves were found to be lacerated.[106] Further, delayed repair of the radial nerve 6 to 16 weeks after injury appears to be nearly as successful in restoring radial nerve function as primary repair.[46,106,120]

The most compelling reason to delay exploration of the nerve is that the overall functional result is not different for patients treated with early or delayed exploration.[14] A special case is made for persistent radial nerve palsy in which the radial nerve is entrapped in fracture callus. This may be seen radiographically with a radiolucent tunnel within the radial shaft.[32] One case has been reported in which the nerve was extracted from an osseous tunnel.[106] In another case the nerve was transected at both ends of the tunnel and primary repair performed.[32] Both patients reportedly regained full

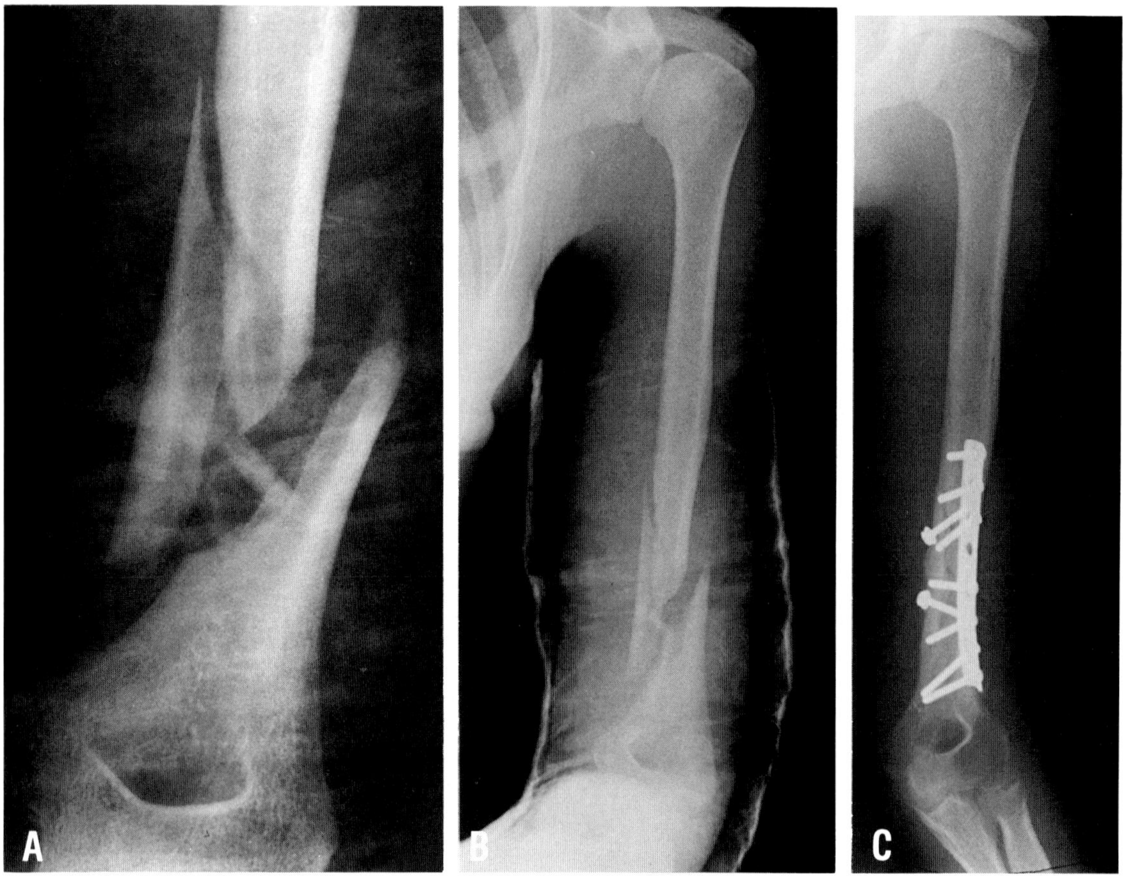

Figure 44–1. **(A)** *This patient had a closed distal humeral fracture with radial nerve injury.* **(B)** *Cast immobilization failed to align the fracture adequately.* **(C)** *At the time of open reduction, a lacerated radial nerve was repaired. If open reduction is necessary, an injured nerve should be explored.*

neurological function. A third patient, treated with a sural nerve graft, had partial nerve recovery.[39] However, it has been noted that not all radial nerves enveloped in fracture callus cause symptoms of nerve loss.[99]

Authors' Preferred Method

In summary, for radial nerve palsies associated with open humeral shaft fractures, or fractures in which open reduction and internal fixation is indicated, the nerve is explored. For extremities treated with primary nerve repair, internal or external fixation is used to protect the nerve. Radial nerve palsies in the presence of closed humeral shaft fractures are observed; exceptions are those developing after closed reduction, or when there is high suspicion that the radial nerve is entrapped between the fracture fragments. If there is no return of nerve function after 4 months, by clinical or electromyographic examination, the nerve is explored and repaired. If the nerve is trapped within fracture callus, neurolysis or nerve transection and repair are carried out.

Tendon transfers are not performed primarily in children. In general, the functional results of nerve repair, primary or delayed, are better than those following tendon transfers.[46]

SUPRACONDYLAR HUMERUS FRACTURES

Supracondylar humerus fractures are the most common elbow fractures in children.[15,80,81,145] Numerous articles about this fracture have drawn attention to associated nerve injuries.[3,15,27,139,145]

A typical displaced (Type III) supracondylar humerus fracture is shown in Figure 44-2. These fractures result from hyperextension forces applied to the skeletally immature elbow.[58,86] Nerve injuries occur in 7% of these fractures.[143] In most studies, the most common nerve injured is the radial nerve, followed by the median nerve and then the ulnar nerve.[3,15,29,34,48,51,73,75,82,93,108,143] Isolated anterior interosseous nerve palsies have also been reported.[63,82,83,86,87,126,128] Some authors report a similar rate of injury of the median and radial nerves.[30,31,40,61,103,122,140,141] Other authors, similar to our experience, have found median nerve injuries to be most common, with anterior interosseous nerve palsy predominating.[35,42,70]

Radial nerve injuries are most often associated with supracondylar humerus fractures in which the distal fragment is posteromedially displaced. The radial nerve is tented across the lateral spike of the proximal fragment. Partial[39] or complete[9,78,82] transections of the radial nerve have been reported. The tendency of these fractures to displace posteromedially accounts for the high incidence of radial nerve injury.

Median nerve injuries are associated with posterolateral displaced fractures. Nerve injury occurs when the proximal humeral spike is driven forward into the neurovascular bundle. Neurapraxia or complete median nerve transection may occur.[36] In these cases the clinician should be alert

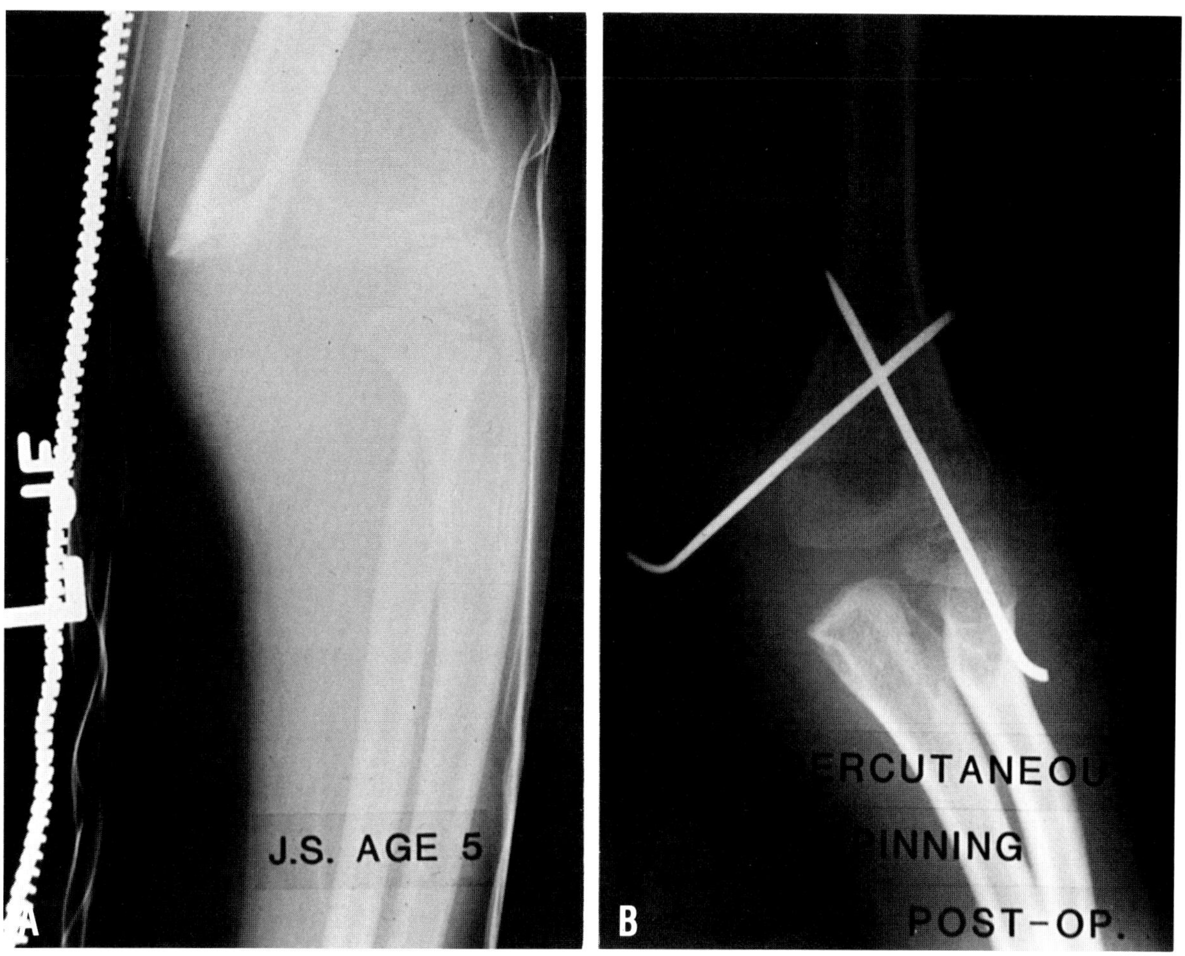

Figure 44–2. **(A)** *This type III supracondylar fracture shows posterior displacement of the distal fragment with obvious trauma to the neurovascular bundle from the proximal fragment.* **(B)** *Optimal treatment is closed reduction and percutaneous pin fixation.*

for a possible associated brachial artery injury.[35,65,66,75,130] The anterior interosseous nerve may be selectively involved with no other evidence of median nerve palsy.[42] Figure 44-2 demonstrates the forward movement of the proximal fracture fragment in type III supracondylar humerus fracture, where the humeral spike is driven into the neurovascular bundle.[98] The brachial artery, tethered by a supratrochlear branch, is predisposed to injury at the time of fracture.[117]

Only 2.5% of supracondylar humerus fractures are of the flexion type,[143] and associated ulnar nerve palsies are more common with this pattern. These injuries usually cause traction on the nerve over the posterior medial spike of the proximal fragment.[40] Injuries to the median and radial nerves have been reported in only one case.[3]

Generally, type III supracondylar humerus fractures are easily reduced. The finding of an irreducible fracture in association with a nerve palsy suggests possible nerve entrapment, most frequently involving the ulnar nerve as illustrated in Figure 44-3. Entrapment of the median nerve and the brachial artery have been reported also.[65,66,130] The finding of an irreducible fracture in association with a neurological injury represents an indication for nerve exploration.[130]

Recovery of nerve function may occur immediately after reduction or may take several weeks to months. Continued improvement in neurological

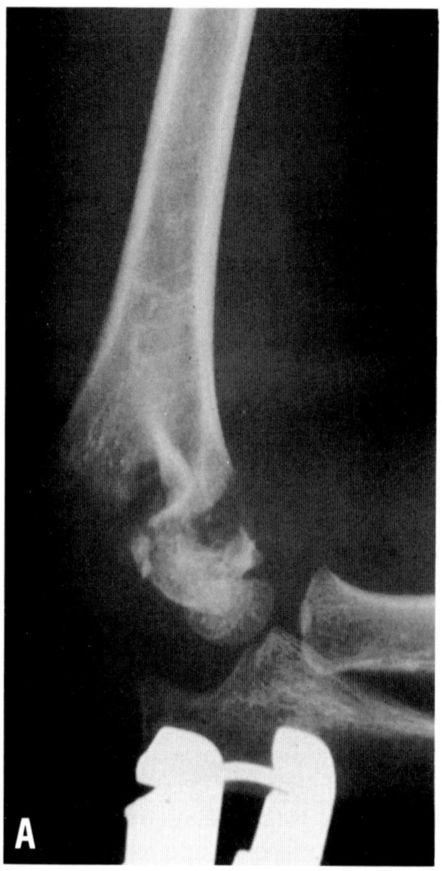

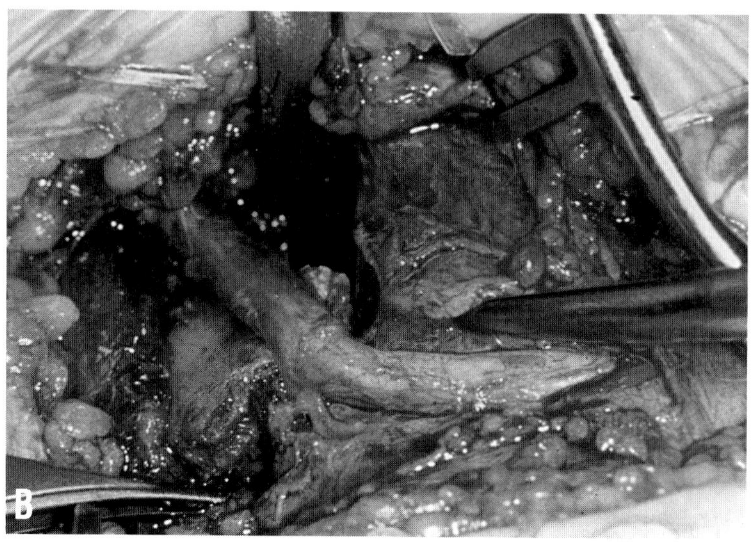

Figure 44–3. **(A)** *This supracondylar fracture was irreducible and was placed in traction. In traction, progressive ulnar neuropathy occurred, indicating a need for open reduction and internal fixation of this fracture.* **(B)** *At the time of open reduction, the ulnar nerve was found to be in the fracture site. An irreducible supracondylar fracture with associated nerve deficit represents an indication for open reduction and exploration.*

function has been reported to occur for as long as 9 months following injury.[82] Prolonged delay in recovery, or delayed onset of nerve palsy following fracture healing, alerts the clinician to the potential of entrapment of the nerve in fracture callus. Nerve palsies occurring secondary to entrapment by fracture callus have been reported for the median,[107] radial,[32,136] and ulnar nerves.[69] In the single case of ulnar nerve entrapment, symptoms of ulnar nerve palsy did not occur until 2 months after fracture. Either freeing the nerve from osseous tunnels and neurolysis, or transecting it at its entry to and exit from the fracture callus and accomplishing nerve repair, are acceptable options, depending on the extent of structural nerve damage.

The treatment of supracondylar humerus fractures may also be associated with nerve injuries. Closed reduction followed by immobilization in excessive flexion, or missed brachial artery injuries, may lead to inadequate perfusion of the forearm, with resulting Volkmann's ischemic contracture. This is the most devastating complication of this fracture, and all attempts should be made to prevent it. Olecranon pin traction has been associated with a high rate of ulnar nerve palsy, an injury occurring with treatment, rather than the injury.[33,54,129] Although we do not routinely use overhead olecranon pin tracture, we feel it is appropriate in some cases and can be used safely if attention is paid to the pin insertion site and excessive traction force is avoided.

At this time the standard treatment in most centers for supracondylar humerus fractures in children is closed reduction with percutaneous pin fixation.[4,5,50,64,85,93,103,135] Availability of intraoperative fluoroscopy has improved the clinician's ability to examine the reduction and has aided in the correct placement of the pins. Despite these advances, the incidence of iatrogenic nerve palsies is 2.8% when this technique is used. In a series of 143 supracondylar humerus fractures treated with percutaneous pin fixation, three ulnar nerve palsies and one radial nerve palsy resulted. All four injuries occurred with the placement of a medial pin. The authors concluded that two lateral pins should be used for stabilization whenever possible. When a medial pin is necessary for fracture stabilization, a small incision is made to expose the medial epicondyle in order to allow proper pin placement. All four reported nerve palsies resolved in 4 months.[118]

Indications for Operative Treatment of Nerves That Do Not Recover Spontaneously

In a retrospective review of displaced extension-type supracondylar fractures of the humerus, Culp and associates recommended that external neurolysis be carried out on nerves that do not improve spontaneously, 5 months following injury. Nine of 18 nerves in their series did not demonstrate clinical or electrophysiological evidence of return within that time. If the exposed nerve was in-continuity, the prognosis following neurolysis was excellent.[29a]

LATERAL CONDYLE FRACTURES

Fractures involving the lateral condylar or capitellar epiphysis of the humerus are common in children. One case of a transient radial nerve palsy occurring at the time of fracture has been reported. The nerve recovered spontaneously a few weeks after open reduction.[81] We have treated two patients with radial nerve palsies associated with lateral condylar fractures (Fig. 44-4). Both fractures were treated with open reduction of the lateral condyle. Exploration revealed that the radial nerves were intact, and both recovered spontaneously.

The radial nerve courses adjacent to the brachioradialis muscle anterior to the lateral condyle of the humerus. At the time of fracture, the lateral condyle is pulled laterally and spun anteriorly secondary to the pull of the extensor musculature. The spike of the lateral humeral metaphysis may be driven forward into the brachioradialis muscle mass, injuring the radial nerve.

Lateral condylar fractures, being intra-articular and often unstable, have a high rate of non-union. When the fracture fragments are displaced, open reduction and internal fixation is carried out. Displaced lateral condyle fractures, such as the one shown in Figure 44-5, are reduced and stabilized in an effort to prevent non-union and subsequent

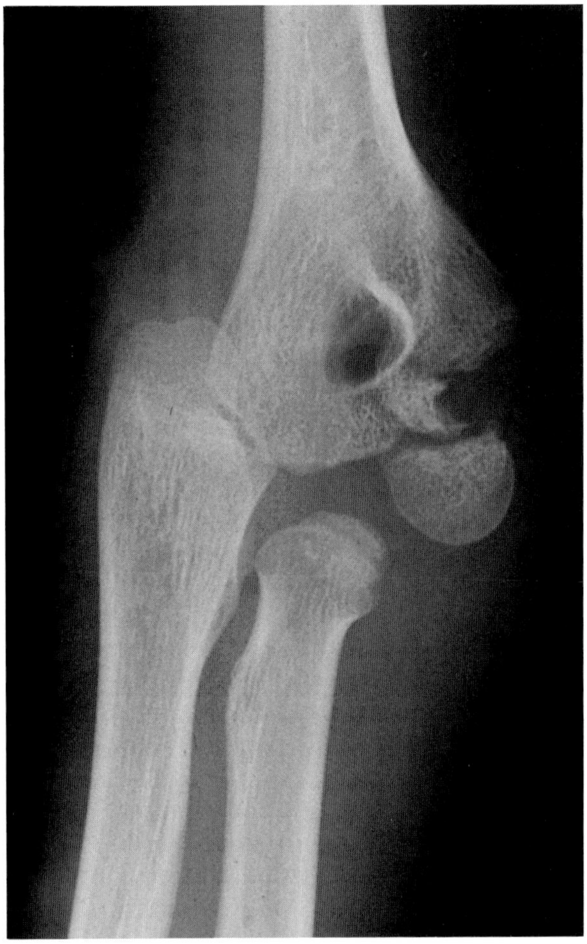

Figure 44–4. *In a displaced lateral condylar fracture, the metaphyseal fragment is generally spun anteriorly and may cause direct trauma to the radial nerve. In this case, open reduction and internal fixation were accomplished, and the radial nerve was explored and found to be intact. Displaced lateral condylar fractures should always be opened and internally fixed.*

valgus elbow deformity. If fracture non-union occurs, lateral growth diminishes and valgus elbow deformity results, increasing the risk of tardy ulnar nerve palsy (Fig. 44-6).[26,81,104,147]

Panas,[100] in 1878, first reported the association of cubitus valgus and tardy ulnar nerve palsy, although he credited Duchenne with prior knowledge of the condition.[67] Of the four cases Panas reported, one was a 40-year-old cobbler who had fractured an elbow as a child. Aside from an elbow deformity, he had had no problems with his upper extremity until 6 months prior to presenting for treatment. At that time he noticed increasing difficulty using his hammer in mending shoes. On examination it was evident that he had a complete ulnar nerve palsy.[84]

In 1898, Mouchet, in his doctoral thesis, first conceptualized the whole clinical picture with its most common cause, ensuing cubitus valgus and late ulnar nerve palsy.[91] Also in 1898, Curtis reported on ulnar nerve transposition after splitting the sheath.[37] Murphy, in 1916, described the procedure of ulnar nerve transposition commonly used today.[92] That same year Hunt termed the entity "tardy ulnar nerve paralysis."[59]

Following an established non-union of a lateral condyle or capitellar fracture in a child, the ulna is noted to slowly migrate laterally as the non-united capitellum migrates proximally. Resulting cubitus valgus leads to increased stretch on the ulnar nerve during elbow flexion. The nerve is compressed in the ulnar groove of the distal humerus.[138] Although symptoms of tardy ulnar nerve palsy may be noted as soon as 2 years after injury, in one patient symptoms were first noted 59 years after injury.[67] Forty percent of patients develop symptoms 20 to 30 years after injury.[67,84] Patients may present with a variety of symptoms, from intrinsic atrophy with sensory changes to intermittent paresthesias.[44]

Authors' Preferred Method

The treatment of choice is ulnar nerve transposition (see Chap. 78).[44] Decompression and transposition are recommended as soon as symptoms are noted. Recovery of nerve function is variable. Some authors recommend prophylactic ulnar nerve transposition in cases of established lateral condylar non-union, and we consider this a reasonable option when accompanied with fusion of the lateral condyle in situ.

MEDIAL CONDYLE AND EPICONDYLE HUMERUS FRACTURES

Forces that result in medial condyle and epicondyle humerus fractures in children are the same ones that result in elbow dislocations. The presence of

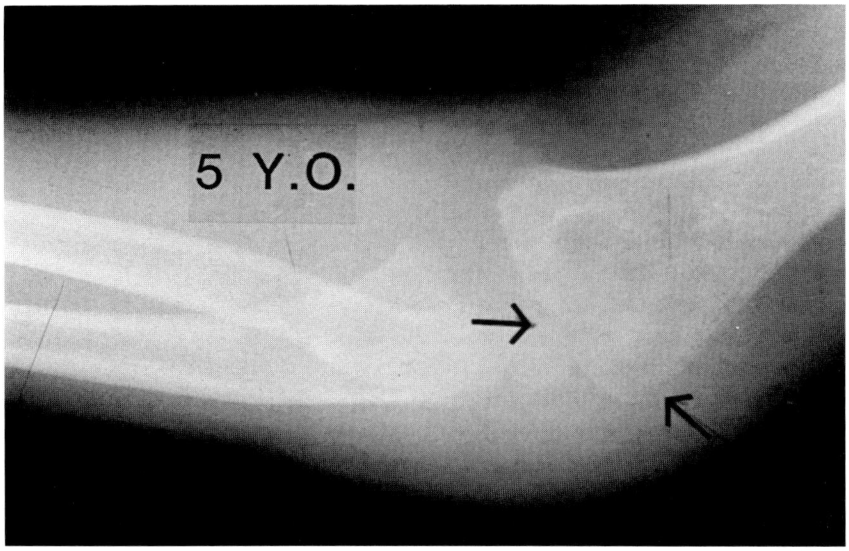

Figure 44–5. *Even minimally displaced lateral condylar fractures (2 mm) should be treated with pin fixation to prevent displacement and facilitate union.*

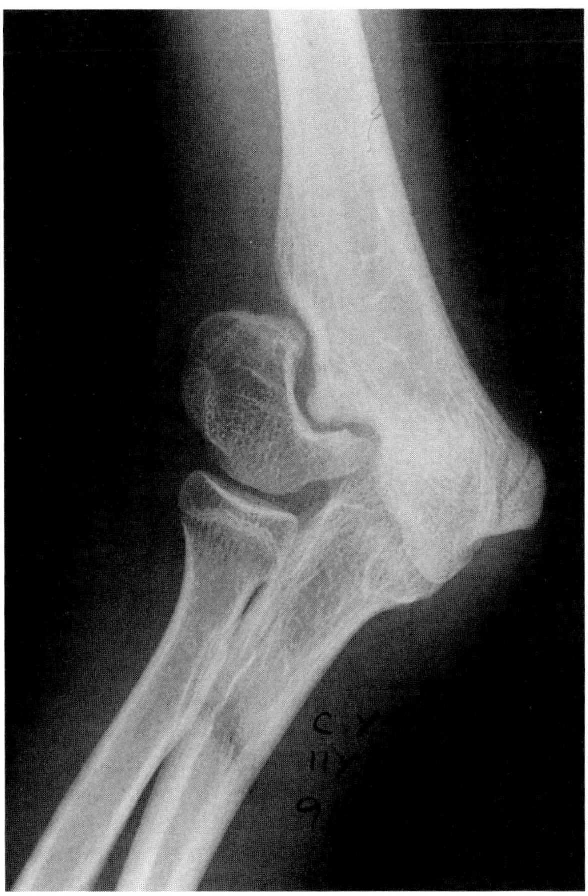

Figure 44–6. *A lateral condylar non-union will result in progressive valgus deformity and will often be accompanied by a tardy ulnar nerve palsy.*

a medial condyle or epicondyle fracture alerts the physician to the possibility of elbow subluxation or dislocation. Median nerve, ulnar nerve, and combined nerve palsies have been observed in these patients.

In 1818 Granger provided the first descriptions of medial condyle and epicondyle fractures in children. One case was associated with a dislocated elbow and one with a dislocated radial head. Of the five cases reported, three were associated with symptoms of ulnar nerve injury. While symptoms improved over time, they did not completely resolve. Granger concluded that the forces that lead to medial condyle and epicondyle fractures are the same forces that cause elbow dislocations, that concomitant ulnar nerve palsy is the result of local pressure, and that the nerve, although injured, is not disrupted.[47]

Ulnar nerve injuries are three times more common than median nerve injuries in association with elbow dislocations. The incidence of ulnar nerve palsy is 14%.[52,74] The incidence of medial epicondylar fracture or medial condyle fracture in patients with elbow dislocations is about 12% and is evenly distributed between adults and children.[74] Displacement of the medial epicondyle into the elbow joint in children following dislocation is common and is often associated with ulnar nerve injury.[2,19,28,42,49,74,101,116,145] In cases in which the medial epicondyle has been displaced into the joint, the incidence of ulnar nerve injury is reported to be as high as 60%.[101]

If closed reduction of the elbow is successful, the accompanying ulnar neuropathy generally resolves immediately.[94] If there is an associated medial epicondylar fracture and the fragment is within the joint, and if it cannot be reduced by closed means, open reduction is performed. Most authors recommend that ulnar nerve transposition be performed at the time of reduction.[2,6,28,74,145] The prognosis for recovery is good in patients who are treated promptly.

Median nerve injury is a well-described but unusual complication of dislocation of the elbow. It may be noted in association with ulnar nerve injury or, more seriously, with brachial artery injury.[74,109] It may be present on initial presentation or following closed reduction. If the injury is caused by a traction mechanism, successful closed reduction of the dislocated elbow generally results in immediate relief of median nerve symptoms.[94,116] One patient with isolated anterior interosseous nerve palsy had symptoms that persisted for 10 weeks before full function was regained.[12]

Persistent pain, paresthesias, or weakness in the median nerve distribution following reduction of an elbow dislocation alerts the clinician to the possibility of median nerve entrapment (Fig. 44-7). This is rare; only 18 cases are described in the literature.[49,52,77,113] In children ranging in age from 5 to 13, delays in diagnosis ranging from 7 days to 5 years have occurred.

Three types of median nerve entrapment have been described:[12]

1. Type 1: The nerve dislocates behind the medial epicondyle and is entrapped in the ulnar–humeral joint.
2. Type 2: The nerve is embedded in medial epicondyle fracture callus.
3. Type 3: The nerve is looped and trapped anteriorly in the ulnar–humeral joint.

In order to have entrapment of the type 1 or 2 variety, there must have been a medial epicondyle fracture at the time of elbow dislocation or disruption of the medial collateral ligament complex.[119] For type 1 entrapment to occur, the median nerve dislocates posteromedially behind the humerus. For type 2 entrapment to occur, the nerve subluxes posteromedially and becomes trapped by the medial epicondyle. It becomes engulfed in fracture callus as healing occurs. Following osseous healing, with types 1 and 2 median nerve entrapment, a characteristic X-ray finding, Matev's sign, is seen (Fig. 44-8).[52,79,119] In 1976, Matev described lucency with sclerotic margins on the ulnar side of

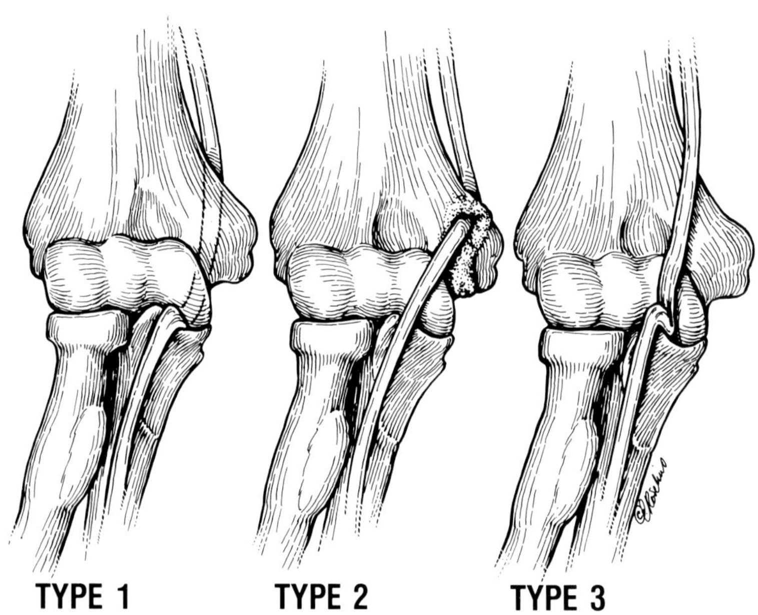

Figure 44–7. *This diagram demonstrates median nerve entrapment in the elbow joint after reduction of an elbow dislocation. Incongruous appearance on x-ray, in association with progressive median nerve symptoms, should alert the surgeon to this infrequent complication of dislocation of the elbow.*

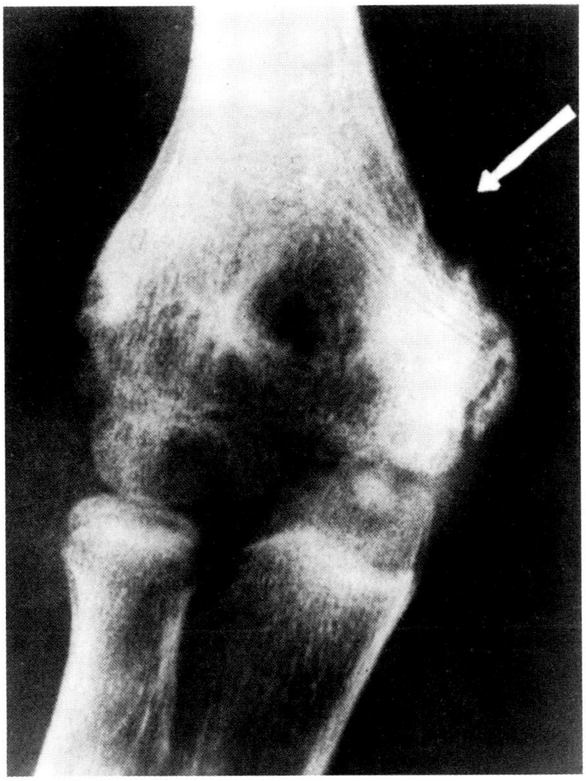

Figure 44–8. *Matev's sign, a lucency over the medial distal humeral metaphysis (arrow), indicates chronic posterior displacement of the median nerve seen in Type I and II median nerve entrapment.*

the distal humeral metaphysis seen on anteroposterior radiographs of two elbows.[79] The same X-ray finding had been noted by Roaf 19 years earlier.[113] In type 3 median nerve entrapment, the nerve may be transected[111] or may remain in continuity.[52,77,109,131]

Treatment of all three types, by neurolysis or by transecting the nerve followed by primary suture, have been reported with varying degrees of return of function.[52,77,79,109,111,131]

Authors' Preferred Method

In summary, the presence of a medial condyle or epicondyle fracture in a child alerts the clinician to the possibility of elbow subluxation or dislocation. The ulnar nerve is most commonly injured. If the elbow is reduced acceptably, ulnar neuropathy generally resolves quickly. If the medial epicondyle remains trapped in the elbow joint, open reduction with ulnar nerve exploration and transposition is carried out. Median nerve injuries are rare with elbow dislocations, with or without medial epicondyle or medial condyle fractures. Reduction of the elbow also results in rapid resolution of the median neuropathy.

Persistent median neuropathy, or worsening of symptoms following reduction, alerts the clinician to the possibility of median nerve entrapment, and early exploration is indicated.[6] If the nerve is in continuity and can be freed from surrounding tissue, external neurolysis generally provides satisfactory return of function. If the nerve is transected or engulfed in fracture callus, dividing the nerve ends at the edges of the bone with primary suture can also be expected to provide satisfactory results. Even in cases where the diagnosis of median nerve entrapment is delayed, operative exploration and repair is performed. Useful sensory recovery occurs, even after entrapment of 2 years or longer, but motor recovery is unlikely after a delay of 18 months (see Chap. 24).[52]

MONTEGGIA FRACTURES

In 1814, Monteggia described two cases of fractures of the proximal ulna associated with anterior dislocation of the radial head.[88] Bado subsequently included all cases of ulnar fractures with radial head dislocation into a classification of "Monteggia lesions."[8] He noted that lateral dislocation of the radial head was occasionally associated with radial nerve palsy. The radial nerve generally recovered spontaneously after 6 to 8 weeks.

Monteggia fractures are relatively uncommon. The incidence of nerve palsies with this injury ranges from 3% to 24%.[16,123] Nerve injuries are found in those types in which anterior,[20,41,132] posterior,[20,127,132] and lateral[20,124,125,127] dislocation of the radial head occurs. Radial[20,41,42,132] and posterior interosseous[42,124,125,127] nerve palsies are most common, but ulnar[20,132] and median[62] nerve injuries have been reported also.

The radial nerve is easily injured by anterior dislocation of the radial head. With this hyperextension injury, the anteriorly dislocated radial head places stretch on the radial nerve as the latter courses anterior to the elbow joint (Fig. 44-9). Because the nerve injury is associated with a dislo-

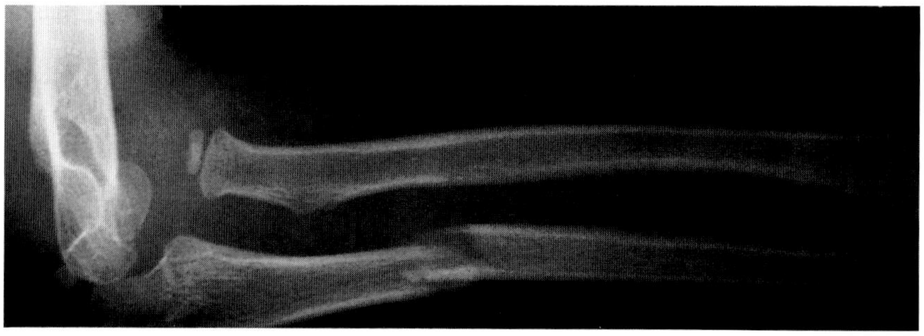

Figure 44–9. *Anterior displacement of the radial head occurs in association with mid or proximal ulnar fractures. This is known as the anterior Monteggia fracture and may be associated with radial nerve palsy.*

cation, in the absence of fracture, there are no sharp edges present to transect the nerve; thus, these injuries are most often neurapraxias.

Initial treatment is reduction of the Monteggia fracture and dislocation. Once the reduction is accomplished, the nerve palsy almost always resolves within 8 weeks.[16,123,125] One report noted recovery of posterior interosseous nerve palsy 12 months after injury.[124] There are two reports of Monteggia lesions that could not be reduced by closed means. At exploration the posterior interosseous nerve was found to be wrapped around the neck of the radius. In one case an anterior dislocation was present,[90] and in the other an anterolateral one.[124] Both patients regained full neurological function after the nerve was released at surgery.

Explorations of radial and ulnar nerves have been performed in nerve palsies persisting 5 to 18 weeks following Monteggia lesions.[132] Release of the radial nerve at the arcade of Frohse and the ulnar nerve at the cubital tunnel has resulted in full return of neurological function. An exception was noted in one patient with a posterior interosseous nerve palsy in whom the nerve was noted to be transected at the level of the radial head.

Two cases of tardy radial nerve palsy following unreduced Monteggia lesions have been reported. These occurred 39 and 65 years after the original injury.[7,72] Both patients were treated with operative exploration, neurolysis, and radial head excision. Both had significant improvement of radial nerve function postoperatively but did not regain full function.

Authors' Preferred Method

While neurological injuries in association with Monteggia fractures may involve the ulnar and median nerves, the radial nerve is most commonly injured. The vast majority of nerve palsies resolve within 8 weeks of successful closed reduction. If the Monteggia lesion cannot be reduced by closed means, open reduction is performed; the surgeon pays particular attention to the possibility that the posterior interosseous nerve may be wrapped around the radial neck. Persistent nerve palsy 8 weeks after reduction is an indication for electromyographic evaluation. Operative exploration and neurolysis is reserved for longstanding nerve palsies (4–6 months post-injury).

Unreduced Monteggia lesions may lead to the development of a tardy radial nerve palsy. These should be treated aggressively with operative exploration, neurolysis, and radial head excision. Significant, if incomplete, return of function in these limbs can be expected.

FOREARM FRACTURES

Diaphyseal fractures of both bones of the forearm in children are common, but the abundant soft-tissue protection and the low energy mechanisms make associated nerve lesions rare. In 1885, Puzy was the first to report a nerve injury associated with a forearm fracture.[110] The patient had a persistent ulnar neuropathy after the fracture healed. Six months after the injury, the ulnar nerve was found to trapped in fracture callus. The nerve was freed and full neurological function was regained by 8 months following surgery.

The only other reported injury was that of a partial transection of the ulnar nerve by a closed middle-third ulna fracture. Treatment consisted of neurolysis and partial nerve suture 4 months after injury. Full neurological recovery was reported.[49]

We treated a patient with a type 1 open ulna fracture in which the ulnar nerve was noted to have been completely transected by the sharp edge of one of the fracture fragments. Following debridement and irrigation of the fracture and intramedullary fixation of the ulna, primary nerve repair was performed. The patient regained considerable neurological function.

There are two reports of entrapment of the median nerve in greenstick fractures of the forearm; one was with a fracture of the radius[146] and the other with a fracture of the ulna.[97] In the patient with the greenstick radius fracture, closed reduction was required. Persistent complete median neuropathy was reported during the healing phase of the fracture. The patient came to operative exploration 39 days after injury. The median nerve was found to be trapped in fracture callus. The exposed ends of the nerve were transected and primary suture performed. The patient regained full motor and sensation function within 2 years.

In the patient with a greenstick fracture of the ulna, reduction was not required. Persistent partial median neuropathy was recorded during and after the healing phase. The forearm was explored 9 months after injury. The median nerve was found to be partially engulfed in the healed fracture. The nerve was partially transected and a fascicular repair performed. Neurological function improved but did not return to normal.

Authors' Preferred Method

Nerve injuries occurring with diaphyseal fractures in children are rare. When such a lesion presents, the clinician considers the possibility of nerve transection or entrapment. If nerve function does not improve rapidly following reduction, early exploration is justified. Late release and repair of median nerves entrapped in fracture callus have given varying results. Nerve palsies occurring after fracture reduction are an indicator for operative exploration.

WRIST AND HAND FRACTURES

Displaced distal radius fractures in children are common. Although median and ulnar nerve paresthesias are often encountered on initial examination in the emergency room, relief of symptoms is expected following successful closed reduction. Cases of persistent neuropathy following closed reduction are rare and should alert the clinician to the presence of potential nerve entrapment or laceration. While median nerve injuries are more common than ulnar nerve injuries, the precise incidence in children is unknown.[1]

The first case of nerve entrapment was reported by Gensoul in 1836.[45] He reported the case of a young girl with a complete median nerve palsy associated with a distal forearm fracture. The patient died of tetanus and, at autopsy, the median nerve was found to be caught between the fractured ends of the radius. Lewis and Miller reported a case of complete ulnar nerve transection by the sharp ends of an open distal radius fracture.[71]

Displaced distal radius fracture fragments may cause median nerve injuries in 2 ways. First, a dorsally displaced distal fragment may carry with it the median nerve, stretching it over the sharp proximal radial fragment (Fig. 44-10). The pronator quadratus may provide a cushion of sorts between the median nerve and the osseous fragments, but a significant stretch injury may occur. Transection of the nerve is rare.

The second method of median nerve injury in association with a distal radius fracture is acute carpal tunnel syndrome (see Chap. 65). The commonly recommended position following reduction is with the wrist in palmar flexion and ulnar deviation. While this position may help maintain reduction, significant increases in the interstitial pressure in the carpal canal occur. If there is a progressive median nerve lesion at presentation, acute carpal tunnel syndrome is suspected and pressure is measured within the carpal canal. Elevated carpal canal pressure in association with this fracture is an indication for carpal tunnel release. Excessive wrist volar flexion (>40°) is not recommended in the immobilization of these fractures, as the risk of median nerve compression is increased substantially in that position.

Fractures of the hand in children are rarely associated with nerve injuries, although nerve injuries have been noted in children with severe crush injuries or other major trauma.[57] Treatment of these injuries follows the same principles as for similar injuries in adults (see Chap. 43).

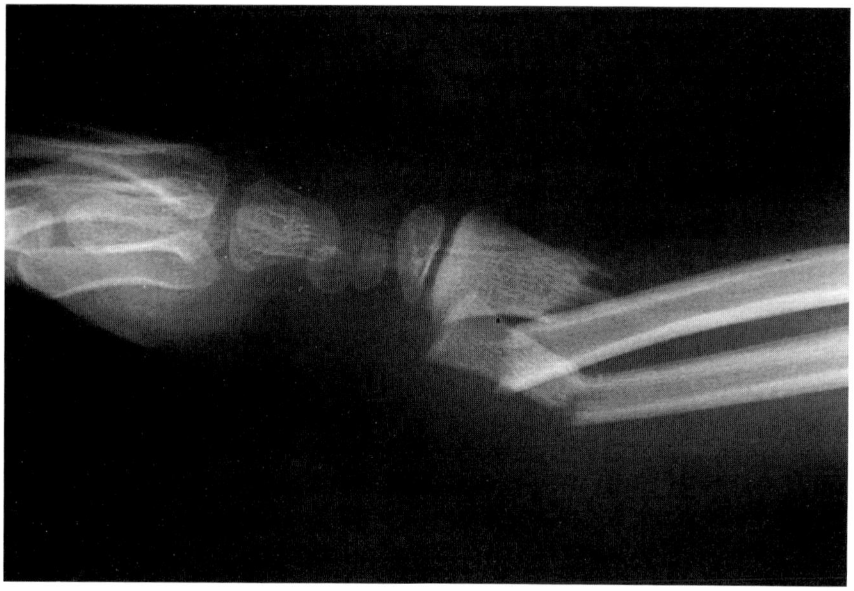

Figure 44–10. *Displaced distal radius fracture is the most common fracture in childhood. Median nerve dysfunction may result from direct trauma and stretch to the median nerve or an acute carpal tunnel syndrome.*

HIP FRACTURES

Fractures of the femoral neck and intertrochanteric region, even though they are often the result of high-energy trauma, are rarely associated with nerve injuries. In a review of 61 hip fractures in children, there were no associated nerve injuries reported.[25,89]

Hip dislocations in children are reportedly more common than hip fractures.[112] As in adults, posterior dislocation is more common than anterior dislocation.[10,102,144] In the case of a posteriorly dislocated hip, sciatic nerve palsy may be encountered.[102] Prompt reduction of the hip is performed, which relieves pressure on the sciatic nerve.

DISTAL FEMUR FRACTURES

While distal femoral epiphyseal separations in children are uncommon, they alert the clinician to a potential associated nerve injury. This was first recognized by Hutchinson, in 1893.[60] The mechanism of injury determines the direction of displacement of the distal femoral epiphysis. The distal femoral metaphysis, left uncovered, may transect or stretch an adjacent nerve.

Hyperextension injuries result in anterior displacement of the distal femoral epiphysis. This forces the distal femoral metaphysis into the popliteal fossa, where both nerve and vascular structures may be injured.[60,105,115] In the presence of a closed fracture with an associated nerve injury, treatment is directed at immediate reduction and casting. Internal fixation is done when stability is not achieved by closed treatment alone.

In an open fracture, the popliteal fossa is explored to visualize the neurovascular structures. Immediate repair is performed if an artery or neural injury is discovered. Suspicion of vascular injury warrants arteriographic examination. When vascular repair is required, four compartment distal fasciotomies are performed. The knee is immobilized in a position of flexion to relieve tension on neurovascular structures.

Valgus stress on the skeletally immature knee may result in medial displacement of the distal femoral epiphysis. The distal femoral metaphysis, displaced laterally, may injure the peroneal nerve.[76,114,133] Treatment of these fractures, when there are associated nerve injuries, is identical to that for hyperextension fractures, discussed above. As return of peroneal nerve function may be delayed for several months,[76,114] conservative treatment is initiated with appropriate splinting. Electromyographic studies are performed if there is no evidence of nerve recovery at 6 months.

PROXIMAL TIBIA FRACTURES

Hyperextension injuries of the knee in children may result in proximal tibial fractures through the proximal growth plate. In these cases the proximal tibial epiphysis displaces anteriorly. The most feared complication of this fracture is popliteal artery injury, as the proximal tibial metaphysis is displaced posteriorly into the popliteal space.[22,24,95] Neurological injury may occur also. Both transient and permanent peroneal nerve palsies have been reported in association with proximal tibial epiphyseal separations.[24]

Principles of treatment for these injuries are the same as for distal femoral epiphyseal separations associated with neurovascular injuries. Prompt reduction is obtained and vascular reassessment carried out.

We have treated one very unusual case of a teenager with an anteriorly angulated proximal tibial epiphyseal separation sustained while playing basketball. At presentation the patient's fracture was anteriorly angulated 45° and there was a complete peroneal nerve palsy. The fracture was reduced in the emergency room, and full peroneal function was noted after 30 minutes.

DISTAL TIBIAL FRACTURES

Except for severe open fractures of the ankle in children, such as lawn-mower injuries, an associated nerve injury accompanying a distal tibial fracture has not been reported in the literature. However, a nerve palsy may be detected in a severely displaced fracture in which the distal tibial metaphysis is pushed anteriorly against the superficial peroneal nerve or posteromedially against the tibial nerve. These nerve palsies generally resolve with fracture reduction.

FOOT FRACTURES

Nerve injuries associated with foot fractures in children occur in cases of crush injuries, high-energy trauma, and severe open injuries such as lawn mower accidents. In these cases, if nerve repair is impossible, reconstructive surgery is based on functional deficits.

REFERENCES

1. Abbott LC, Saunders JB de CM. Injuries of the median nerve in fractures of the lower end of the radius. Surg Gynecol Obstet 1933; 57:507–516.
2. Aitken AP, Childress HM. Intra-articular displacement of the internal epicondyle following dislocation. J Bone Joint Surg 1938; 20:161–166.
3. Aitken AP, Smith L, Blackette CW. Supracondylar fractures in children. Am J Surg 1943; 59:161–171.
4. Arino VL, Lluch EE, Ramirez AM, Ferrer J, Rodriguez L, Baixauli F. Percutaneous fixation of supracondylar fractures of the humerus in children. J Bone Joint Surg [Am] 1977; 59:914–916.
5. Aronson DD, Prager BI. Supracondylar fractures of the humerus in children. Clin Orthop 1987; 219:174–184.
6. Asher MA. Dislocations of the upper extremity in children. Orthop Clin North Am 1976; 7:583–591.
7. Austin R. Tardy palsy of the radial nerve from a Monteggia fracture. Injury 1976; 7:202–204.
8. Bado JL. The Monteggia lesion. Clin Orthop 1967; 50:71–86.
9. Banskota A, Volz RG. Traumatic laceration of the radial nerve following supracondylar fracture of the elbow. Clin Orthop 1984; 184:150–152.
10. Barquet A. Traumatic hip dislocation in childhood. A report of 26 cases and a review of the literature. Acta Orthop Scand 1979; 50:549–553.
11. Bateman JE. Trauma to nerves in limbs. Philadelphia: WB Saunders, 1962:.
12. Beverly MC, Fearn CB d'A. Anterior interosseous nerve palsy and dislocation of the elbow. Injury 1984; 16:126–128.
13. Bohler L. Conservative treatment of fresh closed fractures of the shaft of the humerus. J Trauma 1965; 5:464.
14. Bostman O, Bakalim G, Vainionpaa S, Wilppula E, Patiala H, Rokkanen P. Radial palsy in shaft fracture of the humerus. Acta Orthop Scand 1986; 57: 316–319.
15. Boyd HB, Altenberg AR. Fractures about the elbow in children. Arch Surg 1944; 49:213–224.
16. Boyd HB, Boals JC. The Monteggia lesion. a review of 159 cases. Clin Orthop 1969; 66:94.
17. Boyes JH. Bunnell's surgery of the hand, ed 5. Philadelphia: JB Lippincott, 1970:.
18. Brauniger H. Munchen Med Wchuschr 1900; 9: 290–291.
19. Broca A, Mouchet A. Complications nerveuses de

l'extremite inferieure de l'humerus. Rev Chir Orthop 1899; 19:701–744.

20. Bryan RS. Monteggia fracture of the forearm. J Trauma 1971; 11:992–998.
21. Bunnell S. Hand surgery: The surgery of the nerves of the upper extremity. American Academy of Orthopaedic Surgeons Instructional Course Lectures 1956; 13:101.
22. Burkhart SS, Peterson HA. Fractures of the proximal tibial epiphysis. J Bone Joint Surg [Am] 1979; 61:996–1002.
23. Byer BF. Management of humeral shaft fractures. Arch Surg 1960; 81:914.
24. Canale ST. Fractures and dislocations in children. In: Crenshaw AH, ed. Campbell's operative orthopaedics, ed 7. St. Louis: CV Mosby, 1987: 1833–2013.
25. Canale ST, Bourland WL. Fracture of the neck and intertrochanteric region of the femur in children. J Bone Joint Surg [Am] 1977; 59:431.
26. Conway FM. Traumatic ulnar neuritis. Ann Surg 1933; 97:425–432.
27. Cotton FJ. Elbow fractures in children. Ann Surg 1902; 35:75.
28. Cotton FJ. Elbow dislocation and ulnar nerve injury. J Bone Joint Surg 1929; 11:348–352.
29. Coventry MB, Henderson CC. Supracondylar fractures of the humerus: 49 cases in children. Rocky Mountain Med J 1956; 53:458–465.

29a. Culp RW, Osterman AL, Davidson RS, Skirven T, Bora FW. Neural injuries associated with supracondylar fractures of the humerus in children. J Bone Joint Surg [Am] 1990; 72:1211–1215.

30. D'Ambrosia RD. Supracondylar fractures of humerus: Prevention of cubitus varus. J Bone Joint Surg [Am] 1972; 54:60–66.
31. Dodge HS. Displaced supracondylar fractures of the humerus in children: Treatment by Dunlop's traction. J Bone Joint Surg [Am] 1972; 54:1408–1418.
32. Duthie HL. Radial nerve in osseous tunnel at humeral fracture site diagnosed radiographically. J Bone Joint Surg [Br] 1957; 39:746–747.
33. Edman P, Lohr G. Supracondylar fractures of the humerus treated with olecranon traction. Acta Chir Scand 1963; 126:505–516.
34. Eid AM. Reduction of displaced supracondylar fracture of the humerus in children by manipulation in flexion. Acta Orthop Scand 1978; 49:39–45.
35. El-Ahwany MD. Supracondylar fractures of the humerus in children with a note on the surgical correction of late cubitus varus. Injury 1974; 6: 45–56.
36. El-Sharkawi AH, Fattah HA. Treatment of displaced supracondylar fractures of the humerus in children in full extension and supination. J Bone Joint Surg [Br] 1965; 47:273–279.
37. Feindel W, Stratford J. Cubital compression in tardy ulnar palsy. Can Med Assoc J 1958; 78:351.
38. Fenton RL. Radial nerve transplant and internal fixation in cases of humerus fracture with radial nerve injury. Bull Hosp Joint Dis 1964; 25:71.
39. Fisher TR, McGeoch CM. Severe injuries of the radial nerve treated by sural nerve grafting. Injury 1985; 16:411–412.
40. Fowles JV, Kassab MT. Displaced supracondylar fractures of the elbow in children. J Bone Joint Surg [Br] 1974; 56:490–500.
41. Freundlich BD, Spinner M. Nerve compression syndrome in derangements of the proximal and distal radial ulnar joints. Bull Hosp Joint Dis 1968; 29:38–47.
42. Galbraith KA, McCullough CJ. Acute nerve injury as a complication of closed fractures or dislocations of the elbow. Injury 1979; 11:159–164.
43. Garcia A, Maeck BH. Radial nerve injuries in fractures of the shaft of the humerus. Am J Surg 1960; 99:625.
44. Gay JR, Love JG. Diagnosis and treatment of tardy paralysis of the ulnar nerve. J Bone Joint Surg 1947; 29:1087–1097.
45. Gensoul M. Arch Gen de Med 1836; 11:198.
46. Goldner JL, Kelley JM. Radial nerve injuries. South Med J 1958; 51:873–883.
47. Granger B. On a particular fracture of the inner condyle of the humerus. Edinburgh Medical and Surgical Journal 1818; 14:196–201.
48. Gruber MA, Hudson OC. Supracondylar fracture of the humerus in childhood. J Bone Joint Surg [Am] 1964; 46:1245–1252.
49. Gurdjian ES, Smathers HM. Peripheral nerve injury in fractures and dislocations of long bones. J Neurosurg 1945; 2:202–219.
50. Haddad RJ, Saer JK, Riordan DC. Percutaneous pinning of displaced supracondylar fractures of the elbow in children. Clin Orthop 1970; 71:112–117.
51. Hagen R. Skin traction treatment of supracondylar fractures of the humerus in children. Acta Orthop Scand 1964; 35:138–148.
52. Hallett J. Entrapment of the median nerve after dislocation of the elbow. J Bone Joint Surg [Br] 1981; 63:408–412.
53. Hanlon CR, Estes WL. Fractures in childhood, a statistical analysis. Am J Surg 1954; 87:312–323.

54. Henrikson B. Supracondylar fracture of the humerus in children. Acta Chir Scand 1966; supp 369:67–72.
55. Hohl JC. Fractures of the humerus in children. Orthop Clin North Am 1976; 7:557–582.
56. Holstein A, Lewis GB. Fractures of the humerus with radial-nerve paralysis. J Bone Joint Surg [Am] 1963; 45:1382–1388.
57. Howard FM. Ulnar-nerve palsy in wrist fractures. J Bone Joint Surg [Am] 1961; 43:1197–1201.
58. Hoyer A. Treatment of supracondylar fracture of the humerus by skeletal traction in an abduction splint. J Bone Joint Surg [Am] 1952; 34:623–637.
59. Hunt JR. Tardy or late paralysis of the ulnar nerve. JAMA 1916; 66:4.
60. Hutchinson J Jr. Lectures on injuries to the epiphyses and their results. Br Med J 1894; 1:669–673.
61. Jacobs RL. Supracondylar fracture of the humerus in children. Illinois Med J 1967; 132:696–704.
62. Jessing P. Monteggia lesions and their complicating nerve damage. Acta Orthop Scand 1975; 46:601–609.
63. Jones ET, Louis DS. Median nerve injuries associated with supracondylar fractures of the humerus in children. Clin Orthop 1980; 150:181–186.
64. Jones KG. Percutaneous pin fixation of fractures of the lower end of the humerus. Clin Orthop 1967; 50:53–69.
65. Kamal AS, Auston RT. Dislocation of the median nerve and brachial artery in supracondylar fractures of the humerus. Injury 1981; 12:161–164.
66. Karlsson J, Thorsteinsson T, Thorleifsson R, Arnason H. Entrapment of the median nerve and brachial artery after supracondylar fractures of the humerus in children. Arch Orthop Trauma Surg 1986; 104:389–391.
67. Keschner M, Berman W. Tardy or late ulnar neuritis. Med J Rec 1930; 132:480–483.
68. Kettelkamp DB, Alexander H. Clinical review of radial nerve injury. J Trauma 1967; 7:424–432.
69. Lalanandham T, Laurence WN. Entrapment of the ulnar nerve in the callus of a supracondylar fracture of the humerus. Injury 1984; 16:129–130.
70. Laurence W. Supracondylar fractures of the humerus in children. Br J Surg 1956; 44:143–147.
71. Lewis, Dean, Miller EM. Tr Am Surg Assoc 1922; 40:489–581.
72. Lichter RL, Jacobsen T. Tardy palsy of the posterior interosseous nerve with a Monteggia fracture. J Bone Joint Surg [Am] 1975; 57:124–125.
73. Liddell WA. Neurovascular complications in widely displaced supracondylar fractures of the humerus (abstract). J Bone Joint Surg [Br] 1967; 49:806.
74. Linscheid RL, Wheeler DK. Elbow dislocations. JAMA 1965; 194:1171–1176.
75. Lipscomb PR, Burleson RJ. Vascular and neural complications in supracondylar fractures of the humerus in children. J Bone Joint Surg [Am] 1955; 37:487–492.
76. Lombardo SJ, Harvey JP Jr. Fractures of the distal femoral epiphyses: Factors influencing prognosis. A review of 34 cases. J Bone Joint Surg [Am] 1977; 59:742–751.
77. Mannerfelt L. Median nerve entrapment after dislocation of the elbow. J Bone Joint Surg [Br] 1968; 50:152–155.
78. Martin DF, Tolo VT, Sellers DS, Weiland AJ. Radial nerve laceration and retraction associated with a supracondylar fracture of the humerus. J Hand Surg [Am] 1989; 14:542–545.
79. Matev I. A radiological sign of entrapment of the median nerve in the elbow joint after posterior dislocation. J Bone Joint Surg [Br] 1976; 58:353–355.
80. Maylahn DJ, Fahey JJ. Fractures of the elbow in children. JAMA 1958; 166:220–228.
81. McDonnell DP, Wilson JC. Fractures of the lower end of the humerus in children. J Bone Joint Surg [Am] 1948; 30:347–358.
82. McGraw JJ, Akbarnia BA, Hanel DP, Keppler L, Burge RE. Neurological complications resulting from supracondylar fractures of the humerus in children. J Pediatr Orthop 1986; 6:647–650.
83. Meya U, Hacke W. Anterior interosseous nerve syndrome following supracondylar lesions of the median nerve: Clinical findings and electrophysiological investigations. J Neurol 1983; 229:91–96.
84. Miller EM. Late ulnar nerve palsy. Surg Gynecol Obstet 1924; 38:37–46.
85. Millis MB, Singer IJ, Hall JE. Supracondylar fracture of the humerus in children. Clin Orthop 1984; 188:90–97.
86. Mitchell WJ, Adams JP. Supracondylar fractures of the humerus in children. JAMA 1961; 175:573–577.
87. Moehring HD. Irreducible supracondylar fracture of the humerus complicated by anterior interosseous nerve palsy. Clin Orthop 1986; 206:228–232.
88. Monteggia GB. Istituzioni Chirurgiche J 1814.
89. Moore RW, Canale ST. Hip fractures in children: Update. Presented at the American Academy of

Orthopaedic Surgeons Annual Meeting, Los Angeles, 1989.
90. Morris AH. Irreducible Monteggia lesion with radial-nerve entrapment. J Bone Joint Surg [Am] 1974; 56:1744–1746.
91. Mouchet A. These de Doct. Paris, 1898.
92. Murphy JB. Cicatricial fixation of ulnar nerve from ancient cubitus valgus—release and transference to new site. Clin John B Murphy 1916; 5:661–670.
93. Nacht JL, Ecker ML, Chung SMK, Lotke PA, Das M. Supracondylar fractures of the humerus in children treated by closed reduction and percutaneous pinning. Clin Orthop 1983; 177:203–209.
94. Neviaser JS, Wickstrom JK. Dislocation of the elbow: A retrospective study of 115 patients. South Med J 1977; 70:172–173.
95. Nicholson JT. Epiphyseal fractures about the knee. American Academy of Orthopaedic Surgeons Instructional Course Lectures 1967; 18:74–83.
96. Nilsson S, Svartholm F. Fracture of the upper end of the humerus in children. Acta Chir Scand 1965; 130:433–439.
97. Nunley JA, Urbaniak JR. Partial bony entrapment of the median nerve in a greenstick fracture of the ulna. J Hand Surg 1980; 5:557–559.
98. Ottolenghi CE. Acute ischemic syndrome: Its treatment; prophylaxis of Volkmann's syndrome. Amer J Orthop 1960; 2:312.
99. Packer JW, Foster RR, Garcia A, Grantham SA. The humeral fracture with radial nerve palsy: Is exploration warranted? Clin Orthop 1972; 88:34–38.
100. Panas. Sur une cause peu connue de paralysie du nerf cubital. Arch Gen de Med 1878; 2:5.
101. Patrick J. Fracture of the medial epicondyle with displacement into the elbow joint. J Bone Joint Surg 1946; 28:143–147.
102. Pearson DE, Mann RJ. Traumatic hip dislocation in children. Clin Orthop 1973; 92:189–194.
103. Pirone AM, Graham HK, Krajbich JI. Management of displaced extension-type supracondylar fractures of the humerus in children. J Bone Joint Surg [Am] 1988; 70:641–650.
104. Platt H. The pathogenesis and treatment of traumatic neuritis of the ulnar nerve in the postcondylar groove. Br J Surg 1926; 13:409–431.
105. Poland J. Traumatic separation of the epiphyses. London: Smith, Elder, 1898.
106. Pollock FH, Drake D, Bovill EG, Day L, Trafton PG. Treatment of radial neuropathy associated with fractures of the humerus. J Bone Joint Surg [Am] 1981; 63:239–243.
107. Post M, Haskell SS. Reconstruction of the median nerve following entrapment in supracondylar fracture of the humerus. J Trauma 1974; 14:252–264.
108. Prietto CA. Supracondylar fractures of the humerus. J Bone Joint Surg [Am] 1979; 61:425–428.
109. Pritchard DJ, Linscheid RL, Svien HJ. Intra-articular median nerve entrapment with dislocation of the elbow. Clin Orthop 1973; 90:100–103.
110. Puzy. Lancet 1885; :979.
111. Rana NA, Kenwright J, Taylor RG, Rushworth G. Complete lesion of the median nerve associated with dislocation of the elbow joint. Acta Orthop Scand 1974; 45:365–369.
112. Rang M. Children's fractures. Philadelphia: JB Lippincott, 1974:
113. Roaf R. Foramen in the humerus caused by the median nerve. J Bone Joint Surg [Br] 1957; 39: 748–749.
114. Roberts JM. Fracture separation of the distal femoral epiphysis, in proceedings of the American Academy of Orthopaedic Surgeons. J Bone Joint Surg [Am] 1973; 55:1324.
115. Roberts JM. Fractures and dislocations of the knee. In: Rockwood CA, Wilkins KE, King RE, eds. Fractures in children. Philadelphia: JB Lippincott, 1984:891–982.
116. Roberts PH. Dislocation of the elbow. Br J Surg 1969; 56:806–815.
117. Rowell PJW. Arterial occlusion in juvenile humeral supracondylar fracture. Injury 1974; 6:254–256.
118. Royce RO, Dutkowsky JP, Kasser JR, Rand FR. Neurological complications following K-wire fixation of supracondylar fractures in children. Accepted for publication in J Pediatr Ortho, 1990.
119. St. Clair Strange FG. Entrapment of the median nerve after dislocation of the elbow. J Bone Joint Surg [Br] 1982; 64:224–225.
120. Shah JJ, Bhatti NA. Radial nerve paralysis associated with fractures of the humerus. Clin Orthop 1983; 172:171–176.
121. Shaw JL, Sakellarides H. Radial-nerve paralysis associated with fractures of the humerus. J Bone Joint Surg [Am] 1967; 49:899–902.
122. Skolnick MD, Hall JE, Micheli LJ. Supracondylar fractures of the humerus in children. Orthopedics 1980; 3:395–406.
123. Smith F. Monteggia fractures. Surg Gynecol Obstet 1947; 85:630.
124. Spar I. A neurologic complication following Monteggia fracture. Clin Orthop 1977; 122:207–209.
125. Spinner M. The arcade of Frohse and its relation-

ship to posterior interosseous nerve paralysis. J Bone Joint Surg [Br] 1968; 50:809.

126. Spinner M. Injuries to the major branches of peripheral nerves of the forearm, ed 2. Philadelphia: WB Saunders, 1972:

127. Spinner M, Freundlich BD, Teicher J. Posterior interosseous nerve palsy as a complication of Monteggia fractures in children. Clin Orthop 1968; 58:141–145.

128. Spinner M, Schreiber SN. Anterior interosseous nerve paralysis as a complication of supracondylar fractures of the humerus in children. J Bone Joint Surg [Am] 1969; 51:1584–1590.

129. Staples OS. Supracondylar fractures of the humerus in children. JAMA 1958; 168:730–734.

130. Staples OS. Dislocation of the brachial artery. J Bone Joint Surg [Am] 1965; 47:1525–1532.

131. Steiger RN, Larrick RB, Meyer TL. Median-nerve entrapment following elbow dislocation in children. J Bone Joint Surg [Am] 1969; 51:381–385.

132. Stein F, Grabias SL, Deffer PA. Nerve injuries complicating Monteggia lesions. J Bone Joint Surg [Am] 1971; 53:1432–1436.

133. Stephens DC, Louis DS, Louis E. Traumatic separation of the distal femoral epiphyseal cartilage plate. J Bone Joint Surg [Am] 1974; 56:1383–1390.

134. Sunderland S. Nerves and nerve injuries. London: Churchill-Livingstone, 1968:.

135. Swenson AL. Treatment of supracondylar fractures of the humerus by Kirschner-wire transfixion. J Bone Joint Surg [Am] 1948; 30:993–997.

136. Symeonides PP, Paschaloglou C, Pagalides T. Radial nerve enclosed in the callus of a supracondylar fracture. J Bone Joint Surg [Br] 1975; 57:523.

137. Vogt P. Dtsch Z Chir 1877; 7:144–159.

138. Wadsworth TG. Injuries of the capitular (lateral humeral condylar) epiphysis. Clin Orthop 1972; 85:127–142.

139. Watson-Jones R. Primary nerve lesions in injuries of the elbow and wrist. J Bone Joint Surg 1930: 12:121–140.

140. Webb AJ, Sherman FC. Supracondylar fractures of the humerus in children. J Pediatr Orthop 1989; 9:315–325.

141. Weiland AJ, Meyer S, Tolo VT, Berg HL, Mueller J. Surgical treatment of displaced supracondylar fractures of the humerus in children. J Bone Joint Surg [Am] 1978; 60:657–661.

142. Whitson RO. Relation of the radial nerve to the shaft of the humerus. J Bone Joint Surg [Am] 1954; 36:85–88.

143. Wilkins KE. Fractures and dislocations of the elbow region. In: Rockwood CA, Wilkins KE, King RE, eds. Fractures in children. Philadelphia: JB Lippincott, 1984:363–576.

144. Wilson DW. Traumatic dislocation of the hip in children: A report of four cases. J Trauma 1966; 6:739–743.

145. Wilson PD. Fractures and dislocations in the region of the elbow. Surg Gynecol Obstet 1933; 56:335–359.

146. Wolfe JS, Eyring EJ. Median-nerve entrapment within a greenstick fracture. J Bone Joint Surg [Am] 1974; 56:1270–1272.

147. Zeier FG. Lateral condylar fracture and its many complications. Orthop Review 1981; 10:49–55.

45

Nerve Injuries Associated With Gunshot Wounds of the Extremities

George E. Omer, Jr.

AUTHOR'S KEY POINTS

- Impacting projectiles, rather than weapons, are classified into velocity ranges that correlate with wound severity: low (<1200 feet [370 meters] per second), medium (1200–2500 feet [372–760 meters] per second), and high (> 2500 feet [760 meters] per second).
- The potential for tissue disruption depends on projectile mass and projectile striking velocity; the actual amount, type, and location of disruption depend on projectile shape, construction, and target tissue type. For non-military gunshot wounds, information is obtained about the type of weapon used and the distance from which the weapon was fired.
- The frequency of injury to peripheral nerve in the upper extremity in armed conflict has been, in descending order, ulnar, median, radial, and musculocutaneous nerves. In the lower extremity, the sciatic nerve is most commonly injured, followed by the peroneal, tibial, and femoral nerves.
- Appropriate management of gunshot wounds of the perforating or penetrating types is based on early operative intervention. The operative technique of *debridement* has two objectives: the excision of necrotic tissue and the incision of fascial sheaths that impede the circulation of edematous tissue.
- A striking decline in the incidence of clostridial myositis (from 5% of those wounded in World War I to 0.7% in World War II and 0.08% in the Korean War) correlates more closely with the use of antibiotics on the battlefield than with changing techniques in debridement, since debridement techniques remained essentially unchanged during that time.
- As transected nerve stumps shorten following nerve transection, the epineurium of the proximal and distal stumps is sutured with very fine monofilament wire to adjacent soft tissue to prevent retraction. The location of the neural stumps can be identified later on roentgenograms.
- A clean wound, fracture stability, restoration of adequate circulation, and skin closure over neurovascular structures have priority over peripheral nerve repair. After optimal wound care is accomplished, neurorrhaphy is indicated as soon as possible. A variable loss of neural function is seen with a delay to suture (about 1% of maximal performance for every 6 days of delay).
- The return of useful function depends as much on the total response of the extremity to the injury as on the regeneration of the injured nerve. Spontaneous regeneration may be delayed for up to 11 months.

- In a prospective study of gunshot wounds during the Vietnam War, spontaneous recovery was noted after 69% of low-velocity gunshot wounds; 69% of high-velocity gunshot wounds follow the same pattern. Neurapraxia lesions recover in 1 to 4 months, axonotmesis lesions in 4 to 9 months.
- About three fourths of causalgia cases from gunshot wound injuries of peripheral nerves involve the median or sciatic–tibial nerves. The lower extremity is involved more often than the upper extremity, and the onset of pain occurs within 24 hours of injury in half the cases. Gunshot wounds are particularly likely to provoke causalgia.
- The results of two recent series from Vietnam indicate that in only 40% to 45% of cases does nerve repair result in progressive functional return over the first 1 to 2 years after repair.

HISTORY

Gunshot wounds were first recorded in Europe during the Hundred Years War (1337–1453). One of the first detailed accounts of gunshot wound therapy was published in 1497 by Hieronymus Brunschwig, an Alsatian army surgeon who considered gunshot wounds poisonous.[17] This was not an individual idiosyncrasy, as a book entitled "Fifty Strange and Wonderful Cures of Gunshot Wounds" was published in 1693. The most popular treatment recorded consisted of ignoring the patient's wound and generously applying magic salve to the gun that had fired the missile. If the patient died, it was concluded that the wrong gun had been treated.[34]

There were more reasonable approaches: The outstanding surgeon of the Renaissance, Ambroise Paré, in his 1545 treatise on gunshot wounds, emphasized the need for cleanliness in all operative work.[3,4] Removal of badly traumatized tissue was advocated as early as 1563 by the Elizabethan surgeon Thomas Gale.[19] William Clowes, the greatest surgeon of Elizabethan England, emphasized the removal of contaminated and traumatized tissue in his treatise on gunshot wounds published in 1588, about 250 years after gunpowder began to be used in warfare.[15] The same procedure was recommended by Henry Gray in 1915 and gained fame as the "debridement" technique of World War I.[19]

WOUND BALLISTICS

Wound ballistics is the study of the effects on the body produced by penetrating projectiles.[15] In 1894, Horsley identified the explosive pattern of gunshot wounds and concluded that the cause of tissue disruption was the high velocity and spin of the bullet.[1] Woodruff reported in 1898 that during the missile's passage, a cavity was created in the target medium into which air was sucked. Borrowing a marine engineering term, he called this effect "cavitation."[1] The theory was correct and was later confirmed by high-speed photography.

The caliber (bore diameter) of small arms does not usually exceed 0.60 inch or 15.24 mm.[16] American and British authorities indicate small-arms caliber in millimeters or in hundredths or thousandths of an inch (Table 45-1), while the caliber of shotguns is expressed as gauge or bore (Table 45-2). Impacting projectiles, rather than weapons, are classified into velocity ranges that correlate with wound severity: low, less than 1200 ft/sec (370 m/sec); medium, 1200 to 2500 ft/sec (370–760 m/sec); and high, above 2500 ft/sec (760 m/sec).[47] The energy transferred from the missile, in foot-pounds of energy absorbed, can be quantitated by the formula

$$KE = W(V_1^2 - V_2^2)/2g,$$

Table 45-1. *Some Common Designations of Small Arms Calibers*

Inches	Millimeters
.22 (.222, .223)	5.56
.243 (.244)	6.00
.25	6.35
.264	6.50
.30 (.308)	7.62
.32	7.65
.357 (.38)	9.00
.45	11 (11.43)
.50	12.7

(From Finck PA. Ballistic and forensic pathologic aspects of missile wounds. Conversion between Anglo-American and metric system units. Milit Med 1965;130:545.)

where W is bullet weight in pounds, g is gravitational acceleration (32.2), and

$$(V_1 - V_2)$$

is the effective velocity of the injury (striking velocity minus residual velocity, if the bullet leaves the target) (Table 45-3).[1,47]

Studies done at the wound ballistics laboratory of the Letterman Army Institute of Research have demonstrated the location along the tissue path at which projectiles cause tissue disruption and the type of disruption (crush from direct contact with the projectiles, or stretch from temporary cavitation).[14,15] Comparison of wound profiles illustrates the fallacy of attempting to judge wound severity using velocity alone.[26] It is widely believed that high-velocity projectiles cause wounds that must be treated by extensive excision of tissue around the missile path,[61] and low-velocity missile wounds need little or no treatment.[31] Tissue disruption studies done at penetration depths of 12 and 24 cm emphasize that increased velocity is pertinent only with greater tissue penetration.[14,15] The M-16 has far more potential for damage than the .22 long rifle, but this potential generally is realized only with greater tissue penetration. In most soft-tissue extremity wounds, with less than 12 cm of penetration, the high-velocity M-16 bullet would not be expected to cause more tissue disruption than the low-velocity .22 long rifle bullet. The potential for tissue disruption depends on projectile mass and projectile striking velocity; the actual amount, type, and location of disruption depends on projectile shape and construction and target tissue type.[14] Therefore, marked tissue disruption is typical on abdominal perforations with the M-16 bullet, while extremity wounds may be minimal.

ENVIRONMENT

Gunshot wounds are on the increase around the world. An average of more than 2.5 million new handguns are legally sold in the United States each year. The number of nonfatal shooting injuries unintentionally inflicted has been estimated at 50,000 annually, with 59,000 fatal injuries per year.[51] In the nonmilitary situation, information is obtained concerning the type of weapon used and the distance from which the weapon was fired. For example, a hunting accident usually involves a weapon with known velocity, but there often is a delay in reaching the hospital, and the wound carries a risk of contamination with soilborne or gas-forming organisms. Contact wounds are produced when the barrel of a gun is held against the skin. Close-range wounds are defined as those in which

Table 45-2. *Calibers of Shotguns*

Bore or Gauge	Inches	Millimeters
4-gauge	.935	23.75
8-gauge	.835	21.21
10-gauge	.775	19.68
12-gauge	.729	18.52
16-gauge	.662	16.81
20-gauge	.615	15.62
28-gauge	.550	13.97
.410-bore	.410	10.41
67.5-gauge		

(From Finck PA. Ballistic and forensic pathologic aspects of missile wounds. Conversion between Anglo-American and metric system units. Milit Med 1965;130:545.)

Table 45–3. *Handgun and Rifle Ammunition in Order of Velocity*

Velocity Category	Caliber	Bullet Wt. (grains)	Muzzle Velocity (ft/sec)	Energy (ft/lb)
LOW	.38 special	148 WC	740	180
	.25 auto	50 FJ	810	70
	.45 long Colt	255 LRN	820	380
	.38 spec	158 LRN	920	300
	9 mm	115 FJ	1130	330
	.22 LR	40 LRN	1180	120
MEDIUM	.357 magnum	158 LRN	1230	530
	.44 magnum	240 SWC	1330	940
	.30 (M-1)	111 FJ	1970	960
	.30-30	170	2200	1830
HIGH	.30-06	180	2710	2940
	.375	270	2720	4440
	7.62 mm (M-14)	150 FJ	2750	2520
	.270	130	3140	2850
	5.56 mm (M-16)	55 FJ	3200	1250

LR, long rifle; WC, wadcutter; FJ, full metal jacket; LRN, lead round nose; SWC, semi-wadcutter; M-1, M-14, M-16, all US military rifles.
(Data from Ragsdale BD. Gunshot wounds: a historical perspective. Milit Med 1984;149:301–315.)

the weapon was fired from 2.5 feet or less; the bullet and the expelled gases, smoke, and gunpowder particles are driven inside the skin.

Shotgun injuries, often with extensive tissue damage and contamination, are common. Range is a key variable in determining the severity of this wound, but in one study it was difficult to obtain an accurate history of such important data as the distance of the patient from the weapon at the time of injury, the stance of the patient at the time of injury, or even the type of weapon involved.[25] Wounds sustained in urban areas are even less predictable; in only one third of patients with gunshot wounds seen on the Louisiana State University Surgical Service in New Orleans was the weapon identified.[12]

The modern soldier sustains extremity injuries that range from poisoned-stick puncture wounds to high-velocity missile wounds. His occupation has most likely produced an endocrine imbalance and a chronic stress reaction long before he is injured, and his environment enhances the probability of infection. Treatment of extremity injuries must be secondary to care of more lethal injuries, such as wounds of the chest or abdomen. While management of the injury usually is interrupted by successive evacuations away from the battlefield, definitive treatment is done by a series of secondary medical teams that did not perform initial care, may have lost documentation data, and therefore may not comprehend the full extent of injury.

INCIDENCE OF PERIPHERAL NERVE INJURIES ASSOCIATED WITH GUNSHOT WOUNDS

After World War I, the incidence of peripheral nerve injuries in all nonfatal wounds was estimated to be 2%.[10] Total peripheral nerve injuries in World War II were about 40,000,[64] representing 6.6% of all wounds requiring hospitalization.[5] Final disposition data from Army hospitals in Vietnam indicate an incidence of peripheral nerve injuries of about 7.3% of the nonfatal wounds from 1964 to 1973.[5,50]

In World War II the ulnar nerve was the most commonly injured peripheral nerve in the upper extremity, followed by the median, radial, and musculocutaneous nerves in descending order. In the lower extremity, the sciatic nerve was the most commonly involved, followed by the peroneal, tibial, and femoral nerves.[64] Data from Army hospitals in Vietnam from 1964 through 1973 indicate that 61% of 7138 peripheral nerve injuries involved the upper extremity.[57,64]

Multiple nerve injuries are more common in the upper extremity. In 102 successive casualties observed during World War II, 18 patients had multiple nerve injuries. In 14 of the 18 cases, the injuries involved the upper extremity.[10] Of the patients with injuries of the upper extremity admitted to Brooke Army Medical Center from Vietnam between January 1966 and September 1970, 22% had lesions of major peripheral nerves.[35]

The Vietnam Vascular Registry recorded concomitant nerve injury in 42.4% and fractures in 28.5% of 1000 acute major arterial injuries.[49]

PRINCIPLES FOR INITIAL CARE

Gunshot wounds are managed in the same manner as any other traumatic injury in that the location and extent of tissue disruption are determined by physical examination and radiographic studies. Tissue disruption caused by a gunshot wound is no more mysterious than that caused by an automobile or the paddle of a washing machine.[14,26] Appropriate management of gunshot wounds of the penetrating or perforating type hinges on early operative intervention.

The operative procedure termed *debridement* has two objectives: to excise necrotic tissue and to incise fascial sheets that inhibit the circulation of edematous muscle.[62] The earlier French definition of the procedure (from the verb *débrider*, to unbridle) was the cutting of parts (fascia) that, like a bridle, constrict or strangulate the organs they cover and prevent the discharge of pus and hematoma.[47] In the American usage begun in World War II, debridement is the macroscopic cleaning of wounds by operative removal of nonviable tissue, foreign matter, and even tissue of questionable viability, with provision for ample drainage.

Development of life-threatening gas gangrene is the complication most often cited to justify "radical debridement" or wide excision of muscles. A precipitous decline in the incidence of clostridial myositis, from 5% of those wounded in World War I to 0.7% in World War II and 0.08% in the Korean War, correlates closely with the increasing use of antibiotics on the battlefield, since debridement techniques remained essentially unchanged during that time.[7,15]

Debridement should be rational rather than radical. The surgeon aggressively incises the wound, but does not empirically excise tissue more widely than clinical judgment normally dictates.[7] The incision for fasciotomy includes the overlying skin and is extensive. Debridement includes the direct observation of potentially involved neurovascular structures. The nature of the nerve deficit, such as total or partial transection vs contusion, is documented. Magnification is indicated for evaluation of the injury, and only those portions of peripheral nerves that are obviously damaged are excised. Remaining nerve is replaced in the best available bed of soft tissue. Because transected nerves shorten with joint motion, the epineurium of the proximal and distal stumps is sutured to adjacent soft tissue with very fine monofilament wire to prevent retraction. The level of disruption of nerve is identified later with roentgenograms.[42]

Miniaturization of existing components of external fixation devices has been a significant step toward solving problems such as maintenance of length, alignment, and mobility.[9,51] While microvascular composite flap reconstruction may be an appropriate alternative to conventional staged skin flaps and cancellous bone grafting,[30,53] it is done only when the tissues are receptive to the transfer and the wound is clean. Unless done well, such surgery will further jeopardize a wound with marginal circulation.

A clean wound, fracture stability, restoration of adequate circulation, and skin closure over neurovascular structures have priority over peripheral nerve repair. However, the appropriate treatment for a severed nerve, neurorrhaphy, should be performed as soon as the clinical situation permits. World War II studies of 3418 nerve sutures established that delay in suture involves a loss that averages about 1% of maximal performance for every 6 days of delay.[64] Severe peripheral nerve deficits are the ultimate determinant of poor function in surviving extremities.

SPONTANEOUS RECOVERY

The more extensive and severe the injury to the involved extremity, the longer the time required for homeostasis of tissues. Nerves are only as functional as the pertinent sensory receptors and muscle-tendon motors. Multiple nerve involvement is a more serious problem for functional recovery of the entire extremity than is an isolated nerve injury. Clinical studies of neural recovery in the human show considerable variation, because return of useful function depends as much on the total response of the extremity to the injury as on the regeneration of the injured nerve.[35] Rakolta and Omer observed that spontaneous regeneration could be delayed for as long as 11 months with subsequent clinical recovery.[48]

Seddon introduced a simple classification for traumatic nerve injuries (see Chap. 7).[54] The minimal injury (*neurapraxia*) may result from localized ischemic demyelination. Moderate injury (*axonotmesis*) is characterized by interruption of axons and their myelin sheaths, but the endoneural tubes remain intact and guide the regenerating axons to their appropriate peripheral connections. Severe injury (*neurotmesis*) occurs when a nerve either has been completely severed or is so seriously disorganized that spontaneous regeneration is impossible. Gunshot wounds can result in any one of the three types of injury (Table 45-4).[48,55]

In a retrospective report on 2915 cases of extremity motor paralysis during World War I, Forester found that 1980 (67%) improved sufficiently under expected treatment to obviate operative intervention.[6] Sunderland studied retrospectively a series of World War II military patients and documented spontaneous recovery in 68%.[58] In a prospective study of 595 gunshot wounds during the Vietnam War, I found that spontaneous recovery occurred in 227 of 331 low-velocity gunshot wounds (69%) and 183 of 264 high-velocity gunshot wounds (69%) (Table 45-5; Figs. 45-1, 45-2).[35,36,38,39]

The prognosis is more accurate if the time required for return of clinical function is known. In a 1974 study, I selected two parameters for a time frame: the interval after injury at which half of the nerves had recovered function, and the interval after injury at which only 10% of nerves recovered function.[35] This established a time frame of 3 to 9 months in 90% of the nerves that demonstrated

Table 45-4. *Interval Between Injury and Spontaneous Recovery in Gunshot Wounds*

Nerve	Neurapraxia (0–4 months)	Axonotmesis (4–9 months)	Axonotmesis (9+ months)
Radial	20	9	2
Median	10	7	
Ulnar	9	13	4
Sciatic and popliteal	14	14	3
Femoral	1	4	1
Total (111)	54	47	10

(From Seddon HJ. Surgical disorders of peripheral nerve, ed 2. Edinburgh: Churchill-Livingstone, 1975, except for femoral nerve information, from Rakolta GC, Omer GE. Combat-sustained femoral nerve injuries. Surg Gynecol Obstet 1969; 128:813–817.)

Table 45-5. *Time Frame for Spontaneous Recovery in Gunshot wounds*

	Isolated Nerve Lesions	
	Above-Elbow	*Below-Elbow*
Low-velocity	4–7 months (48)	3–6 months (90)
High-velocity	3–6 months (31)	3–6 months (32)
	Multiple Nerve Lesions	
	Above-Elbow	*Below-Elbow*
Low-velocity	5–8 months (41)	3–7 months (48)
High-velocity	5–9 months (65)	5–8 months (55)
Total nerves (410)	(185)	(225)

(From Omer GE Jr. Injuries to nerves of the upper extremity. J Bone Joint Surg [Am] 1974;56: 1615–1624.)

spontaneous recovery. Proximal (high) extremity injuries took longer to show clinical function than distal (low) injuries. Extensive injuries producing multiple nerve lesions needed longer to show clinical function than isolated nerve injuries. The prognosis for spontaneous recovery of clinical function was the same for low-velocity as for high-velocity gunshot wounds. Both types of wounds demonstrated neurapraxic lesions, which recovered in 1 to 4 months, and axonotmetic lesions, which recovered in 4 to 9 months (Table 45-5).

CAUSALGIA

The recognition of pain is subjective and depends on the intensity of the peripheral stimulus, central summation, and the personality of the patient.[40,41] Many clinical syndromes have been described that include burning pain, abnormal vasomotor response, and dystrophy (see Chap. 102). The dreadful pain associated with penetrating injuries of nerves was best described by Mitchell, Morehouse, and Keen in their 1864 monograph,[32] al-

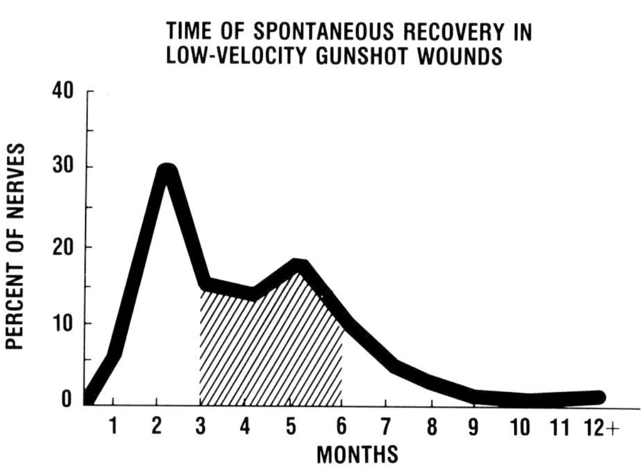

Figure 45-1. *Time of spontaneous recovery in low-velocity gunshot wounds.*

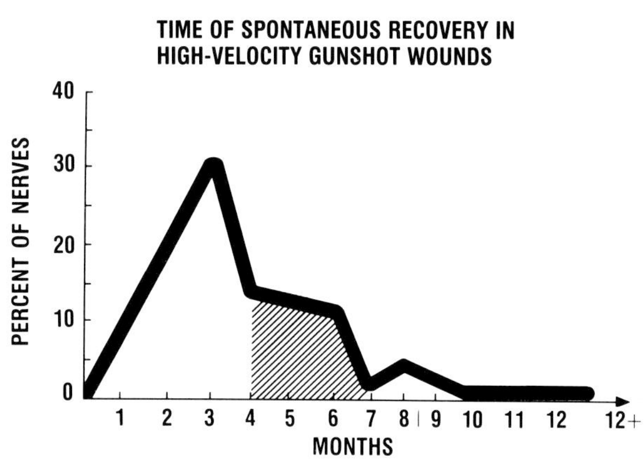

Figure 45-2. *Time of spontaneous recovery in high-velocity gunshot wounds.*

though the condition had been described in 1813 by Denmark, another military surgeon.[58] Variants of classical causalgia include Leriche's post-traumatic pain syndrome, Sudek's atrophy, or shoulder-arm-hand syndrome.[24]

The incidence of causalgia has varied with the criteria used for diagnosis. Data from World War I and II indicated that causalgia occurred in 2% to 4% of wounds involving major nerves.[50] Final disposition records from U.S. Army hospitals from 1964 through 1973 diagnosed causalgia in 1.5% of nerve injuries.[50] In a series of 77 Vietnam cases from 1966 to 1970, Thomas and I found that 74% of causalgia cases involved the median or sciatic-tibial nerves.[42] There was a high incidence of multiple nerve injuries in these cases, with only 21% due to wounds distal to the elbow or knee (Table 45-6). The lower extremity was involved more often than the upper extremity (Table 45-7). The onset of pain was within the first 24 hours after injury in 49% of cases and within the first week in 70%. Gunshot wounds provoked 87% of these cases (Table 45-8).

While a precise definition of causalgia has not been accepted, characteristics of the syndrome have been outlined by the British Medical Research Council: the pain is spontaneous; it is hot and burning, intense, diffuse, persistent, and subject to exacerbations; it can be elicited by stimuli that do not necessarily have a physical effect on the limb; and it is aggravated by disturbance to the patient's emotional or physical environment.[55] It tends to lead to profound changes in the patient's mental state and dominates the patient's life, prohibiting effective rehabilitation.

There are two principles in the treatment of an established pain syndrome involving the extremities: relieve the patient's symptoms, and institute active use of the involved extremity.[37,45] The source of the pain may be due to nociceptive peripheral increased stimulus, summation of the reflex sympathetic overflow, and central pain.[40]

Peripheral nociceptive stimuli enhance pain for many reasons. A peripheral nerve responds to injury, either partial or complete, with proliferation of connective tissue and regeneration of damaged

Table 45–6. *Causalgia: Nerves Involved*

		Level of Injury	
Nerve	**Number of Cases**	*Above Elbow or Knee*	*Below Elbow or Knee*
UPPER LIMB			
Brachial plexus	8	8	0
Median	25	15	10
Ulnar	2	1	1
Radial	1	0	1
LOWER LIMB			
Sacral plexus	7	7	0
Sciatic	24	24	0
Tibial	8	4	4
Peroneal	1	1	0
Femoral	1	1	0
TOTAL	77	61	16

(From Omer GE Jr. War wounds of the hand. In Tubiana R (ed). The hand, vol. 3. Philadelphia: WB Saunders, 1988:903–924.)

Table 45–7. *Causalgia: Time of Onset of Symptoms*

Time of Onset	Upper Extremity	Lower Extremity	Total
Day of injury	18	20	38
1st week post-injury	9	7	16
1–3 weeks post-injury	5	9	14
3–6 weeks post-injury	3	2	5
Over 6 weeks post-injury	1	3	4
Total	36	41	77

(From Omer GE Jr. War wounds of the hand. In: Tubiana R (ed). The hand, vol 3. Philadelphia: WB Saunders, 1988:903–924.)

axons to form neuromas. The neuromas, which become symptomatic depending on the quality of regeneration, are influenced by the extent of fibrosis, infection, foreign material, and external adhesions. The compressed nerve has venous stasis, capillary leakage, and perineural edema.[52] Decreased blood flow is associated with pain, as in any compression syndrome (see Chap. 59).[18] The patient characteristically has extreme sensitivity directly over the neuroma, altered sensibility in at least part of the area supplied by the nerve, and sustained pain that is widely distributed and poorly localized. Percutaneous injection about the painful neuroma provides local anesthesia.

A peripheral chemical sympathetic block may be performed for an identified site of peripheral nociceptive neuroma. A 16-gauge needle is inserted just proximal to the "trigger point," and a flexible 18-gauge polyethylene intravenous catheter is inserted through the needle. The needle is removed, leaving the catheter in place. A solution of 0.5 mL of lidocaine hydrochloride, 0.5%, is injected. If the pain is relieved, the catheter is capped and taped in place, allowing exercise activity. Additional periodic injections of lidocaine solution are based on the length of pain-free activity. Periodic infusion is continued for a few days up to 2 weeks. If there is more than one "trigger point," separate

Table 45–8. *Causalgia: Causative Agent*

Agent	Upper Extremity	Lower Extremity	Total
GUNSHOT WOUND			
High-velocity	18	23	41
Fragment wounds	12	14	26
CRUSH WOUNDS	3	2	5
AIRCRAFT ACCIDENT	1	2	3
STAB WOUND/PENETRATION	2	0	2
Total	36	41	77

(From Omer GE Jr. War wounds of the hand. In Tubiana R (ed). The hand, vol 3. Philadelphia: WB Saunders, 1988:903–924.)

catheters should be used. This method was used for injuries in Vietnam (Table 45-9) but has not been as effective in patients in whom the pain has been untreated for 3 or more months.[42–45]

In patients with Raynaud's symptoms associated with pain, it is appropriate to measure digital blood flow.[40,46] Chuinard and associates have reported the use of intravenous reserpine to relieve pain in large vessel spasm and sympathetic overflow.[11] The technique is the same as that used for intravenous regional anesthesia. One milligram of reserpine diluted in 50 mL of normal saline solution is injected, and the tourniquet is released after 15 minutes. Hannington-Kiff introduced the intravenous regional sympathetic block technique with guanethidine.[20]

In most patients with causalgia, specific peripheral nociceptive stimuli cease after a few days because the reflex sympathetic overflow increases to dominate the clinical picture. Treatment for these cases includes chemical central interruption of the abnormal sympathetic reflex. A cervical sympathetic block is performed as a diagnostic test as well as a therapeutic procedure.[2,40] I use either 1% lidocaine hydrochloride or 1% mepivacaine hydrochloride to produce peripheral warming and cessation of sweating, as well as relief of pain. A series of four or five blocks is given on consecutive days; the introduction of one placebo of normal saline solution during the series will confirm the value of the sympathetic block.

Leffert and colleagues have developed a technique for continuous sympathetic blockade that uses an indwelling catheter for injection about the stellate ganglion.[40] The initial technique for periodic chemical sympathetic blocks involved the lumbar area.[60]

The sympathetic block can have the following effects:

1. One block may give total relief.
2. One block may give tolerable relief.
3. The duration of the first block may exceed that expected, and subsequent blocks may give progressively longer relief.
4. The duration of the first block may exceed that expected, but subsequent blocks may give progressively shorter relief.
5. The block may give relief only for the duration expected from the anesthetic agent used.[45]

For the first three responses, a series of chemical central sympathetic blocks should lead to resolution of the pain syndrome, and further treat-

Table 45–9. *Causalgia: Results of Treatment*

		Improved		***Failure***	
Method	***Cases***	*Upper Extremity*	*Lower Extremity*	*Upper Extremity*	*Lower Extremity*
CHEMICAL SYMPATHECTOMY					
Central block	43	7	11	11	14
Epidural (spinal cord)	4	0	4	0	0
Peripheral periodic infusion	30	5	9	2	14
Total	77	36 (47%)		41 (53%)	
SURGERY (41 failures)					
Central sympathectomy	37	20	14	1	2
Destruction of nerve	2	0	0	2	0
Neurolysis	1	0	0	1	0
Removal of foreign body	1	0	1	0	0
Total	41	35 (85%)		6 (15%)	

(From Omer GE Jr. War wounds of the hand. In: Tubiana R (ed). The hand, vol 3. Philadelphia: WB Saunders, 1988:903–924.)

ment, other than physical medicine, may not be necessary.

Surgery is performed when the burning pain responds completely to central chemical sympathectomy but requires repeated blocks for long-term relief of pain. The effectiveness of surgical sympathectomy is related not to interrupting a sensory pathway from the extremity, but to eliminating the sympathetic efferent discharge to the peripheral arteries and sweat glands. I prefer the transaxillary approach, with removal of the sympathetic chain from the fourth thoracic level superior to include the lower half of the stellate ganglion. In the lower extremity, a retroperitoneal approach through a lateral flank incision allows removal of sympathetic ganglia from the second to fifth lumbar level. For a satisfactory result, precise postoperative sudomotor function tests should demonstrate complete sympathetic denervation of the involved extremity.

Baker and Winegarner reported improvement in 59 of 65 Vietnam patients (91%) following surgical sympathectomy.[33] Thomas and I reported similar results in a series of 77 patients, using chemical and surgical procedures (Table 45-9).[44]

For responses 4 and 5 (above) to the chemical cervical block, permanent improvement by surgical sympathectomy is not expected.[45] While transcutaneous electrical nerve stimulation is considered, pain relief is complete in fewer than one third of patients, and for the best results transcutaneous electrical stimulation must be initiated within 3 months of the onset of pain.[27] Nashold and associates reported on 38 peripheral nerves in 35 patients stimulated with electrodes placed directly on peripheral nerves.[33] There was successful pain relief in 53% of patients with upper extremity pain.

Current researchers are implanting electrodes to stimulate cells in the periaqueductal periventricular gray matter to release beta-endorphins, obtaining analgesia for both peripheral nerve pain and central pain.[28]

Central pain is generally hyperpathic, paroxysmal, and spontaneous. Beneficial medical treatment has resulted with the use of anticonvulsants or tricyclic antidepressants.[40,63] Mesencephalic tractotomy may give lasting pain relief in nerve root avulsion.[65]

The patient's physical condition may deteriorate due to inadequate sleep, improper diet, lack of exercise, or other complications. Depression may progress to the point of hopelessness. These patients often become addicted to narcotics, as characterized by symptoms of increased dose tolerance, psychic craving, withdrawal syndrome, and an inability to sustain abstinence. Drug dependency must be reversed. Optimal management requires a multifaceted and highly individualized program.

The second goal in all treatment programs for pain is functional use of the involved extremity. Physical modalities may be divided into passive and active ones. Passive activities improve circulation, decrease edema, prevent contracture, and prepare the patient for active voluntary participation in the active exercise program. Passive modalities include elevation, traction, plaster casts, static splints, vibrators, faradic muscle stimulation, microwaves, ultrasound, ice packs, hot paraffin packs, contrast baths, massage, and inflatable splints with positive-negative pressure. It may be necessary to precede these passive modalities by very delicate techniques in the apprehensive patient. The skin may be lightly stroked with a feather, followed by very gentle massage, and progressing to warm paraffin packs. Other desensitization techniques include contact with foam rubber chips, jelly beans, navy beans, and rice to provide progressively greater contact pressure.[41]

The more important phase is active exercise, which can be assisted with dynamic splints, supportive exercise slings, and special handles for tools. Special care is directed to major circulation areas, such as the rotator cuff muscles in the shoulder. General body conditioning is important, and the patient should be ambulatory, if at all possible, to meet the environment. Function is encouraged with diversional games, assigned work, and activities of daily living. It is most important for physicians, physical therapists, occupational therapists, and all other attendants to be compassionate and yet to encourage maximal effort by the patient. Ultimately, patients "cure" themselves by returning to normal functional activity.

Elective surgery is undertaken when the patient has successfully performed an extensive physical medicine program. Elective surgery performed under less stable conditions is ill advised.

OPERATIVE TECHNIQUES FOR PERIPHERAL NERVES

All peripheral nerve repairs have only two technical principles. The first is longitudinal alignment or matching of the fascicular bundles within the nerve, and the second is minimal tension at the suture line, both longitudinal and circumferential (see Chap. 18). The only factor affecting the return of function that is fully under the surgeon's control is the technique of nerve suture.

An associated problem in terms of prognosis is the nerve gap. Sharp lacerations without loss of nerve tissue that are allowed to persist for a number of weeks create nerve gaps. In the complex injury, with fractures and soft-tissue loss, the nerve gap is associated with extensive scarring. World War II studies indicate an average loss of about 6% per centimeter from optimal motor recovery following suture of the shortest gaps, until the critical limit when suturing becomes impossible is reached.[64] A nerve gap of 7.5 cm is the maximal distance that can be approximated without requiring rigid immobilization of the extremity in flexion (see Chap. 10).

During the Vietnam War, the techniques used to overcome a nerve gap associated with a gunshot wound included the following:

1. Mobilization of nerve trunks. A longitudinal release requires that the nerve survive on its internal longitudinal circulation. In addition, the surgical bed is often severely scarred, providing little segmental recirculation.
2. Shortening the skeleton. This is potentially dangerous because all soft-tissue structures, such as muscle-tendon units, are relatively lengthened and weakened.
3. Bulb suture. This technique is unacceptable because it produces acute stretch of the nerve. Functional failure has been reported with stretching as little as 5% of the length of the nerve.[29]
4. Transposition and rerouting. An example is transferring the ulnar nerve from the extensor to the flexor surface at the elbow. If a choice is available, the distal portion of a nerve is rerouted because the proximal portion contains the regenerating axons and needs immediate blood supply.
5. Flexion of joints. The elbow or knee is not flexed beyond 90%. After the initial healing period of 3 to 6 weeks, joints are extended only 10% per week to prevent intrinsic ischemia (see Chap. 36).[21]
6. Nerve grafts. Autogenous tissue is preferred for grafts; the sural nerve and the medial or lateral antebrachial cutaneous nerves are the best sources. The nerve pedicle graft was introduced in World War II in an attempt to maintain adequate circulation in a full-thickness graft. The first procedure involved the median and ulnar nerves in the forearm, with the ulnar nerve filling a gap in the median nerve.[56] The result was reported long after the time of surgery.

Of the few nerve grafts performed during the Vietnam era, almost all were free cable or pedicle grafts, done without microscopic assistance for precise longitudinal alignment of the groups of fascicles. There is no information concerning either the nerve gap that was overcome or the longitudinal tension on the nerve graft. I found that only 4 of 34 grafts followed for at least 12 months (12%) demonstrated return of functional activity.[35] A long-term follow-up study of combat-incurred peripheral nerve injuries was done at Fitzsimons Army Medical Center from 1967 to 1983.[13] A few patients with injuries of the median and ulnar nerves in the forearm had pedicle grafts to bridge a gap of the median nerve. The pedicle nerve graft, when appropriate, is preferred over free nerve grafts.[13]

Neurolysis is recommended when an intact nerve is found during exploration of a nonfunctioning nerve. During World War II, external neurolysis was done in 70% of cases, saline injection in 25%, and fascicular dissection in 5%. Evidence indicates that internal and external neurolysis differ in their effects on recovery.[64] I performed external neurolysis in 59 cases from Vietnam in which the injured nerve was found in continuity but bound in scar tissue.[35] Nine of these cases were excluded for short follow-up (less than 3 months), but the neurolysis procedure was successful in 60% of the remaining 50 nerves. When function of the extremity returns within the time frame for spontaneous recovery after injury, there is doubt concerning the efficacy of neurolysis, as the intact nerve in such a case might have recovered spontaneously without surgery.

In the same study, of 45 gunshot wounds followed for 12 months or longer, 25 demonstrated clinical return of function. Ten of the nerves recovered during the time frame allotted for spontaneous recovery. Therefore, neurolysis was successful in restoring function in only 15 (33%) of 45 gunshot wounds.[35] Kline's subsequent studies indicated that in vivo nerve action potential studies should be performed during neurolysis procedures (see Chap. 42).[22,23]

While appropriate treatment for a severed nerve is neurorrhaphy, many factors prevent ideal treatment of gunshot wound injuries. The condition of the whole extremity, the level and extent of the nerve injury, and the time until definitive care is provided influence the results of operation.

In addition, motor and sensory performance are greatly improved by practice and experience. In evaluating results, it is important to consider that final function is improved by retraining that is directed at increasing the patient's ability to use new and altered patterns of motor and sensory innervation. It is difficult to put a time limit on this phase of recovery, since it depends on nerve regeneration plus other factors such as intelligence, patience, perseverance, and motivation. It is a slow process that certainly continues for at least 5 years following neurorrhaphy.[59]

During the Vietnam era, the use of magnification, delicate instruments, and less reactive suture material improved the techniques of nerve suture. An effort was made to perform suture as early as possible in the clinical situation. I reported the results of 143 epineural sutures of upper extremity nerves,[35] and Brown reported the results of 135 epineural sutures followed for 6 to 24 months[8] (Tables 45-10, 45-11). Neither study had adequate follow-up, and the results are not fully graded. Brown stated "some return," and I had two criteria for "clinical return": for an above-elbow lesion, progressive motor return with independent movement and point localization of 3.84 von Frey monofilament without overresponse (M3–S2); for a below-elbow lesion, progressive motor return with independent movement and two-point discrimination less than 20 mm (M3–S3). In addition, I found that none of my patients with above-elbow neurorrhaphy showed recovery of function of the

Table 45–10. *Neurorrhaphy Related to Etiology and Level of Injury*

Etiology	Number	Adequate Follow-Up	Clinical Return	Percentage
LACERATIONS				
Above-elbow	9	8	3	37
Below-elbow	90	67	30	45
HIGH-VELOCITY GUNSHOT				
Above-elbow	24	21	6	28
Below-elbow	24	14	6	43
LOW-VELOCITY GUNSHOT				
Above-elbow	19	18	9	50
Below-elbow	16	14	6	43
FRACTURE-DISLOCATIONS				
Above-elbow	1	1	0	0
Below-elbow	1	0	0	0
Total	184	143	60	42

(From Omer GE Jr. Injuries to nerves of the upper extremity. J Bone Joint Surg [Am] 1974;56:1615.)

Table 45–11. *Results of Secondary Suture of Specific Nerves*

Nerve	Number Repaired	No Return		Some Return	
		Number	Percentage	Number	Percentage
Ulnar	68	44	65	24	35
Median	38	19	50	19	50
Radial	5	3	60	2	40
Digital	24	10	40	14	60
Total	135	76	56	59	44

(From Brown PW. The time factor in surgery of upper extremity peripheral nerve injury. Clin Orthop 1970;68:14–21.)

intrinsic muscles of the hand during the period of study.

The results of these two series from Vietnam indicate that in only 40% to 45% of cases does suture of nerves result in progressive function return over the first 1 to 2 years after surgery. However, the continued long-term study on these cases demonstrated higher percentages of functional return.[13] In several well-studied cases, a return of interosseous muscles with intrinsic function was clearly demonstrated more than 2 years after above-elbow suture of the ulnar nerve. The longest time elapsed before functional return was 8 years after nerve suture.

REFERENCES

1. Adams DB. Wound ballistics: A review. Milit Med 1982; 147:831–835.
2. Barnes R. The role of sympathectomy in the treatment of causalgia. J Bone Joint Surg [Br] 1953; 35: 172–180.
3. Berry FB. Editorial. United States Armed Forces Medical Journal, 1954; 5:9.
4. Bick EM. Source book of orthopaedics. New York: Hafner Publishing Co., 1968 (original published 1948):37–44.
5. Bjik KD, Bellamy RF. Editorial: A note on combat casualty statistics. Milit Med 1984; 149:229–230.
6. af Bjorkesten G. Suture of war injuries to peripheral nerves. Clinical studies of end results. Acta Chir Scand [Suppl 119] 1947.
7. Bowen TE, Bellamy RF, eds. Emergency war surgery, ed 2. 2nd US Revision of Emergency War Surgery NATO Handbook. Washington DC: US Govt. Printing Office, 1988:231–238.
8. Brown PW. The time factor in surgery of upper extremity peripheral nerve injury. Clin Orthop 1970; 68:14–21.
9. Calkins MS, Burkhalter WE, Reyes F. Traumatic segmented bone defects in the upper extremity. J Bone Joint Surg [Am] 1987; 69:19–27.
10. Campbell EH Jr. The Mediterranean (formerly North African) theater of operation. In: Coates JB Jr, Spurling RG, Woodhall B, eds. Surgery in World War II. Washington DC: Office of the Surgeon General, Department of the Army, 1959:231–238.
11. Chuinard RG, Dabezies EJ, Gould JS, Murphy GA, Mathews RE. Intravenous reserpine for treatment of reflex sympathetic dystrophy. ASSH Proceedings. J Hand Surg 1980; 5:289.
12. Dugas R, D'Ambrosia R. Civilian gunshot wounds. Orthopaedics 1985; 8:1121–1125.
13. Eversmann WW Jr. Long-term follow up of combat-incurred nerve injuries. In: Omer GE Jr, ed. Peripheral nerve problems. In: Burkhalter WE, ed. Orthopedic surgery in Vietnam. Washington, DC: US Govt. Printing Office, in press.
14. Fackler ML. Ballistic injury. Ann Emerg Med 1986; 15:1451–1455.
15. Fackler ML. Wound ballistics, a review of common misconceptions. JAMA 1988; 259:2730–2736.
16. Finck PA. Ballistic and forensic pathologic aspects of missile wounds. Conversion between Anglo-American and metric system units. Milit Med 1965; 130:545–569.

17. Garrison FH. An introduction to the history of medicine, ed 3. Philadelphia: WB Saunders, 1921:193–194.
18. Gelberman RH, Hergenroeder PT, Hargens AR, Lundborg GH, Akeson WH. The carpal tunnel syndrome. A study of carpal tunnel pressure. J Bone Joint Surg [Am] 1981; 63:380–383.
19. Gray HMW. Treatment of gunshot wounds by excision and primary suture. Br Med J 1915; 2 (28 August):317–320.
20. Hannington-Kiff JG. Relief of Sudek's atrophy by regional intravenous guanethidine. Lancet 1977; 1: 1132–1133.
21. Highet WB, Sanders FK. The effects of stretching nerves after suture. Br J Surg 1943; 30:355–369.
22. Kline DG. Evaluation of the neuroma-in-continuity. In: Omer GE Jr, Spinner M, eds. Management of peripheral nerve problems. Philadelphia: WB Saunders, 1980:450–461.
23. Kline DG, De Jong BR. Evoked potentials to evaluate peripheral nerve injuries. Surg Gynecol Obstet 1968; 127:1239–1248.
24. Lankford LL. Reflex sympathetic dystrophy. In: Omer GE Jr, Spinner M, eds. Management of peripheral nerve problems. Philadelphia: WB Saunders, 1980:216–244.
25. Letts RM, Miller D. Gunshot wounds of the extremities in children. J Trauma 1976; 16:807–811.
26. Lindsey D. The idolatry of velocity, or lies, damn lies, and ballistics. J Trauma 1980; 20:1068–1069.
27. Lolser JD, Black RG, Christman A. Relief of pain by transcutaneous stimulation. J Neurosurg 1975; 43:308–314.
28. Long DM. Neuromodulation for the control of chronic pain. Surgical Rounds 1982; 5:25–34.
29. Lui CT, Benda CE, Lewey FH. The tensile strength of human nerves: Experimental, physiologic, and histologic study. Arch Neurol Psychiatr 1948; 59: 332–336.
30. MacKennon SE, Weiland AJ, Godina M. Immediate forearm reconstruction with a functional latissimus dorsi island pedicle myocutaneous flap. Plast Reconstr Surg 1983; 71:706–710.
31. Marcus NA, Blair WF, Shuck JM, Omer GE Jr. Low-velocity gunshot wounds to extremities. J Trauma 1980; 20:1061–1064.
32. Mitchell SW, Morehouse GR, Keen WW. Gunshot wounds and other injuries of nerves. Philadelphia: JB Lippincott, 1864.
33. Nashold BS, Goldner JL, Mullen JB, Bright DS. Long-term pain control by direct peripheral nerve stimulation. J Bone Joint Surg [Am] 1982; 64:1–10.
34. Omer GE Jr. The early management of gunshot wounds of the extremities. South Dakota J Med Pharm 1956; 9:340–346.
35. Omer GE Jr. Injuries to nerves of the upper extremity. J Bone Joint Surg [Am] 1974; 56:1615–1624.
36. Omer GE Jr. The results of untreated traumatic injuries. In: Omer GE Jr, Spinner M, eds. Management of peripheral nerve problems. Philadelphia: WB Saunders, 1980:502–506.
37. Omer GE Jr. Nerve, neuroma, and pain problems related to upper limb amputations. Orthop Clin North Am 1981; 12:751–762.
38. Omer GE Jr. Results of untreated peripheral nerve injuries. Clin Orthop 1982; 163:15–19.
39. Omer GE Jr. Fractures and major nerve injuries in the fractured extremity. In: Meyers MH, ed. The multiply injured patient with complex fractures. Philadelphia: Lea & Febiger, 1984:156–161.
40. Omer GE Jr. Management techniques for chronic pain of the upper extremity. Bull Hosp Jt Dis Orthop Inst 1984; 44:381–405.
41. Omer GE Jr. Present thoughts on the management of pain in the upper extremity. Clin Plast Surg 1984; 11:85–93.
42. Omer GE Jr. War wounds of the hand. In: Tubiana R, ed. The hand, vol. 3. Philadelphia: WB Saunders, 1988:903–924.
43. Omer GE Jr, Thomas SR. Treatment of causalgia. Review of cases at Brooke General Hospital. Tex Med 1971; 67:93–96.
44. Omer GE Jr, Thomas SR. Peripheral periodic infusion sympathectomy for the treatment of causalgia. Proceedings of the American Society for Surgery of the Hand. J Bone Joint Surg [Am] 1972; 54: 898–899.
45. Omer GE Jr, Thomas SR. The management of chronic pain syndromes in the upper extremity. Clin Orthop 1974; 104:37–43.
46. Porter JM, Snider RL, Bardana EJ, Rosch J, Eidemiller LR. The diagnosis and treatment of Raynaud's phenomenon. Surgery 1975; 77:11–23.
47. Ragsdale BD. Gunshot wounds: A historical perspective. Milit Med 1984; 149:301–315.
48. Rakolta GG, Omer GE Jr. Combat-sustained femoral nerve injuries. Surg Gynecol Obstet 1969; 128: 813–817.
49. Rich NM, Spencer FC. Vascular trauma. Philadelphia: WB Saunders, 1978:125–155.

50. Rothberg JM, Tahmoush AJ, Oldakowski R. The epidemiology of causalgia among soldiers wounded in Vietnam. Milit Med 1983; 148:347–350.
51. Russotti GM, Sim FH. Missile wounds of the extremities: A current concept review. Orthopaedics 1985; 8:1106–1116.
52. Rydevick B, Lundborg G, Bagge U. Effects of graded compression on intraneural blood flow. J Hand Surg 1981; 6:3–12.
53. Salibian AH, Anzel SH, Mallerick M, Tesoro VE. Microvascular reconstruction for close-range gunshot injuries to the distal forearm. J Hand Surg [Am] 1984; 9:799–804.
54. Seddon HJ. Three types of nerve injury. Brain 1946; 66:237–288.
55. Seddon HJ. Surgical disorders of peripheral nerve, ed 2. Edinburgh: Churchill-Livingstone, 1975:32–36.
56. Strange FG St. C. An operation for nerve pedicle grafting. Br J Surg 1947; 34:423–425.
57. Sunderland S. Nerve and nerve injuries. Edinburgh: Churchill-Livingstone, 1972:785, 837, 923, 1075.
58. Sunderland S. Nerve and nerve injuries, ed 2. Edinburgh: Churchill-Livingstone, 1978:505–507.
59. Sunderland S. End result assessment following nerve repair and its implications. In: Tubiana R, ed. The hand, vol 3. Philadelphia: WB Saunders, 1988:528–537.
60. Thomason JR, Moritz WH. Continuous lumbar paravertebral sympathetic block maintained by fractional installation of procaine. Surg Gynecol Obstet 1949; 89:447–453.
61. Whelan TJ Jr, Burkhalter WE, Gomez A. Management of war wounds. Adv Surg 1968; 3:227–350.
62. Whelan TJ Jr. Emergency war surgery. Washington DC: US Govt. Printing Office, 1975:198–203.
63. Wiley AM, Poplawski ZB, Murray J. Post-traumatic dystrophy of the hand. Orthop Rev 1977; 6:59–61.
64. Woodhall B, Beebe GW, eds. Peripheral nerve regeneration. VA medical monograph. Washington DC: US Govt. Printing Office, 1956:5, 191, 311–340, 498.
65. Zorub DS, Nashold BS Jr, Cook WA Jr. Avulsion of the brachial plexus. I. A review with implications on the therapy of intractable pain. Surg Neurol 1974; 2:347–353.

46

Thermal Injury of Peripheral Nerve

C. Andrew Salzberg
Roger E. Salisbury

AUTHORS' KEY POINTS

- Most burn-induced nerve injuries result from compression by circumferential eschar. These effects are treatable, avoiding irreversible nerve injury.
- The median and ulnar nerves are most commonly injured in electrical burns.
- Escharotomy is performed early in the course of management to avoid irreversible neural changes.
- Escharotomy incisions are extended well into unburned tissue; the ulnar cubital tunnel and fibular head regions are avoided.
- Definitive nerve reconstruction is delayed due to the indeterminate nature of the extent of nerve injury at the time of initial treatment.

There are various causes of burn-induced injury that directly or indirectly affect peripheral nerve. Neural management is specific to the acute, subacute, and chronic phases of burn wound care. Direct thermal injury, chemical burns, radiation, electrical injuries, and compression from noncompliant burn eschars cause a variety of injuries to peripheral nerve, ranging from transient neurapraxias to irreversible injuries due to ischemia. The goals of management are to identify peripheral nerve problems early and to prevent irreversible neural damage.

THERMAL INJURY

Thermal injuries result from fire, steam, or scalding liquids. Nerve damage occurs by coagulation necrosis due to direct heating or by ischemic necrosis secondary to unyielding compression of nerve due to overlying full-thickness circumferential burn eschar. It has been demonstrated that nerves and blood vessels conduct heat readily, while bone is relatively nonconductive (Fig. 46-1). A "fourth-degree" burn from direct injury causes coagulation necrosis in subcutaneous fat and its underlying structures. Because of the nerves' relatively protected position beneath the skin and subcutaneous structures, direct thermal injury of nerve is uncommon. Only a few nerves, because of their superficial locations, are susceptible to this type of injury: the ulnar nerve at the elbow, the superficial branch of the radial nerve on the dorsum of the hand, and the peroneal nerve as it courses around the fibula head.

Patients who present with direct deep thermal injury usually have been involved in a high-velocity accident (eg, automobile or airplane) leading to loss

Resistance of Tissue to Electric Current

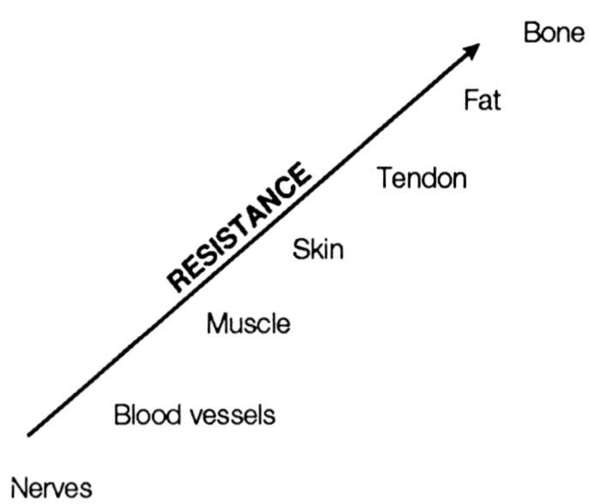

Figure 46–1. *This graph demonstrates the progressive increased resistance of different tissues to electrical current.*

of consciousness and prolonged direct exposure to hot metal. The extensive nature of these burns, which cause deep penetration necrosis, requires immediate management of other more life-threatening conditions. Primary treatment of peripheral nerve injury is rarely indicated. Life-threatening burn injuries are treated initially, and the management of peripheral nerve is delayed until wounds are healed. If the injury is localized to one extremity, early attention to burn wound management with eschar removal is indicated in order to assess the neural injury. In this situation, primary repair of small segmental injuries or nerve grating is indicated. Commonly, fourth-degree burns are associated with severe extremity injuries that ultimately may require amputation of the affected part.

More commonly, significant thermal burns involve more than 25% total body surface area, creating a nondistensible, unyielding burn eschar. Capillaries of both burned and uninjured tissues become abnormally permeable, and plasma escapes into interstitial spaces, causing large amounts of edema. While the normal elasticity of unburned tissue allows dissipation of large amounts of hydrostatic pressure, circumferential burn eschars result in an unyielding barrier, causing tourniquet effects to the extremity. As edema increases, exacerbated by the large volumes of resuscitation fluid required to support the intravenous volume depleted by burn shock, blood flow in the extremity is compromised. This occurs initially because of venous insufficiency. Poor outflow due to collapsing veins decreases perfusion, thereby increasing arterial ischemia. Gangrene or Volkmann's contracture of the upper or lower extremities quickly develops. This must be corrected rapidly if irreversible damage to underlying neurovascular structures of the extremity is to be prevented.

The major indication for escharotomy is evidence of ischemia distal to a circumferential burn. This is the most easily and effectively treated mechanism of injury to peripheral nerve. Clinically, the decision for operative intervention is made when there is evidence of poor tissue perfusion. A bounding radial or dorsalis pedis pulse and Doppler confirmation of palmar arch flow are good indications that perfusion is adequate. If, however, edema increases due to circumferential injury and the pulse weakens, escharotomy is indicated. The presence of faint Doppler pulse indicates that there is perfusion of soft tissues. However, the perfusion of vital small muscles (intrinsics) may be inadequate. Recording compartment pressures has been found to be a valuable way of determining limb perfusion, as long as the catheter is in the appropriate position and the readings are reliable. Likewise, the attending surgeon and nurse must watch for adequate hourly urine output, indicative of good systemic perfusion. Diminished flow from an injured extremity is a sign of inadequate intravenous resuscitation. A decision-making stepwise algorithm for treatment is useful (Fig. 46-2).

ESCHAROTOMY

Author's Preferred Technique

Escharotomy is performed in the emergency room, at the bedside, or in the operating room. The procedure requires adequate lighting, nursing assistance, and electrocautery. Anesthesia, although usually not required, may be achieved by local infiltration of 0.5% Xylocaine into proposed incision sites. More often, the patient's anxiety level requires intravenous administration of morphine and benzodiazepines. The pulse oximeter, placed on an unburned extremity, provides an adequate assessment of tissue oxygen saturation, which should remain above 95%.

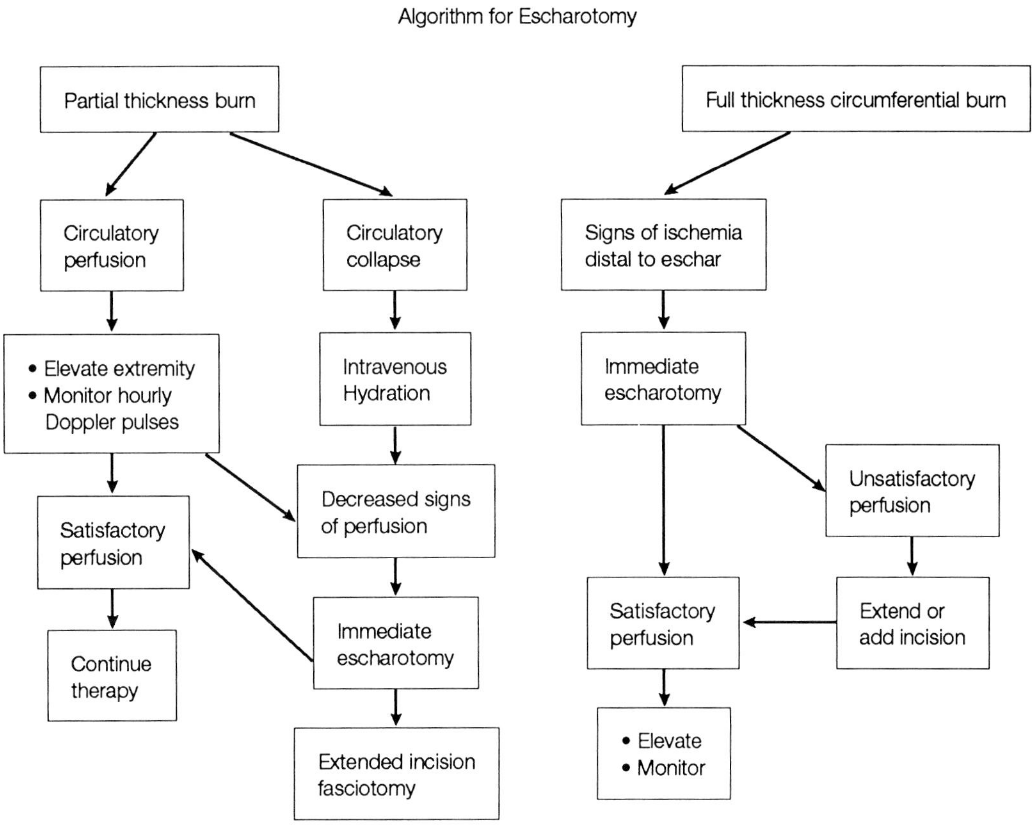

Figure 46–2. *Steps for care of partial and full thickness burn injuries.*

If, despite adequate hydration and intravenous resuscitation, pulses are not detectable, an incision (for the upper extremity) is begun along the radial aspect of the arm on a line extending from the tip of the acromion to the antecubital flexion crease and further extended to the radial side of the wrist flexion crease. The incision begins proximally at the site of the circumferential burn. It is continued across the wrist onto the thenar eminence, extending into unburned tissue (Fig. 46-3). Following elevation of the arm, pulses are again evaluated by palpation or Doppler examination. If pulses are not detectable after a few minutes, a determination of the adequacy of operative incision is made. If arterial flow in the digital vessels is inadequate, medial (ulnar) decompressive escharotomy is carried out through an incision that runs from mid-axilla to the ulnar side of the antecubital flexion crease, and is extended to the ulnar border of the wrist flexion crease. The incision is carried proximally from the beginning of the circumferential burn across the wrist flexion crease. With this approach anatomical structures are at minimal risk, as the incisions are lateral, extending only to the interval between burned and viable tissues. Particular caution is used around the elbow to avoid the ulnar nerve in the cubital tunnel. The incision in this region is anterior to the medial epicondyle (see Fig. 46-2).

After restoration of pulses, the arm is elevated to minimize edema and to encourage venous drainage. The extremity is dressed with appropriate topical antimicrobial therapy.

If the patient has an intrinsic minus digital posture, intrinsic compartmental ischemia is diagnosed and prompt decompression of the dorsal interosseous muscles is performed. Longitudinal incisions are made on the dorsum of the hand on a course paralleling the extensor tendons. These are extended onto the fingers at the mid-axial plane to

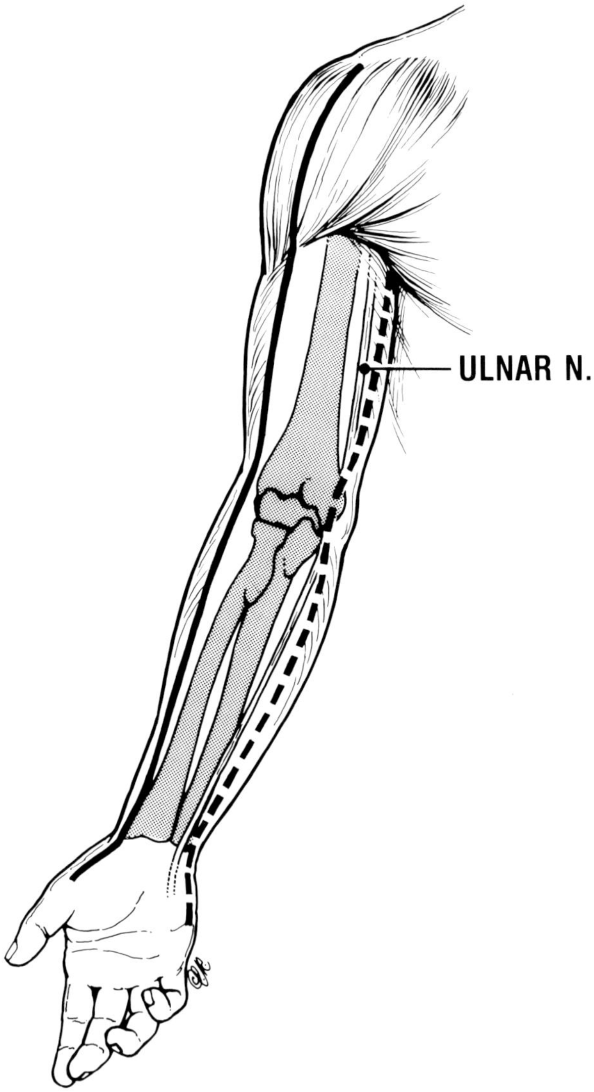

Figure 46–3. *The solid line indicates the upper extremity location for lateral escharotomy; the dotted line indicates the location for medial escharotomy. Note the ulnar nerve passing behind the medial epicondyle; the incision must be anterior to the condyle.*

decompress tight eschar of the digits. Digital pulses should now be audible via Doppler flow examination.

Usually, escharotomy without fasciotomy is sufficient for restoration of adequate pulses in the extremity. However, with high-voltage electrical injury where tissue injury is often subfascial, fasciotomy is required. Lower-extremity escharotomy, performed at lateral and medial mid-lateral points, avoids the fibular head, as the peroneal nerve is superficially located at this point. The escharotomies extend to the base of the large and small toes if the foot has deep full-thickness burn injuries (Fig. 46-4).

Infection of the escharotomy site or burn wound is not a common complication if these wounds are treated with topical chemotherapeutic agents on a regular and timely basis.

Iatrogenic injury to peripheral nerve occurs during escharotomy when landmarks are obscured or when treatment has been left to the least experienced member of the burn team. A localized nerve injury with electrocautery usually resolves spontaneously. However, a short segment injury of the peripheral nerve may be amenable to resection and primary repair. Other causes of iatrogenic injury related to the burn wound include improperly placed skeletal pin traction and stretch neuropathy caused by traction devices (especially on the brachial plexus). Circumferentially tight dressings over superficially located nerves (the ulnar nerve at the cubital tunnel and peroneal nerve at the fibular head) may induce neurapraxias. As axillary or sciatic nerve injuries from intramuscular injections are not unusual, these types of injections are avoided in burn patients.

Reconstruction

Consideration of reconstruction is delayed until the burn wound has healed. Immediate nerve reconstruction is usually impossible due to necrotic tissue, high bacterial counts, the necessity for early splinting and aggressive range-of-motion exercises, and, most importantly, the indeterminate nature of the nerve lesion. In cases of direct thermal injury, the wound bed for nerve reconstruction is not well vascularized. Flap coverage with delayed nerve grafting may be required. Generally, nerve reconstruction with interpositional cable grafts has a poor prognosis due to the relatively poor vascular environment induced by the burn. Unless intermediate coverage is provided with local or distant flaps, long-term failure due to fibrosis results. The

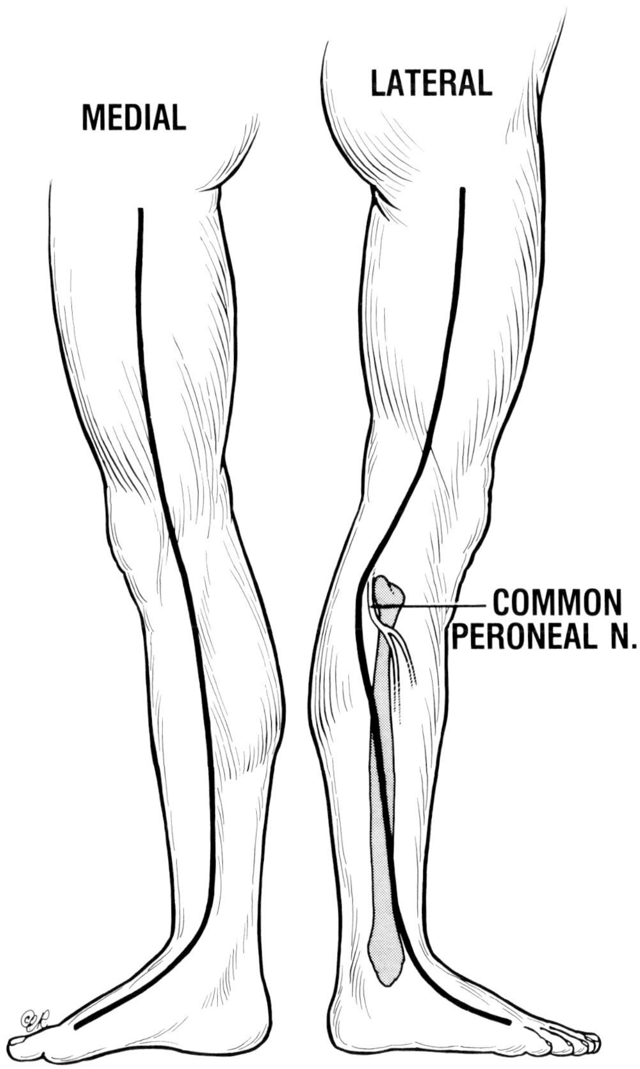

Figure 46–4. *Location of medial and lateral escharotomies in the lower extremity. Note the location of the common peroneal nerve behind the fibular head. The incision must avoid the bony prominence.*

most appropriate treatment, especially in high motor lesions of upper and lower extremity, is early tendon transfer. This will facilitate early range of motion and exercises rehabilitation.

The chronic phase of burn management peripheral polyneuropathy has been reported frequently. In patients with burn wounds of 20% total body surface area or more, the incidence is higher. These patients may show slowing of conduction velocities in multiple peripheral nerves; the cause of these lesions is undetermined.[2,3] Those presenting with associated encephalopathy have been related to metabolic disturbances. In a recent series, Helm indicted poor patient positioning, heavy bulky dressings over superficial nerves, and failure to rotate intramuscular injections.[6] Frequent injections into the deltoid cause muscle and, in particular, nerve injury by a combination of toxicity of the drugs, pressure from the volume injected, the physical trauma of needles, and associated inflammatory reactions. Helm emphasized that neuropathies are also produced by faulty positioning. The ulnar nerve is easily injured in the cubital canal if the extremity is flexed, pronated, and placed on a pillow. Staff education is critical to preventing iatrogenic injuries. Treatment is specific to the nerve at risk; no single remedy has been effective.

A late cause of peripheral nerve injury in burn patients is heterotopic bone formation. This a crippling complication of thermal injury is seen following full-thickness injuries. The specific cause is unknown, but the impaired motion of joints has been implicated. While the elbow is most often affected, ossification can occur anywhere, most often in periarticular locations.[11] The ulnar nerve may become entrapped, requiring operative decompression and anterior transposition. Dissection and release is difficult due to the intraosseous position of the nerve. A meticulous osteotomy, performed in small increments, is required to expose the nerve within the heterotopic bony canal. Even with these operative measures, recurrence is common.

ELECTRICAL INJURY

Electrical burns directly affect nerve tissue, accounting for the highest incidence of nerve injury. Alterations in nerve begin with change in current density at approximately 45°C. Damage occurs in nerves before surrounding tissues because of the increased current they convey per unit area.[4] Because electrical current follows the path of least resistance, it often destroys neurovascular bundles first, resulting in permanent, irreversible damage. Relative tissue resistance to electric current varies, with the lowest values in nerve and the highest in bone. The extent of tissue destruction is directly proportional to energy and duration of contact.[4] Laboratory studies on the changes in action potentials of nerves indicate that direct neuronal damage occurs secondary to current. The destruction of local and regional blood flow compounds the problem.

Patients sustaining high-voltage electrical burns are stabilized with the same aggressive management as those with thermal injuries. More attention is focused during acute resuscitation to decompression of muscular compartments. After the patient is stabilized hemodynamically, early treatment of the extremity involves intraoperative exploration and decompression with debridement of dead muscle in an effort to maintain perfusion and reduce the risk of gas gangrene from nonviable muscle and necrotic tissue.

The hallmarks of electrical injury are the propensity for spotty injuries, evidence of skip areas of necrosis within muscle compartments, and progression of cellular death over the first few days of injury. In addition to escharotomy, early fasciotomy, followed by thorough exploration of muscle compartments, is required in the treatment of extensive electrical injuries.

This initial aggressive approach may expose peripheral nerves with undetermined viability. Wounds are managed temporarily with biological dressings (allograft or xenograft), wet antibiotic dressings, or skin grafting. It is imperative to leave wounds so that it is possible to inspect them regularly, because it often becomes apparent within 72 hours that nerve is nonviable, requiring debridement.

Because of the highly erratic and unpredictable nature of electrical injury, management is conservative initially. Reconstruction is delayed until viability of tissue is finally determined. Cut ends of nerve are temporarily transfixed with wire sutures placed through the epineurium for the purposes of preventing retraction and easing identification.

After complete stabilization of the wound, coverage is obtained with split-thickness skin grafts, local or distant flaps, or, if necessary, free tissue transfers. The obvious advantage of flap coverage is the provision of a well-vascularized, pliable bed for subsequent nerve reconstruction.

Most frequently encountered electrical nerve injuries are to the median and ulnar nerves, reflecting the high proportion of hand injuries. In electrical injuries where muscle mass is small, debridement is initially conservative, as all attempts are made to preserve viable tissue. In the case of isolated digital involvement in the hands and feet, salvage is achieved by effective debridement, preservation of digital length, and coverage with grafts after granulation tissue has formed.[5] If the digit is useless and salvageable only through heroic efforts, amputation is advisable.

Nerve reconstruction of the stable wound involves cooperation between the patient and the reconstructive surgeon. The armamentarium includes resection and primary repair, cable grafting, and vascularized microvascular nerve transfers.

RADIATION INJURY

Peripheral nerve tends to be relatively radioresistant due to its protected position and tissue depth, low metabolic rate, and low reproductive capabilities. Tissues exposed to high-energy sources such as X-ray or gamma radiation can be injured lethally. Initially, tissue is hyperemic. This is followed by arteritis with thrombosis, obstructive endothelial proliferation, and fibroplasia. These wounds often progress to complete ischemic necrosis. If they epithelize, they are pale, ischemic, atrophic, and friable, making them more susceptible to ulceration from minor trauma or mechanical injury.

Management of radiation wounds with nerve injury begins with meticulous debridement, administration of antibiotics, and advancement of a vascular bed for grafting. The major difference between radiation burns and other thermal wounds is the chronic ischemia induced by radiation. Wide excision of injured tissue usually is required to reach a well-vascularized bed. Vascularized tissue is required for coverage of these large wounds.

Healing can be achieved with local or distant myocutaneous flaps or free tissue transfer, especially where reinnervation and neovascularization to a specific area is critical. Peripheral neuritis and wound pain due to ischemia are commonly associated with more severe injuries.[5] Nerve reconstruction by way of neurorrhaphy, nerve grafting, or vascularized nerve grafting is delayed until wound revascularization has been achieved. If nerve reconstruction is impossible, patient reeducation and mechanical assistance to denervated areas are required.

CHEMICAL INJURY

Although chemical burns do not usually cause full-thickness loss, they can cause substantial nerve injury. Initial treatment begins with copious lavage with water. Selected agents are used to neutralize specific acids and alkali.

Phosphorus causes extensive tissue destruction. Particles erode skin and subcutaneous tissue, inducing a deep chemical burn and occasionally leading to localized nerve trunk destruction. White phosphorus produces both chemical and thermal injury after exposure to air, with oxidation to phosphorus pentoxide. Operative debridement of the particles is indicated. If doubt exists regarding the presence of particulate matter, the wound is washed with 1% copper sulfate to produce readily visible black particles.

More commonly, these caustic agents produce a large amount of edematous eschar, producing nerve injury by compression. After lavage, a full examination of the extremity is performed. Escharotomy is carried out if necessary; the limb is then splinted and elevated.

The long-term effects of injury to peripheral nerve include decreased sensation, constant itching (which may resolve within 12 months), and intolerance to heat and cold. These complaints are best treated symptomatically with lubrication of healed wounds, pharmacologic treatment with antihistamines, and overall support by the burn management team. The team's support is essential because these complaints may not be alleviated completely, and regeneration of cutaneous nerves may be incomplete.

Although not well established at present, a future role for microneurovascular nerve transfer in the reconstruction of thermally injured tissues is possible. The technical difficulties encountered with a poorly vascularized bed may be avoided with vascularized transfer. The effect of the ischemic environment on axonal regeneration may be reduced substantially (see Chap. 40).[21]

CONCLUSION

Early recognition and treatment of *vascular* injury in the burned extremity is critical in the acute phase. Prevention of infection and timely wound closure hastens rehabilitation. Subsequent reconstruction is carried out; operative alternatives are outlined in Chapters 49 through 54.

REFERENCES

1. Berger A. Nerve lesions due to electrical current and thermal damage. Hefte-Unfallheilkd 1974; 0(117):394–398.
2. Blom S, Ugland OM. Peripheral nerve injuries in electrical burns. Scand J Plast Reconstr Surg 1967; 2:45.
3. Carver N, Logan A. Critically ill polyneuropathy associated with burns: A case report. Burns 1989; 15:179–180.
4. Cohen BE, Cukier J. Simultaneous posterior and anterior interosseous nerve syndromes. J Hand Surg [Am] 1982; 7:398–400.
5. Curreri WP, Morris J, Pruitt BA Jr. The treatment of chemical burns: Specialized diagnostic therapeutic and prognostic considerations. J Trauma 1970; 10:634.
6. Helm PA, Pondian G, Heck E. Neuromuscular problems in the burn patient: Causes and prevention. Arch Phys Med Rehab 1985; 66:451–453.
7. Helme RD, Andrews PV. The effect of nerve lesions on the inflammatory response to injury. J Neurosci Res 1985; 13:453–459.
8. Henderson B, Koepke GH, Feller I. Peripheral polyneuropathy among patients with burns. Arch Phys Med Rehab 1971; 52:149–151.
9. Krupp S, Nigst H. Deep burns of hands (with affected tendons, nerves, musculature, joints and

bones). Klinische Medizin Osterreichische Zeitschrift-Gur Wissenschaftliche Und Praktische Medizin (Vienna) 1967; 22:396–400.

10. Monafo WW, Eliasson SG. Sciatic nerve function following hindlimb thermal injury. J Surg Res 1987; 43:344–350.
11. Munster AJ, Bruck HM, Johns LA. Heterotopic calcification following burns: A prospective study. J Trauma 1972; 12:1071.
12. Ponder E. The coefficient of thermal conductivity of blood and various tissues. J Gen Physiol 1962; 45:545.
13. Poticha SM, Bell JL, Mehn WH. Electrical injuries with special reference to the hand. Arch Surg 1962; 85:172.
14. Rouse RG, Dimic AR. The treatment of electrical injury compared to burn injury: A review of pathophysiology and comparison of patient management protocols. J Trauma 1978; 18:43.
15. Salisbury RE. Burns of the upper extremity. In: Salisbury RE, Pruitt BA. Burns of the upper extremities. Philadelphia: WB Saunders, 1976:36.
16. Salisbury RE, Bevin AG. Management of peripheral nerve problems. In: Omer GE Jr, Spinner M, eds. The management of peripheral nerve problems. Philadelphia: WB Saunders, 1980:755.
17. Salisbury RE, Dingeldein GP. Peripheral nerve complications following burn injury. Clin Orthop 1982; 163:92–97.
18. Salisbury RE, Hunt JL, Glenn D, Pruitt BA. Management of electrical burns of the upper extremity. Plast Reconstr Surg 1973; 51:648.
19. Sances A Jr, Myklebust JB, Larson SJ, et al. Experimental electrical injury studies. J Trauma 1981; 21:589–597.
20. Solen L, Fischer R, Strute RG. The natural history of electrical injury. J Trauma 1977; 17:487.
21. Taylor I, Ham F. The free vascularized nerve graft: A further experimental and clinical application of microvascular techniques. Plast Reconstr Surg 1976; 57:413.
22. Ugland OM. Electrical burns. A clinical and experimental study with special reference to peripheral nerve injury. Scand J Plas Reconstr Surg Suppl 1967; 2:1–74.

47

Nerve Injury Associated with Devascularizing Trauma

Jesse B. Jupiter

AUTHOR'S KEY POINTS

- Nerve injury associated with devascularizing trauma is a complex injury that produces symptoms of cold intolerance and pain, despite adequate vascular reconstruction.
- In the replanted digit, there is a strong correlation between failure to achieve discriminatory sensibility and significantly reduced vascularization.
- When combined nerve and noncritical arterial injury occur in the forearm, the surgeon should place more emphasis on performing tension-free nerve repair rather than on arterial repair.
- When the injury is at knee level, the association of a complete tibial nerve injury with a vascular injury has a very poor prognosis. Primary amputation is often warranted.

The relationship and outcome of nerve injury associated with devascularizing trauma has been the subject of considerable scrutiny. Several questions confront clinicians faced with these complex injuries. While some have suggested that arterial interruption is a critical factor that adversely affects recovery from concomitant major nerve injury,[10,29,30,38] others have not found this to be so.[7,26,32] More often than not, devascularizing trauma represents the sequelae of complex, high-energy injuries. It should not be surprising that the outcome of any or all of the injured structures (ie, neural, vascular, or skeletal) would be intertwined and subject to a host of factors, including the level and mechanism of the injury, the duration of ischemia (both warm and cold), and the quality of the operative repairs.

An important consideration is the influence that arterial revascularization has on neural regeneration.[4,5,9,15,23] This becomes most apparent when acute neurovascular injury exists in a limb that retains sufficient arterial inflow for survival. Considerable effort has been made to determine the relationship between arterial repair, neural regeneration, and other associated symptoms. Clinicians have sought to determine how best to evaluate combined neurovascular injuries, what the relationship is between arterial inflow and cold intolerance, and how standard sensory tests values such as moving touch,[3] two-point discrimination,[22,25] tuning fork, or sharp–dull discrimination are affected by arterial pulse pressure. Does cold stress testing provide an adequate measure of the relationship of arterial inflow and neurological injury and recovery?[17]

DEFINITIONS

The literature has not always clearly defined what is meant by a "devascularizing" injury. Similarly, differentiation between injuries requiring vascular repair, revascularization, or replantation has been inconsistent.[20] This chapter uses the following definitions:

- Amputation ("replantation"): those limbs or parts completely severed without any residual attachment.
- Incomplete amputation ("revascularization"): those limbs or parts whose circulation has been so disrupted that immediate vascular repair is required for survival.
- Noncritical vascular injury ("repair"): those injured extremities or parts that include an arterial disruption but have sufficient vascularity for survival.

RESEARCH

The relationship of vascular injury and neural regeneration has been the subject of several experimental and clinical studies. The rabbit ear has served as an excellent animal model, as its central artery has been shown to be innervated by a uniform population of sympathetic postganglionic norepinephrine-releasing axons located near the medial–adventitial border of the artery.[2,11,13,19] It would appear from previous studies that the vascular response to norepinephrine is exceedingly complex, involving both extraluminal and intraluminal factors.[2] Lassmann and Piza, using the autotransplanted rabbit ear model, found a rapid regeneration of the central arterial nerve supply following revascularization.[19] The regenerating nerves, however, were observed to be poorly attached to the vascular wall and did not become incorporated into the Schwann cells of the distal parts of the transected and repaired vessels. These investigators concluded that defects in the restoration of the adrenergic vascular plexus could account, to some degree, for altered vasomotor function following combined neurovascular injury.

The replanted digit represents a completely denervated, sympathectomized, and devascularized structure without any possibility of cross-innervation by anatomical variations. As such, it has provided an excellent clinical model to study the relationship of reestablished blood flow to functional nerve regeneration.[5,9,15,23] Gelberman and coworkers observed a strong correlation between blood flow (as measured by comparing the pulse pressure of the replanted digit with the contralateral uninjured digit) and both two-point discrimination and the response to cold stress.[9] Diminished blood flow (pulse pressure $< 75\%$ of the control digit) correlated statistically with a poor sensory return, although enhanced vascular inflow did not guarantee good sensory function, suggesting that other factors, such as the mechanism of injury or the length of nerve defect, may be equally important. The investigators also noted a strong correlation with improved sensibility and tolerance to cold stress.

Freelander, using laser Doppler flowmetry,[5] Kay, using venous occlusion plethysmography,[15] and Nylander and associates, using finger systolic pressure measurement,[23] also confirmed improved sensibility with tolerance to cold stress, but could not document a strong correlation with either vascular inflow and sensibility or response to cold stress.

Although cold intolerance is a common feature of combined neurovascular injury as well as nerve injuries alone,[4,7,12,17,26] its exact mechanism has not been clearly defined. Cold intolerance appears to represent a disorder of vasoregulation of the digital vascular tree rather than the absolute degree of the reestablished blood flow.[4] Both local and central mechanisms are involved in regulating the peripheral circulation. The vasoconstrictor input of the sympathetic nervous system is one of a number

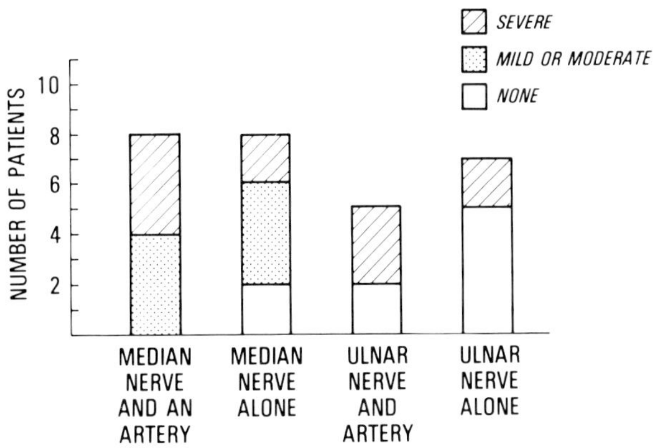

Figure 47–1. *Cold intolerance was observed by Gelberman and coworkers following isolated forearm nerve injury as well as combined nerve and artery trauma. (From Gelberman RH, Blasingame JP, Fronek A, Dimick MP. Forearm arterial injuries. J Hand Surg 1979;4:401–408, with permission.)*

of central factors, including humeral control by circulating catecholamines[33] and chemical mediators such as serotonin, histamines, and prostaglandins.[36] Locally, there exists myogenic control related to perfusion pressure, which, in the presence of operative or chemical denervation, may react directly to cold by vasoconstriction.[34] Following nerve repair, regeneration of both somatic and automatic function occurs, yet control over arteriovenous shunting in the digital pulp varies widely.

The observations found in the replanted digits were also confirmed in a study of forearm arterial and nerve injuries carried out by Gelberman and associates.[7] While the combination of arterial and nerve injury led to symptoms of pain and cold intolerance, those symptoms were also noted in patients with isolated forearm median nerve injuries (Fig. 47-1). These investigators found no correlation between the rate or completeness of sensory and motor return and the patency of the adjacent artery. In addition, there was no evidence that arterial repair would offset the symptoms of cold intolerance (Fig. 47-2).

In a study of cold stress testing, Koman and coworkers observed three distinct patterns of response:[17]

1. Type I: baseline digital temperature 30° to 32°C; 3° to 4°C drop with cooling, with prompt rise during rewarming
   a. Normal hand
   b. Isolated upper extremity arterial injuries with good collateral circulation
   c. Early stages post-sympathectomy
2. Type II: digital temperature between 2° and 6°C cooler than Type I; more dramatic drop with cooling and slower rewarming
   a. Isolated peripheral nerve injury
   b. Isolated arterial injury with fair collateral circulation
   c. Arterial injury with good collateral circulation, but combined with peripheral nerve injury.
3. Type III: baseline temperature below 28.5°C; drop

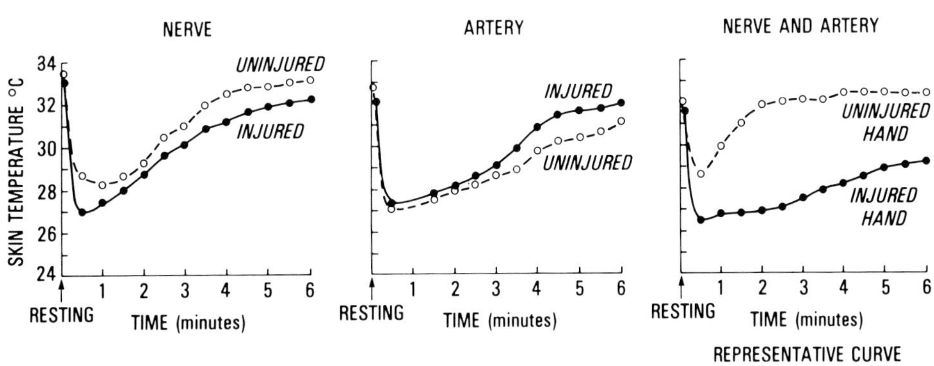

Figure 47–2. *Representative rewarming curves comparing uninjured to injured hands following forearm arterial repair alone and combined arterial and nerve repair. Significant delays in rewarming were observed only in the combined nerve and artery group. (From Gelberman RH, Blasingame JP, Fronek A, Dimick MP. Forearm arterial injuries. J Hand Surg 1979;4:401–408, with permission.)*

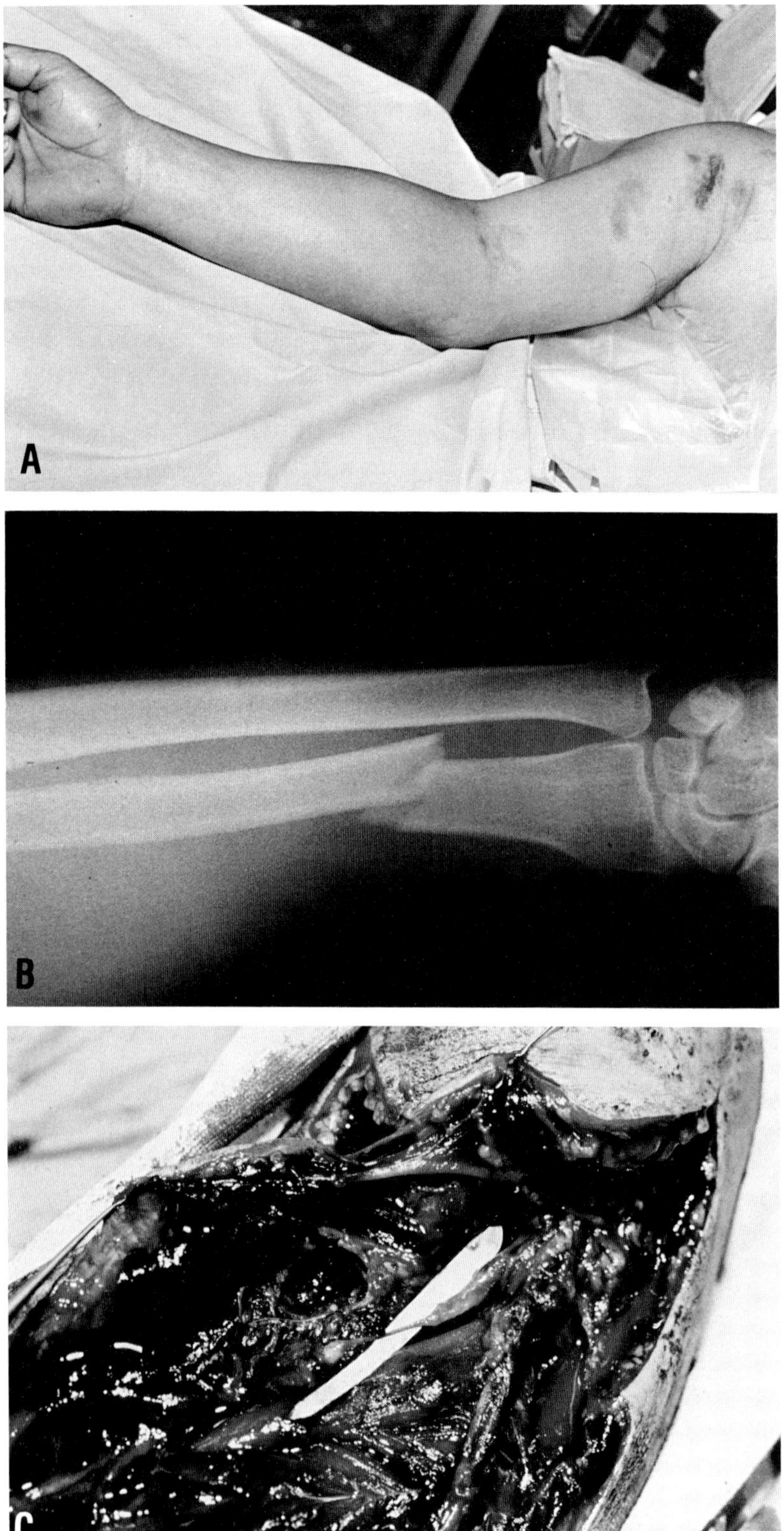

Figure 47–3. A 60-year-old fisherman's right dominant arm was caught in a winch on a boat. (***A, B***) Upon arrival at the hospital, loss of sensibility was noted in his median nerve distribution, no radial or ulnar nerve pulses could be palpated, and a fracture of his humerus and radius was noted on X-ray. (***C***) At surgery, following wide fasciotomy of the forearm, the brachial artery was found to be disrupted and the median nerve, although intact, was stretched over a distance of 8–10 cm.

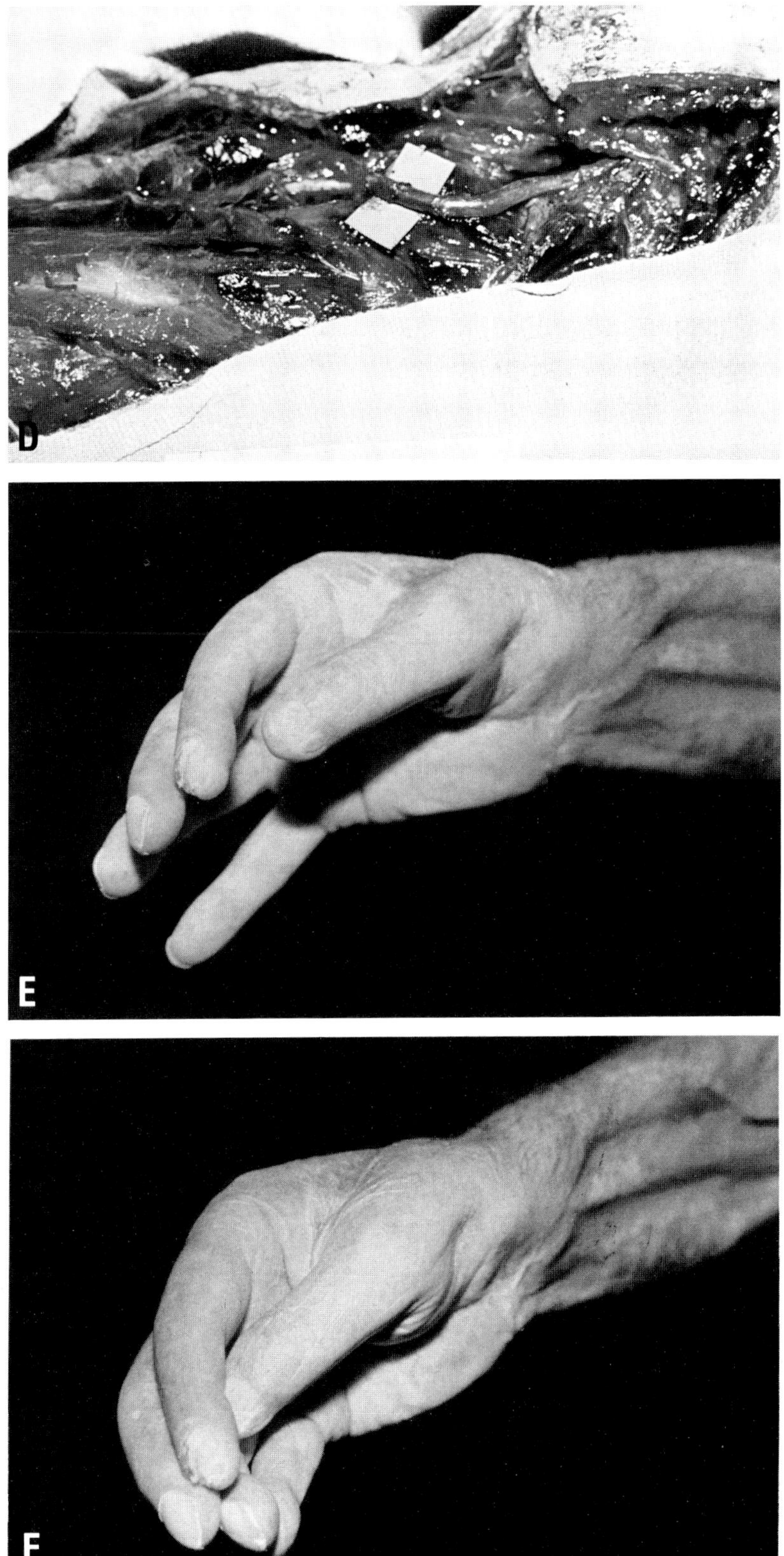

Figure 47–3. (Continued) (**D**) Repair of the brachial artery was performed using a reversed vein graft and the fractures were stabilized with internal fixation. (**E, F**) At a follow-up exam of 1 year, excellent arterial perfusion was seen, but the patient had only protective sensibility in the median nerve distribution and experienced extreme cold intolerance. Limited mobility was noted in his hand.

of 8° to 13°C with rapid cooling followed by slow rewarming
a. Arterial insufficiency
b. Combined arterial and peripheral nerve injury
c. Vasospastic disease.

In a separate investigation, Koman and associates used cold stress testing to investigate thermoregulatory control after upper extremity replantation.[16] They observed a return of two-point sensibility and intrinsic motor nerve recovery accompanied by a return of normal thermoregulatory patterns and loss of cold intolerance. When neurological function did not return, cold intolerance persisted along with an abnormal response to cold stress testing.

UPPER EXTREMITY

Revascularization of severely traumatized or amputated limbs continues to be commonplace because of the ability to shorten the upper extremity skeleton and the limited prehensile function offered by a prosthetic hand or terminal unit. Replantation offers the most extreme example of combined neurovascular trauma. The outcome is related to a number of factors, including the level and type of injury, duration of warm ischemia, type and extent of nerve injury, and age of the patient.

With replantation proximal to the carpus, return of sensibility as measured by two-point discrimination generally diminishes as the level of injury extends proximally. Young patients, sharp nerve division, and short ischemia times are factors associated with more favorable sensory outcomes (see Chap. 24).[1,21,27,28,35,37] Of interest is the fact that cold intolerance, hyperesthesia, or tropic ulceration is rarely recorded in the major upper extremity replantations, regardless of the quality of sensory return.

While the quality of motor recovery appears more variable, in most series intrinsic muscle function rarely recovers.[1,27,35,37] This probably reflects the level of nerve injury as well as damage due to anoxia. Above-elbow replantations often recover elbow flexion, providing the patient with an improved assistive limb.

The outcome of upper extremity "revascularizations" has a wider spectrum of functional recovery. This is due, in part, to the fact that associated nerve injury can extend from contusion to stretch to transection. In addition, the collateral circulation in the upper extremity course is relatively parallel to the path of the dominant vessel.[14,31] This is in sharp contrast to the lower limb, particularly around the knee, where collateral branches run in a perpendicular plane to the dominant popliteal artery. Thus, it is not uncommon to find occlusion of the brachial artery in the setting of a viable hand (Fig. 47-3).

When a major nerve has been lacerated and one or both arteries in the forearm have been injured, Gelberman and coworkers found no evidence to suggest that arterial patency will offset the symptoms of cold or stress intolerance.[8] Rather, they observed these to be related primarily to the associated nerve injury. Using a timed Allen test[6] to determine the extent of arterial support of the hand from each artery individually, the authors recommended the following:

1. Laceration of both arteries with distal ischemia: Repair both vessels.
2. Laceration of both arteries without distal ischemia: Repair both vessels.
3. Laceration of one artery: Repair if timed Allen test suggests incomplete support of the hand through the intact artery.

LOWER EXTREMITY

Devascularizing trauma in combination with peripheral nerve injury in the lower extremity (most commonly the sequelae of fracture-dislocations about the knee or high-energy open tibia fractures) often presents a difficult decision for the surgeon.[24] Accurate clinical assessment of the neural deficit is difficult in the emergency department when arterial insufficiency of the involved limb gives rise to signs and symptoms of neural dysfunction. By the same token, the nature and extent of the nerve injury correlates well with the ultimate functional result.[18]

Despite advances in the surgical salvage of mangled lower extremities, it has become increasingly apparent that some of these revascularized limbs are a functional liability. Further, a below-the-knee prosthesis effectively provides the functional needs of the lower limb (a stable stance and functional gait) in sharp contrast to the upper extremity, where sensibility of the terminal unit is critical to function. Several investigators, recognizing the complexities involved in assessing functional outcome in these difficult lower extremity combined neurovascular injuries, have established guidelines to help the surgeon decide which limbs should be salvaged. Lange and associates have presented guidelines to suggest which limbs are best treated by primary amputation in open tibia fractures with vascular injury:[18]

1. Absolute indications for amputation
   a. Anatomically complete disruption of the posterior tibial nerve in the adult
   b. Crush injury with warm ischemia beyond 6 hours
2. Relative indications
   a. Serious associated polytrauma
   b. Severe ipsilateral foot trauma
   c. Anticipated protracted course to obtain soft-tissue coverage and tibial reconstruction

Primary amputation is recommended if either of the absolute indications or two or three of the relative indications are present.

It appears that devascularizing trauma associated with nerve injury represents not only a difficult surgical problem but also a clinical entity that is not well understood. Current information suggests that blood flow depends not only on an efficient readaptation and new formation of vessels, but also on the reinnervation of the pre-existing vascular system by the efferent and afferent constituents of the nervous system.

REFERENCES

1. Berger A, Millesi H. Functional results from replantation surgery: A 5-year report from the Viennese replantation team. Aust N Z J Surg 1980; 50:244–247.
2. De la Lande IS. Adrenergic mechanisms in the rabbit ear artery. Blood Vessels 1975; 12:137–160.
3. Dellon AL, Curtis RM, Edgerton MT. Evaluating recovery of sensation in the hand following nerve injury. Johns Hopkins Med J 1972; 130:235–243.
4. Engkvist O, Wahren LK, Wallin G, Torebjork E, Nystrom B. Effects of regional intravenous guanethidine block in post-traumatic cold intolerance in hand amputees. J Hand Surg [Br] 1985; 10:145–150.
5. Freelander E. The relationship between cold intolerance and cutaneous blood flow in digital replantation patients. J Hand Surg [Br] 1986; 11:15–19.
6. Gelberman RH, Blasingame JP. The timed Allen test. J Trauma 1977; 21:477–479.
7. Gelberman RH, Blasingame JP, Fronek A, Dimick MP. Forearm arterial injuries. J Hand Surg 1979; 4:401–408.
8. Gelberman RH, Nunley JA, Koman LA, et al. The results of radial and ulnar arterial repair in the forearm. J Bone Joint Surg [Am] 1982; 64:383–387.
9. Gelberman RH, Urbaniak JR, Bright DS, Levin LS. Digital sensibility following replantation. J Hand Surg 1978; 3:313–319.
10. Gilliat RW, Wilson TG. Ischaemic sensory loss in patients with peripheral nerve lesions. J Neurol Neurosurg Psychiatry 1954; 17:104.
11. Grant RT, Thompson RWS. Cholinesterase and the nerve supply to blood vessels in the rabbit's external ear. J Anat 1963; 97:7–22.
12. Guttmann E, Guttmann L. Factors affecting recovery of sensory function after nerve lesions. J Neurol Neurosurg Psychiatry 1942; 5:117.
13. Hume WR, Waterson JG. The innervation of the rabbit ear artery. Blood Vessels 1978; 15:348–364.
14. Jupiter J, Kleinert HE. Vascular injuries in the upper extremity. In: Tubiana R, ed. The hand, vol 3. Philadelphia: WB Saunders, 1988; 593–611.
15. Kay S. Venous occlusion plethysmography in patients with cold-related symptoms after digital salvage procedures. J Hand Surg [Br] 1985; 10:151–154.
16. Koman LA, Nunley JH. Thermoregulatory control after upper extremity replantation. J Hand Surg [Am] 1986; 11:548–552.
17. Koman LA, Nunley JA, Goldner JL, Seaber AV, Urbaniak JR. Isolated cold stress testing in the assessment of symptoms in the upper extremity. J Hand Surg [Am] 1984; 9:305–313.
18. Lange RH, Bach AW, Hansen ST Jr, Johansen KH. Open tibial fractures with associated vascular injuries: Prognosis for limb salvage. J Trauma 1985; 25:203–208.
19. Lassmann G, Piza H. The nerve response after au-

totransplantation of the rabbit ear. J Hand Surg [Am] 1984; 9:121–124.

20. May JW Jr. Letter to the editor. Digital replantation. J Hand Surg 1980; 5:515.
21. Meyer VE. Hand amputations proximal but close to the wrist joint: Prime candidate for reattachment (long-term functional results). J Hand Surg [Am] 1985; 10:989–991.
22. Moberg E. Evaluation and management of nerve injuries in the hand. Surg Clin North Am 1964; 44: 1019–1029.
23. Nylander G, Nylander E, Lassvik C. Cold sensitivity after replantation in relation to arterial circulation and vasoregulation. J Hand Surg [Br] 1987; 12:78–81.
24. O'Donnell TF Jr, Brewster DC, Darling RC. Arterial injuries associated with fractures and/or dislocations of the knee. J Trauma 1977; 17:775–782.
25. Omer GE Jr. Injuries to nerves of the upper extremity. J Bone Joint Surg [Am] 1974; 56:1615–1624.
26. Richards RL. Neurovascular lesions. In: Seddon HJ, ed. Peripheral nerve injuries. Medical Research Council Special Report Series No. 282. London: Her Majesty's Stationery Office, 1954.
27. Russell RC, O'Brien B, Morrison WA, Pamamull G, MacLeod A. The late functional results of upper limb revascularization and replantation. J Hand Surg [Am] 1984; 9:623–633.
28. Schlenker JD, Kleinert HE, Tsai TM. Methods and results of replantation following traumatic amputation of the thumb in 64 patients. J Hand Surg 1980; 5:63–70.
29. Seddon HJ. Surgical disorders of the peripheral nerves. Edinburgh: Churchill-Livingstone, 1972.
30. Shumaker HG, Boone R, Kunkler A. Studies of combined vascular and neurologic injuries. Arch Surg 1953; 67:753.
31. Strandness DE Jr, ed. Collateral circulation in clinical surgery. Philadelphia: WB Saunders, 1969.
32. Sunderland S. Nerves and nerve injuries, ed 2. Edinburgh: Churchill-Livingstone, 1978.
33. Trendelenberg U. Mechanisms of supersensitivity and subsensitivity to sympathetic amines. Pharmacol Rev 1966; 18:629–640.
34. Vanhoutte PM. Physical factors of regulations. In: Bohr DF, ed. Handbook of physiology, vol 2. Bethesda: American Physiological Society, 1983.
35. Wang SH, Young KF, Wei JN. Replantation of severed limbs: Clinical analysis of 91 cases. J Hand Surg 1981; 6:311–318.
36. Witzleb E. Functions of the vascular system. In: Schmidt RF, Thews G, eds. Human physiology. New York: Springer-Verlag, 1983.
37. Wood MB, Cooney WP. Above-elbow limb replantation: Functional results. J Hand Surg [Am] 1986; 11:682–687.
38. Yahr MD, Beebe GW. Recovery of motor function. In: Woodhall B, Beebe GW, eds. Peripheral nerve regeneration: A follow-up study of 3,656 World War II injuries. Washington DC: US Government Printing Office, 1956.

X

OPERATIVE RECONSTRUCTION FOR IRREPARABLE PERIPHERAL NERVE INJURIES (Excluding Brachial Plexus)

48 Principles of Tendon Transfers
49 Tendon Transfer for Radial Nerve Palsy
50 Median Nerve Palsy
51 Ulnar Nerve Palsy
52 Tendon Transfers for Combined Nerve Injuries
53 Lower Extremity Nerve Palsies
54 Free Muscle Transfer for Functional Reconstruction
55 Direct Muscular Neurotization
56 Free Flaps for Providing Sensibility to the Hand

48

Principles of Tendon Transfers

Edward E. Almquist

AUTHOR'S KEY POINTS

- Muscle *force* is directly proportional to the cross sectional area of all of a muscle's fibers (the physiological cross section).
- *Work* is force multiplied by distance. *Work capacity* is related to the physiological cross section and length of a muscle's fibers.
- *Power* is a measurement of work over time. The transferred muscle must have adequate power; its strength should compare with that of the one being replaced.
- *Amplitude* is the amount a muscle can be stretched from its resting position, plus the amount it contracts. A muscle contracts to approximately 40% of its resting length, at which point it stops exerting force.
- The major principles of tendon transfer are the following:
  1. Deformities due to contracture are corrected prior to transfer.
  2. Muscles with actions similar to the ones they are replacing are used.
  3. The line of pull is as straight as possible.
  4. In the lower extremity, tendons are commonly inserted into bone. In the upper extremity, distal attachment to tendon is most often satisfactory.

Surgery is the ability to intervene directly into the workings of the body, and transplanting tendons is a very specific mechanical manifestation of that ability. The development of surgery required anatomical knowledge, anesthesia, and an acceptance of the idea that one human could or should intervene into the workings of another, an action that had previously been permitted only to God. Because the principles of tendon transplant surgery originate in the early days of medicine, it is appropriate to examine briefly the evolution of medicine.

BRIEF HISTORY OF SURGERY

Historically, medicine has been a mixture of specific treatments, such as herbs, potions, and surgery, and divine intervention. Ancient physicians played a role in both of these forms of treatment: as far back as the Paleolithic era (10,000–7000 B.C.), skulls clearly show signs of trephination and cave drawings depict supernatural powers of healing and strength.[13] Codified medical knowledge in Mesopotamia dates back to about 4000 B.C.; surgical tools have been found, and tablets depict diseases, their symptoms, and treatment.

Greece became the dominant culture in Europe in the 6th century B.C. Greek philosophy was a mixture of inductive logic, mysticism, and divine intervention. Illness was thought to be caused by an imbalance of four elements—air, water, fire, and earth—and treatment was directed at bringing these elements back into harmony. Techniques consisted primarily of diet, hygiene, and rest, but surgery also was performed. Fractures were reduced and splinted; cautery was used, as was drainage for infection; and herbs were applied directly to enhance wound healing. The Greek temples of Aesculapius, each with its own medical staff, became known as centers of healing throughout the eastern Mediterranean region. Itinerant physicians were drawn to these temples, which could be considered forerunners of the modern hospital system.

Galen, who lived in the 1st century A.D., may have been the most influential physician of all time. Among his 500 treatises was the first medical book about the hand, in which he wrote:

> Thus man is the most intelligent of the animals and so, also, hands are the instruments most suitable for an intelligent animal. For it is not because he has hands that he is the most intelligent, as Anaxagoras says, but because he is the most intelligent that he has hands, as Aristotle says, judging most correctly.[8] Indeed, not by his hands, but by his reason has man been instructed in the arts. Hands are an instrument, as the lyre is the instrument of the musician, and tongs of the smith.

Galen urged readers to be wary of relying on the written word, saying that someone who wished to observe the works of nature should "put his trust not in books of anatomy but in his own eyes."[8] Galen's philosophy and writings dominated medical thought for 1500 years, but the teaching that direct observation is better than relying on previous writings was not actually followed until the Renaissance (Fig. 48-1).

Medicine, like the rest of society, stagnated during the Middle Ages. There was virtually no knowledge of internal anatomy; dissection was forbidden by the church. Healing was thought to take place by divine intervention, and any medical expertise came from the writings of Galen.

During the Renaissance, Galen's principle of gaining knowledge through experimentation was rediscovered. In the 16th century Vesalius wrote a treatise on anatomy that displayed detailed drawings of the human body.[25] A Swiss physician, Paracelsus, made accurate medical observations and concluded that the body was a chemical machine. He thought, quite accurately, that a specific entity, not imbalance of the humors, caused disease, but he believed that this entity came from the stars.

Paré,[20] born in 1510, is considered the father of surgery. As an army surgeon in France, he applied the newly developing knowledge of anatomy to the practice of surgery, particularly to the treatment of war wounds. He is perhaps best remembered for initiating the gentle cleansing of wounds and closure by suture rather than by cautery. He described devices to facilitate setting fractures and

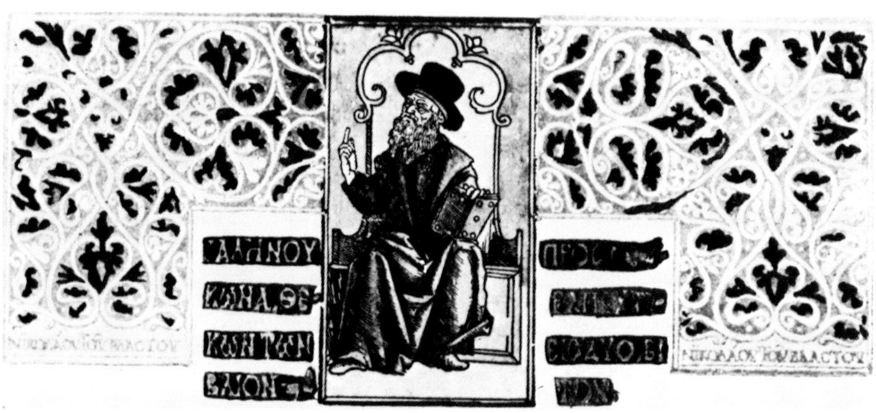

Figure 48–1. *Galen teaching (medieval manuscript, c. 1500).*

even described an artificial hand for use by amputees (Fig. 48-2). His 10 books served as the medical texts of the 16th century.

Von Helmont, in the 17th century, disputed the Greek theory of four basic elements: he thought that water was the basic element of the universe, and that all matter could be reduced to water. He believed that disease was an invasive process in the body, rather than a disarrangement of the humors, and rejected the theory that disease was caused by astrological or mystical forces acting on the body. He experimented and formed conclusions, and used chemistry in an attempt to eradicate disease.

The development of microscopy opened another door toward investigation and understanding, dominated by the Italian physician Malpighi. He discovered capillaries and their relationships, but his detailed findings in anatomy and physiology were challenged by his contemporaries and were only slowly understood.

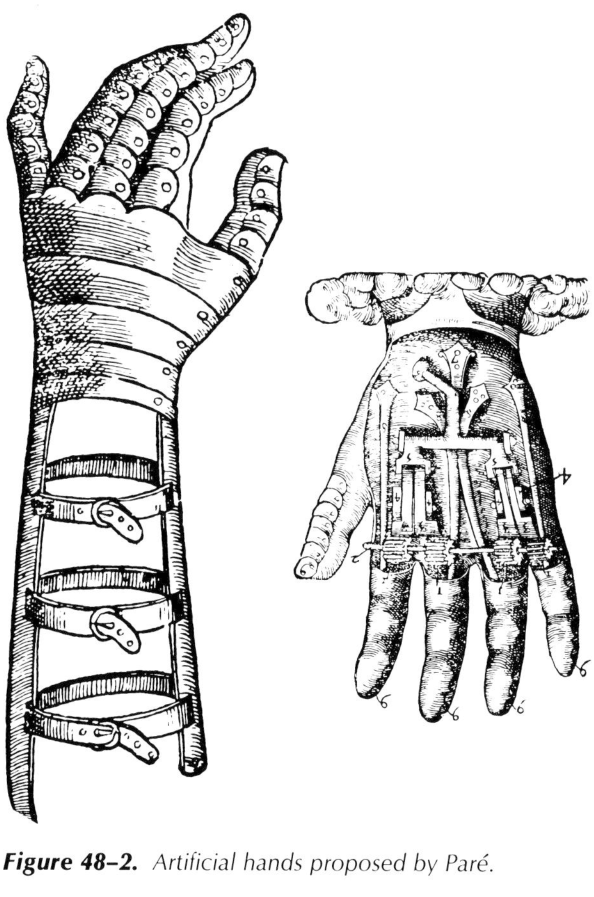

Figure 48–2. *Artificial hands proposed by Paré.*

The 18th century saw a steady advance in science but relatively little change in medicine. The two great philosophers of that century, Descartes and Bacon, were immensely influential, and the wisdom of the ancients was almost totally set aside. The body was seen more mechanically, making it easier to understand as a direct product of calculable forces and activities. Surgery, however, remained undeveloped. Although detailed anatomy and rudimentary physiology and biochemistry were developing, the technical problems of infection and the uncontrollability of unanesthetized patients ruled out any but the most basic surgery.

Modern surgery was launched by two quite different discoveries in the 19th century: the development of the cell theory of matter and the development of anesthesia (although alcohol and opiates had been used to sedate patients since antiquity). The cell theory soon led to the realization that bacteria cause infection, a theory first proposed 4000 years earlier in Babylonia. The development of anesthesia and the control of infection by antisepsis were prerequisites for the era of reconstructive surgery.

HISTORY OF TENDON TRANSFER SURGERY

The burgeoning surgical experience of the last half of the 19th century provided the foundation of knowledge necessary to support the development of specific techniques for repair and transfer of tendons. Nicoladoni, working in the second half of the 19th century, is credited with popularizing the use of tendon transfers to counter motor imbalance.[18,19] Most of these procedures were performed in the lower extremity, primarily for aftereffects of poliomyelitis, which had become rampant during the mid-19th century. Vulpius also wrote extensively about tendon transfers, and by the end of the 19th century hundreds of cases were reported.[26]

A classic clinical report on tendon transplants was published by the Italian orthopedist Codavilla in 1899.[7] He introduced four basics of tendon transplant surgery:

1. Recognizing before surgery the degree of functional capacity in the active muscles, and distinguishing between functional loss caused by paralysis from functional loss from misuse alone
2. Gauging accurately the power that could be transferred from one muscle to another
3. Succeeding technically in grafting between distant muscles when the topographical relations otherwise prevent that operation
4. Emphasizing that there are limits of capacity of functional adaptations to the neuromuscular system.

With these principles he introduced the need to balance muscle power. He recognized the possibility of adhesions and advocated early passive motion. He noted that certain adaptations of the muscle would be necessary for its new function, and he described cases of transferring tendons to balance deformity for polio as well as for spastic paralysis. He also noted a decrease in spasticity following these muscle transfers. His description of an opponens transfer in a case of infantile paralysis was probably the first (the flexor digitorum superficialis of the little finger to the insertion of the opponens pollicis through an opening made in the ligament, presumably the transverse metacarpal ligament). Because of adhesions, he noted, 100% return of function was impossible.

There was considerable controversy over the proper technique for tendon transfers. Lange of Munich lengthened tendons with braided strands of silk. He repaired the tendon in a relaxed position, whereas Vulpius sutured the tendon as tightly as possible. Methods of attachment were inconsistent: some advocated suturing into bone, others to tendons.

Within the next two decades, the answer to this controversy came from the laboratory. Bielsalski of Berlin published significant experimental work on tendon transfers in 1910, laying the foundation for future experimental studies. Henze and Mayer reported on methods of tendon transfer and ways to minimize postoperative adhesions.[9] They concluded that artificial methods of preventing adhesions, whether by implanting living tissue or interposing foreign material, were self-defeating, as these methods actually stimulated adhesion formation.

Mayer continued his experimental work, spending 2 years with Bielsalski. On his return to the United States, Mayer published three articles on tendons and tendon transfers.[15–17] He provided a detailed description of the anatomy of the tendon sheath, the paratenon, and the accompanying blood vessels, and established what are still considered the basic rules for tendon transfers:

1. Maintain absolute asepsis, minimal hemorrhage, and minimal trauma.
2. Whenever possible, restore the normal relationship between tendon and sheath.
3. Direct the tendon through tissues adapted to the gliding of tendons.
4. Imitate normal insertion to bone or cartilage of the original tendon.
5. Establish normal tension.
6. Have an effective line of traction.

At about the same time, Jones and Hunt established an orthopedic hospital in England, one of the first in the world. Jones, considered by many the father of orthopedic surgery, was a remarkable personality with extraordinary organizational talents and a worldwide reputation as an orthopedic surgeon. During World War I he organized orthopedic services into specialized centers, providing exceptional opportunities for experience in the treatment of orthopedic injuries. In 1921 he listed four principles of tendon transplant surgery[11]:

1. The joints must be mobile.
2. If possible, the muscles to the tendons must have sufficient strength to carry out the motion.
3. The muscles and tendons must traverse a straight course from origin to insertion, not a course that runs obliquely or around an angle.
4. The transplant must be attached under slight tension.

Bunnell, a San Francisco surgeon, published three famous articles in 1918, 1922, and 1928. The first outlined the principles of tendon surgery in the hand.[4] He recommended the use of a tourniquet to obtain a bloodless field, atraumatic technique, and fat grafts to enhance gliding and preserving pulleys. He condemned the midline palmar incision because it caused a scar contracture similar to Dupuytren's contracture.

In 1922 Bunnell described the use of tendon grafts to replace destroyed tendons, and in tendon transfers. He advocated the use of the palmaris longus, flexor digitorum superficialis, or extensor tendons of the toes as donors. He stressed gentle, progressive splinting to overcome contractures, and suggested using pedicle grafts to place new tendons in soft, pliable beds in cases where cicatrix and scar would otherwise impede the gliding mechanism. He avoided splinting fingers postoperatively and believed that only the wrist should be immobilized and fixed in the flexed position. He encouraged early—but not excessive or overly vigorous—motion.[5]

In 1928 Bunnell discussed tendon transplantation for opposition.[6] He described a pulley at the pisiform insertion of the flexor carpi ulnaris, employing a slip to be used as a loop. A flexor tendon was directed through the pulley, subcutaneously to the distal aspect of the metacarpal of the thumb. He stressed that one tendon transfer could perform only one function and that two opposing insertions of the same tendon could not succeed.

Bunnell also encouraged nerve repair. He believed that wrist, palmar, and digital nerves should be repaired and advocated the use of two stay sutures, atraumatically placed in the periphery of nerve, and then four additional sutures along the margins. He preferred silk suture. Good results were reported with digital, median, and ulnar nerve repairs, and he observed that the more distal the repair, the less complicated the regeneration process. He noted that sensation was as important as movement for hand function and reported that 60% of repaired median nerves restored opposition.

Because these three papers contained case presentations and illustrations of technique, they were quite different from the early reports of tendon transfers by the German and Swiss schools of Vulpius, Nicoladoni, Lange, and others. The earlier accounts described how the procedure should be performed and how satisfactory the results were, but gave no verification.

In 1922 Starr's landmark article on tendon transfers appeared in the *Journal of Bone and Joint Surgery*.[23] It outlined nine principles of tendon transfer:

1. As far as possible, muscles with action similar to the ones they are replacing should be used.
2. If only part of the tendon is to be transferred, it must have the same action as the muscle it is to replace.
3. The line of the pull should be as straight as possible, for mechanically the muscle will work efficiently only if the line between its origin and its new insertion is straight.
4. The fixation of the transferred muscle should be made with a good deal of tension.
5. Any deformity due to contracture of tissue should be overcome before transfer of muscles is attempted.
6. Tendons may be transferred to a new position by using the sheath of the muscle to be replaced and threading the new tendon down the sheath, but for the most part transferred tendons should be in fatty subcutaneous tissue.
7. In the lower extremity, it is common for tendons being transferred to be inserted in the bone or periosteum. In the upper extremity, attachment of tendon to tendon has been quite satisfactory.
8. Care should be taken to fix tendon to tendon adequately, as many cases have failed and required subsequent repair because the union slipped. The tendon should be split, and the transferred tendon should be denuded of its sheath. Linen should be used; catgut is not strong enough.
9. The limb must be placed in a splint, preferably of plaster of Paris, and all motion that would strain the suture line prevented for 3 weeks. Then a removable splint that can be removed for daily training is substituted. The patient should be in the hands of an expert therapist who has thorough knowledge of anatomy and has seen the operation performed so as to appreciate the aims of the surgeon. After 2 months, all splints should be discarded.

Starr described a muscle transfer for loss of the musculospiral (radial) nerve, which in his experience was the most common nerve loss of the upper extremity. The palmaris longus was transferred to the extensor pollicis longus and the adductor longus; the flexor carpi radialis to the extensor digitorum communis; and the pronator teres to the extensor carpi radialis longus or brevis. Starr summarized the results of 52 cases and noted that "the poor results seen in tendon surgery at the time were the result of the physicians' not learning the principles [of tendon transplantation] and sticking to them. . . . The principles seem obvious, but one sees cases in which these are so grossly violated that return of function is impossible."[23]

Steindler published a monumental book on surgery of the upper extremity in 1938 and a classic article on tendon transfers in the upper extremity in 1939.[24] He outlined the principles of tendon transfers and illustrated their use in specific clinical conditions. He stressed that any previous contracture must be completely corrected, because tendons cannot overcome established shortened muscles or soft tissues. The muscle selected for replacement should have a similar or related action, but he noted that some re-education was necessary, particularly in the upper extremity. The integrity of the muscle unit must be respected, he wrote: it is impossible to educate a portion of the same muscle to act as an antagonist against itself. The transferred muscle must have adequate muscle power—that is, its strength should compare with that of the one that being replaced. The mechanical arrangement of the transplanted tendon must be in a straight line or, if the line of pull changes direction, it must be deflected by pulleys through which the tendon may glide freely. The tendon is transferred under suitable tension, meaning that, under anesthesia, a moderate tension should be applied in the position in which a tendon is sutured. Decisions on degrees of tension are critical, he wrote. When it is impossible to attach to bone, tendon-to-tendon transfer is possible. Steindler stressed the necessity for preserving the gliding apparatus of tendon, since tendon deprived of its gliding surface is nonfunctional. He credited Codavilla with originating the so-called tendon sheath method.

Both Bunnell and Steindler emphasized the evaluation of the patient prior to tendon transfers. They advocated scheduling tendon transfers for a time when tissues were in a suitable condition, swelling had subsided, and joints were supple and soft.

Tendon transplantation had evolved to a high degree by the first half of the 20th century. Experimentation in the laboratory led to new clinical applications. Scientists and clinicians of this period began documenting clinical results with detailed follow-up studies.

World War II caused a great increase in the number of hand injuries seen by surgeons. Regional centers for hand surgery were founded in the United States, the first one supervised by Bunnell. Ultimately this stimulated interest in treatment of hand problems. The American Society for Surgery of the Hand was formed in 1946, and its yearly meetings provided a forum for discussion of the growing research on tendon transplants and clinical results.

Force, Work, and Power

The language and principles of bioengineering were introduced into hand surgery and applied to tendon transfers. The *force* of a muscle is directly proportional to the cross-sectional area of *all* its muscle fibers (the physiological cross section). Blix found that the greatest force of contraction is exerted when muscle is at its resting length.[1] *Work* is force multiplied by distance. The work capacity of a muscle relates to its physiological cross section and the length of its muscle fibers; work relates to the total volume of the muscle and force to its cross-sectional area. *Power* is a measurement of work over a period of time (Tables 48-1, 48-2).

The *amplitude* of a muscle is the amount it can be stretched from its resting position, plus the amount it contracts from its resting position. A muscle can contract to about 40% of its resting length, at which point it stops exerting force. The effective amplitude of a muscle varies by changing position of any intercalated joints across which the muscle–tendon unit works (eg, digital flexion is enhanced by wrist extension). Electrical stimulation and electromyographic evaluation demonstrate how muscle functions.

A more detailed appreciation of functional anatomy led to more detailed applications to the clinical problems of muscle loss. Intrinsic transfers were advocated by Zancolli[27] and Riordan.[22] Brand's vast experience with leprosy patients led to further refinement of tendon transplantation.[3]

RECENT ADVANCES

The construction of fine swaged needles in the late 1960s made microvascular surgery possible and led ultimately to the free transplantation of muscle.

Table 48-1. *Excursion of Muscles in the Adult Forearm and Hand*

Muscle	Excursion (cm)
Brachioradialis	4.0
Flexor digitorum profundus	7.0
Flexor digitorum superficialis	6.5
Extensor pollicis longus	6.0
Extensor digitorum communis	5.0
Extensor indicis proprius	5.0
Flexor pollicis longus	5.0
Flexor carpi ulnaris	3.0
Flexor carpi radialis	3.0
Extensor carpi radialis longus	3.0
Extensor carpi radialis brevis	3.0
Extensor carpi ulnaris	3.0
Extensor pollicis brevis	3.0
Abductor pollicis longus	3.0
Lumbrical	3.8
Thenar	3.8
Interossei	2.0

Manktelow pioneered this work, which is a further tool in our armamentarium of tendon transplantation.[14]

In the last 10 to 15 years, research on tendon transfers has focused primarily on the biology of tendon healing and the ability to control adhesions. Bielsalski noted in 1910 that transferred tendons had fewer adhesions when transferred into a recipient tendon sheath, but this sheath could not be artificially created until 1968. Hunter described the silicone rod mechanism for creating a synovial sheath by placing a nonreactive implant as a spacer and later replacing it with a functioning unit. This allowed the gliding necessary to make tendon transfers possible in previously scarred tissue.[10]

The exact mechanism of tendon healing is controversial. In 1962 Potenza described the necessity for tendon healing to occur by cells migrating from the peripheral tendon sheath to repopulate in transgressional tendons.[21] This concept has been challenged, however, by reports of intrinsic healing of tendon. This was demonstrated conclusively by Lundborg, who observed healing in tendons transferred to a synovial joint.[12] It was surmised that tendon could heal by synovial fluid nutrition alone. This led to the idea of encapsulating tendon repairs within synovial sheaths, allowing contact healing while limiting extrinsic cellular ingrowth. Thus, closing a tendon sheath over a repair was suggested. Whether the clinical results are improved over non-encased repairs remains inconclusive.

CONCLUSION

This chapter has reviewed the principles of tendon transfer from a historical perspective. Ten thousand years ago humans realized that they could control their environment, could create their own food source, and could affect their health. The progress of medicine and its permission to intervene with the divine waxed and waned through the Mesopotamian, Hellenistic, and medieval times. The ability to understand and control the environment awakened in the 16th century and blossomed in the 17th century, when medical experimentation began and understanding of anatomy, biology, and physiology prospered. Surgery remained primitive before the advent of anesthesia in 1846 and the control of germs by antisepsis.

The last two decades of the 19th century saw the birth of tendon transplant surgery, primarily in the lower extremities for polio. In the early 20th century, the principles of transplant surgery were

Table 48-2. *Relative Strengths of Muscles in the Forearm and Hand*

Muscle	Strength Relative to FCR Muscle
Brachioradialis	2.0
Flexor carpi ulnaris	2.0
ECRL, ECRB, ECU, PT, FPL, FDS, FDP	1.0 (each tendon)
EDC, EIP, EDQ	0.5 (each tendon)
APL, EPB, PL	0.1 (each tendon)
Interossei	2.7 (total/combined)
Lumbricals	0.5 (total/combined)

established in the laboratory and verified by clinical experience.

REFERENCES

1. Blix M. Die Lange und dei Spannung des Muskels. Skand Arch Physiol 1891; 3:295–318.
2. Boorstin DJ. The discovers. New York: Vintage, 1983:338–383.
3. Brand PW. Paralytic claw hand. J Bone Joint Surg [Br] 1958; 40:618–632.
4. Bunnell S. Repair of tendons in the fingers and description of two new instruments. Surg Gynecol Obstet 1918; 26:103–110.
5. Bunnell S. Repair of tendons in the fingers. Surg Gynecol Obstet 1922; 35:88–97.
6. Bunnell S. Repair of nerves and tendons of the hand. J Bone Joint Surg 1928; 10:1–26.
7. Codavilla A. Tendon transplants in orthopaedic practice, 1899. Translated by Ferrara JD. Clin Orthop 1976; 118:2.
8. Galen. On the usefulness of the parts of the body. (Translated by May MT). Ithaca: Cornell University Press, 1968:69–70.
9. Henze C, Mayer L. An experimental study of silk-tendon plastics with particular reference to the prevention of postoperative adhesions. Surg Gynecol Obstet 1814; 19:10.
10. Hunter JM. Artificial tendons. Early development and application. Am J Surg 1965; 109:325.
11. Jones R. Tendon transplantation in cases of musculospiral injuries not amenable to suture. Am J Surg 1921; 35:333.
12. Lundborg G. Experimental flexor tendon healing without adhesion formation—a new concept of tendon nutrition and intrinsic healing mechanism. A preliminary report. Hand 1976; 8:235.
13. Lyons AS, Petrucelli RJ. Medicine, an illustrated history. New York: Harry N. Abrams, 1978:22, 23, 65.
14. Manktelow RT, Zuher RM, McKee NH. Functioning free muscle transplantation. J Hand Surg [Am] 1984; 9:32–39.
15. Mayer L. The physiological method of tendon transplantation. Surg Gynecol Obstet 1916; 22: 182–197.
16. Mayer L. The application of the physiological principle to tendon transplantation. Am J Surg 1918; 32:1.
17. Mayer L. The free transplantation of tendons. Am J Surg 1921; 35:271.
18. Nicoladoni C. Uber Sehnentransplantation. Samml Dtsch Naturforsch Artze Salzburg 1880; 54.
19. Nicoladoni C. Nachtrag zum Pes calcaneus and zur transplantation der Peronealsehnen. Arch Klin Chir Berlin 1881; 27:660.
20. Paré A. The workes of that famous chirurgion Ambrose Paré. Translated by Johnson T. London, 1634.
21. Potenza AD. Healing tendons within the flexor digital sheath in the dog. J Bone Joint Surg [Am] 1962; 44:49.
22. Riordan DC. Tendon transplantations in median nerve and ulnar nerve paralysis. J Bone Joint Surg [Am] 1953; 35:312–320.
23. Starr CL. Army experiences with tendon transference. J Bone Joint Surg 1922; 4:3–21.
24. Steindler A. Tendon transplantation in the upper extremity. Am J Surg 1939; 44:260–271.
25. Vesalius A. De corporis humani fabrica. Basel, 1543.
26. Vulpius O. Der heutige Stand der Sehnenplastik. Z Orthop Chir 1904; 1.
27. Zancolli EA. Structural and dynamic bases of hand surgery. Philadelphia: JB Lippincott, 1968.

49

Tendon Transfer for Radial Nerve Palsy

Lawrence H. Schneider

AUTHOR'S KEY POINTS

- If wrist extension is desired early (while awaiting radial nerve recovery), pronator teres to extensor carpi radialis brevis transfer can be carried out.
- Recommended tendon transfers for *high radial nerve palsy* are pronator teres to extensor carpi radialis brevis; flexor carpi ulnaris (well mobilized proximally) to extensor digitorum communis; and palmaris longus to re-routed extensor pollicis longus.
- As wrist flexor tendon amplitude (30 mm) is insufficient for substitution for the digital extensors (amplitude: 50 mm), tenodesis action using wrist flexion is required for full digital extension when wrist flexor to digital extensor transfers are used.
- Commonly used alternative transfers include flexor carpi radialis or flexor digitorum superficialis (long finger) to the extensor digitorum communis and flexor digitorum superficialis (ring finger) to extensor indicis proprius and extensor pollicis longus.

Loss of radial nerve function, manifested by inability to extend the fingers and thumb, is a severe impairment to hand function. The loss of wrist extension, particularly, greatly reduces grasping function, due mainly to a lack of stability of the wrist. With the wrist falling into flexion, grasp and use of the fingers is greatly weakened. When nerve repair is either not feasible or unsuccessful, tendon transfers successfully palliate the problem. Tendon transfers are more effective following radial nerve palsy than any other peripheral nerve palsy.

Patients with paralysis of the muscles supplied by the radial nerve present with one of two clinical pictures: High or low radial (posterior interosseous) nerve paralysis. When the lesion is above the elbow, prior to the innervation of the brachioradialis and wrist extensors, it is referred to as a *high* radial nerve injury. The patient loses function of the brachioradialis, all wrist extension, and finger and thumb extension, as well as long thumb abduction. A *low* radial nerve lesion, below the elbow and involving only the posterior interosseous nerve, spares the brachioradialis and one or both of the radial wrist extensors but still results in paralysis of the long finger extensors, the extensors and abductor of the thumb, and the extensor carpi ulnaris

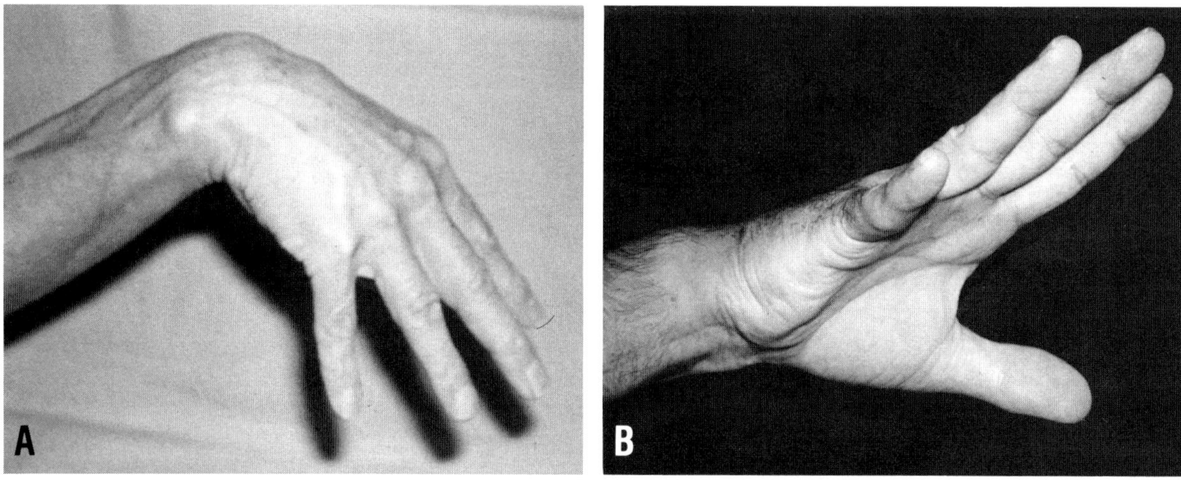

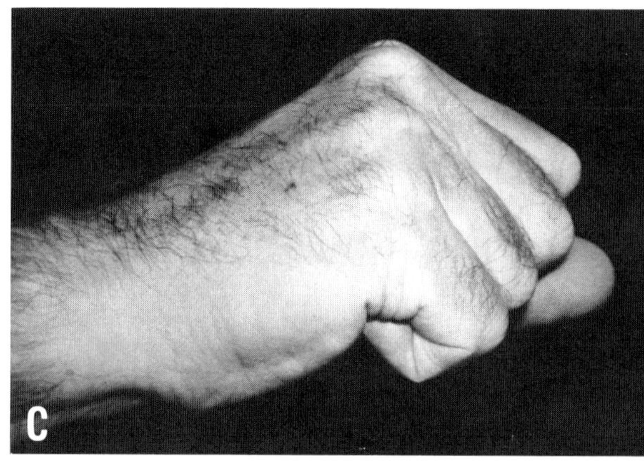

Figure 49–1. *High radial nerve paralysis. (**A**) Preoperative photo shows loss of wrist and finger extension. (**B, C**) Three years after the standard transfer was carried out, successful functional result is seen.*

(ECU) (Fig. 49-1). While wrist extension is possible in the low lesion, there may be a radial deviation posture on wrist extension because of the overpull of the radial wrist extensors in the absence of an ECU to balance the wrist.

Tendon transfers are performed to restore wrist extension and finger and thumb extension and abduction. Tendon transfers are not performed to replace the paralyzed brachioradialis and supinator muscles, as other motors (the biceps and other elbow flexors) are present to carry out their functions. Since the sensory area supplied by the radial nerve is not a critical one insofar as hand function is concerned, and the motor loss is significant, radial nerve paralysis presents an ideal problem for restoration of function by tendon transfer (Fig. 49-2).

PERTINENT ANATOMY

The radial nerve originates in the posterior cord of the brachial plexus, which has received fibers from cervical roots 5, 6, 7, and 8.[34] In the arm the nerve travels posterior to the humerus in the musculospiral groove, becoming anterior and lateral in the distal arm after penetrating the lateral intermuscular septum. High in the arm, it supplies the triceps and also provides sensory branches, the posterior cutaneous nerves of the forearm and arm. In the distal arm it innervates the brachioradialis and the extensor carpi radialis longus (ECRL) and brevis (ECRB). At the elbow level the nerve divides into sensory (superficial radial) and motor (posterior interosseous) divisions. While the ECRL and

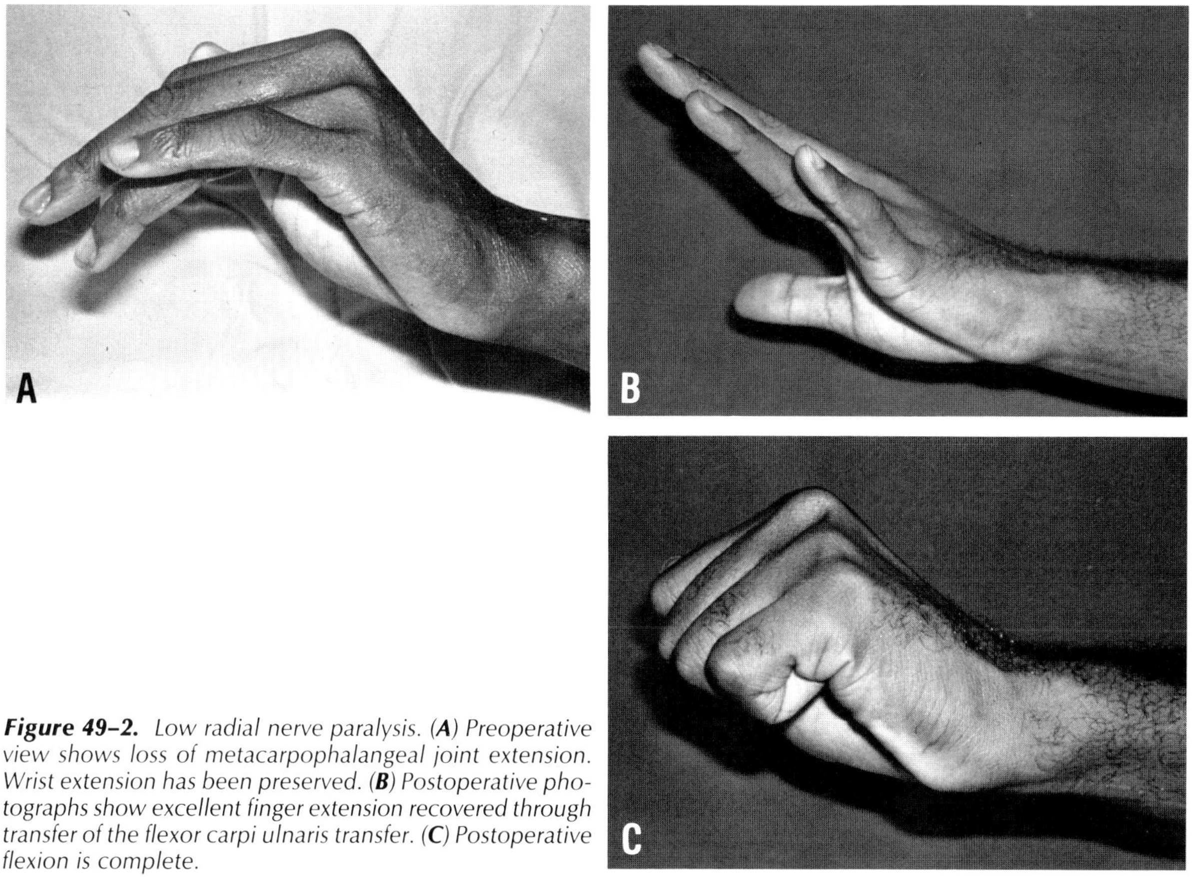

Figure 49–2. *Low radial nerve paralysis. (**A**) Preoperative view shows loss of metacarpophalangeal joint extension. Wrist extension has been preserved. (**B**) Postoperative photographs show excellent finger extension recovered through transfer of the flexor carpi ulnaris transfer. (**C**) Postoperative flexion is complete.*

ECRB are innervated by the radial nerve itself, in about one half of cases the ECRB receives its innervation from a branch traveling in the superficial sensory branch of the radial nerve.[34] The posterior interosseous nerve supplies all the remaining muscles: extensor carpi ulnaris (ECU), extensor digitorum communis (EDC), extensor digiti minimi (EDM), abductor pollicis longus (APL), extensor pollicis longus (EPL) and brevis (EPB), and extensor indicus proprius (EIP). In high radial nerve lesions, there is a variable area of sensory loss on the dorsum of the hand, but this is not of major importance.

TENDON TRANSFERS

History

The history of tendon transfer for paralysis of the radial nerve is an interesting segment in upper-extremity reconstruction.[42] Transfers have used median- and ulnar-innervated wrist extensors to substitute for the paralyzed radial innervated muscles. White[43] mentions that Murphy[21] originated this type of transfer, although Robert Jones[16–18] is usually given credit. In fact, others described these transfers much earlier. Franke appears to be the originator of these procedures, having described cases in 1892 in which the first "transplantation" for complete radial nerve paralysis was performed.[3,30,42] Franke shortened the paralyzed extensors at the wrist to create a tenodesis and transferred the flexor carpi ulnaris (FCU) to the digital extensors. Franke also transferred part of the flexor carpi radialis (FCR) to the thumb. Jones developed the procedure in several clinical cases and made a significant additional contribution by using the pronator teres (PT) as a separate motor to the radial wrist extensors in order to provide wrist extension.[16–18] The PT transfer has become a standard method for restoring wrist extension in radial nerve paralysis. Jones also transferred the FCU to extensors of the long, ring, and small digits and the FCR to EPL and EIP. For thumb extension, Stiles[37] and later Dunn[14] published papers that described the use of the palmaris longus (PL) transferred to the EPL to provide extension of the thumb.

While transfer of both wrist flexors must have caused extension deformities at the wrist, early authors did not mention this as a problem. Starr first described a technique that left one of the wrist flexors behind.[35] He used the FCR to extend the digits and the PL to extend the thumb but did not disturb the FCU. In patients who lacked the PL, Starr used a portion of the FCR for transfer to the thumb tendons. Starr did not stress this point in his paper, which caused Green to conclude that he may not have realized the significance of this contribution.[15] This point was overlooked by most authors until it was definitively addressed by Zachary, who stated clearly that one wrist flexor must be left behind, in its original location, to avoid extension contractures at the wrist.[44]

Scuderi reported in 1946 on his considerable experience with this problem.[32] He modified the PL to EPL transfer, which formerly had been done on the dorsum of the wrist. He rerouted the EPL to the volar aspect, where it was sutured to the PL. This improved the transfer by providing an abduction vector, in addition to providing thumb interphalangeal joint extension. This modification was quickly adopted by others.[27,28]

An approach then was designed to address the problem of inadequate amplitude for simultaneous wrist and finger extension. This involved the use of the flexor digitorum superficialis (FDS) as a motor for the EDC. The FDS, with an amplitude of 60 to 70 mm, is the only available tendon with sufficient excursion. While Fiori was the first clinician to use the FDS (through the interosseous membrane) to motor the EDC, Boyes popularized this transfer.[3] Later Chuinard and Boyes stressed the importance of preserving the FCU as a wrist stabilizer, pointing out the problems of wrist control when the FCU was sacrificed.[11] This provided further impetus for the use of the FDS as a finger extensor.

The treatment for this problem has taken several pathways. Wrist extension is now generally restored with the PT transfer. The tendon is sutured into the ECRB alone to reduce the tendency for radial deviation. The surgeon has several options for restoring finger extension. When using a wrist flexor for finger extension, the choice is between FCU and FCR, each of which has its advocates. Boyes stressed that leaving the FCU behind is better for stabilization of the wrist in the ulnar deviation of power grip.[3]

Use of the FDS not only allows both wrist flexors to stay in place, but is the only transfer with sufficient potential amplitude for complete finger extension when the wrist is in extension. However, I have had difficulty in obtaining good finger extension using the FDS transfer. An additional concern is radial deviation at the wrist. I feel that it is rarely a problem and not sufficient cause, in itself, for using the FDS for finger extension. Moberg has made the same observation.[20] Others have questioned the efficacy of the FDS transfer.[15] If concern for sparing the FCU is a consideration, perhaps more liberal use of the FCR is indicated. On the other hand, many surgeons have expressed satisfaction with the superficialis transfer for restoring digital extension.[1,25,33,38–41]

General Rules

The general rules of tendon transfer have evolved through the years.[13] The patient must have sparable muscles and must be able to cooperate in the operative and postoperative program.[31] The essential criteria for successful tendon transfer (see Chapter 48) were considered in the development of the basic tendon transfers for radial nerve palsy.[4–6] A major deficiency in these transfers, however, is the shortage of amplitude when using wrist flexors as substitutes for finger extensors. Simultaneous full extension of fingers and wrist requires an amplitude of 50 mm by the motor tendon. The wrist flexors, provide, at best, 30 to 35 mm of amplitude.[13] In order to improve the excursion of the transfer, when a wrist flexor is used to motor a finger extensor, the use of tenodesis action by the patient using wrist flexion is necessary for good finger extension. For this reason it is inadvisable to fuse the wrist in these patients, as wrist motion is key to effective extension of the fingers. Important classical work on tendon transfers has been provided by Boyes,[3] Brand,[5] Bunnell,[8] Curtis,[13] Mayer,[19] Omer,[22,23] Riordan,[27,28] Steindler,[36] and White.[43]

Preoperative Considerations

All wounds are healed and soft tissues are pliable prior to surgery. Joint motion is passively maintained through passive motion exercises and splinting.[12] At times, when contractures do not respond to therapy, additional operative procedures are needed to release contracted joints. Soft tissues may need revision or flap coverage to provide gliding tissues through which tendons are passed. In general there should be no hope for spontaneous recovery of nerve function prior to tendon transfer, although, as we shall see later in this chapter, this point is controversial.

Timing

After repair of the radial nerve, time is allowed for muscular reinnervation. In ideal conditions surgeons have been able to obtain good recovery after repair of this motor nerve. If the repair is in the lower third of the arm, some evidence of recovery in the brachioradialis or the radial wrist extensors should be seen within 4 to 6 months of repair. Because of the time needed for recovery of nerve function after radial nerve repair, some surgeons have advocated that nerve repair be combined with immediate tendon transfer. Burkhalter, making a case for the importance of wrist extension in gripping function of the hand, transfers the pronator teres, end-to-side, to the ECRB at or soon after nerve repair, to provide active wrist extension.[9,10] This makes the hand useful to the patient much earlier. This plan has been supported by Omer.[24] I have not done this tendon transfer at the time of radial nerve repair but recognize an indication for this in patients with specific needs.

Bevin advocated early transfers, even suggesting that the nerve not be repaired at all.[2] Certainly this has allowed his patients to return to work at a much earlier date. Bevin compared 12 radial nerve repairs with 13 similar cases treated only by tendon transfer. He emphasized that not only did all patients with transfers do well but that the group of patients with transfers returned to work in 8 weeks, compared to a return-to-work date that averaged 8 months in the nerve repair group.

Brown has stated that tendon transfers should be considered from the outset when the surgeon feels that the conditions of nerve repair are unfavorable,[7] and I agree with that.

Closed injuries to the radial nerve, such as those seen in "Saturday night palsy," are managed nonoperatively, with recovery occurring within 8 weeks. It has become clear also that radial nerve injuries occurring in association with closed fractures of the humerus are treatable without exploration, with expectation of full motor recovery (see Chap. 43).[15]

As a general rule I commit the patient with a good nerve repair done under favorable conditions to a period of 6 months of observation prior to proceeding to tendon transfers. When adequate time has been allowed for recovery and such recovery has not occurred, a decision regarding tendon transfers is made. Electrodiagnostic studies aid in the decision-making process.

The patient with a radial nerve paralysis needs wrist extension, finger extension, and thumb abduction and extension. The muscles available for transfer are those innervated by the median and ulnar nerves. Use of wrist flexors as transfers for finger extension is not a perfect situation, as the tenodesis effect provided by wrist motion is needed to achieve extension of the fingers at the metacarpophalangeal (MP) joint.

OPERATIVE PROCEDURES

General Principles

As a rule, when doing multiple tendon transfers, the donor muscles and recipient tendons are exposed initially. The motors are freed from their insertions (unless a side-to-side transfer is planned) and transferred via subcutaneous tunnels (or through the interosseous membrane) to the new location. The tourniquet is deflated and hemostasis obtained. Wounds no longer needed are now closed. Transfers are completed by suturing the tendons into the new insertions and closing the remaining wounds.

The Standard Transfer

For wrist extension, the standard transfer is the pronator teres to the ECRB. All techniques for high radial nerve palsy now include this transfer. A vertical incision, 6 cm long, is made on the radial–volar aspect of the mid-forearm (Fig. 49-3). The PT tendon is found at its insertion into the radius, freed, and lengthened with a 2- to 3-cm extension of periosteum (Fig. 49-4). The forearm is pronated, and the PT is passed subcutaneously over the brachioradialis (BR) and the ECRL. The tendon of the ECRB is obtained in the same wound, tagged, and set aside for later completion of the transfer (see Fig. 49-4).

The FCU is obtained through a wound created along the volar–ulnar aspect of the forearm with an extension at right angles in the wrist crease, which extends to the mid-volar region, to the tendon of the PL (see Fig. 49-3*A*). The insertion of the tendon, on the pisiform, is transected, and the tendon is freed from surrounding tissue. The FCU is mobilized proximally, protecting the ulnar vessels and nerve. Mobilization of this muscle requires extensive dissection, as the muscle's origin extends almost completely to its insertion. It is dissected off the ulna as well as from the overlying fascia from which it takes origin.

A third incision is made obliquely across the ulnar aspect of the proximal forearm overlying the belly of the FCU in such a way as to cross at right angles the pathway of the muscle belly in its transferred position (see Fig. 49-3*A*). The muscle is freed subcutaneously beneath the skin bridge between the second and third incisions.

A fourth incision, which is curvilinear (see Fig. 49-3*B*), is made on the dorsum of the forearm, proximal to the transverse dorsal retinaculum. The EDC and EPL are isolated proximal to the retinaculum. A subcutaneous tunnel is created around the ulnar border of the forearm and the FCU passed into the wound for later suturing to the EDC (Fig. 49-5).

The EPL is now transected at the musculotendinous junction. This tendon is obtained through a curvilinear incision at the MP joint of the thumb and pulled distally. It is rerouted subcutaneously over the thenar eminence into wound 1 at the wrist, where the PL has been transected at its insertion (Fig. 49-6). All tendons are then tagged with 4-0 silk sutures. The tourniquet is released, bleeding is controlled, and the wounds no longer needed are closed.

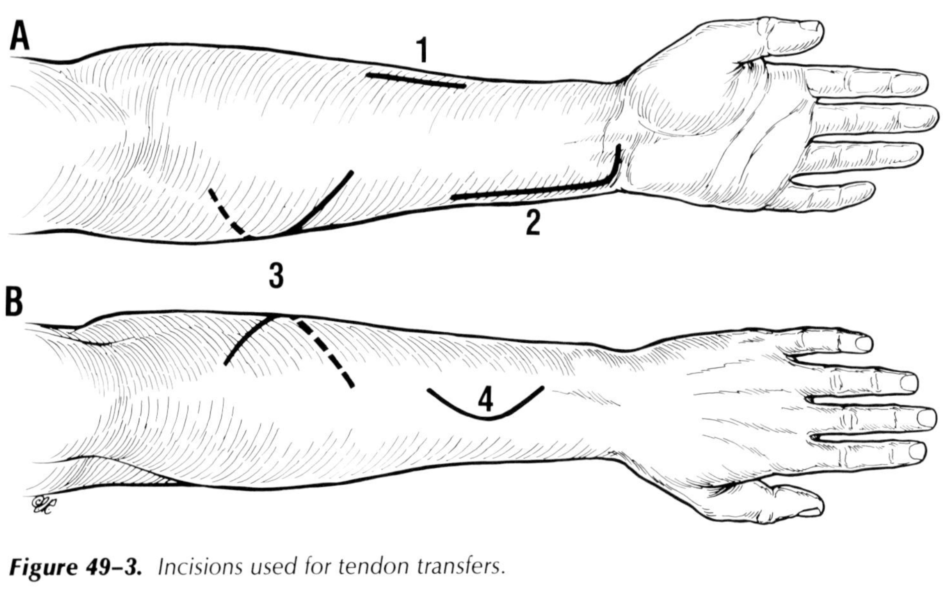

Figure 49–3. *Incisions used for tendon transfers.*

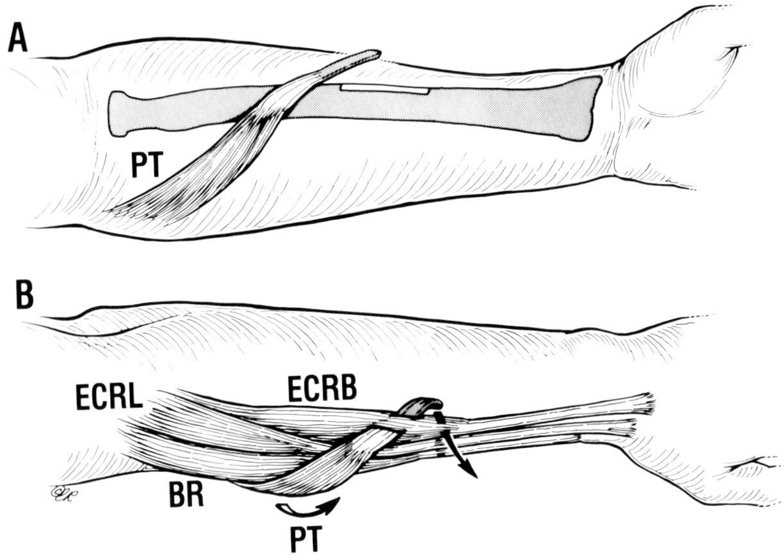

Figure 49–4. *The pronator teres (PT) transfer to the extensor carpi radialis brevis (ECRB). The pronator teres is removed from its insertion on the radius and lengthened by a periosteal extension. It is then passed over to the extensor carpi radialis brevis in the same wound. BR, brachioradialis; ECRL, extensor carpi radialis longus.*

Tendon suture is now carried out. While some authors recommend attaching tendons to the finger extensors first,[1,41] I agree with those[40] who perform the wrist extensor transfer first. The PT is interwoven into the ECRB at sufficient tension to hold the wrist at 45° of extension.

The transfer of the FCU to the EDC is then completed. An end-to-side juncture is created first by using an interweave suture of 4-0 nonabsorbable suture in the EDC tendons to bind them together side to side (see Fig. 49-5A). The FCU is woven into the tendons of the EDC at a tension sufficient to maintain the MP joints at 0° with the wrist in 25° of extension. As this is difficult to accomplish, it is helpful to supinate the forearm to bring the tendons together at this tension. Some authors[20] recommend that the EDC be transected and an end-to-end juncture created, but I have not used this modification. The wounds no longer needed are closed and the PL-to-rerouted-EPL transfer completed along the volar aspect of the wrist (Fig. 49-6). The last transfer is interwoven in tension sufficient to keep the thumb extended at the interphalangeal (IP) joint and abducted at the carpometacarpal (CMC) joint with the wrist in 25° of extension.

Tension determination is not absolutely definable in a scientific manner. I prefer to err on the tight side; if sutured too loosely, there will be inadequate extension.

Postoperative Management

A long arm plaster splint is applied with the elbow in flexion, the forearm in slight supination, the wrist in 40° extension, and the thumb in abduction at the basilar joint with extension at the MP and IP joints. The splint extends distal to the IP joint of the thumb and distal to the proximal interphalangeal (PIP) joints of the fingers, all of which (including the MP joints) are in 0° extension. Two plaster slabs are used: one extends from above the elbow to the middle phalanges of the fingers, and a second is added to control the thumb.

At 10 to 14 days, sutures are removed and a long arm cast is applied. The wrist is maintained at 45° extension and the fingers in 0° at the MP joints. The PIP joints are mobilized. At 4 weeks, active therapy is initiated with intermittent splint protection for an additional 2 weeks.[26] In therapy, active motion exercises are stressed. The patient may require passive assistive exercises at 6 weeks if passive motion is difficult to regain. Functional recovery using the tenodesis action at the wrist is learned spontaneously.

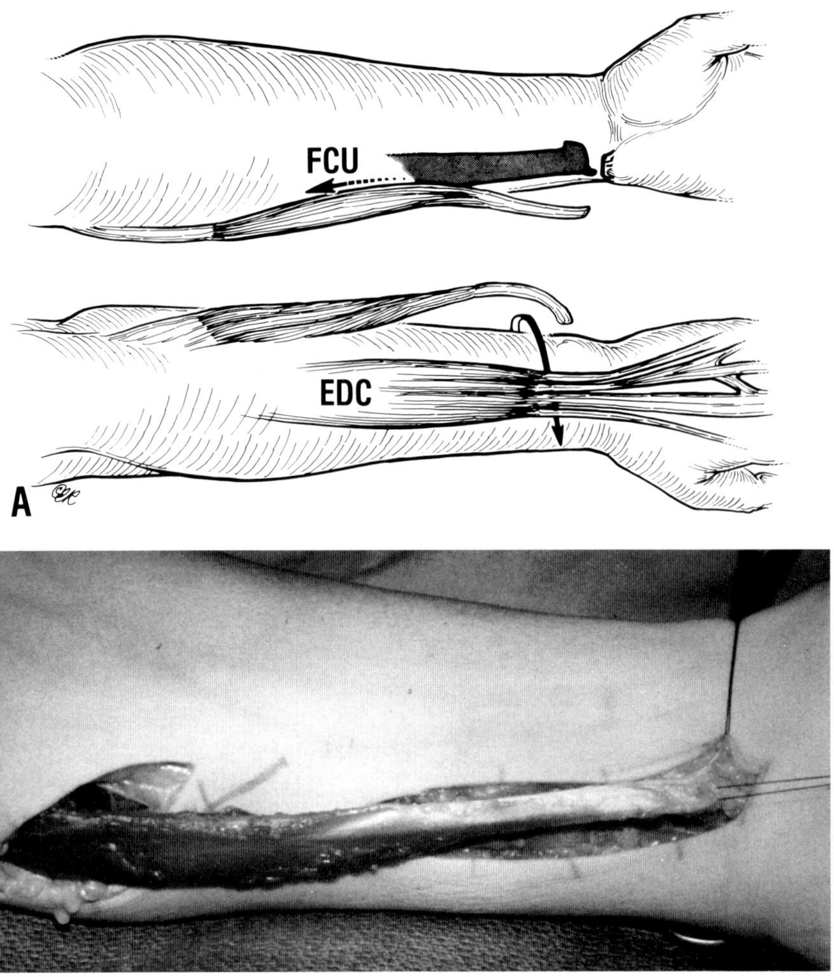

Figure 49–5. *Transfer of the flexor carpi ulnaris (FCU) to the extensor digitorum communis (EDC). (**A**) The transfer is mobilized proximally to give it a straight approach to the recipient tendons. It is then woven into the extensor digitorum communis. (**B**) The flexor carpi ulnaris has been mobilized into the proximal forearm wound. Excess muscle that runs almost down to the insertion is removed from the distal tendon. (**C**) The flexor carpi ulnaris tendon has been passed around the ulnar border of the forearm and is ready for juncture with the extensor digitorum communis tendons.*

OTHER TECHNIQUES

The FCR Transfer

The FCR can be substituted for the FCU (Fig. 49-7). Use of the FCR allows the FCU to remain in its functional position and answers the objections of those who are hesitant to use the FCU. The FCR is exposed through a longitudinal incision on the volar–radial aspect of the forearm. The tendon is divided at the wrist and mobilized into the forearm. It is passed around the radial border of the forearm, where it is interwoven into the EDC as described for the FCU transfer (see Fig. 49-7). Tsuge has modified the FCR transfer by passing it through the interosseous membrane so that the tendon takes a straighter course to its insertion.[40]

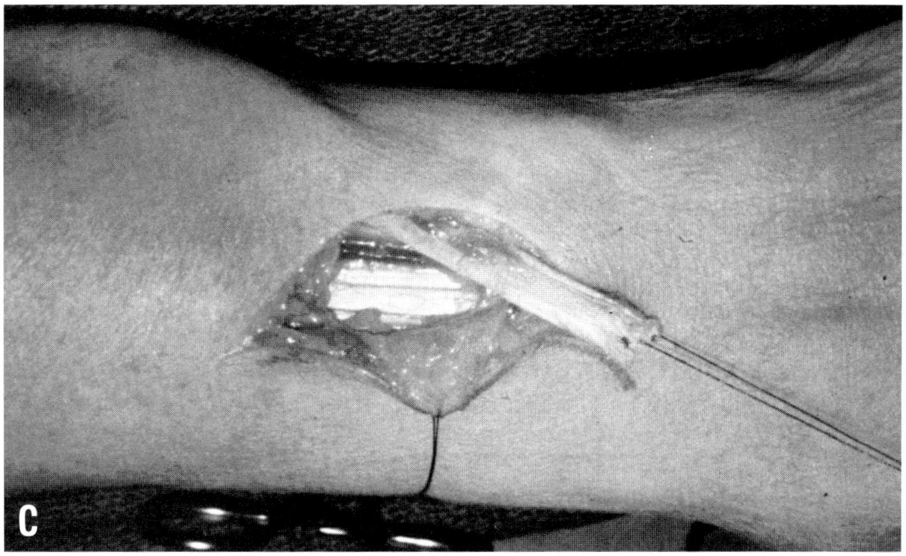

Figure 49-5. (Continued)

Use of the FDS for Finger Extension[3,12,15,33]

The tendons of the PT and the ECR are exposed, as described earlier. The forearm wound is extended more proximally. Chuinard recommends Boyes' technique of transferring the PT to both radial wrist extensors.[11] The FDS of long and ring fingers are exposed through transverse incisions at the base of each finger. The FDS tendons are divided and pulled into the vertical volar distal forearm wound. Just proximal to the pronator quadratus (PQ) two openings of 1 × 2 cm are created in the interosseous membrane, one on each side of the anterior interosseous artery. Green mentions that it takes a larger hole in the interosseous membrane to freely pass these muscle bellies from volar to dorsal.[11,15] The EDC, EIP, and EPL are exposed through a dorsal inverted L–shaped incision. The FDS tendons are passed through to the dorsum via the openings in the interosseous membrane, with the FDS of the long finger on the radial side of the profundus mass and between it and the FPL. The FDS of the ring finger is passed to the ulnar side of the FDP mass. The FDS-ring is transferred to the EIP and EPL while the FDS-long is transferred to the EDC. The median nerve is protected during these manipulations.

In addition, in this procedure the FCR is exposed through a transverse incision at the base of the thumb and divided sharply at the wrist.[11] It is then sutured to the APL and EPB in this same wound. The tourniquet is released prior to completion of the transfers. The junctures located on the dorsum of the forearm are proximal to the transverse dorsal retinaculum. The retinaculum is narrowed if its proximal edge impinges on the junctures. Smith, using this procedure, preferred passing the superficialis tendons subcutaneously around the forearm rather than through the interosseous membrane.[33]

Some have criticized this procedure because it weakens flexion and reduces independence of flexion of the two donor fingers[41]; however, it is the only transfer that can ensure adequate amplitude for full finger extension. Is its use justified? I have used these tendons, passed through the interosseous membrane and subcutaneously around the forearm, but have not been able to produce consistent results. I attribute the difficulties to problems in retraining the FDS to function as a digital extensor.

Author's Preferred Method

My first option is to transfer the PT to the ECRB. The FCU is then sutured end-to-side to the EDC as described. The rerouted EPL is sutured to the PL

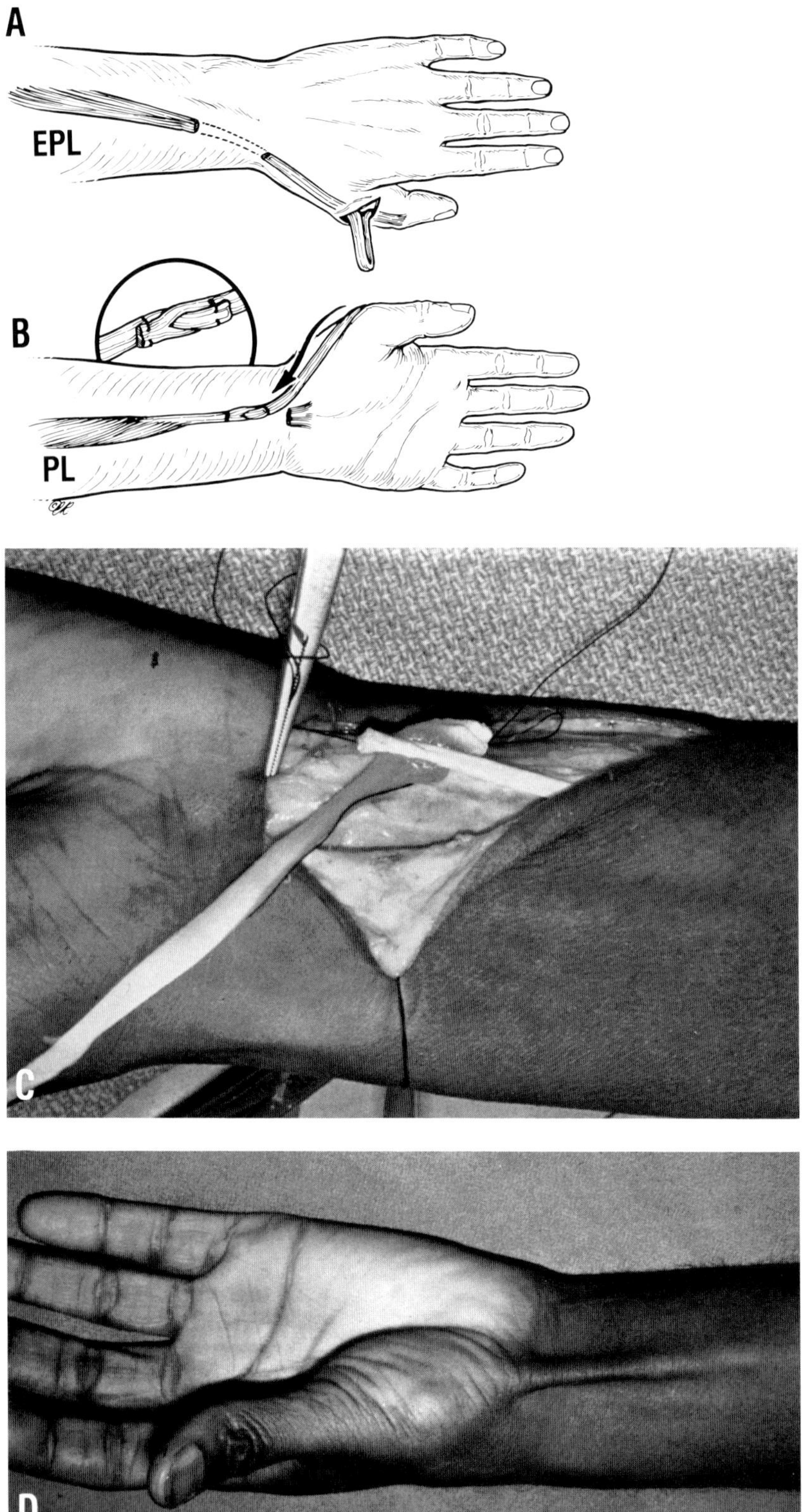

Figure 49–6. *The palmaris longus (PL) to rerouted extensor pollicis longus (EPL) transfer. (**A, B**) The EPL is transected at the musculotendinous junction, pulled distally through an incision at the MP joint of the thumb, and then rerouted subcutaneously to the palmaris longus. An interweave juncture is created at the volar aspect of the distal forearm. (**C**) The EPL will be passed subcutaneously over the thenar eminence to the wrist wound where the palmaris longus awaits. (**D**) Abduction and extension provided by the palmaris longus transfer in the patient seen in Fig. 49–6C.*

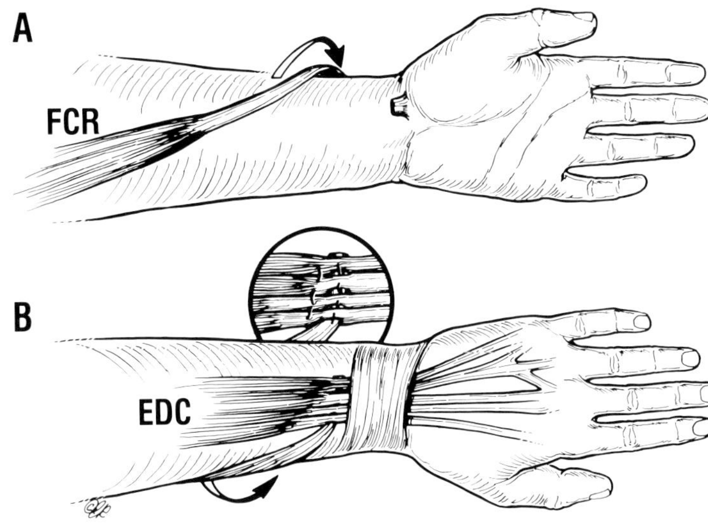

Figure 49–7. *The flexor carpi radialis (FCR) transfer. (**A**) The motor tendon is mobilized in the forearm and passed around the radial border. (**B**) It is then interwoven into the tendons of the extensor digitorum communis (EDC).*

with an interweave juncture in front of the wrist. This provides abduction as well as extension of the thumb. If there is no PL, the FDS-ring is transferred in a similar manner to the rerouted EPL.

As a second option, the FCR is used as the motor for the EDC instead of FCU. I have used the FCR in cases where heavy scarring on the ulnar side of the forearm precludes use of the FCU. It appears to be as effective as the FCU, and its use obviates the objections posed by those who stress the value of maintaining the FCU in its normal location. I also consider using the FCR in patients with low radial nerve lesions and markedly radially deviated wrists.

Overall these procedures have produced good results (see Figs. 49-1 and 49-2). One point of occasional dissatisfaction has been the inconsistency of the PL tendon transfer to the rerouted EPL. Although abduction has been good, some patients have not achieved satisfactory thumb extension. To provide better extension I have recently modified the procedure by transferring the FCU, side-to-side, to the EPL as well as the EDC on the dorsum of the distal forearm. In addition, the FDS-ring is brought into the volar distal forearm wound and passed subcutaneously to the thenar eminence, where it is sutured to the extensor apparatus at the MP joint of the thumb. This provides excellent thumb function.

I have used the standard FCU transfer to the EDC in over 30 patients. Like Moberg,[20] I have not found the radial deviation posture a major problem. Another technique is available, however, if one is concerned about radial deviation at the wrist. Said's operative modification transfers the PT to the ECU as well as the ECRB in high radial nerve palsy.[29] I believe this may also be useful following low radial nerve injuries if there is severe radial deviation prior to surgery. In this procedure the ECU is severed at its musculotendinous juncture and the distal segment transferred, end-to-side, to the functioning ECRB. I have no experience using this technique.

COMPLICATIONS

Complications specific to these operations include the adherence of sutured tendons to the surrounding tissues with inadequate gliding. This is avoidable to some degree by applying the general rules of tendon transfer, which require good skin cover and pliable soft tissues. Full passive motion is obtained prior to tendon transfer. Supervision by a trained hand therapist in the pre- and postoperative periods is helpful. Transfers that are sutured too loosely do not function well; I prefer to suture them on the tight side. With excessive tension, there will be difficulty regaining wrist flexion. This is further aggravated by the fact that the PT does not have adequate amplitude to provide good wrist extension and also allow full wrist flexion. Thus, some loss of wrist flexion is inevitable. While difficulty in regaining digital flexion at the MP joints may be a problem, this will usually respond to passive stretching therapy. I have had to release the dorsal capsule of the MP joint of the little finger in one patient. Breakdown or disruption of sutured tendons at their insertions is another unusual complication that is preventable with reasonable attention to the appropriate techniques of tendon suture.

REFERENCES

1. Beasley RW. Tendon transfers for radial nerve palsy. Orthop Clin North Am 1970; 1:439–445.
2. Bevin AG. Early tendon transfer for radial nerve transection. Hand 1976; 8:134–136.
3. Boyes JH. Tendon transfers for radial palsy. Bull Hosp Jt Dis 1960; 21:97–105.
4. Brand PW. Mechanics of tendon transfers. In: Hunter JM, Schneider LH, Mackin EJ, Callahan AD, eds. Rehabilitation of the hand, ed 2. St. Louis: CV Mosby, 1984:457–469.
5. Brand PW. Clinical mechanics of the hand. St. Louis: CV Mosby, 1985:11–29.
6. Brand PW. Biomechanics of tendon transfer. Hand Clin 1988; 4:137–154.
7. Brown PW. The time factor in surgery of upper extremity peripheral nerve surgery. Clin Orthop 1970; 68:14–21.
8. Bunnell S. Surgery of the hand, ed 3. Philadelphia: J B Lippincott, 1956:457–465.
9. Burkhalter WE. Early tendon transfer in upper extremity peripheral nerve injury. Clin Orthop 1974; 104:68–79.
10. Burkhalter WE. Tendon transfers as internal splints. In: Omer G, Spinner M, eds. Management of peripheral nerve problems. Philadelphia: WB Saunders, 1980:798–804.
11. Chuinard RG, Boyes JH, Stark HH, et al. Tendon transfers for radial palsy: Use of superficialis tendons for digital extension. J Hand Surg 1978; 3:560–570.
12. Colditz JC. Splinting for radial nerve palsy. J Hand Ther 1987; 1:18–23.
13. Curtis R. Fundamental principles of tendon transfer. Orthop Clin North Am 1974; 5:231–242.
14. Dunn N. Treatment of lesion of the musculospiral nerve in military surgery. Am J Orthop Surg 1918; 16:258–265.
15. Green DP. Radial nerve palsy. In: Green DP, ed. Operative hand surgery. New York: Churchill-Livingstone, 1988:1479–1498.
16. Jones R. On suture of nerves, and alternative methods of treatment by transplantation of tendon. Br Med J 1916; 1:641–643.
17. Jones R. On suture of nerves, and alternative methods of treatment by transplantation of tendon. Br Med J 1916; 1:679–682.
18. Jones R. Tendon transplantation in cases of musculospiral injuries not amenable to suture. Am J Surg 1921; 35:333–335.
19. Mayer L. The physiological method of tendon transplantation. Surg Gynecol Obstet 1916; 22: 182–197;298–306;472–481.
20. Moberg E, Nachemson A. Tendon transfers for defective long extensors of the wrist and fingers. Acta Chir Scand 1967; 133:31–34.
21. Murphy JB. Tenoplasty; tendon transplantation; tendon substitution; neuroplasty. Surgical Clinics of John B. Murphy 1914; 3:467.
22. Omer GE. Evaluation and reconstruction of the forearm and hand after acute peripheral nerve injuries. J Bone Joint Surg [Am] 1968; 50:1454–1478.
23. Omer GE. Tendon transfers for reconstruction of the forearm and hand following peripheral nerve injuries. In: Omer G, Spinner M, eds. Management of peripheral nerve problems. Philadelphia: WB Saunders, 1980:817–846.
24. Omer GE. Early tendon transfers as internal splints after nerve injury. In: Hunter JM, Schneider LH, Mackin EJ, eds. Tendon surgery in the hand. St. Louis: CV Mosby, 1987:413–418.
25. Reid RL. Radial nerve palsy. Hand Clinics 1988; 4: 179–186.
26. Reynolds CC. Preoperative and postoperative management of tendon transfers after radial nerve injury. In: Hunter JM, Schneider LH, Mackin EJ, Callahan AD, eds. Rehabilitation of the hand, ed 3. St. Louis: CV Mosby, 1990:696–704.
27. Riordan DC. Surgery of the paralytic hand. American Academy of Orthopaedic Surgeons Instructional Course Lectures 1959; 16:79–90.
28. Riordan DC. Radial nerve paralysis. Orthop Clin North Am 1974; 5:283–287.
29. Said GZ. A modified tendon transference for radial nerve paralysis. J Bone Joint Surg [Br] 1974; 56: 320–322.
30. Saikku LA. Tendon transplantation for radial paralysis. Acta Chir Scand 1947; 96(suppl 132):1–121.
31. Schneider LH. Tendon transfers in the upper extremity. In: Hunter JM, Schneider LH, Mackin EJ, Callahan AD, eds. Rehabilitation of the hand. St. Louis: CV Mosby, 1990:669–675.
32. Scuderi C. Tendon transplants for irreparable radial nerve paralysis. Surg Gynecol Obstet 1949; 88:643–651.
33. Smith RJ. Tendon transfers to restore wrist and digit extension. In: Smith RJ. Tendon transfers of the hand and forearm. Boston: Little, Brown, 1987:35–56.

34. Spinner M. Injuries to the major branches of peripheral nerves of the forearm, ed 2. Philadelphia: WB Saunders, 1978:79–157.
35. Starr CL. Army experiences with tendon transference. J Bone Joint Surg 1922; 4:3–21.
36. Steindler A. A textbook of operative orthopedics. New York: Appleton, 1925;89–105.
37. Stiles HJ. Operative treatment of nerve injuries. Amer J Orthop Surg 1918; 16:351–363.
38. Tagima T. Tendon transfers in radial nerve palsy. In: Hunter JM, Schneider LH, Mackin EJ, eds. Tendon surgery in the hand. St. Louis: CV Mosby, 1987: 432–438.
39. Thomsen M, Rasmussen KB. Tendon transfers for defective long extensors of the wrist and fingers. Scand J Plast Reconstr Surg 1969; 3:71–78.
40. Tsuge K. Tendon transfers for radial nerve palsy. Aust NZ J Surg 1980; 50:267–272.
41. Tubiana R. Our experience in tendon transfers for radial palsy. Ann Chir Main 1985; 4:197–210.
42. Waterman JH. Tendon transplantation: Its history, indications and technique. Med News 1902; 12:54–61.
43. White WL. Restoration of function and balance of the wrist and hand by tendon transfers. Surg Clin North Am 1960; 40:427–459.
44. Zachary RB. Tendon transplantation for radial paralysis. Brit J Surg 1946; 33:358–364.

50

Median Nerve Palsy

William W. Eversmann

AUTHOR'S KEY POINTS

- Attempts to restore the continuity of the median nerve precede attempts to reconstruct the forearm or hand by tendon transfer in median nerve palsy.
- End-to-end suture of the median nerve at or above the elbow usually results in some beneficial flexor function in the extrinsic flexors innervated by the median nerve.
- Restoration of the continuity of the median nerve, when it is lacerated in the proximal forearm or more proximally, rarely results in functional reinnervation of the intrinsic muscles innervated by the median nerve in the hand. Accordingly, early tendon transfer for intrinsic median nerve palsy often provides the best functional result for the thumb by preventing long delays in treatment and adduction and supination contracture of the thumb.
- The two major reasons for failure of opponens transfer to the thumb are adduction contracture of the thumb and poor motor selection for tendon transfer.

Paralysis of the median nerve is most commonly associated with penetrating, lacerating, or severe crush injuries to the arm, forearm, or wrist. Although median nerve laceration can occur in the absence of associated injuries to muscles, tendons, major vascular channels, or even the skeleton, it is more likely to occur in conjunction with injury to other major tissues in the arm and forearm. Regardless of the level of median nerve laceration and because of the overwhelming importance of the restoration of median nerve sensibility to the function of the hand, nerve suture is emphasized, as early as the wound will accept the repair. Restoring sensibility to the fingers and thumb augments the function of both extrinsic and intrinsic muscles of the fingers and thumb, and facilitates the retraining of tendon transfers to replace lost function.

Initial Care

Innervation of the intrinsic muscles of the hand by the median nerve occurs distal to the wrist flexion crease by at least 2 or 3 cm. The only notable branch of the median nerve between the junction of the proximal and middle third of the forearm and the wrist flexion crease is a purely sensory branch innervating the skin of the thenar eminence of the palm, the palmar cutaneous branch of the median nerve. Consequently, all other innervation of extrinsic flexor muscles by the median nerve occurs between the elbow flexion crease and the junction of the proximal and middle thirds of the forearm. Within this 8-cm segment of the proximal forearm, the median nerve provides innervation to the pronator teres, flexor carpi radialis, flexor digitorum superficialis, and palmaris longus. In addition, the major branch of the median nerve to the deep volar compartment of the forearm arises, is joined by a branch of the ulnar artery, and proceeds to the deep volar compartment innervating the flexor digitorum profundus of the index and middle fingers and, in the mid-portion of the forearm, the flexor pollicis longus and, still more distally, the pronator quadratus muscle.

It is important for the surgeon performing the initial surgery to be aware of the level of injury and whether or not nerve transection is proximal or distal to the branching of the anterior interosseous nerve. If the injury is distal to the anterior interosseous nerve branch, the surgeon determines if that nerve was transected separately. The anterior interosseous nerve, a pure motor nerve, should be repaired in addition to the median nerve proper so that extrinsic flexor tendon function is restored. Proximal to the elbow flexion crease, laceration of the median nerve results in both extrinsic and intrinsic median nerve palsy. Distal to the proximal third of the forearm, laceration of the median nerve results solely in intrinsic median nerve palsy, unless there has been concomitant laceration to the anterior interosseous nerve in the deep volar compartment, or concomitant severe muscle injury. Restoration of the continuity of the median nerve by direct suture or nerve graft is a prerequisite to further reconstruction by tendon transfer.[19,24]

EXTRINSIC RECONSTRUCTION FOR MEDIAN NERVE PALSY

Paralysis of median nerve–innervated muscles extrinsic to the hand results in loss of active pronation of the forearm, flexion of the thumb by the flexor pollicis longus, and flexion of the index finger by loss of the flexor digitorum superficialis and profundus to that finger. Nearly complete flexion of the middle finger is usually retained by virtue of the crossover innervation by the ulnar nerve to the medial two flexor digitorum profundus muscles. However, the strength of flexion of the middle finger is compromised, providing little strength against resistance. In addition, there is severe loss of strength by loss of the function of the flexor digitorum superficialis muscles to all fingers. Loss of strength in wrist flexion occurs due to paralysis of the palmaris longus and flexor carpi radialis. The patient retains little pronation against resistance, but rarely develops a supination contracture of the forearm.

The timing of tendon transfer for the extrinsic muscles innervated by the median nerve is influenced by two factors: the type of nerve repair of the median nerve,[19] and the return of tissue equilibrium of the forearm and hand following injury. When the median nerve has been repaired by end-to-end suture, either at the time of initial surgery or within several weeks, the likelihood of reinnervation of one or more of the flexor muscles necessary to accomplish flexion of the thumb (the flexor pollicis longus) or index finger (the flexor digitorum superficialis or profundus of the index) is likely. In addition, significant reinnervation of muscles to provide some active pronation and some additional strength of grip is likely. Supplemental reconstruction by tendon transfer is delayed until such time as the degree of reinnervation provided by direct suture of the median nerve can be assessed. When the continuity of the median nerve has been restored by nerve grafting (using the pedicle technique[61,62] or free grafting), the reinnervation of forearm flexor muscles is far less certain, and reconstruction by tendon transfer is undertaken as soon as tissue equilibrium is reached. The achievement of tissue equilibrium, which is necessary for success of tendon transfer surgery, is a physiological process in which the tissues of the forearm become softened and more supple, the resistance of scar is lessened, and the nutrition of the tissues of the forearm is returned to a more normal state. After reinnervation of the forearm flexors, in the case of end-to-end suture or nerve grafting, reconstruction by tendon transfers for extrinsic flexors of the forearm is indicated.[1,3,4,10,16]

Initially, functional loss is assessed. Donor muscles considered for tendon transfer in extrinsic median nerve palsy include the extensor carpi radialis longus and the brachioradialis. If the extensor carpi ulnaris is used, one may also consider the extensor carpi radialis available. Undesirable radial deviation deformity occurs if the extensor carpi ulnaris is used, leaving the extensor carpi radialis intact. This deformity is lessened when the extensor carpi radialis longus tendon is also transferred. Flexion of the middle finger is usually nearly complete, without tendon transfer, due to crossover function between the ulnar nerve–innervated flexor digitorum profundus of the middle finger. This crossover gives little or no strength of grasp to the middle finger, however. Accordingly, a side-to-side tendon transfer of the middle to ring and little finger profundi improves the function of the middle finger (Fig. 50-1). If the middle finger tendon is sutured to the ring finger tendon in slightly greater than normal resting posture (usually about 1–1.5 cm is sufficient), the strength provided to the middle finger profundus augments grasp and provides the necessary excursion desired for a profundus mechanism.

Provided the wrist is mobile and has an active wrist extensor, the extensor carpi radialis longus or the brachioradialis is used to complete the tendon transfers for extrinsic median palsy through the mechanism of dynamic tenodesis (see Fig. 50-1).[19] Contraction of short excursion muscles that are transferred to the flexor mechanism (eg, brachioradialis or extensor carpi radialis longus) is augmented by extension of the wrist. Transfer of the extensor carpi radialis longus to the index finger flexor digitorum profundus (avoiding excessive tension, so as not to create a flexion contracture of the index finger with the wrist in 20° of flexion and the muscle–tendon unit at resting length) provides, with combined muscle contraction of the transferred motor and extension of the wrist, sufficient flexion strength to provide reasonable grasp.

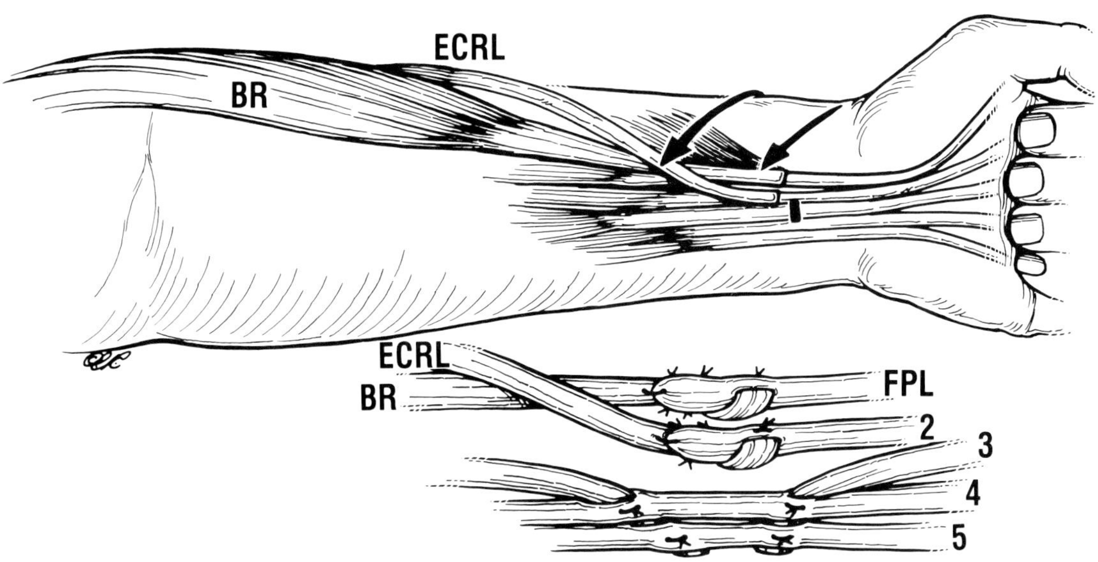

Figure 50–1. The brachioradialis is transferred to the flexor pollicis longus. The extensor carpi radialis longus is transferred to the flexor digitorum profundus of the index, and the profundus of the middle finger is divided and interwoven into the ring and little fingers in slightly greater tension than normal to provide full flexion of the middle finger with some strength.

The principle of dynamic tenodesis also works effectively when the brachioradialis is transferred to the flexor pollicis longus (Fig. 50-1). Through it, stability is promoted and some flexion of the interphalangeal joint of the thumb is regained, augmenting pinch and grasp. Transfer of the brachioradialis to the flexor pollicis longus requires extensive dissection of the brachioradialis muscle, freeing it from its bony insertion on deeper tissues of the forearm. This is carried out sufficiently proximally so that 4-cm passive stretch of the brachioradialis motor–tendon unit is achieved. This requires dissection to the junction of the proximal and middle thirds of the forearm, completely freeing the muscle–tendon unit so that, from a resting position, the muscle can be drawn distally approximately 4 cm. With this degree of passive stretch, the brachioradialis is satisfactory for tendon transfer to the flexor pollicis longus. It is sutured to the thumb flexor in the distal third of the forearm. This transfer provides interphalangeal joint stability and, with practice and training, some interphalangeal joint flexion for pinch and grasp.

The extensor carpi radialis longus does not require dissection into the proximal forearm; it is passed proximal to the abductor pollicis longus and extensor pollicis brevis. It is then rerouted subcutaneously to its insertion in the index flexor digitorum profundus tendon. It crosses over the brachioradialis tendon (which is transferred to the flexor pollicis longus). If there is some possibility of reinnervating either the flexor pollicis longus or the index and middle finger profundus tendons, possibly through a nerve graft more proximal in the arm or forearm, it is prudent to perform the tendon transfers in an end-to-side fashion with an interlocking weave. Under these circumstances, if there is some reinnervation of the paralyzed muscle, the function of that muscle augments the function of the transferred tendon.[18] If there is no possibility of reinnervation of paralyzed muscles, either because of irreparable median nerve injury or irreparable proximal muscle damage, end-to-end repair using a modification of the tendinous weave initially described by Pulvertaft is indicated. This repair technique allows a more accurate adjustment of tension of the transferred tendon.

If wrist mobility is limited, either because of primary injury to the wrist joint or limitation of muscle–tendon function, it is desirable to transfer the brachioradialis to the flexor pollicis longus tendon, tightening the transfer slightly to provide some interphalangeal joint flexion with the wrist in neutral position. Interphalangeal joint flexion should not exceed 10° and should be neutralized by flexion of the wrist to 20°. With limited motion of the wrist, the index and middle finger profundi are transferred to the profundi of the ring and little fingers, which are innervated by the ulnar nerve. This method achieves full, or nearly full, excursion of the profundus tendons without the added function of wrist extension.

It is important to establish greater tension in the index finger than in the middle finger as the side-to-side tendon transfers are performed. It is also advisable to detach the distal segment of the profundus tendons of the index and middle fingers and weave them into the profundus tendons of the ring and little fingers in order to set tension accurately. It is ill-advised to suture the tendons of the index and middle fingers side-to-side to those of the ring and little fingers without dividing the tendons of the index and middle fingers. Such side-to-side suturing techniques, depending on scar created between the long flexor tendons for continued function, generally fail. As the scar lengthens, index and middle finger flexion is lost.

When the extensor carpi radialis longus or brachioradialis is used for transfer, full extension of the thumb and index fingers at the distal two joints of each digit is achieved when the wrist is positioned in 20° of flexion.[17] It is desirable to deflate the tourniquet when setting tension so that muscle ischemia does not contract the muscle to a degree that causes the surgeon to set the tension too loosely.

It is extremely disabling, particularly with extrinsic median nerve palsy, to be unable to extend the thumb and index fingers in the process of grasp. The permanent flexion contracture produced by establishing tension too tightly reduces thumb and index finger functions significantly.[17] As long as the extensor carpi radialis longus and brachioradialis tendons are available for transfer, their use is preferred to that of the extensor carpi ulnaris. Only when one of the primary tendons is unavailable for tendon transfer is the extensor carpi ulnaris used.

RESTORATION OF INTRINSIC MUSCLE FUNCTION

Opposition of the thumb is a composite function that requires rotation of the thumb into pronation so that pulp-to-pulp pinch between thumb and index and middle fingers can be achieved.[25] A second motion, abduction of the thumb away from the palm, is required to position the thumb for pulp-to-pulp pinch.[19] To achieve optimal function, the two motions (abduction and rotation) are combined with extension of the metacarpophalangeal (MP) joint during abduction and rotation. These motions are combined with strong, short flexor function at the MP joint to achieve pulp-to-pulp pinch of the thumb to the index and middle fingers.[13–15,53]

Restoration of true opposition of the thumb is required if the thumb has a very high level of sensibility. Patients with normal sensation in the thumb, as well as the index and middle fingers, require a thumb for precision pinch activities and full opposition for pulp-to-pulp pinch. Conversely, in patients with impaired thumb sensibility, index and middle fingers achieve maximal use with end-to-side pinch with the thumb (Fig. 50-2). Satisfactory function is achieved by restoring short thumb flexor function combined with extension of the MP joint and abduction from the palm.[26] In these thumbs, full rotation of the thumb for true pulp-to-pulp pinch is unnecessary (this is not to say that restoration of full rotation is impossible; however, it is unnecessary for maximal function).

Because of variations in the innervation of the flexor pollicis brevis,[23,43,55,63] particularly the superficial head, about one third of hands with median nerve palsy have excellent extension at the MP joint and sufficient pulp-to-side pinch of the thumb to index or middle fingers so that additional tendon transfers are not indicated.[43] Unless the quality of sensibility is superior, these thumbs do require an opponens transfer. Two thirds of patients (those who lack ulnar nerve innervation of the superficial head of the flexor pollicis brevis) require an additional tendon transfer for opposition.[26] The transfer creates either a functional su-

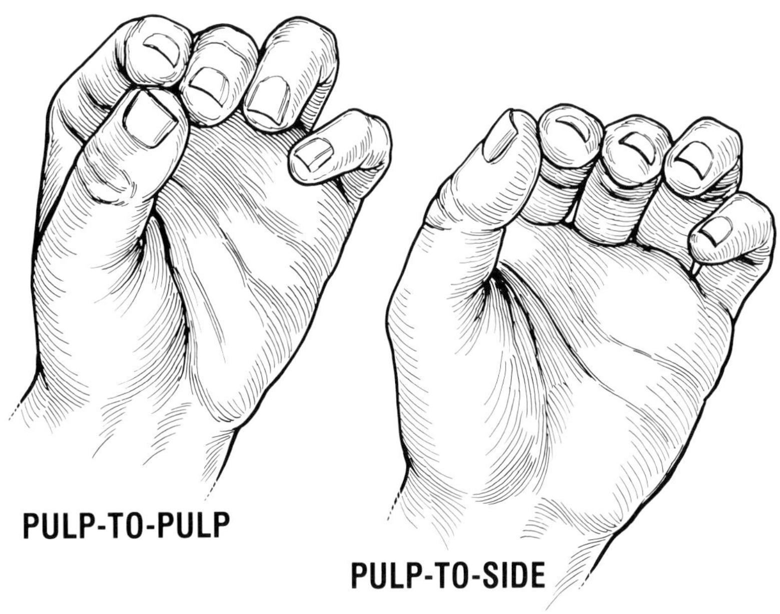

Figure 50–2. *In a normal sensate hand, pulp-to-pulp pinch must be sought in order to accomplish fine motions of the hand and thumb in pinch, but in a hand deprived of some sensibility, pulp-to-side pinch, mitigated largely through short flexor function, will be adequate.*

perficial short flexor or a combined short flexor and abductor of the thumb so that pulp-to-side or pulp-to-pulp pinch is achieved (Fig. 50-3).

Before undertaking an abduction opposition transfer, certain prerequisites must be satisfied in order to have a reasonable chance of obtaining maximal function. The most important of these is the relief of web-space contractures.[1,12,38,47,58] Two deformities create the web-space contracture: an adduction contracture of the thumb metacarpal, and a supination contracture. The combination of adduction and supination contractures negate the effects of opposition transfer regardless of the motor, tendon, or technique used.[44,45] Mayer emphasized that failure of opposition transfer was almost certain if surgery was performed in the face of a first web space contracture in either adduction or adduction–supination.[45] Accordingly, the relief of the adduction or adduction–supination contracture is a prerequisite for undertaking opponensplasty to improve function of the hand. The techniques for the relief of this contracture are well documented in the literature and include release of joints (even the carpometacarpal joint of the thumb), lengthening or mobilizing muscle groups (usually the intrinsic muscles of the thumb), and using rotation flaps or distant pedicle flaps to lengthen the web between the thumb and index finger, thereby improving abduction and the ability to rotate into opposition.[1,12,38,46]

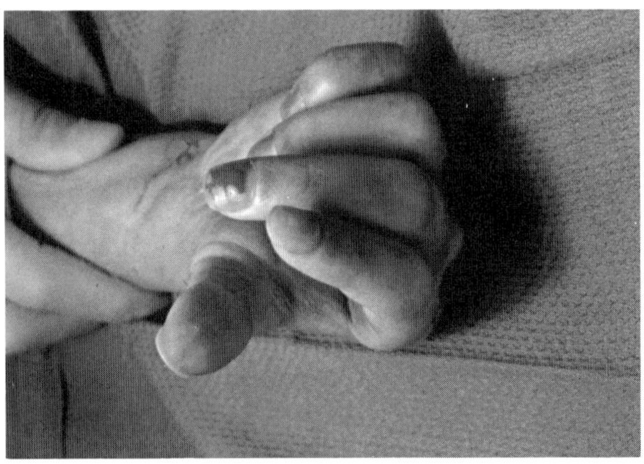

Figure 50–3. *Postoperative opponensplasty, illustrating the position and rotation of the thumb with a functioning opponensplasty transfer.*

A second prerequisite for opponensplasty is adequate thumb sensibility. If nerve suture or grafting has not yet reinnervated the thumb and the palmar surface is nonsensate, it is important to have some retained dorsal sensibility, provided by the superficial branch of the radial nerve, for some degree of position sense. Radial sensibility on the thumb is of considerable help in rehabilitation of tendon transfers. Without both position sense, provided by the radial nerve, and palmar sensibility, it is necessary to select an opponensplasty technique that requires minimal retraining for maximum use. In my experience, the extensor indicis proprius opponensplasty serves this purpose in the nonsensate thumb.[20]

The third prerequisite for opponensplasty is extension of the MP joint. If there is limited extension of the MP or interphalangeal (IP) joint of the thumb, it is important to recognize this before opponensplasty so that either extension of the MP joint can be gained with opponensplasty insertion into the extensor of the thumb, or fusion of the MP joint in the usual position of extension is performed at the time of opponensplasty.

But the most important prerequisite for opponensplasty is to evaluate the patient's specific needs from the standpoint of hand and thumb function. Functional needs (from the standpoint of thumb position, pinch, and grasp) and others dictate the selection of type of opponensplasty.[26] I have already mentioned that reduced sensibility, particularly of position sense of the thumb, dictates the selection of an appropriate motor for opponensplasty in order to minimize the difficulty of retraining and rehabilitation of the tendon transfer. The nonsensate thumb requires an opponensplasty, after which retraining and rehabilitation can be most easily undertaken. For the nonsensate thumb, a synergistic muscle such as the extensor indicis proprius is desirable.

In a patient with a high median nerve laceration in whom the superficialis muscles have been reinnervated by nerve suture, the surgeon is discouraged from selecting the ring finger superficialis as an appropriate motor and tendon for opponensplasty.[19] The reinnervated muscle lacks the specificity of function that it had prior to nerve laceration. In addition, it regains less strength with reinnervation than it had prior to injury. Accordingly, it makes an unsatisfactory motor for opponensplasty.

The patient with generalized polyneuropathy, particularly if it is a progressive process that can be expected to worsen, requires an opponensplasty that has increased inherent strength and is proximally innervated.[5,40,67] Accordingly, a patient with Hansen's disease,[5,67] amyotrophic lateral sclerosis, multiple sclerosis, or Charcot-Marie-Tooth disease is a candidate for an extensor carpi radialis longus opponensplasty or palmaris longus opponensplasty rather than an opponensplasty with a more distal, and weaker, motor.

Timing of Opponensplasty

Restoration of abductor pollicis brevis function with nerve suture is unlikely with laceration of the median nerve at a site proximal to the junction of the proximal and middle thirds of the forearm. If the abductor pollicis brevis is reinnervated by nerve suture at the level of the elbow, its function is usually weak and insufficient to provide adequate positioning of the thumb. Accordingly, following high median nerve laceration, tendon transfer for the intrinsic function of the thumb is indicated and even desirable to prevent long-term splinting or the associated deformities of web-space contracture and supination contracture of the thumb.[6,11,18,19] However, tendon transfer for the extrinsic muscles innervated by the median nerve may be delayed, anticipating return of long flexor function. It is desirable, although not mandatory, that the patient have some position sense of the thumb; this is usually provided by the superficial radial nerve.

Lacerations of the median nerve distal to the mid-portion of the forearm, which cause paralysis of intrinsic muscle function of the thumb, require additional information in order to appropriately plan opponensplasty. The surgeon can anticipate some return of abductor pollicis brevis and opponens pollicis function if a more distal median nerve laceration has been treated with a fascicular isolation and repair technique (as described by Hakstian), accompanied by fascicular repair of the motor fascicle of the median nerve (see Chap. 15). It is then preferable to delay opponensplasty to allow reinnervation of the intrinsic muscles of the thumb. If the patient has had a partial laceration of the median nerve, accompanied by intrinsic paralysis of the abductor pollicis brevis and opponens pollicis of the thumb, primary repair could yield some intrinsic function. In this situation, the surgeon is justified in delaying opponensplasty.

In the patient with multiple, sharp tendon lacerations of the distal third of the forearm with loss of the palmaris longus tendon and median nerve, where the palmaris longus tendon has been repaired, I believe that an early tendon transfer of the palmaris longus to the abductor pollicis brevis is indicated. This technique, initially described by Camitz[21] and Ney,[48] is justified to provide the patient with an internal splint, preventing web space contracture while the wrist and hand are positioned for the healing of other tendon lacerations (see Chap. 64).

TYPES OF OPERATIONS

Flexor Digitorum Superficialis Opponensplasty

If tendon transfer to restore opposition for the thumb is the most common tendon transfer in the hand, then flexor digitorum superficialis opponensplasty is the most common opposition transfer. Steindler described the first attempt at opponensplasty using the flexor pollicis longus in 1918.[60] Shortly thereafter, Kruckenberg described an operation in which he divided the flexor digitorum superficialis tendon of the middle finger and inserted the radial half into the insertion of the opponens pollicis muscle.[36] Kruckenberg's operation was the first attempt at flexor digitorum superficialis transfer to provide opponens function. The Royle-Thompson[56,65] opponensplasty evolved after other surgeons[2,14,35,37] had passed the superficialis tendon through portions of the transverse carpal ligament. Initially, Royle passed the ring finger superficialis tendon along the entire length of the sheath of the flexor pollicis longus, attaching it, in two parts, to the tendon of the flexor pollicis brevis and to an insertion site on the dorsum of the thumb metacarpal.[56] Thompson modified Royle's method by passing the tendon around the ulnar border of the palmar fascia (which served as a pulley) to reach the thumb subcutaneously.[65] Once again, the insertion of the transfer included one slip of the tendon of the superficialis fixed distally on the thumb metacarpal and a second slip attached dorsally and ulnarly to the base of the proximal phalanx of the thumb.

Other modifications of the basic Royle-Thompson technique have included the use of a pulley at the distal portion of the transverse carpal ligament, using the tendon of the flexor carpi ulnaris as a pulley, by passing the superficialis tendon deep to the flexor carpi ulnaris tendon in the area of the pisiform. As the superficialis turns volarly, it is passed subcutaneously toward the MP joint of the thumb. Still another modification of the pulley of the flexor digitorum superficialis was suggested by Brand, who used the canal of Guyon lying just radial to the pisiform bone as a natural pulley for the superficialis, passing the tendon through the canal, then subcutaneously to the MP joint of the thumb (Fig. 50-4).[7,8] Curtis, in an unpublished series of 25 opponensplasties, used the flexor digitorum superficialis of the ring finger and a Guyon's canal pulley. This did not cause ulnar tunnel syndrome, and excellent short flexor–opponens function of the thumb occurred. Palazzi suggested using the origin of the abductor digiti quinti as a pulley by drawing the flexor superficialis tendon beneath the abductor muscle origin after traversing the palmar aspect of the pisiform, and using that bone as a fulcrum in the passage of the tendon toward the MP joint of the thumb [51]

Bunnell established the classical elements of an opposition transfer.[14] He called attention to motor selection and to the observation that certain muscles require an additional tendon graft to make them long enough to act as opposition transfers. He emphasized the importance of the direction of pull of the muscle–tendon unit, using a fixed pulley located in the area of the pisiform for the most efficient abductor pollicis brevis transfer. His method of attachment on the dorsal ulnar aspect of the proximal phalanx of the thumb ensured that the opponensplasty would act as a rotator–abductor of the thumb.

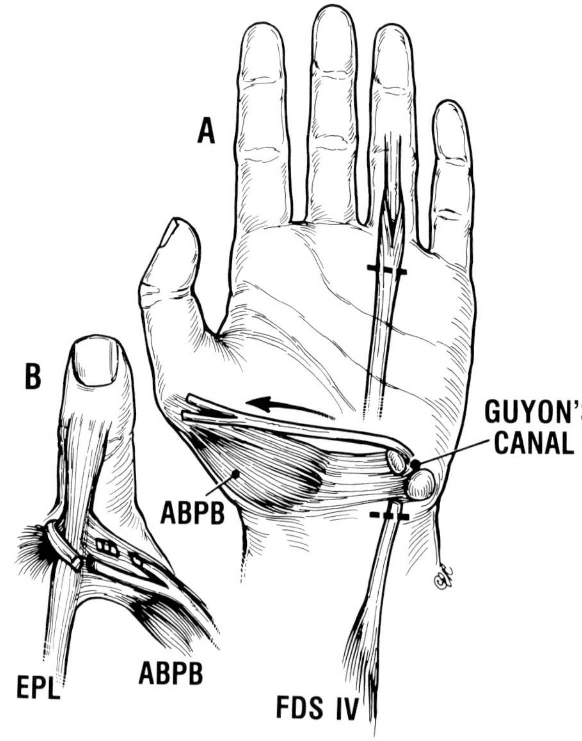

Figure 50–4. *The flexor digitorum superficialis transfer, having been detached from the ring finger, is passed through Guyon's canal, acting as a pulley in its course to the thumb.*

The operative technique for a flexor digitorum superficialis opponensplasty begins with harvesting the tendon to be transferred from the ring finger. Use of the middle finger superficialis is discouraged because, although it provides a satisfactory opponensplasty, it causes a greater loss of strength on the radial side of the hand. The incision for removal of the ring finger superficialis is positioned in the area between 1 cm distal to the distal palmar crease and the proximal finger crease of the ring finger. Through this incision, the superficialis tendon is identified at the flexor tendon sheath. It is pulled as far into the wound as possible with the finger in maximum flexion, and divided either at the proximal or distal borders of the A1 pulley. Either division provides stability for the proximal IP joint of the finger, preventing hyperextension and (by not violating the flexor sheath over that joint) eliminating the possibility of flexion contracture of the proximal interphalangeal (PIP) joint. Adequate length is achieved by dividing the flexor superficialis at this level.

Depending on the pulley to be used, a more proximal incision is made at the distal extent of Guyon's canal or the palmar fascia, if either is to be used as a pulley, and at the level of the wrist flexion crease extending proximally 2 cm if the flexor carpi ulnaris is to be used as a pulley. Rerouting the flexor superficialis begins subcutaneously just proximal to the wrist flexion crease. If the palmar fascia is to be used as a pulley, the tendon is tunneled subcutaneously along the ulnar border of the palmar fascia and rerouted radially 1.5 cm distal to the wrist flexion crease around the ulnar border of the palmar fascia. The passage is subcutaneous to the MP joint of the thumb. By using Guyon's canal as a pulley, the flexor digitorum superficialis is drawn into Guyon's canal just distal to the wrist flexion crease, through a transverse incision that allows it to be redirected toward the MP joint.

With a pulley constructed at the flexor carpi ulnaris just proximal to the pisiform, the tendon can be passed around the flexor carpi ulnaris, passing deep to the tendon, then volarly across the base of the palm to the MP joint of the thumb. If a loop pulley of the flexor carpi ulnaris is constructed, the distal 4 to 5 cm of flexor carpi ulnaris are divided longitudinally, and the radial half is allowed to remain attached distally to the pisiform. The proximal extent of the radial half is looped in a circle and anchored firmly in place to the remaining flexor carpi ulnaris with multiple nonabsorbable sutures. The flexor superficialis is passed through the loop and then extended subcutaneously across the base of the palm to the MP joint of the thumb.

My preference for a pulley for the flexor superficialis is the canal of Guyon as described by Brand. It does not scar, does not produce ulnar tunnel syndrome, and allows for an excellent, short flexor–abductor opponensplasty (see Fig. 50-4).

The method of attachment of the opponens transfer to the thumb is an important part of the procedure. Bunnell's method of attachment to bone along the ulnar–dorsal border of the proximal phalanx provides excellent rotation of the thumb into an opponens position but, if the attachment is too distal on the proximal phalanx, may provide excessive flexion force at the MP joint, and a deformity known as a "crank" thumb may occur.[14,19,54] A more proximal attachment on the proximal phalanx jeopardizes the motion of the MP joint by creating scar about its dorsal–ulnar border. Riordan's technique, using a two-tailed attachment interweaving one slip of the flexor superficialis into the abductor pollicis brevis muscle and tendon, and continuing the second slip into the hood over the MP joint and extensor pollicis longus, on the ulnar–dorsal portion of the MP joint, provides excellent rotation of the thumb (Fig. 50-5).[26,54] This attachment creates an extensor moment for the MP and

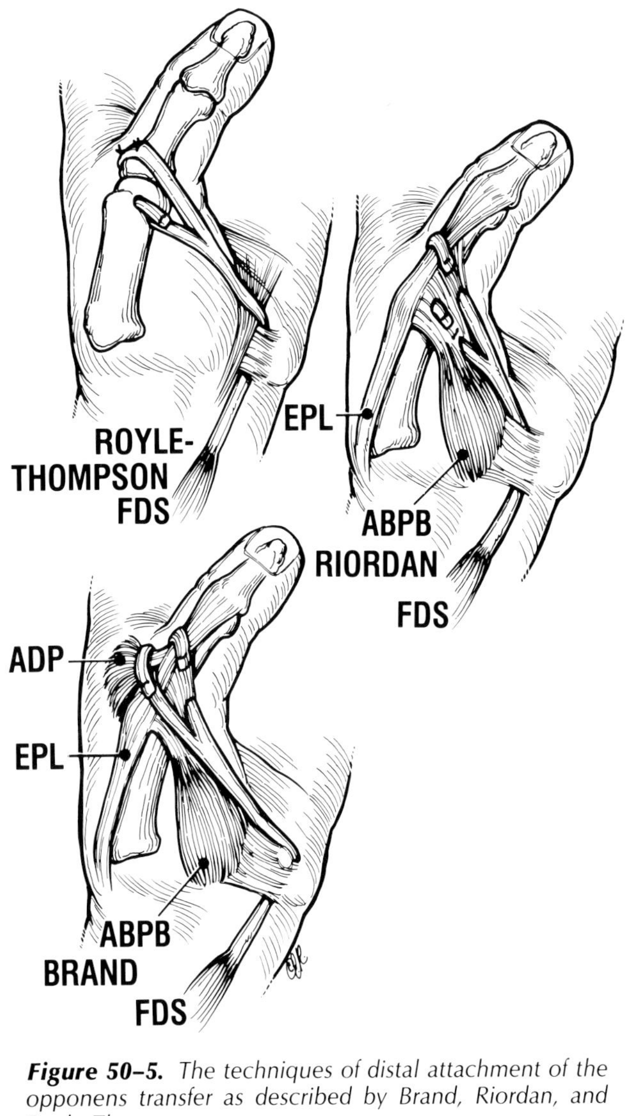

Figure 50–5. *The techniques of distal attachment of the opponens transfer as described by Brand, Riordan, and Royle-Thompson.*

IP joints of the thumb, which is desirable (except when there is an extremely weakened flexor pollicis longus).

Brand's method of distal attachment of the tendon (see Fig. 50-5) requires interweaving one slip of the tendon through the tendon of the abductor pollicis brevis, continuing it to the extensor pollicis longus in a manner similar to Riordan's technique.[26] The other slip, however, provides an additional rotation moment for the thumb by extending across the extensor muscle, even attaching as far ulnar on the adductor pollicis. Brand's attachment, if there is sufficient tendon available, provides excellent rotational position of the thumb and provides extensor stability of the MP joint.[26]

An advantage of a flexor superficialis opponensplasty is the excursion that is available, making the setting of tension less complex than with other donors. The tension is adjusted so that, with the wrist in neutral position, the thumb is brought to nearly full opposition. With wrist flexion, it is relaxed. The thumb lies against the palm with 20° to 25° of wrist flexion. Another distinct advantage, again attendant on the generous excursion of the flexor superficialis, is the ability to flatten the hand, necessary for a patient using crutches or a wheelchair or one who must transfer from bed to wheelchair or wheelchair to walker. This is an important feature: a muscle–tendon unit with a shorter amplitude stretches out with these maneuvers.

One of the disadvantages of the flexor superficialis opponensplasty is the relative difficulty in retraining the muscle. Retraining is begun with opposition motions toward the ring finger as the ring finger is brought into flexion. This can be difficult for the patient with limited muscular coordination. Certain pulley selections of this transfer (particularly pulleys at the flexor carpi ulnaris) seem less desirable. The loop pulley of Bunnell at the flexor carpi ulnaris is difficult to adjust and seems to result in scar that limits tendon excursion. The passage of the tendon around the flexor carpi ulnaris inevitably leads to proximal migration of the tendon. This weakens the transfer, providing more abduction than flexion. Using the canal of Guyon as a pulley for the flexor superficialis transfer, as recommended by Brand and Curtis, seems to be the most desirable pulley for this transfer.[7,26]

Another disadvantage is that the flexor superficialis cannot be used in the patient with a high median nerve laceration due to paralysis of the muscle. Also, it is not used if the muscle has been reinnervated after nerve suture.

Palmaris Longus Opponensplasty

The direction of pull of the palmar longus, from its origin in the proximal forearm transferred to an attachment at the MP joint of the thumb or in the tendon of the abductor pollicis brevis, provides an excellent internal splint and abductor force.[9,21,48] The technique is not complex (Fig. 50-6).

The palmaris longus tendon is identified in the distal third of the forearm and is dissected free of fascial attachments in the distal 2 inches of the

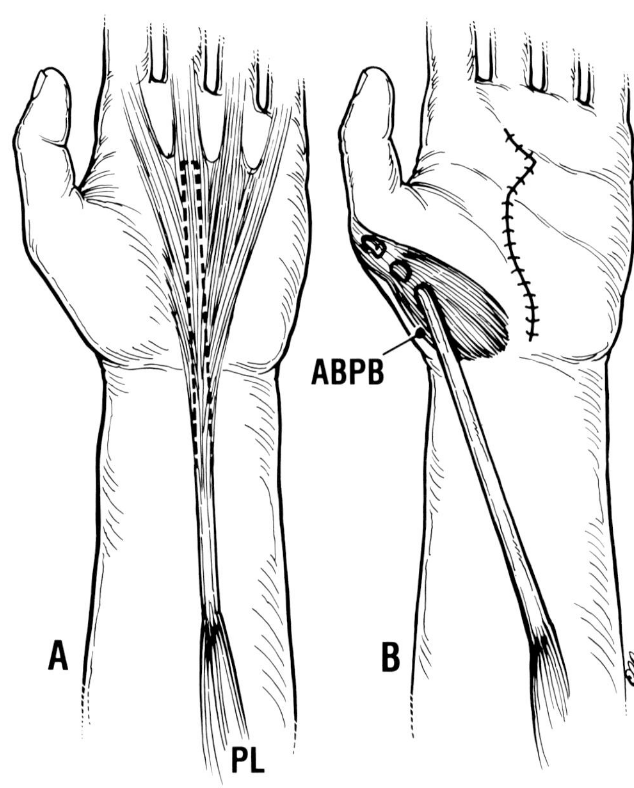

Figure 50–6. *(**A**) The dissection of the palmaris longus opponensplasty into the palm follows the direction of fibers. (**B**) The motor tendon unit is directed in a straight line to the abductor pollicis brevis insertion on the thumb.*

forearm, proximal to the wrist flexion crease. As the tendon is not long enough at this level, dissection is continued into the palm, prolonging a strip of palmar fascia as originally described by Camitz.[21] The width of tendon and fascia provided is equal to that of the palmaris longus at the wrist. Dissection is directed to the bases of the index or middle fingers. The entire dissection is performed under direct visualization. The palmaris longus, with its attached strip of palmar fascia, is retracted to the mid-portion of the distal third of the forearm and then rerouted subcutaneously toward the MP joint of the thumb. Attachment at the MP joint of the thumb is by interweaving into the tendon of the abductor pollicis brevis. Excess palmar fascia is looped around the extensor tendon or dorsal hood at the MP joint to secure the attachment.

The main advantages of the palmaris longus opponensplasty are its simplicity, its function as an internal splint, preventing contracture of the first web space, and the fact that a pulley is not needed.

The disadvantages of the palmaris longus opponensplasty include its limited use, since a median nerve laceration proximal to its innervation obviates its use because the muscle is paralyzed. Because of its limited attachment through the abductor pollicis brevis, this opponensplasty provides neither rotation nor flexion of the thumb. With the tendon in place, the palm cannot be flattened for bed-to-wheelchair transfer or for the use of crutches. In addition, the palmaris longus is not easily re-educated.

Opponensplasty Using a Wrist Extensor

Although the extensor carpi radialis brevis has been mentioned by Henderson as an adequate motor for opponensplasty,[30] most authors prefer either the extensor carpi ulnaris (as described by Phalen and Miller,[52] and later by Iselin[33]), or the extensor carpi radialis longus (as discussed by Henderson[30] and White[66]). The opponensplasties using wrist extensors require prolongation with tendon grafts; usually the palmaris longus is used. The extensor tendon, prolonged with the tendon graft, is passed around the ulnar border of the forearm (using the ulnar border at the base of the palm as a fulcrum) subcutaneously across the base of the palm to the thumb. When the extensor carpi radialis longus is used, the tendon is detached from the base of the index metacarpal, withdrawn proximally through a separate incision to the mid-portion on the dorsal surface of the forearm, and then rerouted distally and ulnarly, prolonging the muscle–tendon unit with a tendon graft and routing the tendon along the base of the palm toward the MP joint of the thumb.

The extensor carpi ulnaris opponensplasty is freed sufficiently proximally (usually 4 to 5 cm) to allow a smooth curve from its origin, the proximal ulna, to the thumb. The extensor carpi ulnaris, with its tendon graft, is routed subcutaneously along the base of the palm to the MP joint of the thumb.

One technique of prolonging the wrist extensor described by Burkhalter requires harvesting the extensor pollicis brevis muscle at its musculotendinous junction in the first dorsal compartment.[19] That tendon remains attached to its insertion at the MP joint of the thumb. It is divided at its musculotendinous junction and rerouted across the base of the palm toward the pisiform. The tendon is usually long enough to be sutured to the wrist extensor tendon motor, either the extensor carpi ulnaris or the extensor carpi radialis longus.

The creation of a repair site along the fulcrum of the tendon transfer, at the ulnar border of the palm, is an undesirable feature of this method. This technique provides a ready-made insertion in a good position on the thumb for the opponensplasty. In the process, however, the function of two muscles is sacrificed. When an arthrodesis of the MP joint of the thumb has been carried out, this is an acceptable technique. However, it must be considered in perspective in other clinical situations.

When the wrist extensor is prolonged with a palmaris longus tendon graft, any of the insertions previously described for the flexor superficialis by Bunnell, Riordan, or Brand, in addition to the insertion described by Littler, is satisfactory. Tension is adjusted so that, with the wrist in a neutral position, the thumb is brought to full opposition.

The advantages of the wrist extensor opponensplasty are its strength, its proximal innervation, and its usefulness in cases of progressive polyneuropathy. The disadvantages relate to the use of a second tendon as a graft to prolong the motor to the thumb. These tendon grafts have a tendency to scar, particularly at the site where the tendon graft is interwoven into the donor muscle tendon. The excursion of these muscles is adequate but not excessive, and in the case of the extensor carpi ulnaris the loss of function to balance the wrist in neutral may result in radial deviation deformity. This is normally an undesirable posture for function of the hand.

Extensor Indicis Proprius Opponensplasty

The proper extensors of the index and little fingers provide excellent donor muscles and tendons for opponensplasty. The technique for the extensor digiti minimi starts with a small incision over the MP joint of the little finger. After verifying the tendinous slip to the little finger from the ring finger for extension of the MP joint of the little finger, the extensor digiti minimi can be divided and passed to a second incision just distal to the extensor retinaculum on the dorsum of the wrist and hand.[57,64] The extensor tendon is then passed to a third incision on the proximal edge of the dorsal retinaculum and, after a generous fasciotomy along the extensor surface of the forearm, is rerouted around the ulnar border of the wrist and across the subcutaneous area of the proximal palm toward the MP joint of the thumb. The attachment can be accomplished through a modified Riordan or Brand technique, and the tendon is usually long enough to accomplish any reasonable insertion into the thumb.

The technique for the extensor indicis proprius is only slightly more complex (Fig. 50-7).[17,22] The initial incision is made over the MP joint of the index finger, and the extensor indicis proprius lying on the ulnar side of the MP joint is detached from the index finger with a small slip of tissue extending into the extensor hood of the index MP joint. The extensor hood is then meticulously repaired so as not to result in an extensor lag at the index MP joint. The indicis proprius is then passed proximally to a second incision just distal to the dorsal retinaculum and then across the extensor retinaculum to its proximal border and a third and somewhat larger incision. At this point in the dissection, it is important to ensure that the extensor indicis proprius can be rerouted in a straight line through a generous extensor fasciotomy over the indicis proprius. The indicis proprius is freed from the common extensor to the index finger and rerouted along the ulnar border of the hand in the area of the pisiform, where a fourth incision is helpful in subcutaneous passage of the transfer across the base of the palm toward the MP joint of the thumb. The tendon of the indicis proprius, if properly rerouted at the proximal edge of the extensor retinaculum, will be long enough to attach to the abductor pollicis brevis or a combined attachment to the abductor pollicis brevis and extensor pollicis longus or brevis. Any of the previously described insertions to the thumb can be used successfully, except those that require additional tendon length to attach to tissues on the ulnar side of the thumb.

The opponensplasty of the extensor digiti minimi, although it provides adequate opposition, is not often used. That of the extensor indicis proprius, however, has several distinct advantages, and it is often used with excellent results. The extensor indicis proprius has no distinct pulley as an opponensplasty, using instead the ulnar border of the wrist as a very simple pulley mechanism. It is always available with volar injury, does not reduce the strength of the hand the way a superficialis opponensplasty does, and above all is extremely easily retrained even in the most uncoordinated patient.

The retraining of the opponensplasty of the extensor indicis proprius starts simply by extending the index finger and thumb simultaneously, at which point the patient will nearly immediately notice that the thumb comes into a position of opposition with the extension of the index finger. This motion is natural and allows the patient to position the thumb to the index finger for pinch in the most natural fashion.

The disadvantage of the extensor indicis proprius opponensplasty is that the patient who must flatten the palm for transfer from bed to wheelchair or wheelchair to walker cannot do so without stretching out the transfer. Accordingly, an alternate method of opponensplasty should be selected in a patient who is paraplegic or whose injuries to the lower extremities require transfer using the hands.

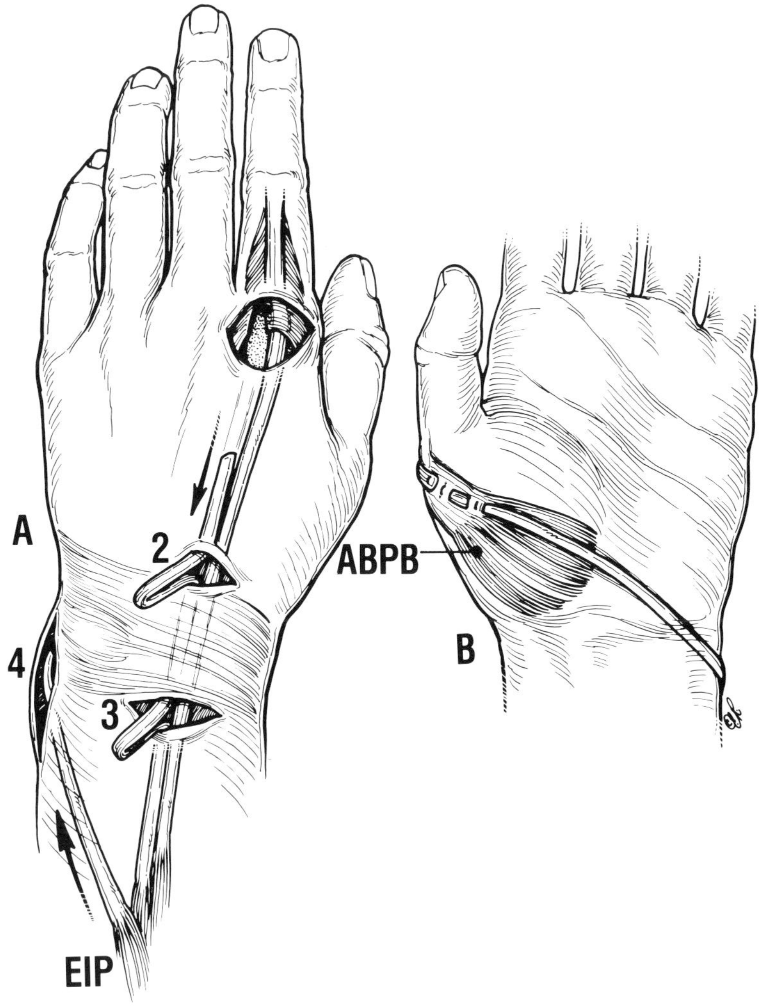

Figure 50–7. *The technique of extensor indicis proprius opponensplasty with detachment of the tendon from the metacarpophalangeal joint of the thumb and retraction of the tendon proximal to the dorsal retinaculum (**A**). The tendon transfer is then redirected around the ulnar border of the wrist to the area of the pisiform and from there traverses the base of the palm toward the metacarpophalangeal joint of the thumb (**B**).*

Abductor Digiti Minimi Opponensplasty

Huber[32] in 1921 and Nicolaysen[49] a year later described the restoration of opposition of the thumb by transfer of the abductor digiti minimi muscle. This procedure, popularized by Littler and Cooley in 1963,[39] is predicated on the use of the abductor digiti quinti, which remains viable on a thin neurovascular pedicle despite the fact that its entire insertion and its entire origin are detached and repositioned across the base of the palm. The fragile neurovascular pedicle of the abductor digiti quinti provides one of the major disadvantages of this procedure, since loss of this neurovascular pedicle will result in loss of the muscle and its function, and failure of the procedure.

The distal tendon of the abductor digit quinti is exposed through an incision along the radial border of the hypothenar muscles and curving to the ulnar border of the little finger at the MP joint (Fig. 50-8). Through this incision, the entire abductor digiti quinti muscle can be detached from its distal insertion on the little finger. After dissection from distal to proximal, taking care to protect the neurovascular bundle to the muscle, the muscle can then be turned so that the superficial surface of the muscle as it was initially exposed becomes the deep surface as the muscle is transferred to the thumb; the corresponding deep surface containing the neurovascular bundle to the abductor digiti quinti is then reflected to be superficial with the transfer of the muscle.

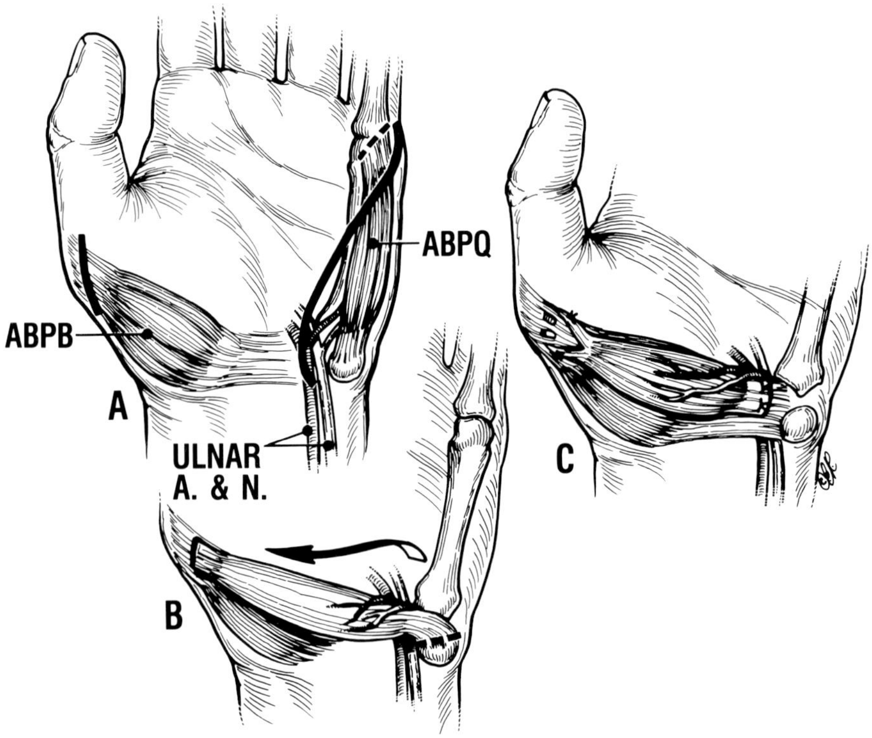

Figure 50–8. *The incisions required for the transfer of the abductor digiti quinti include a larger ulnar incision for the mobilization of the muscle and a smaller radial incision over the abductor pollicis brevis for the attachment of the distal extent of the muscle to the thumb. The muscle tendon unit is rotated as if turning the page of a book and reinserted to the abductor pollicis brevis.*

After isolating the neurovascular bundle and protecting it and turning the muscle toward the thumb as one would turn a page in a book (essentially rotating the muscle on its own axis by 180°), the proximal origin of the muscle is detached and transposed toward the thumb, taking care again to protect the neurovascular bundle. The transposition or shifting of the origin of the muscle is very limited and is resutured into place at the base of the palmar fascia. The distal insertion of the abductor digiti quinti is then tunneled subcutaneously toward the MP joint of the thumb, and the distal tendon of that muscle is attached to that of the abductor pollicis brevis tendon.

It would seem that there are more disadvantages than advantages to the Huber procedure. There can be no question that the fragile neurovascular bundle to the abductor digiti quinti is at risk throughout the dissection and in the early postoperative period. This small muscle does not provide sufficient thrust to oppose some thumbs and does not sufficiently rotate the thumb to position it in an ideal posture for pinch. The removal of the abductor digiti quinti from the hypothenar area creates cosmetic deformity and weakens the power grip of the little finger. The restoration of muscle bulk in the thenar eminence with the transposition of the abductor digiti quinti does not constitute a sufficient advantage to recommend this procedure. The use of other ulnar nerve–innervated intrinsic muscles of the hand has been described by DeVecchi[27] (using the adductor pollicis) and Ortiochea[50] (using an innervated portion of the flexor pollicis brevis to create opposition of the thumb). Neither of these procedures has gained wide acceptance, and neither restores true opposition of the thumb.

Opponensplasty Using Extrinsic Muscles of the Thumb (Fig. 50-9)

Three muscles extrinsic to the thumb have been described as providing, with repositioning, adequate opponens function. Using the abductor pollicis longus tendon, Sherb detached the insertion of the tendon and reinserted this tendon more distal and ulnar along the thumb metacarpal in order to provide abduction and rotation to the thumb.[53] Edgerton and Brand in 1965 rerouted the abductor pollicis longus, rerouting the tendon across the brachioradialis and using the palmaris longus as a pulley, tunneling subcutaneously back toward the thumb and inserting the tendon distal to the original insertion.[29]

A variety of authors have suggested the use of the flexor pollicis longus as an opponensplasty. Although various methods[31,41,42,53,59] have been suggested since Steindler's first opponensplasty in 1918,[60] the simplest method seems to be that described by Williams[67] in which the flexor pollicis longus is divided just proximal to its insertion and withdrawn proximal to the wrist flexion crease. After the flexor pollicis longus is withdrawn from its sheath, it is then rerouted through the carpal tunnel beneath the transverse carpal ligament. At the distal border of the transverse carpal ligament, it is tunneled subcutaneously to the area of the MP joint of the thumb. The IP joint of the thumb is treated with either tenodesis of the stump of the flexor pollicis longus or arthrodesis of the IP joint.

Burkhalter has used the extensor pollicis longus as an opponensplasty in those patients who have progressive neurological disease and an extended and supinated thumb, and who cannot bring the thumb to an opponens posture.[19] His concept is a simple one: removing the deforming force of the extensor pollicis longus and converting it to a corrective force as an opposition transfer. With his technique, the central portion of the extensor pollicis longus is harvested through the hood at the MP joint on the dorsum of the thumb and withdrawn to a proximal incision at the proximal border of the dorsal retinaculum at the wrist, removing the extensor pollicis longus from the third dorsal compartment. The extensor pollicis longus tendon is then rerouted from an area proximal to the dorsal retinaculum along the ulnar border of the wrist, where a third incision is used to tunnel subcutaneously across the base of the palm to the area of the MP joint of the thumb. Arthrodesis of the MP joint of the thumb is performed, the lateral bands are approximated, and the opponens transfer of the rerouted extensor pollicis longus is sutured into the lateral portions of the extensor mechanism from which it was earlier dissected. The IP joint of the thumb is stabilized with a single Kirschner wire to allow healing of the extensor mechanism but is neither arthrodesed or tenodesed.

The use of the extrinsic muscles of the thumb to provide opposition has relatively narrow indications. There can be no doubt that the usual median palsy with intact thumb extensors, long abductors, and ulnarly innervated intrinsics is not a case in which the extrinsic muscles of the thumb will provide the best opposition transfer. Conversely, in a hand with limited motors and in which

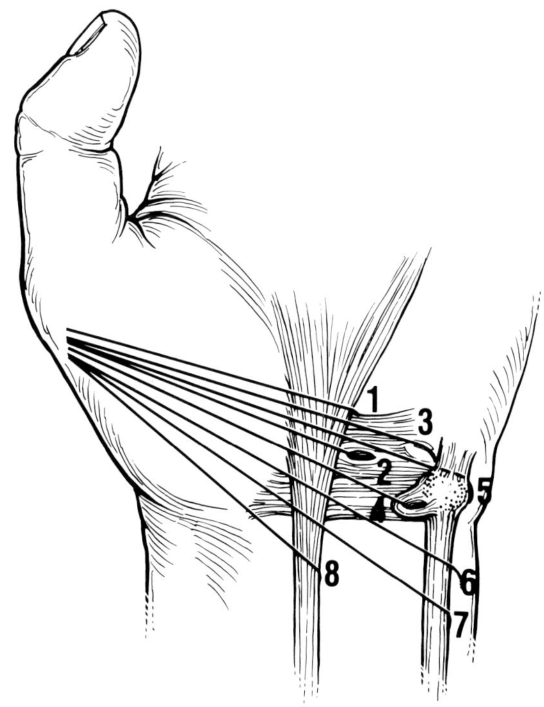

Figure 50–9. *The positions of the multiple pulleys used by various surgeons for the opponens transfer. (1) Ulnar margin of the palmar fascia Thompson pulley using superficialis of the ring finger. (2) A window in the distal portion of the transverse carpal ligament, Roeren using superficialis of ring finger. (3) Guyon's tunnel, Brand's superficialis of ring finger. (4) Flexor carpi ulnaris sling after the technique of Bunnell, superficialis of the ring finger. (5) Pisiform bone and the abductor digiti quinti origin; method of Palazzi using ring finger superficialis. (6) Ulnar margin of the wrist used for wrist extensor opponensplasties as well as opponensplasty of the extensor digiti quinti and extensor indicis proprius. (7) Ulnar margin of the flexor carpi ulnaris used by Littler and Bunnell for the ring finger superficialis. (8) Ulnar margin of the palmaris longus tendon used by Edgerton and Brand for the abductor pollicis longus.*

neurological improvement cannot be anticipated or in a patient in whom neurological deterioration is likely, the use of a flexor pollicis longus or extensor pollicis longus opponensplasty may be indicated.

Special Techniques for Opponensplasty

The transfer of the flexor digitorum profundus of the little finger has been performed to create an opponensplasty of the thumb.[34] Most hand surgeons would see little justification in removing an essential tendon from any digit to create an opponensplasty of the thumb when that essential tendon must then be reconstructed to restore the digit from which it was removed.

Many opponensplasties traverse the base of the palm subcutaneously. With volar injuries—particularly volar injuries at the wrist or the base of the palm—this area to be traversed may be involved with previous surgical incisions or even fixed, immovable scars. Under these circumstances, the preparation of the base of the palm with the insertion of a Silastic rod to create a tunnel through which the opponens transfer can be routed has proven helpful in reducing the scarring and improving excursion of the opponens transfer. The Silastic rod should be placed approximately 3 months before the anticipated opponens transfer and will provide an adequate channel for the transfer at the time of opponensplasty.

The postoperative management of opponens transfer requires at least 4 weeks of immobilization with the wrist in 30° of flexion and the thumb held in full opposition for most opponens transfers. The wrist can then be brought to a neutral position and rehabilitation started with retraining of the transfer to provide opposition to the thumb. Tenolysis of the opponens transfer should be delayed for at least 4 to 6 months, and after tenolysis immediate motion of the tendon transfer with the wrist supported should be instituted to guarantee the transfer's continued function.

Author's Preferred Method

The extensor indicis proprius opponensplasty as described by Burkhalter provides most patients with a natural opponens transfer that is easily retrained. When the extensor indicis proprius is unavailable in a patient with a distal median nerve injury, the flexor digitorum superficialis with Guyon's canal as a pulley provides excellent short flexor–opponens function. In patients with multiple, sharp lacerations of the flexor tendons in the distal half of the flexor surface of the forearm and with a palmaris longus that has normally been lacerated with the median nerve, the Camitz technique for the palmaris longus to reconstruct an internal splint for opposition of the thumb is useful. It prevents web space contracture and supination of the thumb.

SUMMARY

The continuing lack of median nerve sensibility on the radial side of the hand reduces the functional potential of the median nerve palsy hand. Restoring high-quality sensibility is the first reconstructive method addressed. Subsequently, tendon transfers improve function further but only simulate, never reproduce, normal function. Optimal functional results from opponensplasty require careful consideration of the method of transfer and selection of motor and elimination of adduction or adduction–supination contractures of the thumb web space.

REFERENCES

1. Beasley RW. Principles of tendon transfer. Orthop Clin North Am 1970; 1:433–439.
2. Bohr HH. Tendon transposition in paralysis of opposition of the thumb. Acta Chir Scand 1953; 105: 45.
3. Bowden REM, Napier JR. The assessment of hand function after peripheral nerve injuries. J Bone Joint Surg [Br] 1961; 43:481.
4. Boyes JH. Bunnell's surgery of the hand. Philadelphia: JB Lippincott, 1964.
5. Brand PW. Tendon grafting, illustrated by a new operation for intrinsic paralysis of the fingers. J Bone Joint Surg [Br] 1961; 43:444.
6. Brand PW. The hand in leprosy. In: Pulvertaft RG, ed. Clinical surgery of the hand. London: Butterworth & Co, 1966:279.
7. Brand PW. Tendon transfer for median and ulnar nerve paralysis. Orthop Clin North Am 1970; 1: 447.
8. Brand PW. Biomechanics of tendon transfers. Orthop Clin North Am 1974; 5:204.

9. Braun RM. Palmaris longus tendon transfer for augmentation of the thenar musculature in low median palsy. J Hand Surg 1978; 3:488–491.
10. Brooks DM. Treatment of the paralytic hand. In Pulvertaft RG, ed. Clinical surgery of the hand. London: Butterworth & Co, 1966:269.
11. Brown PW. The time factor in surgery of upper extremity peripheral nerve injury. Clin Orthop 1970; 68:14–21.
12. Brown PW. Adduction–flexion contracture of the thumb. Correction with dorsal rotation flap and release of contracture. Clin Orthop 1972; 88:161.
13. Bunnell S. Reconstructive surgery of the hand. Surg Gynecol Obstet 1924; 39:259.
14. Bunnell S. Opposition of the thumb. J Bone Joint Surg 1938; 20:269–284.
15. Bunnell S. Surgery of the intrinsic muscles of the hand other than those producing opposition of the thumb. J Bone Joint Surg 1942; 24:1.
16. Bunnell S. Surgery of the hand, ed 3. Philadelphia: JB Lippincott, 1956.
17. Burkhalter WE. Tendon transfer in median nerve paralysis. Orthop Clin North Am 1974; 5:271.
18. Burkhalter WE. Early tendon transfer in upper extremity peripheral nerve injury. Clin Orthop 1974; 104:68–79.
19. Burkhalter WE. Median nerve palsy. In: Green DP, ed. Operative hand surgery, ed 2. Philadelphia: JB Lippincott, 1988:1499–1532.
20. Burkhalter WE, Christensen RC, Brown PW. Extensor indicis proprius opponensplasty. J Bone Joint Surg [Am] 1973; 55:725–732.
21. Camitz H. Über die Behandlung der Oppositionslähmung. Acta Chir Scand 1929; 65:77.
22. Chouhy-Aguirre S, Caplan S. Sobre secuelas de lesion alta e irreparable di nervio mediano y cubital y su tratamiento. Prensa Med Argentina 1956; 43: 2341–2346.
23. Clifton EE. Unusual innervation of the intrinsic muscles of the hand by median and ulnar nerves. Surgery 1948; 23:12.
24. Cooney WP. Tendon transfer for median nerve palsy. Hand Clin 1988; 4:155–164.
25. Cooney WP, Lucas MJ, Chao EYS, et al. The kinesiology of the thumb trapeziometacarpal joint. J Bone Joint Surg [Am] 1981; 63:1371.
26. Curtis RM. Opposition of the thumb. Orthop Clin North Am 1974; 5:305–321.
27. DeVecchi J. Oposición del pulgar fisiopatologia una nerva operactíon transplante del aductor. Bol Soc Cir Uruguay 1961; 32:423.
28. Duchenne GBA. Physiology of motion (translated by Kaplan EB). Philadelphia: WB Saunders, 1959.
29. Edgerton MT, Brand PW. Restoration of abduction and adduction to the unstable thumb in median and ulnar paralysis. Plast Reconstr Surg 1965; 36:150.
30. Henderson ED. Transfer of wrist extensor and brachioradialis to restore opposition of the thumb. J Bone Joint Surg [Am] 1962; 44:513–522.
31. Howell BW. A new operation for opponens paralysis of the thumb. Lancet 1926; 1:131.
32. Huber E. Hilfsoperation bei median Uslähmung. Dtsch Arch Klin Med 1921; 136:271.
33. Iselin M. Chirurgie de la main, ed 2. Paris: Masson et Cie, 1955:314.
34. Jacobs B, Thompson TC. Opposition of the thumb and its restoration. J Bone Joint Surg [Am] 1960; 42:1015–1026.
35. Kochs J. Opponens-Plastik. Chirug 1932; 4:67.
36. Kruckenberg H. Ueber Ersatz des M. opponens pollicis. Z Orthop Chir 1921; 42:178.
37. Littler JW. Tendon transfers and arthrodesis in combined median and ulnar nerve paralysis. J Bone Joint Surg [Am] 1949; 31:225–234.
38. Littler JW. Principles of tendon transfer. In: Converse JM, ed. Reconstructive plastic surgery. Philadelphia, WB Saunders, 1964:1674–1695.
39. Littler JW, Cooley SGE. Opposition of the thumb and its restoration by abductor digiti quint transfer. J Bone Joint Surg [Am] 1963; 45:1389–1396.
40. Luckey CA, McPherson SR. Tendinous reconstruction of the hand following irreparable injury to the peripheral nerves and brachial plexus. J Bone Joint Surg 1947; 29:560.
41. Makin M. Translocation of the flexor pollicis longus tendon to restore opposition. J Bone Joint Surg [Br] 1967; 49:458–461.
42. Mangus DJ. Flexor pollicis longus tendon transfer for restoration of opposition of the thumb. Plast Reconstr Surg 1973; 52:155.
43. Mannerfelt L. Structures of the hand in ulnar nerve paralysis. A clinical experimental investigation in normal and anomalies of innervation. Acta Orthop Scand 1966 (suppl):87.
44. Mayer L. The physiological method of tendon transplantation; operative technique. Surg Gynecol Obstet 1916; 22:298.
45. Mayer L. Operative reconstruction of the paralyzed upper extremity. J Bone Joint Surg 1939; 21:377.
46. Moberg E. Methods for examining sensibility of the hand. In: Flynn JE, ed. Hand surgery. Baltimore: Williams & Wilkins, 1966:435.
47. Mutz SB: Thumb web contracture. Hand 1972; 4: 236–246.
48. Ney KW. A tendon transplant for intrinsic hand

muscle paralysis. Surg Gynecol Obstet 1921; 33: 342.
49. Nicolaysen J. Transplantation des M. Abductor dig. V. Die Fenlender Oppositions Fehigkeit des Daumens. Dtsch Z Chir 1922; 168:133.
50. Orticochea M. Use of the deep bundle of the flexor pollicis brevis to restore opposition of the thumb. Plast Reconstr Surg 1971; 47:220.
51. Palazzi AS. On the treatment of the loss of opposition. Acta Orthop Scand 1962; 32:396.
52. Phalen GS, Miller RC. Transfer of wrist extensor muscles to restore or reinforce flexion power of the fingers and opposition of the thumb. J Bone Joint Surg 1947; 29:993–997.
53. Ramselaar JM. Tendon transfer to restore opposition of the thumb. Leiden, Holland: HE Stenfert, Kroese NV, 1970; 26–33, 36.
54. Riordan DC. Tendon transfers for nerve paralysis of the hand and wrist. Curr Pract Orthop Surg 1964; 2:17.
55. Rowntree T. Anomalous innervation of the hand muscles. J Bone Joint Surg [Br] 1949; 31:505–510.
56. Royle ND. An operation for paralysis of the intrinsic muscles of the thumb. JAMA 1938; 111:612.
57. Schneider LH. Opponensplasty using the extensor digiti minimi. J Bone Joint Surg [Am] 1969; 51: 1297–1302.
58. Smith RJ, Hastings H II. Principles of tendon transfer to the hand. AAOS Instr Course Lect 29, 1980; 129–152.
59. Snow JW, Fink GH. Use of transverse carpal ligament window for the pulley in tendon transfers for median nerve palsy. Plast Reconstr Surg 1971; 48: 238.
60. Steindler A. Orthopaedic operations on the hand. JAMA 1918; 71:1288.
61. Strange FGSC. An operation for nerve pedicle grafting; preliminary communication. Br J Surg 1947; 34:423.
62. Strange FGSC. Case report on pedicled nerve-graft. Br J Surg 1950; 37:331.
63. Sunderland S. Nerves and nerve injuries. Edinburgh: E&S Livingston, 1968:683.
64. Taylor TR. Reconstruction of the hand: A new technique in tenoplasty. Surg Gynecol Obstet 1921; 32: 237–248.
65. Thompson TC. A modified operation for opponens paralysis. J Bone Joint Surg 1942; 24:632–642.
66. White WL. Discussion on paper of ED Henderson. J Bone Joint Surg [Am] 1962; 44:513.
67. Williams HWG. The leprosy thumb. Br J Plast Surg 1966; 19:136.

51

Ulnar Nerve Palsy

William E. Burkhalter

AUTHOR'S KEY POINTS

- One third to one half of the strength of the hand and 80% of pinch strength are lost in ulnar nerve paralysis.
- The ring and long flexor digitorum superficialis tendons are unsuitable motors for transfer in the intrinsic-minus hand if the goal is to improve strength.
- The extensor carpi radialis longus and flexor carpi radialis are the major motors available to improve strength in the ulnar-palsied hand.
- Tendon transfers are done at any time as long as significant attenuation of the central extensor tendons over the proximal interphalangeal joints of the ring and small fingers has not occurred.
- Adding a new motor to the proximal phalanx of any digit improves strength and closure pattern and controls the collapse pattern.

DIGITAL MOTION

Tendon transfers for irreparable ulnar nerve paralysis cover the area from thumb to small finger. The major deficits are paralysis or weakness of the muscles that control flexion of the metacarpophalangeal (MCP) joints of all of the digits, the carpometacarpal (CMC) joints of the small and ring fingers, and the thumb. Because there is total intrinsic paralysis of only two fingers, there is a tendency to concentrate on the claw deformity in the ring and small fingers. However, there is also reduced flexor strength of the CMC joints of the ring and small fingers. Because there are no prime MCP joint flexors of the ring and small fingers, the patterns of closure of those digits become abnormal. The fingers roll up from distal to proximal, with almost full flexion of the distal and proximal interphalangeal (PIP) joints occurring before MCP joint motion occurs. This poor pattern of closure is accentuated by the extension deformity of the CMC joints of the ring and small fingers.

Thus, the lack of prime MCP joint and CMC joint flexors results in an abnormal pattern of closure—from distal to proximal rather than with all four joints flexing simultaneously. If a new motor is added to the proximal phalanx, weakness is reduced and the pattern of closure improved. If the strength of MCP joint flexion improves, the claw deformity, hyperextension of the MCP joint, and hyperflexion of the distal joints disappear. The extensor digitorum communis can provide full PIP joint extension as long as the MCP joints are prevented from going into hyperextension.[7,18] This factor has been used extensively for control of the claw deformity by various sorts of static procedures such as the Zancolli capsulorrhaphy,[44] the Mikhail bone block,[29] and various static tendon transfers through the intermetacarpal spaces. While they control the claw deformity of the ring and small fingers, static procedures do not address the major problem in ulnar nerve paralysis, the lack of strength of MCP joint flexion.

The only joints other than the MCP joints of the ring and small fingers that are completely unstable because of intrinsic paralysis are the CMC joints of the same digits (Fig. 51-1). Although Masse's sign (the inability to cup the hand to hold objects in the palm) has not been considered a profound disability, it is certainly a problem for some patients.[28] The extension deformity of the CMC joints is accentuated by certain tendon transfers located more distally in the finger.[36]

While both high and low ulnar nerve lesions cause intrinsic paralysis, only the high lesion denervates the flexor carpi ulnaris (FCU) and the ulnar side of the flexor digitorum profundus (FDP). Loss of the FCU is rarely a functional problem.[37] Compensation for the FCU, a muscle of considerable bulk, is provided by the digital flexors, which become ulnar deviators and flexors of the wrist. They have a much smaller moment arm than the FCU and must be under tension in order to create a flexion and ulnar deviation force. In high lesions, the digital flexors on the ulnar side are also partially paralyzed. In spite of this, tendon transfers to replace the function of the denervated FCU are rarely needed in isolated high ulnar nerve paralysis.

When the muscle bellies of the FDP of the ulnar fingers are tethered in the presence of a functional flexor digitorum superficialis (FDS), there is rarely an indication for suture of the ring and small FDP to the long profundus. I feel that there is little functional difference between high and low ulnar nerve lesions and thus have not performed tendon transfers for extrinsic digital flexion or wrist flexion and ulnar deviation.

The flexor carpi radialis (FCR) should not be used when a high ulnar nerve paralysis exists, even when there is a functioning palmaris longus muscle.

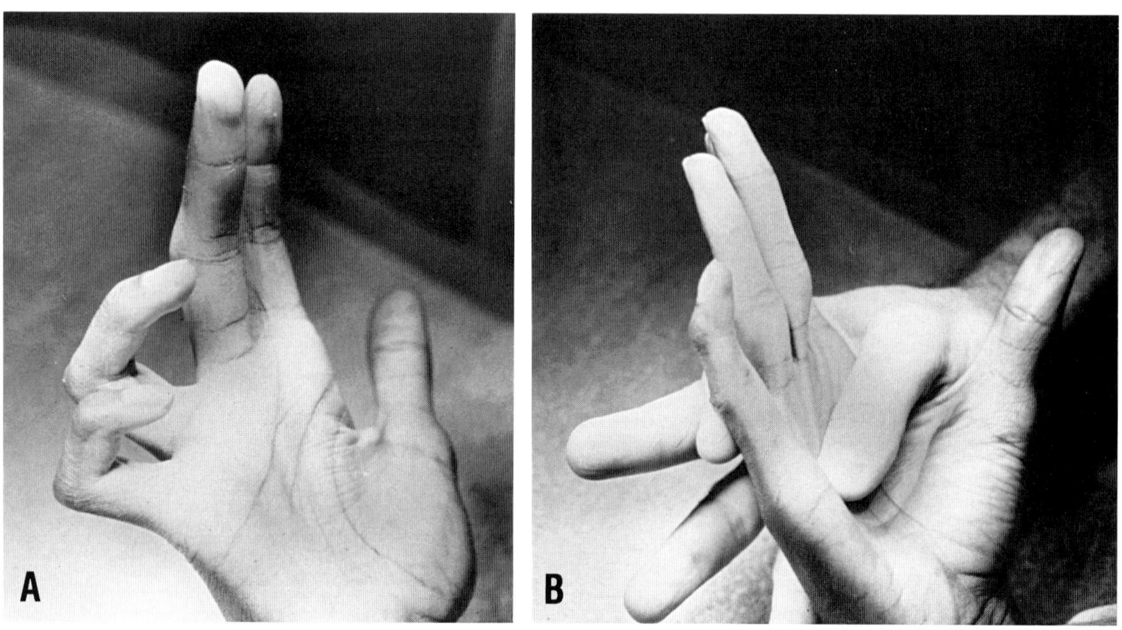

Figure 51–1. **(A)** *The claw deformity in this patient demonstrates, in addition to hyperextension of the metacarpal joints, hyperextension of the carpometacarpal joints of the ring and small fingers as well.* **(B)** *The examiner's hand demonstrates the Fowler or Bouvier test of limiting hyperextension of metacarpophalangeal joints. It is simultaneously limiting hyperextension of the carpometacarpal joints and maintaining the normal transverse arch of the hand.*

Although a partial transfer of the FCR in certain leprosy patients has been suggested, it is not advisable to use a muscle tendon unit for more than one function.[1,2]

THE PINCH MECHANISM

Three areas of weakness do not involve complete paralysis: the MCP joints of the index and long fingers, the MCP joint of the thumb, and the CMC joint of the thumb. The radial side of the hand (that is, the thumb and index and long fingers) has normal sensation and has a fairly normal appearance when the fingers are used without resistance. However, when the joints are put under load, a zigzag collapse pattern occurs. Lack of MCP joint stability becomes obvious only with load applications. The lumbrical muscles to the index and long fingers, innervated by the median nerve, control the claw deformity in the radial digits. With loads, though, they cannot maintain MCP joint flexion against resistance. The thumb collapses similarly, with the MCP joint going into extension. Jeanne's sign exists because only half of the flexor pollicis brevis is innervated by the median nerve.[25] Thus, while the median nerve-innervated flexor pollicis brevis and index and long lumbricals allow the thumb and index and long fingers to look relatively normal, they are not strong enough to keep the pinch mechanism from collapsing under loads. While the index and long fingers have stable CMC joints, they have only weak MCP joint flexion through the lumbrical muscles.

During precision pinch, the index finger is prevented from ulnar deviation by the adjacent digits in a cascade fashion. The loss of the abducting function of the first dorsal interosseous muscle is compensated for relatively well by the adjacent digits; however, there is no substitute for the lack of flexor strength of the MCP joint. During precision pinch, the PIP joint of the index finger is relatively hyperflexed and the distal interphalangeal (DIP) joint hyperextended (Fig. 51-2). There is pseudoparalysis of the FDP to the index. If the FDP becomes active, the patient senses that the fingernail of the index is presented to the thumb for pinch. Without proximal MCP joint strength and stability, there is functional paralysis of the profundus.

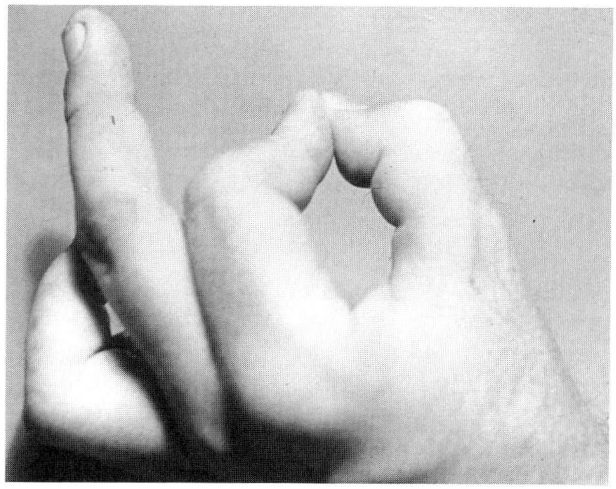

Figure 51–2. *Two-digit pinch in ulnar palsy demonstrating pseudoparalysis of the index profundus as well as hyperextension of the MPJ of the thumb (Jeanne's sign) and hyperflexion of the IPJ (Froment sign).*

To reverse this phenomenon, the examiner may place a finger over the proximal phalanx of the patient's index finger, maintaining 30° of MCP joint flexion. Then, as the patient pinches the thumb against the index finger, the pseudoparalysis of the profundus, another cause of pinch weakness in ulnar paralysis, disappears. Many patients sense this and, to compensate, position the thumb inside the flexor arc of the index finger so that the profundus can be used during power pinch. The thumb and index rarely function alone for power pinch. The index finger is almost always supported by the long finger. If increased strength of MCP joint flexion of the index finger is important, the same is true for the long finger.[30] If intrinsic replacement in the digits in ulnar nerve paralysis, either high or low, is being done, transfer to all four fingers should be performed.

The thumb in ulnar paralysis loses CMC joint as well as MCP joint flexor power. In an attempt to overcome this weakness, the flexor pollicis longus (FPL), which becomes very active, actually hyperflexes the interphalangeal joint preferentially. The patient positions the basal joint of the thumb in as much extension as possible to increase the tension on the FPL. In order to improve function to the thumb, MCP joint as well as CMC joint flexion must be strengthened.

AVAILABLE MOTORS

There are many lost motions in the combined median and ulnar, and isolated ulnar intrinsically minus hand. In addition to loss of dexterity and fine control, there is enormous loss of strength: Björkesten and Bunnell estimated that one third to one half of the strength of the hand is lost in ulnar nerve paralysis[3,4,8] and Mannerfelt stated that 80% of pinch strength is lost.[27] While fine control and dexterity cannot be restored by tendon transfers, strength and joint stability can be obtained.

What extrinsic tendons are available to be transferred for a patient with ulnar nerve paralysis? The FDS of the ring or long fingers immediately come to mind, but I do not believe that these should be used. If the major problem in the hand is a lack of flexor strength, redistribution of these forces may not result in increased strength at all, but may simply rebalance a weakened hand.[23,24] It has been shown that using the FDS as an intrinsic replacement actually weakens the hand to testing, despite improving balance.[24] Therefore, eliminating the superficialis of the ring and long fingers, the list includes only the FCR (in a low ulnar nerve paralysis with an intact FCU), brachioradialis, extensor carpi radialis longus (ECRL), and perhaps the palmaris longus and the extensor indicis proprius and extensor digiti quinti. Without the familiar FDS, the list of motors is relatively small. Because of this, arthrodesis is included as a treatment option.

The brachioradialis is a difficult muscle to use even if it is extensively freed from the forearm fascia to the elbow. The muscle remains extremely elbow position–dependent, and attempts to move the origin distally have been frustrated by short vascular branches. For bulk, the ECRL and FCR remain. Both of these muscle tendon units are excellent motors with good control. The FCR, however, is not used unless a functioning FCU is present, even when the palmaris longus is strong.

The other extrinsic motors, such as extensor indicis proprius, extensor digiti quinti, or extensor carpi ulnaris (ECU), also must be considered. While the proprius tendons are expendable and have adequate excursion, they lack sufficient bulk. The ECRL and extensor carpi radialis brevis (ECRB) are both radial deviators of the wrist. The ECU should be left in place in case high paralysis occurs when the FCU is paralyzed.

The most attractive reasons for using the FDS in any type of tendon transfer are that it is relatively available, it is easy and convenient for the surgeon, the muscle tendon unit has considerable excursion, and there is a good margin for error in adjusting tension. However, convenience should not be a major reason for choosing this motor; specific defects and loss of power occur in the donor finger. The major motors that should be used to improve strength in the ulnar palsied hand are the ECRL by itself, or the FCR and perhaps the ECRB with the ECRL and ECU carefully maintained in position.

TIMING AND CHOICE OF PROCEDURE

The timing of tendon transfer surgery is relatively easy in irreparable lesions. Once the patient has recovered from the injury and has resumed normal or near-normal use of the hand, it is time to consider the functional problems that have occurred in the extremity. Transfers are carried out at any point as long as there has been no significant attenuation of the central extensor tendons over the PIP joints of the ring and small fingers. With attenuation, prolonged splinting is required until the extensor digitorum communis becomes capable of PIP joint extension. Even when extension is restored, the overall result is reduced. It is important to avoid an extensor lag due to central slip attenuation leading to a contracture of the PIP joint.[10]

Many tendon transfers are available to the surgeon treating a patient with either a high or a low lesion of the ulnar nerve, and no single operation is appropriate for all patients. If cosmesis is a consideration, from the standpoint of both surgical scars and claw deformity, the choice of operations is narrowed considerably. Does the patient need power grip or better pinch? Does the patient complain of being unable to hold things in the palm of the hand? Since intrinsic atrophy does not disappear with tendon transfer, thin patients are advised that transfers will be visible beneath the skin. Is the involved hand dominant or non-dominant? In the case of a high ulnar nerve paralysis in the nondominant hand of an older sedentary individual, surgery may not be indicated. The surgeon must consider how much improvement can be expected, not in pinch in terms of pounds per square inch with specific transfers, but in the functional improvement that can be expected. Can activities of daily living be improved by the transfer? Will more than one operation be required (ie, one for the thumb and one for the ulnar side of the hand)?

The patient's problems are identified, and the operative procedures are designed specifically to solve them. Many patients with high ulnar nerve paralysis complain only of inability to put the hand in a pocket because of an abducted small finger.[5,43] While leaving the superficialis intact is important from the standpoint of strength, it may be necessary to split the ring finger FDS tendon and transfer its slips down the lumbrical canals to the lateral bands of the ring and small finger or to the A1–A2 pulley area of the same fingers. This will control the claw and improve the pattern of closure of the patient concerned about cosmesis. There will be no dorsal scars (Fig. 51-3). A good balancing cosmetic operative procedure will not improve strength but may alleviate the patient's complaints by solving the claw problem and improving the pattern of closure.[6]

FDS TRANSFER FOR INTRINSIC-MINUS DEFORMITY

Once the motor has been selected and the procedure chosen, the route of transfer and the distal method of attachment are determined. Although it is better not to use the FDS to improve intrinsic function of the fingers, it can be used to improve closure pattern and cosmesis. Two routes and three methods of distal attachment are available. The FDS is removed from the ring finger between the A1 and A2 pulleys, with the finger in flexion, by placing tension on the proximal portion of the tendon.[31] The tendon is split longitudinally down its raphe, and a subcutaneous route is created to the base of the ring and small fingers (Fig. 51-4). The A1–A2 interval of the small finger is then identified. The tendon sheath is opened, and another transverse incision is made 2 mm distal to this interval. This allows the split superficialis tendon of the ring finger to be looped through the base of the A2 pulley of both the ring and small fingers and sutured onto itself. The tension is adjusted so that passive MCP joint hyperextension is prevented when the wrist is placed in neutral.[12,45]

An alternative to this route is the lumbrical canal of the ring and small fingers. The distal attachment, once the tendon enters the finger, is to the lateral band or to the bone of the proximal phalanx. A straight dorsal incision is made in the finger, or an incision along the mid-axial line of the finger on its radial aspect over the proximal phalanx is created. While dorsal incisions are easier to close after distal attachment of the tendon, either incision is acceptable. With lateral band attachment, the split FDS is interwoven and anchored with interrupted sutures. The tension is somewhat difficult to adjust because the transfer affects two reciprocal joints.

With removal of the FDS, there is always concern about the development of a swan-neck deformity, especially in the ring finger. Because of this, and because the extensor digitorum communis is capable of PIP joint extension if hyperextension of the MCP joint is avoided, tension is adjusted with the PIP joint partially flexed (that is, tension is adjusted with the PIP joint and MCP joint flexed equally). In this way, less tension occurs at the PIP joint, and more is centered over the MCP joint. With motion of the FDS transfer, more tension is applied one joint proximal, avoiding the problem of swan neck.

A bony attachment distally requires creation of a unicortical drill hole in the radial aspect of the proximal phalanx in the mid-axial line. The opening must be large enough to accept the split superficialis tendon. In the case of a bony attachment, a dorsal incision should be used because the surgeon must get to both sides of the proximal phalanx. Kirschner wires are used to create two holes in the ulnar cortex through the large radial unicortical opening. Tension of the FDS is adjusted so that MCP joint extension with the wrist in neutral is impossible.

Once this has been done, the tendon is marked and two sutures are passed through the FDS in either a horizontal mattress or a Kessler-type configuration. The two straight needles are placed through the previously made holes in the ulnar cortex and the tendon pulled into the medullary

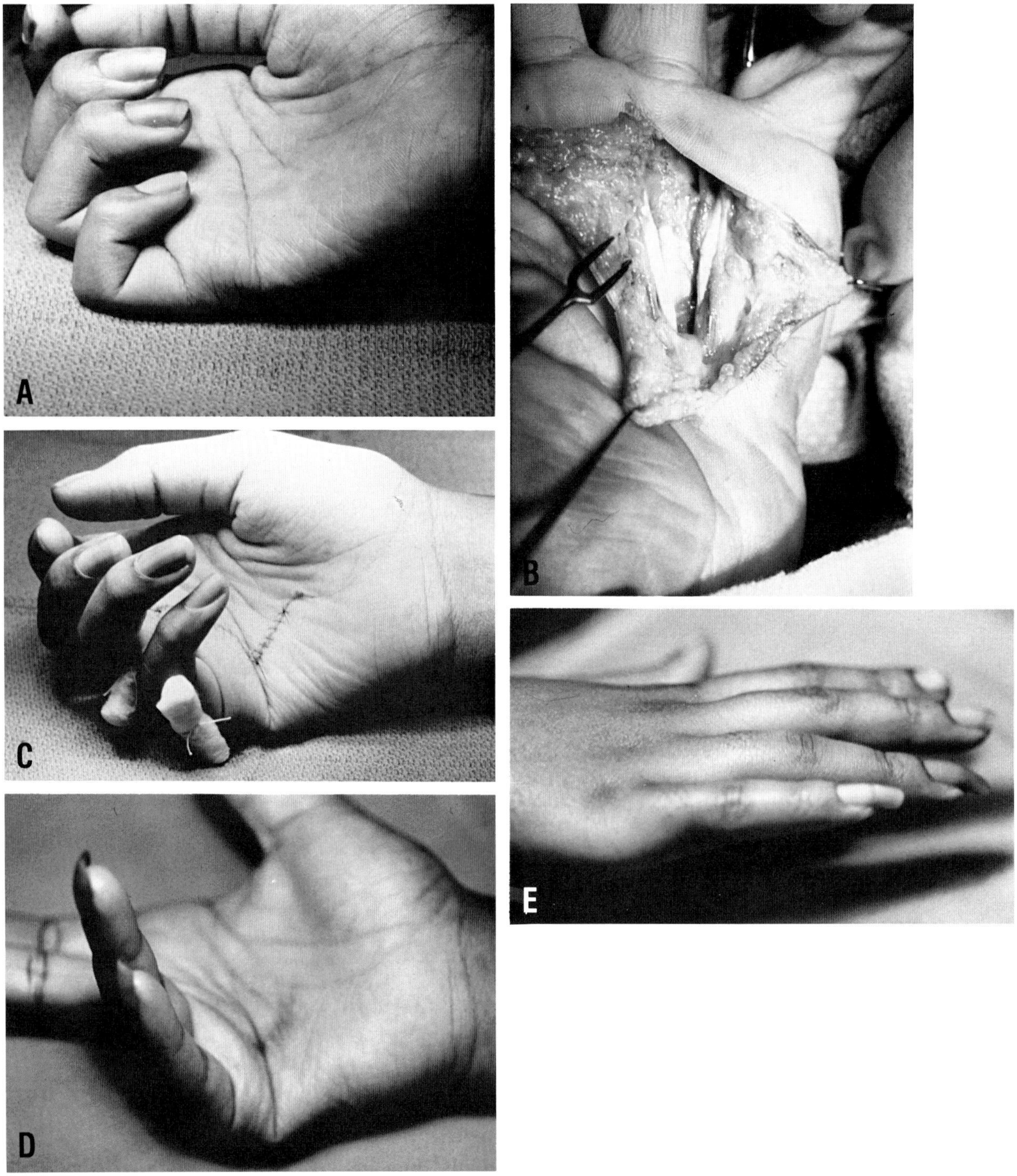

Figure 51–3. **(A)** *The resting posture of the ulnar palsied hand, with hyperflexion of the middle and distal joints and extension of the MPJ.* **(B)** *A split ring finger superficialis is passed down the lumbrical canal of the ring and small finger and attached to the bone of the proximal phalanx.* **(C)** *At the conclusion of the procedure, the resting position is changed to a more normal configuration with less distal joint flexion and more MPJ flexion.* **(D)** *The patient gains control of MPJ flexion postoperatively and can achieve the intrinsic plus position.* **(E)** *There is no claw deformity. There is also no loss of PIPJ flexion, because the transfer acts only to flex the MPJ.*

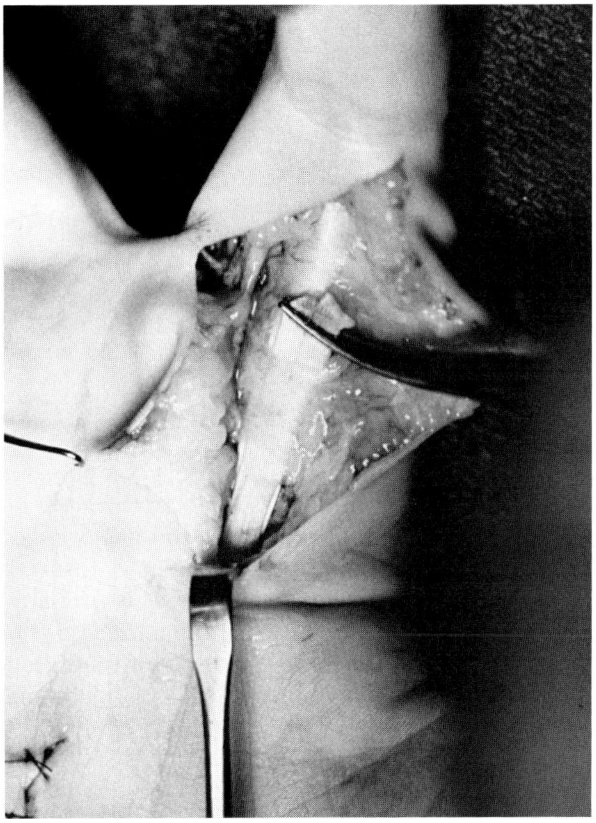

Figure 51–4. *The Zancolli loop transfer using the Brooks method of attachment to the A_2 pulley can be done using a single superficialis split into four tails, a single superficialis split into two tails, or a superficialis for each digit.*

canal. The sutures are tied using the ulnar cortex of the proximal phalanx as a "button" (Figs. 51-5, 51-6). In this way exposed tendon suture and dental rolls are avoided.

Among the methods of distal attachment, the volar loop methods of Zancolli or Brooks are easiest, the bony attachment most difficult, and the lateral band attachment most likely to produce swan-neck deformity. The Zancolli loop or Brooks attachment is preferred when the FDS is used as a motor (Fig. 51-7).[6,39]

What should be done when there has been attenuation of the central extensor at the PIP joint? Even with extensive splinting, both static and dynamic, the PIP joint may not extend easily when the MCP joints are maintained in flexion. While this problem can be avoided by early surgery or splinting, patients with central slip attenuation will be seen.

If improvement by splinting has plateaued and full PIP joint extension is impossible with the MCP joint blocked in flexion, PIP joint extension can be improved at the time of surgery if there is no contracture and there is a lag at the middle joint only. The distal method of attachment is critical. Obviously, a bony or pulley attachment will do nothing to improve PIP joint extension. A lateral band insertion will probably not aid PIP joint extension once there has been central slip attenuation.

The transfer goes superficial to the extensor mechanism after entering the finger through the lumbrical canal and is attached directly to the central extensor tendon. When using a superficialis tendon, tension should be adjusted with the wrist in neutral, the MCP joint flexed to 45°, and the PIP joint in about 20° to 30° of flexion. Concern is necessary about postoperative development of a swan-neck deformity after removal of an FDS and the resulting increase in tension on the central tendon. If another motor is being used, there is little need for concern about swan neck unless the PIP joint is placed in full extension at the time of tension adjustment.

As with any tendon attachment in the finger, postoperative immobilization must include both the MCP joint in flexion and the PIP joint in extension. This may give considerable postoperative stiffness.

WRIST EXTENSORS OR BRACHIORADIALIS TRANSFERS FOR INTRINSIC FUNCTION

The ECRL is a better motor than the brachioradialis. In order to reach the fingers and act as an intrinsic substitute, it must be prolonged with a tendon graft. The plantaris is removed from the leg and used to lengthen the muscle tendon unit. Once the ECRL has been divided distally, it is removed from the second compartment and brought to the midline of the forearm dorsally in a subcutaneous location. The plantaris tendon is woven into the distal end of the ECRL using the Pulvertaft side-weave configuration, with at least two passes, 90° to each other. The plantaris tendon is sutured

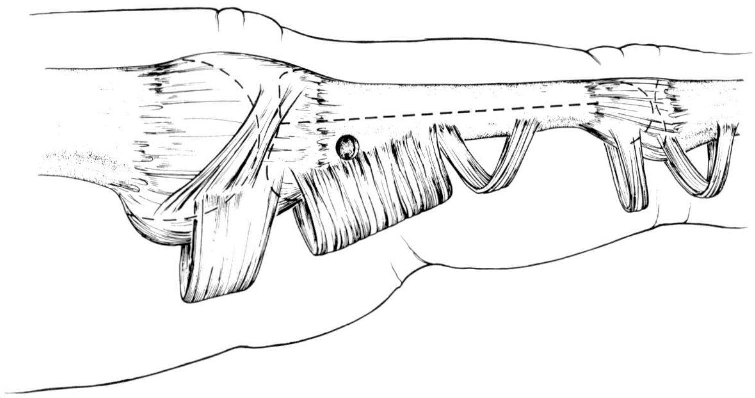

Figure 51–5. *If a bony attachment is elected for MPJ flexor replacement, the tendon attachment should be volar to the rotational axis of the digit. The tendon transfer should not add a significant rotational moment to the digit, which it would do if it were placed dorsal to the rotational axis.*

to the midportion of the ECRL. The tendon sutures must be strong, located in the distal forearm rather than the wrist or hand. Each limb of the plantaris that exits from the ECRL is longitudinally divided so that four "tails" are created from the single tendon unit. Incisions are made over the dorsum of the second metacarpal and fourth metacarpal shafts, and the fascia over the intermetacarpal spaces is excised. Incisions in the finger over the dorsum are preferable to mid-axial incision because of ease of closure after the transfer has been completed. The radial side of each proximal phalanx is exposed.

A curved tendon passer, either Carroll or Brand type, is tunneled from the finger in a proximal direction, with the MCP joint held in full flexion. The instrument is passed down the lumbrical canal with the MCP joints flexed. The surgeon palpates the motion of the tunneler as it moves through the palm. In this way the location of the passer volar to the deep intermetacarpal ligament is ensured. If the instrument moves too easily, it is probably dorsal to the intermetacarpal ligament. If the transfer is placed dorsal to the deep intermetacarpal ligament, only deviation of the fingers will occur and the desired MCP joint flexion will not be obtained.

Once the tendon passer is felt volarly in the palm, its direction is directed dorsally toward the appropriate intermetacarpal space. The tendon is directed to the radial side of each digit. In the index finger it is tunneled subcutaneously. Dorsal subluxation of the tendon to the index finger is prevented by the strong fascial extensions between

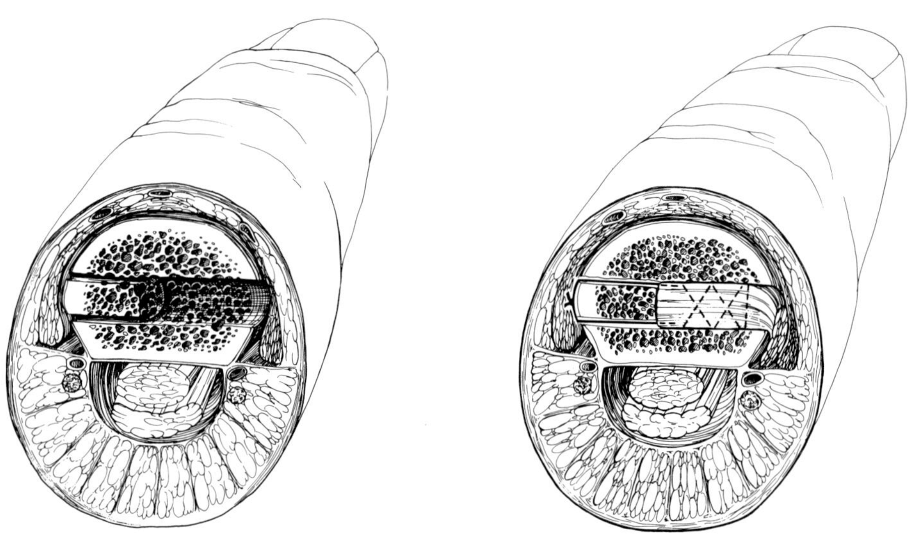

Figure 51–6. *By pulling the tendon or tendon graft into the medullary cavity of the proximal phalanx, the opposite cortex can be used as the "button" with no exposed sutures.*

skin and deeper structures. Once the tendon passer exits the intermetacarpal space, it is used to grasp one of the four tails of the transfer proximally. The tendon is then pulled into the digit.

With the wrist in 30° of dorsiflexion and the MCP joints flexed 45°, the course of the transfer from dorsal to volar becomes a straight line. An osseous attachment distally requires a radial unicortical drill hole of sufficient size to accommodate the tendon graft. Two 0.045-inch K-wires are passed through the unicortical hole and drilled through the ulnar cortex of the proximal phalanx. A 2-0 nonabsorbable suture with two straight needles anchors the tendon graft distally once tension has been adjusted. Locking stitches at 90° to each other are preferable in these relatively small tendon grafts.

The two straight needles are then passed through the drill holes on the ulnar border of the finger and tension is applied, bringing the tendon graft into the medullary canal. Tension is adjusted beginning at the index and ending with the small finger. Tension is adjusted so that MCP joint extension with the wrist in neutral is prevented. Again, the ulnar cortex of the proximal phalanx is used as a "button" so that there is no exposed suture material.

At the conclusion of surgery, prior to closure, all fingers should demonstrate flexion of the MCP joints. The index finger should be flexed the least and the small finger the most (Fig. 51-8).[15]

In another method of tendon routing, the ECRL is passed volarly around the radial aspect of the forearm in a subcutaneous location. It is then passed through the carpal tunnel and attached distally to the A1 or A2 pulleys, lateral band, or bone of the proximal phalanx. This route, volar to the axis of the wrist, through the carpal tunnel, is of some concern as the patient may develop carpal tunnel syndrome. However, although some nerve compression symptoms may be seen early, long-term carpal tunnel syndrome has not been observed.[11]

Another worrisome feature of this route is its volar position in relation to the axis of wrist motion. Initially, the patient must learn to control the tendon transfer by wrist extension only. Since the transfer is active only with the wrist in dorsiflexion, the patient must learn digital extension with wrist dorsiflexion rather than digital extension with wrist volar flexion. This is not a problem in patients with recent nerve paralysis, but in patients with longstanding injuries, when flexor habitus of the wrist has developed, the wrist is maintained in flexion constantly both for digital flexion and extension. In these cases the transfer is nonfunctional.[38]

OTHER TRANSFERS FOR INTRINSIC FUNCTION

Other motors, primarily the palmaris longus and FCR, have been prolonged with tendon grafts and brought through the carpal tunnel to the digits. The palmaris longus, a small muscle, adds little strength to the hand but may improve the pattern of closure and control the claw deformity.[1,19] If a wrist flexor is selected, the FCR is prolonged with a four-tailed tendon graft and extended through the carpal tunnel to each of the digits.

In longstanding ulnar nerve paralysis, the flexor habitus of the wrist may be improved by transferring the FCR to the digits. If this motor is selected, it may be brought either through the carpal tunnel (preferred) or around the radial side of the forearm. In either case the muscle–tendon unit is prolonged with a four-tailed tendon graft similar to that used with wrist extensor transfers (Fig. 51-9). The suture line is made in the distal forearm rather than the wrist so that the tendon grafts can be placed deep in the carpal tunnel, away from the median nerve. The graft-motor suture line must not impinge on the carpal tunnel.

After the plantaris or toe extensor graft has been interwoven into the FCR proximally, the palm is exposed through a lazy oblique incision, generously removing the palmar fascia and exposing the lumbrical muscle to each finger and the A1–A2 pulley area. The surgeon determines whether the tendon transfer is to be attached to the A2 pulley, the lateral band, or the bone of the proximal phalanx. In cases when the FDS is intact, the transfer is not added to the lateral band if the patient has passed the Bouvier[7] or Fowler's tests[18] preoperatively. That is, if the patient's extrinsic extensors are capable of full PIP joint extension when the MCP joints are held in less than full extension, little is gained by securing the transfer to the lateral bands. Powerful PIP joint extension is unnecessary and, even with an intact FDS, swan-neck deformity

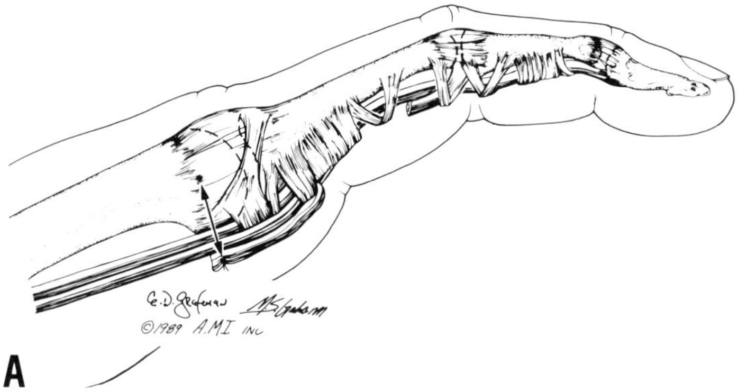

A

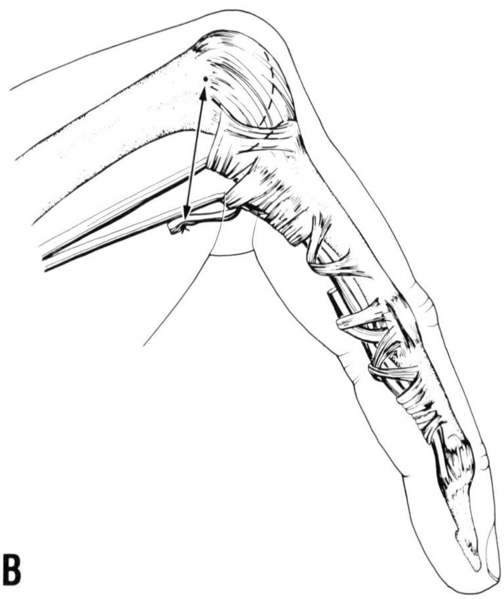

B

Figure 51–7. **(A)** *With a pulley attachment to the A_2 area, the moment arm for MPJ flexion increases with MPJ flexion.* **(B)** *In the normal individual this does not occur because of the intact deep intermetacarpal ligament.* **(C)** *With a bony attachment this increase in the moment arm is not seen to the same extent as with MPJ flexion.* **(D)** *An increase in moment arm may contribute to MPJ flexion contractures.*

can occur. Attachment to the A2 pulley or bone of the proximal phalanx is preferred. A2 pulley attachment is easiest, as proximal phalangeal attachment through the volar approach requires additional mid-dorsal digital incisions. A2 pulley attachment requires a palmar incision only.

Anita[1] and Fritschi[19] have had extensive experience with use of the palmaris longus transfer volarly in patients with leprosy. These authors differentiate between the hyperextensible Asian type of hand and the heavier Western hand and select the palmaris longus transfer for the former. In high ulnar nerve paralysis, just as in leprosy, the FCU is paralyzed, so the other prime flexor of the wrist should not be taken as a transfer. This use of the palmaris longus as a transfer adds little strength and probably has little usefulness in the heavier Western hand except to control the claw deformity and improve the pattern of closure.

SEMI-ACTIVE TENODESIS TO CORRECT CLAW DEFORMITY

In addition to static procedures designed to improve claw deformity of the ring and small fingers, and transfers of active motors, a number of procedures create semi-active tenodeses. These procedures improve the pattern of closure and control the claw deformity but do not add appreciably to strength. A retinacular ligament is created that extends volar to the axis of flexion of the MCP joints

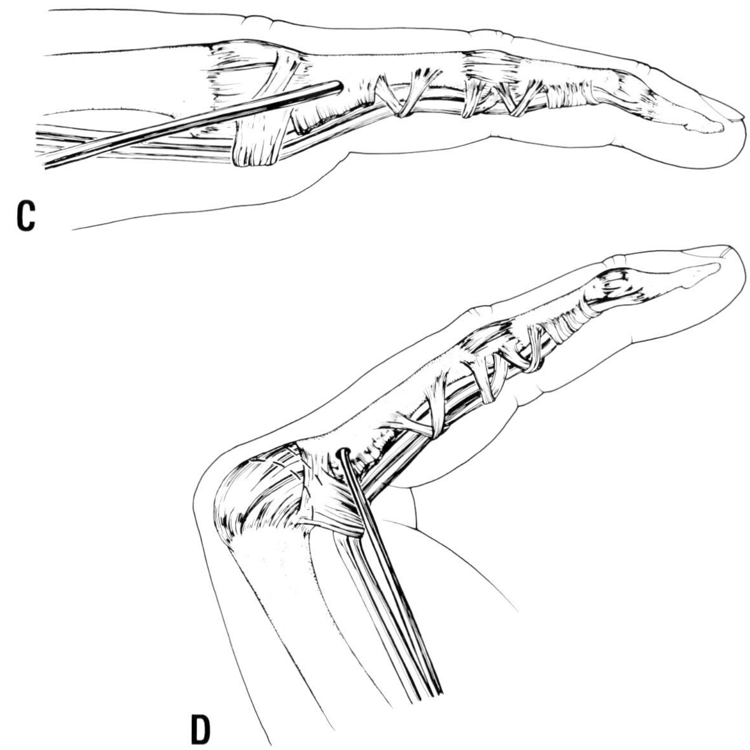

Figure 51-7. *(Continued)*

of the fingers and dorsal to the PIP joints of the same digits. It may be created from tendon grafts, as proposed by Parks[21,34] and Smith,[41] or available extensor tendons, as described by Carneiro.[14]

Parks recommended anchoring the grafts proximally in the palm to the flexor retinaculum. They are passed through the lumbrical canals to the radial lateral bands of each digit. Tension is adjusted so that the PIP joints and DIP joints cannot flex unless the MCP joints also flex. Likewise, as the digits are brought into extension, the MCP joints cannot extend completely until the PIP joints come into extension. The action is much like that of the oblique retinacular ligament of the fingers extended one joint proximally.

Smith used a tendon graft looped around the deep intermetacarpal ligament, sutured either to the central tendon or lateral bands of two adjacent digits to create a retinacular ligament of the MCP joints and PIP joints. The grafts pass volar to the axis of the MCP joint and dorsal to the axis of the PIP joint.

Carneiro, rather then using grafts, used structures already in place. He advocated use of a Littler boutonnière procedure, carrying the centralization proximally as far as possible until a flexion contracture of the MCP joint occurs. An extensor tenotomy is done over the middle phalanx. In this technique, PIP joint extension is made possible through the extensor digitorum communis, but DIP joint extension through the oblique retinacular ligament is incomplete. Full three-joint flexion is made possible by the tenotomy over the midphalanx.

FLAT PALM

Tendon transfers are occasionally required to improve CMC joint flexion of the small finger, overcoming the deformity that creates Masse's sign. The flat palm is not a problem in many ulnar-palsied hands. In very supple hands, however, especially when tendon transfers to the digits are passed dorsally through the intermetacarpal spaces, problems may be seen (Fig. 51-10).[36] Hyperextension of the

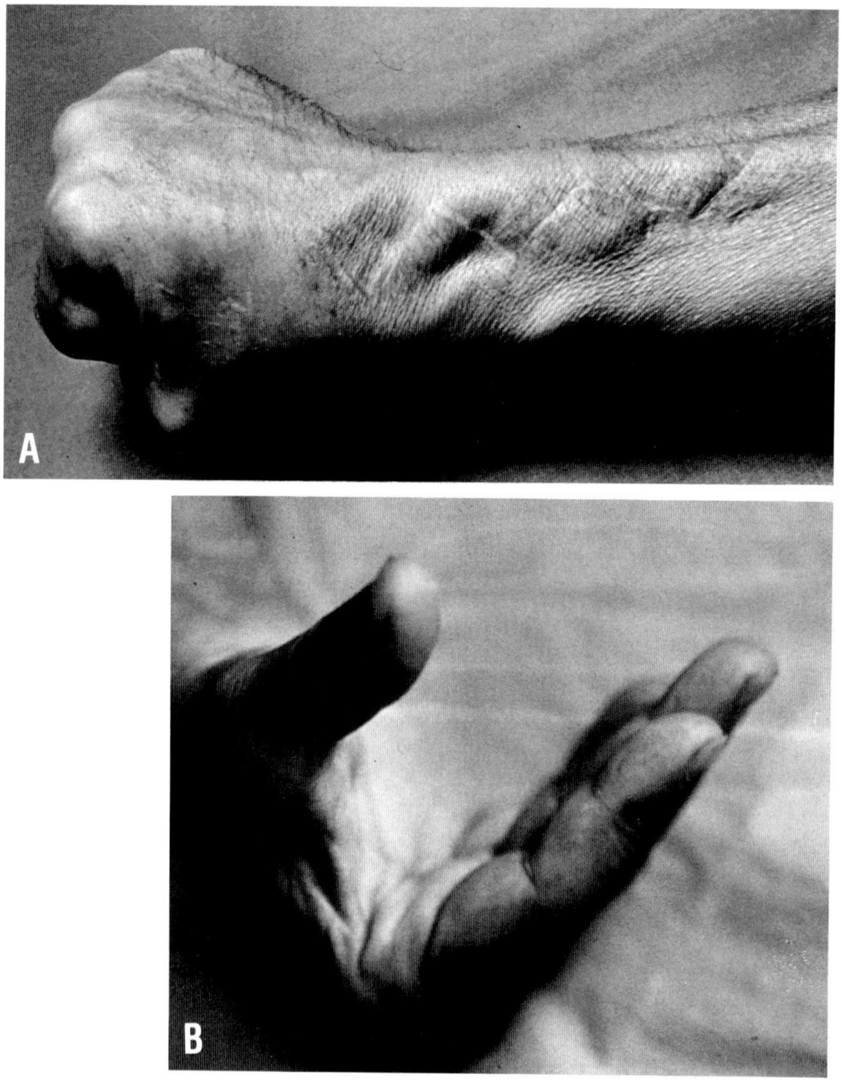

Figure 51–8. **(A)** *In a high ulnar nerve lesion, no flexor digitorum superficialis tendons should be sacrificed. A Brand-type transfer using the extensor carpi radialis longus prolonged with tendon grafts is preferred. The suture line is subcutaneously dorsal at the distal forearm area.* **(B)** *The grafts go to all fingers in order to add strength to index and long fingers as well as the more involved ring and small fingers.*

CMC joints of the ulnar digits may occur, and the flat palm may become almost convex. Both the extensor digiti quinti and FDS of the small finger have been used to provide active flexors to the CMC joint of the small finger. Ranney rerouted the extensor digiti quinti around the radial side of the wrist and superficially across the palm and back to the small finger.[35] Transfer of the FDS to the capsule of the MCP joint of the small finger is another alternative. Because of indifferent results with both transfers, there has been little enthusiasm for controlling the instability of the basilar joint in this way.

I have had experience with arthrodesis of the CMC joint of the small finger in a position of maximal flexion in patients who have had dorsal tendon transfers. As pointed out by Clendenin and Smith, considerable compensatory motion occurs proximal to the arthrodesis, but true hyperextension is impossible.[16] If a volar transfer is used, such as a split flexor superficialis or FCR prolonged with grafts through the carpal tunnel, hyperextension of the basilar joint of the small finger is not seen. It is likely that Masse's sign requires treatment only in patients with lax hands who have had dorsal tendon transfers.

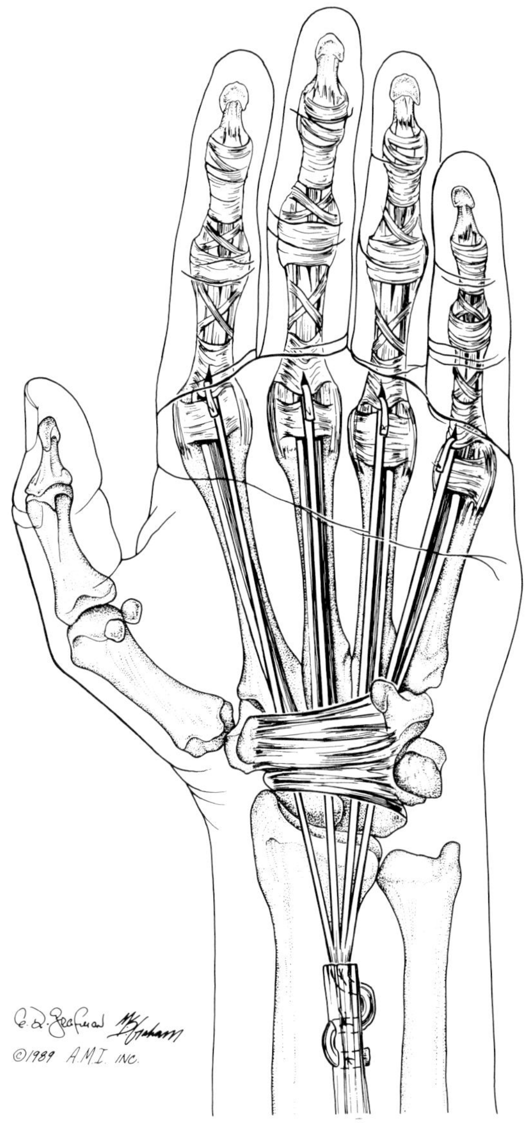

Figure 51–9. The flexor carpi radialis prolonged with tendon grafts to the A_2 pulley of each digit is an excellent MPJ flexor replacement. A new motor is added to the proximal phalanx without increased PIPJ extensor force while maintaining the flexor digitorum superficialis in position.

IMPROVING PINCH WITH TENDON TRANSFERS

Strengthening the thumb is just as important as adding strength to the fingers. Loss of strength in the thumb is demonstrated clinically with Froment's and Jeanne's signs.[20,25] Hyperextension of the MCP joint from the deformity seen in claw fingers and hyperflexion of the distal interphalangeal joint occurs. The only difference is that in the fingers the claw is an extension phenomenon while in the thumb the collapse occurs with loaded flexion. Adding MCP joint flexor power controls hyperextension of the MCP joint. Most adductorplasties, which attempt to obtain MCP joint flexion as well as flexion of the CMC joint, reproduce the action of the adductor pollicis. The most commonly used motors and routes are:

1. Ring flexor FDS across the palm deep to the flexor tendons of the index finger to the bony attachment of the adductor pollicis.[22,26]
2. ECRB prolonged with a tendon graft through the intermetacarpal space of index and long fingers, deep to the flexor tendons of the index finger, to the osseous attachment of the adductor pollicis.[40]
3. Similar to 2 (above), using either the ECRL or brachioradialis.[8,33]
4. The extensor indicis proprius through the index–long finger intermetacarpal space deep to the flexor tendons of the index finger to the adductor tubercle on the thumb.[13,17]

The use of the flexor tendons of the index as a pulley is common to all of these transfers. However, Brown has shown that even without this pulley, adductorplasties improve pinch power.[13]

Other motors may be used to strengthen the pinch mechanism between the thumb and index finger or index and long fingers. The extensor digit minimi[46] and extensor pollicis brevis[17] both have been used but are felt to be too weak to add much strength to the pinch mechanism.[42]

METACARPOPHALANGEAL AND INTERPHALANGEAL JOINT FUSION IN THE THUMB

Arthrodesis of either the MCP joint or interphalangeal (IP) joint of the thumb may be indicated in ulnar nerve paralysis. The standard MCP joint arthrodesis improves the stability of the MCP joint but does not add flexor power to either the MCP joint or the CMC joint.[32] Performing an adductorplasty without MCP joint fusion may add only flexor power to the MCP joint. Combining adduc-

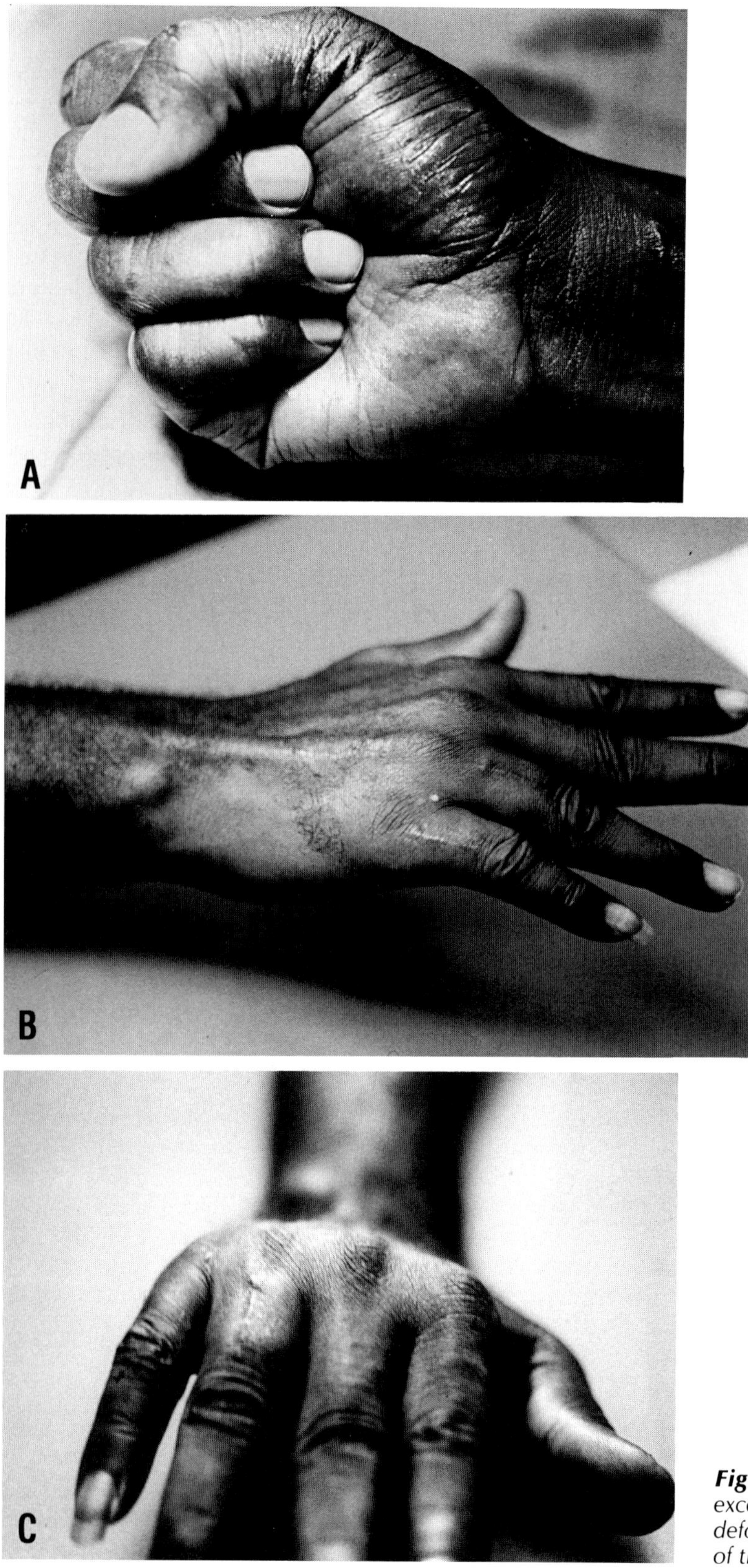

Figure 51–10. *Although this patient has* **(A)** *excellent flexion and* **(B)** *good control of the claw deformity,* **(C)** *hyperextension of the CMC joints of the ring and small fingers is not controlled.*

torplasty with arthrodesis of the MCP joint adds strength as well as improved CMC joint flexion. Patients may still overuse the FPL, with resulting hyperflexion of the IP joint of the thumb. This, however, occurs only when relatively large loads are applied to the thumb.[24]

An IP joint arthrodesis transfers the excursion of the FPL proximally to the MCP joint and the CMC joint of the thumb. This creates a true short flexor of the thumb, one that does not increase supination through the basilar joint. While most adductorplasties add a supination moment to the thumb, the FPL has no rotational moment, even when combined with IP joint arthrodesis.[9] Thus, IP joint arthrodesis improves the pinch pattern and negates the Froment sign, but increases the strength of the thumb only slightly.[24]

The efficacy of arthrodesis is determined preoperatively by applying a splint to stabilize the IP joint of the thumb with most of the pulp free. The patient uses the splints in daily activities to determine the positive and negative aspects of IP joint arthrodesis. An advantage of IP joint arthrodesis is that a tendon transfer is not required. IP joint fusion alone is superior to any combination of arthrodesis or transfer to improve thumb strength in patients who note improved function with the splint (Fig. 51-11).

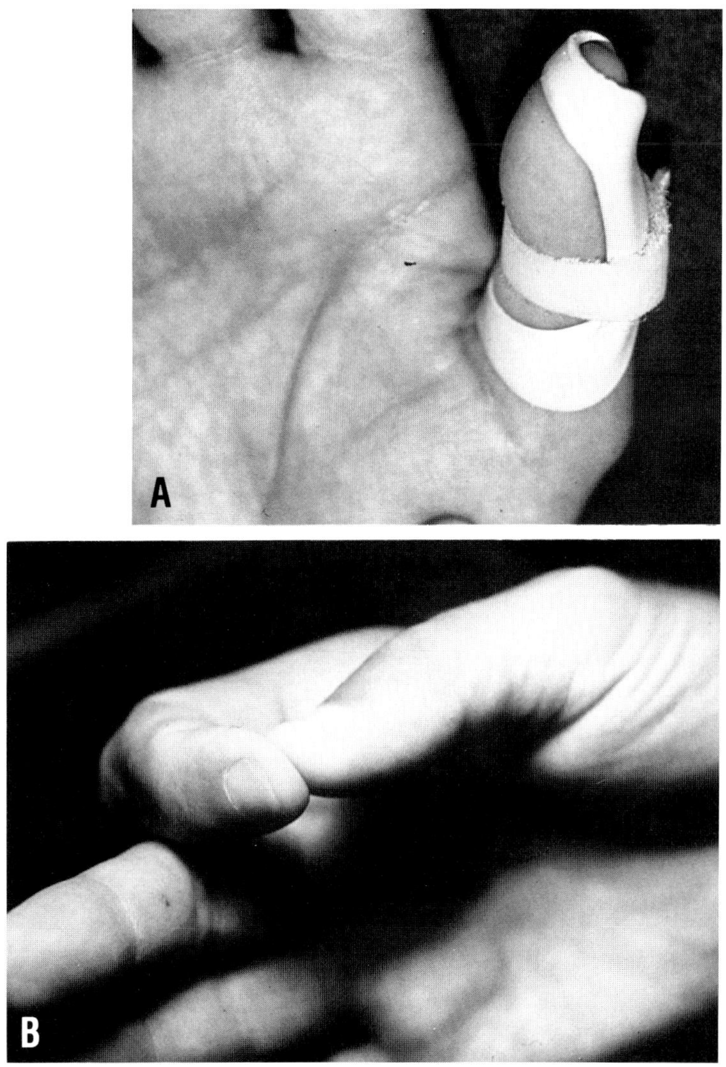

Figure 51–11. **(A)** *This splint simulates an arthrodesis of the IPJ of the thumb.* **(B)** *A stable pinch is seen following arthrodesis of the IPJ.*

Alternatives to IP joint arthrodesis include arthrodesis of the MCP joint of the thumb plus an adductorplasty. This combination adds considerable strength to the thumb, even though the Froment's sign may not be relieved completely.[23,24] The ECRB or ECRL prolonged with a tendon graft, to an osseous attachment, as described by Smith,[40] or to the tendon of the adductor pollicis, is an excellent choice. This adds a new motor to the thumb that coincides directly with the action of the adductor pollicis. The intermetacarpal route from dorsal to volar leaves the palm free for tendon transfers to the fingers. If one of the wrist extensors has been used for another purpose, the brachioradialis, with the same route and method of attachment, is preferred.

Author's Preferred Method

In attempting maximal strengthening and rehabilitation of the ulnar-palsied hand, three things are required:

1. MCP joint flexor strength in all four fingers
2. Improved short flexor action in the thumb
3. Flexor stability of the small finger CMC joint.

Can all of these be achieved in one operative procedure?

Operative procedures are available that will add flexor strength to the CMC joint of the small finger. A disadvantage is the necessity of performing another operative procedure at a time when other transfers are not being done, which adds another stage to the myriad of transfers required for ulnar nerve paralysis. Arthrodesis in maximal CMC joint flexion is preferred to stabilization of the basilar joint of the small finger by transfer. Although there is some compensatory motion through the hamate–triquetral joint, hyperextension is prevented and the palm maintains the cup effectively. The procedure is carried out at the same time as other operative procedures to either the thumb or fingers.

Next, it is necessary to evaluate the need for an operative procedure to the thumb. Prehension is weak and may require treatment. The surgeon determines whether the patient presents with a problem rather than searching for one. If there is a complaint of thumb weakness, a splint is applied to limit IP joint flexion, leaving as much of the pulp surface uncovered as possible; this simulates an IP joint arthrodesis, giving the patient a chance to see if pinch strength improves sufficiently. The splint also is used to determine whether arthrodesis of the IP joint of the thumb, a procedure that can be performed easily at the time of the other operative procedures on the fingers, is a good substitute for tendon transfer.

If IP joint arthrodesis is not elected and an adductorplasty is to be carried out, arthrodesis of the MCP joint of the thumb is performed as well. The arthrodesis is done at the same time as the transfer.

For maximum strength, transfer of a wrist extensor prolonged with a tendon graft through the intermetacarpal space is preferred. This cannot be done if the ECRL has been used for digital MCP joint flexion, however, since at least one wrist extensor must be left in place. In this case, the FDS of the ring finger is transferred across the palm. While this transfer adds less strength to the thumb than a wrist extensor, it frees the ECRL to use as an MCP joint flexor in the digits. If the ECRB is used as the motor, both the ECRL and ECU are left in place in order to maintain a stable, balanced wrist.

Some compromises are necessary. In a recent palsy without a flexor wrist habitus, either the ECRB or ECRL prolonged with a graft is transferred through the intermetacarpal space to the fused MCP joint of the thumb. The ECRL is preferred because of its longer potential excursion. This is particularly important considering that the worst complication of adductorplasty is an adduction contracture of the thumb.[41] In this case the four fingers are motored by the FCR, which is passed through the carpal tunnel with tendon grafts to the A1–A2 pulley area. This combination will require two separate operative procedures because the wrist must be positioned in dorsiflexion for the wrist extensor adductorplasty and in flexion for the FCR digital MCP joint flexorplasty. Attempting to carry out both procedures at the same time by placing the wrist in neutral compromises the result, as MCP joint flexor control is not obtained and an adducted thumb occurs.

If the surgeon elects to perform CMC joint arthrodesis of the small finger, it is carried out at the same time as the adductorplasty. With a longstanding palsy and a flexed wrist, the ECRL is prolonged with grafts over the dorsum of the wrist through the intermetacarpal spaces to the proximal phalanges of all four fingers. Thumb strength will not be improved as much with this combination as when a wrist extensor is transferred to the thumb. I prefer to use the ring finger FDS across the palm to a fused MCP joint of the thumb, if IP joint arthrodesis of thumb alone is insufficient. While using the FDS is convenient for the surgeon, it requires two separate operative procedures. As mentioned earlier, the reason for two operative procedures is the requirement for different positions of the wrist for postoperative immobilization.

The only combination of procedures that can be performed easily at one operative sitting is the following:

1. IP joint arthrodesis to the thumb
2. Arthrodesis of the CMC joint of the little finger
3. Either FCR or ECRL prolonged with tendon grafts to the digits.

POSTOPERATIVE CARE AND REHABILITATION

With attachment of transfers for MCP joint flexion either to bone of the proximal phalanx or to the A1–A2 pulley area, there is no reason to immobilize the PIP joint in the postoperative period. Early motion of the PIP joint is important, especially following pulley insertion, to avoid loss of middle joint motion.

When the surgical dressing is removed, the MCP joint is maintained in 60° to 70° of flexion. When the cast is applied, the wrist is in 45° dorsiflexion in the case of the dorsal, wrist extensor intermetacarpal route and only 30° volar flexion in the case of the FCR—carpal tunnel route. Using more flexion postoperatively may cause carpal tunnel syndrome. These positions are maintained for 4 to 6 weeks, with emphasis on full PIP joint and DIP joint motion in the cast.

After cast removal, a splint is used until the patient demonstrates good automatic control of the transfer. Without such control, even with 6 to 8 weeks of immobilization in a postoperative cast, attenuation of the tendon graft occurs. In the case of the dorsal intermetacarpal route, simultaneous wrist dorsiflexion and isolated MCP joint flexion is emphasized. MCP joint splinting is continued, having the patient carry out further MCP joint flexion out of the splint while the wrist is held in dorsiflexion. In this case the distal joint is maintained in near-full extension to avoid substitution of extrinsic flexion for intrinsic flexion. Once the patient can achieve the intrinsic-plus position, he or she has control of the transfer and splintage can be gradually discontinued. The patient must be discouraged from attempting to passively achieve full MCP joint extension.

With the FCR transfer volarly through the carpal tunnel to the A1–A2 pulley area, wrist dorsiflexion is stressed. While the MCP joints are maintained in flexion, the wrist is gradually brought into dorsiflexion. A natural tenodesis results at the MCP joints, the PIP joints, and the DIP joints. In the intrinsically minus hand, the PIP joints and DIP joints are hyperflexed and the MCP joints are hyperextended in the resting state. Early in rehabilitation, MCP joint flexion with wrist dorsiflexion is stressed. Once this has been achieved, isolated MCP joint flexion, with the wrist immobilized, is begun. When control is obtained, active flexion and extension of the fingers is started, with the wrist held in a splint in neutral or slight dorsiflexion. In either case, splinting of the MCP joints in flexion is maintained for 3 months postoperatively in order to avoid recurrence of MCP joint hyperextension due to overactivity of the extrinsic flexors and extensors.

REFERENCES

1. Anita NH. The palmaris longus motor for lumbrical replacement. Hand 1969; 2:139.
2. Beine A. Partial flexor carpi radialis many-tailed transfer for correction of claw fingers. Indian J Leprosy 1985; 57:624.
3. Björkesten G. Position of the fingers and function defined in ulnar paralysis. Acta Chir Scand 1946; 93:99–110.
4. Björkesten G. Suture of war injuries to peripheral nerves: Clinical studies of results. Acta Chir Scand 1947; 27:52–54.
5. Blacker G, Lister G, Kleinert H. The abducted little finger in low ulnar nerve palsy. J Hand Surg 1976; 1:190.
6. Boucher P, Vandroogenbroeck J, Hirzel C. Correction of the Hansen claw hand using direct Zancolli lasso procedures and two of its variations. Acta Leprologia 1986; 100:73–78.
7. Bouvier M. Note sur une paralysie partielle des muscles de la main. Bull Acad Nat Med (Paris) 1851; 18:125.
8. Boyes J. Bunnell's surgery of the hand, ed 4. Philadelphia: JB Lippincott, 1964:514.
9. Brand P. Clinical mechanics of the hand. St. Louis: CV Mosby, 1985:141–149.

10. Brand P. Tendon transfers for correction of paralysis of the intrinsic muscles of the hand. In: Hunter J, Schneider L, Mackin E, eds. Tendon surgery in the hand. St Louis: CV Mosby, 1987:439–449.
11. Brandsma J, Brand P. Median nerve function after tendon transfer for ulnar paralysis. J Hand Surg [Br] 1985; 10:30–32.
12. Brooks AL. A new intrinsic tendon transfer for the paralytic hand. J Bone Joint Surg [Am] 1975; 57: 730.
13. Brown P. Reconstruction for pinch in ulnar intrinsic palsy. Orthop Clin North Am 1974; 5:233.
14. Burkhalter W, Carneiro R. Correctional of attritional boutonnière deformity in high ulnar nerve paralysis. J Bone Joint Surg [Am] 1979; 61:131.
15. Burkhalter W, Strait J. Metacarpophalangeal flexor replacement for intrinsic muscle paralysis. J Bone Joint Surg [Am] 1973; 55:1667.
16. Clendenin MB, Smith RJ. Fifth metacarpal hamate fusion for post-traumatic osteoarthritis. J Hand Surg [Am] 1984; 9:374.
17. DeAbreu LB. Early restoration of pinch grip after ulnar nerve repair. J Hand Surg [Br] 1989; 14:309.
18. Fowler S. Extensor apparatus of the digits. J Bone Joint Surg [Br] 1949; 31:477.
19. Fritschi E. Reconstructive surgery in leprosy. Baltimore: Williams & Wilkins, 1971:42–65.
20. Froment J. La paralysie de l'adducteur du pouce et le signe de la prehension. Rev Neurol 1914; 28: 1236.
21. Galal Abdel-Halim M. Claw hand evaluation of peripheral nerve suture and Parkes graft-tenodesis. Thesis for M Ch Orthop, Liverpool, 1977.
22. Hamlin C, Littler J. Reconstruction of power pinch. J Hand Surg 1980; 5:396.
23. Hastings H. Low ulnar nerve palsy: Evaluation and treatment consideration. In: Strickland J, Steichen J, eds. Difficult problems in hand surgery. St. Louis: CV Mosby, 1982:285.
24. Hastings H, Davidson S. Tendon transfers for ulnar nerve palsy: Evaluation of results and practical treatment considerations. Hand Clin 1988; 4:167–178.
25. Jeanne M. La deformation du pouce dans la paralysie cubitale. Bull Mem Soc Chir 1915; 41:703.
26. Littler J. Reconstruction of thumb pinch strength with loss of flexion adductor muscle function. In: Hunter J, Schneider L, Mackin E, eds. Tendon surgery in the hand. St. Louis: CV Mosby, 1987:450–453.
27. Mannerfelt L. Studies on the hand in ulnar nerve paralysis. Acta Orthop Scand (Suppl) 1966; 87:4.
28. Masse L. Contribution a l'étude de l'achon des interosseous. J Med (Bordeaux) 1966; 46:198.
29. Mikhail L. Bone block operation for claw hand. Surg Gynecol Obstet 1964; 118:1077.
30. Nevaiser R, Wilson JN, Gardner MM. Abductor pollicis longus transfer for replacement of first dorsal interosseous. J Hand Surg 1980; 5:53–57.
31. North ER, Littler JW. Transferring the flexor superficialis tendon: Technical considerations in the prevention of proximal interphalangeal joint disability. J Hand Surg 1980; 5:498–501.
32. Omer G Jr. Tendon transfers for reconstruction of the forearm and hand following peripheral nerve injuries. In: Omer G, Spinner M, eds. Management of peripheral nerve problems. Philadelphia: WB Saunders, 1980:817–846.
33. Omer G Jr. Tendon transfer in ulnar palsy. In: Green D, ed. Operative hand surgery, ed 2. New York: Churchill-Livingstone, 1988:1535.
34. Parkes A. Paralytic claw fingers—a graft tenodesis operation. Hand 1973; 5:192.
35. Ranney DA. Reconstruction of the transverse metacarpal arch in ulnar palsy by transfer of extensor digiti minimi. Plast Reconstr Surg 1973; 52:406.
36. Ranney DA. The mechanism of arch reversal in the surgically corrected claw hand. Hand 1974; 6:266.
37. Raskin KB, Wilgis S. Flexor carpi ulnaris transfer for radial nerve palsy. Functional testing of long-term results. Presented at American Society for Surgery of the Hand: Annual Meeting, Seattle, Washington, 1989.
38. Riordan D. Tendon transplantation in median nerve and ulnar nerve paralysis. J Bone Joint Surg [Am] 1953; 35:312.
39. Riordan D. Intrinsic paralysis of the hand. Bull Hosp Jt Dis Orthop Inst 1984; 44:435.
40. Smith R. Extensor carpi radialis brevis tendon transfer for thumb adduction. J Hand Surg 1983; 8:4–15.
41. Smith R. Metacarpal ligament sling tenodesis. Bull Hosp Jt Dis Orthop Inst 1984; 44:466.
42. Solonen K, Bakalim G. Restoration of pinch grip in ulnar palsy. Hand 1976; 8:39.
43. Wartenberg R. A sign of ulnar palsy. JAMA 1939; 112:1688.
44. Zancolli EA. Claw hand caused by paralysis of the intrinsic muscle: A simple surgical procedure for its correction. J Bone Joint Surg [Am] 1957; 39:1076–1080.
45. Zancolli EA. Structural and dynamic basis of hand surgery, ed 2. Philadelphia: JB Lippincott, 1978: 168.
46. Zweig J, Rosenthal S, Burns H. Transfer of the extensor digit quinti to restore pinch in ulnar palsy. J Bone Joint Surg [Am] 1972; 54:51.

52

Tendon Transfers for Combined Nerve Injuries

George E. Omer, Jr.

AUTHOR'S KEY POINTS

- Muscles with temporary loss of function due to a nerve injury generally do not regain sufficient strength for elective tendon transfer.
- Skin incisions used in tendon transfer are transverse to the subcutaneous paths of transferred tendons.
- If a transferred tendon has a split insertion, the motor acts primarily on the attachment placed under greatest tension.
- Procedures to restore sensibility are delayed until all tendon transfers have been completed and supple tissues have been restored with adequate range of motion.
- Distal median–ulnar nerve palsy is the most commonly encountered combined nerve palsy. The requirements for restoration of wrist and hand function are improved key pinch provided by an adductor transfer, restoration of abduction of the thumb for opposition, improved strength for pinch between thumb and index fingers, improved flexion power of the proximal phalanx, restoration of the palmar transverse arch and correction of the abduction deformity of the little finger, and provision of sensibility to the tip regions required for key pinch.

The objective of reconstructive surgery in the extremity with combined nerve injuries is balanced performance, because tendon transfers redistribute existing assets rather than creating new ones. Tendon transfers either eliminate deforming forces that produce further imbalances or replace single motions to assist grasp, pinch, or release. Specific composite tissue transplantation is useful in sensory-depleted glabrous skin areas required for precise pinch and grasp.

- Surgeons reconstructing extremities with combined nerve injuries should be experienced enough to select appropriate procedures based on individual cases.
- Precise sensibility requires precise motion.
- Additional strength in a palsied power train requires a new muscle–tendon unit.
- Tendon transfers in combined nerve injuries are more complicated than those in isolated nerve palsy because of complex extremity injuries, including poor proprioception, weakness of muscles for

potential transfer, and the need for multiple operations.

GENERAL PRINCIPLES

When multiple nerves are injured in a single extremity, the functional loss is severe. Circulation is usually impaired, which results in ischemic pain and increased fibrosis. The skeleton may be unstable, with loss of normal joint stability and motion. Muscle–tendon units are often lacerated and sometimes avulsed, increasing the neuromotor impairment, and resulting scar complicates the technical transfer of remaining intact tendons. Unhealed or chronic wounds are contraindications to elective surgery. As joints stiffen and muscles atrophy, maintaining a mobile extremity without deforming contracture demands persistent therapy and meticulous splinting. The most important aspect of a rehabilitation program is the patient's acceptance of the responsibility and initiative for recovery. Reconstructive procedures should not be undertaken until normal joint motion has been established and skeletal alignment is stable.[25]

In addition to the physical condition of the involved extremity, the success of tendon transfers depends on the cause and prognosis of motor imbalance. The cause of motor imbalance is important in predicting the further involvement of additional muscle–tendon units with progressive functional impairment. The extent of muscle imbalance is usually static after traumatic injury, but is often unstable in upper motor neuron problems, such as a series of cerebrovascular accidents. The prognosis for progressive muscle imbalance may be a contraindication for elective surgery.

A major problem in multiple nerve palsy is sensory loss coupled with a loss of position sense and other normal feedback mechanisms. Spinal reflex arcs coordinate with the ventral horn motor neurons to produce a pattern of motor function. For each muscle there is an optimal tension at which force and motion are efficient.[10,35] In addition, the surgeon considers the potential for excursion of each muscle in a new position.[6] Muscles with only temporary loss of function (due, for example, to a neurapraxia lesion) do not regain normal strength for elective transfer procedures.[20] Sensibility loss is more profound in combined nerve palsies, and motor return rarely passes two major joints distal to the injury.[23]

The motion expected after tendon transfer cannot exceed the passive movement present preoperatively. However, the longer the surgeon waits for nerve recovery, the more difficult it is to prevent deformity. Combined nerve palsies are further complicated because there are fewer motor tendons available to stabilize residual function[14] or to provide additional function while awaiting potential nerve recovery following neurorrhaphy.[28] Therefore, it is difficult to use muscle–tendon units as internal splints to enhance patterns of motion in combined nerve palsies.

SELECTION OF THE MOTOR MUSCLE FOR TRANSFER

The surgeon should use as few transfers as necessary to meet the objective, because all tendon transfers potentially complicate the basic imbalance.

The motor muscle selected must have more than enough strength for its new task because it will have to pull itself free of the postoperative healing process and usually will lose one grade of strength on Lovett's clinical scale.[33] Paralyzed muscles that have regained function following nerve structure usually lack the individualized control and strength desirable for successful transfer.[20]

The polyarticulated system of longitudinal arches may demand simplification by carefully selected arthrodesis if transfers are to be effective.[15] This is particularly important with severe deficits when one or two transfers are required in combined palsies. For example, the opponens transfers for combined median and ulnar palsy are often much more functional if combined with thumb metacarpophalangeal (MCP) joint arthrodesis.

The present action of the selected motor muscle should be synergistic with the anticipated action, or at least retrainable by conscious control. Electromyographic studies indicate that a new activity pattern can be developed to correspond with the new mechanical function, but the old activity pattern is not lost.[13]

The motor muscle–tendon units should have adequate excursion for the anticipated motion. For example, measured amplitude approximates 33 mm for wrist movers, 70 mm for finger flexors, and 50 mm for finger extensors and the thumb motor muscles.[3] Brand suggested that these excursion figures should be termed *required excursion* because they refer to the tendon excursion necessary for the total joint movement associated with a given muscle. Brand emphasized the *potential excursion* of the tendon, which refers to the excursion possible in a new position for the muscle–tendon unit. The potential excursion is directly related to the mean fiber length of a muscle. Mean resting fiber length for forearm muscles varies from 16.1 cm for the brachioradialis to 7.2 cm for the flexor digitorum superficialis to the index, 6.0 cm for the extensor digitorum communis to the middle finger, and 4.2 cm for the flexor carpi ulnaris.[6]

The motor muscle selected should have a work capacity equal to that of the antagonist of the anticipated motion. Work for a muscle equals force times distance (where force is 3.6 kg × the physiological cross-sectional area of the muscle). The "normal" work capacity has been listed for some forearm muscles as follows:

Flexor carpi ulnaris, 2.0 kg
Extensor carpi radialis brevis, 0.9 kg
Flexor digitorum profundus, 4.5 kg
Extensor digitorum communis, 1.7 kg

However, the mass of muscle is proportional to an individual's strength at the time of measurement and is variable. Brand has developed the concept of a *tension fraction* for each muscle, defined as the percentage contribution of that muscle to the contraction tension capability of all muscles within an anatomic unit, such as the forearm and hand.[6] The tension fraction is derived by converting each muscle mass to volume and dividing by the mean fiber length of that muscle to obtain the physiologic cross section of each muscle. The tension fraction of each muscle is then a percentage of the total. For the flexor carpi ulnaris, it is 6.7%; for the extensor carpi radialis brevis, 4.2%; for the adductor pollicis, 3.0%; and for the flexor carpi radialis, 4.1%. The tension fraction indicates the relative work capacity of two muscles within the same individual.

Other considerations are as follows:

- The principle of dynamic tenodesis is used to enhance amplitude, but joints involved in the dynamic tenodesis must be mobile and stable.
- The motor unit should have a line of pull as straight as possible to the new insertion. Pulleys may be necessary to enforce a proper vector, and if so, the angulation of the tendon must be minimized.
- The soft-tissue bed for the transferred musculotendinous unit must be as free as possible from scar and other "fixed tissue" (such as raw bone surface or fibrous septa).
- To be certain that secondary dysfunction is avoided, the available motor transfer should be listed along with retained muscle power.
- Patient evaluation is factored into the final decision. The patient who has developed the cerebral imprint for the proposed function will be able to comprehend what is to be done and will be ready to accept the postoperative discipline necessary for reeducation.

OPERATIVE TECHNIQUES

Incisions are placed so that tendon repair sites are beneath skin flaps and free of subcutaneous scar. *As a rule, incisions are transverse to the subcutaneous path of the transferred tendon.* The subcutaneous pathway glides with the transferred tendon.

The motor muscle is mobilized to protect its neurovascular bundle, which usually enters the proximal third of the muscle. The texture, vascularity, and excursion of the muscle–tendon unit should be evaluated under direct vision at the operating table.[35]

The transferred tendon should not cross raw bone. Muscle–tendon units that must move through fascial planes, such as an interosseous membrane, should have a larger opening in the fascia than the cross-section of the muscle. The muscle must be placed in the fascial window because the exterior muscle fibers will "freeze" to the fascia while the interior muscle fibers will retain motion; if the tendon is placed in the fascial window, it will bind fast and motion will be lost.[26]

The direction of pull for the transferred tendon is in as straight a line as practicable. In addition, most muscle–tendon units are parallel to bone, and the angle of approach between the transferred tendon and its insertion should be small. The greater the angle of approach of the tendon to its insertion point, the greater the force the muscle can exert, but this creates a bowstring effect, which may be uncomfortable. In addition, a pulley is required to increase the approach angle, and the result is actually a loss of force secondary to friction when the angle is greater than 45°. Eventually a bowstrung tendon will shift to a straight-line pull and then will become too slack for effective force.

The more distal to the axis of motion of a joint the tendon is anchored, the more force the muscle exerts on the joint, but also the more excursion required of the tendon to provide a normal range of motion in the joint. *If a transferred tendon has a split insertion, the motor acts primarily on the slip under greater tension.*

A tendon transfer is most effective when it crosses only one joint. If a tendon bowstrings across a proximal joint, its mechanical advantage at that joint will be so great that it may force that joint into unwanted motion or use up all its fiber excursion so that it cannot move the distal joint. An example of this last point is the tendon transfer of the brachioradialis into the flexor pollicis longus: when the elbow and wrist are extended, the patient can hold an object tightly, but when the elbow is flexed, the muscle–tendon power is dissipated at the elbow, and the patient drops the object.[32]

There is considerable interconnection in the forearm between the individual finger elements of the flexor digitorum superficialis, especially the index and little fingers. If the flexor digitorum superficialis muscle–tendon unit of either the index or little finger is transferred to the dorsum of the hand, the other muscle–tendon unit should be transferred also, or the intermediate connecting fibers will severely limit excursion.[6]

Suture material for tendon fixation is monofilament steel or synthetic material that causes minimal tissue reaction. To prevent tendon necrosis, the suture is inserted through the center of the tendon and should then circle only half the tendon; sutures along the length of the tendon are placed so that the circle to be tied alternates from side to side in order to protect circulation further. "Lacing" a transferred tendon into a group of paralyzed muscle–tendon units is avoided because it creates bulk, twist, and friction and increases scar. A precise insertion point is selected, but at that point a short length of paralyzed and transferred tendon is sutured side to side to prevent "whip-sawing." The paralyzed tendon can be disconnected from its fibrosed muscle and sutured directly to the transferred tendon. However, excision of the paralyzed muscle may bring unwelcome hemorrhage and should not be done unless the muscle mass is causing deformity. When the transferred tendon is attached to bone, the surrounding periosteum is elevated as a flap and then closed over the insertion.

The appropriate tension of the tendon transfer depends upon muscle mean fiber length, cross-sectional area, and total volume.[9] Tension has been evaluated by electrical stimulation[35] and laser light diffraction techniques.[10] If there has been appropriate evaluation of tissue homeostasis, then tendon tension can be determined adequately at the operating table. The tension of the tendon transfer is judged best while the extremity is placed in the position it will assume when the new muscle–tendon unit has actively contracted. For extensor transfers, resting tendon tension should be adequate to hold the extremity passively in the usual functional position against gravity. In those cases in which extensive re-education is likely to be required, it is better to attach the transferred tendon under greater-than-normal tension. This brings perception of the new muscle more readily into consciousness, as stretch reflexes and other feedback mechanisms are stimulated when opposing muscles restore the neutral position of the extremity.[4]

Procedures to restore sensibility are delayed until all indicated tendon transfers have been accomplished and the patient has supple tissues with an established range of motion. The design of any neurovascular free flap requires that the vascular and neural distribution overlap to ensure both viability and potential reinnervation. The vascular supply of the flap should be accessible for dissection and should be of appropriate diameter and available length for anastomosis. The arterial distribution may be confirmed by arteriogram. Specific nerves should provide the primary sensory innervation of the flaps and should be accessible for dissection and subsequent suture to the proximal stump of the original sensory nerve to the recipient area. Neural distribution may be surveyed by preoperative nerve blocks of the surrounding nerves.

Selection of the donor site for a neurovascular free flap is based on the sensibility requirements of the recipient cutaneous area. In an elective procedure to reinnervate an area of sensory importance, such as the pulp of the thumb, the surgeon should always try to use glabrous rather than hairy skin. The cortical representation of glabrous skin areas is much greater than the cortical areas representing hairy skin. The central processing involved in encoding the afferent sensation from glabrous skin may be different from the central processing required for sensibility related to the hairy skin. The density of innervation of glabrous skin is greater than that of hairy skin. Pulp tissue of the toes compares better with the pulp tissue of the fingers than with any nonhand tissue in the body. The toe pulp's histology and skin-wear characteristics are similar to those of the pulp tissue of the fingers. The donor site is immediately resurfaced with a split-thickness skin graft. If the foot has been the donor site, a Jobst foot stocking is used for compression.

The foot is more variable in its blood supply than the hand, and arteriography or a Doppler probe is most helpful in previewing the anatomic variations. Preoperative planning is essential, but the surgeon must be prepared to insert segmental grafts into arteries, veins, or nerves as the situation dictates at the time of surgery.

The key to success in operative technique is simplicity; complexity invites failure.

SENSORY DEFECTS

Tactile gnosis is very important as a "sensory feedback" for precise function,[19] but voluntary motor activity is an essential component of tactile gnosis.[34] Tendon transfers should be done before sensory reconstruction is undertaken because abnormal patterns of motor activity enhance the distortion of sensibility that accompanies a peripheral nerve deficit.

Operative procedures to restore sensibility following irreparable nerve loss have usually been neurovascular pedicle island flaps from one finger to another.[34,39] Neurovascular cutaneous island pedicle flaps for the reconstruction of peripheral nerve defects have been used primarily to restore median nerve sensation. If the ulnar nerve is to be the donor, only the common digital nerve between the ring and little fingers is available, since sensibility along the ulnar aspect of the little finger is essential in total medial nerve loss. The usual technique is to transfer a cutaneous island, with its neurovascular pedicle, from the ulnar aspect of the ring finger to the ulnar–volar aspect of the thumb pulp.[27] A large island should be dissected from the ulnar–volar aspect of the ring finger. The superficial vascular arch may have to be interrupted and the radial portion freed to swing with the cutaneous island. A double island along the ulnar border of the ring finger, across the distal edge of the palm, and along the radial border of the little finger has been transferred to the thumb–index web space.[27] As an alternative, the radial-innervated cross-finger flap from the dorsum of the proximal index to the thumb pulp will provide a critical area with sensation.[11]

Omer and associates reported their findings in 15 patients with high (proximal) median nerve loss who were followed with evaluation tests of sensibility after neurovascular island pedicle flaps.[34] There was a gradual reduction from normal sensation to merely protective sensation. This loss of sensibility was related to the associated motor loss for the radial side of the hand, and without adequate motion and power, sensibility for precise prehension is lost. There is disorientation of sensitivity in all neurovascular island pedicle flaps.[29] For several months after transplant, the patient recognizes stimulation in the island as originating from the original donor site. Later, sensation is interpreted in both the recipient and donor sites. In an emergency, such as a flame burn, the patient loses interpretation ability and first moves the original donor site. There is also a high incidence of cold intolerance, and paresthesia is common at the margin of these flaps.

Littler now believes that neurovascular island pedicle flaps that transfer sensation from one digit to another are anachronistic procedures.[17] Current techniques include free vascularized nerve grafts and free neurovascular sensory flaps.

Taylor has demonstrated that a nerve graft can be isolated with an intact arteriovenous system by dissecting a neurovascular bundle with a sleeve of areolar connective tissue to preserve the direct and recurrent vasa nervorum.[37] The graft consists of a long unbranched conducting length of nerve, with a blood supply emanating from a single arteriovenous system that parallels the nerve. Taylor has used a free superficial radial nerve vascularized graft to fill a gap in a median nerve and has used segments of median and ulnar nerves, vascularized by the brachial vessels, from an amputated right arm stump to fill nerve gaps in the left arm.

The microsurgical composite free flaps includes donor skin that approximates the quality of the recipient skin, and the pattern of the donor skin is predictable for precise sensibility. In addition to free sensory neurovascular flaps from the first web space of the foot, Morrison and coworkers have described a modification of the toe-to-thumb transfer that is a free neurovascular wrap-around flap from the big toe for thumb reconstruction after amputation.[21] The trimmed nail and nail bed, as well as subcutaneous tissue, are included to prevent pulp swivel. The thumb skeleton is sculpted from the iliac crest if there has been avulsion of the thumb; otherwise the flap is added to the existing bony base. The dorsalis pedis artery and the long saphenous vein are left long enough to anastomose to the radial artery and the cephalic vein at the level of the snuffbox of the wrist. The deep peroneal nerve is joined to the superficial radial nerve, and the plantar digital nerves must join the proximal median nerve. A long gap in the median nerve eliminates the possibility of this type of transfer.

POSTOPERATIVE RE-EDUCATION AND EVALUATION

The extremity is immobilized in rigid dressings in the proper position to achieve the desired result. For example, after tendon transfers for an intrinsic-minus thumb and the clawed fingers of ulnar palsy, the wrist and hand are positioned with the wrist extended, the finger MCP joints flexed, and the interphalangeal joints straight (the so-called hoe hand, position of protection, or safe position). Rigid dressings are more extensive in cases where two joint-length tendons have been transferred and in children. Flexor tendon transfers are immobilized for 3 to 4 weeks and then protected with a removable splint for 1 more week. Extensor tendon transfers work against the stronger flexor units and thus are immobilized for 5 weeks and then protected with a removable volar splint for 2 weeks more.

The results of tendon transfers are assessed only after a follow-up period of at least 6 months. Many aspects of function are considered:

1. Power with a voluntary muscle test
2. Range of active motion
3. Balance, or the passive equilibrium between opposing myotonic forces
4. Stability, or the positive action between antagonist muscles
5. Synergistic balance, such as the action between wrist flexors and finger extensors or wrist extensors and finger flexors
6. Coordination, the smooth transfer of force from one synergistic muscle group to another group.

Re-education is more important than the operative procedure in the final result. Postoperative re-education does not terminate with a demonstration to the patient that attempting a former active motion now produces a new, more desirable action. The new action becomes an integrated part of a coordinated multimuscle functional pattern. Prolonged daily therapy is extremely important in a child, uncomprehending adult, or patient who is easily inhibited by pain. Function of the extremities is patterned in the brain as coordinated multimuscle action patterns, not as individualized muscle–tendon motion. The ultimate control of movement is related to tactile, proprioceptive, and visual sensory input as well as to available individual muscle power.

In contrast, clinical observation demonstrates that precise sensibility depends upon precise motor activity.[24] Sensory re-education programs depend on movement as an important factor in appropriate stimulation of cutaneous receptors.[40] The patient alters motor patterns to obtain the best available sensory function. For example, the patient with loss of volar pulp sensibility of the index finger secondary to median palsy adapts by "divorcing" the index finger and extending it out of the pinch pattern, which then will be altered to a chuck between the thumb and the ring or middle finger. The Moberg pick-up test is a good check of functional motor patterns if one of the objects is a short length of soft chalk.[18] The chalk will rub against the fingers and leave a visible trail of functional surfaces.[30] The abnormal motor function that usually accompanies nerve palsy exacerbates the distorted sensibility patterns and contributes to dysesthesia. These problems are the basis for an aggressive motor re-education program.

UPPER EXTREMITY

Low (Distal) Median–Ulnar Nerve Palsy

In late distal median–ulnar nerve palsy, the most common combined nerve palsy, the complete loss of volar sensation and intrinsic motor muscles produces an almost useless claw hand (Fig. 52-1).[15] Reconstruction of the thumb is extremely important, and special efforts must be made to prevent adduction contractures of the thumb–index web. There is a flat transverse palmar arch (metacarpal arch), with hyperextension at the MCP joints and hyperflexion at the proximal interphalangeal (PIP) joints. An abducted little finger may be associated with the flat transverse metacarpal arch. The patient flexes the wrist to obtain greater finger extension, a functional tenodesis, but with prolonged use this often results in a fixed flexion contracture of the wrist. Following individualized transfers, the residual loss of sensibility may well be a greater functional problem than patterns for motion (Table 52-1).

The basic requirements for restoration of wrist and hand function are:

1. Improved key pinch provided by a stronger adductor of the thumb
2. Restored abduction of the thumb for opposition
3. Strengthened tip pinch between the thumb and index fingers
4. Improved power flexion of the proximal phalanx
5. Restored metacarpal (palmar) transverse arch and correction of the associated abduction deformity of the little finger
6. Specific sensory area for tip or key pinch.

When the superficial radial nerve is used for restoration of sensibility, it is advisable to perform a preoperative evaluation of the distribution of the nerve over the dorsal aspect of the index finger. A V-shaped incision is made, with one limb of the V at the level of the midlateral line on the radial side of the index finger and the other limb at the midlateral line on the ulnar side of the thumb.[11] The proximal point of the V incision is near the first dorsal metacarpal branch of the radial artery. Dissection will demonstrate the longitudinal branches of the superficial radial nerve and vascular structures dorsal to the second metacarpal. If the vessels can be followed distally to the area of the proximal phalanx, a racket-shaped cutaneous island with a neurovascular pedicle is dissected from the dorsal–radial surface of the index finger. The neurovascular island is then fitted into the volar–ulnar aspect of the thumb pulp. The procedure is precarious

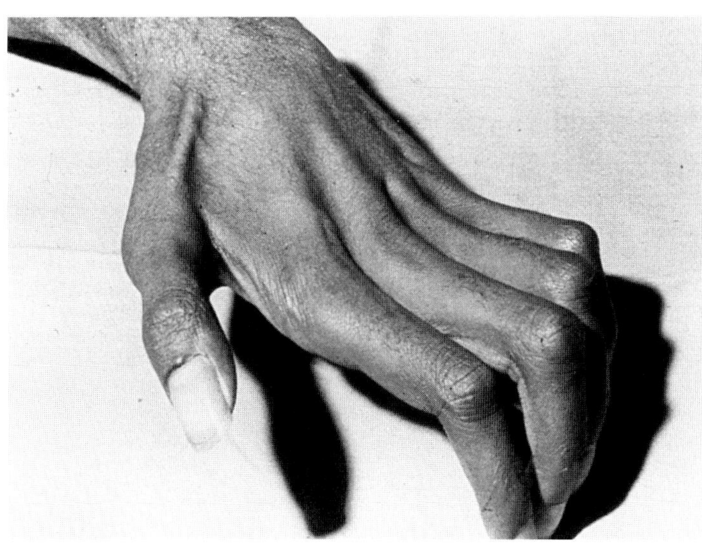

Figure 52-1. *Combined median–ulnar palsy with intrinsic motor atrophy. There is an adduction contracture of the thumb and atrophy of the pulp of the fingers.*

Table 52–1 Combined Low (Distal) Median and Ulnar Palsy

Needed Function	Preferred Transfer	Alternate Transfer
Thumb adduction (key pinch)	Brachioradialis with free tendon graft between third and fourth metacarpals to abductor tubercle of first metacarpal	Flexor digitorum superficialis (middle) to abductor tubercle of first metacarpal with palmar fascia and flexor tendons as pulleys
Thumb abduction (opposition)	Extensor indicis proprius to insertion of abductor pollicis brevis and extensor pollicis longus tendon	Palmaris longus tendon transfer or Extensor carpi ulnaris with free graft
Thumb–index tip pinch	Abductor pollicis longus slip to first dorsal interosseous tendon and Arthrodesis, MCP joint of thumb	Extensor pollicis brevis and Arthrodesis, MCP joint of thumb
Metacarpal (palmar) transferse arch, and active abduction for little finger	Extensor digiti minimi to proximal phalanx or dorsal apparatus (extensor digitorum communis to little finger must be active)	Flexor digitorum superficialis of little finger to deep transverse metacarpal ligament between fourth and fifth metacarpals or Should be combined as single transfer with thumb adduction transfer
Power flexion—proximal phalanx and Integration of MCP and interphalangeal motion	Extensor carpi radialis longus to all four fingers, using four-tailed free graft to either flexor sheath insertion or dorsal apparatus	Flexor carpi radialis (if wrist) flexion contracture with four-tailed graft and flexor sheath insertion (A2 pulley)
Volar sensibility	Free neurovascular cutaneous island flap	Cross-finger—index-to-thumb neurocutaneous flap

(From Omer GE Jr. Combined nerve palsies. In: Green DP, ed. Operative hand surgery, ed 2. New York: Churchill-Livingstone, 1988: 1556, with permission.)

because the arterial supply to the cutaneous island is not constant, and the operation must often be modified by constructing a cross-finger flap from the index finger to the thumb that contains the transposed nerve.[1]

High (Proximal) Median–Ulnar Nerve Palsy (Late)

The hand rarely will be used for precision activity following the severe injury of late proximal median–ulnar nerve palsy, even if minimal muscle balance is restored. Atrophy of the finger pulps will discourage both power and precise grip. If the other hand is normal, it is best to direct the surgical endeavor toward establishing a key pinch and a simple grasp (Table 52-2).

The extensor carpi radialis brevis has the best mechanical advantage for wrist extension and should remain in place, but all other wrist extrinsic muscles on the extensor aspect can be used. There is no wrist extensor muscle with adequate amplitude for full flexion of the digits unless the motion is reinforced by active wrist extension. Since the brachioradialis has the greatest "potential excursion," this muscle can provide finger flexion (Fig. 52-2).[6] Goldner has extended the biceps brachii with a free tendon graft.[12] Abduction of the thumb for opposition does not require great strength, and the thumb extensor muscles can be rerouted to clear the thumb from the palm.[38,42]

The loss of simultaneous MCP joint flexion with either interphalangeal extension or interphalangeal flexion prevents the rhythm necessary to hold large and small objects. There are no available motors to provide dynamic integration of motion, so static techniques must be used. Parkes has devised a tenodesis by placing a free tendon graft between the radial lateral band of the dorsal apparatus of the finger and the flexor retinaculum (deep transverse metacarpal ligament) in the palm.[36] The grafts function independently for each finger. Zancolli approaches the MCP joint through a volar longitudinal incision.[41] It is necessary to open the proximal pulley of the flexor sheath. A short flap with a distal base is cut from the volar plate and drawn proximally to be sutured with the joint in 20° of flexion. The result is a flexor pulley advancement with capsulodesis and a mild flexion contracture.

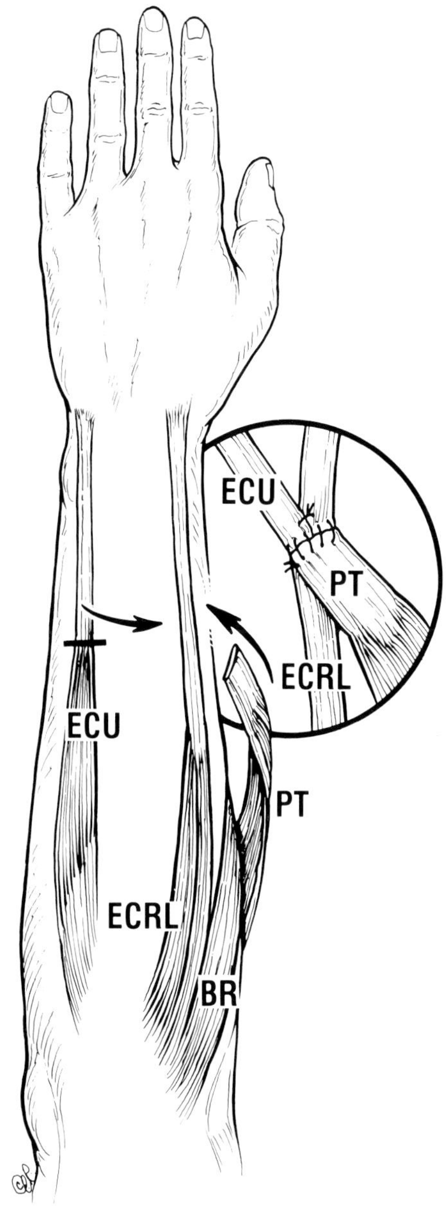

Figure 52–2. *Transfer of the pronator teres (PT) to a balanced yoke insertion into the extensor carpi ulnaris (ECU) and extensor carpi radialis longus (ECRL) for wrist extension. The pronator teres should pass subcutaneously over the brachioradialis (BR).*

Long-term results of the capsulodesis procedure have demonstrated indifferent results,[8] and there have been several modifications of the technique.[22]

Sensation can be transferred to the radiovolar aspect of the hand.[27] Careful testing of the super-

Table 52–2 Combined High (Proximal) Median and Ulnar Palsy

Needed Function	Preferred Transfer	Alternate Transfer
Thumb adduction (key pinch)	Extensor carpi radialis longus with free tendon graft between third and fourth metacarpal to abductor tubercle of first metacarpal	Extensor indicis proprius between third and fourth metacarpal
Thumb flexion (interphalangeal joint)	Extensor indicis proprius to flexor pollicis longus	Tenodesis of flexor pollicis longus distal to MCP joint
Thumb abduction (opposition)	Extensor pollicis brevis around tendon of flexor carpi radialis (if thumb MCP joint is fused)	Extensor pollicis longus rerouted around pisiform (if thumb MCP joint fused and no active thumb flexion at interphalangeal joint)
Thumb–long (index) pinch (tip pinch)	Arthrodesis, thumb MCP joint and Abductor pollicis longus slip to first dorsal interosseous tendon	Extensor digitorum communis of index to first dorsal interosseous tendon (if index fillet flap is used or sensation)
Finger flexion	Brachioradialis to tendons of flexor digitorum profundus and Tenodesis DIP joint, three ulnar fingers	Biceps brachii extended with flexor carpi radialis tendons of flexor digitorum profundus
Clawed fingers—power flexion proximal phalanx and Integration of MCP and interphalangeal motion	Tenodesis of all digits with free tendon graft from dorsal apparatus to deep transverse metacarpal ligament	Capsulodesis of MCP volar capsule or Arthrodesis of PIP joints
Metacarpal (palmar) arch and adduction for little finger	Extensor digiti minimi to proximal phalanx or dorsal apparatus (extensor digitorum communis of little finger must be active)	

(continued)

Table 52–2 *(continued)*

Needed Function	**Preferred Transfer**	**Alternate Transfer**
Wrist flexion	Extensor carpi ulnaris to insertion of flexor carpi ulnaris	
Radiovolar sensibility	Superficial radial innervated index fillet flap to palm	Free vascularized nerve graft

(From Omer GE Jr. Combined nerve palsies. In: Green DP, ed. Operative hand surgery, ed 2. New York: Churchill-Livingstone, 1988: 1557, with permission.)

ficial radial nerve will demonstrate the distal level of sensibility on the dorsum of the index finger. The skeleton of the index finger is removed distal to the proximal third of the second metacarpal. The index ray is excised through a racket incision at the distal end of good dorsal index sensibility and a longitudinal palmar incision between the second and third metacarpals. The insensitive distal index skin is discarded. The fillet index finger flap is then fitted into an additional volar defect created for it in the insensitive palmar skin. This broad-based finger flap is innervated by the superficial radial nerve and provides protective palmar sensibility for key pinch (Fig. 52-3).

High (Proximal) Ulnar–Radial Nerve Palsy (Late)

Patients with late proximal ulnar–radial nerve palsy retain radiovolar sensibility, and reconstruction is a useful investment to improve function (Table 52-3). Although more than 30 different procedures are described for isolated radial nerve palsy, the combination of ulnar and radial palsy leaves few expendable muscle–tendon units for transfer.[2]

Because transfer of the pronator teres to the extensor carpi radialis brevis for wrist extension in a high ulnar–radial nerve palsy may result in radial deviation of the hand, a balanced yoke insertion

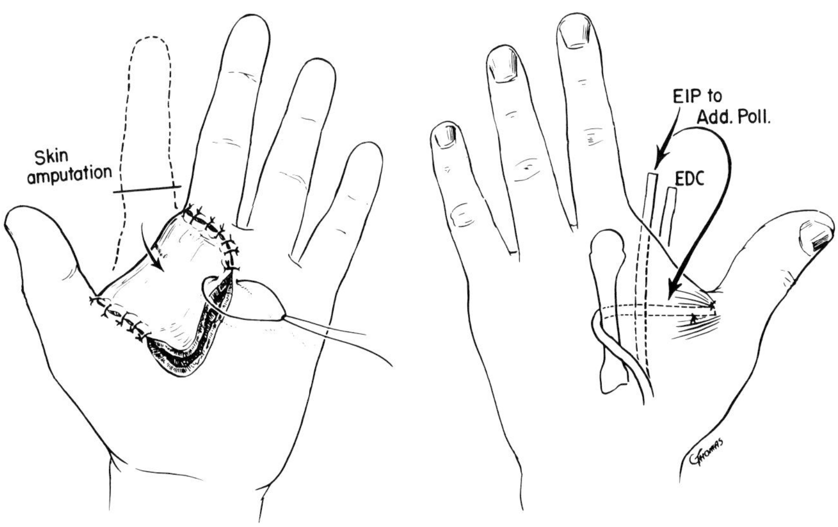

Figure 52-3. *(**A**) The broad based fillet index finger flap created by using radial innervated dorsal skin to provide protective sensibility for simple grasp in reconstruction in high median–ulnar palsy. The index ray is excised and the skin is amputated distal to the radial nerve innervation. (**B**) Fillet of the index ray allows use of the extensor indicis proprius tendon as a transfer for adduction of the thumb. (From Omer GE Jr. Tendon transfers in combined nerve lesions. Orthop Clin North Am 1974;5:383, with permission.)*

Table 52–3 *Combined High (Proximal) Ulnar and Radial Palsy*

Needed Function	Preferred Transfer	Alternate Transfer
Wrist extension	Pronator teres (yoke insertion) to extensor carpi radialis longus and extensor carpi ulnaris	
Thumb adduction (key pinch)	One half flexor digitorum superficialis (middle) as split transfer to abductor tubercle of the thumb	
Clawed fingers: Metacarpal (palmar) transverse arch and Power flexion—proximal and Integration MCP and interphalangeal motion	One half flexor digitorum superficialis (middle) in two slips to A2 pulley as flexor sheath insertion to ring and little fingers and, later Arthrodesis, PIP joint of ring and little fingers if unable to extend fully	Tenodesis with free tendon graft from radial lateral band of dorsal apparatus to deep phalanx metacarpal ligament or Capsulodesis of MCP volar capsule
Thumb–index tip pinch	Arthrodesis, MCP joint of thumb	
Proximal thumb abduction stability and Wrist flexion (radial aspect)	Flexor carpi radialis (yoke insertion) to abductor pollicis longus and extensor pollicis brevis	Tenodesis, abductor pollicis longus to radius
Wrist flexion (ulnar aspect)	Palmaris longus to insertion of flexor carpi ulnaris	
Finger and thumb extension	Flexor digitorum superficialis (index and little) through interosseous membrane to extensor digitorum communis and extensor pollicis longus	Flexor carpi radialis to extensor digitorum communis and Palmaris longus to extensor pollicis longus
Finger flexion (ring and little)	Tenodesis of flexor digitorum profundus index and middle (active motors) to ring and little flexor digitorum profundus and Tenodesis of DIP joint ring and little fingers, using flexor digitorum profundus	

(continued)

Table 52–3 (continued)

Needed Function	Preferred Transfer	Alternate Transfer
Volar sensibility—ring and little fingers		Free vascularized nerve graft

(From Omer GE Jr. Combined nerve palsies. In: Green DP, ed. Operative hand surgery, ed 2. New York: Churchill-Livingstone, 1988: 1560, with permission.)

into both the extensor carpi ulnaris and extensor carpi radialis longus is preferable (Fig. 52-4).[4] The extensor carpi ulnaris tendon is cut at the muscle–tendon junction, and the proximal (high) end of the tendon is sutured to the extensor carpi radialis longus tendon to provide balanced extension. A low ulnar–radial nerve palsy retains ulnar wrist flexion, and the yoke insertion should not be done; instead the pronator teres should insert into the tendon of the extensor carpi radialis brevis. The middle and ring superficialis tendons are usually transferred to provide thumb and finger extension, but the middle finger tendon may be needed for thumb adduction (the superficialis of the little finger is often congenitally absent).

The loss of balanced power across the PIP joints may result ultimately in either a flexion contracture or a swan-neck deformity of these joints. The sur-

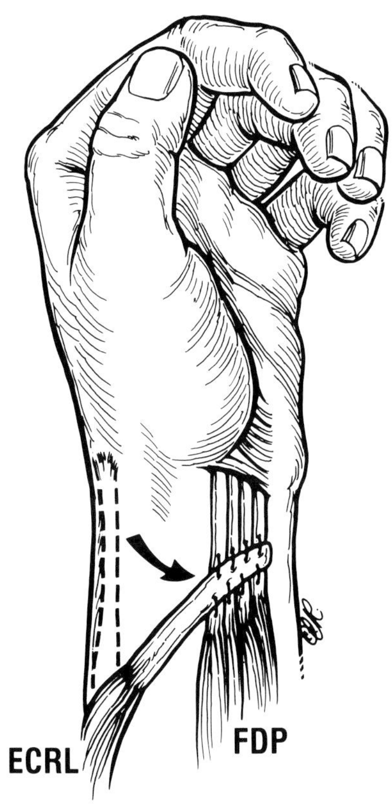

Figure 52–4. *Transfer of the extensor carpi radialis longus (ECRL) around the radial aspect of the forearm to the tendons of the flexor digitorum profundus (FDP) for finger flex ion. The anastomosis should be proximal to the carpal tunnel. The range of finger motion is less than normal.*

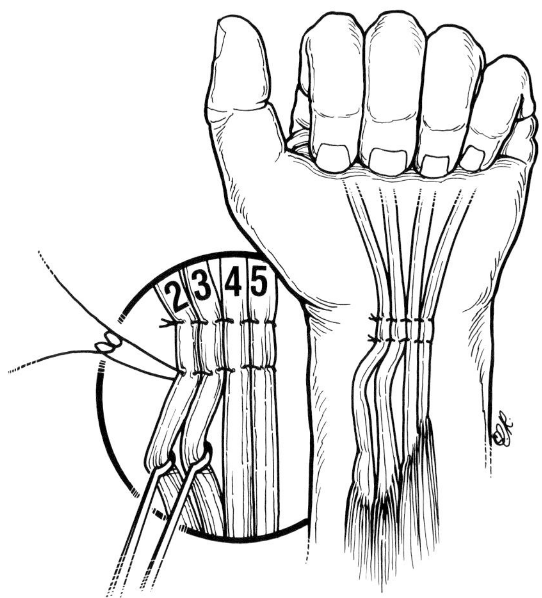

Figure 52–5. *Tenodesis of the denervated index and long tendons to the innervated ring and little tendons of the flexor digitorum profundus (FDP) for flexion of all four fingers. A double line of sutures is important to prevent "whipsawing" of the tendons with power grip. The index profundus has been tenodesed across the DIP joint to eliminate one joint in the arc of motion.*

Table 52–4 *Combined High (Proximal) Median and Radial Palsy*

Needed Function	***Preferred Transfer***	***Alternate Transfer***
Forearm pronation	Biceps brachii tendon rerouting around the radius	
Wrist extension and flexion	Radial–carpal arthrodesis	
Finger flexion	Tenodesis of flexor digitorum profundus ring and little finger (active motors) to index and middle flexor digitorum	
Finger extension and Thumb extension	Flexor carpi ulnaris to tendons of extensor digitorum communis and extensor pollicis longus	
Proximal thumb abduction stability	Arthrodesis, MCP joint of thumb and Tenodesis abductor pollicis longus to radius	
Thumb abduction (opposition)	Abductor digiti quinti to the insertion of abductor pollicis brevis (Huber operation)	Adductor pollicis tendon from adductor tubercle to abductor tubercle (de Vecchi operation)
Thumb flexion	Tenodesis of flexor pollicis longus across interphalangeal joint of thumb	Biceps brachii extended with flexor carpi radialis tendon to tendon of flexor pollicis longus
Sensibility—radiovolar area	Free neurovascular cutaneous island flap	Free vascularized nerve graft

(From Omer GE Jr. Combined nerve palsies. In: Green DP, ed. Operative hand surgery, ed 2. New York: Churchill-Livingstone, 1988: 1565, with permission.)

geon should observe for the onset of the deformity before electing to perform an arthrodesis.

High (Proximal) Median–Radial Nerve Palsy (Late)

Tendon transfers in combined median–radial nerve palsy lesion will result in a hand that functions only slightly more effectively than a prosthesis.[7] All wrist motors are lost except the flexor carpi ulnaris, and radial–carpal arthrodesis is indicated for the patient needing stability for even basic tasks, such as wheelchair ambulation. However, wrist motors will not provide adequate finger excursion when the carpus is fused. The flexor profundi tendons are sutured side to side for ulnar-innervated finger action.[26,32] The profundus tendons to the index and middle fingers must be under greater tension at the suture line to obtain appropriate flexion (Fig. 52-5).

The transfer of the abductor digiti quinti for thumb abduction (Huber operation) should not be attempted until the wrist is stabilized and there is normal thumb adduction power. The neurovascular pedicle to the abductor digiti quinti is proximally situated, and the muscle should be freed distally to proximally, then turned like the page in a book to its new position (Fig. 52-6).[16] This muscle has inadequate excursion but will provide functional opposition. Transfer of the insertion of the adductor pollicis from the adductor tubercle of the first metacarpal to the abductor tubercle is almost as effective (de Vecchi operation) (Table 52-4).[5]

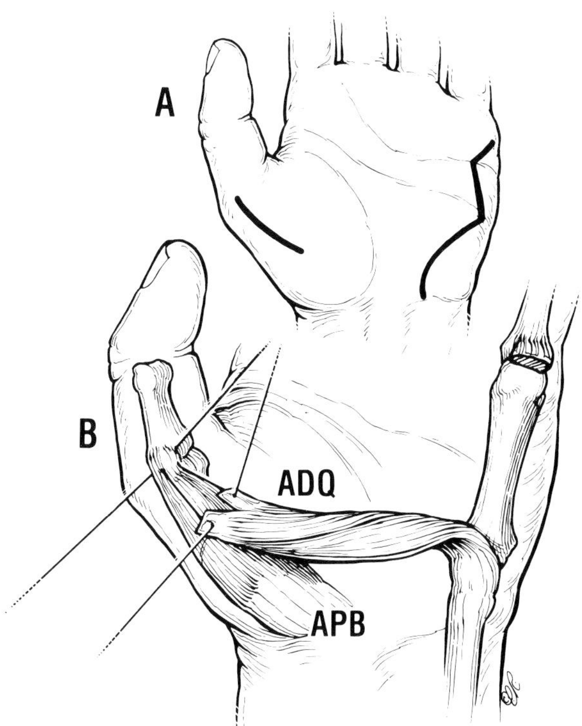

Figure 52-6. *Transfer of the abductor digiti quinti (ADQ) from its hypothenar position to the thenar area for abduction. Two incisions are made to minimize damage to the superficial nerves and grasping surface of the palm. The muscle is folded over 170° and passed subcutaneously to be inserted into the tendon of the abductor pollicis brevis (APB).*

LOWER EXTREMITY

Tendon transfers may enhance the rehabilitation of patients with paralysis of the lower extremity. The successful tendon transfer should have only one basic objective: to eliminate a deforming force that will produce further imbalance, to replace a single lost motion, or to produce stability. In contrast to the upper extremity, stability against gravity is much more important than mobility and range of motion in the lower extremity. With combined nerve injuries, it becomes very difficult to restore stability through tendon transfers.[31] In most combined nerve injuries of the lower extremity, the best reconstructive procedure is an effective orthosis.

REFERENCES

1. Adamson JE, Horton CE, Crawford HH. Sensory rehabilitation of the injured thumb. Plast Reconstr Surg 1967; 40:53.
2. Boyes JH. Tendon transfers for radial palsy. Bull Hosp Joint Dis Orthop Inst 1959; 21:97–105.
3. Boyes JH. Bunnell's surgery of the hand, ed 4. Philadelphia: JB Lippincott, 1964.
4. Brand PW. Tendon transfers in the forearm. In: Flynn JE, ed. Hand surgery. Baltimore: Williams & Wilkins, 1966:331–342.
5. Brand PW. Tendon transfers for median and ulnar nerve paralysis. Orthop Clin North Am 1970; 1: 447–454.
6. Brand PW, Beach RB, Thompson DE. Relative tension and potential excursion of muscles in the forearm and hand. J Hand Surg 1981; 6:209–219.
7. Brown PW. The time factor in surgery of upper extremity peripheral nerve injury. Clin Orthop 1970; 68:14–21.
8. Brown PW. Zancolli capsulorrhaphy for ulnar claw hand. J Bone Joint Surg [Am] 1970; 52:868–877.
9. Cooney WP, Linscheid RL, An KN. Opposition of the thumb: An anatomic and biomechanic study of tendon transfer. J Hand Surg [Am] 1984; 9:777–786.
10. Fleeter TB, Adams JP, Brenner B, Podolsky RJ. A laser diffraction method for measuring muscle sarcomere length in vivo for application to tendon transfers. J Hand Surg [Am] 1985; 10:542–546.
11. Gaul JS Jr. Radial-innervated cross-finger flap from index to provide sensory pulp to injured thumb. J Bone Joint Surg [Am] 1969; 51:1257–1263.

12. Goldner JL. Tendon transfer for irreparable peripheral nerve injuries. Orthop Clin North Am 1974; 5:343–375.
13. Ilbert M, Trauner M, Waller E, Wiedemann E. Forearm muscles of man can reverse their function after tendon transfers; an electromyographic study. Neurosci Lett 1986; 67:129.
14. Labosky DA, Waggy CA. Apparent weakness of median and ulnar motors in radial nerve palsy. J Hand Surg [Am] 1986; 11:528–533.
15. Littler JW. Tendon transfers and arthrodesis in combined median and ulnar nerve paralysis. J Bone Joint Surg [Am] 1949; 31:225–234.
16. Littler JW, Cooley SGE. Opposition of the thumb and its restoration by abductor digiti quinti transfer. J Bone Joint Surg [Am] 1963; 45:1389–1396.
17. Littler JW. In: Burton RI, ed. The thumb: Applications and Reconstructions. American Society for Surgery of the Hand Symposium. May 14–16, 1981.
18. Moberg E. Objective methods for determining the functional value of sensibility in the hand. J Bone Joint Surg [Br] 1958; 40:454–476.
19. Moberg E, Nachemson A. Tendon transfer for defective long extensors of the wrist and fingers. Acta Chir Scand 1967; 133:31–34.
20. Moneim MS, Omer GE Jr. Latissimus dorsi muscle transfer for restoration of elbow flexion after brachial plexus disruption. J Hand Surg [Am] 1986; 11: 135–139.
21. Morrison WA, O'Brien BM, MacLeod AM. Thumb reconstruction with a free neurovascular wraparound flap from the big toe. J Hand Surg 1980; 5: 575–583.
22. Omer GE Jr. Evaluation and reconstruction of the forearm and hand after acute traumatic peripheral nerve injuries. J Bone Joint Surg [Am] 1968; 50: 1454–1478.
23. Omer GE Jr. Injuries to nerves of the upper extremity. J Bone Joint Surg [Am] 1974; 56:1615–1624.
24. Omer GE Jr. Sensation and sensibility in the upper extremity. Clin Orthop 1974; 104:30–36.
25. Omer GE Jr. The technique and timing of tendon transfers. Orthop Clin North Am 1974; 5:243–252.
26. Omer GE Jr. Tendon transfers in combined nerve lesions. Orthop Clin North Am 1974; 5:377–387.
27. Omer GE Jr. Neurovascular sensory island transplants. In: Fredericks S, Brody GS, eds. Neurologic aspects of plastic surgery. Educational Foundation of the American Society of Plastic and Reconstructive Surgeons. St. Louis: CV Mosby, 1978:17:52–60.
28. Omer GE Jr. Tendon transfers as early internal splints following peripheral nerve injury in the upper extremity. In: Hunter JM, Schneider LH, Mackin EJ, Bell JA, eds. Rehabilitation of the hand. St. Louis: CV Mosby, 1978:292–296.
29. Omer GE Jr. Neurovascular cutaneous island flaps. In: Omer GE Jr, Spinner M, eds. Management of peripheral nerve problems. Philadelphia: WB Saunders, 1980:779–790.
30. Omer GE Jr. Sensory evaluation by the pick-up test. In: Jewett DL, McCarroll HR Jr, eds. Nerve repair and regeneration, its clinical and experimental basis. Philadelphia: WB Saunders, 1980:250–251.
31. Omer GE Jr. Tendon transfers as reconstructive procedures in the leg and foot. In: Omer GE Jr, Spinner M, eds. Management of peripheral nerve problems. Philadelphia: WB Saunders, 1980:873–880.
32. Omer GE Jr. Tendon transfer for reconstruction of the forearm and hand following peripheral nerve injuries. In: Omer GE Jr, Spinner M, eds. Management of peripheral nerve problems. Philadelphia: WB Saunders, 1980:817–846.
33. Omer GE Jr. Evaluation of the extremity with peripheral nerve injury and timing for nerve suture. In: American Academy of Orthopedic Surgeons Instructional Course Lectures, vol 33. St. Louis: CV Mosby, 1984:463.
34. Omer GE Jr, Day DJ, Ratcliff H, Lambert P. Neurovascular cutaneous island pedicles for deficient median nerve sensibility. J Bone Joint Surg [Am] 1970; 52:1181–1192.
35. Omer GE Jr, Vogel JA. Determination of physiological length of a reconstructed muscle-tendon unit through muscle stimulation. J Bone Joint Surg [Am] 1965; 47:304–310.
36. Parkes A. Paralytic claw fingers: A graft tenodesis operation. Hand 1973; 5:192–199.
37. Taylor GI. Nerve grafting with simultaneous microvascular reconstruction. Clin Orthop 1978; 133:56–70.
38. Tubiana R. Anatomic and physiologic basis for the surgical treatment of paralysis of the hand. J Bone Joint Surg [Am] 1969; 51:643–660.
39. Tubiana R, Duparc J. Restoration of sensibility in the hand by neurovascular skin island transfer. J Bone Joint Surg [Br] 1961; 43:474–480.
40. Wynn-Parry CB. Rehabilitation of the hand, ed 3. London: Butterworth, 1973.
41. Zancolli EA. Claw hand caused by paralysis of intrinsic muscles. A simple surgical procedure for its correction. J Bone Joint Surg [Am] 1957; 39:1076–1080.
42. Zancolli E. Tendon transfer after ischemic contracture of the forearm. Amer J Surg 1965; 109:356–360.

53

Lower Extremity Nerve Palsies

John M. Siliski
Frank Voss

AUTHORS' KEY POINTS

- Deformity caused by irreparable *peroneal* nerve palsy is reconstructed by a combination of triple arthrodesis, posterior bone block, and tibialis posterior tendon transfer.
- Deformity caused by irreparable *tibial* nerve palsy is reconstructed by a combination of triple arthrodesis with posterior calcaneal displacement, plantar fascia release, and tibialis anterior tendon transfer.
- Deformity caused by irreparable *sciatic* nerve palsy is reconstructed by a combination of triple arthrodesis, posterior bone block, and correction of toe deformities.
- Deformity caused by irreparable *femoral* nerve palsy is reconstructed by transfer of the biceps femoris to the patella, with or without transfer of the semitendinosus.

Reconstruction for unrepaired or irreparable lower extremity nerve injuries involves both joint-stabilization procedures and tendon transfers. These procedures were first performed for anterior poliomyelitis and only later for paralytic deficits related to trauma. This chapter focuses on techniques for the management of common peroneal, tibial, sciatic, and femoral nerve deficits not amenable to nerve repair.

The mechanisms of nerve injury in the lower extremity are diverse, and their precise incidences are difficult to define. The number that fail to recover (ie, those associated with neurotmesis) is substantially less than the total. More specifically, traumatic injuries can be classified as complete disruption, traction, and compression/ischemia. Sunderland reviewed many series that studied war injuries and noted that the common peroneal nerve was much more commonly injured than the tibial nerve, due to its more superficial course, its fixed position at the fibular head, and the decreased content of connective tissue.[28] A summary of his series suggested that sciatic injury was even more common than injury of its branches. (The frequency of femoral nerve injury was not mentioned in his series.)

In their large series of sacral fractures, Denis and coworkers found that 51 of 236 (22%) patients had nerve deficits attributable to fracture.[7] Six percent of alar fractures were associated with L5 deficits. Their second category, foraminal fractures, usually involved the L5, S1, and S2 roots. About half of these deficits resolved with conservative management.

In addition to fractures as a cause of nerve injury (see Chap. 43), numerous other causes have been described, including dislocations, operative complications, tumor resections, injection injuries, aneurysms, hematomas, compression during anesthesia, and traction during delivery.[28] Omer cites a 13% incidence of sciatic or peroneal nerve injury associated with posterior dislocation of the hip.[21] Similarly, knee dislocations have been noted to have an 18% incidence of peroneal nerve palsy.[21]

In total hip replacements, the reported incidence of postoperative sciatic nerve dysfunction is 1% to 3% in primary surgeries and 3% to 8% in revisions, according to Stone's review.[27] Rose and coworkers reported a 0.87% incidence of peroneal palsy after total knee replacement; most of these, attributed to traction, partially improved with time.[24] In general, open wounds had a poorer prognosis for nerve recovery than closed wounds, and dislocations associated with nerve palsies had a poorer prognosis than fractures with nerve palsies.[21]

APPLIED ANATOMY

A review of the anatomy of the nerves and their muscular and cutaneous innervations better defines the deficits associated with these lower extremity palsies (Fig. 53-1). The sciatic nerve (L4, L5, S1, S2, S3) divides into anterior and posterior divisions, the tibial (L4, L5, S1, S2, S3) and common peroneal (L4, L5, S1, S2) branches, which separate distal to the sciatic notch. In the thigh, the sciatic nerve innervates the biceps femoris, the semitendinosus, the semimembranosus, and part of the adductor magnus. The only cutaneous branch in the thigh is the posterior femoral cutaneous. Muscular branches of the tibial nerve supply the gastrocnemius, soleus, tibialis posterior, flexor digitorum longus, flexor hallucis longus, plantaris, popliteus, and intrinsic muscles of the foot. Almost the entire plantar surface of the foot and the posterolateral calf are innervated by the tibial nerve via the calcaneal, plantar, and medial sural branches.

The common peroneal nerve gives rise to superficial and deep branches. The former supplies the peroneus longus and brevis muscles and sensation to the anterolateral calf and dorsal foot. The latter innervates the tibialis anterior, extensor digitorum longus, extensor hallucis longus, and peroneus brevis and supplies sensation to the first dorsal web space.

The femoral nerve (L2, L3, L4) supplies the vastus medialis, intermedius, and lateralis, as well as the rectus femoris muscles. Its cutaneous branches supply the anterior thigh and the medial calf and foot via the saphenous nerves.

Deformities Associated with Lower Extremity Nerve Loss

A total sciatic nerve palsy leaves a major deficit. While hip motion and knee extension are preserved, knee flexion and ankle, foot, and toe motion are lost. Also, all regions of decreased sensation are susceptible to trauma and ulceration, especially the plantar surface of the foot. For the same reason, tibial palsies lead to ulceration more often than do common peroneal palsies.

In tibial nerve palsy, dorsiflexion and eversion of the foot and extension of the toes are preserved, but plantar flexion is not. Conversely, a common peroneal nerve palsy is associated with the ability to plantar-flex and invert the foot but not the ability to evert and extend the foot and toes.

A femoral nerve deficit lacks only knee extension and a small cutaneous deficit. The resultant deformities are variable and depend on the amount of splinting and range of motion achieved with prior therapy. The management of sensory deficits is discussed in Chapter 35.[10,20]

Historical Aspects of Lower Extremity Tendon Transfer

The history of tendon transfers for lower extremity nerve palsies dates back to 1882, when Viennese surgeon Karl Nicoladoni transferred the peroneal tendons to the Achilles tendon to generate plantar flexion in a patient with a calcaneus deformity secondary to poliomyelitis.[18] Mayer, a pioneer of tendon transplantation, subsequently outlined the guidelines for successful tendon transfer:[17]

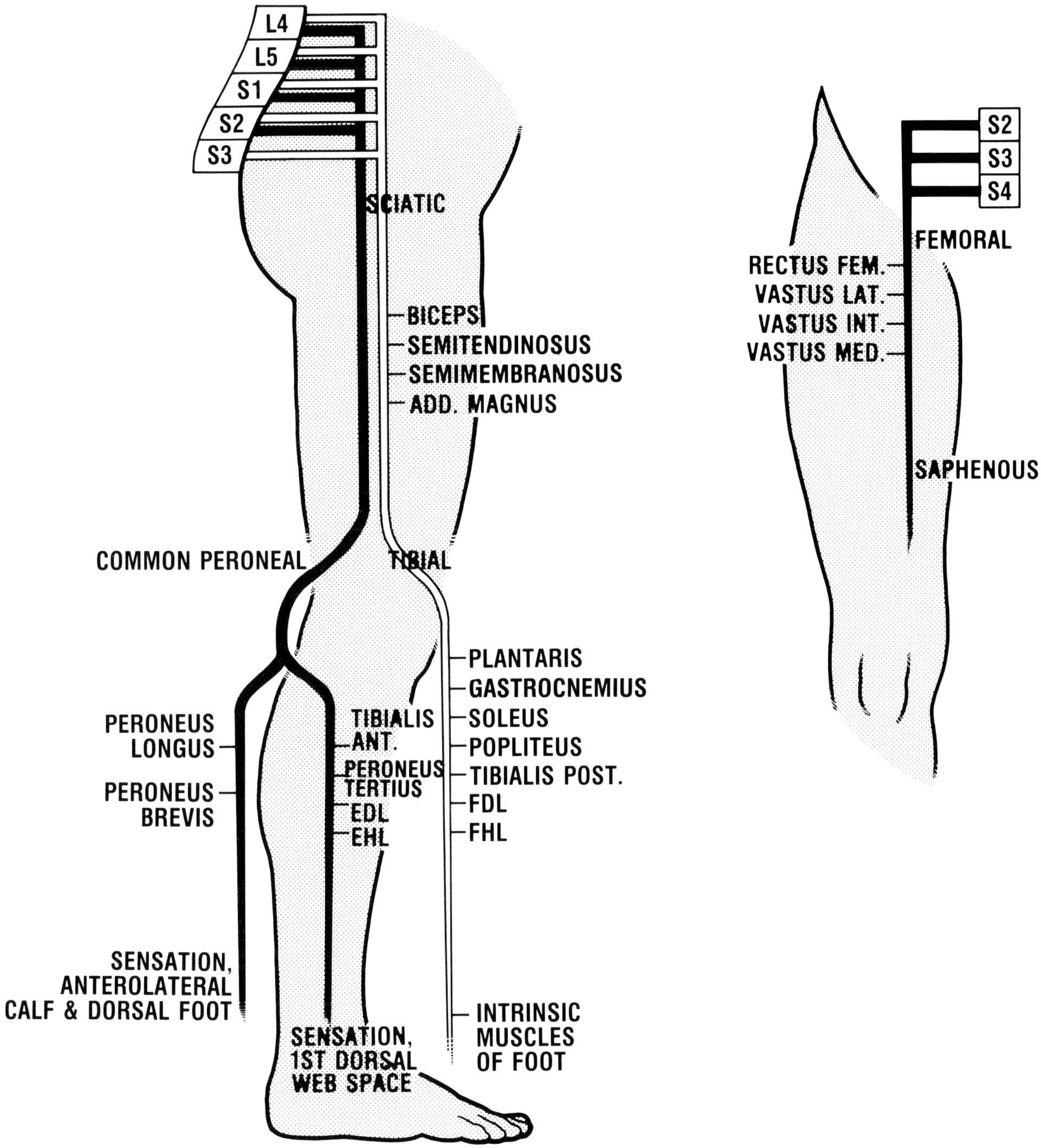

Figure 53–1. *Schematic diagram of the motor nerves and their muscles in the lower extremity.*

1. Deformity must be corrected first.
2. The line of action should be mechanically efficient and direct.
3. The transferred muscle must be strong enough to perform the desired function.
4. Stability of the foot is crucial.
5. Tendons are attached to bone.
6. Therapy begins when the tendon is firmly anchored and the bone has healed.

Many procedures have been described for palsies of the common peroneal, tibial, femoral, and sciatic nerves. This chapter's goal is to describe those techniques and offer guidance in the selection of one for selected irreparable nerve deficits.

COMMON PERONEAL PALSY

An irreparable common peroneal nerve palsy leads ultimately to an equinus or equinovarus deformity secondary to the deforming force of the tibialis posterior muscle. An ankle-stabilizing procedure, lengthening of a tight Achilles tendon, and anterior transfer of the tibialis posterior muscle are the mainstays of therapy for this palsy. The ankle-stabilizing procedures both correct deformity and allow transfer of muscles previously required for medial and lateral movement of the foot.

There are many techniques of stabilizing the ankle. Davis is credited with recognizing, in 1913, that fusing the major bones of the hindfoot to the talus prevents medial and lateral deviation.[6] In 1921 Hoke described talocalcaneal and calcaneonavicular arthrodesis, which involved removal and reshaping of the talar head.[14] In the same year, Dunn described a similar procedure with excision of the navicular, combined with talocuneiform fusion that effectively transferred the calcaneus posteriorly.[8] In 1923 Ryerson described the triple arthrodesis (talocalcaneal, talonavicular, and calcaneocuboid) via two skin incisions.[25] Subsequent variations were designed to minimize the deformity when it was associated with foot drop. In 1927 Lambrinudi suggested that a wedge removed from the head of the talus be inserted into the posterior portion of the talocalcaneal arthrodesis to maintain the talus in a relatively plantarflexed position, thereby minimizing the risk of recurrent equinus deformity.[15] In an alternative solution, the posterior bone block technique, a bone block is attached to the posterior dome of the talus to prevent further plantar flexion.[3] Pan-talar arthrodesis (ie, triple arthrodesis and tibiotalar fusion) is reserved as a salvage procedure, as it nearly eliminates plantar flexion and dorsiflexion of the foot.

Triple Arthrodesis

Authors' Preferred Method

This arthrodesis, based on Ryerson's method,[25] is best performed under tourniquet control via two incisions, although a single lateral incision may be sufficient. The medial incision begins about 1 to 2 cm inferior to the medial malleolus, extending over the tuberosity of the navicular to the proximal portion of the first metatarsal. The skin flaps are made as thick as possible, and the saphenous vein and nerve are preserved with the upper flap. By retracting the posterior tibial tendon dorsally, access to the subtalar joint is gained through the tendon sheath. Careful retraction is required to avoid injuring the flexor tendons, posterior tibial artery, and tibial nerve. Debridement of the cartilage surface and bone, as needed to correct deformity, is performed with curets, osteotomes, saws, or power burrers (Fig. 53-2). After opening the talonavicular joint capsule, cartilage is debrided. Once bony correction has been obtained, fixation is performed with staples, or plates and screws.

On the lateral side, a similar incision is made beginning 1 to 2 cm inferior to the lateral malleolus and extending distally toward the fourth toe, ending at the base of the fourth metatarsal. The sural nerve travels with the lesser saphenous vein and crosses this incision to the lateral side of the foot. The fat pad over the sinus tarsi is elevated with the medial skin flap. The origin of the extensor digitorum brevis is sharply removed from bone and reflected distally. The peroneal tendons are reflected anteriorly in the same manner as the posterior tibial tendon was managed on the medial side. These maneuvers allow access to both subtalar and calcaneocuboid joints. If this lateral approach is the only one used, the talonavicular joint is approached by elevating the flap medially onto the dorsum of the foot. Bony fixation is obtained, and then the tendon sheaths are reconstructed, the

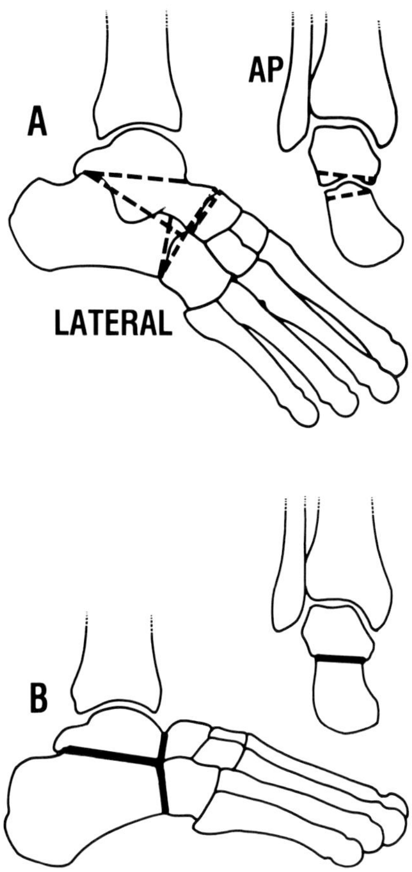

Figure 53–2. Triple arthrodesis for stabilization of the hindfoot. When needed, nonparallel bone cuts permit correction of fixed deformities.

origin of the short extensors is reattached to bone, and the skin edges are reapproximated atraumatically.

Two variations are designed specifically for foot drop. The Lambrinudi technique requires, first, resection of the head of the talus with an oblique osteotomy nearly perpendicular to the shaft of the tibia. Second, a notch is made in the posteroinferior region of the navicular. Third, the bone removed from the head of the talus is wedged in the posterior portion of the subtalar fusion to plantar-flex the talus. Then, the new anterior edge of the talus is inserted into the notch in the navicular. The goal is to leave the foot at 95° to the leg. Although the original description does not describe talonavicular or calcaneocuboid fusions, these are now usually included with this procedure.

The other procedure, the posterior bone block technique, requires a 10-cm vertical incision over the medial tendo calcaneus. This provides access to the posterior calcaneus and talus. Reflecting the flexor hallucis longus anteriorly and medially, the space over the posterior–superior surface of the calcaneus and the posterior dome of the talus are identified and cleared with an elevator. Decortication of these two bones and formation of a small notch prepares this space for the bone block. The block is constructed from the bony fragments removed as part of the triple arthrodesis or as grafts harvested from a separate site (such as the iliac crest). The block is large enough to extend at least 1 cm above the edge of the tibia (Fig. 53-3). Fixation is achieved with a screw or wires, so that the foot is blocked at an angle of 95° to the tibia. As a variation, Gill recommended removing the wedge of bone from the posterior calcaneus and securing

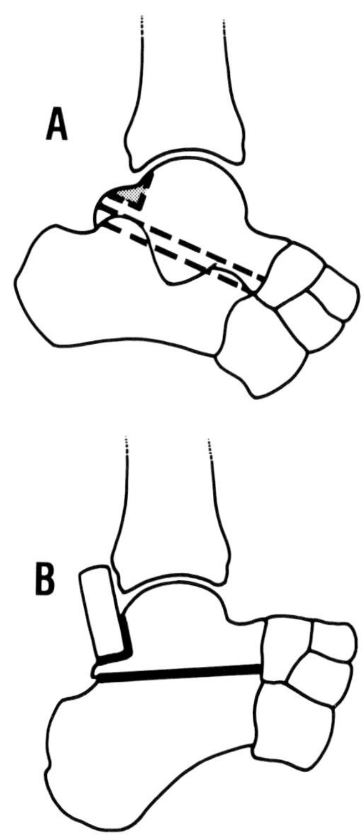

Figure 53–3. Posterior bone block to limit ankle plantar flexion may be combined with a triple arthrodesis.

it under a thin bony flap of the posterior dome of the talus.[9] Abrasion of the posterior surface of the tibia increases the risk of tibiotalar fusion.

If lengthening the Achilles tendon is required, this is performed using the same posteromedial incision along the edge of the Achilles tendon. The lengthening is performed using a Z-type cut and repair as described in most standard texts.

Forward transfer of the tibialis posterior via a superficial route is attributed to Ober. He suggested transfer so that the muscle belly lies in contact with the tibia and the tendon passes through the anterior compartment to the third metatarsal.[19] Lipscomb modified this by suggesting that fewer adhesions form if the entire transfer route is subcutaneous.[16] Searching for a more direct line of action, Putti transferred the posterior tibialis through the interosseous membrane to the dorsum of the foot; this technique is described in a series by Watkins.[30] Carayon added transfer of the flexor digitorum longus to the extensor hallucis longus and extensor digitorum longus to correct clawtoe deformity and augment ankle dorsiflexion.[4]

Anterior Transfer of Tibialis Posterior

Authors' Preferred Method

The tendon-retrieving incision is the same one used for the medial portion of the triple arthrodesis. The tendon is released at its bony insertion on the first cuneiform and navicular. It is wise to place either a whip stitch or a Kessler-type stitch at the distal end of the tendon in order to facilitate its transfer and subsequent anchoring. The second (rerouting) incision is made 1 to 2 cm lateral to the tibial crest, from just above the midshaft of the tibia to several centimeters above the ankle joint. After incising the deep fascia, the tibialis anterior muscle is retracted laterally, protecting the deep peroneal nerve (nonfunctional) and the anterior tibial artery. Adhesions to the tibia are minimized by leaving the periosteum intact. At about the midshaft of the tibia, the origin of the tibialis anterior muscle on the tibia begins; this is retracted or debrided as necessary. Staying on the lateral side of the tibia, the interosseous membrane is exposed and a large window made in it. The tibialis posterior muscle, the only muscle that lies directly behind the interosseous membrane, bulges into the anterior compartment. Injury to the posterior tibial artery, peroneal artery, and tibial nerve is avoided by carefully bringing the muscle and its tendon through the window.

Initially, the tendon is passed under the anterior tibial tendon and then subcutaneously to the dorsum of the foot (Fig. 53-4). The anchoring incision is the distal end of the lateral incision required for the arthrodesis. The site of anchoring the tendon is variable: Watkins favored the cuboid, Turner the third cuneiform.[29] Both agreed that it is anchored in a bony tunnel and that it is fixed by a Bunnell-type pull-out wire to the plantar surface of the foot. Ideally, the tendon is brought through a bony tunnel and then sutured to itself, avoiding a tract to the skin. Watkins recommended a cast for 6 weeks and further bracing for 3 additional months.

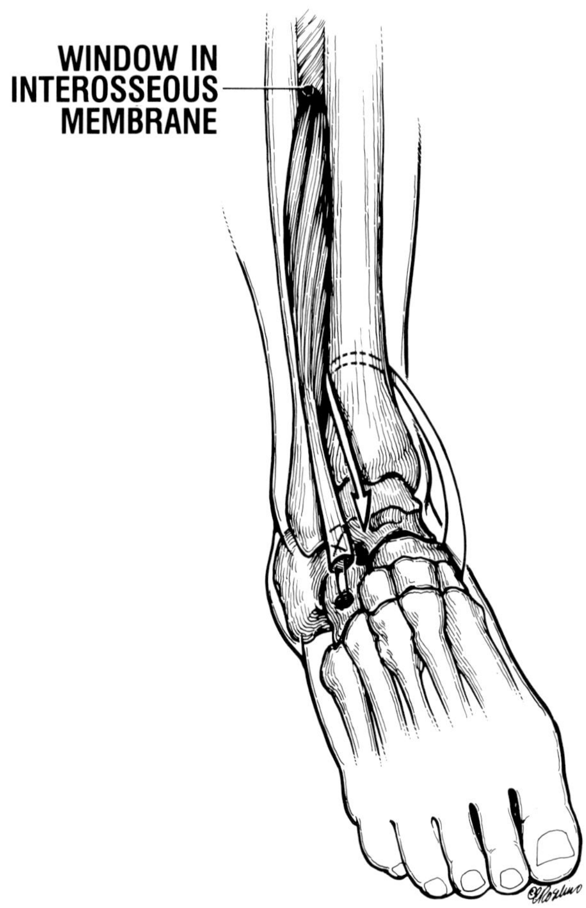

Figure 53–4. *Transfer of the posterior tibialis tendon to the dorsum of the foot (third metatarsal) as described by Ober. The tendon may also be passed through the interosseus membrane as described by Watkins and Barr.*

Arguing that subcutaneous transfer was easier and caused less adhesions, Lipscomb recommended that the transfer be performed via a medial route.[16] He agreed that a two-incision arthrodesis should be performed, but his technique required that the rerouting incision be made over the posteromedial portion of the calf. This incision is made 1 cm posterior to the palpable, medial border of the tibia in the middle third of that bone. In the subcutaneous portion of this incision, the saphenous nerve, which travels with the greater saphenous vein, is preserved. The upper limit of this incision is the muscle innervation by the tibial nerve. A tendon-passer is then used to pass this tendon around the medial border of the tibia to the dorsum of the foot. No attempt is made to bring the tendon through the extensor retinaculum. Bony insertions are made in the second or third cuneiform or occasionally into the base of the third metatarsal. Postoperative immobilization is carried out for 3 months in a short leg cast.

Carayon transferred the posterior tibial tendon anteriorly via the interosseous membrane, attaching it to the anterior tibial tendon.[4] (Leprosy was the cause of the nerve palsy in most of his cases.) In addition, the flexor digitorum longus was transferred to the extensor hallucis longus and the extensor digitorum longus tendons. His procedures were not performed with an ankle-stabilization procedure. The transfers were performed via two incisions: one posteromedial to the tibia down to the medial malleolus, where the tendons were divided, and a second over the anterolateral portion of the calf to the lateral malleolus. No incisions were made in the foot. Immobilization was carried out for 2 weeks.

Complications

The complications of the ankle-stabilizing procedures are many, including recurrence of deformity, excess varus or valgus, arthritis of the ankle or tarsal joints, osteonecrosis of the talus, and pseudarthrosis. The long-term results of triple arthrodeses were reviewed most recently by Angus.[1] With an average 13-year follow-up, 62% had residual deformity, 22% pseudarthrosis, 14% severe degenerative changes, and 25% pain. Correction of an equinovarus deformity was the procedure most commonly associated with a poor result. In addition, varus deformity of the arthrodesis was often poorly tolerated.

Inadvertent laceration of the sural or saphenous nerve can lead to formation of a painful neuroma. In the Lambrinudi technique, resection of a large talar fragment increases the risk of osteonecrosis. Also, preoperative ankle laxity is a contraindication because the plantar-flexed talus is narrower in the mortise. With the posterior bone block, a small block is susceptible to resorption, whereas a large one makes the ankle joint more prone to ankylosis.

Results

Watkins' series reported excellent results in 17 of 25 cases (ie, good foot position, good power of transplant, correction of functional deformity, and improved gait).[30] Using the same technique, Turner noted that even among muscles with 4+ strength, none gained phasic function in normal gait.[29] Lipscomb noted active dorsiflexion to at least -10° in all but one of his transfers.[16] Carayon reported that more than half his patients had active dorsiflexion to 5°.[4]

TIBIAL NERVE PALSY

Tibial nerve palsy is much less common than common peroneal nerve palsy. It responds poorly to attempts at bracing, which result in either a calcaneus or a calcaneocavus deformity, as well as a significant sensory deficit often associated with skin ulceration. Beginning with Nicoladoni's peroneal tendon transfer,[18] numerous approaches have been attempted: Whitman's "astralgectomy" (talectomy), tibial osteotomies, and even transfer of the tensor fascia lata.

More recently, several elements of a successful corrective procedure have been identified. A preliminary ankle-stabilizing procedure corrects deformity while lengthening the lever arm of a transferred muscle, if stabilization has brought about posterior displacement of the calcaneus. Second, plantar release is usually performed to diminish cavus deformity. Ultimately, a tendon transfer of the tibialis anterior or peroneal tendons to the posterior calcaneus is required to correct muscle imbalance. Residual toe deformity is corrected in a separate procedure. When a sensory deficit is associated with chronic ulceration or infection, a neurovascular island pedicle flap is considered.

Triple Arthrodesis with Posterior Displacement

Authors' Preferred Method

Our preferred method is based on Hoke's approach.[14] The standard two-incision approach is used. Osteotomies are made to correct the deformity, and the head of the talus is removed to permit posterior displacement of the calcaneus on the talus (Fig. 53-5). Removal of a large portion of the talar head increases the risk of osteonecrosis.

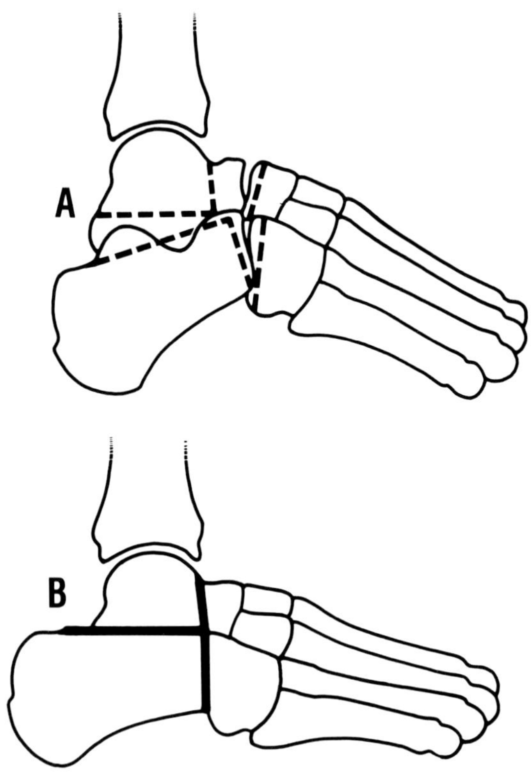

Figure 53–5. *Hoke triple arthrodesis with posterior displacement of the calcaneus achieved by resection of a portion of the talar head and neck. (**A**) Proposed bone resection lines. (**B**) Final position.*

Bony fixation is with staples, wires, or screws. Posterior displacement is also achieved by resecting the navicular bone while performing a triple arthrodesis, as described by Dunn.[8]

Posterior Transfer of Anterior Tibial Tendon[12,13]

The retrieval incision is made along the medial side of the first cuneiform and base of the first metatarsal. This is reached easily at the distal end of the medial incision made for the arthrodesis. The tendon is removed from the first metatarsal and cuneiform subperiosteally. A second (rerouting) incision is made 1 cm lateral to the anterior tibial crest. This 15-cm incision is used to identify the anterior tibial muscle, the deep peroneal nerve, and the anterior tibial artery. After retracting these structures laterally, a large window is made in the interosseous membrane. In the posterior compartment, dissection along the posterolateral surface of the tibia allows the surgeon to avoid injuring the posterior tibial artery. The third (attachment) incision is made over the medial edge of the calcaneus and tendocalcaneus. The inferior end of the tendon is split longitudinally and the tendon anchored in an osteoperiosteal "trapdoor." Alternatively, the tendon is passed through a drill hole in the medial side of the calcaneus and then sutured to itself. The transfer is tensioned with the foot in a position of maximum equinus.

The actions of the tibialis anterior and peroneus longus muscles on the proximal first metatarsal are opposite. Transfer of the former may result in a residual cock-up deformity of the great toe. This can be corrected by transferring the extensor hallucis longus to the first metatarsal head.

For children under 12, Bradley and Coleman described an oblique osteotomy of the calcaneus with posterior–superior displacement of the fragment attached to the tendocalcaneus.[2]

Results

Quantitative evaluation of the results has been difficult because the power of the triceps surae is irreplaceable. Mayer reported that 40% of patients regained tiptoe capability when transferring both peroneal tendons, and the tibialis posterior and flexor digitorum longus tendons.[17]

SCIATIC NERVE PALSY

The most severe nerve deficit in the lower limb is sciatic nerve palsy. While knee extension is possible, active knee flexion and ankle and toe motion are not. In addition, the sensory deficit is extensive, with only the saphenous nerve providing sensation below the knee. Observations made in the era of poliomyelitis suggest that a flail knee is tolerated in the face of a stable hip and ankle.[11] Thus, an ankle-stabilizing procedure may afford these patients a brace-free gait.

Clawson and Seddon described the largest series (329) of patients with this deficit.[5] Numerous problems were confronted: pain (58%), paresthesia (21%), hyperesthesia (35%), vasomotor dysfunction (50%), and pressure sores (14%). Despite this, a surprisingly high level of function was seen in some of these patients, including rock climbing, golfing, and flying aircraft. The primary deformity seen with sciatic nerve palsy is foot drop and claw toes. As an ankle-stabilizing procedure, a posterior bone block or Lambrinudi-type arthrodesis is preferred over pan-talar arthrodesis, because the latter increases the risk of recurvatum at the knee. Aggressive correction of toe deformity through tendon and capsular releases and bony fusions is recommended, because half of the pressure sores are associated with fixed deformity. Amputation often fails to relieve pain. Microsurgical nerve transfers and island flaps for sensation are indicated in selected cases.[10]

FEMORAL NERVE PALSY

Femoral nerve palsy results in loss of active extension of the knee. The deficit is usually not critical for gait, except for climbing stairs or inclines, yet patients often note feelings of knee instability. If this is a problem, several muscles can be transferred from the posterior thigh to the patella to generate active extension. The sensory deficit over the anterior thigh and medial calf and foot does not require intervention.

Restoration of active knee extension requires transfer of posterior muscles anteriorly to the patella. Mayer identified the biceps femoris as the strongest and suggested the sartorius as the second muscle for transfer.[17] He also considered the semitendinosus and gracilis muscles suitable donors. Ober suggested that the tensor fascia lata and sartorius be used.[19] Herndon recommended the biceps femoris and semitendinosus tendons.[12] More recently, Omer[22] recommended transfer of the biceps alone, whereas Wiesseman[31] urged the addition of the semitendinosus.

Anterior Transfer of the Biceps Femoris[12,13]

Authors' Preferred Method

The retrieval incision for the biceps tendon is made over the palpable biceps tendon and extends from the fibular head to above the midshaft of the femur. The proximal extent of this incision is limited by the mobility of the biceps muscle and its neurovascular pedicle (sciatic, profunda femoris). Careful dissection 5 cm proximal to the fibular head allows the surgeon to avoid injuring the common peroneal nerve, which travels medial to the biceps tendon in the posterior thigh. The short head of the biceps is separated from the femur and linea aspera. Several perforating arterial branches from the profunda femoris are ligated. The distal insertion of the biceps tendon is then separated from the fibula and tagged. A large window is made in the lateral intermuscular septum and fascia lata. The route of the tendon is through this window, under the vastus lateralis, and through the quadriceps tendon to the superior patella (Fig. 53-6A).

The second, or anchoring, incision is a short vertical incision over the superior patella and quadriceps tendon. Fixation is either through an osseous tunnel from the superior pole of the patella to the anterior surface, or into an osteoperiosteal flap.

The leg is held in extension for 4 weeks, after which re-education is begun. A brace preventing acute flexion is then used for 3 to 6 months.

If the biceps femoris muscle has inadequate strength or causes lateral subluxation of the patella, the semitendinosus tendon should also be

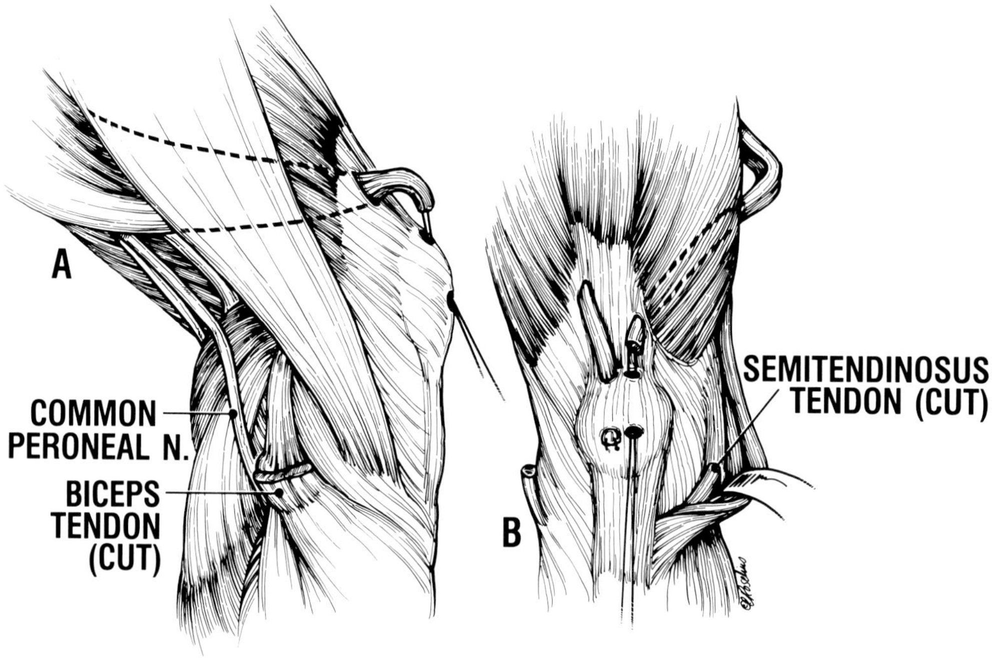

Figure 53–6. *Transfer of the biceps femoris and semitendinosus to the patella in femoral nerve palsy with quadriceps paralysis.*

transferred (Fig. 53-6B). The retrieval incision is over the medial, proximal tibia near the tibial tubercle and can be quite small. The surgeon should recall that the semitendinosus tendon is the most inferior of the tendons of the pes anserinus and that its insertion flares. A good rule of thumb is that the pes anserinus begins about 5 cm below the joint line. The upper end of the tendon sheath is very thin and lies directly over the distal end of the medial collateral ligament of the knee. The upper tendons are those of the sartorius and gracilis muscles. A second incision over the posteromedial hamstrings, at about midfemur, is used to reroute the tendon. The new course of this tendon is initially subcutaneous, then under the vastus medialis, and through the quadriceps tendon to the patella. It can be anchored by the same technique described above.

Complications

Complications of these procedures are numerous, including injury to the common peroneal, tibial, sciatic, and saphenous nerves and injury to the lateral collateral ligament. Genu recurvatum is uncommon. Transfer of the biceps femoris tendon alone is associated with lateral subluxation or dislocation of the patella. Other technical errors can lead to an incorrect line of pull for these transferred muscles. The evaluation of results reveals that extension of the knee against gravity is often attainable, although progressive stair climbing is not. The more common practical goal is ambulation without fear of buckling.[31] Schwartzmann and Crego's review of their initial results using only biceps femoris tendon revealed a 29% rate of lateral patellar dislocation in polio patients.[26]

REFERENCES

1. Angus PD, Cowell HR. Triple arthrodesis. A critical long-term review. J Bone Joint Surg [Br] 1986; 68: 260–265.
2. Bradley GW, Coleman SS. Treatment of the calcaneocavus foot deformity. J Bone Joint Surg [Am] 1981; 63:1159–1166.

3. Campbell WC. An operation for the correction of "drop-foot". J Bone Joint Surg 1923; 5:815.
4. Carayon A, Bourrel P, Bourges M, Touze M. Dual transfer of the posterior tibial and flexor digitorum longus tendons for drop foot. J Bone Joint Surg [Am] 1967; 49:144–148.
5. Clawson DK, Seddon HJ. The late consequences of sciatic nerve injury. J Bone Joint Surg [Br] 1960; 42:213–225.
6. Davis GG. The treatment of hollow foot (pes cavus). Am J Orthop Surg 1913; 11:231.
7. Denis F, Davis S, Comfort T. Sacral fractures: An important problem. Retrospective analysis of 236 cases. Clin Orthop 1988; 227:67–81.
8. Dunn N. Stabilizing operations in the treatment of paralytic deformities of the foot. Proc R Soc Med 1921; 15:15–22.
9. Gill AB. An operation to make a posterior bone block at the ankle to limit foot-drop. J Bone Joint Surg 1933; 15:166–170.
10. Hall EJ, Buncke HJ. Microsurgical techniques to reconstruct irreparable nerve loss. Orthop Clin 1981; 12:381–401.
11. Hallock, H. Arthrodesis of the hip for instability and pain in poliomyelitis. J Bone Joint Surg [Am] 1950; 32:904.
12. Herndon CH. Tendon transplantation at the knee and foot. In: American Academy of Orthopaedic Surgeons. Instructional Course Lectures. St. Louis: CV Mosby, 1961; 18:145–168.
13. Herndon CH, Strong JM, Heyman CH. Transposition of the tibialis anterior in the treatment of paralytic talipes Calcaneus. J Bone Joint Surg [Am] 1956; 38:751–760.
14. Hoke M. An operation for stabilizing paralytic feet. Am J Orthop Surg 1921; 3:494–507.
15. Lambrinudi C. New operation on drop-foot. Br J Surg 1927; 15:193–200.
16. Lipscomb PR, Sanchez JJ. Anterior transplantation of the posterior tibial tendon for persistent palsy of the common peroneal nerve. J Bone Joint Surg [Am] 1961; 43:60–66.
17. Mayer L. Tendon transplantation on the lower extremity. In: The American Academy of Orthopaedic Surgeons, Instructional Course Lectures. Ann Arbor; J W Edwards, 1949; 6:189–200.
18. Nicoladoni K. Nachtragzum Pes calcaneus und zur Transplantation der peronealsehnen. Arch Klin Chir 1881; 27:660.
19. Ober FR. Tendon transplantation in the lower extremity. N Engl J Med 1933; 209:52–59.
20. Omer GE. Tendon transfers as reconstructive procedures in the leg and foot. In: Omer GE, Spinner M, eds. Management of peripheral nerve problems. Philadelphia: W B Saunders, 1980:873–880.
21. Omer GE. Results of untreated peripheral nerve injuries, Clin Orthop 1982; 163:15–19.
22. Omer GE. Reconstructive procedures for extremities with peripheral nerve defects. Clin Orthop 1982; 163:80–91.
23. Reidy JA, Broderick TF, Barr, JS. Tendon transplantations in the lower extremity. J Bone Joint Surg [Am] 1952; 34:900–914.
24. Rose HA, Hood RW, Otis JC, Ranawat CS, Insall JN. Peroneal-nerve Palsy following total knee arthroplasty. J Bone Joint Surg [Am] 1982; 64:347–351.
25. Ryerson EW. Arthrodesing operations on the feet. J Bone Joint Surg 1923; 5:453–471.
26. Schwartzmann JR, Crego CH. Hamstring-tendon transplantation for the relief of quadriceps femoris paralysis in residual poliomyelitis. A follow-up study of 134 cases. J Bone Joint Surg [Am] 1948; 30:541–549.
27. Stone RG, Weeks LE, Hajdu M, Stinchfield FE. Evaluation of sciatic nerve compromise during total hip arthrosplasty. Clin Orthop 1985; 201:26–31.
28. Sunderland S. Nerves and nerve injuries, ed 2. Edinburgh: Churchill Livingstone, 1978:967–991.
29. Turner JW, Cooper RR. Anterior transfer of the tibialis posterior through the interosseous membrane. Clin Orthop 1972; 83:241.
30. Watkins MB, Jones JB, Ryder CT, Brown TH. Transplantation of the posterior tibial tendon. J Bone Joint Surg [Am] 1954; 36;1181–1189.
31. Wiesseman GJ. Tendon transfers for peripheral nerve injuries of the lower extremity. Orthop Clin 1981; 12:459–467.

54

Free Muscle Transfer for Functional Reconstruction

Ralph T. Manktelow

AUTHOR'S KEY POINTS

- Patient selection is important to successful outcome of muscle transplantation. The ideal extremity for finger reconstruction has intact median and ulnar nerves providing hand sensation, intrinsic muscle function, and adequate finger extensor function.
- The operative technique is precise. An appropriate, undamaged motor nerve and insertion of the muscle at proper tension are critical steps in the procedure.
- This procedure is complex and requires significant time before maximal functional return.
- Alternate techniques of tendon transfers are used if available.

Functioning muscle transplantation involves the transfer of all of a skeletal muscle from one site to another by means of microneurovascular techniques. Circulation and survival of the muscle are ensured by microvascular anastomoses between the muscle's artery and vein and vessels in the recipient site. Useful function occurs through reinnervation with the motor nerve.

The quality of muscle function depends on the muscle selected, the adequacy of reinnervation, fixation of the muscle's origin and insertion at optimum tension, the quality of the muscle-tendon bed, and the postoperative exercise program.

Muscle such as the gracilis, latissimus dorsi, tensor fascia lata, and pectoralis major can be transplanted reliably with good expectation of survival and function.

Tamai demonstrated in 1970 the feasibility of transplanting muscle in the experimental animal.[8] Subsequently, Harii used the gracilis muscle to reconstruct the face following facial nerve paralysis,[1] and a surgical team of the Sixth People's Hospital in Shanghai successfully transplanted the lateral portion of the pectoralis major muscles to provide finger flexion in a patient with Volkmann's ischemic contracture.[7] We have had clinical experience with 98 functioning muscle transplantations in Toronto: 60 for facial reanimation for smile reconstruction and 38 to the upper extremity and leg for functional reconstruction.[4–6]

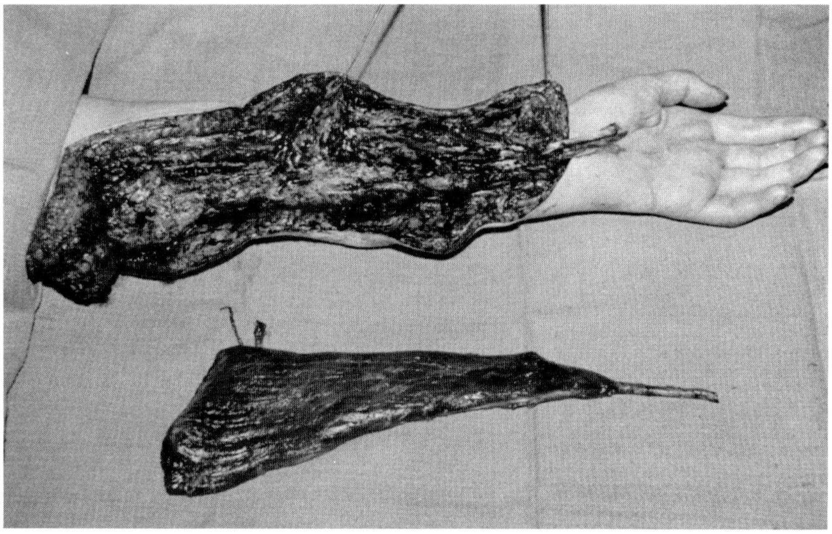

Figure 54-1. *The forearm and muscle after both have been prepared for muscle transplantation. The gracilis muscle is used to provide finger flexion.*

In the upper extremity, transplantation to the forearm provides very useful mass flexion or extension of the fingers or elbow or shoulder flexion (Figs. 54-1, 54-2). The purpose of this chapter is to outline our experience with muscle transplantation to the extremities and to review the factors important for the success of this procedure.

INDICATIONS

Muscle transplantation is considered for patients with significant functional deficits because of a major loss of skeletal musculature. Since this is a relatively complex procedure, and the patient must wait until reinnervation has occurred before useful

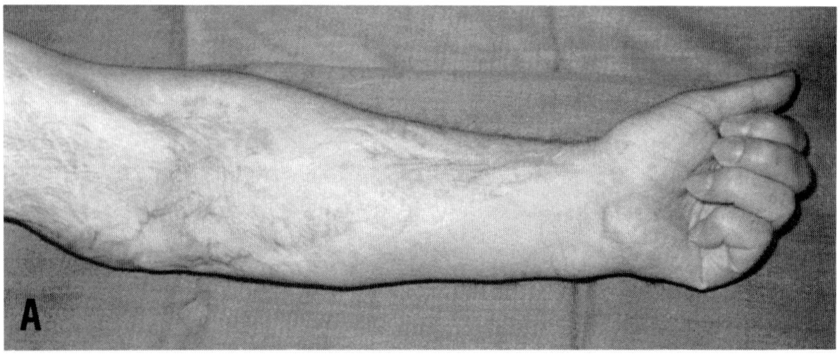

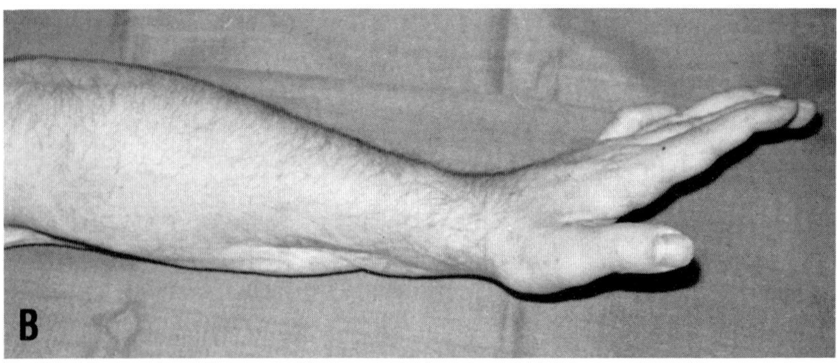

Figure 54-2. *(**A**) This patient sustained a severe injury to the forearm, with loss of all the finger flexors, in an industrial accident. The flexor carpi ulnaris, a portion of the flexor pollicis longus, and the median and ulnar nerves were spared. A gracilis muscle was used for finger flexor replacement. The muscle provides full finger flexion. (**B**) With relaxation, the muscle allows full finger extension and modest wrist extension.*

function is obtained, simpler procedures such as tendon transfers are used if possible.

The primary application of muscle transplantation to the extremities has been to the flexor and extensor compartments of the forearm. We have used the gracilis, pectoralis major, and latissimus dorsi muscles for this purpose on 28 occasions. Muscle transplantation has a more limited application to the extensor compartment of the forearm, where it is used primarily if there are no flexors available for transfer. The most common causes of muscle loss are direct injury to muscle by trauma and by compartment syndrome leading to muscle necrosis.

SELECTING AN APPROPRIATE MUSCLE

The anatomical structure of the muscle to be used must fit the recipient site. Its length and bulk and the location of the vascular and neural pedicles are determined to be appropriate. The origin and insertion of the muscle should have sufficient tendon structure to allow a strong attachment to recipient structures.

The selected muscle should have adequate strength and a suitable range of motion for the recipient area. A strap muscle is ideal, as its excursion with contraction is greater than that of a pennate muscle. The bulkier the muscle, the more powerful the contraction, since the amount of muscle contractile force is proportional to the cross-sectional area of the muscle fibers.

The gracilis muscle is the most suitable muscle in our experience (Fig. 54-3). It is raised with or without a cutaneous flap, which is quite reliable over the proximal half of the muscle (Fig. 54-4). However, this cutaneous flap tends to be bulky on the forearm and the usual practice is to raise the muscle alone and apply a skin graft to the proximal muscle belly if necessary. The muscle length is suitable for most locations and there is a long tendon of insertion. The range of excursion is more than 10 to 12 cm in most adult muscles. This is much greater than the 6 cm required to replace long finger flexor function (see Chaps. 48 and 50).

OPERATIVE TECHNIQUE

A number of prerequisites must be met for a patient to be judged suitable for muscle transplantation. A good range of passive joint motion at all joints that will be activated by the transplant is achieved preoperatively. In forearm muscle transplantation there should be potential for useful hand function. This requires good intrinsic musculature and good sensibility. Skin flap coverage is available for the distal half of the muscle and muscle tendon junction so that there will be a good gliding bed.

Planning the recipient site requires consideration of five anatomical structures:

1. The site of muscle origin
2. The site of muscle insertion
3. Skin flaps that will house the muscle
4. Vessels for microvascular anastomoses
5. A pure motor nerve for reinnervation.

The known extent of injury allows the surgeon to anticipate the location and condition of these

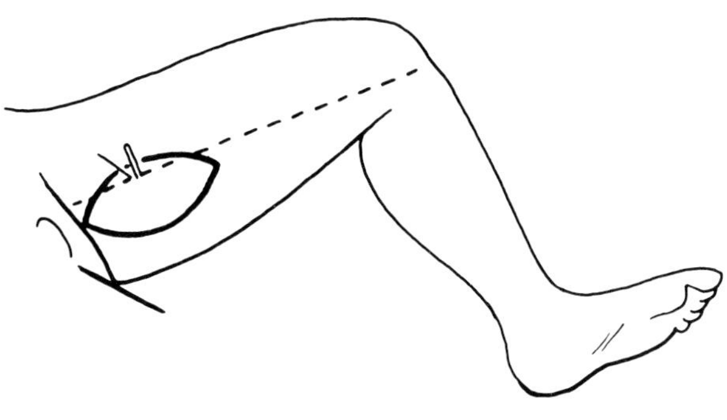

Figure 54–3. *The gracilis muscle is found below a line extending from the pubic tubercle to the tibial tubercle. (From Manktelow RT. Microvascular reconstruction. New York: Springer-Verlag, 1986:44, with permission.)*

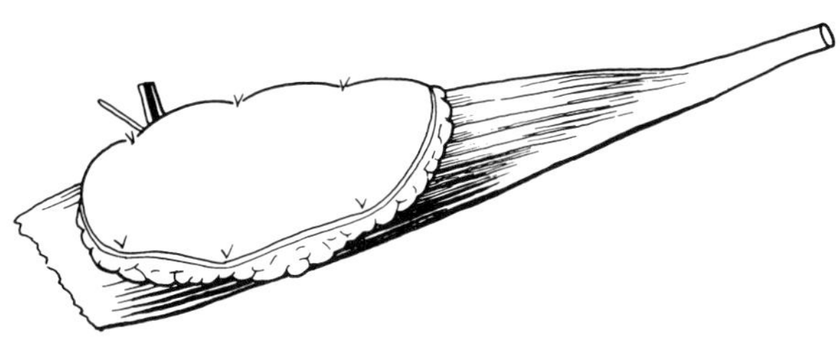

Figure 54–4. *When a skin flap is required, it is outlined below this line and centered over the dominant pedicle, which identifies the constant cutaneous perforator that supplies the skin paddle. (From Manktelow RT. Microvascular reconstruction. New York: Springer-Verlag, 1986:44, with permission.)*

structures. Usually an arteriogram is used to confirm the condition of the recipient artery. Venous repairs to either the superficial vein or the venae comitantes of the chosen artery are planned. An undamaged motor nerve is chosen for reinnervation. If the nerve is a mixed nerve, it creates a significant problem in identifying the motor component of the nerve. For forearm flexor reinnervation, the anterior interosseous nerve is often spared from injury because of its deep location and is ideal for reinnervating long finger flexors. If a mixed nerve is used (such as the musculocutaneous nerve for biceps reconstruction), the motor fascicles are chosen on the basis of awake stimulation, histochemical studies, or the surgeon's anatomical knowledge of the location of the motor component (see Chaps. 14, 15, and 16). If there is a question about the quality of the motor nerve, preliminary operative exploration and histologic evaluation of the nerve is carried out.

Good skin flap coverage is required at the site of tendon insertion to cover the distal portion of the muscle. This allows good tendon gliding and, if necessary, facilitates subsequent tenolysis procedures. Flap coverage is provided by the skin that is present, augmented by tissue expansion, preliminary flap coverage, or transferring the muscle as a myocutaneous flap.

Preparing the Muscle

Before surgery, recipient sites are marked with the expected positions of vessels, motor nerve, and the location of muscle origin and insertion. A pattern of the desired muscle with the location of the vessels and nerve identified is then drawn and applied to different parts of the patient's body in an effort to determine the optimal muscle. In practice we have found the gracilis muscle to be suitable for all locations in the upper extremities.

Safe excision of the selected muscle depends upon a clear understanding of the muscle's anatomy.[3] The muscle is separated from its surrounding structures and the pedicle is dissected free from its branches and the surrounding tissues. Secondary vascular attachments are severed so the muscle can be assessed when it is supplied by its single dominant pedicle. Adequate signs of muscle viability are color, contractility, and bleeding.

To facilitate insertion of the muscle at optimal tension, the muscle is marked prior to its transfer. The muscle is placed at the maximal physiological tension before separating origin and insertion. In the case of the gracilis muscle, this tension is accomplished by abducting the thigh and extending the knee. Suture markers, placed at 5-cm intervals along the muscle's surface, assist in inserting the muscle at the correct tension in the arm (Fig. 54-5).

Preparing the Recipient Site

Before removing the muscle from its donor site, the recipient site is prepared completely (Fig. 54-6). This often is one of the most technically demanding parts of the procedure, particularly if there has been severe trauma and the recipient vessels and nerves are encased in scar tissue. Each

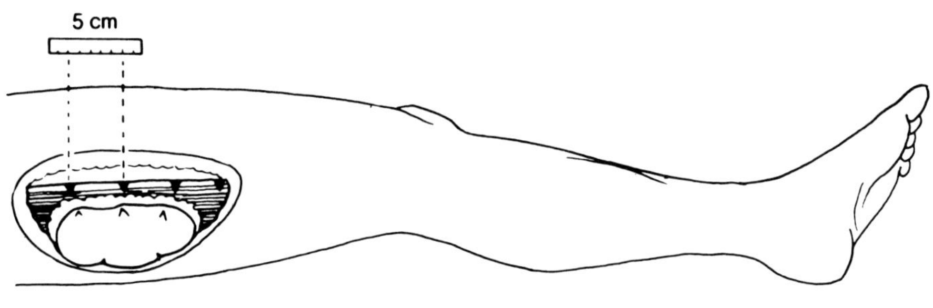

Figure 54–5. *In repairing the gracilis for transfer, it is stretched to its physiological extended maximum length by abducting the thigh and extending the knee. Suture markers are placed every 5 cm on the surface of the muscle. (From Manktelow RT. Microvascular reconstruction. New York: Springer-Verlag, 1986:157, with permission.)*

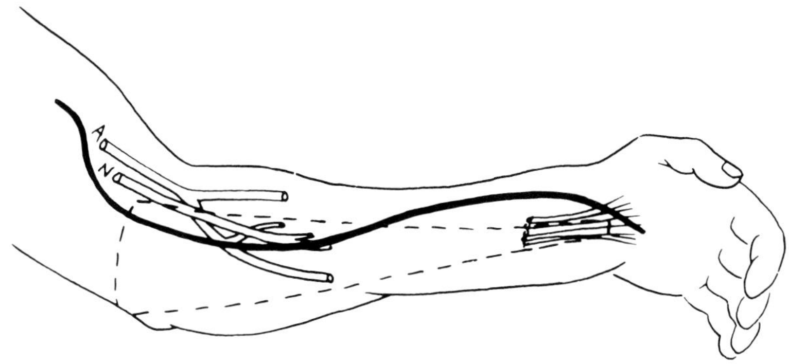

Figure 54–6. *The incision (heavy line) is outlined after identifying the expected location of the recipient's vessels, motor nerve, and tendons. The incision should allow good coverage of the flexor tendon repair in the wrist. (From Manktelow RT. Microvascular reconstruction. New York: Springer-Verlag, 1986:156, with permission.)*

of the structures to be used in the transfer, including the origin, tendons of insertion, motor nerve, veins, arteries, and skin flaps, is prepared before separating the muscle.

Muscle Transplantation

The muscle is first loosely tacked with sutures in the recipient site to visualize the proper position of the muscle with respect to the vessel and nerve repairs. To avoid placing undue tension on the vessel repair sites, the muscle is stretched and allowed to relax through the normal range it performs. This maneuver allows visualization of possible tension on vessel and nerve repair sites.

Usually the transplantation is carried out in the following order:

1. Revascularization
2. Nerve repair
3. Positioning of origin and insertion at optimal tension
4. Flap or graft coverage.

The experimental work of Kuzon, and our own clinical experience, suggest that 3 hours of warm ischemia time is not damaging to the eventual functional return of muscle.[2] Therefore, there is adequate time to perform the anastomosis carefully and precisely to minimize the possibility of subsequent thrombosis. Usually the venous repair or repairs are done first, followed by the arterial repair. Following completion of the vascular anastomoses, the muscle turns pink and bleeds from the perimysium. Occasionally the distal portion of the muscle remains dark; this portion is trimmed if it does not "pink up" after 5 to 10 minutes.

A technically perfect nerve repair with end-to-end fascicle apposition is then carried out. The gracilis motor nerve has considerable fatty connective tissue, which is trimmed away so that individual fascicles are repaired. The repair is placed as close as possible to the neuromuscular junction in order to minimize denervation time and atrophy of the muscle.

When muscle is used to provide motion to more than one structure, as in four fingers, the fingers are placed in a functional position throughout their ranges of excursion. To ensure this, individual finger tendons are sutured together so that all fingers flex in parallel, giving a balanced grip or balanced extension (Fig. 54-7). For finger flexor reconstruction, only the profundus tendons are used. The muscle's tendon is then woven into the profundus tendons en masse and fixed with multiple mattress sutures. Satisfactory tension is required in the transplanted muscle for maximal muscle strength. As the most powerful contraction occurs when the muscle is almost fully stretched, it is important that adequate tension be used when inserting the muscle. For forearm flexor reconstruction, the muscle is attached to the medial epicondyle and surrounding fascia. The muscle is then stretched until the markings previously made with sutures are once again 5 cm apart. Then, with the fingers and wrist in extension, the position of the profundus tendons relative to the gracilis tendon is noted. This is the site at which the tendon repair is done. This placement allows full finger and wrist extension within the most powerful range of the muscle's contraction. The actual tendon repair is done with the wrist

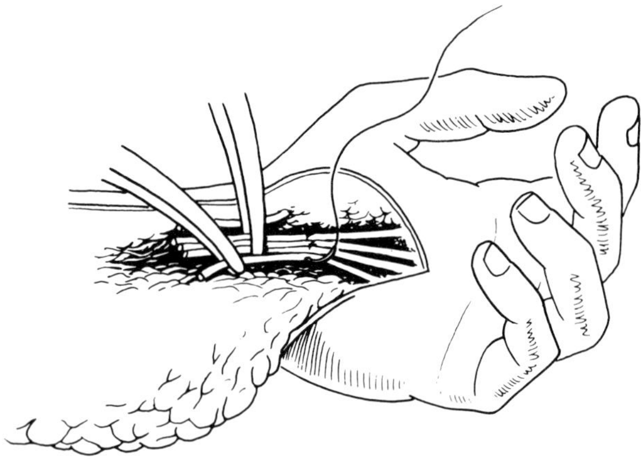

Figure 54–7. *The four flexor tendons are sutured to each other so that the fingers will flex in a balanced position to provide a firm grip with all fingers in contact with the gripped object. (From Manktelow RT. Microvascular reconstruction. New York: Springer-Verlag, 1986:160, with permission.)*

and fingers flexed, so that undue tension at the site of repair is avoided (Fig. 54-8).

Usually, adjacent forearm or upper arm skin is available for coverage of the distal part of the muscle and the muscle tendon junction and nerve and vessel pedicles. If necessary, a skin graft is applied to the proximal portion of the muscle. This does not limit the muscle's useful range of excursion.

Postoperative Care

Good blood flow is necessary to maintain patency of anastomoses in the immediate postoperative period. The patient is kept warm and given adequate intravenous fluids both during and after the operation.

Tension is minimized in the suture repairs at the origin and insertion by flexing the extremity suitably and splinting it for 3 weeks. After this time, passive stretching exercises are carried out. In the case of a finger flexor muscle transfer, these involve passively extending the fingers and wrist. Passive excursion prevents muscle and tendon adherence to the surrounding tissues. Once a satisfactory range of passive tendon gliding is developed, when reinnervation occurs the muscle is able to produce the desired motion. After a good range of active motion is developed, a program of resisted exercises is carried out daily at the level of the muscle's maximal strength in order to maximize the contractile capability of the muscle.

RESULTS

Muscle transplantation to the extremities has been used in a variety of locations, primarily in the upper extremity. We have performed muscle transfer for reconstruction of finger flexion in 32 cases, finger

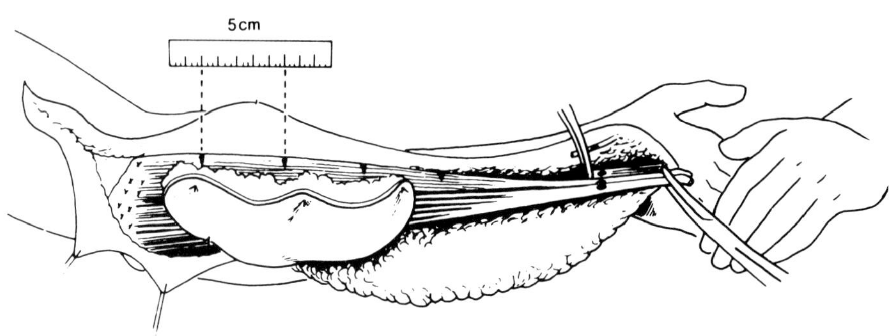

Figure 54–8. *After neurovascular repairs and attachment of the gracilis to the medial epicondyle and common flexor fascia, the tension is determined. With the fingers and wrist in full passive extension, the gracilis is stretched distally until the previously placed sutures on the surface are 5 cm apart. The dots are placed opposite each other on the flexor digitorum profundus and the gracilis tendon, to locate the point at which the tendons should be sutured together. This provides adequate tension to the muscle to allow maximum grip strength and a full range of motion. (From Manktelow RT. Microvascular reconstruction. New York: Springer-Verlag, 1986:160, with permission.)*

extension in six cases, upper arm biceps reconstruction in one case, and upper arm deltoid reconstruction in three patients. In the lower leg, muscle transplantation has been used on three occasions for dorsiflexion of the ankle.

Twenty-two patients with finger flexor transfers were available for long-term follow-up of more than 2 years. Twelve showed excellent results, seven had good results, one was fair, and two were poor.

We have classified our results in terms of range of motion and grip strength. Range of motion has been classified as follows:

Excellent: Full finger flexion and extension with the wrist in a stable functional position
Good: A useful range of motion that allows gripping of large and small objects
Fair: A small amount of motion that provides some useful cupping function of the fingers
Poor: No movement

Fourteen patients, some of them children, were available for grip strength evaluation. The results were expressed as a percentage of the individual's grip strength on the opposite arm. The range of strength varied from 11% to 69% of the normal arm (average, 33.3%).

Of the 22 patients, 19 felt the procedure was successful and 3 (those with fair and poor range-of-motion results) felt that it was a failure.

The gracilis muscle was used in 18 cases, the pectoralis major in two, and the latissimus dorsi in one. With this small series, it is impossible to give a firm opinion with respect to the value of different muscles. However, the advantages of obtaining extra cross-sectional area seem to be outweighed by the increased technical difficulty of inserting the pectoralis major and latissimus dorsi muscles into the flexor tendons.

Five patients had long-term follow-up for finger extension. Four of these were double transfers, with a gracilis muscle used for finger flexion and a gracilis used for finger extension. Using the same range-of-motion criteria, three were rated excellent, one good, and one fair. Poor patient selection was the reason for the single fair result, as this was a badly scarred forearm with poor passive range of finger motion. One patient had a vascular thrombosis and muscular necrosis shortly after surgery. This patient rejected further muscle transplantation. The other failure occurred in a man who was doing well until he was involved in an altercation 9 months postoperatively, traumatizing his forearm. This trauma probably produced an arterial thrombosis, as his arteriogram failed to visualize the arterial pedicle.

The relative tension of the four fingers and thumb is critical for good grip and pinch function. With finger flexion, all fingers should flex into the palm in a symmetrical fashion so that they grip objects evenly. One of the patients with a good result would have been rated as excellent if the fingers had flexed in a balanced fashion.

CONCLUSION

In carefully selected patients, functioning microneurovascular muscle transplantation is a useful operation. The disadvantages of the procedure are its complexity and the time required before maximal return of function is achieved.

REFERENCES

1. Harii K, Ohmorik T. Free gracilis muscle transplantation with microneurovascular anastomoses for the treatment of facial paralysis. Plastic Reconstr Surg 1976; 57:133.
2. Kuzon WM, McKee NH, Fish JS, Pynn BR, Rosenblatt JD. The effect of intraoperative ischemia on the recovery of contractile function after free muscle transfer. J Hand Surg [Am] 1988; 13:263.
3. Manktelow RT. Functioning muscle transplantation. In Manktelow RT. Microvascular reconstruction. New York: Springer-Verlag, 1986:151–164.
4. Manktelow RT, McKee NH. Free muscle transplantation to provide active finger flexion. J Hand Surg 1978; 3:416.
5. Manktelow RT, Zuker RM, McKee NH. Functioning free muscle transplantation. J Hand Surg [Am] 1984; 9:32.
6. Manktelow RT, Zuker RM. Muscle transplantation by fascicular territory. Plast Reconstr Surg 1984; 73:751.
7. Shanghai Sixth People's Hospital. Free muscle transplantation by Microsurgical neurovascular anastomoses. Chinese Med 1976; 2:47.
8. Tamai S, Komatsu S, Sakamoto H, et al. Free muscle transplants in dogs with microsurgical anastomoses. Plast Reconstr Surg 1970; 46:219.

55

Direct Muscular Neurotization

Giorgio A. Brunelli

AUTHOR'S KEY POINTS

- There is a biological basis for denervated muscle accepting reinnervation in a new nerve/muscle zone. The efficacy of innervation with foreign nerve has also been demonstrated.
- New motor end plates form as functional modifications at the junction of new axons and muscle.
- Based on encouraging experimental studies in which trophism of muscle fibers has been reestablished, a human experimental series has been undertaken in which more than 80% of patients have regained M4 or better muscle strength.

PHYSIOLOGICAL BASIS FOR DIRECT MUSCLE NEUROTIZATION

The first experiments on the technique of direct muscular reinnervation (reimplanting the original nerve or foreign nerve into muscle) were done by Heineke in 1914.[15] Subsequently, Erlacher, Steindler, and Elsberg reported on the technique.[6,8,9,22] Early research was designed to determine the effects of neurotizing paralyzed muscles rather than reinnervating denervated, paralyzed muscles. The clinical applications that followed, mainly for muscle affected by poliomyelitis, had such inconsistent results that enthusiasm for the technique was lost and the method was not used for the next half-century. In retrospect, the unsatisfactory results of early experiments may have been due to the limited equipment available at that time as well as to poor operative techniques.

Recently, several researchers have performed physiological studies on the effects of placing a nerve directly on the surface of denervated muscle.[1,13,14,17] In these experiments, the nerve was stimulated postoperatively and produced weak contractile responses from muscle. Formation of new synapses at the contact of nerve with denervated muscle was thought to have been responsible.

In 1970, experimental studies were performed in which some nerves were placed in contact with muscle and others were implanted directly into muscle.[5] Physiological muscle responses were obtained, and the formation of new motor end plates in aneural zones of muscle was noted. In 1972, Sakellarides, Sorbie, and James published similar results from experiments performed in dogs.[21]

In 1973, the experimental model was modified, as the nerve was placed within muscle in several fascicles to obtain a larger area of reinnervation.

In 1976, after obtaining encouraging experimental results, human studies were begun in my clinic. Clinical research was started to determine whether it was feasible and practical to reinnervate denervated muscle by direct implantation of nerve. Operative techniques were based on modifications made over 8 years of animal research and were considerably different from those used earlier. These experiments showed that placing nerve on the surface of the denervated muscle brought about weak contraction of the muscle fibers surrounding the nerve. This phenomenon, not seen in control muscles, appears to be due to the formation of new motor end plates between nerve and denervated muscle fibers.[18,19]

Other studies demonstrated that denervated muscle was sensitive all over to acetylcholine, although normally innervated muscle was not.[2–4,11,15,16,17,20] The response of normally innervated muscle to acetylcholine was confined to its motor end plates; denervated muscle accepted stimulation de novo in ectopic places. Similarly, new motor end plates formed in aneural ectopic sites in innervated muscle as functional adaptations of nerve endings where they came into contact with muscle membranes.[12]

Further experimental studies were performed in rabbits. The distal portion of the tibial nerve with its intramuscular branches was removed to denervate the gastrocnemius muscle, and the peroneal nerve was reimplanted in the proximal portion of the lateral head of that muscle in an aneural zone. This zone would not, under normal conditions, show motor end plates (Fig. 55-1). At 1- and 2-month intervals, 21 rabbits operated on with this technique were sacrificed. The distal end of the transplanted nerve was identified and studied by light and transmission electron microscopy. When the nerve/muscle junction was stained in an effort to detect acetylcholinesterase and motor end plates, the formation of new motor end plates was noted; this was thought to be a functional adaptation of nerve branches where they came into contact with the muscle surface.

A subsequent animal study used a modified technique in which the epineurium in the peroneal nerve was removed and groups of fascicles were created under the operating microscope. These small branches were implanted directly into muscle through small slits. The nerve branches were spread and the nerves distributed as widely and deeply as possible in order both to supply new innervation to the largest area of muscle and to increase the number of neurotized muscular fibers (Fig. 55-2). Small branches were sutured to muscle with 10-0 or 11-0 nylon suture, and the epineurium was anchored to the muscle with 6-0 suture to prevent nerve regression. A greater quantity of motor end plates was noted histologically; the amount, in different microscopic fields, appeared to depend on the distance of the muscular field from the nerve implant.[7]

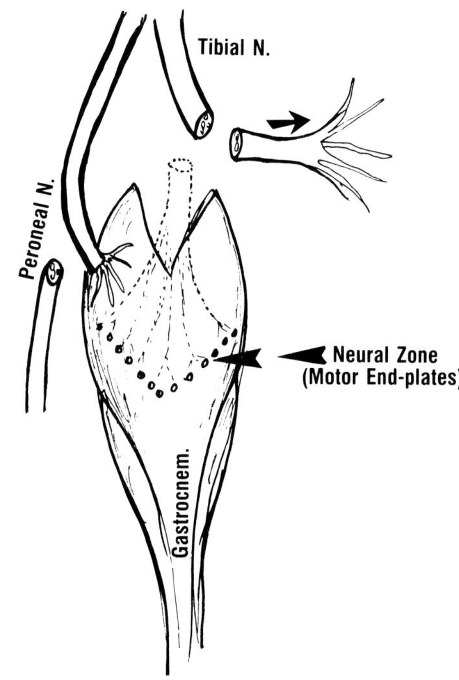

Figure 55–1. *Removal of the tibial nerve from the gastrocnemius muscle and insertion of the peroneal nerve into the denervated muscle.*

Prior to sacrifice, electrical stimulation of the peroneal nerve demonstrated good functional reinnervation as early as 1 month after surgery. Muscle fibers in which new motor end plates had formed regained trophicity and showed normal morphology; in contrast, the non-reinnervated fibers showed a typical dystrophic appearance (Figs. 55-3, 55-4). Transmission electron microscopy demonstrated a normal end plate with bare axon branches rich in presynaptic vesicles in direct contact with membranes of muscle fibers that had normal-appearing folds (Fig. 55-5). Presynaptic

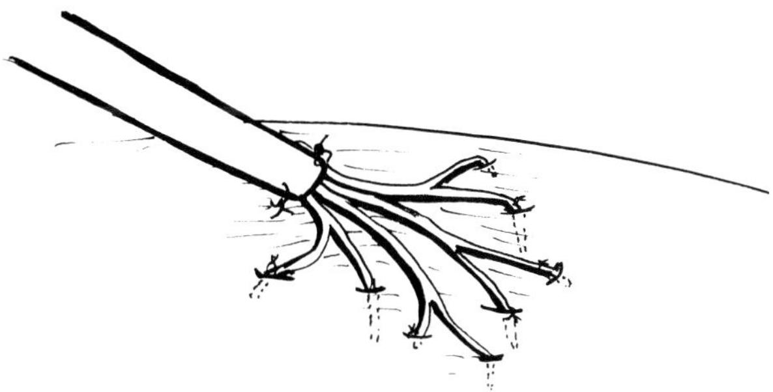

Figure 55–2. *The graft is divided into many thin slips, which are atraumatically introduced into the muscle. The epineurium of the graft and the slips are sutured to the muscle.*

vesicles and mitochondria were noted in the axon branches, whereas only a single layer of Schwann cytoplasm was present over the axon on the opposite side of the muscle. There was an absence of connective tissue elements between the axon branches and muscle.

In subsequent research, nerve specimens have been stained for acetylcholine using the technique described by Koelle and Tsuge. The fact that some of the fibers of the newly implanted nerve did not take up the stain is indirect evidence that both afferent and efferent fibers have been preserved following this procedure.

Several conclusions can be drawn from this series of studies. It appears that the sensitivity of normally innervated muscle to acetylcholine is limited and that it is confined to the motor end plates. When new nerve fibers are inserted within normal muscle, they are not accepted. However, a denervated muscle is sensitive to acetylcholine spread throughout its fibers, and new motor fibers inserted into denervated muscle *are* accepted. They provoke a functional adaptation that takes place at the nerve fiber's point of contact with the muscle, and a new motor end plate is formed.

Encouraging results may also have been due to an "adoption phenomenon." Branching of a pre-motor end plate fiber or extension of a post-motor end plate fiber has been observed. These branches extend further into muscle, adopting new muscle fibers two to three times larger than those seen normally. These *giant motor units* constitute a large part of the new functioning muscle unit.

INDICATIONS FOR NEUROTIZATION

Clinical experiments with direct muscular neurotization were begun in 1975. Candidates were those patients who had sustained injuries in which the proximal nerve stump was available but the distal stump had been destroyed by either avulsion of terminal muscular branches, avulsion of branches directly from muscle, or traumatic or op-

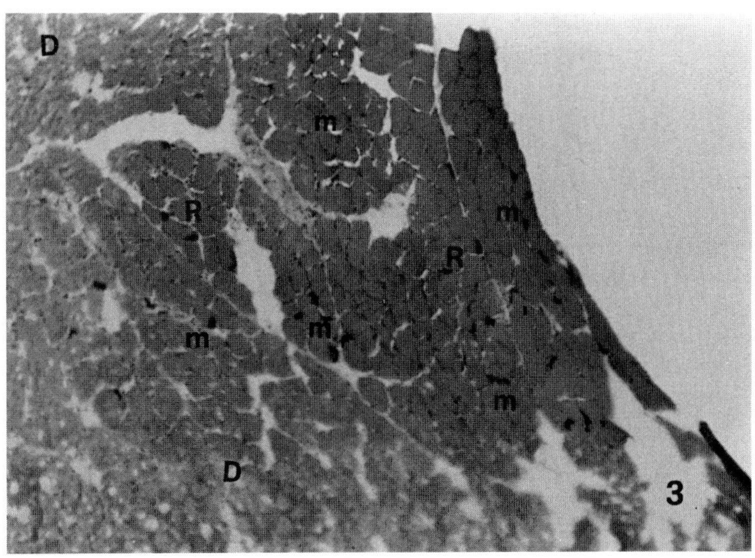

Figure 55–3. *The reinnervated fibers, showing motor end-plates, are trophic. Those not yet innervated are distrophic. m, newly formed motor end-plates; R, reinnervated muscle fibers; D, degenerated muscle fibers that have degenerated because they are not yet reinnervated.*

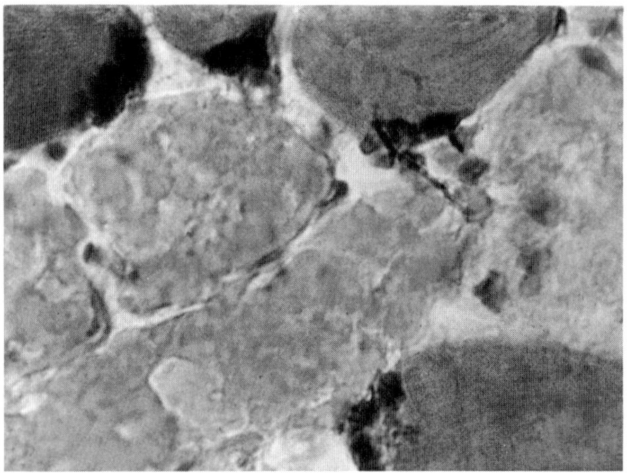

Figure 55–4. *Light microscopy of a muscle near the implantation of a slip of nerve. The motor end-plates demonstrate functional reinnervation.*

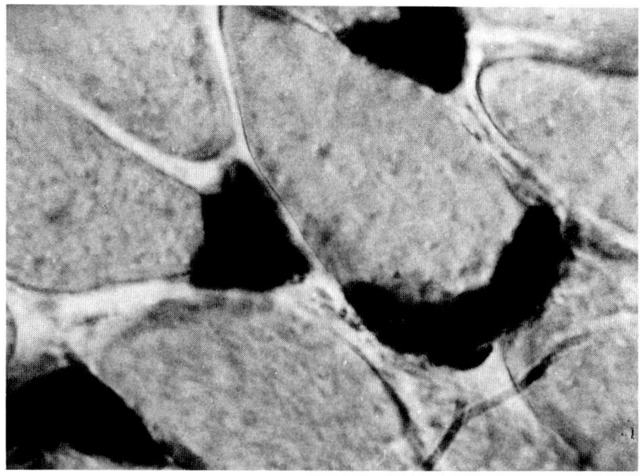

Figure 55–5. *Appearance of motor end-plates after complete formation.*

erative removal of that portion of muscle in which motor nerve branches and motor end plates were located.

Contraindications include a long interval of denervation such that the reparative ability of anterior horn cells has been exhausted. The procedure is also considered inappropriate if a large portion of muscle has been destroyed, if the remaining muscle is extremely fibrotic, or if other extramuscular limiting conditions, such as marked joint stiffness, exist.

OPERATIVE TECHNIQUE

The original nerve is dissected initially from normal tissue into scar and is prolonged by means of nerve grafts to muscle. As many grafts as necessary are performed to match the fascicles of the proximal nerve stump. The grafts must be long enough to extend to a normal-appearing zone of muscle belly. The distal ends of the grafts are divided into thin slips of fascicles, which are introduced into muscle through longitudinal slits made as atraumatically

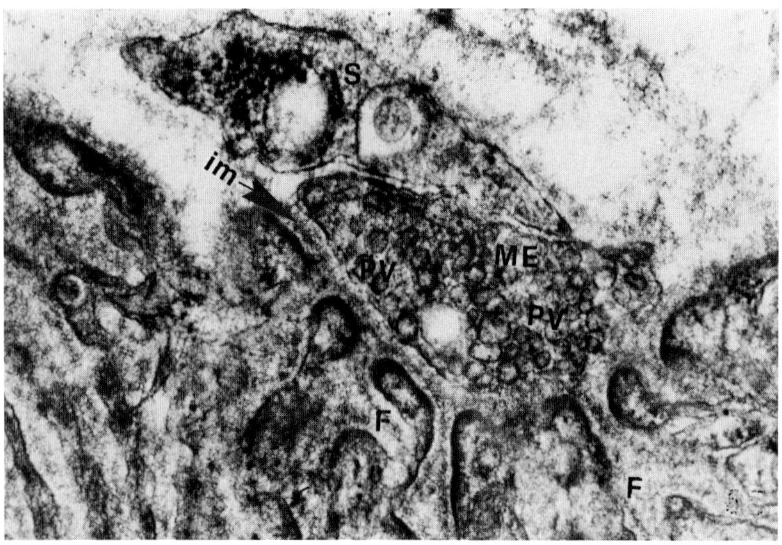

Figure 55–6. *Typical motor end-plate formed experimentally by muscle fiber and nerve ending in touch with each other in an "aneural" zone of the muscle. S, Schwann cell elongation; ME, motor fiber ending; PV, presynaptic vesicles; F, folding of the muscular fiber; im, intersynaptic dense substance, expression of function.*

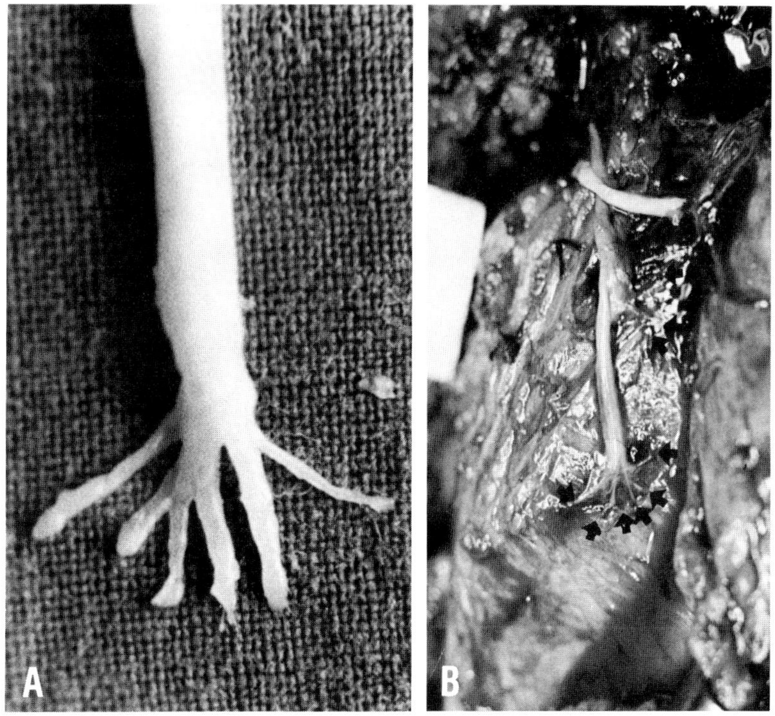

Figure 55–7. (***A***) Under the operating microscope the distal end of the graft is divided into as many slips as possible. (***B***) Operative example of how direct muscular neurotization is done.

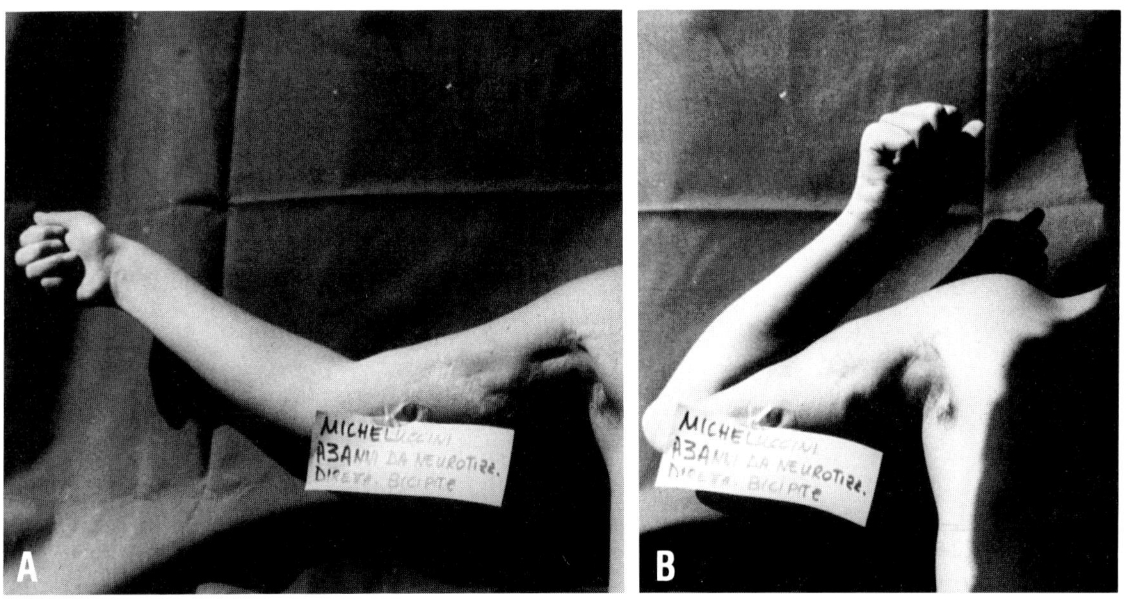

Figure 55–8. *Result of distal direct neurotization after traumatic removal of the proximal third of extensor muscles.*

Table 55–1. *Results of Direct Muscle Neurotization*

Muscle	Number of Cases	M-5*	M-4*	M-3+*	M-3* or Less
Extensor muscles, forearm	13	10	2	1	0
Extensor muscles, leg	13	10	2	1	0
Trapezius	6	3	2	1	0
Biceps	5	4	1	0	0
Thenar	3	2	1	0	0
Extensor pollicis longus	1	0	1	0	0
Deltoid	6	1	3	1	1
Tongue (hypoglosseal)	2	1	1	0	0
Total	49	31	13	4	1

* *British Medical Research Council grade*

as possible in the distal portion of the damaged muscle. If bleeding is noted following creation of a slit, a new atraumatic slit is created in another area. Bleeding is avoided to limit the formation of scar.

The nerve branches are implanted in as wide an area as possible to increase the volume of reinnervated muscle. The epineurium is sutured to muscle fascia with 6-0 nonabsorbable suture, and the grafts are sewn individually with 11-0 nylon suture (Fig. 55-6).

Alternate Techniques

There are no current techniques by which reinnervation can be obtained when the distal segment of nerve has been completely destroyed and reinsertion of the proximal nerve stump is impossible. In these cases, procedures such as tendon transfers and arthrodeses are indicated.

In three cases in which the proximal stump was unavailable for reinnervation (due to a direct avulsion of the brachial plexus from the spinal cord) a foreign donor nerve was used. In one case a radial nerve branch of the triceps was transferred to the biceps.

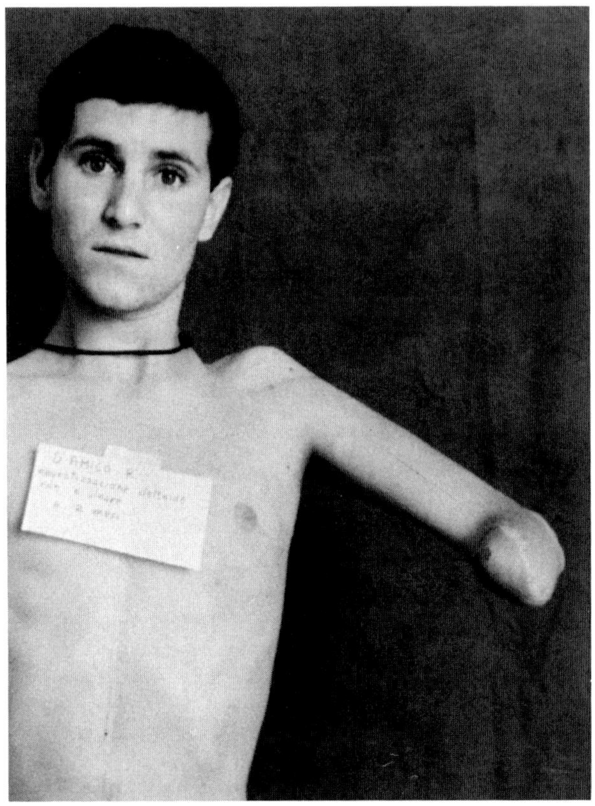

Figure 55–9. *Result of deltoid direct muscular neurotization by means of ulnar nerve in a case of C5, C6, C7 avulsion.*

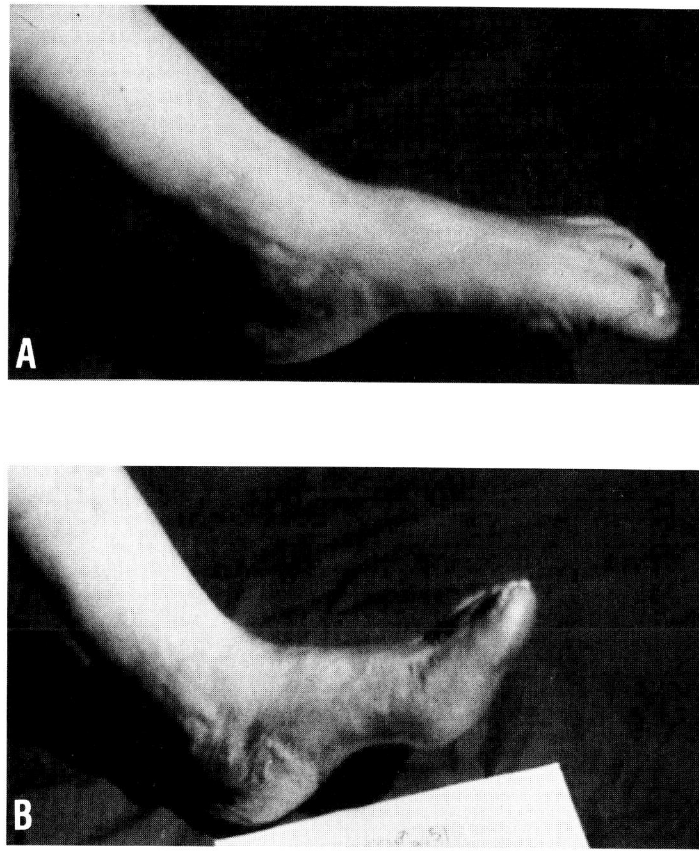

Figure 55–10. *Result of direct neurotization of the extensors of the foot.*

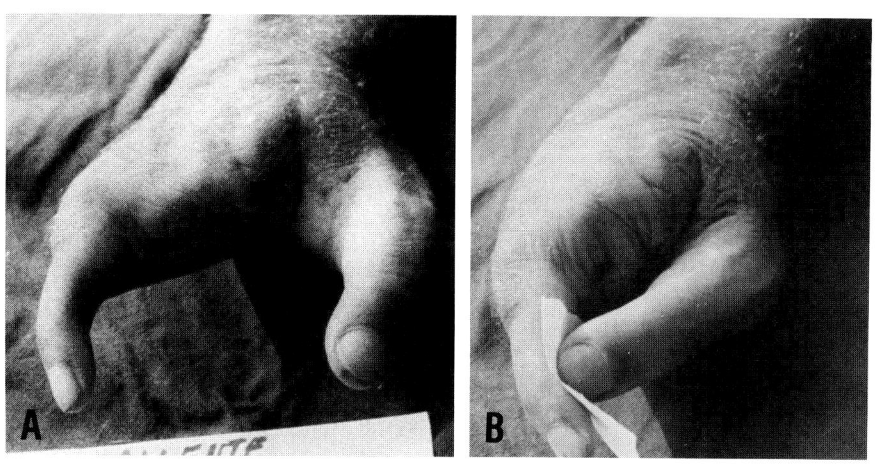

Figure 55–11. *Result of direct neurotization of thenar muscles in a mutilated hand.*

Postoperative Care

The time for reinnervation depends on the distance from the proximal nerve stump to the point of implantation. Nerve regenerates an average of 1 mm/day.[10] The limb is immobilized, and the reinnervated muscle is kept at rest for 15 days after surgery. Passive motion is then initiated, and electrical stimulation is begun. Other techniques, such as local radiation therapy to avoid scar formation, steroids, and ganglioside administration, have been used.

Complications

Avulsion of implanted grafts due to insufficient protection during the early postoperative period must be avoided. Careful anchoring of nerve and initial immobilization are essential. In addition, bleeding at the insertion site should be avoided to discourage scar formation between nerve and muscle. To avoid constriction of donor nerves and grafts, care must be taken to ensure that both the donor nerve and grafts lie within as healthy and wide a bed as possible.

CLINICAL RESULTS

The most common indications have been reinnervation of extensor muscles of the forearm and extensor muscles of the leg; respectively, 13 and 12 cases have been performed. In addition, the operation has been performed in six trapezius muscles (five of them iatrogenic injuries), six deltoid muscles (four were due to avulsion of the C5–C6 roots of the brachial plexus, and one was due to avulsion of the muscular branches of the axillary nerve), and five biceps muscles (two of which had implantation of foreign nerve [eg, radial nerve]). Three thenar muscles, two muscles of the tongue, and one extensor pollicis longus reinnervation have also been done.

On the whole, results have fallen into the good to very good category (Figs. 55-7, through 55-12). Results were good or very good in 44 of 48 operative cases (Table 55-1).

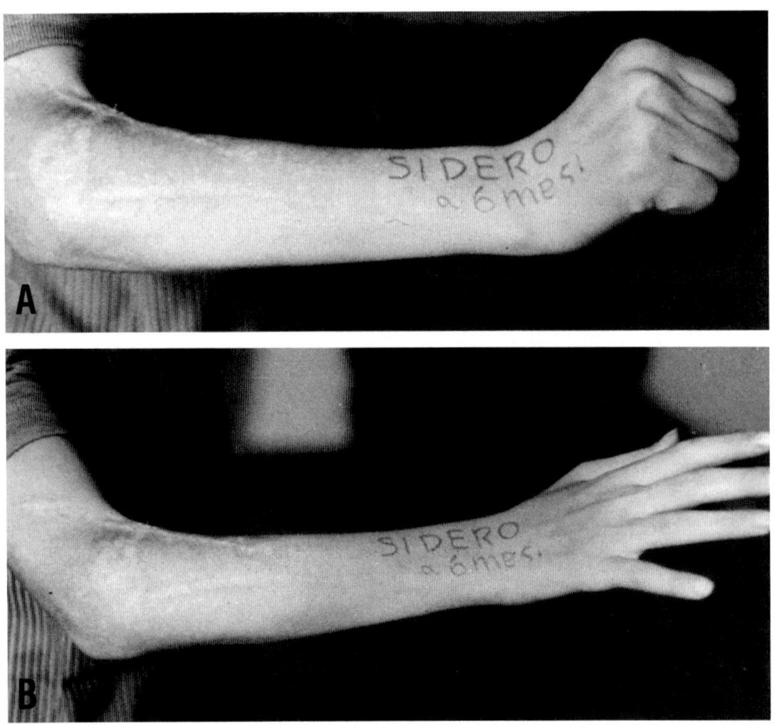

Figure 55–12. *Result of direct neurotization of the forearm muscles.*

In a recent survey of cases of direct muscular neurotization operated on by one group of surgeons, the percentage of good and very good results was not as high as that reported here. This may have been due to the fact that the procedure was being performed for the first time by this group and details of the technique were not adhered to precisely.

SUMMARY

Meticulous microsurgical technique and the "adoption phenomenon" have accounted for promising results with direct muscular neurotization. The results have been encouraging enough to warrant extending indications to cases where traditional repair by direct nerve suture or nerve graft is impossible because of the lack of a distal nerve segment or because of destruction of the neural portion of one or more of a group of muscles. Prerequisites include a satisfactory volume of muscle with sufficient vascularity and adequate preoperative joint mobilization.

REFERENCES

1. Aitken JT. Growth of nerve implants in voluntary muscle. J Anat 1950; 84:38.
2. Bennet MR, Pettigrew G. The formation of neuromuscular synapses. Cold Spring Harbor Symp Quant Biol 1976; 40:409.
3. Bradley R. The morphology of the normal end plate in lambs as revealed by silver impregnation and light microscopy. Res Vet Sci 1977; 23:250.
4. Brenner HR, Sakmann B. Gating properties of acetylcholine receptor in newly formed neuromuscular synapses. Nature 1978; 271:366–368.
5. Brunelli G, Monini L, Antonucci A, Maraldi N. Neurotizzazione in zona aneurale di muscoli denervati. Il Policlinico 1976; 83:611–616.
6. Elsberg CA. Experiments on motor nerve regeneration and the direct neurotization of paralysed muscles by their own and by foreign nerves. Science 1917; 45:318.
7. Engel G. Locating motor end plates for electron microscopy. Mayo Clin Proc 1970; 45:450.
8. Erlacher P. Ueber die motorischen nervendigungen. Z Orthop Chir 1914; 34:561.
9. Erlacher P. Direct and muscular neurotization of paralysed muscles. Amer J Orthop Surg 1915; 13: 22.
10. Fex S, Thesleft S. The time required for innervation of denervated muscles by nerve implants. Life Sci 1967; 6:635.
11. Frank E, Jansen JKS, Lomo T, Westgaard RH. The interaction between foreign and original motor nerves innervating the soleus muscle of rats. J Physiol 1975; 247:725–742.
12. Gozenbach HR, Waser PG. Electron microscopic studies of degeneration of rat neuromuscular junctions. Brain Res 1973; 63:167.
13. Guth L, Zalewski AA. Disposition of cholinesterase following implantation of nerve into denervated muscle. Exp Neurol 1963; 7:316.
14. Gutmann E, Hanzlikova V. Effects of accessory nerve supply to muscle achieved by implantation into muscle during regeneration of its nerve. Phisiol Bohemostaw 1967; 16:244.
15. Heineke D. Die directs einpflanzung des nerve in den muskel. Zentralb Chir 1914; 41:465.
16. Hoffman H. A study of the factors influencing innervation of muscles by nerves implanted. Aust Exp Biol Med Sci 1951; 29:289.
17. Katz B, Miledi R. The development of acetylcholine sensitivity in nerve free segments of skeletal muscle. J Physiol 1964; 170:389.
18. Korneliussen H, Sommerschild H. Ultrastructure of the new neuromuscular junctions formed during reinnervation of rat soleus muscle. Cell Biol Proc 1975; 6:321.
19. Korneliussen H, Sommerschild H. Ultrastructure of the new neuromuscular junctions formed during reinnervation of rat soleus muscle by a "foreign" nerve. Cell Tissue Res 1976; 167:439.
20. Lomo T, Slater CR. Acetylcholine sensitivity of developing junctions in adult rat soleus muscle. J Physiol 1980; 303:173–187.
21. Sakellarides HT, Sorbie C, James L. Reinnervation of denervated muscles by nerve transplantation. Clin Orthop 1972; 83:194.
22. Steindler A. The method of direct neurotization of paralysed muscles. Amer J Orthop Surg 1915; 13: 33.

56

Free Flaps for Providing Sensibility to the Hand

Alain Gilbert
Francesco Brunelli

AUTHORS' KEY POINTS

- Well-defined anatomy, the presence of glabrous skin, and a high density of sensory receptors make the foot the best donor site for providing sensibility to the hand.
- In 88% of cases, the first dorsal metatarsal artery is of sufficient size and anatomic consistency to allow dissection via a dorsal operative approach.
- Patients are carefully selected for these difficult procedures, particularly in light of the considerable risks of failure. Physical impairment, actual and biological age of the patient, and the desired activities are taken into account.

DESCRIPTION OF THE CONDITION

While noninnervated flaps and cutaneous grafts are important in the treatment of acute lesions, particularly in the preservation of exposed tissues, they do not restore critical sensibility to the hand. Neurovascular free flaps, introduced in 1975 by Daniel, Terzis, and Midgley, allow successful soft-tissue reconstruction and provide the sensibility required to avoid new injuries and burns.[3] The advantages of these flaps are as follows:

- Good-quality sensory restoration according to the appropriate physiologic cortical scheme results from connection of the flap's nerve directly to the nerve of the injured area
- Possibility of elevation of large cutaneous areas, if necessary, by associating areas of different innervation vascularized by the same system (eg, foot flaps)
- Minimal donor site deficiencies, from both aesthetic and functional points of view.

Technical complications and the possibility of failure, accompanied by a scarred post-traumatic operative site, confine the performance of such operations to well-selected cases.

It is difficult to standardize indications for these procedures, as the choice for reconstruction depends on factors such as anatomic deficiency, actual and biological age of the patient, and the activities carried out, professional or otherwise. General guidelines can be provided, however. In cases of severe impairment of the hand with complete loss of sensibility, the only possibility for restoring sensible pinch is by using a free neurovascular flap. Less severe lesions, however, especially those that are homo-digital, represent debatable indications. Neurovascular free flaps are required in particular professions (eg, musicians, surgeons) for which it is not advisable to impair the hand further, for both functional and aesthetic reasons, and in patients in whom full restitution of function is sought. A variety of complex lesions require the elevation of fingernails and of the extensor or osteoarticular apparatus, making careful evaluation of specific cases mandatory.

In the final analysis, absolute indications do not exist. Reconstruction of the tip of a ring finger with a microneurovascular pulp flap may be suitable in a 50-year-old piano player, but not in a 20-year-old football player.

The quality of sensibility provided by different flaps varies according to their source. The ability to localize a stimulus accurately runs more or less parallel to the ability to discriminate two points from one. According to Moberg, only a two-point discrimination of less than 15 mm can provide "tactile gnosis," defined as "a quality of sensation that makes a precision sensory grip possible, such as that necessary to screw a nut on a bolt, wind up a wristwatch, sew with a needle, knot a string, and button and unbutton without the help of the sight."[15] Beyond that limit, only "gross grip" and "cutaneous protective function" are possible.

Bossy noted that an external cutaneous nerve of the thigh is the same size as a digital nerve but covers a sensory territory of about 600 cm^2, in comparison to 15 cm^2 in the digit.[18] Sherrington fixed two-point discrimination at 45 mm at the anterior thoracic region, 67 mm at the arm and thigh, 41 mm at the forearm and leg, 41 mm at the dorsum of the foot, and 11 mm at the toes.[19] Other authors report more selective discriminations at the foot, with values of about 20 mm for the dorsum of the foot, 15 mm for the first web, and 6 to 8 mm for the pulpar areas.

No flap can attain the accuracy of the digital pulps, where discrimination is 2 to 3 mm. Sensibility may, however, be improved with practice, and several authors report sensibility restoration of pulpar or web free flaps that is close to normal.

In the last 20 years many neurovascular free flaps have been suggested, but the only ones capable of restoring tactile gnosis in the hand are those elevated from toes (Fig. 56-1); all others restore only a cutaneous protective function or, at most, sensibility that is good enough for gross grip (Fig. 56-2). It is clear that only "cutaneous protective function" can be attained when innervating a region normally supplied by a digital nerve by the anterior skin of the thigh.

FLAPS TO RESTORE TACTILE GNOSIS

In 1975 the first description was given of a neurovascular flap elevated from the first web of the foot, vascularized by the first dorsal metatarsal artery, and innervated by the deep peroneal nerve and by the first common digital plantar nerve (Fig. 56-3).[8] Many variants have been derived from this initial description, using different subunits elevated from the first and second toe block.

One or both of the hemipulps, the web skin, the nail, the dorsal skin, bone segments, or tendons are elevated singularly or in association with the same vascular system. Usually the dorsal system is elevated, but anatomic abnormalities (an acquaintance with which is important) may compel the surgeon to base a flap on the plantar arterial system at the cost of performing much more difficult and tedious dissections.

The three subunits most commonly used are neurovascular flaps from the first web, pulpar flaps, and wrap-around flaps.

Neurovascular Flaps From the First Web (Fig. 56–4)

This flap, described by Gilbert and Morrison in 1975, includes the hemipulps of the first and second digits, the web skin, and if required a cutaneous part elevated from the dorsum of the foot.[8] The flap is reinnervated by reconnecting the deep peroneal nerve, which innervates the web area, and the common digital plantar nerve, which innervates the two hemipulps. The precise technique for this flap is discussed under "Author's Preferred Method."

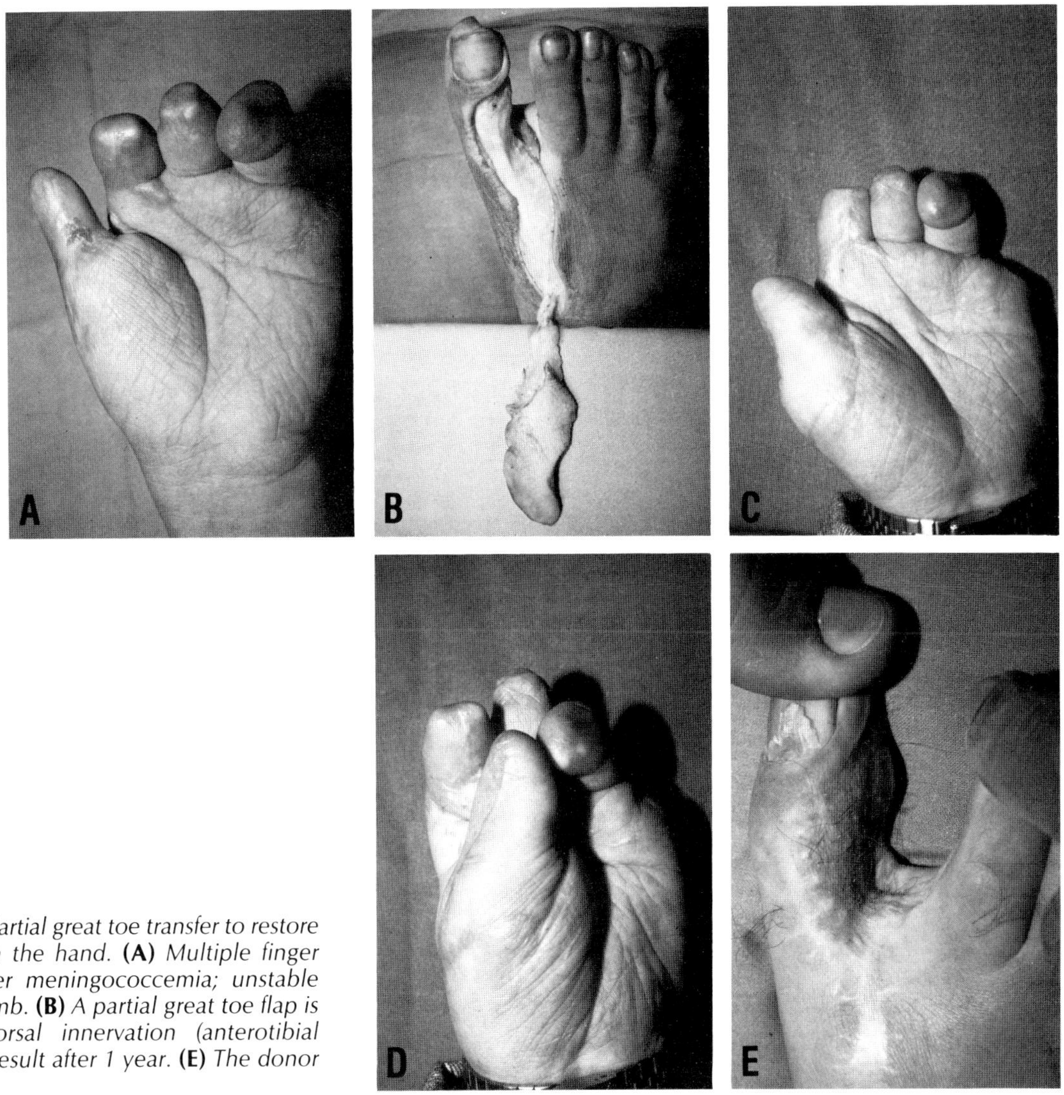

Figure 56–1. *Partial great toe transfer to restore tactile gnosis in the hand.* **(A)** *Multiple finger amputation after meningococcemia; unstable scar on the thumb.* **(B)** *A partial great toe flap is raised with dorsal innervation (anterotibial nerve).* **(C, D)** *Result after 1 year.* **(E)** *The donor area.*

Pulpar Flap

Theoretically, the pulpar flap may be elevated from any toe, but practically, for anatomical reasons, the first two toes are chosen. According to the original description by Buncke, the external hemipulp of the hallux or most of the pulp of the second toe is used.[2] The sensory surface of the flap may be increased by elevating the more proximal cutaneous portions and continuing on the pulp, thus obtaining a large flap that can completely cover the anterior areas of the thumb or digit. The nerve used in the reconnection is the digital nerve of the corresponding hemipulp or, in the case of complete elevation from the second finger, both digital palmar nerves.

The main indication for the transfer of this flap is a degloving lesion that involves several digits and cannot be covered with local flaps. The indication for single-finger reconstruction by such complicated methods is debatable, because the inferior capacity for sensory return will inevitably mean that the patient will use another finger for pinch grip.

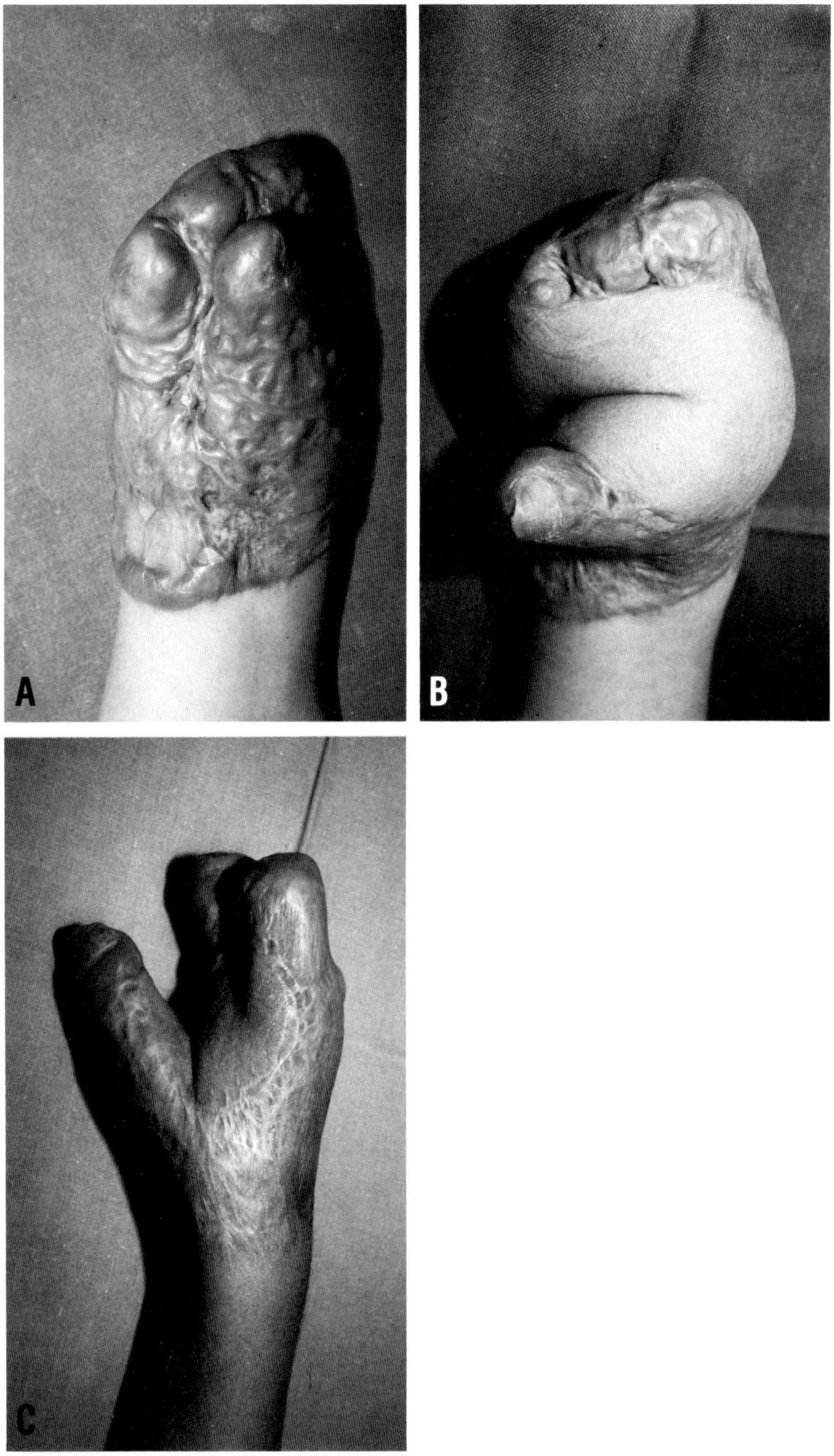

Figure 56–2. *Using a noninnervated flap.* **(A)** *Severe burn of the hand in a 4-year-old girl.* **(B)** *Microvascular transfer of a groin flap.* **(C)** *Hand after defatting and finger separation.*

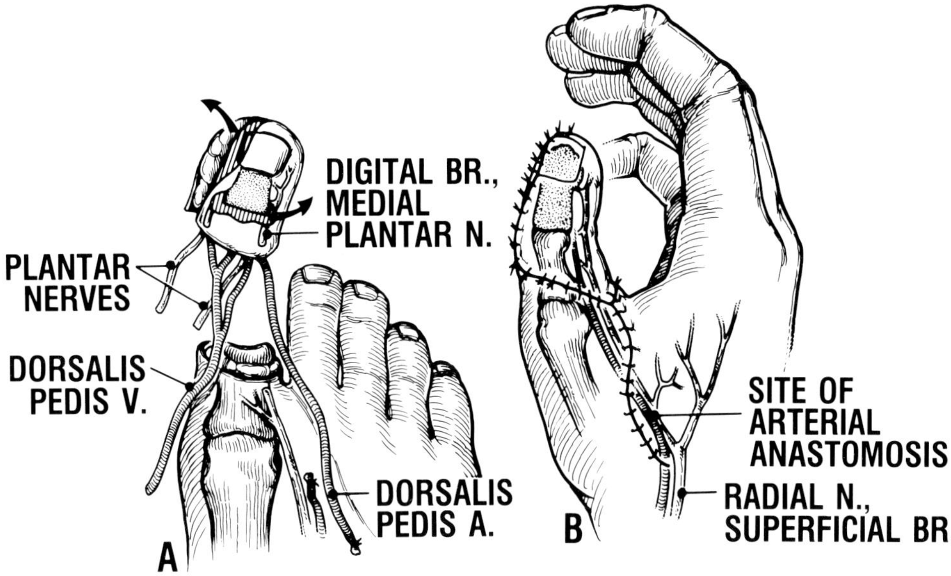

Figure 56–3. *Great toe transfer.*

Wrap-Around Flap (Figs. 56-5, 56-6)

This flap, described by Morrison in 1980, is the most elegant method of reconstruction of the thumb.[17] In the original description it is a composite flap including skin, pulp, and the thumbnail covering a bone graft of iliac crest cut into the shape and length of the missing thumb. Better aesthetic results may be obtained by elevating the nail and skin partially so as to obtain the same size as the contralateral thumb. At present most authors also agree on the elevation of the distal phalanx of the hallux, which makes dissection easier and eliminates the problem of bone graft reabsorption.

Loss of substance at the donor site is partially covered by the medial cutaneous flap, which is left in place at the time of elevation. This flap covers the area that undergoes most shoe trauma. Loss of external and plantar substance is replaced by a cutaneous graft, while the dorsal region, where bone is exposed at the base of the nail, is covered by a "cross-toe" flap elevated from the second digit.[9] This flap is divided under local anesthesia after 4 weeks. The transferred flap is reinnervated by reconnecting the two plantar nerves of the hallux to the two palmar nerves of the thumb. The deep peroneal nerve is sutured to the terminals of the radial nerve in order to restore dorsal sensibility.

FLAPS TO SUPPLY PROTECTIVE SENSIBILITY OR GROSS GRIP

Neurovascular flaps that can supply only protective sensibility or gross grip are suggested when toes are unavailable or when restoration of tactile gnosis is unnecessary. In the last 20 years, many microsurgeons have carried out anatomic studies accurately defining the operative anatomy necessary for microsurgical anastomosis. Unlike the flaps previously described, in this group it is difficult to find the ideal flap with the following characteristics:

- The skin of the flap is similar to that of the hand (ie, thin, sensible, and glabrous).
- The neural and vascular anatomy of the flap is reliable and constant.
- The flap vessels are of adequate diameter and length for anastomosis.
- The flap innervation comes from only one nerve, allowing minimal "overlapping sensation" and only one nerve reconnection.
- The donor site results in minimal morbidity, both aesthetic and functional, and allows direct cutaneous closure.
- The elevation site is convenient and does not compel the surgeon to change the patient's position.
- Dissection is performed under pneumatic tourniquet ischemia.

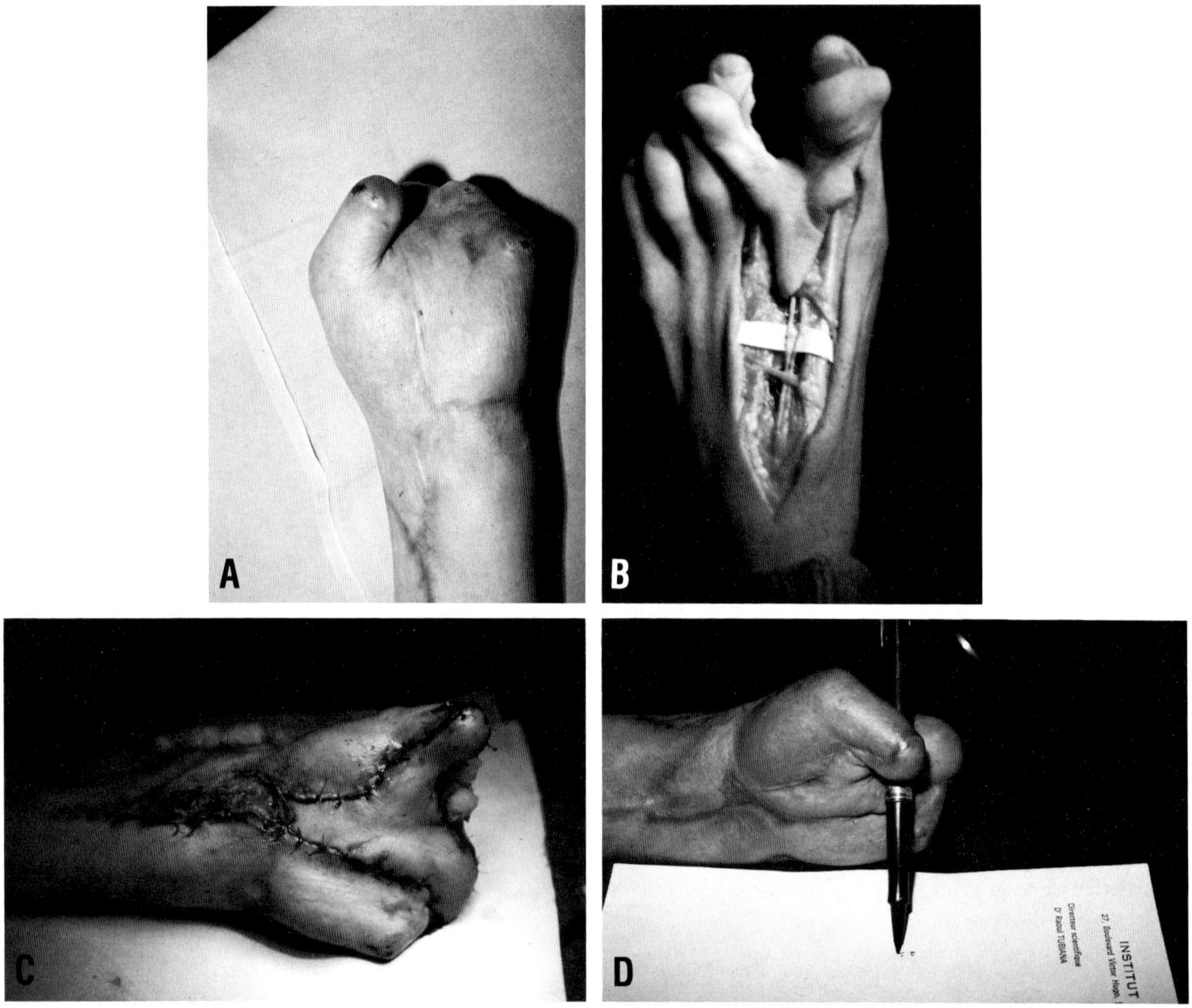

Figure 56–4. *First web transfer.* **(A)** *Crush and multiple amputations in the hand of a 32-year-old man.* **(B)** *Raising a first web space flap with dorsal innervation.* **(C)** *The flap is set in the hand.* **(D)** *Result after 18 months.*

Selection varies from case to case in relation to sex, job, and nature of the skin, which is different in every individual.

Deltoid Flap (Fig. 56-7)

The anatomy and applications of the deltoid flap were described by Franklin in 1983.[5] The deltoid flap is purely cutaneous, is of limited dimensions, and overlies the upper posterolateral aspect of the arm centered over the junction between the posterior border of the deltoid above and the triceps below. While large flaps (27×15 cm) may be elevated, only small flaps (8×10 cm) allow direct closure.

Anatomy

The arterial supply of the flap is from a cutaneous branch of the posterior circumflex artery, which arises from the distal part of the axillary artery and runs backwards with the axillary nerve through the quadrilateral space of Velpeau. The venous drainage of the flap is via the venae comitantes accompanying the artery. Sensory innervation is through

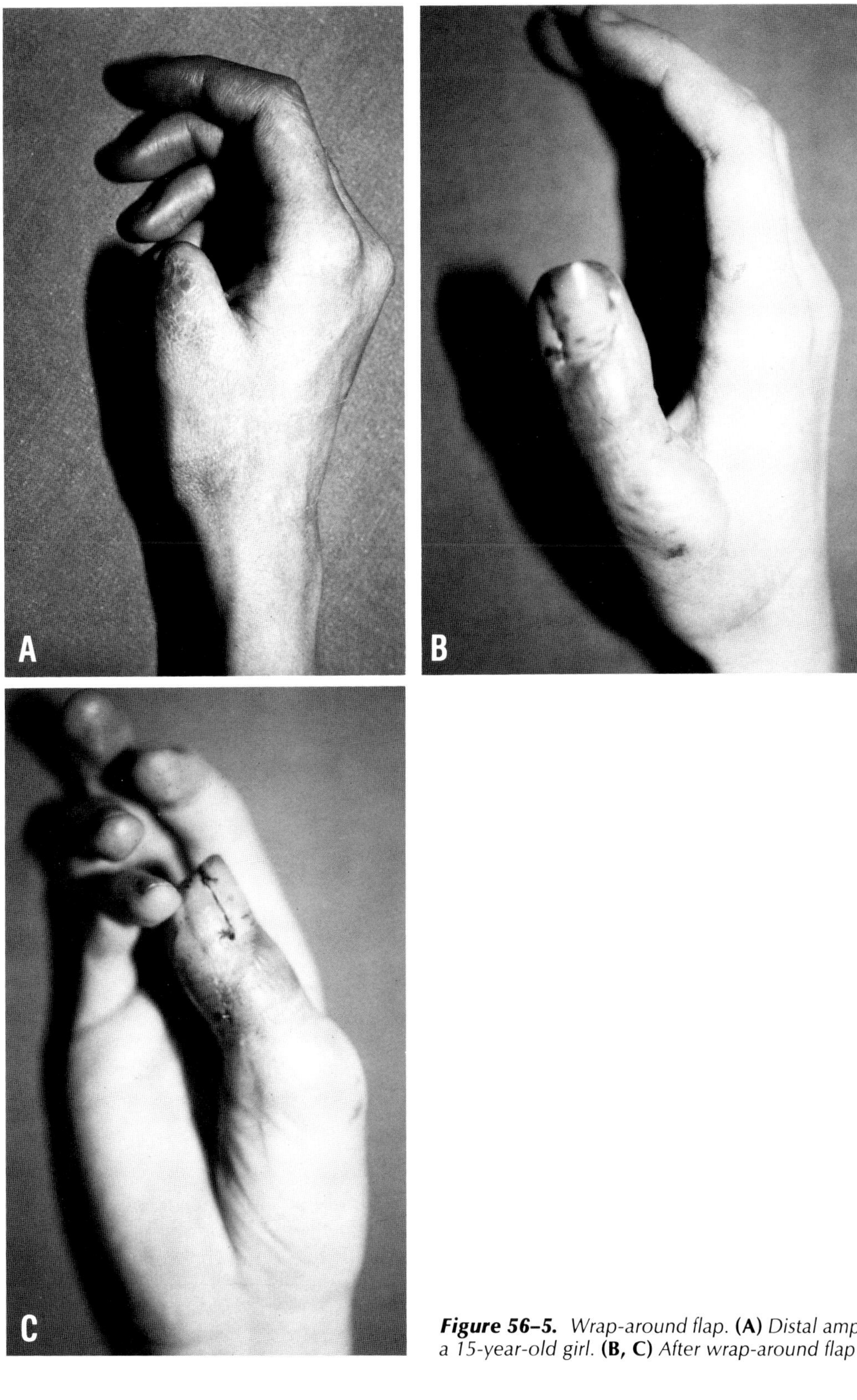

Figure 56–5. *Wrap-around flap.* **(A)** *Distal amputation of the thumb in a 15-year-old girl.* **(B, C)** *After wrap-around flap from the great toe.*

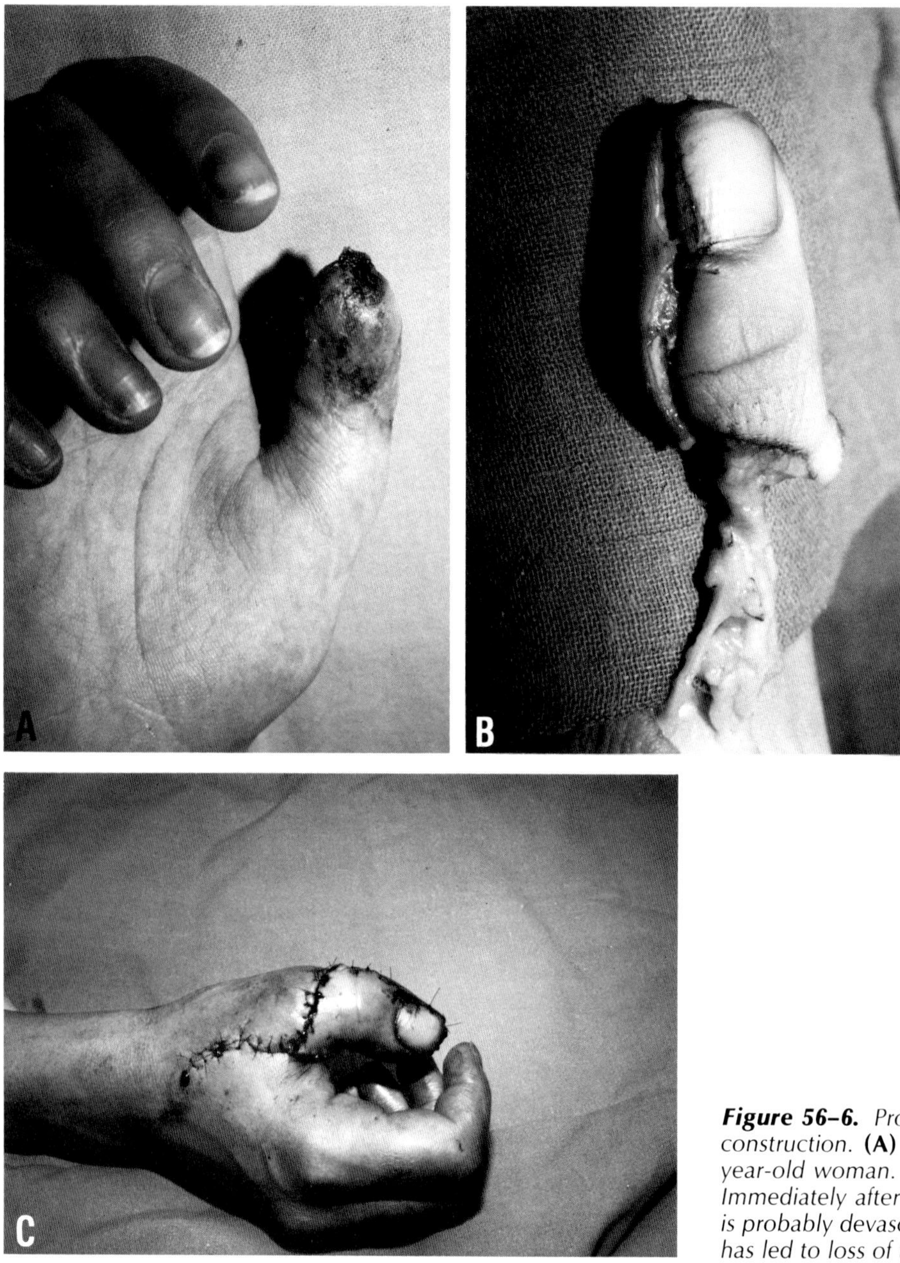

Figure 56–6. *Problems in wrap-around flap reconstruction.* **(A)** *Thumb amputation in an 18-year-old woman.* **(B)** *The wrap-around flap.* **(C)** *Immediately after transfer.* **(D, E)** *After 1 year. It is probably devascularization of the nail bed that has led to loss of the nail.*

the lateral brachial cutaneous nerve, a branch of division of the axillary nerve. This nerve supplies the skin over the lower third of the deltoid muscle and a small area distal to its insertion.

The vessels to the flap are small, with an arterial diameter of only 0.5 mm. To secure a vessel of adequate length and diameter, the artery is dissected to the posterior circumflex humeral artery, and many muscular branches of the deltoid are divided. At the level of the quadrilateral space, the artery is about 2 to 3 mm.

Advantages

The skin area is relatively thin and generally glabrous. The vessels in the quadrilateral space of

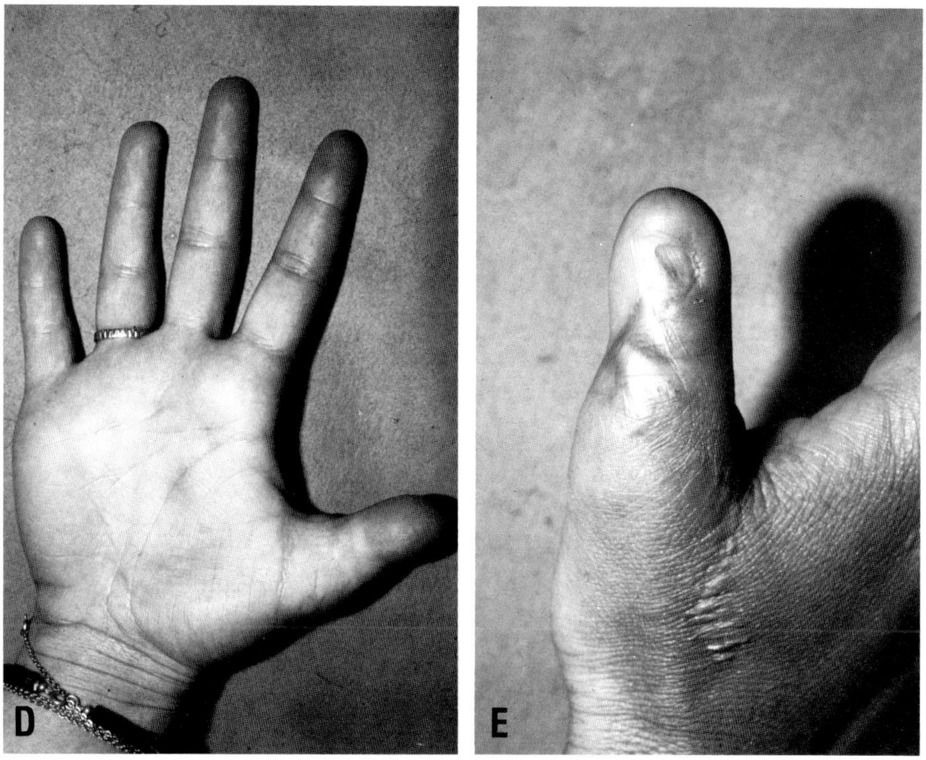

Figure 56-6. *(Continued)*

Velpeau are constant and of adequate diameter. No functional deficiency has been reported after elevation of the flap.

Disadvantages

Only flaps of limited size allow direct closure of the donor site. Skin grafts or closure under tension result in unaesthetic scars. The flap may be fatty, especially in females, or covered by hair in males. Dissection of the neurovascular pedicle is difficult, because its diameter is small at the flap level and because application of a pneumatic tourniquet is impossible.

Medial Upper Arm Flap (see Fig. 56-7)

Transfer of a neurovascular free flap from the medial aspect of the arm was first attempted by Daniel, Terzis, and Schwartz in 1975.[4] This flap is elevated from the middle two fourths of the medial aspect of the upper arm, using skin that is thin and hairless. This region is vascularized from cutaneous branches of the brachial artery and is innervated for the most part by the medial brachial cutaneous nerve.

Anatomy

The arterial supply of the flap is usually from cutaneous branches of the superior ulnar collateral artery, a branch of the brachial artery. At its origin the artery ranges from 0.5 to 1.5 mm in diameter and usually arises from the medial aspect of the brachial artery at the midpoint of the upper arm. It passes posteriorly and inferiorly relative to the brachial artery, and then descends in the subfascial plane, accompanying the ulnar nerve. Both pierce the medial intermuscular septum to enter the posterior compartment on the medial head of the triceps. The artery delivers some branches to the skin and then descends between the medial epicondyle and the olecranon to undergo anastomosis with the

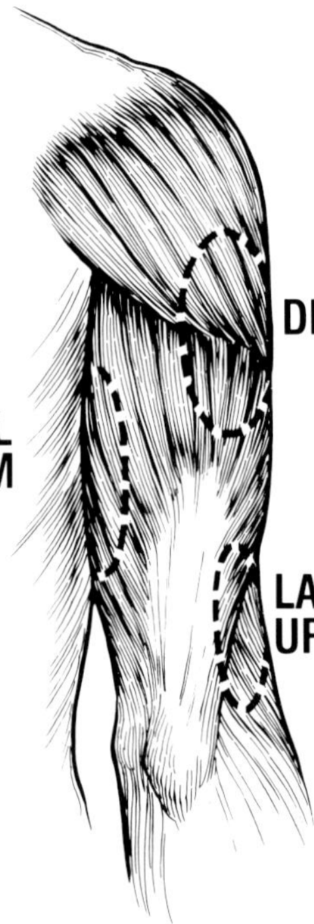

Figure 56–7. *Sources of neurovascular flaps in the upper arm.*

posterior ulnar recurrent and ulnar inferior collateral arteries. Venous drainage is through the venae comitantes of the artery and also through the cephalic and basilic veins. The basilic vein is more central to the flap and is the vessel of choice.

The flap is innervated mainly by the medial cutaneous nerve of the arm, but its most proximal portion encroaches on the territory of the intercostobrachial nerve.

Advantages

The secondary defect on the donor site is relatively hidden, although wide flaps require skin grafting. The skin is thin and hairless, and the elevation site is convenient for the surgeon.

Disadvantages

The major drawback of the medial arm flap is that the diameter of the vessel may vary considerably and in some instances may be unsuitable for microvascular anastomosis. This was noted by Daniel, Terzis, and Schwartz, who, reporting the first clinical case, described an artery with a caliber of 0.6 mm.[4] Dissection must be done without the pneumatic tourniquet. Sensibility is relative to the medial cutaneous nerve of the arm but also to the intercostobrachial nerve, therefore demanding isolation and suture of more nerves.

Lateral Upper Arm Flap (see Fig. 56-7)

A report of this flap was first published by Song in 1982.[20] The lateral arm flap is situated on the lower lateral aspect of the arm, just above the epicondyle. It is based on the lateral intermuscular septum of the arm, receiving its blood supply from the profunda brachial artery and its posterior branch.

Anatomy

The lateral upper arm flap is vascularized mainly by the posterior descending branch of the profunda brachial artery, but sometimes the radial collateral artery appears to contribute to the flap and may be included in the dissection. The posterior cutaneous nerve of the forearm, which is a branch of the radial nerve arising in the spiral groove, accompanies the posterior descending branch of the artery and remains in the intermuscular septum until the level of the lateral epicondyle, where it becomes subcutaneous and descends into the forearm.

The key to dissection is to include the whole of the lateral intermuscular septum with the flap. The vessels within this can ultimately be traced to the profunda artery proper in the spiral groove to allow sufficient length of the pedicle and a large enough diameter. There are both superficial and deep networks of veins draining the flap. The deep veins are the venae comitantes of the profunda brachial artery. The superficial system consists of several large-caliber veins draining into the cephalic vein.

The nerve of the flap is the posterior cutaneous nerve of the arm, a sensory cutaneous branch of the radial nerve.

Advantages

The flap is easy to raise and is usually thin, although it can be fat in females. The lower lateral portion of the shaft of the humerus, underlying the lateral intermuscular septum, can be included to realize a composite flap of bone and soft tissue.

Disadvantages

Only narrow flaps of about 6 cm can be taken and still allow direct closure. The vessels are relatively small (average 1.5 mm) in diameter. Flap sensibility derives not only from the posterior cutaneous nerve of the arm but also from the posterior cutaneous nerve of the forearm, which is usually sacrificed whether it is to be used or not, resulting in a permanent sensory loss to the posterior aspect of the forearm.

Forearm Flap

A skin flap taken from the forearm was introduced in 1978 by Drs. Yang-Guofan, Chen-Baoqui, and Gao Yuzhi in Shenyang Military Hospital in China. This flap, called either the forearm or radial forearm flap, can provide thin and pliable skin of the forearm with few hairs. The large-caliber and long pedicle vessels facilitate microsurgical transfer of the flap.

Anatomy

The arterial supply to the skin is from the radial artery via small cutaneous branches passing along the fascial septum between the extensor muscle group radially and the flexor muscle group ulnarwards, specifically between brachioradialis and flexor carpi radialis. The venous drainage is from the venae comitantes of the radial artery and the superficial veins that run through the flap in the subcutaneous plane.

The flap is innervated by the lateral cutaneous nerve of the forearm radially and the anterior branch of the medial cutaneous nerve of the forearm on its ulnar aspect.

Advantages

This flap is thin and easy to dissect, with large reliable vessels that enter proximally and emerge distally, allowing great facility for anastomosis. The radial artery passing through the flap may be used simultaneously to reconstitute an arterial deficiency at the recipient site. Radius bone may be included for composite skin and bone reconstruction. The flap can be transferred without microvascular anastomosis based on the radial artery and its venae comitantes either proximally for elbow region defects or distally for hand defects. If the distally based flap is used, it can be made sensible by connecting the flap nerve (usually the lateral cutaneous of the forearm) to a nerve of the hand after it has been dissected and severed more proximally to the flap in the forearm.

Disadvantages

Only a limited width of skin can be removed while still allowing linear closure of the defect. Most defects require skin grafting, and, of particular concern to females, this constitutes a significant cosmetic deformity. Aesthetic defects may be reduced by elevating the flap as proximally as possible even if dissection in such a case is more difficult.

One of the major drawbacks of this flap is the sacrifice of the radial artery. However, although some surgeons recommended restoring continuity of the radial artery with a vein graft, this is unnecessary because the remaining ulnar and interosseous arteries can maintain a sufficient blood supply and there are no functional morbidities after removal of the flap.

Dorsalis Pedis Flap

McGraw and Furlow described the dorsalis pedis arterialized flap and suggested its use as a free flap.[14] This technique was subsequently performed by Daniel, Terzis, and Midgley, who reported on the restoration of sensation to an anesthetized hand by a free neurovascular flap from the foot.[3]

Anatomy

The anatomy of this flap is described below under "Foot Flaps."

Advantages

The vessels of the flap are constant and of a caliber and length generally suitable for microanastomosis. Elevation is simple and the skin is thin (although it may be hairy in males). The superficial peroneal nerve responsible for innervating the flap is easy to find and to dissect proximally.

Disadvantages

The major drawback of this flap is the mobility of the donor site. A skin graft is required for closure, and healing in areas of the tarsal bone, extensor hallucis longus tendon, and first metatarsal space may be delayed. Some patients, especially when the entire dorsum of the foot is used, complain of discomfort and pain in the foot when walking. It takes 2 to 3 months for such discomfort to diminish. Recurrent small ulcerations can be observed in some cases. There are non-marked functional disabilities in adult patients, but there may be retardation of development of the foot in children.

FOOT FLAPS

Since the first description of the vascular anatomy of the first web space of the foot,[6] several authors have reported their experiences, either with anatomic dissections[10,13] or clinical findings.[11,12] Basic anatomy has, of course, not changed, but clinical correlation has proved interesting. In many cases the anatomic predominance of the dorsal system was not found clinically, and the plantar system was used. The plantar system seems to be predominant in a large number of cases, and the system of anastomosis between the two systems apparently does not work as well on both sides.

Vascular Anatomy

The vascular supply of the first web space and the first and second toe is derived almost exclusively from the dorsalis pedis artery through the metatarsal arteries, which form a vascular arch around the first dorsal interosseous muscle (Fig. 56-8). Each branch can be extremely variable in size, and the diameters of the two arteries are usually inversely related. In our series, the dorsalis pedis was found in all cases.[7] Its usual diameter was 2 to 3 mm; however, in three cases it was very small and did not exceed 1.5 mm. The diameter of the first dorsal metatarsal artery varies from 1 to 1.5 mm, and the first plantar metatarsal artery is similar in size or slightly smaller. A large plantar metatarsal artery is usually accompanied by a correspondingly slender dorsal vessel.

Dorsalis Pedis Artery

The most common anatomic arrangement involves the dorsalis pedis artery, which lies between the medial cuneiform bone and the base of the second metatarsal before entering the first web space. The extensor hallucis longus lies medially, and the extensor hallucis brevis tendon crosses over the artery. The artery starts to incline in a plantar direction when the first dorsal metatarsal artery branches off. The dorsalis pedis is situated in the intermetatarsal space, limited anteriorly by the arch formed by the first dorsal interosseous muscle and posteriorly by the base of the first two metatarsals and their ligaments. In the middle of the space, the first plantar metatarsal artery arises from the dorsalis pedis artery, which then turns around the base of the second metatarsal and, anastomosing with the lateral plantar artery, forms the plantar arterial arch.

The first dorsal metatarsal artery arises from the dorsalis pedis shortly after this artery begins to incline plantarly. The artery runs toward the web, passing under a muscular arch formed by a belly of the first dorsal interosseous muscle. The arrangement described by Morestin is often found, with the first interosseous muscle having a tendinous insertion into the anterior part of the medial cuneiform.[16] In some cases this tendon is the only medial insertion of the muscle. When the dorsal metatarsal artery is big, this muscle belly is totally separated from the interosseous muscle, inserted on the second metatarsal bone and on the sheet of the extensor of the big toe.

After emerging from this muscular tunnel, which is usually about 15 mm long, the artery again becomes subcutaneous and lies on the interosseous muscle in the subcutaneous fat. It is accompanied by its venae comitantes and the cutaneous branch of the deep peroneal nerve. This nerve lies under the dorsalis pedis artery and the first dorsal metatarsal artery, but it always runs over the muscle belly, never under.

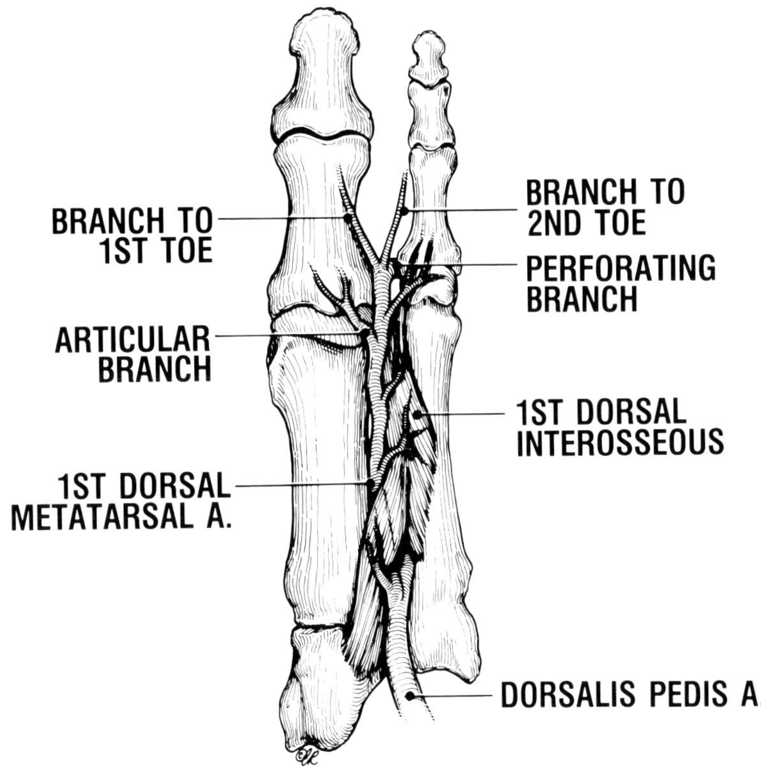

Figure 56–8. *Vascular supply of the first web space and the first and second toe.*

The artery gives branches to the muscle in addition to many small branches to the skin of the dorsum of the foot. These cutaneous branches arise as three main sites: just before the muscular arch, just after the muscular arch, and at the anterior part of the web; at this point the artery is just subcutaneous. The first dorsal metatarsal artery also gives two articular branches to the first and second metatarsal phalangeal joints.

In the anterior part of the web space, the artery gives off a dorsal branch for the second toe and then another dorsal branch for the big toe. Afterwards it takes a plantar direction, branching off to give the plantar collateral arteries to the first and second toes. Just before its division, it is joined by the first plantar metatarsal artery.

The lateral plantar collateral artery of the big toe is large and, by means of anastomosis passing between the flexor tendon and the first phalanx and joining the medial artery, it is responsible for most of the blood supply to the big toe. However, the medial plantar collateral artery of the second toe is quite small, and the medial dorsal collateral artery is often dominant.

First Plantar Metatarsal Artery

The first plantar metatarsal artery branches from the dorsalis pedis at the level of the inferior border of the second metatarsal bone and runs forward medially toward the posterior part of the first plantar ligament. There, between the bone and the flexor tendons, a vascular cross is formed by the junction of the plantar metatarsal artery and the thin medial plantar artery. Two arteries arise directly from this junction: the first re-enters the web space, passes under the deep transverse ligament, and joins the descending part of the dorsal metatarsal artery; the second artery curves around the medial sesamoid bone dorsal medially to form a very thin medial collateral artery. As mentioned, this vessel receives an anatomic branch from the lateral collateral artery at the level of the first phalanx. The first of these two arteries is considered the anterior part of the plantar metatarsal artery. In some cases there is no anastomosis between the plantar metatarsal artery and the medial plantar artery; in these cases, the medial collateral artery to the big toe is merely a branch of the plantar metatarsal artery.

First Dorsal Metatarsal Artery

At our institute we have tried to classify the anatomic variations of the first dorsal metatarsal artery. On lateral view, its two important relations seem to be the first dorsal interosseous muscle and the deep intermetatarsal ligament. Three main variants can be recognized (Fig. 56-9).

In *Type Ia*, the dorsal metatarsal artery is very superficial and is separated from the skin by only the small posterior belly of the interosseous muscle. In *Type Ib* the artery lies in the interosseous muscle but is superficial enough to be easily dissected; 66% of the dissected feet belong to this category (33 of 50 cases).

In *Type IIa*, the artery lies deep under the first interosseous muscle and becomes superficial at the level of the web space. It runs over the deep transverse ligament. Before plunging into the intermetatarsal space, the dorsalis pedis gives off a small superficial branch that lies on the muscle, and this vessel usually anastomoses with the dorsal metatarsal artery at the anterior part of the web. In *Type IIb*, the artery has the same disposition but without a superficial branch. In both IIa and IIb, the plantar metatarsal artery usually branches from the dorsal metatarsal artery beneath the muscle in the middle of the intermetatarsal space. These types were encountered 11 times, in 22% of the specimens.

In *Type III*, the dorsal metatarsal artery is superficial and lies in the interosseous muscle, but the vessel is slender and supplies only the collateral branches to the toes. The plantar collaterals come from the plantar metatarsal branch running under the deep ligament. This type is uncommon; it was found only 5 times (10% of the specimens).

There is no need to stress the anatomic variations of the first plantar metatarsal artery. The course and anatomic location of this artery at the level of the lateral sesamoid bone is fairly constant, but its intricate muscular branches make clinical dissections very hazardous. It may branch from the dorsalis pedis (Type I and III) or the dorsal metatarsal artery (Type II). In one case in our study it was a branch of the plantar arterial arch and in another the terminal branch of the medial plantar artery. The anastomosis with the medial plantar artery behind the sesamoid bones is usual but not constant.

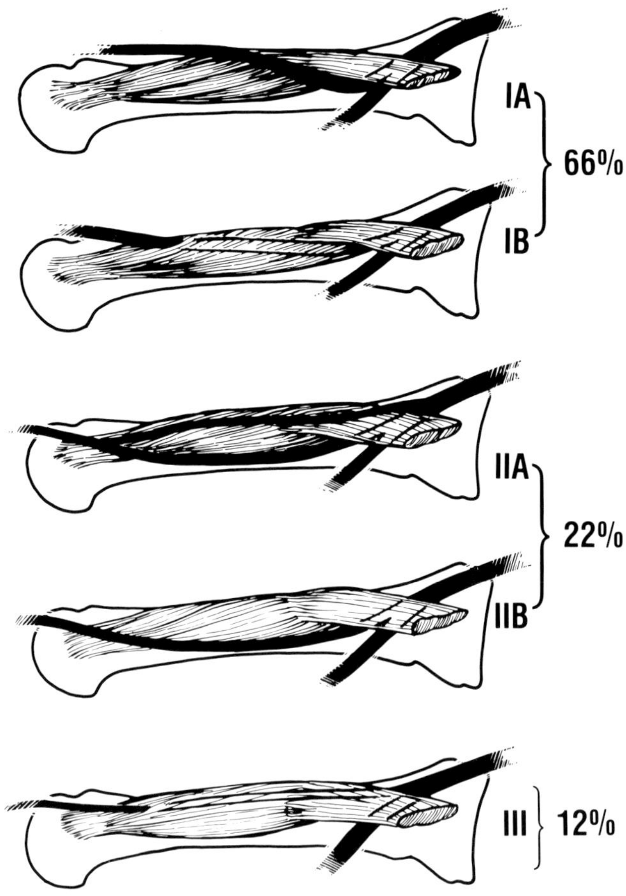

Figure 56–9. *Anatomical variations of the first dorsal metatarsal artery.*

Medial Plantar Collateral Artery to the Big Toe

Inconstant and slender, the medial plantar collateral artery to the big toe usually has two sources: from the anastomosis between the plantar metatarsal artery and the medial plantar artery behind the sesamoid bones and from the anastomosis coming off the lateral plantar collateral artery and passing under the first phalanx of the toe between the bone and the flexor tendons. This vessel may also arise solely from the medial plantar artery (two cases) or may be the terminal branch of the plantar metatarsal artery passing under the first metatarsal bone (one case).

Clinical Correlations

Several large studies have investigated the anatomic variations during surgery. Lister found it impossible to use the dorsal system in 13 out of 38 cases, and the plantar vessels were harvested instead.[11] May and Bartlett were able to use the dorsal system in 31 of 32 cases.[12] A recent study of our cases reviewed 70 transfers in children out of a series of 142 cases.[1] In 65 charts where all information was recorded clearly, the distribution of anatomic situation showed a high percentage of plantar system predominance, with absence of the dorsalis pedis artery in 10% of cases. The disparity between our data and findings from anatomic dissection studies may be due to the fact that the cases were all reconstructions of congenital hand deformities, and some anatomic anomalies in the feet may be associated with them.[12] This led in the clinical transfers to the use of the dorsal pedicle in 59% of cases, slightly lower than predicted.

The surgeon must be cautious in deciding which pedicle will be used and must be prepared to change approaches during the operation.

Authors' Preferred Method
Preoperative Assessment

Palpation of pulses is the first step in the preoperative assessment of anatomic type. Caution should be used if the dorsalis pedis pulse is not felt. In thin patients the first dorsal metatarsal artery may sometimes be felt. Doppler flowmeter studies may be of value in this preoperative assessment; front and side view angiograms of the foot may also be very helpful.

Knowing the area's vascular anatomy helps in interpreting x-ray films. On front view, an artery running straight down the middle of the first intermetatarsal space is always the dorsal metatarsal artery. In contraction, the plantar metatarsal artery describes a sudden curve just behind the sesamoid bones. Spasm is frequent at the foot level, and radiologic diameter is seldom a good indication of anatomic diameter.

A side or slightly oblique view enables the surgeon to categorize the dorsal metatarsal artery into its anatomic type. Angiograms show that the venous return from the big toe is almost completely dorsal and is carried by large superficial channels that are easily dissected. If only one foot has been studied and the vascular disposition is unfavorable, the surgeon should not hesitate to operate on the other foot: it is highly probable that that foot will be of a different anatomic type.

The operation is performed under tourniquet with the patient supine. In the dorsal approach the knee is flexed and the foot is flat on the table.

Approach to the Dorsalis Pedis and First Dorsal Metatarsal Artery

The incision is centered on the dorsalis pedis artery, which has been marked out before surgery. A vertical, slightly curved incision 12 cm long in the middle of the intermetatarsal space is used. Once the skin is opened, dissection should proceed cautiously in order to preserve the dorsal veins. The dorsalis pedis artery should be immediately located at the level of the intermediate cuneiform bone. It is usually found between tendons of extensor hallucis longus and extensor hallucis brevis. The artery is then followed distally. The extensor hallucis brevis tendon is cut, and the most proximal part of the first dorsal metatarsal artery then comes into view. During this dissection, the terminal branch of the anterior tibial nerve should be handled with caution. The artery is followed only to the muscle, after which it is better to carry the dissection more distally. According to the type of operation, the arterial branches are followed during dissection towards the web, the hallux, or the second toe.

Free Sensory Flaps From First Web Space

Several possible flaps are available, including hemipulp, hemipulp plus the dorsolateral aspect of the toe, two hemipulps with the web, and two hemipulps with the web and the flap from the dorsum of the foot.

The operative technique for transfer of the latter flap with a view to reconstruction of a first web space in the hand will be described. It is essential to retain innervation of the forefoot, since reestablishing sensation is the whole aim of the operation. The pulps of the first and second toes are innervated by terminal branches of the medial plantar nerve. In this case, the common digital nerve of the first web space will be used. The first web space and the dorsolateral aspects of the first and second toes are each innervated by the terminal cutaneous branch of the deep peroneal nerve, which is easy to find since it lies close to the artery.

The proposed flap is planned on the skin of the first web space, and the approach to the dorsalis pedis and dorsal metatarsal arteries is the same as that used in a toe transplantation. As soon as the superior border of the flap is reached, the dissection proceeds in a similar manner to that for a flap from the dorsum of the foot, lifting the artery and the flap en bloc. The dissection proceeds from the border of the flap to the center and from the superior border to the web. It is essential to preserve the connections between the artery and the flap and especially the dorsolateral branches to the toes. The plantar approach is necessary for isolation of the plantar common digital nerve. The pulps are dissected out as in a neurovascular digital island flap. This dissection, as well as the dissection for a free toe transfer, takes about 2 hours.

The flap is then transferred to the hand. It is often better to reverse the flap (in other words, to have the dorsum of the foot on the palmar aspect of the hand). The pulp of the second toe will then cover the thumb, and the pulp of the first toe will cover the index finger to the head of the third and fourth metacarpals. All anastomoses can be placed in the palm, especially the nerve sutures with the sensory branches of the median nerve. To avoid difficulties, the plantar nerves should be cut long. The foot defect may be grafted after 1 week, and the aesthetic and functional defect is minimal. In some cases the web space is difficult to graft, and grafts may result in retractions (Fig. 56-10).

POSTOPERATIVE COMPLICATIONS

The main complications of such operations are early postoperative complications that can result in ischemic necrosis of all the structures dependent on the transplanted nutritive pedicle. Even a perfect technique and provisions regarding vasoconstriction and platelet aggregation cannot completely eliminate the risk of vascular thrombosis, which must be recognized immediately.

The tardive complications above are all of the nervous type; they do not threaten survival of the transplanted segment, but the quality of functional restoration depends on them. Infection, the only other complication, has been rare, both in our series and in the literature.

Vascular Complications

Venous thrombosis generally arises during the first 24 hours and is clinically manifested tardively, 3 to 6 hours after its onset, in relation to the possibilities of expansion of the venous bed of the transplanted tissue. The first signs of venous stasis are excessive dark blood outflow from the borders of the surgical wound, acceleration of the capillary pulse, initial congestion of the distal portion of the flap, and a slight decrease of superficial temperature, associated with a darker color. A second immediate surgical intervention is mandatory to re-

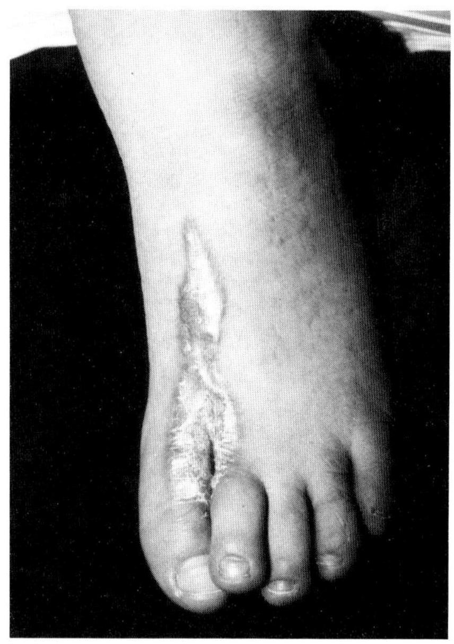

Figure 56–10. *The web space of the foot is sometimes difficult to graft, and grafts may result in retractions.*

store a good venous flow before thrombosis extends to the microvascularity, thus becoming irreversible.

If the second operation is tardive or ineffective, venous flow must be aided with small superficial discharge incisions or by using leeches, which associate a mechanical decongestant effect with a pharmacologic effect through the injection of irudin (a heparin analog) with saliva. Irudin prolongs the bleeding at the puncture site. Formation time of the new venous collateral vascularity is 5 days, and during this period a continuous outflow of blood must be ensured.

Arterial thrombosis is clinically easy to identify because the blocking of arterial flow results in an immediate pallor in the transplanted segment. It is necessary to watch for progressive intramural thromboses, which occur more slowly, alternating periods of acceptable vascularization and periods of almost complete ischemia. The most important clinical signs are color and capillary pulse. Temperature is less reliable, because it often reflects the temperature of the surrounding tissues or of the environment. In case of doubt, a small incision is made; if there is no bleeding, arterial flow is restored immediately with a new anastomosis.

Arterial thrombosis can take place at the end of the operation or later, generally during the first 3 postoperative days. The recovery of arterial anastomosis does not always result in a recovery of blood flow or in survival of the transplanted segment. Obstruction often results in a vicious cycle of relapsing spasms and extensive thrombosis.

Nerve-Related Complications

The quality of functional recovery depends on sensory restoration of the transplanted segment. Generally, if the ground is favorable, sensory reinnervation is obtained, attaining a satisfactory, although incomplete, level. The risk of failure of reinnervation is reduced with a perfect microsuture technique, with a good choice of recipient nerve, and with good local trophism ensured by effective permeability of the anastomoses. No complications such as painful neuroma were observed when free sensible flaps were used. In some painful digital stumps, pain disappeared after a sensible flap transfer in which the flap nerve was sutured to the digital nerve carrying the neuroma (after its resection). Hyperesthesia to cold frequently has been observed, especially in the pulpar flaps, and it persists for as long as several years.

REFERENCES

1. Ben Youssef K: Theše de Médecine: Les Transferts D'Orteil Chez L'enfant. Tunis, 1986.
2. Buncke HJ, Rose E. Free toe to finger tip neurovascular flaps. Plast Reconstr Surg 1979; 63:607–612.
3. Daniel RK, Terzis J, Midgley RD. Restoration of sensation to an anesthetic hand by a free neurovascular flap from the foot. Plast Reconstr Surg 1976; 57:275.
4. Daniel RK, Terzis J, Schwarz G. Neurovascular free flaps: A preliminary report. Plast Reconstr Surg 1975; 56:13.
5. Franklin J. The deltoid flap, anatomy and clinical applications. In: Buncke H, Furnas D, eds. Symposium on clinical frontiers in reconstructive microsurgery. St. Louis: CV Mosby, 1984:63–70.
6. Gilbert A. Composite tissue transfers from the foot: Anatomic basis and surgical technique. In: Daniller A, Strauch B, eds. Symposium on microsurgery, vol 15. St. Louis: CV Mosby, 1976:230–242.
7. Gilbert A. Toe transfers for congenital hand defect. J Hand Surg 1982; 7:118.
8. Gilbert A, Morrison WA. Transfer sur la main d'un lambeau libre sensible. Chirurgie 1975; 101:691–694.
9. Hamilton RB, O'Brien B McC, Morrison WA. The cross toe flap. Br J Plast Surg 1979; 32:213–216.
10. Leung PC. The vessels of the first metatarsal web space. J Bone Joint Surg [Am] 1983; 65;235.
11. Lister G. Reconstruction of the hand with free microvascular toe to the hand transfer: Experience with 54 toe transfers. Plast Reconstr Surg 1983; 71;372.
12. May J, Bartlett S. Great toe to hand free tissue transfer for thumb reconstruction. Hand Clin 1985; 1:271–284.
13. May J, Chait L, Cohen B. Free neurovascular flap from first web of the foot in hand reconstruction. J Hand Surg 1977; 2;387.
14. McCraw JB, Furlow LT. The dorsalis pedis arterialized flap: A clinical study. Plast Reconstr Surg 1975; 55:177.

15. Moberg E. Methods for examining sensibility of the hand. In: Flynn JE. Hand surgery, ed 2. Baltimore: Williams & Wilkins, 1975:295–304.
16. Morestin H. Note sur une bourse séreuse qui existe fréquemment entre le premier cunéiforme et le tendon extenseur propre du gros orteil. Bull Soc Anat Paris, 1894.
17. Morrison WA, O'Brien B McC, MacLeod AM. Thumb reconstruction with a free neurovascular wrap-around flap from the big toe. Hand Surg 1980; 5:575–583.
18. Rabischong P. Les problèmes fondamentaux du rétablissement de la préhension. Ann Chir 1971; 25: 927–933.
19. Sinclair D. Psychophysiology of cutaneous sensation. In: Jarret A. The physiology and pathophysiology of the skin. Academic Press, 1973:429–473.
20. Song R, Song Y, Yu Y, Song Y. The upper arm free flap. Symposium on one-stage reconstruction. In: Song R, ed. Clinics in plastic surgery, vol 9. New York: WB Saunders, 1982:27–36.

XI

REHABILITATION

57 Rehabilitation Following Nerve Repair

58 Sensory Re-Education

57

Rehabilitation Following Nerve Repair

Evelyn J. Mackin
Patricia M. Byron

AUTHORS' KEY POINTS

- For hands with *median nerve injuries*, maintenance of full passive motion, prevention of contractures of the first web space, and preservation of carpometacarpal pronation is accomplished with thumb opposition splinting, passive range-of-motion exercises, and use of a thumb web spacer splint for night wear.
- For *ulnar nerve injuries*, splints that position the ring and little metacarpophalangeal joints in flexion allow the long extensor tendons to transfer power to extend the interphalangeal joints. A figure-eight design is fabricated from doubled thermoplastic material.
- If a *fixed claw deformity* develops in a patient with ulnar nerve paralysis, dynamic splinting or serial plaster splinting is required.
- For *combined median–ulnar nerve palsy*, a figure-eight splint that includes all four digits is used. When clawing requires a stronger counterforce, a "hood"-type splint (one-piece thermoplastic material molded over the proximal phalanges and metacarpals) is indicated.
- For most patients with *radial nerve palsies*, a simple cock-up splint supports the wrist in extension, providing the necessary balance for grasp, manipulation, and prevention of unopposed wrist flexion.
- For functional rehabilitation, exercise sessions that emphasize isolated contraction of reinnervated muscles are initiated as soon as a trace contraction is perceived. Specific sensibility, threshold, and functional tests are carried out at regular intervals.

Rehabilitation of the patient who has sustained a peripheral nerve injury addresses the following areas of dysfunction: sympathetic, motor, functional, and sensibility. Appropriate splinting methods anticipate deformities that can result from nerve injury. A thorough understanding of the mechanics of splinting as it applies to neural injury is required.

SYMPATHETIC DYSFUNCTION

There is an immediate loss of pseudomotor activity in the area of lost skin sensibility when a nerve is severed. Reduced pseudomotor activity results in hand dryness due to loss of sweating and diminished sebaceous secretion. A change in the physical qualities of keratin component (a component of the tough outer layer of the skin) results. Sweat serves not only to moisten the surface of the skin, but also to hydrate the keratin itself. Hydrated keratin is soft and pliable; dry skin becomes hard and does not stretch to accommodate function. The areas of the hand that must flex and stretch sustain damage when they are dry and inelastic. They crack easily and become more prone to injury than normal skin.[11]

A mechanical feature of dry keratin is that it is slippery. The combination of insensitivity and dry, slippery skin seriously limits the mobility and function of the patient's hand despite good muscular control. Dropping objects and lack of strength in the hand are common complaints. Moisturized skin assists gripping and pinching functions.

Nonsweating skin is maintained in a well-hydrated state. Brand recommended the following daily routine[11]: The hand is soaked in water every day for 15 minutes, then blotted lightly with a towel. A massage with petroleum jelly follows; then oil or cream is applied to prevent the water from evaporating. This treatment helps prevent cracking and maintains joint mobility.

To prevent skin injury from excessive forces, overuse, or high temperatures, Brand advocated regular hand inspection during work to check for increased redness, swelling, or warmth.[10,12,15,17]

MOTOR DYSFUNCTION

Early Management

Patients begin therapy 1 to 4 weeks after surgery. Positioning and timing for initiation of motion depends on the degree of involvement of other structures and the magnitude of nerve defect. If there is tension on the repair site, active finger motion is started as soon as possible to avoid stiffness, with the hand maintained in a protected position.

Median and ulnar nerve injuries are generally associated with flexor tendon injuries. Protection is generally in the standard flexor tendon position (30° wrist palmar flexion and 70° metacarpophalangeal joint flexion). Tension on the repair site may require increased wrist flexion to achieve a safe position for the nerve. Even when nerve transection occurs in isolation, a similar positioning splint for median or ulnar injury is used. In this case, active finger motion is started within the 1st postoperative week.

Splinting for Peripheral Nerve Injury

The potential for restoration of function after injury depends on the preservation of passive joint motion and proper positioning of weak or paralyzed muscles. Positioning splints used in conjunction with frequent, careful range-of-motion exercises prevent poor patterns of motion, stiffness, and remodeling of tissue leading to deformities that result from the unopposed action of antagonistic muscles. Overstretching by antagonistic muscles results in contracture of the muscles and of affected joints. If deformities are not prevented, muscles and joints are permanently stretched, leading to inefficient function after reinnervation. Overstretching is prevented by passive range of motion exercises, and a splinting program is designed to reestablish the balance between involved and uninvolved muscles. Splints also position the hand for use while nerve regeneration is occurring, or until tendon transfers are performed.

Splinting for Median Nerve Palsy

The median nerve allows for precision manipulation. It provides sensibility to the working surface of the thumb and index and middle fingers and half of the ring finger. The median nerve–innervated thenar intrinsic muscles position the thumb to the pulp of the index and middle fingers for precise manipulation. The median nerve also innervates the pronator muscles, the radial wrist flexors, the superficialis digital flexors, and the terminal joint flexors of the thumb and index and long fingers.[2]

The deformity caused by median nerve injury at the wrist results from wasting of the thenar muscles and lack of opposition (Fig. 57-1). The thumb is held beside the index finger because the abductor pollicis brevis and opponens pollicis muscles are paralyzed, and therefore their antagonists (the extensor pollicis longus and adductor pollicis) act without opposition. Paralysis of the first and second lumbrical muscles may cause hyperextension of the metacarpophalangeal (MCP) joints of the index and long fingers.

While a high median nerve injury results in paralysis of the flexor muscles of the fingers and wrist and of the pronator muscles, there is no more deformity than that seen after a low median nerve injury. A hand-based splint that positions the thumb in palmar abduction (to counteract the deforming action of the long extensor muscles and to encourage opposition by the long flexor) provides major assistance in activities of daily living (Fig. 57-2). However, many patients achieve satisfactory thumb use without such splints: they rely on the thumb adductor for lateral pinch and on substitution patterns by the abductor pollicis longus and perhaps the flexor pollicis longus tendons to provide adequate thumb function. Patients may elect to use the opposition splint only for certain activities.

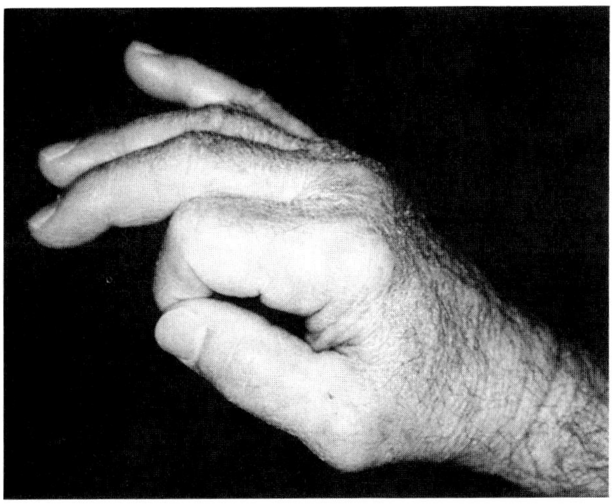

Figure 57–1. *This patient sustained a median nerve injury at wrist level. He compensates for inability to oppose by using lateral pinch.*

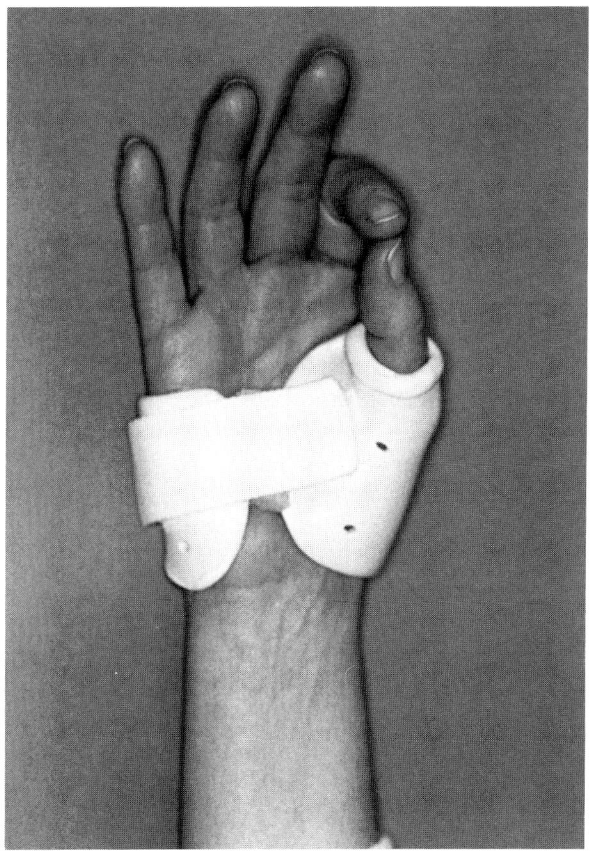

Figure 57–2. *A hand-based thumb spica splint can be used to position the thumb in abduction for activities requiring abduction.*

The goals of splinting hands that have sustained median nerve injuries are to maintain full passive motion, prevent contracture of the first web space, and preserve carpometacarpal pronation. An advantage of thumb opposition splinting is that it maintains the length of the first web space. However, if a thumb opposition splint is not worn, careful passive range-of-motion exercises are carried out and a thumb web spacer splint is provided for night wear. Passive range-of-motion exercises do not exert stress on the collateral ligaments of the MCP joint of the thumb. Exercises also include rotation of the thumb metacarpal into a position of pronation.[17]

If a web space contracture develops, corrective splinting is required. The web space is held in a position of maximum abduction with serial splinting at all times. The splints are removed only to carry out range-of-motion exercises and for certain daily activities (Fig. 57-3).[17]

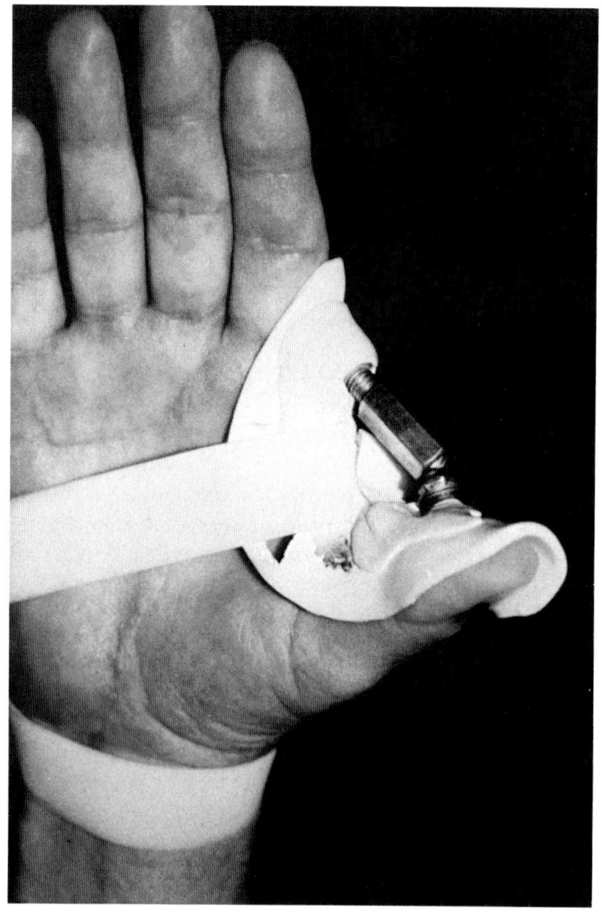

Figure 57–3. *This adjustable web stretcher is adapted from a standard thermoplastic web stretcher. A triangular insert is made in the volar and dorsal surfaces of the splint to allow stretch of the thermoplastic as the nut is extended on the screw. Care is taken to apply stretch to the web space rather than to the metacarpophalangeal joint. (This idea was first introduced in Philadelphia by S. Cheshire of Louisville.)*

Splinting for Ulnar Nerve Palsy

The ulnar-innervated intrinsic muscles are associated with the refined and highly coordinated movements of the hand. Divided into three groups (the thenar group, the hypothenar group, and the interosseous–lumbrical muscle complex), each contributes to finger movements (except for the first dorsal interosseous muscle, which contributes to thumb power pinch).

Following ulnar nerve injury, power is lost or diminished (the higher the level of injury, the greater the loss) and hand function is compromised. There is loss of power for thumb–index pinch and loss of intrinsic muscle power for gross grip. Paralysis of the intrinsic muscles may result in a claw hand deformity with MCP joint hyperextension and interphalangeal (IP) joint flexion of the ring and little fingers. Because the paralyzed intrinsic muscles cannot stabilize the MCP joints on the flexor side, the extensor muscles hyperextend the MCP joints, and in that position cannot extend the IP joints (Fig. 57-4).

Splints that position the ring and little MCP joints in slight flexion prevent MCP hyperextension, thereby allowing the long extensors to transfer power to extend the IP joints. These splints allow full finger flexion so as not to interfere with grasp.[17]

A figure-eight design is made using a ½″- to ¾″-wide piece of doubled thermoplastic material about a foot long. The strip is first molded over the dorsum of the proximal phalanges of the affected digits with the MCP joints in 30° flexion, then brought around to the palm, where it is molded into the

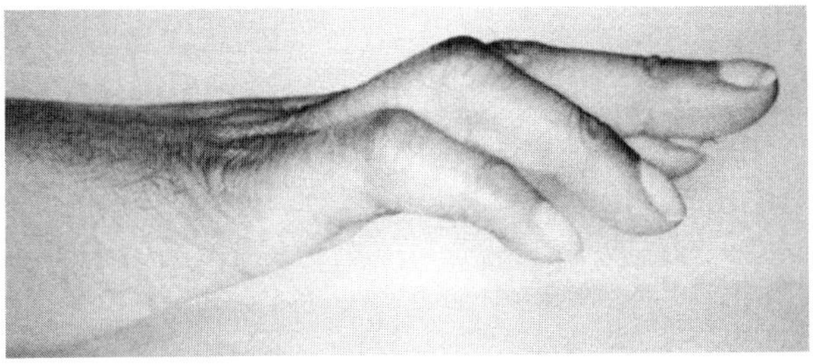

Figure 57–4. A patient who sustained ulnar nerve injury years earlier is unable to extend his interphalangeal joints due to paralyzed ulnar intrinsic muscles. This is a typical position for an individual with ulnar nerve palsy.

distal palmar crease, then brought back to the dorsum of the hand and molded over the metacarpals. The section on the dorsum of the hand is wide enough to distribute pressure over the bony areas of the hand and proximal phalanges. Pressure areas develop as the patient uses the strong power of the extensor digitorum to overcome the splint. Padding applied to the fingers before molding the splint and the secure fit of the palmar section help diminish the high concentration of pressure on the dorsum of the proximal phalanges.

The patient is taught to extend the fingers with the least extension force required to accomplish the task. The section supporting the metacarpal arch is narrow enough so as to avoid restriction of finger flexion and to minimize the area of the palm that is blocked from sensory input (Fig. 57-5).[8,17]

Early attention to clawing is vital. Some hands are naturally so thick and stable that the MCP joints do not hyperextend; these hands may not develop much clawing. Most do not show clawing when first paralyzed because the palmar tissues are tight enough to maintain the MCP joints in a stable position. However, as imbalance becomes more exaggerated over time, clawing develops because unopposed extensor force stretches the volar plate, skin, and other supportive soft tissues.[8]

If a claw deformity develops, with consequent contracted hyperextended MCP joints, flexed IP joints, and shortening of long flexors, corrective splinting (ie, dynamic splinting or serial plaster splinting) is required. Serial plaster splinting is generally necessary due to the fixed nature of the deformities. Circumferential plaster stretchers to increase MCP joint flexion (Fig. 57-6) or cylinder casts (Fig. 57-7) to increase proximal IP joint extension are worn at all times. Plaster splints are

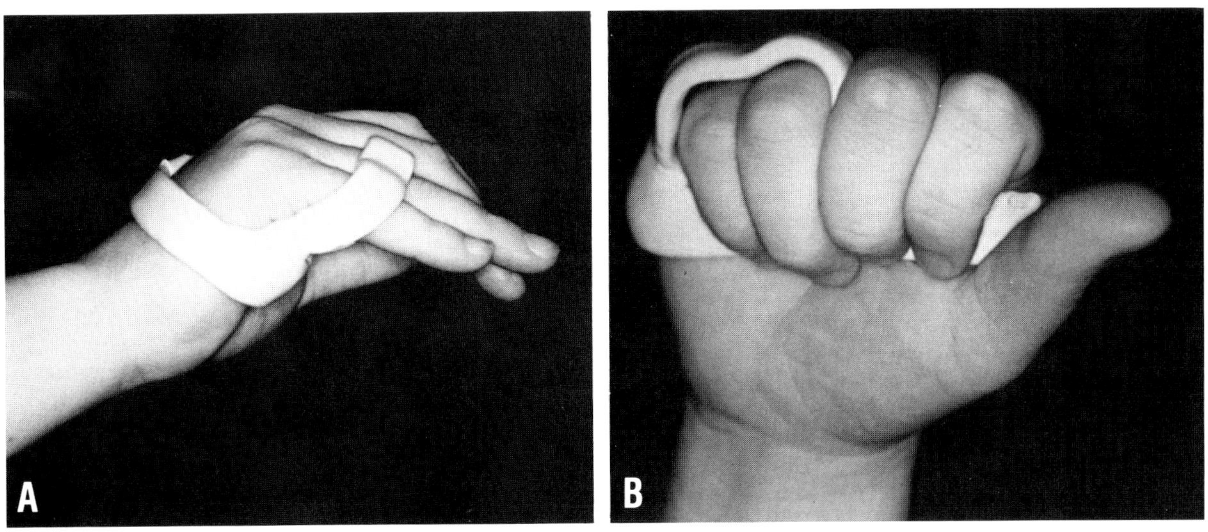

Figure 57–5. (**A**) This patient with ulnar nerve palsy displays active extension without clawing in her figure-eight splint. (**B**) She also displays flexion without hindrance from the splint.

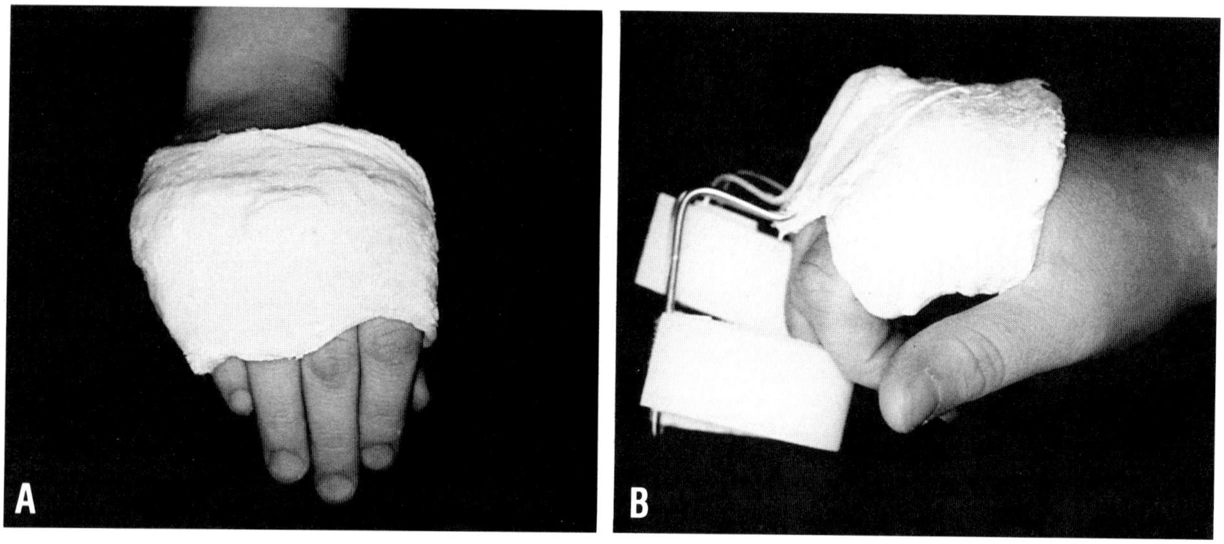

Figure 57–6. *(**A**) This circumferential plaster stretcher is used to increase metacarpophalangeal joint flexion after median or ulnar nerve injury when the metacarpophalangeal joints have stiffened in an extended position. The patient can also exercise in this splint to increase interphalangeal joint extension. Firm volar pressure is necessary to prevent metacarpophalangeal joint hyperextension. (**B**) Static adjustable interphalangeal joint extension outriggers are added to the circumferential serial plaster to increase interphalangeal joint extension.*

usually changed two or three times a week to accommodate tissue elongation. As the contractures become less severe, dynamic splinting replaces the plaster splints.[6,17,36]

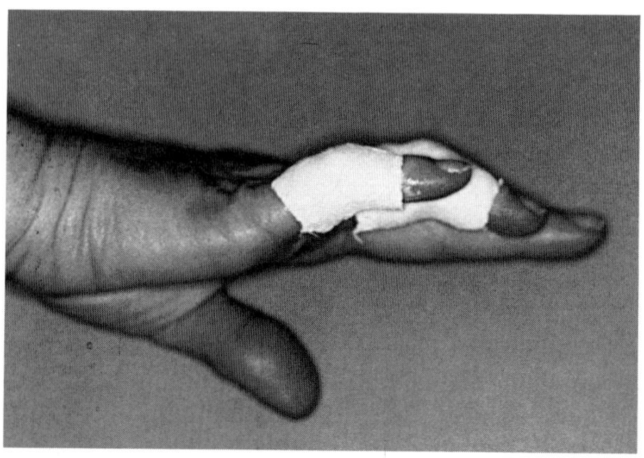

Figure 57–7. *Serial cylinder casting is used to correct proximal interphalangeal joint flexion contractures for this patient with ulnar nerve palsy. Cylinder casts are the treatment of choice for joints with contractures of greater than 35° or joints with a hard end-feel.*

Splinting for Combined Median and Ulnar Nerve Palsy

Patients with combined median and ulnar nerve loss present the most serious rehabilitative challenge, as the dual nerve loss often occurs in conjunction with tendon and vascular damage. The resulting deformity is known as the "ape hand" (Fig. 57-8). It includes full clawing, thenar and hypothenar flattening, and adduction and flexion of the thumb. With this degree of involvement, the incidence of fixed deformity is greater.

A figure-eight splint, as described above, that includes all four digits is used. When clawing requires a stronger counterforce over the proximal phalanges to prevent MCP extension, a "hood"-type splint may be used (Fig. 57-9). A one-piece thermoplastic splint is molded over the proximal phalanges and metacarpals of the involved digits. A palmar section that includes a C-bar is molded into the palm and first web space at the level of the distal palmar crease to prevent movement of the phalangeal heads palmarly when the MCP

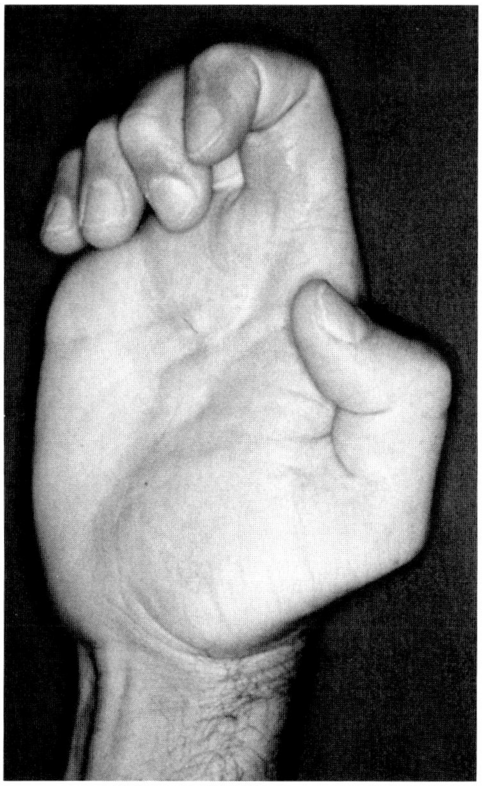

Figure 57–8. *The "ape hand" deformity typical of a hand that has sustained combined median and ulnar nerve laceration.*

joints extend. This splint requires secure strapping through the first web space, across the palm, and around the wrist.[17] Elastic Velcro works well for this purpose.

Splinting for Radial Nerve Injury

Wrist drop is the most obvious deformity in radial nerve paralysis. The wrist is held in varying degrees of palmar flexion because of the overaction of wrist flexors unopposed by wrist extensors. The thumb is held in palmar abduction and slight flexion because of the unopposed action of the short flexor and short abductor muscles working against the long abductor and short and long extensor muscles of the thumb.

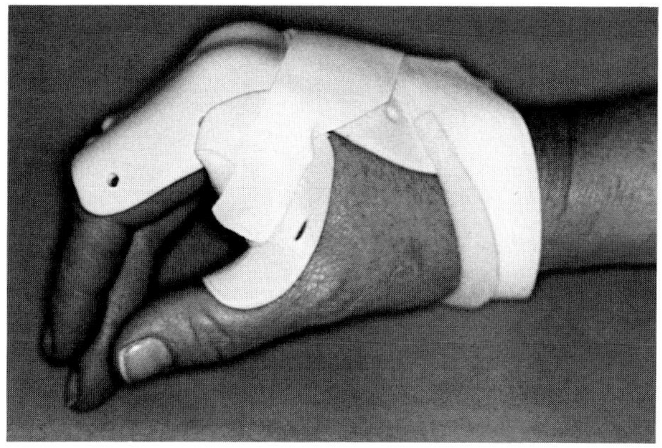

Figure 57–9. *The hood splint is preferable to a figure-eight splint when a strong counterforce is required to prevent clawing.*

Because the wrist provides the key to hand function at the digital level, loss of the ability to position the wrist in extension diminishes coordination and significantly weakens grasp.[2] The deficit of MCP joint extension is a less serious problem. Active IP joint extension is preserved because these joints are extended by the interossei, which are not innervated by the radial nerve.[24]

For most patients a simple cock-up splint (Fig. 57-10) that supports the wrist in extension provides the necessary balance for grasp, manipulation, and prevention of unopposed wrist flexion. A splint that provides the same function as a cock-up splint but allows wrist motion and substitutes for MCP joint extension is the tenodesis splint described by Col-

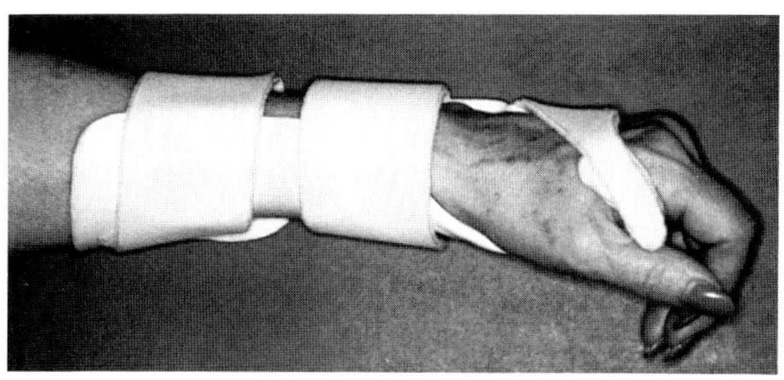

Figure 57–10. *A cock-up splint is used to provide wrist stability for this patient with radial nerve palsy secondary to a humeral fracture.*

ditz.[17,18] To construct this splint, a dorsal trough is molded over the forearm. Firm molding of the trough behind the styloids with appropriate padding prevents distal migration. A low-profile outrigger is based on the trough and extends distally to the midportion of the proximal phalanges. The outrigger is made of ⅛″ brass welding rod. A finger loop is placed around each proximal phalanx. Nylon cord on each finger loop is directed through thermoplastic channels in the outrigger and secured to a hook on the dorsal trough. The length of the cord to each finger loop is adjusted so that when the MCP joints actively flex, the wrist is brought into extension by the tension of the cords (Fig. 57-11). When the wrist actively flexes, cord tension acts to bring the MCP joints into extension. This splint provides a tenodesis function to the hand while maintaining good muscle balance and length.

A forearm palmar pan splint is worn at night to prevent the development of flexor tendon tightness (Fig. 57-12).

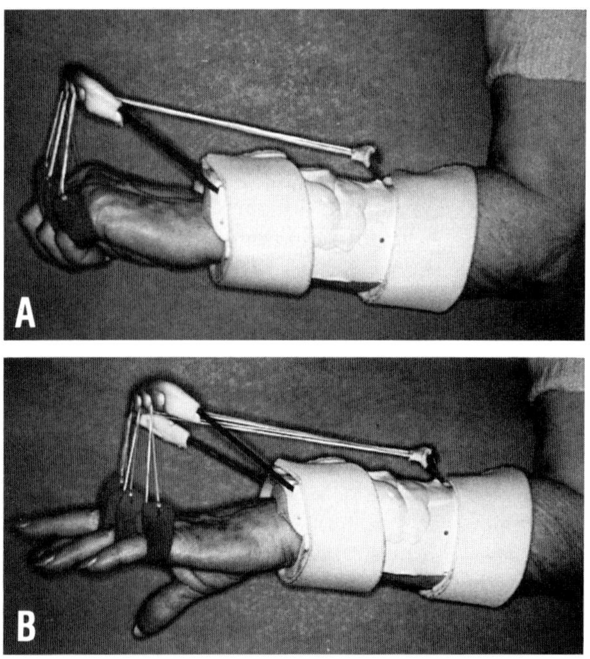

Figure 57–11. *The radial palsy splint designed by Colditz permits (**A**) wrist extension with finger flexion and (**B**) metacarpophalangeal joint extension with wrist flexion.*

FUNCTIONAL REHABILITATION

While splints are used to restore balance externally for imbalances occurring in the hand, active and passive exercise is necessary to influence tendon and nerve excursion and to strengthen the extremity.

Regular testing for motor return is carried out. Exercise sessions that emphasize isolated contraction of reinnervated muscles are initiated as soon as a trace contraction is perceived. Sessions are brief to avoid fatigue. Training begins with isometric exercises and advances to isotonic exercises in gravity-eliminated planes. Biofeedback is often useful in the early stages of retraining for teaching patients to locate the muscle or muscle groups and to document progress.

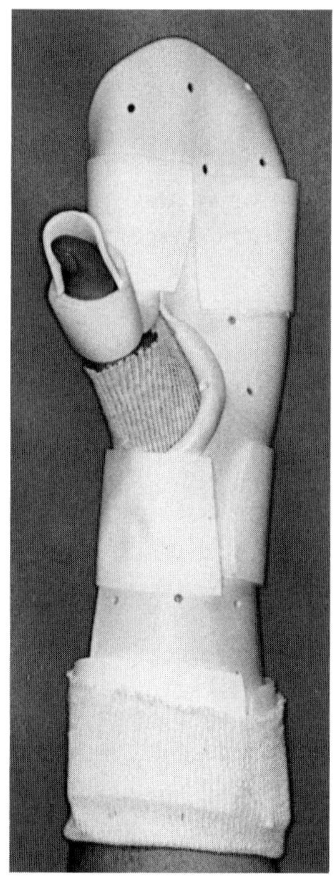

Figure 57–12. *When a wrist extension splint is used for activities, a palmar pan splint worn at night can prevent the development of flexor tendon tightness.*

Carefully selected and purposeful activities, combined with splinting for positioning, are useful because they require muscles to work in groups, which is their natural pattern. This facilitates the development of coordination and strength. In ulnar nerve retraining, activities that require grip, IP joint extension, and thumb lateral pinch are useful. Activities that require precision grip are useful in median nerve palsy. Radial nerve retraining is aided by activities that require a stable wrist during grip.

As nerve recovery progresses, quantitative assessment of hand function is done. In addition to muscle testing, the assessment includes measurement of power grasp (using a dynamometer) and measurement of pinch (using the pinch gauge). Specific standardized tests (eg, Purdue Pegboard, Minnesota Rate of Manipulation, nine-hole peg test) are used to chart functional progress. The BTE Work Simulator is useful in measuring the patient's endurance and ability to perform job-related tasks.

SENSIBILITY EVALUATION

The purpose of sensibility testing is to evaluate recovery on a quantitative and qualitative basis. Such tests can show if axonal regeneration is occurring and, if it is occurring, how well the patient uses the hand with existing return of motor and sensory function.

Sensibility Tests

Sensibility tests are divided into three main categories: threshold tests, functional tests, and objective tests.

Threshold tests, tests for cutaneous function, include pin-prick perception, temperature perception, light touch/deep pressure, and vibration.[4,16,19,23]

Functional tests assess the quality of sensibility. Is it present on a gross level, or on a fine discriminative level? Is it useful for fine prehension tasks? Is it adequate for the patient's activities of daily living and work tasks where the patient must recognize and manipulate objects with vision occluded? Functional tests include two-point discrimination, ridge sensitometer, gnostic rings, the Seddon coin test, and the Moberg pick-up test.[14,16,21,23,28,33,34]

Objective tests require only the passive cooperation of the patient, not subjective interpretation of a stimulus. These tests include the ninhydrin sweat test, wrinkle test, and nerve-conduction studies.[27,30–32] Although these tests do not correlate with functional sensation after nerve repair, the ninhydrin sweat test and the wrinkle test are useful in evaluating nerve function in children and malingerers, and nerve conduction studies provide useful information about fiber regeneration.[1,16,29,35]

Brand emphasized that measurement must be precise and repeatable.[13] Precision requires the therapist's time, but time can be saved by selecting one or two tests to evaluate recovery on a *quantitative anatomical basis* and one or two tests to evaluate recovery on a *functional basis*. The time that is saved is spent ensuring the precision and repeatability of measurements and in measuring the patient's progress more frequently.

Callahan recommends a battery of tests to answer three questions[16]:

1. Is protective sensibility present, as measured by the ability to perceive a sharp object, deep pressure, or hot or cold?
2. Is light touch present?
3. If light touch is present, is it present on a gross level only or on a fine discriminative level?

With these questions in mind, the following tests are used to evaluate nerve recovery on both quantitative anatomical and functional bases.

Threshold Test

Semmes-Weinstein Monofilaments

Semmes-Weinstein monofilaments come in a kit of 20 monofilaments, each attached to a Lucite rod and graded in thickness so that the filaments, except for the very largest, buckle as the examiner presses them against the skin. The stress exerted on the skin is proportional to the length and diameter of the calibrated filament, not to the stress exerted by the examiner, as long as first-order buckling is maintained. First-order buckling is the bowing produced in a properly applied Semmes-Weinstein monofilament when the examiner applies only those lateral forces necessary to keep the top end directly over the lower end when the filament is in contact with the skin.[25]

The stimulus is activated by the mechanical deformation of the skin. The filament bends the skin, and skin deformation causes the firing of nerve endings (see Chap. 8). Despite variables such as callousing and the age of the patient, the Semmes-Weinstein monofilaments are recognized as the best hand-held instrument to monitor sensory change or recovery, especially when the patient is repeatedly tested with the same instrument by the same tester.[5,13] The monofilaments provide controlled, objective, reproducible force stimuli for testing peripheral nerve function.[9] (Implicit in this statement is the assumption that the monofilaments are of correct length and diameter.) If these two measurements have been calibrated by the therapist and are correct, "the application forces of the filaments are repeatable within a predictable range."[9]

Technique

Attention to detail by the examiner will affect the test results. Testing takes place in a quiet room where the patient will not be distracted.

Brand reported that one source of error in testing is that the patient can be given cues other than the intended stimulus.[13] He wrote that even a stimulus as slight as a 1-g fiber will move a finger that is passive and free to move. Movement of the finger is perceived proximally in the forearm by movement of the tendon and muscle even when the finger is insensitive; the patient then points to the totally insensitive finger and says that it has been touched. For this reason, the patient's hand is fully supported in a lump of putty while the finger is being tested.

Visual clues are also helpful to the patient. The tester may observe carefully when touching the digit, but pay less attention when not touching it. Patients respond to facial expressions with a "yes" or "no." To prevent such visual clues, the patient is blindfolded or a screen is used.

Evaluation of sensibility is done more quickly and is more precise when the therapist maps out the area of sensibility dysfunction before testing begins. The therapist draws a probe, such as the blunt end of a pen, lightly over the skin in a radial-to-ulnar and proximal-to-distal manner from an area of normal sensibility to an area of suspected abnormal sensibility. The patient, whose vision is occluded, is asked to say "now" when the sensation produced by the probe feels "different." The area described as "different" is marked with a felt-tip pen. The tester then proceeds to approach the area of dysfunction from another starting point until all boundaries of abnormal sensibility are marked.

When monitoring nerve recovery, testing becomes more systematic and documentation more accurate by using a worksheet that has a grid superimposed on the outline of a hand.[16,22,37] The grid is divided into seven zones. The longitudinal lines parallel the rays of the hand and the horizontal lines correspond to the flexion creases of the IP joints and palmar creases. The tester visualizes the grid on the patient's hand and applies the filament to the center of a particular zone. Correct and incorrect responses are recorded in the corresponding zone on a worksheet.

The uninvolved extremity is tested first, allowing the patient to become familiar with the testing procedure and the tester to establish the patient's normal sensibility range. Testing usually begins with filament 2.83, which is considered normal light touch.[16]

The tester touches a spot, and as soon as the patient feels the applied pressure, he or she says "touch." Delays in response are noted. To attain a repeatable touch threshold measurement, the time of filament application is standardized and the test area varied.[13] Filaments 1.65 through 4.08 are applied three times.[3] Two successive positive responses to a particular filament are required. If the first response is accurate and the second inaccurate, a third trial is made to reach final assessment of that zone. When responses are inaccurate for two trials with a given filament in a given zone, the tester returns to that zone at random intervals with successively thicker filaments until a correct response is elicited. Successive testing is always scattered randomly to prevent the patient from anticipating the next stimulus.

The results of testing are transferred to a color-coded form for quick visual reference and comparable mapping of sensibility. Consistent colors correspond to the sensibility levels; for example, green (1.65–2.83) indicates normal sensibility.

Testing of the monofilament application forces has shown that the 20 monofilaments in the traditional filament kit may not all be necessary. Bell reported that the variation in force range of one monofilament may overlap with its neighbor.[4,7] Brand suggested that no more than five forces need to be used ordinarily in diagnostic tests, and perhaps only one or two for monitoring progress or recovery.[13]

Therefore, the number of monofilaments used can be reduced with no significant loss in sensitivity of the test. Indeed, a mini-kit of five filaments that is considered adequate for most testing is now available. It is less time-consuming and more cost-effective; in fact, Bell reported that unless careful calibration was performed, the complete set was no more sensitive as a test instrument than the mini-kit. The increments between the filaments in the mini-kits are spaced sufficiently far apart so that they never overlap; thus, they can reliably show progressive return or diminution in peripheral nerve function. The five filaments represent the cut-off forces for each functional level of sensibility (normal, diminished light touch, diminished protective, and loss of protective sensation); two filaments are included for loss of protective sensation.

In an effort to eliminate the need for separate test filaments and to place the mini-kit filaments in one instrument, Bell developed Pocket Filaments (Fig. 57-13).[7] The five colored filaments, which correspond to the colors used for mapping peripheral nerve involvement, are arranged in increasing sizes and can be separated and reassembled easily. Telescoping rods allow the filaments to be stored in a small case and extended for use.

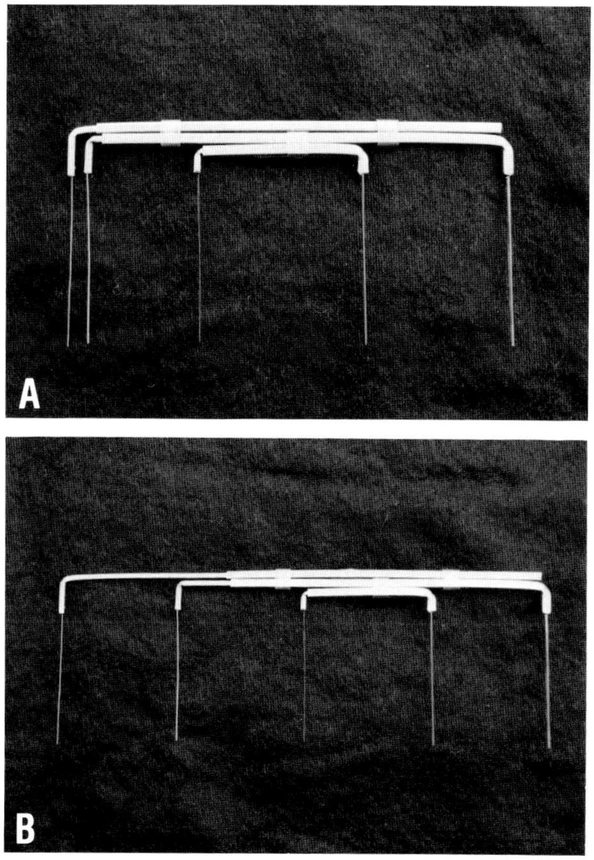

Figure 57–13. *Pocket filaments developed by Bell. (**A**) collapsed for storage; and (**B**) extended for use.*

Functional Tests

Constant Two-Point Discrimination

The Weber two-point discrimination test measures the quality of sensation that has returned and, therefore, assesses the digit's ability to function as a sensory organ.[1,37,38] The test determines the minimal distance at which the patient can discriminate between being touched with one point and being touched with two points.

Although Moberg uses an ordinary paper clip with a diameter of about 0.9 mm as a testing instrument,[27] a paper clip is not recommended because there is a sharp barb on the end of the clip, which stimulates pain receptors. A Boley gauge or other caliper with blunt ends is recommended (Fig. 57-14). The Boley gauge measures the exact distance between the points in millimeters and can be adjusted in 1-mm increments. The tester is careful to avoid applying too much pressure, as the Boley gauge is rather heavy. Although the two-point discrimination test is not a threshold test, the pressure applied should be light (about 5 g). The

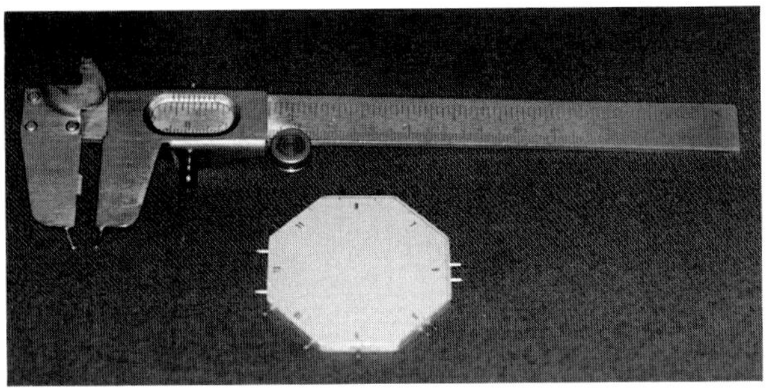

Figure 57–14. *A Boley gauge or Disk-Criminator are recommended two-point discrimination test instruments.*

higher the pressure, the wider is the area of skin that is deformed and stimulated.[13]

The test procedure is explained and demonstrated while the patient observes. The hand is fully supported in putty. During testing, the patient's vision is blocked with a screen or blindfold. The gauge is set with a distance of 5 mm between the two points. One or two points are touched in random sequence along a longitudinal axis in the center of the fingertip. In applying two points, both points touch the skin simultaneously, or the patient will have the obvious clue that pressure builds up in time, even though he or she cannot distinguish separation in space.

The patient responds each time a stimulus is felt. If he or she cannot recognize that the finger has been touched with one or two points, he or she responds, "I don't know." Ten separate stimuli are given. If the patient cannot distinguish seven out of ten stimulations correctly, the distance between the two points is increased and the stimulation is repeated until the patient gives the required accurate responses. Testing is stopped at 15 mm if the response is nondiscriminatory.

The interpretation of scores is based on these recommendations from the American Society for Surgery of the Hand:

Normal: less than 6 mm
Fair: 6 to 10 mm
Poor: 11 to 15 mm
Protective: one point perceived
Anesthetic: no point perceived.

Moving Two-Point Discrimination

Dellon's moving two-point discrimination test provides an earlier means of assessing the return of discrimination than the constant two-point test (see Chap. 8).[21] Moving two-point discrimination depends on quickly adapting fibers, which return sooner and in greater density than slowly adapting fibers, on which constant touch depends.

As with constant two-point discrimination, a Boley gauge is used. Testing is begun with the instrument set at an 8-mm distance between the two points. The gauge is moved proximally to distally on the fingertip, parallel to the long axis of the finger, with the testing ends side by side. The patient is required to respond to seven out of ten stimuli before the distance is narrowed. Testing is stopped at 2 mm, which represents normal moving two-point discrimination.[16]

Dellon reported that moving two-point discrimination returns earlier and is usually 8 to 10 mm better than constant two-point discrimination.[21] Moving two-point discrimination gives a measure of the hand's ability to feel objects, provided hand motion is possible. Constant two-point discrimination indicates the capacity of the hand to be aware of held still objects; this usually returns when constant two-point discrimination is less than 15 mm. This means that a patient whose hand has 10 mm of moving two-point discrimination can detect and identify small objects unseen, but once the object is lifted and held immobile, the patient cannot identify it.[26] The classic two-point discrimination test is still recommended, therefore, to provide this information.[21]

Point Localization

Point localization using the Semmes-Weinstein monofilaments is considered a reflection of higher-level integration than that provided by light touch perception.

With the patient's hand fully supported on putty and his or her vision blocked, the examiner applies a filament to the center of a particular zone. The examiner begins with the lowest-numbered filament that resulted in a positive response during light touch testing. As soon as the patient perceives the stimulus, he or she opens the eyes and points to the area touched. The filament is applied once to each zone. The speed of the response is related to the level of sensibility. If the patient correctly localizes the stimulus, a dot is marked in the corresponding zone on the worksheet. If the stimulus is incorrectly localized, an arrow is drawn on the worksheet from the point of stimulation to the point where the touch is referred. This mapping of responses gives a picture of the patient's level of localization. Serial testing in conjunction with re-education should show fewer and shorter arrows.

Moberg Pick-Up Test

Tactile gnosis is the fine sensibility of the finger pulps that permits recognition of what is being touched without the aid of sight. The Moberg pick-up test assesses general sensibility and tactile gnosis. The advantage of the pick-up test is that it combines sensibility with motion, requiring active manipulation and recognition of an object. The patient must pick up nine objects of different shapes and sizes, one at a time, as quickly as possible, and place them in a container. The objects may be such items as a safety pin, a paper clip, a screw, a key, a marble, coins, and a nut and bolt.

The test is first done with the involved hand and then with the uninvolved hand. When picking up objects with vision blocked, the patient uses whatever sensation he or she has, including the parts of the hand that have not been damaged. The importance of this test is that the examiner can observe the patient's functional aptitude for picking up objects.[27] Dellon modified the test by standardizing test items and by requiring correct object identification.[20]

Objective Test

Nerve Conduction Studies

Nerve conduction studies are valuable for the anatomical localization of a lesion in a peripheral nerve trunk.

SENSORY RE-EDUCATION

Sensory re-education is an integral part of the care of every patient following nerve injury and repair if the patient is to maximize the sensory potential that the repair has provided (see Chap. 58).

The course of treatment for the peripheral nerve–injured patient extends over a long period of time. Unlike a simple fracture, the nerve heals neither quickly nor predictably. The patient's involvement in therapy may vary significantly during this period, from considerable intensity during the early phase, to internal assessment, every few months as nerve function slowly improves. Throughout this process, the skill and encouragement of the therapist are key to a positive outcome.

REFERENCES

1. Almquist E, Eeg-Elofsson O. Sensory nerve conduction velocity and two-point discrimination in sutured nerves. J Bone Joint Surg 1970.
2. Beasley RW. Surgical anatomy of the hand. In: Hand injuries. Philadelphia: WB Saunders, 1981:7–29.
3. Bell JA. Sensibility evaluation. In: Hunter JM, Schneider LH, Mackin EJ, Callahan AD, eds. Rehabilitation of the hand: Surgery and therapy, ed 3. St. Louis: CV Mosby, 1989.
4. Bell JA. Light-touch deep-pressure testing using Semmes-Weinstein monofilaments. In: Hunter JM, Schneider LH, Mackin EJ, Callahan AD, eds. Rehabilitation of the hand: Surgery and therapy, ed 3. St. Louis: CV Mosby, 1984:399–406.
5. Bell JA, Buford WL. The force-time relationship of clinically used sensory testing instruments. J Hand Therapy 1988; 1(2):76–85.
6. Bell-Krotoski JA. Plaster cylinder casting for contractures of the interphalangeal joints. In: Hunter JM, Schneider LH, Mackin EJ, Callahan AD, eds. Rehabilitation of the hand: Surgery and therapy, ed 3. St. Louis: CV Mosby, 1990:1128–1133.
7. Bell-Krotoski JA. Pocket filaments and specifications for the Semmes-Weinstein monofilaments. J Hand Therapy 1990; 3:26.
8. Bell-Krotoski JA. Pre- and postoperative management of tendon transfers after ulnar nerve repair. In: Hunter JM, Schneider LH, Mackin EJ, Callahan AD, eds. Rehabilitation of the Hand: Surgery and therapy, ed 3. St. Louis: CV Mosby, 1990:676–695.

9. Bell-Krotoski JA, Tomancik E. The repeatability of testing with Semmes-Weinstein monofilaments. J Hand Surg [Am] 1987; 12:155–161.
10. Brand PW. Management of the insensitive limb. Phys Ther 1979; 59:8–12.
11. Brand PW. Management of sensory loss in the extremities. In: Management of peripheral nerve problems. Philadelphia: WB Saunders, 1980:862–872.
12. Brand PW. External stress: Effect at the surface. In: Clinical mechanics of the hand. St. Louis: CV Mosby, 1985:88–104.
13. Brand PW. Methods and modalities of clinical assessment of the hand. In: Clinical mechanics of the hand. St. Louis: CV Mosby, 1985:166–191.
14. Brunelli SG. Gnostic rings for assessment of tactile gnosis. ASSH Newsletter, No. 53, 1981.
15. Callahan AD. Methods of compensation and reeducation for sensory dysfunction. In: Hunter JM, Schneider LH, Mackin EJ, Callahan AD. Rehabilitation of the hand, ed 3. St. Louis: CV Mosby, 1990: 611–621.
16. Callahan AD. Sensibility testing: Clinical methods. In: Hunter JM, Schneider LH, Mackin EJ, Callahan AD, eds. Rehabilitation of the hand: Surgery and therapy, ed 3. St. Louis: CV Mosby, 1990:594–610.
17. Callahan AD. Therapist's management of nerve injuries. Presented at Surgery and Rehabilitation of the Hand, Philadelphia, 1986.
18. Colditz JC. Splinting for radial nerve palsy. J Hand Therapy 1987; 1:18–22.
19. Dellon AL. Evaluation of sensibility and re-education of sensation in the hand. Baltimore: Williams & Wilkins, 1981:141–167.
20. Dellon AL. The paper clip: Light hardware to evaluate sensibility in the hand. Contemp Orthop 1979; 1:39.
21. Dellon AL. The moving two-point discrimination test: Clinical evaluation of the quickly-adapting fiber-receptor system. J Hand Surg 1978; 3:474–481.
22. Fess E. Documentation: Essential elements of an upper extremity assessment battery. In Hunter JM, Schneider LH, Mackin EJ, Callahan A, eds. Rehabilitation of the hand, ed 3. St. Louis, CV Mosby, 1990:53–81.
23. Fess E. Evaluation of the hand by objective measurements. In: Hunter JM, Schneider LH, Mackin EJ, Bell JA, eds. Rehabilitation of the hand. St. Louis: CV Mosby, 1978:70–93.
24. Fess EE, Gettle KS, Strickland JW. Exercise and splinting for specific problems. In: Hand splinting. St. Louis: CV Mosby, 1981:204–239.
25. Levin S, Pearsall G, Ruderman RJ. Von Frey's method of measuring pressure sensibility in the hand: An engineering analysis of the Semmes-Weinstein pressure aesthesiometer. J Hand Surg 1978; 3:211.
26. Lister G. Reconstruction. In:. The hand: Diagnosis and indications. New York: Churchill-Livingstone, 1984:107–191.
27. Moberg E. Objective methods for determining the functional sensibility in the hand. J Bone Joint Surg [Br] 1958; 40:454.
28. Moberg E. Criticism and study of methods for examining sensibility in the hand. Neurology 1962; 12:8.
29. Onne L. Recovery of sensibility and sudomotor activity in the hand after nerve suture. Acta Chir Scand [Suppl] 1962; 300:1.
30. O'Riain S. New and simple test of nerve function in the hand. Br Med J 1973; 22:615.
31. Perry GF, Hamilton GF, Lachinbruch PA, et al. Protective sensation in the hand and its correlation to the ninhydrin sweat test following nerve laceration. Am J Phys Med 1974; 53:113.
32. Phelps P, Walker E. Comparison of the finger-wrinkling test results to established sensory tests in peripheral nerve injury. Am J Occup Ther 1977; 31:9.
33. Poppin NK, McCarroll HR, Doyle JR, et al. Recovery of sensibility after suture of digital nerves. J Hand Surg 1979; 4:212–226.
34. Seddon HJ. Surgical disorders of the peripheral nerves, ed 2. New York: Churchill-Livingstone, 1975.
35. Stromberg WB, McFarlane RM, Bell JL, et al. Injury of the median and ulnar nerves: 150 cases with an evaluation of Moberg's ninhydrin test. J Bone Joint Surg [Am] 1961; 43:717.
36. Tribuzi SM. Serial plaster splinting. In: Hunter JM, Schneider LH, Mackin EJ, Callahan AD, eds. Rehabilitation of the hand: Surgery and therapy, ed 3. St. Louis: CV Mosby, 1990:1120–1127.
37. Von Prince K, Butler B. Measuring sensory function of the hand in peripheral nerve injuries. Am J Occup Ther 1967; 21:285.
38. Weber EH. Veber den Tastinn. Arch Anat Physio Wessensch Med 1835:152.

58

Sensory Re-Education

Margaret Carter-Wilson

AUTHOR'S KEY POINTS

- The major persisting deficit following repair of a peripheral nerve is the inability to interpret spatial relationships. This is evidenced both in innervation density testing, such as static two-point discrimination, and in poor functional use of the hand.
- In the first year after repair of a peripheral nerve, the most reliable and helpful means of clinically charting the status of regeneration and sensory re-education is through localization, threshold testing (using both vibration and Semmes-Weinstein monofilaments), and functional testing using time and accuracy object identification.
- Sensory re-education is approached in three stages: desensitization and protection, localization, and discrimination.
- The most significant indicator of success in sensory re-education is functional use of the hand.
- Current neurophysiologic research has established that cortical plasticity exists. Ideally, recent studies on the function of the somatosensory cortex will answer the questions regarding the complex mechanism for perceiving spatial discrimination. Improved functional re-education should follow.

CURRENT STATUS AFTER PERIPHERAL NERVE REPAIR

While efforts to measure sensibility and retrain motor function after nerve transection and repair have received considerable attention, the re-education of sensation is often overlooked.[14,15,68,69]

Between 6 and 9 months after repair of a major nerve at the wrist, the return of protective sensibility to the fingertips can be expected, but localization and tactile gnosis are virtually absent.[65] Hyperaesthesia of some degree is usually present, and normal use of the hand is awkward or purposefully avoided.[27,68,85] The primary method of assessing the status of repaired nerve does not give a complete view of the progress of regeneration. For almost 30 years, the static two-point discrimination test has been used to measure functional sensation in the hand. However, the results of repair cited in the literature indicate that adults with nerve repairs, even under the best circumstances, often have poor values on testing.[7,13,66–68] Although two-point discrimination correlates directly with the ability to execute precise sensory grips,[74] it does not always parallel hand function.[66,68,69] Parry observed that active motion is essential for functional sensation, and that following injury and repair of a major nerve, a static test such as two-point discrimination may be irrelevant to actual performance.[69] Since results obtained by static two-point discrimination are poor, sensory testing methods that assess early levels of return for quantitating regeneration, re-education, and function are essential.[28]

TESTING SENSIBILITY

The parameters used to evaluate sensibility are based on sensory physiological findings that examine the mechanoreceptors, sensory pathways, somatosensory cortex, and the large, myelinated A-beta fibers mediating touch. Mountcastle identified two populations of A-beta fibers, quickly adapting (QA) and slowly adapting (SA), that transmit the perception of touch by response to a constant touch stimulus.[63] QA fibers innervate Meissner's corpuscle in the dermal ridges and Pacinian corpuscles in the dermis.[13,16,20,63] They detect transient touch, movement, and vibration. SA fibers respond to increased indentation of the skin, innervate the Merkel cell-neurite complex, and mediate the sensation of pressure.[13,16,20,63] Clinical tests that evaluate regeneration of both populations include assessment of innervation density (number of nerve fiber/receptors innervating a receptive field) and threshold testing (the intensity of a stimulus necessary to evoke a recognized response).

Since innervation density is related to the amount of cortical representation in the somatosensory cortex, a high level of cortical integration is required to identify a stimulus correctly (Fig. 58-1).[21] Static two-point discrimination is used to assess innervation density of the SA fiber/receptor system, and moving two-point discrimination is used to identify the QA population.[12,13,18,63] Regular progression of receptive field sizes, from small to large, within the somatosensory maps of area 3b has been shown to match the progression of innervation density (Fig. 58-2).[20,76] Following injury and regeneration, sequential reorganization of the cortical representations of involved skin surfaces undergoes several changes, including response to tactile stimulation due to abnormal receptive fields.[20] Since cortical reorganization and reinnervation of peripheral mechanoreceptors occur over

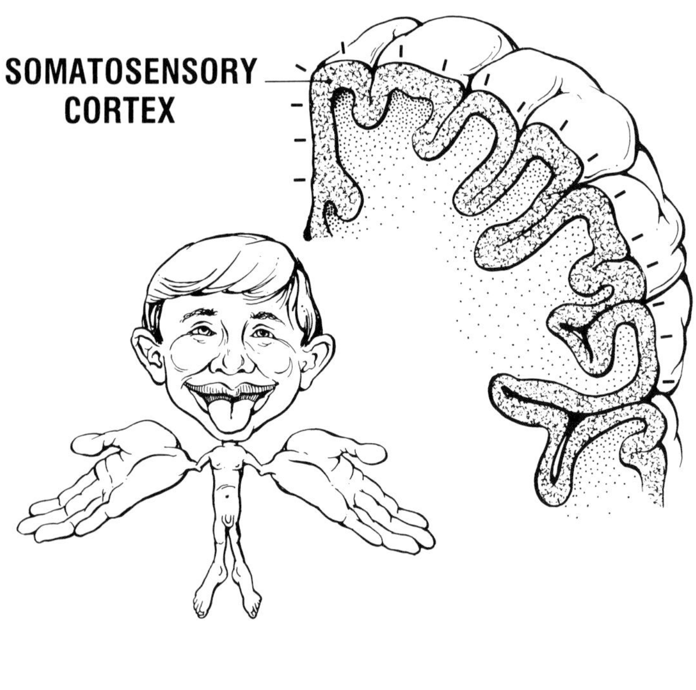

Figure 58–1. *Caricature depicting the significant representation of the hand in the topographically arranged somatosensory cortex in man. The innervation density of the afferent receptors in the periphery is directly proportional to the amount of space allotted to each body part.*

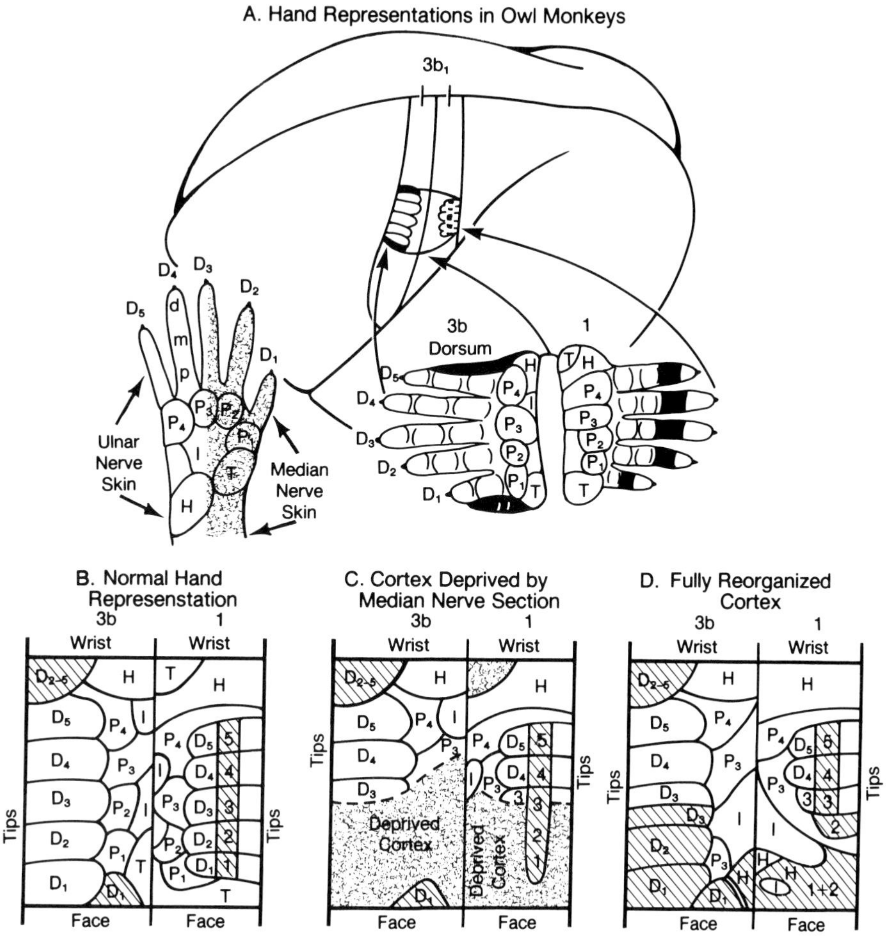

Figure 58–2. *The reorganization of the hand representations in Areas 3b and 1 of somatosensory cortex of monkeys after section of the median nerve.* **(A)** *The location and normal somatotropic organizations of the two hand representations are indicated on a dorsolateral view of the owl monkey brain. The two representations are basically mirror images of each other, adjoined at the 3b/1 border; the major difference is in the representation of dorsal digit and hand surfaces (black). The median nerve subserves the glabrous skin of the medial hand, while the ulnar nerve innervates the dorsal and glabrous surfaces of the lateral hand. The rest of the hand is subserved by the radial nerve. Digits and palmar pads are numbered in order, insular (I), hypothenar (H), thenar (T) pads, and distal (d), middle (m), and proximal (p) phalanges are indicated.* **(B)** *The normal hand representations are schematically portrayed in more detail.* **(C)** *The cortex normally devoted to the median nerve is marked by* ***dots*** *(the deprived cortex).* **(D)** *The organization of the hand representations after complete reactivation following median nerve section. Much of the deprived cortex is activated by stimulation of the dorsal hand and digit surfaces (black). In addition, palmar pads innervated by the ulnar nerve have increased their cortical representation. The ulnar and radial nerves do not grow into the anesthetic skin. (From Kaas JH, Merzenich MM, Killackey HD. The reorganization of somatosensory cortex following peripheral nerve damage in adult and developing mammals. Ann Rev Neuroscience 1983; 6:328, with permission)*

time, results of innervation density testing may not be recordable until late in the regeneration period of a repaired major nerve.[28]

Threshold measurements of sensibility taken early in the sensory recovery period give helpful information regarding the progression of regeneration and re-education.[27] The perception of low-frequency vibration (about 30 cps) and high-frequency vibration (about 256 cps) tests the threshold of the rapidly adapting fiber/receptors.[13,20,47,63] Semmes-Weinstein monofilaments measure the threshold of the SA fiber/receptors and are the most accurate tool for a separate measurement of localization.[3,4,6]

A recent study of 46 adults following median nerve repair at the wrist concluded that Semmes-Weinstein monofilament testing was very useful, especially for assessment of sequential and quantitative sensory recovery within the first postoperative year.[28] The review also determined that object recognition was closely related to the cutaneous pressure threshold within that postoperative year, during which two-point discrimination was seldom recovered. The final conclusion was that the results of Semmes-Weinstein testing of SA threshold improved significantly with sensory re-education and were one of the most valuable measurable parameters in the early stages of sensory recovery.[28]

SENSORY RE-EDUCATION

Sensory re-education programs are based on the assumption that at some point, a patient with a regenerating peripheral nerve begins to demonstrate less recovery of functional sensation than his or her potential. The reason for this underachievement is the patient's inability to interpret the altered impulses he or she perceives.[15] This alteration in perception of precise touch occurs along the entire sensory pathway. At the periphery there are degeneration of receptors,[11,36] reduction in nerve fibers, entrapment of fibers at the repair site, erroneous reinnervation, establishment of receptive fields of discontinuous skin sites, reduced conduction velocity, cross-innervation, and changes in the sizes of the receptive fields.[36,84,88] Centrally, investigation has shown there is significant disorganization in the somatosensory cortex, including abnormalities in receptive fields and topographical organization.[19,25,43,56,57,59,70,73,77] Clinically, the patient demonstrates partial tactile sensitivity, poor ability to localize, and impaired ability to identify patterns, textures, forms, and objects. Hyperaesthesia of varying degrees is usually present.[7,15,68]

The purpose of sensory re-education is to help the patient interpret correctly the pattern of abnormal sensory input through an understanding of the problem, and to provide a structured method of retraining. Two specific findings of sensory physiology have important implications in re-education:

1. There is conclusive evidence that the cortical somatotopic maps in adult mammals are remarkably "plastic" and are not fixed or static in organization (see Fig. 58-2).[19,43,51,56–59,72,73,77]
2. Restructuring of the somatosensory cortex after peripheral nerve injury and repair is use-dependent.[8,37,43] Modification of cortical representation is determined by both the pattern and the frequency of use.[1,8,37,43,57,58]

Methods of sensory re-education focus on specific sensory input to assist in central reorganization, enabling the patient to enhance or even exceed the potential provided by nerve repair.[7,15,53,62]

Historical Perspective

The possibility of improvement of sensation following stroke or peripheral nerve injury has been reported by various clinicians interested in rehabilitation.[7,9,15,69] Stopford introduced this concept in 1926 in an article explaining the two-stage recovery of sensation.[82] In determining the interval between recovery of crude and higher forms of sensibility, he concluded that re-education was necessary to localize a stimulus.[84] Davis in 1949 and Bowden in 1954 noted that functional recovery was better when the tendency to use the hand was stronger and use was started earlier.[5,10] In 1959 Forster and Shields reported on specific sensory retraining in treatment of the hemiplegic hand.[22] Later, Vinograd modified their techniques and described the use of common objects in re-educating sensation.[87]

The first published program of sensory re-education following peripheral nerve repair was that of Parry in 1966.[68] He described a program requiring object identification that was designed to increase in complexity as the patient improved. The rationale offered for the success of his program came from observations of his patients' adaptive behavior; this rationale has now been confirmed by precise neurophysiologic findings. In 1971 Dellon, Edgerton, and Curtis presented a structured sensory re-education program based on Mountcastle's research in sensory physiology.[15–17] Their presentation provided the impetus for development of formal re-education programs, especially in hand rehabilitation. While creative clinicians have expanded on methods of assessment and sources of stimulation, the work of Parry and Dellon remains the foundation of most re-education programs.

STAGES OF RE-EDUCATION

While the technical emphasis of various re-education programs differs, most centers approach retraining in distinct stages: desensitization or protection, early-phase discrimination and localization, and late-phase discrimination or recovery of tactile gnosis.[7,15,62,69] The patient's progress is followed by various methods of sensory assessment designed to determine his or her level and progress.

Stage 1: Desensitization or Protection

In the first period of recovery from peripheral nerve injury, the patient presents initially with an anesthetic hand that is subject to injury due to loss of the most basic elements of sensibility: the patient cannot feel such things as a pinprick, temperature change, deep pressure, or abrading friction. The purpose of re-education at this level is to teach the patient how to compensate for lack of protective sensory input by using both visual and cognitive awareness of hand position and use.[7] The patient is taught to avoid excessive force when gripping or manipulating objects and to use low-grade repetitive pressure and friction instead. The amount of force applied when gripping an object is reduced when necessary by building up handles to disperse pressure. Gripping patterns are changed frequently during a sustained activity to prevent tissue damage, and the skin is observed frequently for such signs of stress as edema and color and temperature changes.[91]

Specific guidelines to compensate for the lack of protective sensation are reviewed with the patient. Exposure to heat, cold, and sharp objects is avoided. The patient is warned that the tips of the thumb, index, and middle fingers (in a median nerve injury) and the lateral border of the palm and little finger (in an ulnar nerve injury) are particularly susceptible. If stress signs, blisters, or lacerations occur, the patient is advised to rest the hand and treat the area to prevent infection. A daily routine of skin care is implemented to keep skin soft and pliable and to remedy the dryness caused by lack of normal sympathetic innervation.[7,15,62,68]

As the repaired nerve begins to regenerate, most patients experience a degree of hyperaesthesia, best described as an unpleasant quality added to cutaneous sensation and associated with an altered sensory threshold.[46,81,86] Stimuli that are pleasant to a normal hand may be perceived as uncomfortable or disagreeable. The precipitating stimulus is often a light, moving touch rather than a firm pressure.[81]

There is a diversity of opinion regarding both the mechanism creating this condition and the methods to resolve it.[46,86] A program of desensitization that applies graded stimuli to decrease discomfort and increase the tolerance for touch is helpful.[2,15] The well-documented techniques are an integral part of the treatment program for a variety of conditions including amputations, painful scar formation, and regenerating nerves.[2,23]

Patients undergoing nerve regeneration often describe their "feeling" as painful burning, pricking, or tingling sensations that interfere with function. Since activity in the A-delta fiber population corresponds with pricking pain and that in the C-fiber correlates with burning, slow, or lingering pain,[20,63,65] it is reasonable to hypothesize that desensitization is the first step in re-education of the immature nociceptor neuronal population. However, several studies have offered another point of view that may better explain the relationship between desensitization and sensory re-education. Large-diameter afferent fibers can create the sensation of pricking pain without stimulation of the nociceptor population.[65] If the non-noxious stimuli producing the discomfort are transmitted by the regenerating fibers mediating touch, an explanation for hyperaesthesia could be found in the reorganizing cortex. An association that has been suggested relates hypersensitivity after peripheral nerve injury to enlarged cortical representations of adjacent skin regions.[88] If repaired and regenerated nerves reactivate only part of their normal cortical space, injury-related cortical enlargements could remain apparent after regeneration. Thus, the hypersensitivity around reinnervated areas may be related to these enlargements, while the hypersensitivity within the reinnervated skin could be related to abnormally large representations of regional patches of skin. This explanation assumes that the quality of sensation is related to the size of the central cell population that is recruited during stimulation of specific skin surfaces. If this association is documented, the techniques and results of desensitization may become identical to those of sensory re-education, since both affect the reestablishment of normal organizational features in the somatosensory cortex.

A recent study of area 1 in the somatosensory cortex, describing the existence of neurons with inhibitory receptive fields, helps explain the effectiveness of desensitization.[32] It was noted that certain activities, such as light rubbing of the palmar skin, evoke an excitatory response. Others, such as continuous and stationary pressing of the fingers or application of a broad, nonmoving object to the finger and palmar surface, are inhibitory to both spontaneous and evoked activity. Further investigations may find a connection between inhibitory receptive fields and the re-education of regenerating afferent fibers through use of inhibitory temporospatial patterns of stimulation, or desensitization.

Most clinicians agree that the early state of intense discomfort patients experience during regeneration must be addressed before more discriminatory sensation can be expected.[7,15] Two schools of thought exist on the timing of retraining. While many clinicians feel that pain relief is essential before advancing to a higher level of re-education, others initiate the re-education process with the assumption that the painful condition will resolve during the process.[27] The reported success of both groups supports the suggestion that hyperaesthesia, usually present following nerve repair, can be resolved in much the same manner as re-education of touch perception.[7,27,68]

Early-Phase Discrimination and Localization

A variety of sensory testing techniques has been used to determine the appropriate time for beginning early-phase discriminatory re-education. The pattern of recovery is charted by evaluating sensibility with 30-cps vibration, moving touch, constant touch, and 256-cps vibration. Dellon found that the ability to perceive these stimuli occurs in a predictable time sequence.[14,16,18] When 30-cps vibration and moving touch return to the palm, early-phase retraining commences. Dellon argued that it is critical for re-education to begin by the time this pattern of recovery reaches the proximal phalanges.[14] Callahan requires the return of touch to the fingertips, as measured by the patient's ability to perceive the touch of the examiner's finger or the touch of the Semmes-Weinstein pressure aesthesiometer at a minimum level of 4.31.[7]

Goals in this early stage are to re-educate specific perception and relearn how to identify the difference between the function of QA and SA fiber/receptor systems. Emphasis is placed on distinguishing between moving touch, constant touch, and pressure, and correction of false localization.[15,54]

The exercises to encourage perception of the QA fiber/receptors or moving touch consist of moving the eraser end of a pencil or a finger across a re-innervating area, proximal to distal. When constant touch is appreciated, the eraser end of a pencil or a finger is used to apply varying pressure to re-educate the perception of the SA fiber/receptor system. In all phases of the re-education process, the patient applies the stimulus with a sequence of visual guidance, vision occluded, and then visual reinforcement.[7,15,53] Since learning requires retention, recognition, and then recall to be effective,[7,62] the sequence of ocular identification followed first by "blind" duplication and then visual affirmation is designed to help establish repeatable cortical interpretation of the stimulus. The pattern of recovery of vibratory sense, moving touch, and constant touch is charted throughout the early phase of retraining.

Incorrect localization of a stimulus responds well to the same method of visual reinforcement, requiring intense repetition to achieve consistent accuracy. Callahan said that the goal of re-education of misreferred stimulus sites is to localize correctly the constant touch stimulus of a Semmes-Weinstein monofilament that is close to or the same as the patient's touch threshold.[7] In her program, correct localization is an ongoing procedure carried out simultaneously with finer discriminatory tasks. With intensive re-education, patients appear to "memorize" consciously a stimulus location different from that tested. This is particularly true in those who have demonstrated a consistent pattern of referred false localization when tested with Semmes-Weinstein monofilaments. After a period of time, they say that because they feel the stimulus in one place, that means that it must be in the new site that they have repeatedly visualized.[67] While the recognition takes time-consuming conscious effort at first, gradually it is performed rapidly and accurately without visual assistance.

Some researchers have suggested that false localization is a simple result of misdirected regeneration of peripheral nerve fibers that disrupts the somatotopy at the level of the sensory cortex.[25,70] A recent study of adult monkeys with median nerve injuries suggests false localization may be related to abnormal patterns of cortical organization. Correct localization could be re-established, despite the underlying abnormality, by effectively improving the use of smaller-than-normal cortical systems that are accurately reconnected to skin surfaces.[88]

Late-Phase Discrimination or Tactile Gnosis

Late-phase re-education begins when moving touch and constant touch are perceived and localized at the fingertips. Callahan and Bell observed that perception of a level of 4.31 on Semmes-Weinstein monofilaments testing is an indication that discriminatory retraining should be initiated.[3,4] A level of 4.31, which is in the diminished protective range, is equivalent to a gross appreciation of two-point discrimination.[3] Weinstein found that accurate localization correlated closely with two-point discrimination, and that this was a positive sign of potential for precise touch.[89]

The goal in late-phase re-education is the recovery of functional tactile gnosis. There appears to be no single correct method, only a common goal.[15] The dynamic process involves object identification with incorporation of movement. Differences in size, shape, texture, and material are maximized initially for ease in identification. As the patient improves, more difficult combinations that require increased ability to discriminate are introduced.[7,15,53,68] Exercises are specific, and they are performed for brief, concentrated periods rather than long sessions to avoid patient frustration. As in the early phase, exercises are performed with an "eyes open, eyes shut, eyes open" sequence. Progress in this period is followed by testing of the cutaneous pressure threshold with Semmes-Weinstein monofilaments and moving and static two-point discrimination.

Overview of Late-Phase Sensory Re-Education Programs

Activities used at the Hand Rehabilitation Center in Philadelphia, reported by Callahan, are graded to require discrimination from gross to fine with three levels of difficulty.[7,62] The patient determines whether stimuli are the same or different, explains how, and identifies the source of stimulation. Tasks are divided into activities requiring minimal motor skills and those that are more difficult because they require greater integration of motor and sensory function. Exercises are designed so that the patient can implement them independently and to encourage follow-up at home.

Re-education begins with texture discrimination using sandpaper or other textures attached to both ends of a dowel. The patient is instructed to "feel" whether the ends are the same or not. As differentiation improves, the grades of sandpaper are made more similar and more difficult to differentiate. The patient matches fabric samples, starting with a small choice and progressing to larger, more diverse groupings. Distinction of roughness and smoothness is accomplished through discriminating between surfaces and edges of objects such as coins, nuts, and washers. If objects cannot be manipulated, they are secured in putty.

Identification of letters, shapes, and figures is implemented through games and puzzles such as recognizing block letters formed from Velcro attached to small wooden blocks or mounted three-dimensionally, identifying Braille designs spaced to determine degree of difficulty, and tracking raised finger mazes from a starting point to the finish. Tasks that require advanced motor skills include picking out and identifying objects in a container filled with a background medium such as rice, beans, or Styrofoam. The items are placed in a box, and the patient first recognizes dissimilar articles and then progresses to objects that are similar in size, shape, and texture.

Finally, activities of daily living and work-simulated skills that are normally performed without vision are incorporated into the program. Assessment of progress is made by recording improvement in ability to localize, the number and timing of correct responses to identification of objects and texture, improvement in two-point discrimination, and the patient's report of increased functional activity.[7,62]

Other programs emphasize movement as a critical factor in object identification.[15,53] Late-phase exercises begin with recognition of large familiar household items that differ distinctly in size, shape, and texture and then progress to more subtle differences. Dellon suggested that various dissimilar stimuli such as vibration, moving two-point discrimination, and static two-point discrimination that are normally used to test sensation should be incorporated in re-education.[15,53]

Parry also uses a program of object training, including wooden blocks of different weights and shapes, cut-out boards, and recognition of objects, shapes, and textures.[68,69] The activities are graded from simple to complex as the patient improves. An interesting aspect of re-education that he mentions is the training and improvement of proprioceptive awareness. While his emphasis is on tactile gnosis, he observed that proprioception advances at the same time through the recognition of weight, size, and shape. Progress is measured by improvement in localization and by time and accuracy in recognition of textures and objects.[68,69]

Imai, Tajima, and Natsuma use a combination of methods originally devised by Dellon and Parry.[27] Initially, patients must differentiate between degrees of roughness of sandpaper and shapes of large wooden blocks. When patients can recognize the difference in more than seven of the 10 wooden plates, they begin working on identification of 12 different small metal objects. Sensory assessment includes testing with Semmes-Weinstein monofilaments, moving and static two-point discrimination, and an object identification test. To eliminate the limitations of motor function, in this test the objects are adhered to a block of wood so that patients can freely run their involved fingers across them.[27]

The Dewey Disc system, an interesting technique used in late-stage sensory re-education, consists of 3-cm plastic discs with $^1/_{16}$-inch and $^1/_{32}$-inch raised numbers from 0 to 9.[15,45] Once the $^1/_{16}$-inch numbers are identified without vision, the patient progresses to the smaller numbers. The discs are small enough that the patient can carry them for frequent practice. Patients are followed by clinic testing for recognition of the discs with vision occluded.[15,45] One drawback mentioned by clinicians using the system is that the technique is effective only after recordable static two-point discrimination is present.

ASSESSMENT OF RESULTS

Most clinicians assess the results of sensory re-education solely by static two-point discrimination testing, but additional means of recording progress are necessary because it is well established that functional two-point discrimination does not return early, if at all, in the course of recovery in adults.[27,28,60,67,68] Most commonly, improvement in localization and time and accuracy of object and texture identification are included, along with a battery of moving and static two-point discrimination and Semmes-Weinstein monofilaments tests.

Parry argued that two-point discrimination is an unfair test of sensory recovery because it does not always correlate with the significant functional recovery seen in the patients trained in re-education.[68,69]

Of the limited number of studies reporting results of sensory re-education, all have demonstrated that patients undergoing a formal program achieved a higher level of functional sensation in less time than those not engaged in retraining. Dellon's series of patients who had sensory re-education were followed with static two-point discrimination so that their results could be compared with prior controls.[15] He used the British Medical Research Council classification, with S4 representing normal (6 mm or less static two-point discrimination) and S3+ being equivalent to 7 to 15 mm. He reported that 54% of patients with re-education achieved a level of S4 for the median nerve and 80% for the ulnar nerve within 2 years of nerve repair at the wrist.[15]

In 1976 Parry noted that 22 of 23 patients recovered normal ability to localize within 3 months of training.[69] Good sensory function was regained by 70% of his patients, as determined by time and accuracy of both object and texture identification. The final measure of progress was the ability of patients to use the hand in work and activities of daily living. He noted that the most impressive functional improvement was seen in patients who actively incorporated the extremity into their daily activities.[68]

Imai, Tajima, and Natsuma studied the effect of sensory re-education in 22 adults with median nerve injuries at the wrist and compared them with 24 adults with similar injuries who did not receive retraining.[27,28] Sensory assessment included Semmes-Weinstein testing, static and moving two-point discrimination, object recognition, and classification of paresthesias. Results showed that sensory re-education significantly diminished the severity of paresthesias, improved moving two-point discrimination significantly over static two-point discrimination, and produced excellent recovery of functional sensation as determined by the ability to recognize nine or more of twelve objects. Semmes-Weinstein testing results showed that a formal program of sensory re-education following median nerve injury at the wrist significantly improved the level of cutaneous pressure threshold and in less time than the program that did not use re-education.[27,28]

Author's Preferred Method

I began using sensory re-education in the treatment of patients with peripheral nerve injuries in 1974. I have measured progress in both regeneration and re-education through a battery of tests including grid mapping of Tinel's sign, moving touch, constant touch, vibration (30 and 256 cps), localization (both point and area), Semmes-Weinstein monofilament testing, and moving and static two-point discrimination. My program is based on the work of Parry and Dellon, expanding to include several newly reported techniques. While observations from my experience confirm many of the findings of other clinicians, some difficult questions have arisen.

The major persisting abnormality in sensory recovery is in the organization of spatial information.[21] Current testing methods reveal a one-dimensional aspect of recovery, while the hand requires the ability to perceive in a three-dimensional plane in order to function. Most studies confirm that a regenerating peripheral nerve re-establishes continuity of classes of sensation,[79] as seen by recovery of pressure, pain, vibration, and temperature.[21] The reason for the persistence of abnormal sensation does not seem to lie in the periphery. Ideally, further study of the somatosensory cortex will provide insight.[21,83,92]

Recently, investigators studying the cortex have made important discoveries that not only help to explain the phenomenon of sensation but also provide the key for retraining it.[43,88] While most agree that the goal of sensory re-education is tactile gnosis, the question is how better to achieve that goal. As neurophysiologists delve further into the role of mechanoreceptors and the somatosensory cortex in the integration of sensation, more effective means for both evaluation and re-education of patients with sensory deficits may be provided. The training program supported by current research findings requires application of stimuli in a specific pattern in order to evoke the maximum desired response.

Dannenbaum and Dykes recently proposed a sensory re-education program based on this concept.[9] While it was designed as a program for stroke victims, the rationale and techniques are equally applicable to patients with peripheral sensory loss. The program is based on four aspects of sensory research:

1. Details of cortical map representation can be modified by specific stimulation of the involved skin surfaces.
2. Classes of sensory messages are specifically conveyed to individual sensory maps attending to that sensory modality.
3. The presence of previously suppressed inputs may be due to changes in inhibitory influences.
4. The reorganization of somatosensory maps is affected by attention, motivation, and use.[9]

Their goal is to gain increased cortical representation so that the involved skin surfaces can improve spatial discrimination or stereognosis.[9]

Electrical stimulation of 100 Hz is applied to the affected skin surfaces initially, both to assess potential and to activate large populations of fiber/receptors. The intensity is set high enough for appreciation, but not to the point of pain.[9] In my experience, electrical stimulation, conventional transcutaneous electrical nerve stimulation, and fluidotherapy are all effective in recruiting maximum responses.[52] Immediately following application, patients often demonstrate a temporarily lower QA and SA threshold, as measured by vibration and Semmes-Weinstein monofilament testing (Fig. 58-3).

When moving touch is present, both QA and SA fiber/receptors are stimulated by stroking across the sensory surface with a grooved irregular article covered with hooked Velcro.[9] Several studies have found that in stroking across the finger pads, both QAs and SAs are stimulated; QAs provide better intensive information about differences in shapes related to sharpness, while SAs provide better spatial information.[42,49,80]

Activities of daily living are encouraged early with holding surfaces adapted to provide increased tactile input (Fig. 58-4). Handles are enlarged, shaped to minimize slipping, and covered with hooked Velcro for activation of receptors. Grip force adjustments in holding activities are fostered by encouraging lateral movements of skin against the object. The thumb and fingertips especially are included to facilitate motor control when grasping.[9] Westling and Johansson found a close interplay between sensory mechanisms related to exploratory function of the fingers and the motor mechanism controlling muscles.[38–41,90,91] Their findings suggest that mechanoreceptors in the skin provide the specific information needed for the adaption of motor performance in precision grip. With anesthesia of the fingers, they found that the capacity to adjust grip with friction was lost, but not the ability to adjust with the weight of the object (Fig. 58-5).[40,90]

The ability to localize is followed by fine form discrimination, achieved by using Velcro on

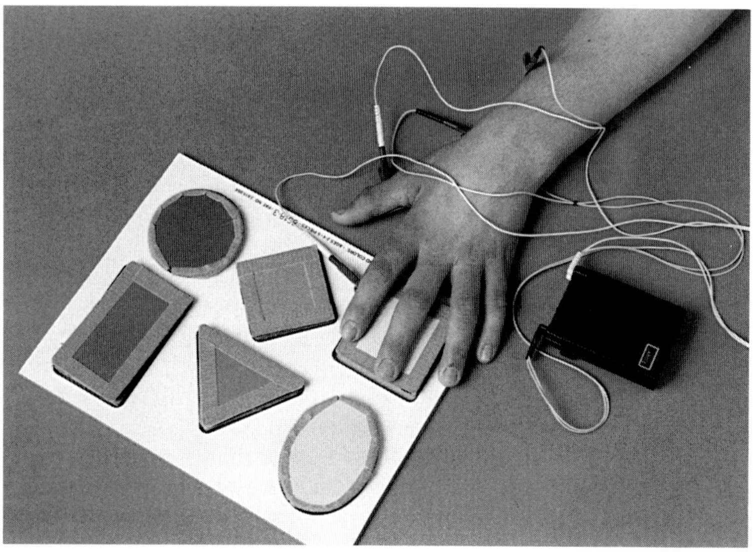

Figure 58–3. *Recognition of shapes with raised edges covered with hook Velcro. TENS is applied to the proximal phalanx of the thumb, the middle phalanx of the index finger, and over the median nerve at the wrist during activity to recruit maximum neuronal population and lower threshold of QA and SA fiber/receptors.*

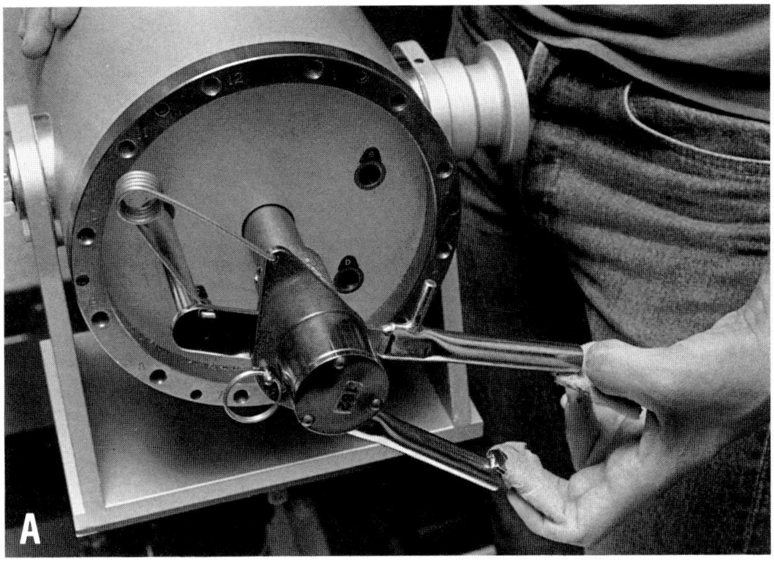

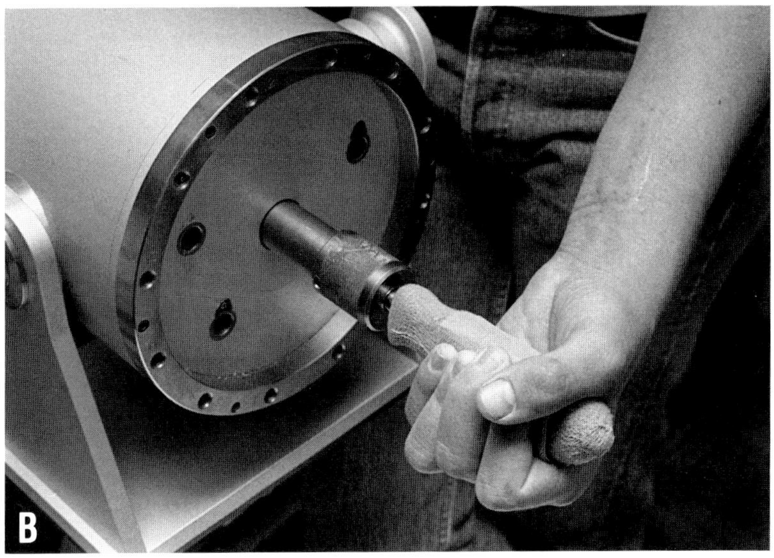

Figure 58–4. *Meaningful functional activities incorporated early in the sensory re-education program are highly motivating and can be structured to include maximum sensory input.* **(A)** *A 33-year-old policeman with a partial median and complete ulnar nerve injury works on the BTE, using tool 162 and pulling index and middle fingers to thumb to simulate the type of precision grip necessary for pulling the trigger of a gun. Contact areas are covered with hook Velcro to increase perception.* **(B)** *The handle of tool 504 is built up and covered with hook Velcro. The patient performs the controlled precision grasp necessary for operating a motorcycle and for holding the tow rope when water skiing. The handle is advanced and then reversed against consistent resistance that allows adjustment of the fingers for manipulating the handle, but is not enough to cause the grip to slip off the tool.*[38–41,90,92]

elevated surfaces with distinct edges for exploring both the site and the form of objects (Fig. 58-6).[9] Since inhibitory influences increase the threshold for activation of cortical neurons, stimulation is applied that has a maximum excitatory potential, such as moving edges of irregular forms in contrast to large smooth surfaces (Fig. 58-7).[29,31,32]

Some clinicians, reporting on the prerequisites for training, have stated that the patient must be motivated,[25,71,85] intelligent, and able to concentrate.[7,53] I believe in placing responsibility on the teacher rather than the patient. Patients are educated initially to help them understand the problem. They respond positively to simplified explanations of the sensory pathways, especially the role of the cortex. With comprehension of the problem, they become much more tolerant of the often frustrating re-education techniques. Education helps them realize that they have some control over final results in recovery. As Dannenbaum and Dykes have stressed, the key is to plan the patient's program from the beginning to

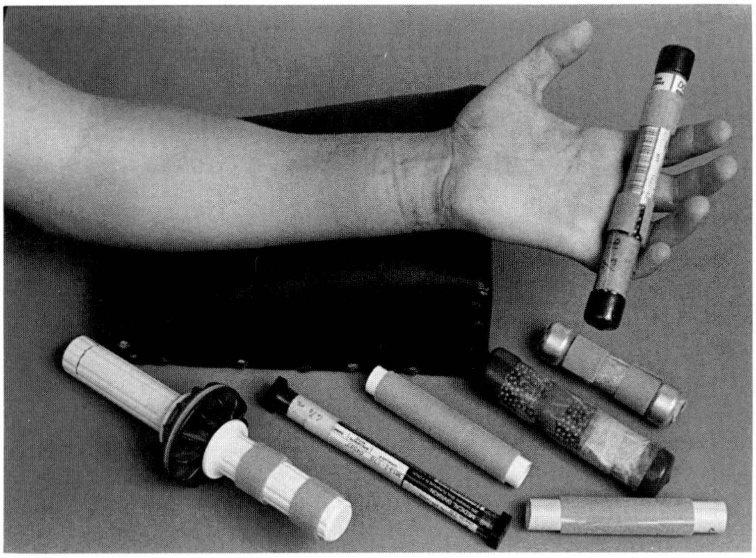

Figure 58–5. *Weighted objects with surfaces of different frictional properties in relation to the skin are used to encourage precision grip adjustments. The bars are rolled out to the fingertips and back into a closed fist in a sequence of loading, maintaining, and releasing the work load. This is repeated with the bars picked up vertically between the thumb, index, and middle fingers with vision occluded. Studies show that the skin afferents provide very specific information that is essential for the adaptation of motor performance in precision grip.*[38–41,90,92]

meet both immediate and long-term goals that the patient finds meaningful, important, and rewarding.[9,85]

A sensory re-education program that attempts to incorporate specific neurophysiologic findings into a well-designed program offers promise for increased success in improving sensation after peripheral nerve injury repair. While the complex mechanism of sensation is incompletely understood, many findings now can be applied directly to clinical techniques of re-education.

For example, in one series of studies on the functional organization of sensory cortex areas 3a, 3b, 2, and 1, based on the receptive fields of single neurons in conscious monkeys, the researchers found that in all areas except 1, most neurons were responsive to very specific stimuli.[24,29–35] In area 1, 40% of neurons investigated had multi-finger or wide-type receptive fields receiving information from more than one finger or the palm, as compared to the single locus receptive fields of neurons in area 3b.[24,32] Specific neurons were

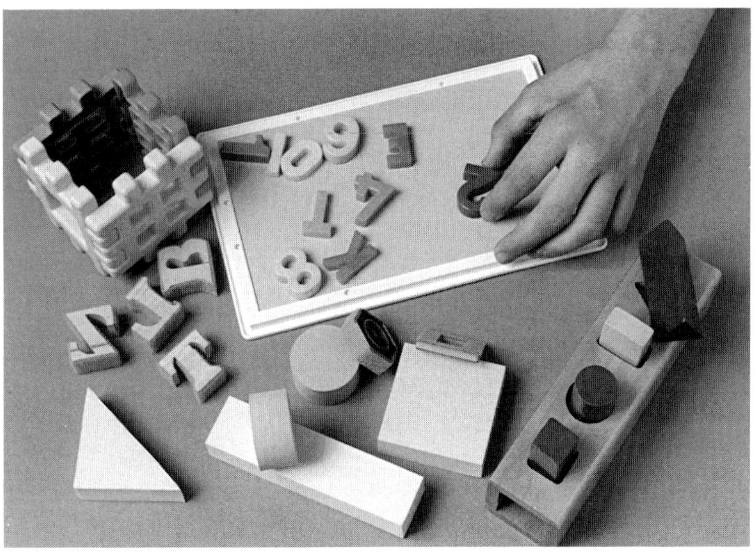

Figure 58–6. *Shapes made of different materials such as dense foam, wood, and plastic are actively explored to foster "feature detection."*[64] *A magnet board semi-stabilizes objects to be scanned by the fingertips. Sharp edges of hook Velcro are added to some shapes to define the edges. The active stroking and distinct edge features are designed to stimulate both QA and SA fiber/receptors.*[48,49]

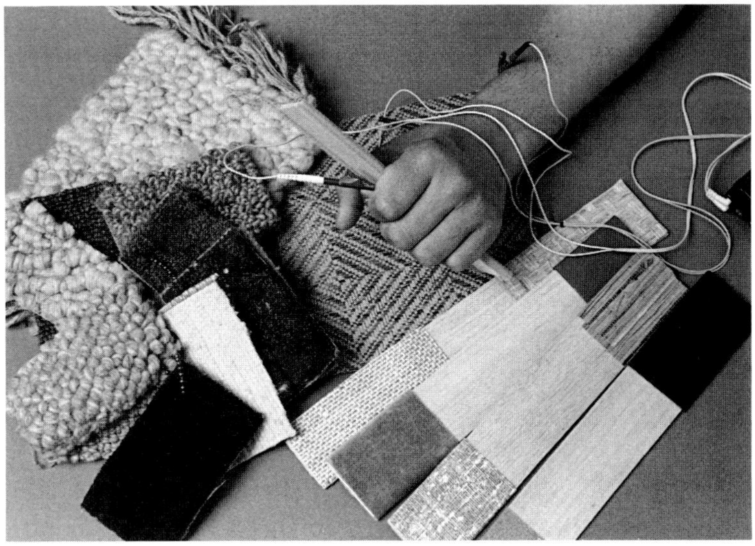

Figure 58–7. *Texture discrimination using dissimilar loose fabric samples for scanning with the fingers to maximize activation of QA receptors through difference in skin vibration set up by surface differences.*[42] *Other textures are mounted on thin wood strips to include sharp edge detection for activation of SA receptors. The wood strips with their different textures are manipulated in various precision and exploratory grips.*[48,49]

activated or inhibited depending on whether the thumb or other fingers were touched. Many had complex patterns of active motion with tactile stimulation necessary for maximum response. All neurons were more responsive to moving stimuli and had directional selectivity (Fig. 58-8).[33] In area 2, it appeared that grasping objects with a particular form, such as a distinct edge, was the only effective mode of stimulation for certain neurons. These same units seemed to use the information from cutaneous and joint sources only in particular combinations.[29,30,33–35]

The significance of these findings to the clinician lies in the correlation between them and the treatment techniques that provide the most effective sensory re-education. Numerous studies have reported on the normal organization of the sensory cortex and its subsequent reorganization following nerve injury. Others continue to study peripheral neural events such as tactile detection,

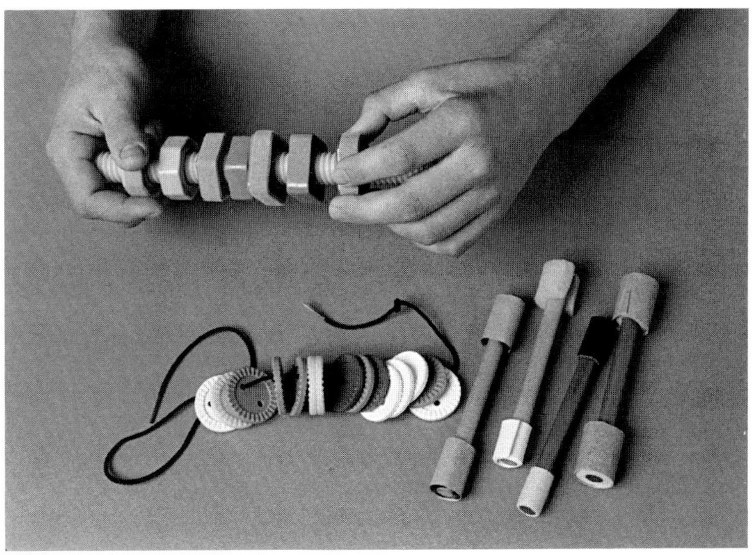

Figure 58–8. *Shape, form, and texture discrimination requiring active movement. With eyes closed, covered dowels are stroked across the skin surfaces to learn differentiation of textures. Forms with distinct edges, some lined with hook Velcro, are explored through movement to provide spatial information.*

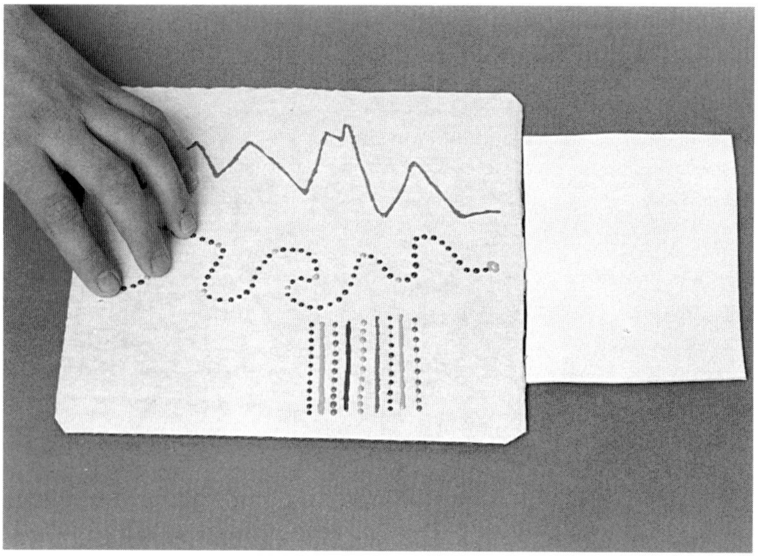

Figure 58–9. *Tracing a finger maze of raised dots and detecting a single raised dot on a smooth surface to evoke response in QA fiber/receptors and provoke varying skin indentation while scanning with the fingertips.*[42,50,55,64,74]

discrimination of shape and texture, and precision grip (Fig. 58-9).[26,38–42,44,48–50,55,71,75,80,90,91]

Two areas of investigation involving control of precision grip, concerning particularly the role of cutaneous afferents in position sense and motor function, have a direct impact on clinicians involved in sensory re-education.[20,38–41,61,78,90,91] Controlling the applied forces while holding an object is of key importance for both exploration and dexterity. The cutaneous receptors in the hand play an important role in kinesthesia. Moberg's experiments with cutaneous anesthesia at different levels suggest that cutaneous receptors in the forearm, activated by the interaction of tendons and muscles, may provide crude position sense for the fingers.[61] Parry[67] and Nakada[64] have observed the important relationship of proprioception to the integration of sensory and motor control necessary for functional sensation (Fig. 58-10).[78]

Continued study of the entire sensory pathway from the periphery to the somatosensory cortex should produce findings that will enable the

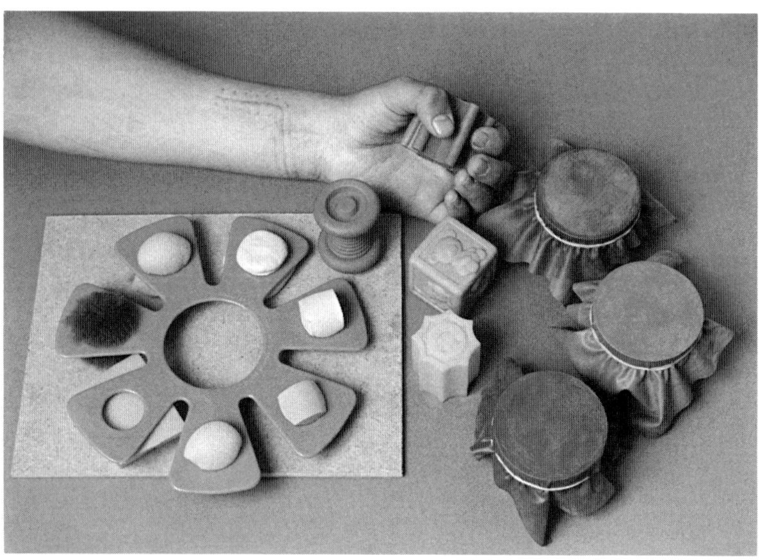

Figure 58–10. *Objects with different consistencies and tensions to help learn necessary precision grip adjustments in holding, manipulating, and pressure-applying activities.*[64] *The four "touch and feel" shapes give audio feedback to help the patient determine and adjust the force applied in grip.*[38,90]

clinician to design the most effective means of restoring functional sensation.[72,83] The interesting possibility has been raised that object recognition requires a highly specific integration across different cortical areas,[44] and that re-establishment of different topographic transformations as seen in the separate cortical areas results in the loss of this integrative capacity.[89] Clinical observation and testing of patients with sensory deficit attest to the fact that the primary missing element in recovery appears to be an integrative component that allows for spatial resolution. I feel that the persisting abnormality in dimensional appreciation can be significantly altered by extrapolating findings from the research laboratory and applying them in the clinic.

REFERENCES

1. Asanuma H, Arissan K. Experiments on functional role of peripheral input to motor cortex during voluntary movements in the monkey. J Neurophysiol 1984; 52:212–227.
2. Barber LM. Desensitization of the traumatized hand. In: Hunter JM, Schneider LH, Mackin EJ, Callahan AD, eds. Rehabilitation of the hand, ed 2. St Louis: CV Mosby, 1984:493–502.
3. Bell JA. Light touch–deep pressure testing using Semmes-Weinstein monofilaments. In: Hunter JM, Schneider LH, Mackin EJ, Callahan AD, eds. Rehabilitation of the hand, ed 2. St. Louis: CV Mosby, 1984:399–406.
4. Bell JA. Sensibility testing: State of the art. In: Hunter JM, Schneider LH, Mackin EJ, Callahan AD, eds. Rehabilitation of the hand, ed 2. St. Louis: CV Mosby, 1984:390–398.
5. Bowden REM. Factors influencing functional recovery. In: Seddon JH, ed. Peripheral nerve injuries. London: Her Majesty's Stationery Office, 1954: 298–354.
6. Callahan AD. Sensibility testing: Clinical methods. In: Hunter JM, Schneider LH, Mackin EJ, Callahan AD, eds. Rehabilitation of the hand, ed 2. St. Louis: CV Mosby, 1984:407–431.
7. Callahan AD. Methods of compensation and re-education for sensory dysfunction. In: Hunter JM, Schneider LH, Mackin EJ, Callahan AD, eds. Rehabilitation of the hand, ed 2. St. Louis: CV Mosby, 1984:432–442.
8. Clark S, Allard T, Jenkins WM, Merzenich MM. Receptive fields in the body-surface map in adult cortex defined by temporally correlated inputs. Nature 1988; 332:444–445.
9. Dannenbaum RM, Dykes RW. Sensory loss in the hand after sensory stroke: Therapeutic rationale. Arch Phys Med Rehabil 1988; 69:833–839.
10. Davis DR. Some factors affecting the results of treatment of peripheral nerve injuries. Lancet 1949; 1:877–880.
11. Dellon AL. Reinnervation of denervated Meissner corpuscles: A sequential histological study in the monkey following fascicular nerve repair. J Hand Surg 1976; 1:98–109.
12. Dellon AL. The moving two-point discrimination test: Clinical evaluation of the quickly adapting fiber/receptor system. J Hand Surg 1978; 3:474–481.
13. Dellon AL. Evaluation of sensation. In: Dellon AL, ed. Evaluation of sensibility and re-education of sensation in the hand. Baltimore: Williams & Wilkins, 1981:95–201.
14. Dellon AL. Re-education of sensation. In: Dellon AL, ed. Evaluation of sensibility and re-education of sensation in the hand. Baltimore: Williams & Wilkins, 1981:203–246.
15. Dellon AL. Sensory rehabilitation after nerve injury. In: Mackinnon SE, Dellon AL, eds. Surgery of the peripheral nerve. New York: Thieme, 1988:521–533.
16. Dellon AL, Curtis RM, Edgerton MT. Evaluating recovery of sensation in the hand following nerve injury. Johns Hopkins Med J 1972; 130:235–243.
17. Dellon AL, Curtis RM, Edgerton MT. Re-education of sensation in the hand after nerve injury and repair. Plast Reconstr Surg 1974; 53:297–305.
18. Dellon AL, Kallman CH. Evaluation of functional sensation in the hand. J Hand Surg 1983; 8:865–870.
19. Donoghue JP, Sanes JN. Organization of adult motor cortex representation patterns following neonatal forelimb nerve injury in rats. J Neurosci 1988; 8: 3221–3232.
20. Dykes RW. Parallel processing of somatosensory information: A theory. Brain Res Rev 1983; 6:47–115.
21. Dykes RW. Central consequences of peripheral nerve injuries. Ann Plast Surg 1984; 13:412–422.
22. Forster FM, Shields CD. Cortical sensory defects causing disability. Arch Phys Med Rehabil 1959; 40:56–61.
23. Hardy MA, Moran CA, Merritt H. Desensitization of the traumatized hand. Va Med 1982; 109:134–137.

24. Hikosaka O, Tanaka M, Sakamoto M, Iwamura Y. Deficits in manipulative behaviors induced by local injections of muscimol in the first somatosensory cortex of the conscious monkey. Brain Res 1985; 325:375–380.
25. Horch KW, Burgess PR. Functional specificity and somatotopic organization during peripheral nerve regeneration. In: Jewett DL, McCarroll HR, eds. Nerve repair and regeneration. St. Louis: CV Mosby, 1979:105–109.
26. Horch KW, Tuckett RP, Burgess PR. Rapid displacements of the skin lack clear positional information. Brain Res 1984; 309:382–383.
27. Imai H, Tajima T, Natsuma Y. Successful re-education of functional sensation after median nerve repair at the wrist. Presented at the 28th Meeting, Japan Society Surg Hand, 1985.
28. Imai H, Tajima T, Natsuma Y. Interpretation of cutaneous pressure threshold (Semmes-Weinstein monofilament measurement) following median nerve repair and sensory re-education in the adult. Microsurg 1989; 10:142–144.
29. Iwamura Y, Tanaka M. Post-central neurons in hand region of area 2: Their possible role in the form discrimination of tactile objects. Brain Res 1978; 150:662–666.
30. Iwamura Y, Tanaka M, Hikosaka O. Overlapping representations of fingers in the somatosensory cortex (area 2) of the conscious monkey. Brain Res 1980; 197:516–520.
31. Iwamura Y, Tanaka M, Sakamoto M, Hikosaka O. Functional subdivisions representing different finger regions in area 3 of the first somatosensory cortex of the conscious monkey. Exp Brain Res 1983; 51:315–326.
32. Iwamura Y, Tanaka M, Sakamota M, Hikosaka O. Converging patterns of finger representation and complex response properties of neurons in area 1 of the first somatosensory cortex of the conscious monkey. Exp Brain Res 1983; 51:327–337.
33. Iwamura Y, Tanaka M, Sakamoto M, Hikosaka O. Functional surface integration, submodality convergence and tactile feature detection in area 2 of the monkey somatosensory cortex. Exp Brain Res 1985; Suppl 10:44–58.
34. Iwamura Y, Tanaka M, Sakamoto M, Hikosaka O. Diversity in receptive field properties of vertical neuronal arrays in the crown of the postcentral gyrus of the conscious monkey. Exp Brain Res 1985; 58: 400–411.
35. Iwamura Y, Tanaka M, Sakamoto M, Hikosaka O. Vertical neuronal arrays in the postcentral gyrus signaling active touch: A receptive field study in the conscious monkey. Exp Brain Res 1985; 58: 412–420.
36. Jabaley ME, Burns JE, Orcutt BS, et al. Comparison of histologic and functional recovery after peripheral nerve repair. J Hand Surg 1976; 1:119–130.
37. Jenkins WM, Merzenich MM. Reorganization of neocortical representations after brain injury: A neurophysiological model of the basis of recovery from stroke. Prog Brain Res 1987; 71:249–266.
38. Johansson RS, Westling G. Roles of glabrous skin receptors and sensorimotor memory in automatic control of precision grip when lifting rougher or more slippery objects. Exp Brain Res 1984; 56:550–564.
39. Johansson RS, Westling G. Signals in tactile afferents from the fingers eliciting adaptive motor responses during precision grip. Exp Brain Res 1987; 66:141–154.
40. Johansson RS, Westling G. Coordinated isometric muscle commands adequately and erroneously programmed for the weight during lifting task with precision grip. Exp Brain Res 1988; 71:59–71.
41. Johansson RS, Westling G. Programmed and triggered actions to rapid load changes during precision grip. Exp Brain Res 1988; 71:72–86.
42. Johnson KO. Neural mechanisms of tactual form and texture discrimination. Federation Proc 1983; 42: 2542–2547.
43. Kaas JH, Merzenich MM, Killackey HD. The reorganization of somatosensory cortex following peripheral nerve damage in adult and developing mammals. Ann Rev Neurosci 1983; 6:325–356.
44. Kang R, Herman D, MacGillis M, Zarzecki P. Convergence of sensory inputs in somatosensory cortex: Interactions from separate afferent sources. Exp Brain Res 1985; 57:271–278.
45. Kiernan-Shultis L. Dewey Disc sensory re-education program. Instructional Sheet, 1986.
46. Lamotte RH. Can the sensitization of nociceptors account for hyperalgesia after skin injury? Human Neurobiol 1984; 3:47–52.
47. Lamotte RH, Mountcastle VB. Capacities of humans and monkeys to discriminate between vibratory stimuli of different frequency and amplitude: A correlation between neural events and psychophysical measurements. J Neurophysiol 1975; 38:539–559.
48. Lamotte RH, Srinivasan MA. Tactile discrimination of shape: Responses of slowly adapting mechanoreceptive afferents to a step stroked across the monkey fingerpad. J Neurosci 1987; 7:1655–1671.
49. Lamotte RH, Srinivasan MA. Tactile discrimination of shape: Responses of rapidly adapting mechano-

receptive afferents to a step stroked across the monkey fingerpad. J Neurosci 1987; 7:1672–1681.
50. Lamotte RH, Whitehouse J. Tactile detection of a dot on a smooth surface: Peripheral neural events. J Neurophysiol 1986; 56:1109–1128.
51. Laurence S, Stein DG. Physiological processes and recovery. In: Finger S, ed. Recovery from brain damage: Research and theory. New York: Plenum, 1978:381–383.
52. Mannheimer JS. Transcutaneous electrical nerve stimulation: Its uses and effectiveness with patients in pain. In: Echternach JL, ed. Pain. New York: Churchill-Livingstone, 1987:213–254.
53. Maynard CJ. Sensory re-education following peripheral nerve injury. In: Hunter JM, Schneider LH, Mackin EJ, Bell JA, eds. Rehabilitation of the hand. St. Louis: CV Mosby, 1978:318–323.
54. Mayumi A, Minoru N. Ability to localize a constant touch and moving touch stimulus in the hand. Presented at the 16th Congress Association of Occupational Therapy, Shizuoka, Japan, 1983.
55. Mei J, Tuckett P, Poulos A, Horch KW, Wei Y, Burgess PR. The neural signal for skin indentation depth: Steady indentation. J Neurosci 1983; 3: 2652–2659.
56. Merzenich MM, Kaas JH. Reorganization of mammalian somatosensory cortex following peripheral nerve injury. Trends Neurosci 1982; 5:434–436.
57. Merzenich MM, Kaas JH, Wall JT, Sur M, Nelson RJ, Felleman DJ. Progression of change following median nerve section in the cortical representation of the hand areas 3b and 1 in adult owl and squirrel monkeys. Neurosci 1983; 10:639–665.
58. Merzenich MM, Nelson RJ, Kaas JH, et al. Variability in hand surface representations in areas 3b and 1 in adult owl and squirrel monkeys. J Comp Neurology 1987; 258:281–296.
59. Merzenich MM, Nelson RJ, Stryker MP, Cynader MS, Schoppmann A, Zook JM. Somatosensory cortical map changes following digit amputations in adult monkeys. J Comp Neurology 1984; 224:591–605.
60. Moberg E. Criticism and study of methods examining sensibility of the hand. Neurol 1962; 12:8–9.
61. Moberg E. The role of cutaneous afferents in position sense kinaesthesia and motor function of the hand. Brain 1983; 106:1–19.
62. Moran CA, Callahan AD. Sensibility measurement and management. In: Moran CA, ed. Hand rehabilitation. New York: Churchill-Livingstone, 1986:45–68.
63. Mountcastle VB. Neural mechanisms in somesthesia. In: Mountcastle VB, ed. Medical physiology, vol 1, ed 14. St. Louis: CV Mosby, 1980:348–390.
64. Nakada M, Tokyo Metropolitan College of Allied Medical Sciences. Personal communication, 1989.
65. Nolon MF. Anatomic and physiologic organization of neural structures involved in pain transmission, modulation and perception. In: Echternach JL, ed. Pain. New York: Churchill-Livingstone, 1987:1–37.
66. Omer GE. The evaluation of clinical results following peripheral nerve suture. In: Omer GE, Spinner M, eds. Management of peripheral nerve problems. Philadelphia: WB Saunders, 1980:431–442.
67. Önne L. Recovery of sensibility and sudomotor activity in the hand after nerve suture. Acta Chir Scand 1962; 300:1–69.
68. Parry CBW. Re-education. In: Parry CBW, ed. Rehabilitation of the hand, ed 3. London: Butterworth, 1973:106–131.
69. Parry CBW, Salter M. Sensory re-education after median nerve lesions. Hand 1976; 8:250–257.
70. Paul RL, Goodman H, Merzenich MM. Alterations in mechanoreceptor input to Brodmann's area 1 and 3 of the postcentral hand area of *Macaca mulatta* after nerve section and regeneration. Brain Res 1972; 39:1–19.
71. Phillips JR, Johnson KO, Hsiao SS. Spatial pattern representation and transformation in monkey somatosensory cortex. Proc Natl Acad Sci USA 1988; 85:1317–1321.
72. Pia HW. Plasticity of the central nervous system—a neurosurgeon's experience of cerebral compensation and decompensation. Acta Neurochir 1985; 77:81–102.
73. Pons TP, Garraghty PE, Mishkin M. Lesion-induced plasticity in the second somatosensory cortex of adult macaques. Proc Natl Acad Sci USA 1988; 85: 5279–5281.
74. Poppen N, McCarroll HR, Doyle J, Niebayer J. Recovery of sensibility after suture of digital nerves. J Hand Surg 1979; 4:212–226.
75. Poulos DA, Mei J, Horch KW, et al. The neural signal for the intensity of a tactile stimulus. J Neurosci 1984; 4:2016–2024.
76. Rasmusson DD. Reorganization of raccoon somatosensory cortex following removal of the fifth digit. J Comp Neur 1982; 205:313–326.
77. Rasmusson DD, Turnbull BG, Leech CK. Unexpected reorganization of somatosensory cortex in a raccoon with extensive forelimb loss. Neurosci Lett 1985; 55:167–172.
78. Roland PE. Metabolic mapping of sensorimotor integration in the human brain. CIBA Foundation Symp 1987; 132:251–268.

79. Sretavan D, Dykes RW. The organization of two cutaneous submodalities in the forearm region of area 3b of cat somatosensory cortex. J Comp Neurol 1983; 213:381–398.
80. Srinivasan MA, Lamotte RH. Tactile discrimination of shape: Responses of slowly and rapidly adapting mechanoreceptive afferents to a step indented into the monkey fingerpad. J Neurosci 1987; 7:1682–1697.
81. Stone LA. Pain in neuromuscular disorders. In: Echternach JL, ed. Pain. New York: Churchill-Livingstone, 1987:179–212.
82. Stopford JSB. An explanation of the two-stage recovery of sensation during regeneration of a peripheral nerve. Brain 1926; 49:372–386.
83. Stryker MP, Jenkins WM, Merzenich MM. Anesthetic state does not affect the map of the hand representation within area 3b somatosensory cortex in owl monkeys. J Comp Neurol 1987; 258:297–303.
84. Sunderland SS. Regeneration of the axon and associated changes. In: Sunderland SS, ed. Nerves and nerve injuries, ed 2. Edinburgh: Churchill-Livingstone, 1978:108–132.
85. Taub E. Somatosensory deafferentation research with monkeys: Implications for rehabilitation medicine. In: Ince LP, ed. Behavioral psychology in rehabilitation medicine. Baltimore: Williams & Wilkins, 1980:371–401.
86. Torebjork EH, Lamotte RH, Robinson CJ. Peripheral neural correlates of magnitude of cutaneous pain and hyperalgesia: Simultaneous recordings in humans of sensory judgements of pain and evoked responses in nociceptors with C-fibers. J Neurophysiol 1984; 51:325–339.
87. Vinograd A, Taylor E, Grossman S. Sensory retraining of the hemiplegic hand. Amer J Occup Ther 1962; 5:246–250.
88. Wall JT, Kaas JH, Sur M, Nelson RJ, Fellman DJ, Merzenich MM. Functional reorganization in somatosensory cortical areas 3b and 1 of adult monkeys after median nerve repair: Possible relationships to sensory recovery in humans. J Neurosci 1986; 6:218–233.
89. Weinstein S. Intensive and extensive aspects of tactile sensitivity as a function of body part, sex and laterality. In: Kenshalo DR, ed. The skin senses: Proceedings of the 1st International Symposium on Skin Senses. Springfield, Ill: Charles C Thomas, 1968.
90. Westling G, Johansson RS. Factors influencing the force control during precision grip. Exp Brain Res 1984; 53:277–284.
91. Westling G, Johansson RS. Responses in glabrous skin mechanoreceptors during precision grip in humans. Exp Brain Res 1987; 66:128–140.
92. Wood CC, Spencer DD, Allison T, McCarthy G, Williamson PD, Goff WR. Localization of human sensorimotor cortex during surgery by cortical surface recording of somatosensory evoked potentials. J Neurosurg 1988; 68:99–111.

Index

Numbers followed by an *f* indicate a figure;
t following a page number indicates tabular material

Abductor digiti minimi
  motor testing of, 164
  opponensplasty using, 723–724, 724*f*
Abductor pollicis brevis
  measuring response time of, 175
  motor examination of, 166–167, 879–880, 881*f*
Abductor pollicis longus
  imbrication of, 1472, 1473*f*
  motor testing of, 163–164
  opponensplasty using, 724–725
Acetylcholine, 75
  degradation of, 77
  and pain response, 1480
  release into synaptic cleft, 76
  sensitivity of denervated muscle to, 784
  synthesization, 76
Acetylcholinesterase, 77
  histochemical materials and methods, 267–268, 268*f*, 269*f*
Acromioclavicular joint pain, following shoulder arthrodesis, 1322
Actin, 5, 62, 64, 67
Action potential, 18, 25
Activation, 37
Active axon, 31–34, 32*f*
Acupuncture, in treating reflex sympathetic dystrophy, 1518
Adaptive therapy, for reflex sympathetic dystrophy, 1514
Adductor pollicis brevis, motor testing of, 167
Adductor pollicis longus, motor testing of, 167
  tendon lengthening of, 1470
A delta fibers, 1480
Adenosine triphosphatase (ATPase), 58
Adenosine triphosphate (ATP), 8
  and pain response, 1480
  synthesis of, 57
Adhesive nerve repair, 328–329
Adoption phenomenon, 785
Adrenergic nerve fibers, 12
Adson maneuver, 1178
Afferent nerve fibers, 89
Age, as factor in peripheral nerve repair, 350–351
Alkaline protease, 64, 67
Allen test, 684, 969, 1139
Allodynia, 1482, 1484, 1499, 1502
Allografts, 528
All-or-none law, 87
Alpha motor neuron regeneration, 221
Ambulation potential, evaluation of, 1420
β-aminopropionitrile, 591
Amitriptyline hydrochloride, for reflex sympathetic dystrophy, 1510, 1511*f*, 1512*f*
Amplitude, of a muscle, 694
Amputation stump, phantom pain in, 1483–1484, 1527
Amyotrophic lateral sclerosis, 717
Analog-to-digital converter, 22
Anastomosis, centrocentral, 1532
Anhydrosis, 1260
Aniline, 86
Ankle and foot deformities, 1441
  fractional lengthening of gastrocnemius, 1445
  open phenol block to tibial nerve, 1441–1442, 1444–1445
  recession of gastrocnemius at knee, 1445–1446, 1445*f*, 1446*f*, 1447*f*
  split anterior tibial tendon transfer, 1445*f*, 1446
  tendo achilles lengthening, 1444–1445
  toe flexor release, 1446, 1446*f*
Ankle-stabilizing procedures, 766
Ankylosis, 1446–1447
Anomalous innervation of the upper extremity, 197–198, 199*f*
    antebrachial cutaneous nerve communication and overlap, 208, 208*f*
    Froment-Rauber communication, 208–209
  lateral pectoral nerve, 198–199
  median nerve variations at wrist and hand, 204–205, 206*f*
  median-ulnar nerve communications, 200–201
    flexor digitorum profundus innervation, 202
    general patterns of anomalous median and ulnar innervation, 201
    Martin-Gruber communication, 201–202
    other median-ulnar nerve variations, 204
    palmar ulnar-median communicating branch of Berrettini, 203–204
    Riche-Cannieu communication, 202–203, 202*f*
  musculocutaneous nerve, 199–200, 200*f*
  ulnar nerve variations at the wrist, 207–208
Ansa of Hyrtl, 1346
Antegrade transport, 5–6, 5*t*, 56, 1212–1215
Anterior interosseous nerve, 237, 370, 983, 984
  compression syndrome
    anatomy in, 984
    cause of, 987–988, 988*t*
    compression of, 370–371
    differential diagnosis of, 986
      electromyography, 986–987

Anterior interosseous nerve, compression syndrome (*continued*)
  electrophysiological testing in, 175
  history of, 984
  operative exposure, 377
  operative technique, 989–990, 990*f*, 991*f*
    complications, 991–992
    postoperative care, 990
  presentation, 984
    atypical presentations, 985–986
    complete syndrome, 985
    incomplete syndrome, 985
  treatment, 988–989
 paralysis of, 987
Anterior intramuscular transposition (ulnar nerve), 1069–1070, 1071*t*, 1113
 anatomy, 1072–1074, 1073*f*, 1074*f*, 1075*f*
 indications for, 1070
 postoperative management, 1074
Anterior subcutaneous transposition (ulnar nerve), 1113
 applied anatomy, 1079–1081, 1079*f*, 1080*f*
 complications, 1083–1084
 history of, 1077–1078
 indications
  primary, 1078, 1078*t*
  secondary, 1078–1079
 operative technique, 1081, 1082–1083*f*, 1083
 postoperative management, 1083
Anterior submuscular transposition (ulnar nerve), 1113–1114
Anterior tarsal tunnel syndrome, 1205
Anterior transfer
 of biceps femoris, 771–772, 772*f*
  complications, 772
 procedures in, 1125–1126
 of tibialis posterior, 768–769, 768*f*
  complications, 769
  results, 769
Anterolateral spinothalamic tract of the spinal cord, 1480
Anterolateral tarsal tunnel syndrome, 1205
Ape hand, 818, 819*f*
Aphasia, 1418
Apolipoprotein E, 59, 63, 65
Apraxia, 1418, 1422
Arcade of Frohse, 400, 1008, 1024–1025, 1031, 1034*f*
Arcade of Struthers, 1072, 1079, 1173
Argon laser, 284, 310, 311, 329
Arm. *See also* Forearm
 median nerve
  anatomy of, 366–367, 368*f*, 366*f*
  in operative exposure, 374
  overcoming defects in, 514, 515*f*
  overcoming musculocutaneous nerve injury at, 521
 radial nerve
  anatomy of, 394–397, 395*f*
  in operative exposure, 401–403, 402*f*, 404*f*
  overcoming injury at, 519
 potential points of neural compression in, 367, 396
 ulnar nerve
  anatomy of, 413–415, 414*f*
  operative exposure, 414*f*, 420–421, 421*f*
  overcoming injury at, 516–517, 517*t*
Arnold's nerve, 465
Arterial ischemia, 672
Arterial thrombosis, 809
Arteriosclerosis, 1416
Arthrodesis
 of carpometacarpal joint, 740, 741
 of interphalangeal joint, 741, 743–744
 of metacarpophalangeal joint, 725, 741, 743, 744, 1470
 of thumb interphalangeal joint, 1438, 1439*f*
 triple, 766–768, 767*f*, 770
 of wrist joint, 1299
Athletes, ulnar nerve compression
  biomechanics of throwing, 1097–1098, 1098*f*
  clinical presentation, 1100–1101
  neuropathy of the ulnar nerve at the elbow, 1099–1100, 1100*t*
  prognosis, 1104
  treatment, 1101–1104
Autogenous neural tissue, 358–359
Autogenous vein graft, 310
Autografts, 528
 with damage due to ischemia, 527–528
Autologous nerve graft, 526–527
Avogadro's number of atoms, 20
Avulsion/crushing injuries, 356
Axillary nerve, 1160
 anatomy of, 440–442, 441*f*, 626, 1157–1158, 1263
 compression of, 1160
 compression and quadrilateral space syndrome, 1157
  diagnosis and treatment, 1160
  operative decompression, 1160–1162
  results of treatment, 1160*t*, 1163
  symptoms of idiopathic quadrilateral tunnel syndrome, 1060*t*, 1158–1160, 1159*f*, 1161*f*, 1162*f*, 1163*t*
 electromyographic evaluation of, 438
 function of, 1155*f*, 1158
 indications and contraindications for surgery, 440
 injury to, 437–438, 439*f*, 440
  following shoulder dislocation
   applied anatomy, 626
   evaluation of deltoid muscle function, 627–628
   incidence of, 626–627
 motor testing of, 162
  results of treatment, 1160*t*, 1163
 palsy, 437
  conservative management of, 438
  types of operations, 442–444
Axolemma, 4, 62
Axon(s), 2, 56, 316. *See also* Nerve fiber
 distal stump, 66
 local response of, to injury, 64–65, 64*f*
 myelination of, 58–59
 orientation of
  end-organ specificity, 122
  tissue specificity, 121
  topographic specificity, 122
 retrograde and regenerative changes in, 65–66
 tips, 58
 tropic and trophic factors, 66–68

Axonal degeneration, 66
Axonal growth
  alteration of microenvironment, 123
  conditioning lesion, 122
  in the distal stump, 116
  electromagnetic fields, 123
  enhancement of, 122
  factors influencing, 117
    chemotaxis, 119
    contact guidance, 119
    hormones, 122
    neurite-promoting factors, 119
    neurotrophic factors, 117–119, 117*f*, 118*f*, 123–124
    neurotropism, 119
Axonal outgrowth
  initiation and organization of, 112, 113*f*, 114
    axonal growth in the distal stump, 116
    compartmentation, 115
    distal nerve stump, 115
    growth cone, 114–115
    non-neuronal cell reactions, 116
Axonal proteins, 56
Axonal regeneration, 63, 66–68
  increasing, 591, 593
Axonal transport, 4–7, 849–850
  antegrade, 5–6, 5t, 849–850
  components of, 5*t*
  effects of compression on, 849–850, 852*f*, 855–856
  retrograde, 5*t*, 5t, 6–7, 850
Axon disaggregation, 66
Axon glycolysis, 62
Axonotmesis, 100, 111, 112, 175, 620, 621, 660, 1232
Axon sprouts, 526
Axon tracing, horseradish peroxidase (HRP) technique of, 225
Axoplasm, 4, 19, 56, 64
Axoplasmic transport, 60, 260
  fast, 60, 61*f*, 62
  slow, 61*f*, 62–63
Axotomy, 66

Bado type injuries, 625–626
Bands of Bungner, 66, 116, 118
Beam splitters, 277, 278*f*
Bell's nerve, 1343
  palsy, 465, 469, 1332
  phenomenon of, 466
  reinnervation, 1349, 1351
Benign tumors. *See under* Tumors
Bernstein's hypothesis, 34, 35*f*
Beta motor neuron regeneration, 221
Biceps
  motor testing of, 164
  tendon transfer, to the ulna, 1366*f*, 1367
Biceps femoris, motor testing of, 168
Bier blocks, in electrical nerve stimulation in the awake patient, 247
Bilateral palsies, 1361
Biofeedback, for reflex sympathetic dystrophy, 1518
Biological membranes, 26
Biomechanical properties, of peripheral nerve, 46–52, 48*f*, 49*f*, 50*f*, 51*f*
Biomechanics, of throwing, 1097–1098, 1098*f*
Biopsy, of soft-tissue sarcomas, 1578–1579
Biphasic action potential, 22, 25
Bipolar electrocautery, 277, 280*f*
Birth injuries, 636
Birth palsies, 1361
  incidence of, 1362
Blepharoplasty, 482
Blepharospasm, use of botulinum toxin in, 486–487
Blood flow determination, in reflex sympathetic dystrophy, 1505
Blood-nerve barrier (BNB), 9, 12–13
  effects of compression on, 856–857
Body neglect, 1418, 1422
  evaluation for, 1419
Boley gauge, 823, 824, 824*f*
Bone grafting, for shoulder arthrodesis, 1320–1321
Bone implantation, for neuromas, 1534
Bone shortening, 514–516, 516*t*
Botulinum toxin, 80
  use of, 486–487
Bowler's thumb, 1527
Brachialis, motor testing of, 164
Brachial plexopathy, 1000
Brachial plexus, 1255
  anatomy, 1257–1263, 1259*f*
  avulsion, pain in, 1484
  cutaneous innervation, 1265, 1266*f*, 1267*f*
  injuries to, 1192–1193
    assessment and monitoring in adult, 1273
      axon reflexes, 1280–1281
      electrodiagnostic studies, 1276–1279, 1278*f*
      history of, 1274
      musculoskeletal examination, 1276
      myelography, 1279–1280
      neurological examination, 1274–1275, 1275*t*
      plain radiography, 1276, 1277*f*
      vascular examination, 1275–1276
    assessment and monitoring in children, 1361–1367
    infraclavicular, 1281–1282
    neurotization in treatment of common patterns of lesions including root avulsions, 1333–1336
      history, 1329–1330
      neurotization according to pathology, 1349, 1351–1352, 1351*f*, 1353*f*, 1354–1355, 1354*f*
      neurotizers and their results, 1336–1349, 1337*t*
      deep cervical plexus, 1341*f*, 1342–1343
      greater occipital nerve, 1336
      intercostal nerves, 1345–1349
      long thoracic nerve, 1343
      phrenic nerve, 1344–1345
      spinal accessory nerve, 1336–1342
      thoracodorsal nerve, 1344
    from patient positioning in operating room, 1234, 1235*f*
      direct compression of, 1236, 1236*f*
      stretching, 1234–1236, 1235*f*
    rationale and principles of nerve repair, 1330–1333
  birth palsies, 636
  intraneural topography, 1265
  lesions in adults
    causes of, 1286–1287
    classification of, 1288–1291
    management of, 1290–1293
  mechanisms of injury, 1287–1288, 1287*f*
    pain, 1300
    postoperative care, 1298–1299
    results, 1300

Brachial plexus (*continued*)
surgery
donor nerves for nerve grafts, 1297–1298
exposure, 1293–1296, 1294*f*, 1295*f*
indications and timing of, 1293
neurotization by nerve transfer, 1297
neurotization of selected distal stumps, 1296–1297
reconstructive, 1299
selection of techniques for, 1298
wound closure and immobilization, 1298
morphology, 1256–1257
motor testing of, 160–161
neuritis, 437, 440
operative repair in infants and children, 1369–1370
evolution of present regimen, 1371–1373
nerve grafts in, 1379
operative technique, 1374–1379, 1375*t*, 1376*f*, 1377*f*, 1378*f*
patient selection, 1370–1371, 1372*f*
postoperative care, 1379
preoperative evaluation, 1373–1374, 1373*f*
preoperative preparation, 1374
results of surgery, 1379–1382, 1380*f*, 1381*f*, 1382*f*
systematic follow up, 1382
operative technique
combined supraclavicular and infraclavicular approach to, 1270
infraclavicular exposure, 1269–1270, 1269*f*
posterior subscapular approach, 1270–1271
preparation, 1265
supraclavicular exposure, 1267, 1269, 1269*f*
operative treatment for irreparable lesions of, 1303–1304, 1304*f*
complete lesions, 1323–1325, 1324*f*, 1325*f*
elbow flexorplasty, 1306
latissimus dorsi transfer, 1311–1312, 1313*f*, 1314*f*
L'Episcopo transfer, 1315–1316, 1316*f*
pectoralis major transfer, 1306–1310, 1306*f*, 1307*f*, 1308*f*, 1309*f*
postoperative care, 1314–1315
shoulder arthrodesis, 1317
complications, 1321–1322
positioning, 1317–1311
results, 1322–1323, 1323*f*
technique, 1318–1321
shoulder stabilization, 1315, 1316*f*
staging of surgery, 1305
Steindler flexorplasty, 1310–1311, 1310*f*, 1311*f*
tendon transfers, 1305–1306
timing of reconstructive procedures, 1304–1305
triceps transfer, 1312–1314
overcoming defects in, 513–514
reconstruction, ulnar nerve as donor nerve in, 581–584, 583*f*
spinal nerve root contributions to, 1258, 1260*f*
sympathetic contributions to, 1260, 1260*f*
Brachioradialis, 1025. *See also* Radial tunnel syndrome
closed phenol block to motor points of, 1427
motor testing of, 162
open phenol block to motor branches of, 1427, 1429
radial motor neurectomy to, 1429
Bradykinin, and pain response, 1480
Brain-derived growth factor, 66
Brain-derived neurotrophic factor, 63
Brain injury and stroke, 1415, 1416*f*. *See also* Spinal cord injury
anatomical correlations, 1416–1418, 1417*f*
epidemiology, 1415–1416
examination and diagnostic procedures, 1418–1422
management, 1423–1424
neurogenic heterotopic ossification, 1446–1449
operative procedures, 1416*f*, 1425–1426, 1425*f*
ankle and foot, 1441–1442, 1444–1446, 1444*f*, 1445*f*, 1446*f*, 1447*f*
elbow, 1427
forearm and hand, 1430–1435, 1433*f*, 1434*f*
hip, 1425*f*, 1438–1440
knee, 1440–1441, 1440*f*, 1442–1443*f*
shoulder, 1416*f*, 1426–1427
thumb, 1435–1438, 1436*f*, 1439*f*
pathophysiology, 1416
potential for rehabilitation, 1421–1423
Brain stem, nonsympathetically maintained pain in, 1484–1485
Bristow procedure, 438
British Medical Research Council classifications, 344, 380–383, 380*t*, 382*t*, 426–430, 835
Brooks attachment, 735, 735*f*
Browlift, 482, 484–485, 484*f*
Brown-Sequard syndrome, 1275, 1335–1336
Buccal branch, 463
Bupivacaine hydrochloride (Marcaine), 1513

Cable equation, 30
Cable grafts, formation of, 574
Cable theory, 31–34
Calcium-activated neutral protease, 67
Calcium ATPase pump, 58
Calcium concentration, regulation of, 58
Calcium-dependent protease, 63–64
Calcium efflux, 58
Calcium ions, influx of, 65
Calmodulin, 6, 58, 62
Calorimetry measurements, 25
Calpain, 59, 64, 66, 67–68
Camitz transfer, 929, 930–931*f*, 933, 936
Camptocormia, 1491
Capacitor, 21
Capsulectomy, 1435
Capsulitis, 1405–1407
Caracoid osteotomy, 374
Carbocaine, 1514
Carbon dioxide laser, 329

Carbonic anhydrase, 243
histochemistry
basis for, 262–263, 263*f*
history, 262
materials and methods, 266–267, 267*f*
Cardiothoracic surgery, and injury to brachial plexus, 1274
Carotid endarterectomy, 448
Carpal tunnel, 889–890. *See also* Carpal tunnel release; Carpal tunnel syndrome
anatomy of, 872, 890–892
flexor retinaculum, 890–892
median nerve, 892–894
branches, 894–896, 894*f*, 896*f*, 897*f*
Carpal tunnel release, 204. *See also* Carpal tunnel syndrome
endoscopic, 913–914, 919*f*
applied anatomy, 915–916, 915*f*, 916*f*, 917*f*
complications and results, 919–920
indications for, 914–915
operative technique, 916–919, 917*f*, 918*f*, 919*f*
open release of transverse carpal ligament, 899
anatomy of, 901–904
changes in the carpal canal following, 909–911
history, 900–901
motor branch of the median nerve, 903–904
operative technique, 904–907, 904*f*, 905*f*, 906*f*, 907*f*, 908*f*, 909*f*
palmar cutaneous branch of the median nerve, 901–903, 902*f*
release of Guyon's canal, 907–909, 907*f*, 908*f*
synovectomy, 909
in patients with peripheral neuropathy, 963–965
technique of, 946
Carpal tunnel surgery, response to, 1220–1221, 1220*t*
Carpal tunnel syndrome, 144, 173–175, 860, 939, 999
and cervical radiculopathy as double crush syndrome, 1216–1221, 1218*t*
characteristic symptoms of, 869
conditions altering fluid balance, 870
conditions causing inflammation, 870
classification of, 874–875
complications in treating, 967–968
adherence of nerve to tendons and bowstringing of flexor tendons, 977
hematoma, 976–977
hypertrophic scar, 969–970, 969*f*
incomplete decompression, 972
incorrect diagnosis, 968–969
injection into the nerve, 968
median nerve injury from neurolysis, 972–973
reflex sympathetic dystrophy, 977–978
and restricted tendon excursion, 975–976
severance of palmar cutaneous branch, 970–971, 970*f*, 971*f*
severance of recurrent motor branch, 971–972
conditions associated with, 964
conservative treatment, 882
carpal tunnel injection, 883–885, 883*f*, 884*f*
and pregnancy, 882
vitamin B_6, 882–883
and cubital tunnel syndrome as double crush syndrome, 1221–1223, 1220*t*
diagnosis of, 875
electrophysiological tests, 880–882
motor examination, 173–175, 879–880, 881*f*
radiographic studies, 875
sensibility tests, 876, 877*t*, 878, 878*f*, 879*f*
underlying conditions and other studies, 875–876
forearm fasciotomy combined with carpal tunnel release, 946–947
as localized compartment syndrome, 940
circular cast, 940, 941*f*
critical pressure threshold for nerve viability, 941–942, 943*f*
effects of wrist position, 940, 941*f*
factors affecting interstitial pressure, 940–942
measuring interstitial pressure, 944*f*, 945–946
as multifactor disease, 963
occurrence of, 869–870
pathogenesis of, 870, 871*t*
anatomy, 872
hemodialysis, 872
paraplegia, 873–874
physical disorders, 872
position and use of wrist, 873
space-occupying lesions, 872–873
postoperative management, 947
tendon transfers for severe, 927
alternative and associated procedures, 935*f*, 936
Camitz transfer, 929, 930–931*f*, 933, 936
formal opponensplasty, 932–933*f*, 934, 936
medical history in, 927–928
operative plan for, 929
physical examination in, 928–929
postoperative care, 933
treating, 204
median nerve injury following wrist trauma, 942–943, 945
workers' compensation claimant with, 954–955
in the workplace, 951–952, 952t
Cathepsins, 64
Causalgia, 661–665, 662*t*, 663*t*, 664*t*, 1483, 1498
effectiveness of stellate ganglion blockade in treating, 1567–1568
Cavitation, 656
Cell membrane, 56, 57–58, 57*f*
Centrocentral anastomosis, 1532
Cerebral palsy, 1455–1456
diagnostic classification, 1459–1460, 1459*t*
examination and diagnostic procedures, 1456
age, 1459
motor evaluation, 1456–1457
sensibility, 1457–1459
operative procedures, 1460
elbow, 1460–1461
flexor origin release, 1461, 1464*f*
musculocutaneous neurectomy, 1461

Cerebral palsy, operative procedures (*continued*)
  forearm, 1461–1462
  shoulder, 1460, 1462–63*f*
  transfer for thumb extension, 1470
  wrist and digits, 1462–1463
    arthrodesis of the metacarphageal joint of thumb, 1470
    digital and thumb extensor transfers, 1469–1470
    flexor carpi ulnaris transfer, 1466–1467
    flexor digitorum superficialis transfer for thumb extension, 1470
    fractional lengthening of wrist and digital flexor tendons, 1463–1466
    imbrication of the abductor pollicis longus and extensor pollicis brevis, 1472, 1473*f*
    pronator teres transfer, 1467, 1468*f*, 1469
  realignment and reinforcement of extensor pollicis longus, 1470, 1473, 1473*f*
  swan-neck deformity, 1472–1474, 1473*f*
  thumb adduction contracture, 1470, 1471*f*
    transfers to the wrist extensors, 1466
  types of, 1455
Cerebral thrombosis, 1416
Cerebrosides, 59
Cerebrovascular accidents. *See* Brain injuries and stroke
Cervical lymph node biopsy, 1148
Cervical radiculopathy, 1000
  and carpal tunnel syndrome as double crush syndrome, 1216–1220, 1218*t*
  and radial tunnel syndrome as double crush syndrome, 1221
Cervical ribs, 1181–1182
Cervical root lesions, 1056–1057
Cervical spondylosis, 964
Cervicofacial division, 463–465
Cervicothoracic sympathectomy, for reflex sympathetic dystrophy, 1514–1515
C fibers, 1480
Chamber models, 120–121
Charcot-Marie-Tooth disease, 717, 1224
Chemical injury, 677
Chemical sympathectomy, in treating causalgia, 663–665, 664*t*
Chemotaxis, 119, 120
Chemotherapy, for malignant soft-tissue tumors, 1583
Cholecystokinin, and pain response, 1480
Cholesterol, 59
Choline acetylase, 243
Choline acetyltransferase, 76
  radioassay
    basis for, 264
    history, 263–264
    materials and methods, 268–269
Cholinesterase, 77
  histochemistry
    basis for, 262
    history, 261–262, 261*f*
Chondrosarcoma, 1575
Choristoma, neuromuscular, 1599, 1599*f*
Chromatolysis, 65, 112
Ciliary neuronotrophic factor (CNTF), 119
Ciliary neurotrophic factor, 63, 66
Circular cast, effects of, on interstitial pressure, 940, 941*f*
Circular nerve-holding forceps, 281–282, 282*f*
Circumferential plaster stretcher, 817, 818*f*
Cis-hydroxyproline, 591
Clathrin, 5, 62
Claviculectomy, 1184
Claw deformity, 729–730, 730*f*
  development of, 817
  semi-active tenodesis to correct, 738–739
Clawing, 433, 1070
Clear-cell sarcoma, 1575
Clenched-fist syndrome, 1492–1493
Close-range wounds, 657–658
CO_2 laser, 310, 311
  in treating neuromas, 1531
Coagulation, 284
Coagulation necrosis, 671
Cock-up splint, 819, 819*f*
Colchicine, 591
Cold gnosis, 90
Cold intolerance, 680–681
Cold stress testing, patterns of response in, 681, 684
Collagen, 58
Collagen scar (neuroma), 65
Collateral sprouts, 112
Colles' fracture, 860
  interstitial pressure in patient with, 941
  malunited, 872
  and median nerve compression, 943
  treatment of, 940
Combined median-ulnar nerve palsy, 813
Common peroneal nerve palsy, 764, 766
  anterior transfer of tibialis posterior, 768–769, 768*f*
  complications, 769
  results, 769
  triple arthrodesis, 766–768, 767*f*
Compartmentation, 115
Compartment syndrome, 940. *See also* Carpal tunnel syndrome
Composite tissue transfers, technique of, 179–180, 181*f*
Compound nerve action potential (CNAP), 22–23, 51–52
  electrophysiology of, 603–605, 605, 605*f*
    equipment, 610–612, 611*f*
    practical considerations, 608–610, 609*f*, 610*f*
    technique, 612–614, 615*f*, 616
    theoretical considerations, 606–608, 606*f*, 607*f*
Compressive femoral neuropathy, 1200
Compressive lateral femoral cutaneous neuropathy (Meralgia Paresthetica), 1201–1202, 1201*f*
Compressive lumbosacral plexopathy, 1198
Compressive neuropathies, 1198. *See also* Carpal tunnel syndrome; Double crush syndrome
  applied anatomy and operative exposure, 1199–1200, 1200*f*
  of axillary nerve, 1157
    anatomy, 1157–1158

diagnosis and treatment, 1160
function of, 1155*f*, 1158
operative decompression, 1160, 1162
quadrilateral tunnel syndrome, 1158–1160, 1159*f*, 1160*t*, 1161*f*, 1162*f*, 1163*t*
results of treatment, 1160*t*, 1163
symptoms and signs of idiopathic quadrilateral tunnel syndrome, 1158–1160
electrophysiological testing in evaluation of, 173
anterior interosseous nerve compression syndrome, 175
carpal tunnel syndrome, 173–175, 174*f*, 880–882, 969
compressive neuropathy in the lower extremity, 177, 178*f*
cubital tunnel syndrome, 176
posterior tibial nerve compression, 177
pronator syndrome, 176
thoracic outlet syndrome, 176–177
ulnar nerve compression at Guyon's canal, 176
of femoral nerve, 1200
and interdigital neuroma, 1207–1208
of lateral femoral cutaneous nerve, 1201–1202
of long thoracic nerve, 1163, 1164*f*
of the lower extremity, 177
electrophysiological testing in, 173, 177, 178*f*
of lumbosacral plexus, 1198
of median nerve, 1170
anomalous muscles and tendons, 1170
anomalous vessels, 1171–1172
congenital bands and fractures of humerus, 1172
Cruveilhier's canal, 1172
deltopectoral fascia, 1172
pathology, 1170
supracondyloid process and ligament of Struthers, 1172–1173
of musculocutaneous nerve, 1165
anatomy and function, 1165–1166
pathophysiology, symptoms and signs, 1166
of obturator nerve, 1200–1201
of peroneal nerve, 1202–1205, 1203*f*, 1204*f*, 1206*f*
of posterior tibial nerve, 1202, 1203*f*
of radial nerve, 1166
anatomy and function, 1167–1168, 1167*f*
operative treatment, 1169–1170
symptoms, signs, and diagnosis, 1168–1169
of sciatic nerve, 1198–1199
of suprascapular nerve
anatomy of, 1152–1153, 1156*f*
function of, 1151–1152, 1152*f*, 1154*f*
operative technique, 1155–1157
pathology, 1153
symptoms and diagnosis, 1153–1154
treatment, 1154–1155
symptoms and signs, 1151*f*, 1163–1164
and tarsal tunnel syndrome, 1206–1207, 1207*f*
treatment and results, 1164–1165
of ulnar nerve, 1173
Computed tomography (CT)
in assessing facial nerve paralysis, 468
in diagnosis of carpal tunnel syndrome, 875
Conditioning lesion, 122
Conductance (g), 20–21
Conduction, 235
Connectin, 67
Constant field assumption, 28
Constant two-point discrimination test, 823–825, 824*f*, 828
Contact guidance, 66, 119
Contact recognition, 216, 222, 226
Contact wounds, 657
Continuous axillary (brachial) blockade, for reflex sympathetic dystrophy, 1514, 1516*f*
Continuous stellate blockade, for reflex sympathetic dystrophy, 1515
Contractures, in spinal cord injury, 1388–1389
Contralateral myectomy, 486
Conversion disorders, 1490
Coracobrachialis muscle, anatomy of, 1262
Cortex, nonsympathetically maintained pain in, 1485
Corticosteroids
for carpal canal syndrome, 883–885, 968
for neuromas, 1529
for reflex sympathetic dystrophy, 978, 1511–1512
Costoclavicular maneuver, 1178
Costoclavicular passage, 1180
Coulomb (C), 20
Counterstimulation, 87
C protein, 64, 67
Cranial nerve branches, and patient positioning in operating room, 1237, 1237*f*, 1238*f*
Creatinine phosphokinase, 62
Creep phenomenon, 46, 49
Cross-sectional mapping, 242–243
Cross-union technique, 1532
Crushing, in treating neuromas, 1529
Cruveilhier's canal, 1172
Cryptogenic brachial plexus neuropathy, 1150
Cubital tunnel, 1080
Cubital tunnel syndrome, 238, 1221–1223, 1222*t*
anatomy in, 1122
and carpal tunnel syndrome as double crush syndrome, 1221–1223, 1222*t*
causes of, 1072
clinical assessment, 1056–1059
clinical presentation, 1056
conservative treatment, 1059–1060
decompressive management, 421, 422*f*, 423, 1117, 1121–1122, 1123, 1123*t*
anterior transposition procedures, 1102, 1125–1126
intramuscular, 1069–1075, 1112, 1113
subcutaneous, 1077–1084, 1112, 1113
external neurolysis, 1117

Cubital tunnel syndrome, decompressive management (*continued*)
failures of, 1111–1112, 1122–1123
implantable electrode stimulation, 1116
internal neurolysis, 1117–1118, 1126
local procedures, 1123–1124
medial epicondylectomy, 1087–1095, 1124–1125,
revision ulnar nerve decompression, 1127–1128
silicone sheathing in, 1118, 1126–1127
in situ decompression, 1063–1066, 1124
submuscular transposition, 1099–1104, 1107, 1113–1116
diagnosis of, 1070
and elbow flexion contractures, 1108
and elbow instability, 1109
electrophysiological testing in, 176
history of, 1055
and neurolysis, 1112
and neuromas, 1108–1109
nonoperative treatment of, 1122–1123, 1122*f*
pathophysiology of, 1055–1056
and persistent motor and sensory deficits, 1110–1111, 1110*t*
release, 1112
presence of perineural scarring following, 1114
Cumulative trauma, 873. *See also* Carpal tunnel syndrome
carpal tunnel syndrome as, 954–952, 952*t*, 957–960
investigations testing hypothesis of, 953, 954**t**
median neuropathy associated with, 957–958
evaluation of, 959
management of, 960
pathology and pathophysiology, 958–959
treatment of, 959
and worker's compensation, 953–954
Current (I) flows, 20
Cutaneous nerve, 528
innervation of, 1265, 1266*f*, 1267*f*
in nerve grafting, 538–539
Cutaneous pressure threshold, 136, 147
Cutaneous sensation, 86
Cutaneous vibratory threshold, 144, 146*f*, 147
Cybex testing, 1094
Cylinder casting, 817, 818*f*
Cytogenetics, 1589
Cytomegalovirus infection, as cause of anterior interosseous nerve paralysis, 988
Cytoplasm, 19, 56
Cytoskeleton, 56, 59–60

Dead arm syndrome, 626
Debridement, 659
Decompression, 442
Deep cervical plexus, as neurotizer, 1341*f*, 1342–1343, 1342*f*
Deep penetration necrosis, 672
Dejerine-Klumpke palsy, 162
Dejerine-Sottas neuropathy, 1224
Deltoid flap, 798, 800–801, 802*f*
Deltoid muscle
atrophy of, 440
function of, 1151
motor testing of, 162
paralysis of, 438
Deltopectoral fascia, 1172
Demagnetization of microinstruments, 280
Demyelinating disease, pain in, 1484–1485
Dendrites, 19*f*
Denervation following fractures and dislocations, 620–621
management, 621–622
reinnervation and recovery, 621, 621*f*
secondary nerve injury, 622
Deoxyribonucleic acid (DNA), 56
Depression, chronic pain in, 1485
deQuervain's tenosynovitis, 1528
Dermal papilla, 137
Desensitization, 154
Desmin, 67
Devascularizing trauma
nerve injury associated with, 679–680
definitions, 680
in lower extremity, 684–685
research, 680–681
in upper extremity, 682–683*f*, 684
de Vecchi operation, 761
Developmental factors, 63
Dewey Disc system, 834
Diabetes mellitus, 30
and carpel tunnel syndrome, 964
neuropathy in, 193–194, 964, 1215, 1224–1225
susceptibility of nerves to compression in, 861–862, 862*f*
Diamond knife, 281
Diffuse neurofibroma, 1601
Diffusion, 27
Diffusion barrier, perineural, 8–9
Digastric transfer, 481–482
Digital and thumb extensor transfers, 1469–1470
Digital clawing, 434
Digital flexors, Z-lengthening of, 1432
Digital motion, 729–731, 730*f*
Digital nerve
applied anatomy, 453–454
grafting of, 558–559, 558*t*
indications for repair, 454
modes of injury, 454
overcoming defects, 455–457, 457*f*, 458*f*
repair of, 353, 353*t*, 356
results, 457–459, 458*f*
treatment for lipofibromatous hamartoma in, 1598–1599
types of operations, 454–455, 455*f*, 456*f*
Digital plethysmography, 1179
Digital swan-neck deformities, 1472–1474, 1473*f*
Digital vibrogram, 878
Diisopropyl fluorophosphate, 79
Diphtheria, 964
α-dipyridyl, 591
Direct current (DC), effect of, on outgrowth, 123
Direct neurorrhaphy
for femoral nerve injury, 494
for peroneal nerve injury, 499–500, 499*f*
for posterior nerve injury, 496, 496*f*
Disk–Criminator, 147*f*, 151
Dislocations, denervation following, 620–621
Disodium etidronate, in prevention of heterotopic ossification, 1449
Dispersive fibrosis, 1527

Dissection distance, 236
Distal femur fractures, nerve injuries associated with, in children, 648
Distal hamstring release or lengthening, 1441, 1442*f*
Distal humerus fracture, open reduction of, 1079
Distal intrinsic muscle release, 1435
Distal median-ulnar nerve palsy, 747
Distal motor latency (DML), in studying carpal tunnel syndrome, 175
Distal quadriceps release, 1440–1441, 1440*f*, 1442*f*
Distal sensory latency (DSL), in studying carpal tunnel syndrome, 174–175
Distal stump, 66, 115
  axonal growth in, 116
  importance of, 121
  neurolization of selected, 1296–1297
Distal tibial fractures, nerve injuries associated with, in children, 649
Distal tissues, reinnervation of, by nerve reconstruction, 509
Distal ulnar nerve repairs, 356
Donor nerve(s). *See also* Nerve graft(s)
  dorsal antebrachial cutaneous nerve, 531
  dorsal cutaneous branch of ulnar nerve, 549
  lateral antebrachial cutaneous nerve, 531, 548–549
  lateral femoral cutaneous nerve, 551
  medial antebrachial cutaneous nerve, 531, 547, 547*f*
  for nerve grafting, 528, 530–532
    requirements for, 545–546
      cross-sectional area, 546
      donor site morbidity, 546–547
      length of donor grafts, 546, 547*t*
  posterior interosseous nerve, 549
  saphenous nerve, 532
  superficial radial nerve, 531
  sural nerve, 530–531, 550–551, 550*f*
Dorsal antebrachial cutaneous nerve, as donor nerve, 531
Dorsal cutaneous branch of ulnar nerve, 238
  as donor nerve, 549
Dorsal horn, as pain pathway, 1480–1481, 1481*f*
Dorsal interosseous
  motor testing of, 165
  release of the first, 1436*f*, 1438
Dorsalis pedis flap, 803–804
Dorsal root ganglia, 1480
Dorsal scapular nerve, motor testing for, 161
Double compressive neuropathy, 1212
Double crush neuropathy, 859, 870, 964, 1070, 1223–1224
  combined median and ulnar neuropathy at, 1225
  diabetic and uremic neuropathies, 1224–1225
  experimental basis, 1212, 1213*f*
    altered nerve elasticity, 1216
    generalized connective tissue abnormalities, 1213*f*, 1216, 1217*f*
    impairment of axonal flow, 1212–1215, 1214*f*
    intraneural blood flow, 1215
    nerve to compression, 1215
  hereditary neuropathy and pressure palsies, 1224
  median nerve, 1216–1221
  multiple entrapment, 1224
  other, 1223–1224
  phenomenon of, 1057
  radial nerve, 1221
  thoracic outlet syndrome and distal compression lesions, 1221–1223
  ulnar neuropathy at elbow and wrist, 1224
Double limb support standing test, 1420
Droopy shoulder syndrome, 177
Drug action
  junctional, 79–80
  postjunctional, 77–79
  prejunctional, 80
Ducker-Hayes cap, 1532
Dupuytren's contractures, 1526
Durable swaged-on microneedles, 282
Dynein, 62
Dysesthesias, 1039
Dystrophy, reflex sympathetic, 977–978

Ectodermal derivatives, 316
Edema
  effect of, on compression, 854–855
  endoneural, 7, 8, 13, 852–853, 1215
Edge effect, 854
Edrophonium (Tensilon), 79
Elbow. *See also* Cubital tunnel syndrome
  arthroplasty, 1079
  median nerve
    operative exposure at, 375, 376*f*, 377
    overcoming injury at, 515, 516*t*
  restoration of extension, 1394–1395, 1395*f*
  ulnar nerve
    anatomy of, 415–419
    neuropathy of at, 1099–1100, 1100*t*
    overcoming injury at, 517
Elbow flexion, 144, 1427, 1428*f*
  closed phenol block
    to motor points of brachioradialis muscle, 1427
    to musculocutaneous nerve, 1427
  contracture, 1108
    operative procedures, 1460
    flexor origin release, 1461, 1464*f*
    musculocutaneous neurectomy, 1461
  open phenol block
    to the motor branches of brachioradiolis muscle, 1427, 1429
    to musculocutaneous nerve, 1427
  test for, in diagnosing ulnar nerve compression, 1101
Elbow flexorplasty, 1306, 1365
Electrical injury, 675–676
Electrical nerve stimulation, 243–244

Electrical nerve stimulation (*continued*)
in the awake patient, 241–242
clinical examples, 249–252, 250*f*, 251*f*, 252*f*, 253*f*, 254*f*, 255
cross-sectional mapping, 242–243
electrical stimulation and recording, 243–244
histologic staining, 243
direct inspection, 242
technique of
anesthetic technique, 246–247
history, 244–245, 244*f*
operative procedure, 247–249
premedication and sedation, 245
preoperative counseling, 245
tourniquet in, 246
value of, 255–256, 256*t*
for chronic pain, 1551–1552
clinical experience with, 1552, 1553*f*, 1554–1555, 1554*f*
effects of, 123
evaluation, 1560
results, 1557–1559, 1559*f*
technique of, 1555, 1556*f*, 1557, 1557*f*
Electrodiagnostic studies, 1276–1279
agreement of results with clinical sensibility testing, 151, 153–154, 155*f*
of brachial plexus injury, 1276–1279, 1278*f*
in diagnosing pronator syndrome, 998
in identifying malingering, 141
of partial nerve injuries, 338–339, 338*f*
Electromagnetic fields, 123
Electromyography, 171, 468, 1239, 1273
in assessing
anterior interosseous nerve compression syndrome, 986–987
axillary nerve, 438
brachial plexus injury, 1273, 1278, 1278*f*
cerebral palsy patient, 1457
hip impairment, 1250
motor function, 1420
operating room injuries, 1239
radial sensory nerve entrapment, 1046–1047
Electroneurography, 468
Electronic amplification and display, 21
Electronic responses, 30
Electron spin resonance, 26
Electrophysiology, 171–172
of compound nerve action potential
practical considerations, 608
electrodes, 603*f*, 608–610, 609*f*, 610*f*
equipment, 610–612, 611*f*
technique, 612–614, 615*f*, 616
theoretical considerations, 606–608, 606*f*, 607*f*
definitions in, 172–173
equipment in, 177, 179
in evaluation of compressive neuropathies, 173
anterior interosseous nerve compression syndrome, 175
carpal tunnel syndrome, 173–175, 174*f*, 880–882, 969
compressive neuropathy in the lower extremity, 177, 178*f*
cubital tunnel syndrome, 176
posterior tibial nerve compression, 177
pronator syndrome, 176
thoracic outlet syndrome, 176–177
ulnar nerve compression at Guyon's canal, 176
intraoperative stimulation and recording, 180–181, 183, 183*f*
of nerve lesions in continuity, 603–605, 604*f*
nerve stimulation techniques, 179
motor fascicle territory, 179–180, 181*f*
sensory identification, 179, 180*f*
pitfalls in interpreting, 185–187, 186*ft*, 187*ft*, 188*f*, 189*ft*, 190*f*, 191*f*, 192*t*
multiple compression sites versus distal axonopathy, 193–194
thoracic outlet syndrome, 193
Encapsulated receptors, 101
Endoneural capillaries, 12
Endoneural connective tissue, 1
Endoneural edema, 7, 8, 13, 852–853
Endoneural fibrosis, 13, 1290
Endoneural fluid pressure (EFP), 9, 12–13
Endoneural space, 8, 8*f*, 10, 12
Endoneural tissue, fibrosis of the, 1290
Endoneural tube, 4, 111
Endoneurium, 316
Endoplasmic reticulum, 56, 74
Endoscopic carpel tunnel release, 913–914, 914*f*
and anatomy, 915–916, 915*f*, 916*f*, 917*f*
complications and results, 919–920
indications for, 914–915
operative techniques, 916–919
End organ specificity, 216
End-plate potential, 76
End-to-end coaptation, overcoming nerve gaps for, 509–513
End-to-end nerve repair, 526, 527*f*
End-to-end neurorrhaphy, 358
Endurance testing, in reflex sympathetic dystrophy, 1507
Enneking staging system, 1576–1577
Entactin, 59
Entrapment neuropathy, 860, 1216. *See also* Carpal tunnel syndrome
Epicondylitis, lateral, 1221
Epicondylectomy. *See* Medial epicondylectomy
Epidermal growth factor, 63
Epifascicular epineurium, fibrosis of the, 1290
Epineural ligation, 1530–1532
Epineural repair, 290–291, 291*f*, 318
for digital nerve repair, 454–455, 455*f*
Epineural splint, 315–316, 319–321, 320*f*, 321*f*
alternative procedures to, 318
epineural repair, 290–291, 291*f*, 318

interfascicular nerve grafting, 242, 315–316, 319, 493, 554
interfascicular repair, 318, 319
tubulation, 283, 309–310, 319
applied anatomy, 316–318
complications in, 325–326
contraindication to the use of, 316
indications for, 316
postoperative care for, 323–325
technique, 321–323, 322*f*, 323*f*, 324*f*
Epineural suture, 318
Epineurium, 2, 9–10, 233–234, 296–297
Epineurotomy of the anterior interosseous or median nerve, 990
Epithelioid sarcoma, 1575
Erb-Duchenne palsy, 162, 1362
reconstruction for, 1364–1365
Escharotomy, 672–674, 674*f*, 675*f*
iatrogenic injury during, 674
reconstruction, 674–675
Ethanolamine phosphatides, 59
Ewing's sarcomas, 1575, 1618
chemotherapy for, 1583
Excision, for recalcitrant nerve pain, 1545, 1548
Excitation, ionic basis of, 34–39, 35*f*, 36*f*
Exocytosis, 57
Experimental regeneration in chamber models, 120
Extensor carpi radialis brevis, 397, 1024. *See also* Radial tunnel syndrome
motor testing of, 162
transfer of, 714–715
Extensor carpi radialis longus
motor testing of, 162
transfer of, 713, 714, 735–737, 740*f*
Extensor carpi ulnaris, 398
motor testing of, 163
opponensplasty using, 721–722
Extensor digiti minimi, 398
motor testing of, 163
opponensplasty using, 722
Extensor digitorum communis, 398
motor testing of, 163, 169
tenodesis effect of, 1472–1474, 1473*f*
Extensor digitorum longus, motor testing of, 169
Extensor hallucis brevis, motor testing of, 169
Extensor hallucis longus, motor testing of, 169
Extensor indicis proprius
motor testing of, 163
opponensplasty using, 722, 723*f*, 726, 936
Extensor pollicis brevis, 397
imbrication of, 1472, 1473*f*
motor testing of, 163
Extensor pollicis longus, 397
motor testing of, 163
opponensplasty using, 725
realignment and reinforcement of, 1470, 1472, 1472*f*
External neurolysis, 1117, 1117*f*
Exteroceptors, 89
Extracellular recording, 22
Extracranial facial nerve identification, 473–474
Extracranial facial paralysis, 469
Extratemporal course, 462–463
Extratemporal paralysis, 466
Extrinsic potentials, 32
Extrinsic proteins, 26

Facial-hypoglossal transfer, 474, 475*f*
complications in, 476
indications for, 474
technique in, 476
Facial motor paralysis, characteristics of, 466–467
Facial nerve paralysis
anatomy in, 461
cervicofacial division, 463–465
extratemporal course, 462–463, 463*f*
intratemporal course, 461–462, 462*f*
nervus intermedius, 464*f*, 465
temporofacial division, 463, 464*f*
diagnosis, 465–469
myophysiological dynamic muscle transfer, 476
digastric transfer, 481–482
free microvascular transfer of gracilis muscle, 482
masseter transfer, 479–481, 480*f*
temporalis muscle fascial transfer and suspension, 476–479, 477*f*
neurophysiological dynamic repair, 471
facial-hypoglossal transfer, 474, 475*f*, 476
ipsilateral VIIth-to-VIIth repair, 471–474, 473*f*
sural nerve grafts, 474
operative repair
facial incisions, 470
principles, 469–470, 470*t*
static or dynamic facial rehabilitative surgery
adjuvant procedures, 485–487, 485*f*
browlift, 484–485, 484*f*
fascia lata sling, 482–484
Faraday's constant (F), 20
Fascia lata, 483–484
Fascia lata sling, 482–484
incisions for, 483
indications for, 482
Fascia lata suspension, 482
Fascicles, 2
Fascicular nerve repair, 242, 295
anatomy in, 296–297, 296*f*
group, 8, 291–292, 291*f*, 292*f*, 302, 554–556
history of, 295–296
indications for, 297–299
nerve grafting in, 301*f*, 302
for partially severed nerves, 299–302, 299*f*, 300*f*
results, 302
technique for digital nerves, 455, 456*f*
Fasciotomy, forearm, 946–947
Fast axonal transport, 5
Fast axoplasmic transport, 56, 60, 61*f*, 62
Femoral nerve
compression of, 1200
deficit in, 764
injuries to, 493–494, 495*f*
motor testing of, 167
overcoming defects in, 523–524, 523*t*
palsy, 771
anterior transfer of the biceps femoris, 771–772, 772*f*
Femoral neuropathy, 489
Ferrocyanide, 262
Fetal alcohol syndrome, 963
Fibrillation, 80
Fibrillation potential, 171–173

Fibrin glue, 328
autologous preparation, 308
clinical experience, 307–308
historical perspective, 305–306
recent experience, 306–307, 307*f*
in suture repair, 328–329, 328*f*
technique of, 308–309
Fibroblast growth factor (FGF), 63, 119
effect of, on nerve regeneration, 124
Fibronectin, 58, 59, 63, 119, 588
Fibrosis
of endoneural tissue, 13, 1290
of epifascicular epineurium, 1290
of interfascicular epineurium, 1290
Fibular head fractures, 631–632
Figure-eight splint, 816–818
Filopodia, 114–115
Finger extension, use of flexor digitorum superficialis for, 705, 707
Fingerprint, 138
Finkelstein sign, in radial sensory nerve entrapment, 1039
Fixed claw deformity, 813
Flat palm, 739–740, 741*f*
Flexor carpi radialis
motor testing of, 165–166
transfer of
for radial nerve palsy, 704, 707*f*
for ulnar nerve palsy, 730–731, 737
Flexor carpi ulnaris, 238
hiatus, 1080
lengthening, 1431–1432
motor testing of, 164
transfer of, 738, 1466–1467
Flexor digiti minimi, motor testing of, 164–165
Flexor digitorum longus. *See also* Anterior interosseous nerve compression syndrome
motor testing of, 169
Flexor digitorum profundus, 238. *See also* Anterior interosseous nerve compression syndrome
innervation of, 202
motor testing of, 164, 166
opponensplasty using, 726
and pinch mechanism, 731
Flexor digitorum superficialis, 397
for finger extension, 705, 707
opponensplasty using, 717–720, 718*f*, 719*f*
tendon transfer of, 730, 732, 737, 740
for intrinsic-minus deformity, 733, 735, 735*f*
tenodesis of the proximal interphalangeal joint, 1473–1474, 1473*f*
Flexor hallucis longus, motor testing of, 169
Flexor origin release, 1461, 1464*f*
Flexor pollicis brevis
innervation of, 715
motor testing of, 165
Flexor pollicis longus, 397
and development of carpal tunnel syndrome, 873, 874*f*
lengthening, 1437
motor testing of, 166
opponensplasty using, 725
and pinch mechanism, 731
Flexor-pronator aponeurosis, 1069, 1072, 1116, 1116*f*. *See also* Anterior intramuscular transposition
Flexor-pronator origin, 1089–1091, 1090*f*. *See also* Medial epicondylectomy
Flexor-pronator slide, 1431, 1432–1433
Flexor retinaculum, anatomy of, 890–891, 890*f*, 891*f*
Flexor superficialis
motor testing of, 166
operative exposure of, 377
Flexor tendons, bowstringing of, 977
Fluid mosaic model, 25–26
Fluorescence photobleaching, 26
Fluoxetine (Prozac), 1510
for reflex sympathetic dystrophy, 1510
Foot deformities. *See* Ankle and foot
Foot fractures, pediatric nerve injuries associated with, 649
Force, 694
Force-Defined Sensory Discriminator, 147
Forearm. *See also* Arm
atrophy of, 1502
deformities
operative procedures, 1461–1462
pronator teres release, 1462
fasciotomy of, 946–947
flexor-pronator slide, 1432–1433
fractures, pediatric nerve injuries associated with, 646–647
median nerve
anatomy of, 368–371, 369*f*, 370*t*, 372*f*
open phenol block to, 1430–1431
in operative exposure of, 375, 376*f*, 377
overcoming injury at, 516
percutaneous phenol block to the motor points of spastic muscles in, 1430
potential points of neural compression in, 370–371, 398–400
radial nerve
anatomy of, 397–400
operative exposure, 403–406, 405*f*
overcoming injury at, 519–520, 519*t*
ulnar nerve
anatomy of, 415–419
open phenol block to motor branch of, 1433–1435
operative exposure, 422*f*, 423
overcoming injury at, 517
Foream flap, 803
F protein, 67
Frackelton cap, 1532
Fractures
denervation following, 620–621
pediatric nerve injuries associated with
birth injuries, 636
of distal femur, 648
of distal tibial, 649
of foot, 649
of foream, 646–647
of hip, 648
of humeral shaft, 637–638, 638*f*
of lateral condyle, 641–642, 642*f*, 643*f*
of medial condyle and epicondyle humerus, 642–645, 644*f*, 645*f*

of monteggia, 645–646, 646*f*
of proximal humerus, 636–637
of proximal tibial, 649
of supracondylar humerus, 638–641, 639*f*, 640*f*
of wrist and hand, 647
Free nerve endings, 90, 95
Free neurite terminals, 90
F-response, 171, 173
Froment-Rauber communication, 208–209
Froment-Ruber nerve, 401
Froment's sign, 433, 434, 741, 1070
Functional electrical stimulation, 1424
Functional tests, 821
constant two-point discrimination, 823–824
Moberg pick-up test, 381, 752–753, 825, 1390, 1401
moving two-point discrimination, 136, 824, 828
point localization, 824–825
Funicular suture, anchoring of, 329–333, 331*f*, 332*f*

Gallamine, 78
Gamma efferent fusimotor fibers, 95
Gamma motor neuron regeneration, 221
Gangliosides, 64, 66
Gangrene, 672
Gantzer's muscle, 371, 987
Gap, 339
GAP-43, 65
Gas gangrene, as complication in gunshot wounds, 659
Gastrocnemius
fractional lengthening of, 1445
motor testing of, 168–169
recession of, 1445–1446, 1445*f*, 1446*f*, 1447*f*
Gate control theory, 87. *See also* Pain
Generator potential, 97, 97*f*
Genetic control of neural degeneration, 351
Geniculate ganglion, 461–462, 465
Genital end bulb, 94
Giant motor units, 785
Glabrous skin receptors, 90–93
Glia-derived nexin, 63, 64
Glioma, 1526
Glove anesthesia, 1490
Glycerolipids, 59
Glycocalyx, 57
Glycoprotein, 57, 58
GM1, 66
Goldman-Hodgkin-Katz (GHK) equation, 28, 38, 40
Gold weight lid tarsorrhaphy, 485–486, 485*f*
Golgi apparatus, 56
Gracilis muscle
free microvascular transfer of, 482
motor testing of, 167
Granular cell tumor, 1610–1611
treatment of, 1611
Greater occipital nerve, as neurotizer, 1336
Grip
reconstruction of, 1299
testing for, in diagnosing neuromas, 1528–1529
Grip and pinch strength, 434
Group A beta fibers, 89
Group A delta fibers, 89
Group C fibers, 89
Group fascicular repair, 8, 291–292, 291*f*, 292*f*, 302, 554–556. *See also* Fascicular repair
transected, 341–344
Growth-associated proteins, 65
Growth cone, 63, 65–66, 114–115
chemotaxis, 66
Guanethidine, 1483
Guanethidine-sulfate, 1512
Gunshot wounds
causalgia, 661–665
and environment, 657–658
history, 656
incidence of peripheral nerve injuries associated with, 658–659
initial care of, 659–660
operative techniques, 666–668
spontaneous recovery, 660–661, 660*t*
wound ballistics, 656–657, 657*t*, 658*t*
Guyon's canal, 237–238
ulnar nerve at
compression at electrophysiological testing in, 176
entrapment in, 1057
operative decompression of, 1140–1141, 1141*f*
release of, 907–909
Guyon's space, 1131
Hair cells, 90
Hairy skin receptors, 93–94, 94*f*
Hamartoma
lipofibromatous, 1593–1594, 1594*f*, 1595*f*
treatment of, 1594–1595
in digital nerve, 1598–1599
in median or ulnar nerve in the forearm and palm, 1595–1598
neuromuscular, 1599
Hamilton Depression Rating Scale, 1485
Hand. *See also* Wrist; Wrist and digits deformities
median nerve variations at, 204–205, 206*f*
median nerve in, 371, 373
neurovascular free flaps for providing sensibility to the
description of condition, 793–794, 795*f*, 796*f*
flaps to restore tactile gnosis, 794, 797*f*
neurovascular flaps from first web, 794, 798*f*
pulpar flap, 795
wrap-around flap, 797, 799*f*, 800*f*
flaps to supply protective sensibility or gross grip, 797–798
deltoid flap, 798, 800–801, 802*f*
dorsalis pedis flap, 803–804
forearm flap, 803
lateral upper arm flap, 802–803, 802*f*
medial upper arm flap, 801–802, 802*f*
overcoming injury at, 516
foot flaps, 804–808
approach to dorsalis pedis and first dorsal metatarsal artery, 807
clinical correlations, 807
first dorsal mediodorsal artery, 806, 806*f*
free sensory flaps from first web space, 807–808
medial plantar collateral artery to big toe, 806–807
preoperative assessment, 807
nerve injuries associated with pediatric fractures, 647

Hand (*continued*)
points of neural compression in, 373, 401
post-operative complications, 808–809
radial nerve in anatomy of, 400–401
ulnar nerve in anatomy, 417*f*, 419–420, 419*t*
open phenol block to motor branch of, 1432–1435
ulnar nerve neurectomy, 1435
Hands-up test, 1057
Hansen's disease, 717
Hematoma
prevention of, 976–977
treatment of, 977
Hemianopia, 1418, 1423
Hemicholinium, 80
Hemifacial spasm, use of botulinum toxin in, 486–487
Hemiplegic, ambulation potential in, 1420
Hemodialysis, association of carpal tunnel syndrome and, 872
HeNe laser, 329
Henry's mnemonic, 375
Heparin sulfate proteoglycan, 59
Hereditary neuropathy and pressure palsies, 1224
Heterotopic bone formation, 675, 1093, 1094*f*
High-frequency vibration, 148
Highly nonlinear stress-strain behavior, 48–49, 49*f*
Hilgar nerve stimulator, 247–248, 248*f*
Hip, pediatric nerve injuries associated with, 648
Hip arthroplasty (total), 1246
causes for neuropathy following, 1246–1249, 1248*f*, 1249*f*, 1250*f*
diagnosis of injury, 1249–1250
incidence of nerve palsies, 1246
intraoperative monitoring of neural function, 1252–1253
prevention of nerve palsy, 1251–1252
prognosis following, 1250–1251
risk of nerve palsies, 1246
treatment of nerve palsy, 1251
Hip adductor release, 1439
Hip deformities, 1425*f*, 1438–1439
closed phenol block to obturator nerve, 1439
congenital, 1245–1248
hip adductor release, 1439
hip flexor release, 1440
Hip dislocation
sciatic nerve injury with traumatic, 492–493
applied anatomy, 628–629
classification, 629, 630*f*
Hip flexor release, 1440
Histamine, and pain response, 1480
Histochemical and biochemical aids to nerve repair, 259–260
advantages of, 264–265
basis for, 260, 260*f*
carbonic anhydrase histochemistry
basis for, 262–263, 263*f*
history, 262
choline acetyltransferase radioassay
basis, 264
history, 263–264
cholinesterase histochemistry
basis for, 262
history, 261–262, 261*f*
clinical uses, 265–266
nerve fiber physiology and histochemistry, 260
techniques of carbonic anhydrase and acetylcholinesterase histochemistry, 266–267, 267*f*
materials and methods, 267–268, 268*f*, 269*f*
choline acetyltransferase radioassay materials and methods, 268–269
Histologic staining, 243
Homer-Wright rosettes, 1618
Hood splint, 818, 819*f*
Honeymoon paralysis, 999
Horner's sign, 1336, 1373, 1374
Horner's syndrome, 1238, 1260, 1273, 1293, 1362
detection of, 1274–1275
Horseradish peroxidase (HRP), technique of axon tracing, 225
H-reflex, 171, 173, 174*f*
Huber operation, 761
Humeral osteotomy, 519, 520*f*, 1299, 1366–1367
Humeral shaft fractures
pediatric nerve injuries associated with, 637–638, 638*f*
radial nerve palsy with, 623–625
Humeral shortening, 514
Hyperacusis, 467
Hyperalgesia, 1482, 1484
Hyperesthesia, 827, 1482, 1512
Hyperpathia, 1499, 1512
Hypertension, treatment of, 1511
Hyperthyroidism, experimental, 122
Hypertrophic scar, 1050
prevention of, 969, 969*f*
treatment of, 969–970
Hypoglossal nerve
identification, 474, 475*f*
transfer of, 474, 475*f*, 476
complications, 476
indications for, 474
technique of, 475
Hysteria, 1490

Iatrogenic injury, during escharotomy, 674
Iatrogenic ulnar tunnel syndrome, 1137
Idiopathic progressive peroneal nerve palsy, 1203
Idiopathic quadrilateral tunnel syndrome
symptoms and signs of, 1158–1160, 1159*f*, 1160*t*, 1161*f*, 1162*f*, 1163*t*
IGF–1, effect of, on nerve fiber, 124
Iggo dome, 92
Immunohistochemistry, of peripheral nerve tumors, 1588–1589
Immunosuppression, fresh allograft under, 528
Impedance, 21–22
Implantable electrode stimulation, 1116
Impulse conduction, 18–19, 60
active axon, 31–34, 32*f*
concentration gradients, permeabilities, and potentials, 26–28, 27*f*
factors affecting, 39–40
ionic basis of excitation, 34–39
membrane structure, 25–26
origin of the resting potential, 28–30, 29*f*
passive axon, 30–31, 31*f*

physical principles, 20–21
recording techniques, 21–23, 23*f*, 24*f*, 25
system overview, 19–20, 19*f*
Inactivation, 37
Incomplete amputation, 680
Independence relation, 28
Independent gating particles, 37
Infectious mononucleosis, 964
Infraclavicular brachial plexus injuries, 1281–1282
Infraclavicular deficits, motor testing for, 161–162
Infranuclear paralysis, 466
Inhibition, 98–99, 99*f*
Innervation, of sensory receptors, 95–97, 95*t*
Innervation density, 136, 140
tests for, 876, 877*t*, 878*f*
Inositols, 59
Insertional activity, 172
In situ decompression, 1124, 1128
In situ stress and strain, in peripheral nerve, 47
Instrumentation for nerve repair, 275
instruments, 277–282
loupes and microscopes, 276–277, 277*f*, 278*f*
operating room considerations, 275–276, 276*f*
sutureless neurorrhaphy, 283
lasers, 283–284
tubulation, 283
sutures, 282–283
Insulin-like growth factors (IGF I and II), 63, 119
Integral proteins, 57
Intercostal nerves, as neurotizer, 1345–1349, 1348*f*
Intercostobrachial neuralgia, 1192
Intercostobrachial neurotization, unexplained phenomena linked with, 1347–1349
Interdigital neuroma, 1207–1208
Interfascicular epineurium, fibrosis of the, 1290
Interfascicular nerve grafting, 242, 315–316, 319, 493, 554
for peroneal nerve injuries, 500
Interfascicular neurolysis, 922–926, 923*f*, 924*f*, 925*ft*
Interfascicular repair, 318, 319
Interleukin-1, 118
Internal neurolysis, 1117–1118
Interoceptors, 89
Interosseous muscle slide, 1435
Interosseous nerve. *See* Anterior interosseous nerve; Posterior interosseous nerve
Interstitial pressure
effects of circular cast on, 940, 941*f*
measuring, 944*f*, 945–946
Intraarticular elbow fracture, open reduction of, 1079
Intracellular pH, 57
Intracellular recording, 22
Intrafascicular tissue pressure, 9–10
Intrafascicular vascular perfusion, 12
Intramembranous particles, 75
Intramuscular and submuscular transpositional procedures, 1128
Intraneural blood flow, 11
and compression, 1215
Intraneural microcirculation, 11–12
Intraneural microvascular system
architecture, 8*f*, 10–11, 10*f*, 11*f*
blood-nerve barrier, 12–13
intraneural microcirculation, 11–12
nervi nervorum, 12
Intraneural topography, 532, 1265
Intraoperative electroneurography, 443
Intraoperative stimulation and recording, 180–181, 183, 183*f*
Intratemporal course, 461–462
Intratemporal paralysis, 466, 469
Intravenous lidocaine anesthesia (Bier block), 245
Intravital microscopic techniques, in observing capillary function, 11
Intrinsic-minus deformity, flexor digitorum superficialis transfer for, 733, 735
Intrinsic proteins, 26
Intrinsics, motor testing of, 169
Ionic balance, 57–58
Ionic basis of excitation, 34–39
Ionic gradient, 57
I protein, 67
Ipsilateral VIIth-to-VIIth repair, 471–474, 473*f*
Ischemia, 65, 860–861, 940
autograft with damage due to, 527–528
effect of, 77
intracompartmental, 940
Ischemic necrosis, 671
Island flap, 529
Isograft, 528

Jamar grip meter, 1528–1529
Jeanne's sign, 731, 741
Jebsen test, 434
Jeweler's forceps, 277–278, 280
Joint positioning, 513, 513*t*
Joint receptors, 94–95
Junction potential, 27
Juvenile rheumatoid arthritis, 963

Kienbock's disease, 875
Kiloh-Nevin syndrome, 1173
Kinesin, 62
Klippel-Trenaunay-Weber syndrome, lipofibromatous hamartoma in, 1594
Klumpke's palsy, 1335, 1362
Knee
flexion, 1420
hyperextension of, 1420
impairments, 1440
distal hamstring release or lengthening, 1441, 1442*f*
distal quadriceps release, 1440–1441, 1440*f*, 1442*f*
overcoming tibial and peroneal nerve injury at, 523
patient positioning in arthroscopy, 1236
peroneal nerve palsy complicating
fractures and dislocations of
applied anatomy, 629, 631
incidence, 631, 631*f*
treatment, 631–632
recession of gastrocnemius at, 1445–1446, 1445*f*, 1446*f*, 1447*f*
Krause end bulbs, 86, 94
Krebs cycle, 56

Laceration injuries, 489
Lacrimation test, 468
Lambda, 30
Lambrinudi technique, 767, 769
Lamellated mechanoreceptors, 90
Laminin, 58, 59, 63, 119, 588
Lanceolate, 94

Laser technique
experimental and clinical data, 310–311
in nerve repair, 283–284
in nerve suture, 329, 329*f*
Latency, 171, 172
Lateral antebrachial cutaneous nerve, as donor nerve, 531, 548–549, 548*f*
Lateral condyle fractures, pediatric injuries associated with, 641–642, 642*f*, 643*f*
Lateral cord, anatomy of nerves arising from, 1261–1262
Lateral decubitus position
guidelines for, in avoiding nerve injury, 1240
nerve injury in, 1236
Lateral epicondylitis, 1216, 1221
Lateral femoral cutaneous nerve, 1237
compressive neuropathy of, 1201–1202, 1201*f*
as donor nerve, 531, 551
injuries to, 503
and patient positioning in operating room, 1237
Lateral inhibition, 98–99, 99*f*
Lateral neuromas, 1527
Lateral pectoral nerve
anatomy of, 1261
anomalous innervation of, 198–199
Lateral plantar nerves, injuries to, 497, 497*f*
Lateral upper arm flap, 802–803
Latissimus dorsi transfer, 1311–1312, 1313*f*, 1314*f*
Lecithin, 59
L'episcopo transfer, 1315, 1316*f*
Leriche's post-traumatic pain syndrome, 662
Leupeptin, 68
Lidocaine
in electrical nerve stimulation in the awake patient, 247
in reflex sympathetic dystrophy, 1514
Lidocaine hydrochloride nerve blocks, 1423
Ligament of Struthers, 999, 1072
Limb deformity, 1420
Limb stability, 1420
Lipids, role of, in cell membrane, 26
Lip mucosal fold resection, 486
Lipofibromatous hamartoma, 1593–1594, 1594*f*, 1595*f*, 1619
treatment of, 1594–1595
in digital nerve, 1598–1599
in median or ulnar nerve in the forearm and palm, 1595–1598
Lipofibromatous nerve enlargement, 963
Lithotomy position
and nerve injury, 1232–1233
guidelines for avoiding, 1239
Local circuits, 32, 32*f*
Localization, accurate, 96
Lover's palsy, 1166
Lower extremities. *See also nerves in*
donor nerves in, 549
lateral femoral cutaneous nerve, 551
sural nerve, 550–551, 550*f*
internal topography of, as related to repair, 238–239
motor testing in, 167–170
nerve injury associated with devascularizing trauma in, 684–685
problems of spinal cord-injured patients in, 1409–1410
peripheral nerve injuries, 489–490
femoral nerve, 493–494, 495*f*
lateral femoral cutaneous nerve, 503
lumbosacral plexus, 491–492, 491*f*
medial/lateral plantar nerves, 497, 497*f*
obturator nerve, 494–495
peroneal nerve, 497–502
posterior tibial nerve, 495–496, 496*f*
repair of, 355
saphenous nerve, 502, 503*f*
sciatic nerve, 492–493, 492*f*, 494*f*
sural nerve, 503
tendon transfer for paralysis in, 761
Lumbosacral plexus
compression of, 1198
injuries to, 491–492, 491*f*
motor testing of, 167
Lysosomal cathepsins, 66
Lysosomes, 56
Macrophages, 65
Magnetic resonance imaging (MRI)
in assessing facial nerve paralysis, 468
in diagnosis of carpal tunnel syndrome, 875
Magnifying loupes, in nerve repair, 276, 277*f*
Malignant tumors. *See under* Tumors
Malingering, detecting, 141–143
Mandibular branch, 463
Manual muscle grading, 621
Martin-Gruber anastomosis, 1170
Martin-Gruber communication, 192, 197, 201–202, 371, 373
Masse's sign, 730, 739, 740
Masseter transfer, 479, 480*f*
anatomy in, 479–480
complications, 481
indications for, 479
technique in, 480–481
Matev's sign, 644–645, 645*f*
Matter, composition of, 20
McGill-Melzack Pain Questionnaire, 1485
Mechanical and humoral control of specificity in nerve repair, 215–217
discussion, 226–227
mechanical, 222–226, 227*f*
potential mechanisms of specificity generation
contact recognition, 222
neurotropism, 224
neurotropism, 223–224
specificity hierarchy, 216*f*
end organ
motor, 221
sensory, 220–221
nerve trunk, 218
sensory/motor reinnervation, 218–219, 220*f*
tissue, 217–218, 218*f*
topographic
motor, 221
sensory, 219–220
Mechanoreceptors, 89
classification of, 90
Medial antebrachial cutaneous nerve
anatomy of, 1262
as donor nerve, 531, 547, 547*f*
Medial brachial cutaneous nerve, anatomy of, 1262

Medial collateral ligament
  reconstruction of, 1109, 1110*f*
  repairing injuries to, 1079
Medial condyle and epicondyle humerus fractures, pediatric nerve injuries associated with, 642–645, 644*f*, 645*f*
Medial cord, anatomy of nerves arising from, 1262
Medial elbow instability, 1109
  anatomy related to failed treatment, 1111–1112
  anterior intramuscular transposition, 1113
  anterior subcutaneous transposition, 1113
  anterior submuscular transposition, 1113–1114
  cubital tunnel release, 1112
  external neurolysis, 1117
  implantable electrode stimulation, 1116
  internal neurolysis, 1117–1118
  medial epicondylectomy, 1112
  neurolysis, 1112
  operative technique, 1117
  persistent motor and sensory deficits, 1110–1111
  reconstruction of medial collateral ligament, 1109, 1110*f*
  reoperation for failed decompression, 1111
  revision submuscular transposition, 1114–1116
  silastic sheath, 1118
Medial epicondylectomy, 1101–1102, 1112, 1124–1125, 1125*f*, 1128
  advantages of, 1087
  anatomy in, 1088
  complications, 1092–1094
  criticisms of, 1094–1095
  history of, 1087–1088
  indications for, 1088
  presence of perineural scarring following, 1114
  procedures
    epicondyle exposure, 1089–1091, 1090*f*
    incision, 1088, 1088*f*
    nerve decompression, 1088–1089, 1089*f*
    osteotomy, 1090*f*, 1091
    postoperative procedure, 1092
Medial epicondylitis, 1108
Medial intermuscular septum, 1079–1080, 1079*f*
Medial pectoral nerve, anatomy of, 1262
Medial plantar nerves, injuries to, 497, 497*f*
Medial stress syndrome, 1099
Medial upper arm flap, 801–802, 802*f*
Median and ulnar nerve palsy, splinting for combined, 818–819, 819*f*
Median nerve, 165–167, 166*f*, 1170
  action potentials in, 288
  adherence of
    to skin, 973, 974, 977*f*
    to tendons and restricted tendon excursion, 975–976
  anatomy, 366
    in the arm, 366–367, 366*f*, 368*f*
    at carpal tunnel, 892–897
    in the forearm, 368–371, 369*f*, 370*t*, 372*f*
    in the wrist and hand, 371, 373
  anomalous muscles and tendons, 1170
  anomalous vessels, 1171–1172
  and compression of median nerve at wrist. *See* Carpal tunnel syndrome
  compression of ulnar nerve, 1173
  congenital bands and fractures of the humerus, 1172
  Cruveilhier's canal, 1172
  defects in, 514, 514*f*
    at arm level, 514
    at elbow level, 515, 516*t*
    at forearm level, 516
    at wrist level, 516
  deltopectoral fascia, 1172
  double crush syndrome
    cervical radiculopathy and carpal tunnel syndrome, 1216–1220, 218*t*
      response to carpal tunnel surgery, 1220–1221, 1220*t*
  excursion of, 288, 289*f*, 290
  injuries, 813, 814
    from neurolysis, 972–973
    repair of, 356
    treatment of, following wrist trauma, 942–943, 945
  interfascicular neurolysis, 922–926, 923*f*, 924*f*, 925*ft*
  internal topography of, as related to repair, 237
  motor branch of, 903–904
    severance of recurrent, 971–972
  motor recovery, following grafting, 556*f*, 559–560
  neuropathy in cumulative trauma, 957–958
    carpal tunnel release in patients with, 963–964
      conditions associated with, 964
      specific studies, 964–965
    evaluation of patient with, 959
    management of, 960
    pathology and pathophysiology, 958–959
    specific studies, 964–965
    treatment of, 959
    at the wrist, 1225, 1421
  open phenol block to the, 1430–1431
  operative exposure
    in the arm, 374
    at the elbow and in the forearm, 375, 376*f*, 377
  palmar cutaneous branch of, 901–903, 902*f*
    severance of, 970–971
  palsy, 711
    extrinsic reconstruction for, 712–715, 713*f*
    initial care, 712
    restoration of intrinsic muscle function, 715–717
      timing of opponensplasty, 717
    splinting for, 815–816
    types of operations
      abductor digiti minimi opponensplasty, 723–724, 724*f*
      extensor indicis proprius opponensplasty, 722, 723*f*
      flexor digitorum superficialis opponensplasty, 717–720, 718*f*, 719*f*
      opponensplasty using a wrist extensor, 721–722

Median nerve, palsy (*continued*)
opponensplasty using extrinsic muscles of the thumb, 724–726
palmaris longus opponensplasty, 720–721, 720*f*
special techniques for opponensplasty, 726
percutaneous phenol block to recurrent motor branch of, 1437
potential points of compression in, 367, 370–371, 373
pronator syndrome. *See* Pronator syndrome
repair of, 353–354, 379–380
by fascicular alignment and suture, 384
by grafting, 385–386, 387*t*, 388, 388*t*
primary, of lesions in, 383
magnification and other variables in, 384
suture technique in, 384–385
uniform assessment of clinical results, 380–383
vascularized nerve grafts in, 389
sensory recovery following grafting, 560–561, 560*t*
severe compression of the, 921–922, 922*f*
and subcutaneous tender nerve, 973–974, 974*f*, 975*f*, 976*f*
supracondyloid process and ligament of Struthers, 1172–1773
treatment for lipofibromatous hamartoma in, 1595–1598
variations at the wrist and hand, 204–205, 206*f*
Median-ulnar nerve communications, 200–201
Meissner corpuscle, 86, 90, 92, 92*f*, 96, 137*f*, 138–139
innervation of, 98
reinnervation of, 101
Membrane theory, 25
Membranous route, 56
Membranous transport, 60–62
Meralgia paresthetica, 503, 1201–1202, 1201*f*, 1527
Merkel cell-neurite complex, 86, 90, 92–93, 93*f*, 96, 137*f*
reinnervation of, 101
Mesodermal healing, 233
Mesodermal tissue, 316
Metacarpophalangeal and interphalangeal joint fusion in the thumb, 741, 743–745
Methylmethacrylate extrusion, nerve palsies associated with, 1247
Mg-Ca ATPase, 62
Microelectrode, 22
Microfilaments, 4, 59
Microneedles, 280–281, 281*f*
Micropinocytotic vesicles, 8
Micropore tape, 328
Microscopes, in nerve repair, 276–278, 278*f*
Microspikes, 114–115
Microsurgical internal neurolysis, 147
Microtubule-associated protein, 60
Microtubule-dependent transport, 60, 61*f*, 62
Microtubules, 4, 6, 59–60
Microvascular anastomosis, revascularization by, 529
Middle cranial fossa approach, 472
Middle finger test, 1026
Mikhail bone block, 730
Milliwatt CO_2 laser, 284
Miniature closed compartment syndrome, 852
Miniature compartment syndrome, 1215
Minifascicles, 115
Mitochondria, 56, 74
Moberg pick-up test, 381, 752–753, 825, 1390, 1401
Monofascicular nerve, 288
Monophasic action potential, 22, 25
Monteggia fractures, pediatric nerve injuries associated with, 645–646, 646*f*
Monteggia lesions, 628
Morton's metatarsalgia, 1527
Morton's neuroma, 1207–1208
Motor branch of median nerve, 903–904, 903*f*, 904*f*
severance of recurrent, 971–972
Motor dysfunction
for combined median and ulnar nerve palsy, 818–819
early management, 814
for median nerve palsy, 815–816, 815*f*, 816*f*
for radial nerve injury, 819–820, 819*f*, 820*f*
splinting, 814
for ulnar nerve palsy, 816–818
Motor end plate, 74
effects of nerve injury on the, 80–82
acute changes, 80
recovery following injury, 80–81
sprouting, 81–82, 81*f*
histologic appearance of, 74
ultrastructure of, 74–75
Motor innervation, topography of, 221
Motor neurectomy, radial to the brachioradialis muscle, 1429
Motor testing
and brain injury, 1419–1421, 1421*f*, 1422*f*
in cerebral palsy, 1456–1457
clinical uses of, 159–160, 160*t*
in the lower extremity
lumbosacral plexus, 167
peripheral nerves, 167–170
quantitative assessment in, 160
semi-quantitative assessment in, 160
in the upper extremity, 160
axillary nerves, 162
brachial plexus injuries, 160–161, 161*f*
infraclavicular deficits, 161–162, 162*f*
median nerve, 165–167
musculocutaneous nerve, 164
peripheral nerves, 162
radial nerve, 162–163, 163*f*
supraclavicular deficits, 161
ulnar nerve, 164–165, 164*f*
Motor unit, 73–74
Motor unit potential, 171, 172, 173*f*
Moving two-point discrimination test, 136, 824, 828
M protein, 64, 67
Mucocutaneous receptors, 94
Multientrapment syndromes, 859–860
Multiple compression sites versus distal axonopathy, 193–194
Multiple entrapment neuropathy, 1224
Multiple sclerosis, 717

Munchausen syndrome, 1490
Muscle contraction, quantitative assessment of, 159, 160
Muscle fibers, types of, 75–76
Muscle implantation, for neuromas, 1533*f*, 1534, 1534*f*
Muscle receptors, 94–95
Muscle spindle, 95
Muscle transplantation (functioning), 775–776
  indications for, 776–777
  operative technique, 777–780
    postoperative care, 780
    preparing muscle, 778, 778*f*
    preparing recipient site, 778–779, 779*f*
  results, 780–781
  selecting appropriate muscle, 777, 777*f*
Musculocutaneous nerve, 164, 1165, 1262
  anatomy and function, 1165–1166
  anomalous innervation of, 199–200, 200*f*
  closed phenol block to the, 1427
  open phenol block to the, 1427
  overcoming defects in, 520–521, 521*t*, 522*f*
  pathophysiology, symptoms, and signs, 1166
  repair of, 354
Musculocutaneous neurectomy, 1429
Musculoskeletal assessment of brachial plexus injury, 1276
Mushrooming, 9
M-wave, 172, 173, 173*f*
Myelin, 20
Myelin-associated glycoprotein, 59
Myelinated axons, 3, 3*f*, 1480
Myelinated fibers, 20, 39
Myelination, 120
  of axons, 58–59
Myelin basic proteins, 59
Myelin lipids, 59
Myelin sheath, 3, 3f
Myelography, 1273
  in assessing brachial plexus injury, 1279–1280
Myophysiological dynamic muscle transfer, 476
  digastric transfer, 481–482
  free microvascular transfer using gracilis muscle, 482
  masseter transfer, 479–481
  temporalis muscle fascial transfer and suspension, 476–479, 477*f*
Myosin, 64, 67
Myxedema, 872

Nasolabial fold plasty, 486
Needle electromyography, in diagnosing pronator syndrome, 998
Needle holders, 280
Neodymium-YAG laser, 284, 310, 311
Neoplasia, 465
Neostigmine (Prostigmine), 79
Nernst equation, 27–28
Nerve action potential, 57
Nerve block
  in diagnosing neuromas, 1529
  lidocaine hydrochloride, 1423
  phenol, 1423–1424, 1426
    closed, 1427, 1439
    open, 1427, 1429, 1430–1431, 1433–1435, 1441–1442, 1444–1445
    percutaneous, 1426, 1430, 1437
Nerve blood flow (NBF), 11–12
Nerve cell body, effect of compression on morphology and function of, 854, 855*f*
Nerve compression
  degree of, 146–147, 146*t*
  diagnosing, 144, 145*f*, 146, 847–848
  double crush and reversed double crush syndromes, 859
  effects of chronic, 856–857
    on chronic compression and nerve morphology, 857–858
    on chronic compression and neurolysis, 858–859
  effects of locally applied
    on axonal transport and compression, 849–850, 852*f*
    on intraneural microcirculation and edema formation, 854–855
    on morphology and function and structure, of nerve cell body, 854, 855*f*
    on nerve fiber structure and function and axonal transport, 855–856, 856*f*
    on intraneural microvascular flow and compression, 849
    on postcompression phase and edema formation, 851–853, 853*f*, 854*f*
  effects of low-grade compression on human nerves, 860–861, 861*f*
  multientrapment syndromes, 859–860
  nerve microanatomy related to compression injuries, 848–849, 848*f*
  susceptibility of nerves to compression in diabetic neuropathy, 861–862
  treatment of severe in median nerve, 921–926
Nerve conduction velocity (NCV), 176
  in assessing brachial plexus injury, 1276–1277
  evaluation of, 825, 881
Nerve defects, 508, 508*f*
  nerve injuries causing significant gaps, 509, 510*f*
  overcoming nerve gaps for end-to-end coaptation, 509
    joint positioning, 513, 513*t*
    nerve mobilization in situ, 509–511, 512*f*, 513
    nerve rerouting and transposition, 513
  overcoming specific
    bone shortening, 514–516
    brachial plexus defects, 513–514
    femoral nerve defects, 523–524, 523*t*
    median nerve defects, 514, 515*f*
    musculocutaneous nerve defects, 520–521, 521*t*, 522*f*
    peroneal nerve defects, 521–523, 523*f*
    radial nerve defects, 517, 519–520, 519*t*, 520*f*
    sciatic nerve defects, 521, 521*t*, 522*f*
    tibial nerve defects, 521–523, 523*t*
    ulnar nerve defects, 516–517, 517*f*, 518*f*

Nerve elasticity, altered, 1216
Nerve elongation, clinical assessment of, 511, 513
Nerve entrapment, 847. *See also* Nerve compression
Nerve excitability testing, 468
Nerve fiber, 2–4, 2f. *See also* Axon
  function of, 2, 235
  effects of compression on, 851
  physiology and histochemistry of, 260
  types of, 4
Nerve gases, 79
Nerve graft(s), 301*f*, 302, 318, 358, 525. *See also* Donor nerve(s)
  alternatives to
    elongation of nerve tissue, 539
    neuromatous neurotization, 539–540
    providing free space for neuromatous neurotization, 539
  biology in, 526
  bioresorbable, 590–591, 592*f*
  classification of nerve grafts
    circulation, 529
    mechanical aspects, 528–529
    origin of grafts, 528
  in digital nerve defects, 455–457, 457*f*, 458*f*, 556*f*, 558–559, 558*f*
  donor nerves, 528, 1297–1298
  end-to-end nerve repair, 526, 527*f*
    autograft with damage due to ischemia, 527–528
    fresh allograft under immunosuppression, 528
    fresh autologous nerve grafts, 526–527
    neurotization along an empty space, 528
    preserved allografts, 527
  group fascicular, 554, 556
  history of, 526
  interfascicular, 554
    in sciatic nerve injury, 493, 494*f*
  in median nerve repair, 385–386, 387*t*, 388, 388*t*
    motor recovery, 556*f*, 559–560, 559*t*
    sensory recovery, 560–561
  methodology, 557, 557*t*, 558*t*
  in radial nerve repair
    motor recovery, 557*f*, 562–563, 563*t*
    sensory recovery, 563, 564*t*
      lower-extremity nerve grafts, 564, 565*t*
  results, 564–565
  for spinal accessory nerve injury, 450–451
  studies on, 553–554, 554*t*, 555*t*
  technique of free, 530
    donor nerves, 530–532
    exploration and definition of the two nerve stumps, 532
    restoration of continuity, 532–536
    wound closure, 535
  through resorbable tubes
    background, 587–588
    bioresorbable nerve graft, 590–591, 592*f*
    characteristics of the ideal guidance system, 591, 593
    future research, 593–594
    nerve regeneration through tubular prostheses, 588–590, 589*f*
    surgical technique, 593, 593*f*
  of transected fascicular groups, 342–344, 343*f*
  ulnar nerve motor recovery, 556*f*, 561–562, 561*t*
  ulnar nerve sensory recovery, 562, 562*t*
  vascularized, 389, 509, 528, 529, 569–570
    advantages of, 539
    clinical studies of, 577–579
    cutaneous nerves, 538–539
    experimental results, 570–571
    indications for, 571–572
    operative technique, 579–581, 580*f*, 581*f*, 582*f*
      ulnar nerve graft, 581–584, 583*f*
    techniques of, 572, 572*f*, 573*f*, 574–575, 575*f*, 577, 577*f*
    transfer as a pedicle flap, 535, 538
Nerve growth factor (NGF), 6, 59, 63, 66, 117, 224
  autocrine/paracrine function of, 118–119
  and axonal growth, 117–119
  and gangliosides, 64
  and nerve regeneration, 588
Nerve growth protein B50, 63
Nerve injuries
  association with fractures and dislocations, 620
    denervation, 620–621
    management of, 621–622
    reinnervation and recovery, 621, 621*f*
    secondary, 622
  axillary, following shoulder dislocation
    anatomy of, 626
    evaluation of deltoid muscle function, 627–628
    incidence of, 626–627
    nerve exploration, 628
    recovery of, 628
  from chemicals, 677
  classification of, 110–112
  components of, 110, 111*f*
  and devascularizing trauma, 679–681, 681*f*, 682*f*, 683*f*, 684–685
  effects of, on the motor end plate, 80–82
    acute changes, 80
    recovery following injury, 80–81
    sprouting, 81–82, 81*f*
  electrical, 675–676
  initiation and organization of axonal outgrowth, 112, 113*f*, 114
  local response of axons to, 64–65, 64*f*
  partial. *See* Partial nerve injuries
  and patient positioning in operating room, 1231–1232
    compression of superficial peripheral nerves
      cranial nerve branches, 1237, 1237*f*, 1238*f*
      lateral femoral cutaneous nerve, 1237
      peroneal nerve, 1233*f*, 1236
      radial nerve, 1237
      ulnar nerve, 1236–1237
    guidelines for proper positioning, 1239, 1239*f*, 1240, 1240*f*
    incidence, 1232
    injury to the brachial plexus, 1234, 1235*f*

direct compression of, 1236, 1236*f*
stretching of, 1234–1236
pathogenesis of nerve injury, 1232
peroneal nerve palsy complicating fractures and dislocations of the knee
anatomy of, 629, 631
incidence of, 631
treatment of, 631–632
positions associated with, 1232
lithotomy, 1232–1233
prone, 1234
Trendelenburg, 1233
posterior interosseous nerve palsy with Monteggia lesions
anatomy of, 625
classification of, 625
incidence of, 625–626
prognosis for recovery, 1238
thermal, 671–672
treatment, 1238–1239
pediatric. *See* Pediatric nerve injuries
proximal changes, 112
radial nerve palsy with humeral shaft fractures
anatomy of, 622–623
incidence of, 623
and nerve exploration, 623–625, 624*f*
from radiation, 676–677
sciatic, with traumatic hip dislocation and fracture-dislocation
anatomy of, 629, 630*f*
secondary, 622
splinting for, 814
Nerve lesion in continuity, 601–602, 1541–1542
clinical electrophysiology, 603–605, 604*f*
electrophysiology of the CNAP, 605, 605*f*
practical considerations, 608–610, 609*f*, 610*f*
electrodes, 603*f*, 608–610, 609*f*, 610*f*
equipment, 610–612, 611*f*
technique, 612–614, 615*f*, 616
theoretical considerations, 606–608, 606*f*, 607*f*
neuropathology, 602–603, 603*f*
nonoperative management options, 1542, 1544–1545
surgical options in treating, 1542*f*, 1543*f*, 1544*f*, 1545–1548, 1549*f*
Nerve ligation, in treating neuromas, 1529–1530
Nerve microanatomy related to compression injuries, 848–849, 848*f*
Nerve-nerve neurotization, 526
Nerve palsies
axillary, following shoulder dislocation
anatomy of, 626
incidence of, 626–627
evaluation of deltoid muscle function, 627–628
nerve exploration, 628
recovery, 628
in lower extremity, 763–764
applied anatomy, 764, 765*f*
deformities associated with, 764
femoral nerve palsy, 771
anterior transfer of the biceps femoris, 771–772
complications, 772
historical aspects of, 764
peroneal palsy, 766
anterior transfer of tibialis posterior, 768–769, 768*f*
complications, 769
anatomy of, 629, 631
incidence of, 631, 631*f*
treatment of, 631–632
posterior interosseous, with Monteggia lesions
anatomy of, 625
classification of, 625
incidence of, 625–626
posterior transfer of anterior tibial tendon, 770
results, 769, 770
sciatic, 771
with traumatic hip dislocation and fracture dislocation
anatomy of, 628–629
classification of, 629, 630*f*
tibial nerve palsy, 769–770
triple arthrodesis, 766–768, 767*f*
triple arthrodesis with posterior displacement, 770
and total hip arthroplasty, 1246
causes, 1246–1249
diagnosis of injury, 1249–1250
incidence, 1246
and intraoperative monitoring, 1252–1253
prevention, 1251–1252
prognosis following, 1250–1251
risk, 1246
treatment, 1251
variations in, 1257
vascular anatomical relationships to, 1263–1265, 1264*f*
Nerve reconstruction
motor testing following, 160
reinnervation of distal tissues by, 509
Nerve regeneration, 80–81
biology of, 110
experimental, 120–124
testing for, 147–148
Nerve repair. *See also* specific methods
algorithm for, 508*f*
analysis of existing data, 349–350
end-to-end, 526, 527*f*
factors influencing functional recovery, 350, 360*t*
host anatomy and physiology, 350–351
injury
level of, 356–357
mechanics, 355–356
recovery process, 360
specific nerve involved, 352–355
digital nerve, 353, 353*t*
in lower extremity, 355
median nerve, 353–354, 353*t*
ulnar nerve, 354, 354*t*
radial nerve, 354, 354*t*
musculocutaneous nerve, 354
type of nerve, 351–352
histochemical and biochemical aids to, 259–260
advantages of, 264–265
basis for, 260, 260*f*
carbonic anhydrase histochemistry, 262–263, 263*f*
choline acetyltransferase radioassay, 263–264
cholinesterase histochemistry, 261–262, 261*f*
clinical use of, 265–266

Nerve repair, histochemical and biochemical aids to (*continued*)
nerve fiber physiology, 260
techniques of, 266–269
grafting versus repair, 359
instrumentation. *See* Instrumentation for nerve repair
and internal topography of peripheral nerves
applied anatomy, 233–235
history of, 231–233
nerve function, 235
recent studies, 235–240
mechanical and humoral control of specificity in, 215–217
rationale and principles of, 1330–1333
under tension, 509–511, 511*f*, 512*f*, 513
timing of, 357–359
type of, 358–359
Nerve sheath ganglion, 1591, 1619
treatment of, 1591–1593
Nerve stimulation, 1546–1548, 1549
motor fascicle territory, 179–180, 181*f*
sensory identification, 179, 180*f*
Nerve transfer. *See* Neurotization
Nerve transposition, technique of, 513
Nerve trunk specificity, 218
Nerve wrapping
for nerve in continuity, 1546, 1549
for partial nerve injuries, 339–340
Nervus intermedius, 464*f*, 465
Neural cell adhesion molecules, 57
Neural code, 87
Neural compression
points of, in the wrist and hand, 373
potential points of, in arm, 367, 396
potential points of, in forearm, 370–371, 398–400
Neuralgic amyotrophy, 984, 986
Neural regeneration, rate of, 148
Neurapraxia, 100, 110–111, 112, 620, 621, 660, 1232
Neurectomy
musculocutaneous, 1429, 1461
radial motor, 1429
ulnar nerve, 1435
Neurilemmoma, 1606–1608
results, 1608–1609
treatment of, 1608, 1609*f*, 1610*f*
Neurite outgrowth, 67
Neurite-promoting factors, 63, 119
Neurocampsis, 1532
Neurofibroma, 1600
diffuse, 1601
localized, 1600, 1601*f*
treatment of, 1603–1605
plexiform, 1601–1602
treatment of, 1605–1606
solitary, 1619
in von Recklinghausen's disease, 1603
Neurofibrosarcoma, 1575
Neurofilaments, 4, 59, 66, 74
Neurogenic heterotopic ossification, 1446–1449
Neuroleukin, 63
Neurological assessment of brachial plexus injury, 1274–1275, 1275*t*
Neurolysis, 325, 442, 443, 666–667, 1112
external, 1114, 1117, 1117*f*
interfascicular, 922–926
internal, 1117–1118, 1126
median nerve injury from, 972–973
for nerve in-continuity, 1546, 1549
for spinal accessory nerve injury, 450
Neurolytic blockade, in treating reflex sympathetic dystrophy, 1515
Neuroma(s), 1108–1109, 1525–1526
classification of, 1526
following nerve transection, 1527
lateral, 1527
neuromas in-continuity, 1527. *See also* Nerve in-continuity
spindle, 1527
stump, 1527
diagnosis, 1528
grip testing, 1528–1529
nerve blocks, 1529
pain diagrams, 1528
external, 1117, 1117*f*
interdigital, 1207–1208
internal, 1117–1118
nonoperative treatment
local injection, 1529
percussion, 1529
transcutaneous stimulation, 1529
operative treatment
centrocentral anastomosis, 1532
cross-union technique, 1532
crushing, 1529
epineural ligation, 1530–1532, 1530*f*
nerve ligation, 1529–1530
neurocampsis, 1532
pathophysiology, 1526
prevention of, 1527–1528
relocation techniques, 1534
bone implantation, 1534
muscle implantation, 1533*f*, 1534, 1534*f*
translocation, 1535–1536
vascularized island transfer, 1534–1535
traumatic, 1589–1590, 1591*f*
treatment of, 1590–1591
Neuromatous neurotization, 527
providing free space for, 539
providing autologous tissue framework for, 539–540
Neuromuscular choristoma, 1599
treatment of, 1600
Neuromuscular disease, motor testing in, 159
Neuromuscular hamartoma, 1599
Neuromuscular junction, 73
pharmacology, 77
junctional drug action, 79–80
postjunctional drug action, 77–79
prejunctional drug action, 80
physiology of, 76–77
effect of ischemia, 77
impulse transmission, 77
purpose of, 73
structure of, 73–76, 74*f*, 75*f*
Neuronotrophic factors (NTF), 6
Neuropathic pain, 1482
Neuropathy
combined spinal accessory and long thoracic, 1150, 1151*f*
compressive of the spinal accessory, phrenic, and dorsal scapular nerves, 1148, 1149*t*, 1150
diabetic, 1215, 1224–1225
entrapment, 1216

hereditary, 1224
multiple entrapment, 1224
of ulnar nerve at the elbow, 1099–1100, 1100*t*
uremic, 1225
Neuroplasmic organelles, 56
Neurorrhaphy, 291, 442
end-to-end, 358
for gunshot wounds, 659–660
primary, 357, 359
regeneration of sympathetic fibers after, 352
secondary, 357
sutureless, 283–284
in treating gunshot wounds, 667–668, 667*t*
Neurothekeoma, 1611–1612
treatment of, 1612–1613
Neurotization, 1297
along empty space, 528
direct muscular, 783
clinical results, 787*f*, 788*ft*, 789*f*, 790–791, 790*f*
indications for, 785–786
operative technique, 786, 786*f*, 788
alternate techniques, 788
complications, 790
postoperative care, 790
physiological basis for, 783–785, 784*f*, 785*f*, 786*f*
neuromatous, 527, 539–540
of selected distal stumps, 1296–1297
in treating brachial plexus injuries
common patterns of lesions including root avulsions, 1333–1336
history, 1329–1330
neurotization according to pathology, 1349, 1351–1352, 1351*f*, 1353*f*, 1354–1355, 1354*f*
neurotizers and their results, 1336–1349, 1337*t*
deep cervical plexus, 1341*f*, 1342–1343
greater occipital nerve, 1336
intercostal nerves, 1345–1349
long thoracic nerve, 1343
phrenic nerve, 1344–1345
spinal accessory nerve, 1336–1342
thoracodorsal nerve, 1344
rationale and principles of nerve repair, 1330–1333
Neurotmesis, 100, 111–112, 112, 467, 620, 621, 660
Neurotransmitter release, 58
Neurotrophic activity, 68
Neurotrophic capability, 68
Neurotrophic factors, 63
effect of, on nerve regeneration, 123–124
influence of, on axonal growth, 117–119, 117*f*, 118*f*
Neurotrophic generation, 216–217
Neurotrophism, 67, 224
Neurotropism, 66–68, 119, 120, 121, 216, 223–224, 226
definition of, 215
Neurovascular cutaneous island pedicle flaps, 751
Neurovascular free flaps, 793
for providing sensibility to the hand
description of condition, 793–794, 795*f*, 796*f*
flaps to restore tactile gnosis, 794, 797*f*
neurovascular flaps from first web, 794, 798*f*
pulpar flap, 795
wrap-around flap, 797, 799*f*, 800*f*
flaps to supply protective sensibility or gross grip, 797–798
deltoid flap, 798, 800–801, 802*f*
dorsalis pedis flap, 803–804
forearm flap, 803
lateral upper arm flap, 802–803, 802*f*
medial upper arm flap, 801–802, 802*f*
foot flaps, 804–808
approach to dorsalis pedis and first dorsal metatarsal artery, 807
clinical correlations, 807
first dorsal mediodorsal artery, 806, 806*f*
free sensory flaps from first web space, 807–808
medial plantar collateral artery to big toe, 806–807
preoperative assessment, 807
post-operative complications
nerve-related, 809
tardive, 808
vascular, 808–809
Nifedipine, for reflex sympathetic dystrophy, 1510–1511, 1513*f*
Ninhydrin test, to identify malingering, 141
Nissl substance, 56
Nociceptors, 89
Node of Ranvier, 3, 20, 56, 58
Noise, 22
Noncritical vascular injury, 680
Nonlamellated mechanoreceptors, 90
Nonmyelinated axons, 3, 3f
Non-neuronal cell reactions, 116
Nonsympathetically maintained pain
in brain stem, 1484–1485
in cortex, 1485
in nerves and nerve roots, 1483–1484, 1484*f*
in spinal cord, 1484
in thalamus, 1485
Nonvascularized fascicular graft, 509
No reflow phenomenon, 852
Norepinephrine, 1482
Notalgia paraesthetica, 1173
Nuclear paralysis, 466
Nucleus, 56
Nucleus centralis lateralis, 1481
Nucleus parafascicularis, 1481
Nucleus raphe magnus, 1482
Nucleus ventralis posterolateralis, 1481
Nylon monofilament technique, 151

Objective tests, 821
nerve conduction studies, 825
Object training, 834
Obstetrical palsy, 1150
operative intervention for, 1369
Obturator nerve
closed phenol block to, 1439
compressive neuropathies of, 1200–1201
injuries to, 494–495
motor testing of, 167
Ohm's law, 21, 22
Oligofascicular nerve, 288
Open-heart surgery, peripheral nerve injury during, 1238

Operative techniques, for gunshot wounds, 666–668
Opponens digiti minimi, motor testing of, 165
Opponensplasty
  abductor digiti minimi, 723–724, 724*f*
  abductor pollicis longus, 724–725
  extensor indicis proprius, 722, 723*f*, 726, 936
  extensor carpi ulnaris, 771–772
  extensor digiti minimi, 722
  extensor pollicis longus, 725
  flexor digitorum profundus, 726
  flexor digitorum superficialis, 717–720, 718*f*, 719*f*
  flexor pollicis longus, 725
  palmaris longus, 720–721, 720*f*
  prerequisites for, 716
  special techniques for, 726
  timing of, 717
  using extrinsic muscles of the thumb, 724–726
  using wrist extensor, 721–722
Opponens pollicis, motor testing of, 167
Opponens pollicis brevis, motor examination of, 879–880
Orthoses, at the C4 functional level, 1391–1392
Oscilloscope, 22
Osedo technique of laser-assisted nerve repair, 329
Osmosis, role of perineural diffusion barrier in maintaining, 8
Osteoarthritis, risk of nerve palsies following total hip arthroplasty for, 1246
Osteonecrosis, arthroplasty for, 1246
Osteopenia, 1504
Osteosarcoma, 1575
  chemotherapy for soft-tissue, 1583
Osteotomy, 1092
  humeral, 519, 520*f*, 1299, 1366–1367
  in medial epicondylectomy
    complications of, 1092–1093, 1092*f*, 1093*f*, 1094*f*
  upper tibial, 1203
Overstretching, prevention of, 814
Oxidative phosphorylation, 56
Pacinian corpuscle, 86, 90–92, 91*f*, 137*f*, 139
  innervation of, 95, 96–97, 96*f*
  reinnervation of, 101
Pain, 86–87. *See also* Nerve in-continuity; Neuromas; Pain dysfunction syndrome; Reflex sympathic dystrophy
  chronic, 1485, 1551–1552
    clinical experience with electrical nerve stimulation, 1552, 1553*f*, 1554–1555, 1554*f*
    evaluation, 1560
    results, 1557–1559, 1559*f*
    technique of electrical stimulation, 1555, 1556*f*, 1557, 1557*f*
    therapeutic blocks and continuous infusion in treatment, 1563–1564
      applied anatomy in, 1564–1567
      clinical application, 1567–1568
      patient selection for, 1564
  clinical syndromes of, 1482–1483
    nonsympathetically maintained pain
      brain stem, 1484–1485
      cortex, 1485
      nerves and nerve roots, 1483–1484, 1484*f*
      spinal cord, 1484
      thalamus, 1485
    sympathetically maintained pain (SMP), 1483, 1483*f*, 1541
  definition of, 1489
  diagram of, 1528
  masquerading as weakness, 1491
  pathways
    descending, of pain modulation, 1482, 1482*f*
    dorsal horn as, 1480–1481
    peripheral nerve as, 1480
    spinothalamic tract as, 1481–1482, 1481*f*
  psychological aspects of, 1485–1486
  following shoulder arthrodesis, 1322–1323
  in spinal cord injury, 1403–1405
  stimulus, in sensibility testing, 142
  theories of, 87
Pain dysfunction syndrome, 1489. *See also* Reflex sympathetic dystrophy; Sympathetically maintained pain
  diagnosis and treatment planning, 1491–1492
  examples and results, 1492–1493
  patient presentation, 1490
    historical details, 1490–1491
    physical examination details, 1491
  physiological and psychological factors, 1489–1490
  treatment of established, 662–663
Palmar cutaneous branch of median nerve, 237, 370, 901–903, 902*f*
  severance of, 970–971
Palmaris longus tendon
  in Camitz transfer, 929, 930–931*f*, 933
  and development of carpal tunnel syndrome, 872, 973
  opponensplasty using, 720–721, 720*f*
Palmaris profundus, as cause of median nerve compression, 873, 873*f*
Palmar ulnar-median communicating branch of Berrettini, 203–204
Pancoast's tumor and neurilemmoma, 964
Pancuronium, 78
Pan-talar arthrodesis, 766
Paralysie des amoureux, 1166
Paraplegia, and carpal tunnel syndrome, 873–874
Parathion, 79
Paresthetica meralgia, 1201–1202, 1201*f*
Park-bench palsy, 1166
Parsonage-Turner syndrome, 964, 1150, 1163–1164, 1168, 1198, 1541
Partial nerve injuries, 335, 602
  anatomy in, 336, 337*f*
  incidence of, 336
  intraoperative electrodiagnostic evaluation, 338–339

postoperative complications, 344, 344*f*
preoperative examination, 337
repair of, 299–302, 299*f*, 300*f*
surgery for
complete nerve repair, 340–341
completion of, followed by nerve grafting of transected fascicular groups, 342–344, 343*f*
nerve wrapping, 339–340
observation alone, 339
repair of transected fascicular groups, 341–342, 342*f*
tension and repair of partially transected nerves, 339
timing of repair, 336–337
types of, 335–336
Passive axon, 30–31, 31*f*
Passive responses, 30
Pathophysiology, applications of, to sensibility testing, 136*t*, 139–140
Patient positioning in operating room, 1231–1232
compression of superficial peripheral nerves
cranial nerve branches, 1237, 1237*f*, 1238*f*
lateral femoral cutaneous nerve, 1237
peroneal nerve, 1233*f*, 1236
radial nerve, 1237
ulnar nerve, 1236–1237
guidelines for proper positioning, 1239, 1239*f*, 1240, 1240*f*
incidence, 1232
injury to the brachial plexus, 1234, 1235*f*
direct compression of the brachial plexus, 1236
stretching of the brachial plexus, 1234–1236
pathogenesis of nerve injury, 1232
positions associated with nerve injury, 1232
lithotomy, 1232–1233
prone, 1234
Trendelenburg, 1233
prognosis for recovery, 1238
treatment, 1238–1239
Pattern movement, 1419–1420
Pectoralis major, percutaneous phenol block to, 1426
Pectoralis minor tenotomy, 1184–1185
Pectoral nerves, motor testing of, 161
Pediatric nerve injuries, 636. *See also* Nerve injuries
birth injuries, 636
distal femur fractures, 648
distal tibial fractures, 649
foot fractures, 649
forearm fractures, 646–647
hip fractures, 648
humeral shaft fractures, 637–638, 638*f*
lateral condyle fractures, 641–642
medial condyle and epicondyle humerus fractures, 642–645, 644*f*, 645*f*
Monteggia fractures, 645–646
proximal humerus fractures, 636–637
proximal tibia fractures, 649
supracondylar humerus fractures, 638–641
wrist and hand fractures, 647
Pedicle flap, transfer of ulnar nerve as, 535, 538
Pedicle graft, 509
D-penicillamine, 591
Percussion, 325
in treating neuromas, 1529
Percutaneous phenol block
to motor points of spastic forearm muscles, 1430
to pectoralis major, 1426
to recurrent motor branch of median nerve, 1437
Periaqueductal gray region, electrical stimulation of, 1482, 1482*f*
Perikaryon, 56
Perineural cells, 8
Perineural diffusion barrier, 8–9
Perineural membrane, 8
Perineurium, 2, 7–9, 7*f*, 8*f*, 10, 50, 234, 317
Peripheral nerve
anatomy of, 233–235, 296–297, 296*f*, 316–318
axonal transport, 4–7, 5*t*
antegrade, 5–6
retrograde, 6–7
biomechanical properties, 46–52, 48*f*, 49*f*, 50*f*, 51*f*
conduction
in assessing reflex sympathetic dystrophy, 1508–1509
functional changes in, due to stretching, 50–52
internal topography of, 231
applied anatomy, 233–235, 234*f*, 235*f*
history, 231–233, 232*f*, 233*f*
nerve function, 235
recent studies, 235–240
in intraneural microvascular system
architecture, 8*f*, 10–11, 10*f*
blood-nerve barrier, 12–13
intraneural microcirculation, 11–12
nervi-nervorum, 12
motor testing of, 162, 167–170, 169*f*
as pain pathway, 1480, 1480*f*
in situ stress and strain in, 47
stimulation
criteria for, 1552, 1554
technique of, 1555, 1556*f*, 1557, 1557*f*
for treating nerve in-continuity, 1545*f*, 1546–1548, 1546*f*, 1548*f*
structure of, 1–10
epineurium, 2, 9–10, 233–234, 296–297
intrafascicular tissue pressure, 9–10
nerve fibers, 2–4, 2f
perineural diffusion barrier, 8–9
perineurium, 2, 7–9, 7*f*, 8*f*, 10, 50, 234, 317
tensile properties of, 47–49, 48*f*, 49*f*, 50*f*
Peripheral neuropathy, conditions producing, 963–964
Peripheral proteins, 57
Periscapular pain, 1407
Permeability, 27*f*
Peroneal nerve
compression of, 1202–1205, 1203*f*, 1204*f*, 1206*f*
injuries to, 497–502
from positioning in operating room, 1233*f*, 1236
motor testing of, 168*f*, 169
overcoming defects in, 521–523, 523*t*
Peroneal nerve palsy, 489
cause of, 1250

Peroneal nerve palsy (*continued*)
complicating fractures and dislocations of the knee
applied anatomy, 629, 631
incidence, 631, 631*f*
treatment, 631–632
prognosis following, 1251
Peroneal neuropathy, 497
Peroneus brevis, motor testing of, 169
Peroneus longus, motor testing of, 169
Phalen's sign, 144, 147, 1139
in assessment of
carpel tunnel syndrome, 878, 879
pronator syndrome, 996, 1000
Phantom pain, 1483–1484, 1484*f*
Pharmacologic blockade, for reflex sympathetic dystrophy, 1512
Phenol block
closed
to motor points of brachioradialis muscle, 1427
to musculocutaneous nerve, 1427
to the obturator nerve, 1439
open
to median nerve, 1430–1431
to motor branches of brachioradialis muscle, 1427, 1429
to motor branches of the ulnar nerve, 1433–1435
to musculocutaneous nerve, 1427
to the tibial nerve, 1441–1442, 1444–1445
percutaneous
to motor points of spastic forearm muscles, 1430
to pectoralis major, 1426
to recurrent motor branch of the median nerve, 1437
Phenoxybenzamine hydrochloride, in treating reflex sympathetic dystrophy, 1511
Phenytoin, in treating reflex sympathetic dystrophy, 1511
Phosphatidyls, 59
Phospholipid, 57
Photostimulation, 283–284, 310
Phrenic nerve
as neurotizer, 1344–1345
palsies, 1150
Physical therapy, in treating reflex sympathetic dystrophy, 1509
Physostigmine (Eserine), 79
Pinch, improving with tendon transfer, 741
Piriformis syndrome, 1198–1199
Plasma glue, 328
Plasminogen activators, 63–64
Plexiform neurofibroma, 1601
Pneumothorax, 1192
Point localization using Semmes-Weinstein monofilaments, 824–825
Poliomyelitis, 437
Polyarteritis nodosa, as cause of anterior interosseous nerve paralysis, 988
Polyfascicular nerves, 288
Polymodal nociceptors, 1479, 1480
Polymyalgia rheumatica, 963–964
Polyneuropathy, 1000
Positive sharp waves, 173
Postaxial nerves, communication between preaxial nerves, 208–209, 208*f*
Posterior bone block, 766, 767–768, 769
Posterior cord, anatomy of nerves arising from, 1262–1263
Posterior interosseous nerve, 397. *See also* Radial tunnel syndrome
compression syndrome, 1005–1006
applied anatomy, 1007–1009, 1007*f*, 1008*f*
clinical assessment, 1010–1011, 1011*f*
decompression
anterior approach, 1013–1014
brachioradialis-extensor carpi radialis longus interval, 1015–1016
brachioradialis splitting incision, 1014–1015
posterior, or Thompson, approach, 1016–1017, 1016*f*, 1018*f*
differential diagnosis, 1011–1012
history, 1006–1007
indications for operative treatment, 1013
laboratory tests, 1012
nonoperative treatment, 1012
presentation, 1009–1011
as donor nerve, 549
palsy with Monteggia lesions
applied anatomy, 625
classification, 625
incidence, 625–626
nerve exploration, 628
recovery, 628
Posterior polypropylene splint, 502, 502*f*
Posterior tibial nerve
compression of
electrophysiological testing in, 177
compressive neuropathy of, 1202, 1203*f*
injuries to, 495–496, 496*f*
Posterior transfer of anterior tibial tendon, 770
Postjunctional membrane, 77–79
Postoperative complications, 1017
Potassium, and pain response, 1480
Potassium channels, 37–39
Potassium conductance, 37–38
Potassium ferricyanide, 262
Potassium gradient, 57
Potential excursion, 749
Power, 694, 695*t*
Preaxial nerves, communication between postaxial nerves, 208–209, 208*f*
Prednisone, 1511–1512
Pregnancy, and carpal tunnel syndrome, 882
Preserved allografts, 527, 527*f*
Pressure palsies, hereditary neuropathy with susceptibility to, 1224
Pressure-Specifying Discriminator, 144, 146*f*, 151, 155*f*
Primary afferent fibers, 95
Primary neurorrhaphy, 357
Primary synaptic cleft, 74
Primitive neuroectodermal tumor (PNET), 1617–1618
treatment of, 1618–1619
Pronator quadratus
motor testing of, 166
weaknesses of, in anterior interosseous nerve syndrome, 985
Pronator syndrome
cause of, 999, 999*f*
clinical assessment of, 996

electrodiagnostic studies, 998
provocative testing, 996–998, 997f, 998f
differential diagnosis, 999–1000
electrophysiological testing in, 176
history of, 995
operative technique, 1000–1001
complications, 1001
postoperative care, 1001
presentation of, 995–996
release in, 514
Pronator teres
in double crush syndrome, 1224
motor testing of, 165
release of, 1462
transfer of, 1467, 1468f, 1469
Prone position
and nerve injury, 1234
guidelines for avoiding, 1239
Proprioception assessment, 1458
Proprioceptors, 89
Prostaglandins, and pain response, 1480
Protease, 59, 63–64
Protease inhibitors, 63
Proteolysis of actin, 66
Protons, 20
Provocative tests, 154–156, 878–879, 1139, 1178–1179
Adson maneuver, 1178
Phalen's test, 878, 879
for pronator syndrome, 996–998, 997f, 998f
tourniquet test, 878, 879
Proximal humerus fractures, pediatric nerve injuries associated with, 636–637
Proximal intrinsic muscle release, 1435
Proximal joint contractures, 1389
Proximal tibia fractures, pediatric nerve injuries associated with, 649
Proximal tibiofibular joint dislocation, 631
Pseudoanterior interosseous nerve syndrome, 986
Pseudoneuromas, 1527
Pseudoparalysis, 1490
Psychotropic therapy, for reflex sympathetic dystrophy, 1515
Pulpar flap, 795
Pulsed electromagnetic fields, effect of, on outgrowth, 123
Putti-Platt procedure, 438
Pyridostigmine (Nestinon), 79
Pyridoxine (vitamin B_6) and carpal tunnel syndrome, 882–883

Quadriceps, motor testing of, 167
Quadrilateral space syndrome, 437, 440
diagnosis of, 442
Quantal theory of transmitter release, 76
Quantitative assessment of muscle function, 160
Quickly adapting fibers, 136

Radial nerve, 1237
anatomy and function of, 1167–1168, 1167f, 1263
in arm, 394–397, 395f, 396t
in forearm, 397–400
in hand, 400–401
avoiding injury to, 1237
defects in, 517, 519
at arm level, 519
at forearm level, 519–520
double crush
cervical radiculopathy and radial tunnel syndrome, 1221
injury, splinting for, 819–820
internal topography of, as related to repair, 238
motor recovery, following grafting, 557f, 562–563
motor testing of, 162–163
operative exposure
in arm, 401–403, 402f, 404f
in forearm, 403–406, 405f
operative treatment, 1169–1170
palsy, 697–698, 813
and anatomy, 698–699
with humeral shaft fractures, 622–623
tendon transfer for, 699–700
complications in, 707–708
operative procedures, 701–707
potential points of compression, 396, 398–399, 401
repair of, 354, 354t, 409
evaluation of, 412
factors influencing outcome following repair, 410–412
level of injury, 410–411
sensory recovery, following grafting, 563, 564t
studies on, 410
symptoms, signs and diagnosis, 1168–1169, 1169f
Radial recurrent artery, 1025
Radial recurrent leash of Henry, 400
Radial sensory nerve entrapment, 1039, 1040f, 1041f
applied anatomy, 1042–1043, 1044f, 1045, 1046f
differential diagnosis, 1046–1047, 1046t
indications and contraindications for operative intervention, 1039–1040, 1042
operative treatment, 1047f, 1048f, 1049–1050
postoperative complications, 1050–1051
Radial tunnel syndrome, 1006, 1221
and cervical radiculopathy as double crush syndrome, 1221
clinical assessment, 1025–1026
conservative treatment, 1026
history of, 1023–1024
operative technique, 1026–1027
anterior approach, 1027, 1027f, 1029
closure and dressing, 1031
posterior approach, 1028–1029f, 1029, 1030f
postoperative complications, 1036
postoperative management, 1031, 1036
release of the radial tunnel, 1031, 1036f
transmuscular approach through the brachioradialis, 1030–1031, 1032–1035f, 1036, 1036f
pertinent anatomy, 1024–1025
presentation, 1025
Radiation injury, 676–677
Radiculopathy, cervical, 1216–1220, 1218t, 1221
Radiographic assessment, of brachial plexus injury, 1276, 1277f

Ratcheted needle holder, 280
Raynaud's disease, 964
  symptoms in, 664
  treating, 1511
Receptive field, 98, 98*f*
Receptors, specificity of, 97
Recording techniques, 21–23, 23*f*, 24*f*, 25
Recruitment pattern, 172
Referred pain, 1491
Reflex autonomic dystrophy. *See* Pain dysfunction syndrome; Reflex sympathetic dystrophy; Sympathetically maintained pain
Reflex sympathetic dystrophy (RSD), 964, 1407, 1491, 1497–1498, 1564. *See also* Pain dysfunction syndrome; Sympathetically maintained pain
  classification of, 1498*t*
  clinical criteria for, 1499*t*, 1503
  diagnostic evaluation, 1503
    blood flow determination, 1505
    differential diagnosis, 1503
    endurance testing, 1507–1508
    laboratory tests, 1504
      radiologic evaluation, 1504
      three-phase bone scan, 1504
      vasomotor and thermoregulatory assessment, 1504–1505
    peripheral nerve conduction, 1508–1509
    radiologic evaluation, 1504
    stress testing, 1505–1507, 1506*ft*, 1507*f*, 1508*f*
  history of, 1498, 1501–1502
    stage I (acute), 1502
    stage II (dystrophic), 1502–1503
    stage III (atrophic), 1503
  pathophysiology, 1499–1501, 1499*f*, 1500*f*
    central abnormalities, 1500, 1502*f*
    peripheral abnormalities, 1499–1500
  prevention of, 977–978, 1518
  synonyms for, 1498*t*
  treatment of, 978, 1509
    acupuncture, 1518
    adaptive therapy, 1514
    biofeedback, 1518
    oral medications, 1509–1510, 1510*t*
      amitriptyline hydrochloride (elavil hydrochloride), 1510, 1511*f*, 1512*f*
      corticosteroids, 1511–1512
      nifedipine (procardia), 1510–1511, 1513*f*
      phenoxybenzamine hydrochloride (dibenzyline), 1511
      phenytoin, 1511
    pharmacologic blockade, 1512
    physical therapy, 1509
    psychotropic therapy, 1515
    stress therapy, 1509
      continuous axillary (brachial) blockade, 1514, 1516*f*
      continuous stellate blockade, 1513
      stellate ganglion blockade, 1513, 1515*f*, 1516*f*, 1567–1568
    surgical and ablative therapies, 1514
      cervicothoracic ganglion sympathectomy, 1514–1515
      neurolytic blockade, 1515
      neurosurgical therapy, 1515
    sympathetic blockade, 1513
    transcutaneous electrical stimulators, 1518
Regeneration specificity
  operative control of, 224–226
  types of, 216–217, 216*f*, 217*f*
Regeneration unit, 112, 114*f*, 115*f*
Regional musculoskeletal symptoms
  incidence of, 949–950, 950*f*, 951*f*
  and worker's compensation, 952–954
Rehabilitation 814
  functional rehabilitation, 820–821
  motor dysfunction
    early management, 814
    splinting, 814
      for combined median and ulnar nerve palsy, 818–819
      for median nerve palsy, 815–816, 815*f*, 816*f*
      for radial nerve injury, 819–820, 819*f*, 820*f*
      for ulnar nerve palsy, 816–818, 817*f*, 818*f*
  sensibility tests, 821
    functional tests, 823–825
    objective tests, 821, 825
    threshold test, 821–823
  sensory re-education, 825
  sympathetic dysfunction, 814
Reinnervation. *See* Neurotization
Repetitive strain injuries, 963. *See also* Carpel tunnel syndrome
Required excursion, 749
Reserpine, 1512
Resistance, 21
Resorbable tubes
  nerve grafting through
    background, 587–588
    bioresorbable nerve graft, 590–591, 592*f*
    characteristics of the ideal guidance system, 591, 593
    future research, 593–594
    nerve regeneration through tubular prostheses, 588–590, 589*f*
    surgical technique, 593, 593*f*
Resting potential, origin of, 28–30, 29*f*
Retrograde axon reaction, 65
Retrograde flow, 66
Retrograde transport, 5*t*, 6–7, 56
Revascularization, 680, 684
  by microvascular anastomosis, 529
  spontaneous, 529
Reversed double crush syndrome, 859
Revision, submuscular transposition in, 1114–1116
Revision ulnar nerve decompression, 1127–1128
Rhabdomyosarcoma, 1575
  chemotherapy for, 1583
Rheumatoid arthritis
  and posterior interosseous nerve compression syndrome, 1006
  risk of, for ulnar nerve compression, 1137
  risk of nerve palsies following total hip arthroplasty for, 1246

Rhytidectomy, 482
Riche-Cannieu anastomosis, 1170
Riche-Cannieu communication, 197, 202–203, 202*f*, 205, 371, 373, 420
Roos rib cutter, 1187, 1188*f*
Ruffini endings, 86, 90, 93, 97
  innervation of, 95, 96*f*

St. Clair Strange procedure, 389
Saint-Venant, principle of, 320, 321*f*
Salivary flow test, 467
Saltatory conduction, 33
Saltatory movement, 62
Saphenous nerve
  as donor nerve, 532, 574
  injuries to, 502, 503*f*
Sartorius nerve, motor testing of, 167
Saturday-night palsy, 110
  compression neuropathy of the radial nerve, 1166
Scaffold proteins, 67
Scalenotomy, 1184
Schimer test, 468
Schmidt-Lantermann clefts, 58–59
Schwann cells, 3–4, 4f, 20, 58–59, 59, 233
  and mitotic activity, 116
  proliferation of, 65, 116
  role of, in distal stump, 66, 116
Schwann cell tubes, 216–217
Schwannoma, 1606–1608
  malignant, 1613–1615
    treatment of, 1615–1617
  results, 1608–1609
  treatment of, 1608, 1609*f*, 1610*f*
Sciatic functional index (SFI), 225
Sciatic nerve, 489
  compression of, 1198–1199
  diagnosis of impairment, 1249
  injuries to, 492–493, 492*f*, 494*f*
    injection, 493
    with traumatic hip dislocation and fracture-dislocation
      applied anatomy, 628–629
      classification, 629
  motor testing of, 167–168
  overcoming deficits in, 521
  palsy, 764, 771, 1247
    prognosis following, 1251
Sciatic nerve-evoked potential (SNEP) monitoring, 1252
Scintigraphic analysis, in assessing reflex sympathetic dystrophy, 1504
Secondary afferent fibers, 95
Secondary nerve injury, 620, 622
Secondary neurorrhaphy, 357
Segmental regional vessels of extrinsic origin, 10
Selectively permeable, 27
Semimembranosus, motor testing of, 167–168
Semitendinosus, motor testing of, 168
Semmes-Weinstein monofilament testing, 457, 821–823, 823*f*, 830, 833, 834, 835, 908, 1139
  common problems with, 156
Sensation, 85, 87, 136
Sensibility, 87, 136
Sensibility dysfunction, 814
Sensibility tests, 136, 821, 828, 828*f*, 829*f*, 830, 1139, 1418–1419
  actual, 140–154, 141*f*
    diagnosing compression lesions, 144–147
    diagnosing divided nerves, 143
    and malingering, 141–143
    order of sensory recovery, 148–149, 151
  applications of pathophysiology to, 136*t*, 139–140
  for cerebral palsy patient, 1457–1459, 1458*f*
  functional tests, 821
    constant two-point discrimination, 823–824, 824*f*, 828
    Moberg pick-up test, 381, 752–753, 825, 1390, 1401
    moving two-point discrimination test, 136, 824, 828
    point localization, 824–825
  implications of anatomy, 136–139, 137*f*, 138*t*, 139*t*
  innervation density tests, 876, 877*t*, 878*f*
  objective tests, 821
    nerve conduction studies, 825
  recent developments in, 154
  terminology for, 136
  threshold tests, 821, 876, 877*t*, 878, 879*f*
    Semmes-Weinstein monofilaments, 821–822
    technique in, 822–823
Sensory axon regeneration, topographic specificity in, 219–220
Sensory duality, theory of, 87
Sensory end organs
  alterations after denervation, 620–621
  reinnervation of, 220–221
Sensory modality, 86
Sensory/motor reinnervation, 218–219, 220*f*
Sensory receptors, 85
  afferent nerve fibers, 89
  classification of, 89–90
    free nerve endings, 90
    glabrous skin receptors, 90–93, 91*f*, 93*f*
    hairy skin receptors, 93–94
    joint receptors, 94–95
    mucocutaneous receptors, 94
    muscle receptors, 94–95
  definition of, 87
  denervation and reinnervation of, 100–101
    encapsulated receptors, 101
    Meissner corpuscle, 101
    Merkel cell-neurite complex, 101
    pacinian corpuscle, 101
  general characteristics of, 87–88, 88*ft*
  history of, 86–87
  innervation, 95–97, 95*t*, 96*f*
  sensory recovery, 101–102
  sensory transduction
    generator potentials, 97, 97*f*
    inhibition, 98–99, 99*f*
    receptive field, 98, 98*f*
    receptors and their central connections, 99–100
    transformation of stimuli in receptors, 97
Sensory recovery
  order of, 148–149, 151
  pattern of, 149, 149*f*
Sensory re-education
  assessment of results, 834–841
  basis for, 830
  current status after nerve repair, 827–828
  historical perspective, 830–831
  purpose of, 830
  stages of, 831
    desensitization or protection, 831–832

Sensory re-education, stages of (*continued*)
early-phase discrimination and localization, 832–833
late-phase discrimination or tactile gnosis, 833
late-phase sensory re-education programs, 833–834
testing sensibility, 828, 828*f*, 829*f*, 830
Serial casting, 1424
Serine protease, 67
Serotonin, and pain response, 1480, 1482
Serratus anterior, motor testing of, 161
Shotgun injuries, 658. *See also* Gunshot wounds
Shoulder-arm-hand syndrome, 662
Shoulder arthrodesis, 1317, 1332
complications, 1321–1322
positioning, 1317–1318
results, 1322–1323, 1323*f*
technique, 1318
bone grafting, 1320–1321
external fixation, 1320, 1321*f*
extra-articular arthrodesis, 1318
internal fixation, 1319–1320
intra-articular arthrodesis, 1318–1319
Shoulder arthroscopy, positioning of patient for, 1240
Shoulder deformity, 1416*f*, 1426
operative procedures, 1460, 1462–63*f*
percutaneous phenol block to pectoralis major, 1426
shoulder release, 1426–1427
Shoulder dislocation
axillary nerve injury in
applied anatomy, 626
evaluation of deltoid muscle function, 627–628
incidence, 626–627
Shoulder fusion in brachial plexus injuries, 1339–1340
Shoulder-hand syndrome, 1407
Shoulder stabilization, 1315, 1316*f*
tendon transfers for, 1315
Shrug test, 446
Siemens (S), 21
Silicone microprosthetic tube, 283, 283*f*
Silicone sheathing, in cubital tunnel syndrome decompression, 1118, 1126–1127
Skeletal muscle degradation, 67–68, 67*f*, 68*f*
Slit/wick catheter technique for measuring intracompartmental pressure, 944*f*, 945–946
Slow axoplasmic transport, 5–6, 5t, 6f, 61*f*, 62–63
Slowly adapting, 136
Sodium-calcium antiporter, 58
Sodium channels, 38, 39
Sodium conductance, 37
Sodium gradient, 57
Sodium hypothesis, 34–37
Sodium-potassium pump, 57–58
Sodium pump, 28
Soft-tissue osteosarcoma, chemotherapy for, 1583
Soft-tissue tumor. *See under* Tumor
Sole plate, 74
Soleus, motor testing of, 169
Soma, 19*f*
Somatic sensation, 89
Somatization disorders, 1490
Somatoform disorders, chronic pain in, 1485–1486
Somatomedin-C, 119
Somatosensory evoked potentials (SSEP), in assessing brachial plexus injury, 1278–1279
Somatostatin, and pain response, 1480
Space constant, 30
Spastic dysphonia, use of botulinum toxin in, 486–487
Spastic hemiplegia, 1455
Spasticity, phenol blocks for, 1423–1424
Spatial discrimination, accurate, 96
Spatial-temporal progress of nerve regeneration, 120, 121*f*
Special senses, 89
Specific irritability, 86
Specificity
mechanical and humoral control of, in nerve repair, 215–217, 216*f*, 217*f*
end organ—motor, 221
end organ—sensory, 220–221
nerve trunk, 218
sensory/motor reinnervation, 218–219
tissue, 217–218, 218*f*
topographic—motor, 221
topographic—sensory, 219–220
potential mechanisms of contract recognition, 222
neurotropism, 224
neurotropism, 223–224
Sphingomyelin, 59
Spinal accessory nerve
acute compression of, 1148, 1150, 1150*f*
injury, 445
applied anatomy, 449–450
diagnosis of injury, 446–448
etiology and prognosis, 448–449
types of operations
exploration and direct repair, 450
exploration and nerve grafting, 450–451
neurolysis, 450
as neurotizer, 1336–1342
paralysis of, 445
Spinal cord. *See also* Brain injury and stroke
injury to, 1387–1388, 1388*t*
and brachial plexus root avulsion, 1275
C1, C2, C3 functional levels, 1391
C4 functional level, 1391–1392
C5 functional level, 1392–1393, 1393*f*
brachioradialis to wrist extensor transfer, 1395, 1396*f*, 1402*f*
C5 operative reconstruction, 1390*f*, 1393–1394
deltoid to triceps transfer, 1394–1395, 1395*f*
restoration of lateral (key) pinch, 1395, 1397
C6 functional level, 1397–1399, 1398*f*
brachioradialis to flexor pollicis longus transfer, 1401, 1402*f*, 1404–1405*f*
C6 operative reconstruction, 1388*t*, 1399–1400
patient selection, 1400–1401

postoperative care, 1401, 1403
pronator teres to flexor digitorum profundus transfer, 1401, 1406*f*
C7 functional level, 1403
C8 functional level, 1403
classification of neurological levels, 1388*t*, 1389–1391, 1390*f*, 1391*t*
early care, 1388–1389
late complications, 1407–1409, 1408*t*
in lower extremities, 1409–1410
pain in, 1403–1405, 1407
nonsympathetically maintained pain in, 1484
Spinal roots
anatomy of nerves arising from, 1260–1261
contributions to the brachial plexus, 1258, 1260*f*
Spindle neuromas, 1527
Spinothalamic tract, as pain pathway, 1481–1482
Splinting, 814
in brain injury and stroke management, 1423
for carpal tunnel syndrome, 883–885
for combined median and ulnar nerve palsy, 818–819
for median nerve palsy, 815–816, 815*f*, 816*f*
for radial nerve injury, 819–820, 819*f*, 820*f*
for ulnar nerve palsy, 816–818
Split anterior tibial tendon transfer (SPLATT), 1445, 1446
Split trunk graft, 528
Spontaneous revascularization, 529
Sprouting, 81–82, 81*f*, 219
Standard high-energy carbon dioxide (CO_2) laser, 284
Stapedius muscle reflex, 467–468
Static two-point discrimination, 136
Steindler flexorplasty, 1305, 1310
operative technique of, 1310–1311, 1310*f*
results, 1311, 1311*f*
Steindler transfers, 1305
Stellate ganglion, 1564–1565, 1565*f*
blockade of
effectiveness of, 1567–1568
for reflex sympathetic dystrophy, 1513, 1515*f*, 1516*f*
Stereognosis, 87
assessment of, 1458, 1458*f*
Sternocleidomastoid palsy, 448
Steroid injections. *See* Corticosteroids
Stimulation frequency, 172
Stimulation of nerve ends, 611–612
intensity of, 612
technique of, 612–614, 615*f*, 616
Stimulus, adequate, 97
Stimulus duration, 172
Stimulus intensity, 172
Stocking anesthesia, 1490
Straight and angled spring-handled scissors, 281, 281*f*
Stress testing, in reflex sympathetic dystrophy, 1505–1507, 1508*f*
Stress therapy, in treating reflex sympathetic dystrophy, 1509
Stretching, functional changes in peripheral nerve due to, 50–52
Stroke. *See* Brain injury and stroke
Stump neuromas, 1527
Subclavian arteriography, 440
Subcutaneous tender nerve, 973–974, 974*f*, 975*f*, 976*f*
Sublimaze, in electrical nerve stimulation in awake patient, 246
Submuscular transposition, 1107
biomechanics of throwing, 1097–1098, 1098*f*
clinical presentation, 1100–1101
neuropathy of the ulnar nerve at the elbow, 1099–1100, 1100*t*
prognosis in, 1104
treatment, 1101–1104, 1101*f*, 1102*f*, 1103*f*
Subscapular nerve
anatomy of, 1263
motor testing of, 162
Substance P, and pain response, 1480
Substantia gelatinosa, 1480
Substrate binding factors, 63
Succinylcholine, 78–79
Sudeck's atrophy, 662, 1407
Sulfatides, 59
Superficial radial nerve, as donor nerve, 531, 574
Supinator, motor testing of, 162–163
Supraclavicular deficits, motor testing for, 161
Supracondylar humeral fractures
as cause of anterior interosseous nerve paralysis, 987
pediatric nerve injuries associated with, 638–641
treatment of, 988
Supranuclear paralysis, 466
Suprascapular nerve, 1261
anatomy of, 1152–1153, 1156*f*
function of, 1151–1152, 1152*f*, 1154*f*
motor testing of, 161
operative technique, 1155–1157
pathology, 1153
symptoms and diagnosis, 1153–1154
treatment, 1154–1155
Sural nerve
as donor nerve, 474, 530–531, 550–551, 550*f*, 572, 579
injuries to, 503
Survival factors, 63
Suture(s)
basic considerations, 327
leakage of axonal flow, 328
sound soft-tissue environment, 328
suture site tension, 327
topological coaptation, 327
epineural, 290–291
future perspective, 333
for gunshot wounds, 667–668
material for tendon fixation, 750
in nerve repair, 282–283
special techniques
adhesive repair, 328–329
anchoring funicular suture, 329–333, 331*f*, 332*f*
laser-assisted repair, 329
technique in median nerve repair, 384–385
Sutureless neurorrhaphy, 283, 284–285
adhesive repair, 328–329, 328*f*, 331*f*
fibrin glue
autologous preparation, 308

Sutureless neurorrhaphy, fibrin glue (*continued*)
clinical experience, 307–308
historical perspective, 305–306
recent experience, 306–307
technique, 308–309
future for, 311, 333
lasers, 283–284, 329, 329*f*
experimental and clinical data, 310–311
tubulation, 283
clinical data, 310
experimental data, 309–310
Sympathectomy, 1300
cervicothoracic ganglion, 1514–1515
Sympathetically maintained pain (SMP), 1483, 1483*f*, 1541. *See also* Pain; Pain dysfunction syndrome; Reflex sympathetic dystrophy
Sympathetic contributions to the brachial plexus, 1260
Synovectomy, 909
Systemic lupus erythematosus, 963

T_3, 122
T_4, 122
Tactile detection threshold (TDT), 382
Tactile gnosis, 751, 825, 833
definition of, 794
flaps to restore, 794–797, 797*f*, 798*f*, 799*f*, 800*f*
Talocalcaneal and calcaneonavicular arthrodesis, 766
Tarsal tunnel syndrome, 1206–1207, 1207*f*
Tarsorrhaphy, 486
gold weight lid, 485–486, 485*f*
Taste test, 467
Teloglia, 58
Temporalis muscle fascial transfer and suspension, 476
indications for, 476–477
and anatomy, 477
technique in, 477–479, 477*f*
Temporofacial division, 463, 464*f*
Tendo achilles lengthening
open Z-lengthening, 1444–1445
with percutaneous triple hemisection tenotomy, 1444
Tendon transfer
of biceps tendon to ulna, 1366*f*, 1367
for brachial plexus injuries, 1305–1306
brachioradialis
to flexor digitorium profundus, 1399
to wrist extensor, 1395, 1396*f*
for carpal tunnel syndrome, 927
alternative and associated procedures, 935*f*, 936
Camitz transfer, 929, 930–931*f*, 933, 936
formal opponensplasty, 932–933*f*, 934, 936
medical history in, 927–928
operative plan for, 929
physical examination in, 928–929
postoperative care, 933
for combined nerve injuries, 747–748
general principles, 748
high (proximal) median-radial nerve palsy (late), 760–761, 760*t*, 761*f*
high (proximal) median-ulnar nerve palsy (late), 755, 755*f*, 756*t*, 757, 757*f*
high (proximal) ulnar-radial nerve palsy (late), 757, 758–759*t*, 759–760
low (distal) median-ulnar nerve palsy, 753, 753*f*, 754*t*, 755
in lower extremity, 761
operative techniques, 749–751
postoperative re-education and evaluation, 752–753
selection of the motor muscle for, 748–749
sensory defects, 751–752
deltoid to triceps, 1394–1395
digital and thumb extensor, 1469–1470, 1469*f*
in extrinsic reconstruction for median nerve palsy, 712–715, 713*f*
flexor carpi radialis, 704, 707*f*
flexor carpi ulnaris, 1466–1467, 1466*f*, 1467*f*
flexor digitorum superficialis, for thumb extension, 1470
history of tendon transfer surgery, 691–694, 695*t*
latissimus dorsi and teres major, 1365–1366
pectoralis major, 1306–1307, 1309*f*
operative technique, 1306*f*, 1307–1308
for peroneal nerve injuries, 500–501, 501*f*
pertinent anatomy, 698–699
complications, 707–708
general rules of, 700–701
history of, 699–700
operative procedures, 701–703
postoperative management, 703
preoperative considerations, 701
standard transfer, 702–703, 702*f*, 703*f*, 704*f*, 706*f*
timing, 701
use of the flexor digitorum superficialis for finger extension, 705, 707
pronator teres, 1467, 1468*f*, 1469
to flexor digitorum profundus, 1401, 1406*f*
for radial nerve palsy, 697–698
and realignment and reinforcement of extensor pollicis longus, 1470, 1472, 1472*f*
recent advances in, 694–695
and restoration of intrinsic muscle function for median nerve palsy, 715–717, 715*f*, 716*f*
for shoulder stabilization, 1315
for swan-neck deformity, 1472–1474, 1473*f*
for ulnar nerve palsy
available motors, 732
digital motion, 729–731
flexor digitorum superficialis transfer for intrinsic-minus deformity, 733, 735, 735*f*
flat palm, 739–740, 741*f*
improving pinch, 741
for intrinsic function, 735–737, 740*f*
joint fusion in the thumb, 741, 743–745, 743*f*
metacarpophalangeal and interphalangeal joint
other transfers for intrinsic function, 737–738, 741*f*
pinch mechanism, 731, 731*f*
postoperative care and rehabilitation, 745

semi-active tenodesis to correct claw deformity, 738–739
timing and choice of procedure, 732–733, 734*f*
to the wrist extensors, 1466
Tennis elbow, 1023, 1025. *See also* Radial tunnel syndrome
and workers compensation, 953
Tenodesis, semi-active, to correct claw deformity, 738–739
Tenodesis effect, testing for, 986
Tenodesis splint, 819–820, 820*f*
Tenodesis test, 1012
Tenosynovectomy, 905
Tenosynovitis
and carpal tunnel syndrome, 870, 975
of first dorsal extensor compartment, 1040, 1042, 1043*f*
of flexor carpi ulnaris and flexor digitorum superficialis, 1137
Tenotomy, tendo achilles lengthening with percutaneous triple, 1444
Tensile properties, of peripheral nerve, 47–49, 50*f*
Tension, nerve repair under, 509–511, 512*f*, 513
Tension fraction, 749
Teres major transfer, 1365–1366
Teres minor, motor testing of, 162
Teres minor dysfunction, 438
Terminal sprouts, 112
Testing end point, 154
Testing sensibility, 828, 828*f*, 829*f*, 830
Tetraethylammonium (TEA), 38
Tetraplegia. *See* Spinal cord injury
Tetrodotoxin (TTX), 38, 80
Texture discrimination, 833–834
Thalamic syndrome of Dejerine and Roussy, 1485
Thalamus, nonsympathetically maintained pain in, 1485
Thenar muscle atrophy, 928
Thenar origin and adductor pollicis recession, 1437–1438
Thermal injury, 671–672, 673*f*
chemical injury, 677
electrical injury, 675–676
escharotomy, 672–674, 675*f*
reconstruction, 674–675
radiation injury, 676–677
Thermography in diagnosing
carpal tunnel syndrome, 875
reflex sympathetic dystrophy, 1505
Thermoreceptors, 89
Thigh level
overcoming femoral nerve injury at, 523–524, 523*t*
overcoming sciatic nerve injury at, 521, 521*t*
overcoming tibial and peroneal nerve injury at, 522–523
Thiocholine, 262
Thompson-Epstein classification of posterior dislocations and fracture-dislocations, 629
Thoracic nerve (long), 1260–1261
anatomy, 1163, 1164*f*
compression and traction neuropathy
symptoms and signs, 1151*f*, 1163–1164
treatment and results, 1164–1165
injury to, 1193
as neurotizer, 1343
Thoracic outlet syndrome, 154, 193, 1000, 1057
anatomy and pathophysiology, 1179–1181
cervical ribs, 1181–182
clinical correlates, 1179–1181, 1180*f*, 1181*f*
congenital fibrous bands, 1182
first rib, 1183–1184
variations in muscles and vessels, 1182–1183
and brachial plexus injury, 1192–1193
complications of, 1192
description of, 1177
symptoms of, 1177–1178
and distal compression lesions, 1221–1223, 1222*t*
electrophysiological testing in, 176–177
inadequate resection, 1192
and injury to the long thoracic nerve, 1193
operative treatment for, 1184
anterior approaches to, 1188–1189
claviculectomy, 1184
pectoralis minor tenotomy, 1184–1185
posterior approach to, 1190–1192, 1191*f*
scalenotomy, 1184, 1189–1190, 1189*f*
transaxillary first rib resection, 1185–1188
provocative tests for, 1178–1179, 1178*f*
recurrence due to postural abnormality, 1193
vascular injury, 1193
Thoracobrachial orthoses, 1324, 1325*f*
Thoracodorsal nerve
anatomy of, 1263
motor testing of, 161
as neurotizer, 1344
Three-jaw-chuck fingertip palmar pad prehension, 1398
Threshold, 136
Threshold tests, 821, 830, 876, 877*t*, 878, 879*f*
Semmes-Weinstein monofilaments, 821–822
technique in, 822–823
Throwing
biomechanics of, 1097–1098
pathologic abnormalities in extremity, 1098–1099
posture of arm, 1080*f*
Thumb
arthrodesis of metacarpophalangeal joint of, 1470
metacarpophalangeal and interphalangeal joint
fusion in, 741, 743–745
Thumb adduction, contracture, 1470, 1471*f*
Thumb extension
digital and transfers, 1469–1470, 1469*f*
flexor digitorum superficialis transfer for, 1470
Thumb interphalangeal joint, arthrodesis of, 1438, 1439*f*
Thumb spasticity, 1435–1437
arthrodesis of interphalangeal joint, 1438, 1439*f*
flexor pollicis longus lengthening, 1437
percutaneous phenol block to recurrent motor branch of the median nerve, 1437
release of first dorsal interosseous, 1436*f*, 1438
thenar origin and adductor pollicis recession, 1437–1438
L-thyroxine, 122

Tibialis anterior, motor testing of, 169
Tibialis posterior, motor testing of, 169
Tibial nerve
  motor testing of, 168–169
  open phenol block to the, 1441–1442, 1444–1445
  overcoming defects in, 521–523, 523*t*
  palsy, 764, 769–770
    posterior transfer of anterior tibial tendon, 770
    triple arthrodesis with posterior displacement, 770
Tickle and itch sensations, 90
Time constant, 30
Tinel's sign, 438
  in assessment of
    carpal tunnel syndrome, 879
    pronator syndrome, 996, 1000
    ulnar neuropathy, 1100
  and nerve regeneration, 148, 325
  in sensibility testing, 147
Tissue specificity, 121, 217–218
Toe flexor release, 1446, 1446*f*
Topographic specificity, 216
  in sensory axon regeneration, 219–220
Torticollis, use of botulinum toxin in, 486–487
Tourniquet, in electrical nerve stimulation in awake patient, 246, 247–249
Tourniquet test
  in assessing carpal tunnel syndrome, 878, 879
  in free nerve grafting, 535
Toxic neuritis, 437
Traction injuries, 489
Traction neurapraxia, 1069
Traction neuropathies, 492
Tractotomy
  bulbar or mesencephalic, 1484
  trigeminal, 1484
Transaxillary first rib resection, 1185–1188
Transcutaneous electrical nerve stimulation (TENS), 1110, 1116, 1117, 1552
  in treating neuromas, 1529
  in treating reflex sympathetic dystrophy, 1518
Transected fascicular groups
  nerve grafting of, 342–344
  repair of, 341–342, 342*f*
Translocation, in treating neuromas, 1535–1536
Transmastoid cranial fossa approaches, 472
Transport filament model, 62
Trapezius palsy, 448
Trapezius-strengthening exercises, 1155
Traumatic meningoceles, 1279
Traumatic spinal cord injury, 1484
Trendelenburg position
  and nerve injury, 1233, 1233*f*, 1236, 1274
    guidelines for avoiding, 1239–1240
Triceps, motor testing of, 162
Triceps transfer, 1312
  operative technique, 1313–1314
  results, 1314
Tricyclic antidepressants, 1482
Triiodothyronine, 122
Triple arthrodesis, 766–768, 767*f*
  with posterior displacement, 770
Triple-S triangle, 462
Triton tumor, 1599
  malignant, 1615
Tropomyosin, 64, 67
Troponin I, 64
Troponins, 67
Troponin T, 64
d-Tubocurarine, 77–78
Tubular prostheses, nerve regeneration through, 588–590, 589*f*
Tubulation, 309, 319
  clinical data, 310
  experimental data, 309–310
  in nerve repair, 283
Tubulin, 60, 65, 66
α-tubulin, 4, 62
β-tubulin, 4, 62
Tumors, 1587–1588
  classification of, 1588, 1588*t*
  cytogenetics, 1589
  diagnosis of, 1619
  granular cell tumor, 1610–1611, 1610*f*, 1611*f*
    treatment, 1611
  immunohistochemistry of, 1588–1589
  lipofibromatous hamartoma, 1593–1594, 1594*f*, 1595*f*
    treatment, 1594–1599
  malignant schwannomas, 1613–1615, 1614*f*, 1615*f*
    treatment, 1615–1617
  neurofibroma, 1600–1602
    treatment, 1603–1606
  neuromuscular choristoma, 1599, 1599*f*
    treatment, 1600
  neurothekeoma, 1611–1612
    treatment, 1612–1613
  primitive neuroectodermal tumor (PNET), 1617–1618, 1618*f*
    treatment, 1618–1619
  reactive processes
    nerve sheath ganglion, 1591–1593
    traumatic neuroma, 1589–1591, 1590*f*, 1591*f*
  schwannoma, 1606–1608
    results, 1608–1609
    treatment, 1608, 1609*f*, 1610*f*
  soft-tissue, 1573–1575
    axioms, 1575
    biopsy of, 1578–1579
    classification of, 1574*t*
    management of, 1579–1583
      chemotherapy for malignant, 1583
      intralesional, 1580
      marginal procedure, 1580, 1581
      radical procedure, 1580
      wide procedure, 1580, 1581
    staging algorithm, 1577–1578
    staging systems, 1575–1577
  viscoelastic properties of, 49–50, 51*f*
Tuning fork, in sensibility testing, 143–144, 144*f*
Two-point discrimination test, 381, 457, 1458
  constant, 823–824, 828, 835
  moving, 136, 824, 828
  static, 136
Two-point sensory examination, 1139
Tympanic plexus, 465

Ulna, biceps tendon transfer to the, 1366*f*, 1367
Ulnar collateral ligament, injury to, 1093
Ulnar collateral nerve, 394
Ulnar motor neurectomy, 1435
Ulnar nerve, 164–165, 164*f*. *See also* Cubital tunnel syn-

drome; Ulnar tunnel syndrome
anatomy of, 1262
in arm, 413–415, 414*f*
at elbow and forearm, 415–419, 416*f*, 417*f*
in hand and wrist, 417*f*, 419–420, 419*t*
anterior subcutaneous transposition of, 1113
applied anatomy, 1079–1081, 1079*f*, 1080*f*
complications, 1083–1084
history of, 1077–1078
indications, 1078–1079
operative technique, 1081, 1082–83*f*, 1083
postoperative management, 1083
anterior transposition of, 1102
and regional blood flow, 1087–1088
compression of, 1173
electrophysiological testing in at Guyon's canal, 176
as donor nerve, 574
in brachial plexus reconstruction, 581–584
at the elbow
in situ decompression of, 1063–1064
complications, 1065–1066
indications, 1064–1065, 1064*f*, 1065*f*, 1066*f*
treatment and complications of failed decompression of, 1107–1108
anatomy related to, 1111–1112, 1111*f*, 1122
anterior intramuscular transposition, 1113
anterior subcutaneous transposition, 1113
anterior submuscular transposition, 1113–1114
anterior transposition procedures, 1125–1126
cubital tunnel release, 1112
elbow flexion contracture, 1108
elbow instability, 1109, 1110*f*
external neurolysis, 1117, 1117*f*
implantable electrode stimulation, 1116
internal neurolysis, 1117–1118, 1126
local procedures, 1123–1124
medial epicondylectomy, 1112, 1124–1125, 1128
medical epicondylitis, 1108
neurolysis, 1112
neuromas, 1108–1109
nonoperative, 1122–1123
persistent motor and sensory deficits, 1110–1111, 1110*t*
reoperation for, 1111
revision by submuscular transposition, 1114–1116, 1127–1128
silastic sheath, 1118, 1126–1127
entrapment in Guyon's canal, 1057
injury to, 813, 814 from positioning in operating room, 1236–1237, 1237*f*
internal topography of, as related to repair, 237–238
medial epicondylectomy in, 1088
complications, 1092–1094
criticisms of, 1094–1095
history, 1087–1088
procedures, 1088–1092
motor recovery, 431
following grafting, 556*f*, 561–562, 561*t*
open, phenol block to motor branch of, 1433–1435
operative decompression of, in Guyon's canal, 1140–1141, 1141*f*
operative exposure
anterior approach, combined with exposure of the radius and median nerve, 423
in arm, 420–421, 421*f*
in cubital tunnel, 421, 422*f*, 423
in forearm, 422*f*, 423
defects in, 516, 517*f*
at arm level, 516–517, 517*t*
at elbow level, 517
at forearm level, 517, 518*f*
palsy, 433
splinting for, 816–818, 817*f*, 818*f*
tendon transfer for
available motors, 732
digital motion, 729–731
flexor digitorum superficialis transfer for intrinsic-minus deformity, 733, 735
flat palm, 739–740, 741*f*
improving pinch with tendon transfers, 741
joint fusion in the thumb, 741, 743–745, 743*f*
metacarpophalangeal and interphalangeal joint
other transfers for intrinsic function, 737–738, 741*f*
pinch mechanism, 731
postoperative care and rehabilitation, 745
semi-active tenodesis to correct claw deformity, 738–739
timing and choice of procedure, 732–733, 734*f*
transfers for intrinsic function, 735–737, 740*f*
wrist extensors or brachioradialis transfers for intrinsic function, 735–737, 740*f*
potential points of compression, 415, 418, 420
primary decompression of, 1108
repair of, 354, 354*t*, 425
evaluation of, 431, 433–434
historical review, 426–430
results, 430–431, 432*t*
sensory recovery, 431
following grafting, 562, 562*t*
subluxation, 1124
submuscular transposition of, 1097, 1101*f*, 1102*f*, 1103–1104, 1103*f*
biomechanics of throwing, 1097–1098, 1098*f*
clinical presentation, 1100–1101
neuropathy, at elbow, 1099–1100, 1100*t*
pathologic abnormalities in throwing extremity, 1098–1099
prognosis, 1104
treatment of, 1101–1104
transfer of, as pedicle flap, 535, 538
treatment for lipofibromatous hamartoma in, 1595–1598, 1595*f*, 1596*f*, 1597*f*
variations at the wrist, 207–208, 1225

Ulnar tunnel syndrome, 1131
  anatomy in, 1131–1136
  causes of nerve compression, 1136, 1136*t*
    anatomic abnormalities, 1136–1137
    burns, 1137*t*
    fractures and dislocations, 1137
    ganglia and other masses, 1036
    occupational trauma, 1137*t*
    other causes, 1137–1138
  correlation of clinical symptoms and sites of compression, 1138–1139
  evaluation of the patient, 1139
  operative decompression of the ulnar nerve in Guyon's canal, 1140–1141, 1141*f*
  postoperative management, 1141
  treatment of, 1139–1140
Ultrasonography, in diagnosis of carpal tunnel syndrome, 875
Unmyelinated sensory axons, 1480
Upper extremity
  anomalous innervation of, 197–198, 199*f*
    communications between preaxial and postaxial nerves, 208–209
    lateral pectoral nerve, 198–199
    median nerve variations at the wrist and hand, 204–205, 206*f*
    median–ulnar nerve communications, 200–204
    musculocutaneous nerve, 199–200
    ulnar nerve variations at the wrist, 207–208
  donor nerves in, 547
    dorsal cutaneous branch of ulnar nerve, 549
    lateral antebrachial cutaneous nerve, 548–549, 548*f*
    medial antebrachial cutaneous nerve, 547
    posterior interosseous nerve, 549
  motor testing in, 160–167
  nerve injury associated with devascularizing trauma in, 682–683*f*, 684
Upper tibial osteotomy, 1203
Uremic neuropathy, 1224–1225
Urokinase, 64

Van Beek nerve-approximating clamp, 282, 455
Vaporization, 284, 310
Variable-amplitude vibrometer, 878
Vascular anatomical relationships to the brachial plexus, 1263–1265, 1264*f*
Vascular assessment, with brachial plexus injury, 1275–1276
Vascular injury, and thoracic outlet syndrome, 1193
Vascularized island transfer, for neuromas, 1534–1535
Vascularized nerve grafts, 389, 509, 528, 529, 569–570
  advantages of, 539
  clinical studies, 577–579, 579*t*
  cutaneous nerves, 538–539
  experimental results, 570–571
  indications for, 571–572
  operative technique, 579–581, 580*f*, 581*f*, 582*f*
    vascularized ulnar nerve graft, 581–584, 583*f*
  techniques of, 572, 572*t*, 573*t*, 574–575, 575*f*, 577, 577*f*
  transfer as a pedicle flap, 535, 538
Vasoactive intestinal polypeptide, and pain response, 1480
Vasomotor assessment, of reflex sympathetic dystrophy, 1504–1505
Vasomotor disturbance, 1499
Vaughan-Jackson syndrome, 1012
Venous thrombosis, 808–809
Versed, in electrical nerve stimulation in awake patient, 246
Vertebrate nervous system, 18–19
Vibratory detection threshold (VDT), 382
Vibratory testing, 143–144
Video dimensional analyzer (VDA), 47
Viscoelastic properties, of peripheral nerve, 49–50, 51*f*
Vitamin B_6, in treating carpal tunnel syndrome, 882–883
Volar interosseous muscles, motor testing of, 165
Volkmann's contracture, 672
Volkman's ischemia, 389
Voltage clamp, 34–35, 36*f*
Voltage-clamp analysis, 38
Voltage (V), 20
Von Frey pressure test, 140, 879
  with Semmes-Weinstein monofilaments, 876, 878, 879*f*
Von Recklinghausen's disease, 963, 1600–1601, 1601*f*
  and development of malignant Schwannomas, 1613, 1614, 1615, 1619
  lipofibromatous hamartoma in, 1594

Wallerian degeneration, 49, 66, 80, 111, 115, 118, 1276–1277
Warmth receptors, 90
Wartenberg's disease, 1039–1040
Wartenberg's sign, 433, 434, 1070
Wartenberg's traction neuritis, 1039, 1040*f*, 1041*f*
Weber two-point discrimination test, 140, 823–824, 876, 878*f*
Web space contracture, 816
Whole nerve suture, 241–242
Wick catheter technique for measuring interstitial pressure, 943, 943*f*, 944*f*, 945, 945*f*
Work, 694
Work incapacity, 951f, 952
Workplace
  carpal tunnel syndrome in, 954–955, 957–960
  cumulative trauma in, 952–955
  and seeking of medical help, 950–951
Worker's compensation
  and cumulative trauma, 952–955
  and regional musculoskeletal symptoms, 952–954
Wound ballistics, 656–657, 657*t*, 658*t*
Wound closure, following nerve grafting, 535
Wrap-around flap, 797, 799*f*, 800*f*
Wrist. *See also* Hand
  arthrodesis of the, 1299
  combined median and ulnar neuropathy at, 1225
  and digits deformities
    operative procedures, 1462–1463

arthrodesis of metaphalangeal joint of thumb, 1470
digital and thumb extensor transfers, 1469–1470
and extensor pollicis brevis, 1472, 1473*f*
of extensor pollicis longus, 1470, 1472, 1472*f*
flexor carpi ulnaris transfer, 1466–1467
flexor digitorum superficialis transfer for thumb extension, 1470
fractional lengthening of wrist and digital flexor tendons, 1463–1466
imbrication of abductor pollicis longus and extensor pollicis brevis, 1472, 1473
pronator teres transfer, 1467, 1468*f*, 1469
realignment and reinforcement of the extensor pollicis longus, 1470, 1472, 1172*f*
swan-neck deformity, 1472–1474, 1473*f*
thumb adduction contracture, 1470, 1471*f*
transfer for thumb extension, 1470
transfers to wrist extensors, 1466
effects of position on interstitial pressure, 940–941, 942*f*
extensor
opponensplasty using, 721–722
and tendon transfer, 735–737, 740*f*
flexors, 1430
lengthening of, 1431–1432
median nerve cariations at, 204–205, 206*f*
median nerve in, 371, 373
ulnar nerve in
anatomy, 417*f*, 419–420
variations at the, 207–208
Wristwatch neuropathy, 1042–1043, 1044*f*

Xenografts, 528

Yttrium-aluminum-garnet (neodymium-YAG laser), 310

Zancolli capsulorrhaphy, 730
Zancolli loop, 735, 735*f*
Z-lengthening
of biceps, 1429
of digital flexors, 1432
in tendo achilles lengthening, 1444–1445
Z-plasty, for subcutaneous tender nerve, 973
Z protein, 64, 67
Zygomatic branch, 463

ISBN 0-397-51174-4

90000

9 780397 511747